morphine	nalbuphine	pentobarbital	phenobarbital	promethazine	scopolamine	secobarbital	sodium bicarbonate	thiopental	
P	Y	P		P	P				atropine
Y		N		Y	Y				butorphanol
P		N		P	P			N	chlorpromazine
									codeine
N	N	N	N	N	N	N	N	N	diazepam
Y		N		Y	Y	N	N	N	glycopyrrolate
		Y		Y	Y				hydromorphone
P	Y	N	N	P	P				hydroxyzine
N		N		P	P			N	meperidine
■		Y		?	P			N	morphine
	■	N		Y	Y				nalbuphine
Y	N	■		N	Y		Y	Y	pentobarbital
			■				Y		phenobarbital
?	Y	N		■	P			N	promethazine
P	Y	Y		P	■			Y	scopolamine
						■			secobarbital
		Y					■	N	sodium bicarbonate
N		Y		N	Y		N	■	thiopental

Nursing90
DRUG
HANDBOOK

Nursing90
DRUG
HANDBOOK™

NURSING90 BOOKS™
SPRINGHOUSE CORPORATION
SPRINGHOUSE, PENNSYLVANIA

NURSING90 DRUG HANDBOOK™

Staff for this volume

Executive Director, Editorial
Stanley Loeb

Executive Director, Creative Services
Jean Robinson

Editorial Director
Helen Klusek Hamilton

Clinical Director
Barbara F. McVan, RN

Art Director
John Hubbard

Clinical Editors
Joanne Patzek DaCunha, RN, BS;
Helene K. Nawrocki, RN, MSN

Drug Information Editor
George J. Blake, RPh, MS

Editorial Assistants
Beverly Lane, Maree DeRosa

Copy Editors
Diane M. Armento, Jane V. Cray

Designers
Stephanie Peters (associate art director),
Matie Patterson

Art Production
Robert Perry (manager), Donald Knauss,
Anna Brindisi, Bob Wieder, Catherine
Mace

Typography
David C. Kosten (manager), Diane
Paluba (assistant manager)

Manufacturing
Deborah C. Meiris (manager), T.A. Landis

Production Coordination
Aline S. Miller (manager), Colleen M.
Hayman, Susan Hopkins Rodzewich

The clinical procedures described and recommended in this publication are based on research and consultation with nursing, medical, and legal authorities. To the best of our knowledge, these procedures reflect currently accepted practice; nevertheless, they can't be considered absolute and universal recommendations. For individual application, all recommendations must be considered in light of the patient's clinical condition and, before administration of new or infrequently used drugs, in light of latest package-insert information. The authors and the publisher disclaim responsibility for any adverse effects resulting directly or indirectly from the suggested procedures, from any undetected errors, or from the reader's misunderstanding of the text.

NDH-011089
NURSING90 DRUG HANDBOOK
ISSN 0273-320X
ISBN 0-87434-234-1

CONTENTS

Autonomic Nervous System Drugs

Respiratory Tract Drugs

Gastrointestinal Tract Drugs

Hormonal Agents

Agents for Fluid and Electrolyte Balance

Hematologic Agents

Antineoplastic Agents

Immunomodulation Agents

Eye, Ear, Nose, and Throat Drugs

Dermatomucosal Agents

Anesthetic Agents

Nutritional Agents

Miscellaneous Drug Categories

Appendices and Index

CONSULTANTS, REVIEWERS, AND ADVISORS

At the time of publication, the clinical consultants, reviewers, and advisors held the following positions:

Clinical Consultants

Michael J. Booth, RN, MA, CRNA,
Co-Director, Graduate Program of Nurse Anesthesia; Assistant Professor, Department of Anesthesiology, Medical College of Pennsylvania and Hospital, Philadelphia

Charmaine J. Cummings, RN, MSN,
Director, Nursing Education, National Institutes of Health, Clinical Center, Bethesda, Md.

Walter Carl Faubion, RN, MS,
Manager, Parenteral and Enteral Nutrition Team, University of Michigan Medical Center, Ann Arbor

Roseann Hendrickson, RN,
Staff Nurse, Emergency Department, Underwood Memorial Hospital, Woodbury, N.J.

Marcia Jo Hill, RN, MSN,
Manager, Dermatologic Therapeutics, The Methodist Hospital, Houston; Clinical Assistant Professor, Department of Dermatology, Baylor College of Medicine, Tex.

Catharine Keenan Bean, RN, BSN, OCN, Interim Co-Assistant Director of Nursing Education, Dana Farber Cancer Institute, Boston

Karen Landis, RN, MS, CCRN,
Pulmonary Clinical Nurse Specialist, Lehigh Valley Hospital Center, Allentown, Pa.

Chris Platt Moldovanyi, RN, MSN, CDE, Staff Nurse, Operating Room, Endocrinology Clinical Specialist, Cleveland Clinic Foundation, Cleveland, Ohio

Sandra Ludwig Nettina, RNC, MSN, CRNP, Adult Nurse Practitioner, Department of Emergency Medicine, Temple University Hospital, Philadelphia

Marilyn Sawyer Sommers, RN, MA, CCRN, Doctoral Candidate, Ohio State University, Columbus, Ohio

Margaret A. Smellie-Belfield, RN, BSN, CCRN, Clinical Services Director, SICU/PACU, Veterans Administration Medical Center, San Diego

Nancy Baptie Walrath, RN, BSN, CGC, Director, Gastroenterology Department, Daniel Freeman Memorial and Marina Hospitals, Inglewood, Calif.

Special thanks to the following, who contributed to past editions: Jean Marie Amabile-Michiels, RN, MA, MSN; Wendy L. Baker, RN, MS, CCRN; Beverly A. Baldwin, RN, MA; Marjorie Davis Beck, RN; Therese E. Bowman, RN, BSN, MS; Heather Boyd-Monk, SRN, RN, BSN; Paula Brammer-Vetter, RN, BSN, CCRN; Karen E. Burgess, RN, MSN; Nancy Burns, RN, PhD; Carla J. Burton, RN, BS; Priscilla A. Butts, RN, MSN; James J. Claffey, CRNA, BS; Maribel J. Clements, RN, MA; Elizabeth R. DiMeo, RN, MSN; Judy Donlen, RNC, MSN; Gail D'Onofrio, RN, MS; Jeanne Dupont, RN; DeAnn M. Englert, RN, MSN; Joel Glucroft, PhD; Margarethe Hawken, RN, MA, CNRN; Kathleen M. Hawkins, RN; Denise A. Hess, RN, BS; Tobie Hittle, RN, CCRN, BSN; Carolyn Holt, RN, BSEd; Maureen L. Metters, BSN; Kenneth J. Michalko, BSc Phm, PharmD; Margaret E. Miller, RN, MSN; John Nagelhout, CRNA, PhD; Brenda Marion Nevidson, RN, MSN; Elizabeth A. Phillips, RN, BA, BSN; Judith M. Rohde, RN, MS, CNP, CNRN; Dale Elizabeth Schreffler, RN, BSN; Roberta Seifer, RN, CNP, BS; Despina Seremelis, RN, BSN; Barbara Solomon, RN, MS; Robin Tourigian, RN, MSN; Carmen Brochu Wohrle, RN, MS; Patricia H. Worthington, RN, BSN

Pharmacy Reviewers

Steven R. Abel, PharmD, RPh,
Assistant Director of Pharmacy, Clinical/Educational Services, Indiana University Hospitals, Indianapolis

Bruce D. Clayton, BS, PharmD, RPh,
Professor of Pharmacy Practice, College of Pharmacy, University of Arkansas for Medical Sciences, Little Rock

David W. Hawkins, PharmD,
Assistant Dean and Associate Professor, College of Pharmacy, University of Georgia, Athens

Alan W. Hopefl, PharmD,
Assistant Professor of Clinical Pharmacy, St. Louis College of Pharmacy; Assistant Professor of Pharmacy in Internal Medicine, St. Louis University School of Medicine

FOREWORD

Nursing responsibility for administering and monitoring drug therapy is a major professional concern. No wonder. In the United States today, well over 8,000 drugs and drug combinations are available for clinical use. Reportedly, a new chemical entity is approved for human use every two to three weeks. In light of this vast and ever-growing array of drugs, meeting this responsibility with confidence and informed judgment is no easy task; it is possible only with a reliable source of drug information.

The *Nursing90 Drug Handbook* is a comprehensive drug reference that offers practicing nurses all the drug information they need to administer drugs safely and to monitor and counsel their patients during drug therapy. This newest edition of the most comprehensively updated drug reference for nurses offers detailed information on approximately 1,100 generic drugs, including 21 drugs that were recently approved for use in 1990.

As in previous editions, each drug entry is complete in itself, in an easy-to-use format that presents mechanisms of action, indications and dosage, adverse reactions, interactions, and nursing considerations. The clearly defined nursing considerations include contraindications; special precautions; and recommendations for easier administration, prevention of adverse effects, and safe storage. An index that lists trade names, generic names, combination products, and pharmacologic categories helps the reader to quickly find any drug entry. Unlike alphabetical listings, which require the reader to know the drug's generic or trade name, this volume's uniquely helpful organization of chapters by therapeutic use allows the reader to identify an unknown drug simply by knowing its clinical use. Moreover, this organization automatically identifies all drugs of similar use and allows comparison of their dosages and effects—information that can help the nurse anticipate alternative therapy for patients who cannot tolerate or benefit from a particular drug.

New features include a current list of designated orphan drugs and biologicals, a new section covering immunomodulation agents, and a chapter that covers promising investigational drugs; as appropriate, a graphic symbol (an open diamond) identifies generic drugs that are also available in products that do not require a prescription.

Offering meticulous clinical review and the most current drug information, the *Nursing90 Drug Handbook* is an indispensable professional tool for nurses at all levels of practice.

MARY D. NAYLOR, RN, PhD, FAAN
Associate Dean and Director of Undergraduate Studies
University of Pennsylvania School of Nursing
Philadelphia

Drugs and Therapeutic Categories

How to use Nursing90 Drug Handbook

Nursing90 Drug Handbook is meant to fill a very special need. It represents a joint effort by pharmacists and nurses to provide the nursing profession with drug information that focuses on what nurses need to know. With this in mind, it emphasizes clinical aspects and does not attempt to replace detailed pharmacology texts. Also, the information is arranged in a format designed to make it readily accessible.

Introductory information

Following this chapter, Chapter 2 explains, in a general way, how drugs work. It also tells about side effects and adverse reactions and gives general guidelines about drug use in pregnancy and the presence of drugs in breast milk. Chapters 3 and 4 discuss the unique problems of administering drugs to children and elderly patients and offer guidelines to minimize problems in these areas. Chapter 5 discusses drug therapy as it relates to the nursing process.

In the remaining chapters, all drugs are classified according to their approved therapeutic uses. Drugs that have multiple therapeutic uses are classified according to their most common use; they are also listed (with a cross-reference to the major drug entry) in drug groups that share their secondary applications. For example, nadolol, a beta-adrenergic blocker, is described in the chapter that covers antianginals because its major therapeutic application is the management of angina pectoris; because it is less commonly used to treat hypertension, it is listed among the generic drugs grouped as antihypertensives with a cross-reference to Chapter 21, Antianginals.

Such classification by therapeutic use offers several advantages. It helps the reader identify an unknown drug by its clinical application alone. At the same time, it automatically identifies all other drugs that share the same use and provides easy comparison of their dosages and effects. Thereby, it quickly identifies potential pharmacotherapeutic alternatives for patients who cannot tolerate or fail to respond to a particular drug.

Drug information

Each chapter, representing a major therapeutic use, begins with an alphabetically arranged list of the generic names of drugs described in that chapter. This is followed by a list of selected combination products in which these drugs are found. Specific information on each drug is arranged under the following headings: *Mechanism of Action; Indications and Dosage; Adverse Reactions; Interactions;* and *Nursing Considerations.*

In each drug entry, the drug's generic name is immediately followed by an alphabetic list of its brand names. A generic name followed by an open diamond indicates a drug that is also available in preparations that do not require a prescription (◇). Brands available in both the United States and Canada are designated with a diamond (♦); those available *only* in Canada with a double diamond (♦♦).

A brand name with no symbol after it is available only in the United States. If a drug is a controlled substance, that too is clearly indicated (example: Controlled Substance Schedule II). Products listed, although generally available, may not be approved by the Food and Drug Administration. The mention of a brand name in no way implies endorsement of that product or guarantees its legality.

Each systemically absorbed drug has been assigned a pregnancy risk category based upon available clinical and preclinical information. The Pregnancy Risk Category parallels the five Pregnancy Categories (A, B, C, D, and X) assigned by the Food and Drug Administration to reflect a drug's potential to cause birth defects. Although it is generally accepted that NO drugs should be used during pregnancy, this rating system permits rapid assessment of the risk-benefit ratio should drug administration to a pregnant woman become necessary. Drugs in category A are generally considered safe to use in pregnancy; drugs in category X are generally contraindicated.

• A: Adequate studies in pregnant women have failed to show a risk to the fetus in the first trimester of pregnancy—and there is no evidence of risk in later trimesters.

• B: Animal studies have not shown a risk to the fetus, but there are no adequate clinical studies in pregnant women; or, animal studies have shown an adverse effect on the fetus, but adequate studies in pregnant women have not shown a risk to the fetus during the first trimester of pregnancy and there is no evidence of risk in later trimesters.

• C: Animal studies *have* shown an adverse effect on the fetus, but there are no adequate studies in humans. The benefits from use in pregnant women may be acceptable despite potential risks; or, there are no animal reproduction studies or adequate human studies. Pregnancy risk is unknown.

• D: There is evidence of risk to the human fetus, but the potential benefits of use in pregnant women may be acceptable despite risks.

• X: Studies in animals or humans show fetal abnormalities, or adverse reaction reports indicate evidence of fetal risk. The risks involved clearly outweigh potential benefits.

• NR: Not rated.

In this volume, the Pregnancy Risk Category has been omitted if the drug is not rated and if such rating is not applicable.

The section titled *Mechanism of Action* succinctly describes *how* each specific drug provides its therapeutic effect. For example, although all antihypertensives lower blood pressure, they don't all do this by the same pharmacologic process.

The section titled *Indications and Dosage* lists general dosage information for adults (including recommended geriatric dosages, when available) and children, as applicable. Children's dosages are usually indicated in terms of mg/kg daily. Dosage instructions reflect current clinical trends in therapeutics and can't be considered as absolute and universal recommendations. For individual application, dosage instructions must be considered in light of the patient's clinical condition.

The section titled *Adverse Reactions* lists each drug's commonly observed adverse reactions (and selected rare ones if life-threatening). The most common and life-threatening adverse reactions are italicized for easy reference. An exception to this rule is an adverse reaction that, although normally considered hazardous, has been reported to be mild and reversible with the drug in question. For example, thrombocytopenia is considered a life-threatening adverse reaction to mithramycin but a mild and reversible reaction to methyldopa. Hence, thrombocytopenia listed as an adverse reaction to mithramycin is italicized, whereas the same reaction under methyldopa is not. Adverse reactions are grouped according to the body system in which they appear.

The next section, *Interactions,* lists each drug's confirmed, *clinically significant* interactions with other drugs (additive effects, potentiated effects, and antagonistic effects) with specific suggestions for avoiding dangerous drug interactions (for example, by reducing doses). Drug interactions are listed under the drug that is adversely affected. For example, magnesium trisilicate, an ingredient in antacids, interacts with tetracycline to cause decreased absorption of tetracycline. Therefore, this interaction is listed under tetracycline. To check on the possible effects of using two or more drugs simultaneously, refer to the interaction entry for *each* of the drugs in question.

The final section, *Nursing Considerations,* lists other useful information, starting with contraindications and precautions, followed by monitoring techniques and suggestions for prevention and treatment of adverse reactions. Also included are suggestions for patient comfort, for patient teaching, and for preparing, administering, and storing each drug.

Alcohol and tartrazine content

Many liquid drug preparations for oral use contain alcohol. Although the slight sedative effect that alcohol produces is not harmful in most patients—and can sometimes be beneficial—alcohol ingestion can be undesirable and even dangerous in some circumstances. So, alcohol-containing oral drugs should be given very cautiously, if at all, to patients who are:
• concomitantly taking potent CNS depressants, such as barbiturates.

• taking drugs that may produce a disulfiram-type reaction (such as chlorpropamide, metronidazole, and moxalactam).
• taking disulfiram (Antabuse) as part of a treatment program for their alcoholism. Such patients, upon ingestion of alcohol, will exhibit severe symptoms that may include blurred vision, confusion, dyspnea, flushing, sweating, and tachycardia.

To help prevent inadvertent exposure to alcohol, a single asterisk (*) follows the generic name of a drug if its liquid form contains alcohol. In many of the preparations so marked, the alcohol content is small. Nevertheless, these drugs should be avoided in patients who are susceptible to adverse effects upon exposure to alcohol.

Tartrazine dye, also known as FD&C Yellow No. 5, is a common coloring agent in some foods and drugs. Usually harmless, it can provoke a severe allergic reaction in susceptible persons. For this reason, most drug manufacturers have begun to eliminate tartrazine from their products, but many drugs still contain it.

The incidence of tartrazine sensitivity is estimated at approximately 1 in 10,000 in the general population but somewhat higher in persons with asthma and/or sensitivity to aspirin. Why this is so is unknown. The most common symptoms of tartrazine sensitivity are urticaria, rhinorrhea, asthma, and angioedema. Acutely sensitive persons may develop allergic vascular purpura, tachycardia, dyspnea, and chest pain. These allergic symptoms generally subside spontaneously upon discontinuation of the tartrazine-containing drug but occasionally require treatment with antihistamines or epinephrine.

Avoiding exposure to tartrazine is not simply a matter of avoiding yellow-colored drugs because this substance may be present in many other color blends, such as turquoise, green, and maroon. To prevent exposure to tartrazine, this volume signals possible tartrazine content with a double asterisk (**) after each brand that may contain it. If you suspect tartrazine sensitivity in a patient receiving such a drug, inform the doctor and contact the manufacturer to determine which dosage forms contain tartrazine.

A Guide to Abbreviations

AIDS	acquired immunodeficiency syndrome
AV	atrioventricular
b.i.d.	twice daily
BUN	blood urea nitrogen
CBC	complete blood count
CHF	congestive heart failure
CNS	central nervous system
COPD	chronic obstructive pulmonary disease
CV	cardiovascular
CVA	cerebrovascular accident
DNA	deoxyribonucleic acid
EENT	eyes, ears, nose, throat
FDA	Food and Drug Administration
g	gram
G	gauge
GI	gastrointestinal
GU	genitourinary
G6PD	glucose-6-phosphate dehydrogenase
h.s.	at bedtime
I.M.	intramuscular
IPPB	intermittent positive pressure breathing
IU	international unit
I.V.	intravenous
kg	kilogram
m²	square meter
MAO	monoamine oxidase
mcg	microgram
mg	milligram
ml	milliliter
NSAID	nonsteroidal anti-inflammatory drug
OTC	over the counter
P.O.	by mouth
p.r.n.	as needed
q	every
q.i.d.	four times daily
RDA	recommended daily allowance
REM	rapid eye movement
SA	sinoatrial
S.C.	subcutaneous
t.i.d.	three times daily

Drug actions, reactions, and interactions explained

Administration of any drug provokes a series of physiochemical events within the body. The first event, when a drug combines with cell drug receptors, is known as the drug action. What follows as a result of this action of the drug is known as the drug effect. Depending on the number of different cellular drug receptors affected by a given drug, a drug effect can be local, systemic, or both. For example, the antipeptic ulcer drug cimetidine (Tagamet) acts solely by blocking histamine receptor cells in the parietal cells of the stomach. This is known as a local drug effect because the drug action is sharply limited to one area and does not spread to other parts of the body. On the other hand, diphenhydramine (Benadryl) produces a systemic effect in that it blocks histamine receptors in widespread areas of the body. In other words, local drug effects are specific to a limited number of organ systems, whereas systemic drug effects are generalized and affect different and diverse organ systems.

Three factors modify drug action
1. Absorption
Before a drug can act within the body, it must be absorbed into the bloodstream—usually after oral administration, the most frequently used route. Before a drug contained in a tablet or capsule can be absorbed, the dosage form must disintegrate, that is, break into smaller particles. Then, these smaller particles can dissolve in

gastric juices. Only after so dissolving can a drug be absorbed into the bloodstream. Once absorbed and circulated in the bloodstream, it is said to be bioavailable, or ready to produce a drug effect. Whether such absorption is complete or partial depends on several factors: the drug's physiochemical effects, its dosage form, its route of administration, its interactions with other substances in the GI tract, and various patient characteristics. These same factors also determine the speed of absorption. Thus, oral solutions and elixirs, which bypass the need for disintegration and dissolution, are usually absorbed more rapidly. Drugs administered intramuscularly must first be absorbed through the muscle into the bloodstream. Rectal suppositories must dissolve to be absorbed through the rectal mucosa. Drugs administered intravenously are placed directly into the circulation and are completely and immediately bioavailable.

2. Distribution
After absorption, a drug moves from the bloodstream into various fluids and tissues within the body; this is distribution. Individual patient variations can greatly alter the amount of drug that is distributed throughout the body. For example, in an edematous patient, a given dose must be distributed to a larger volume than in a nonedematous patient; the amount of drug must sometimes be increased to account for this. Remember, the dos-

age should be decreased when the edema is corrected. Conversely, in an extremely dehydrated patient, the drug will be distributed to a much smaller volume, so the dose must then be decreased. The total area to which a drug is distributed is known as volume of distribution. Patients who are particularly obese may present another problem when considering drug distribution. Some drugs—such as digoxin, gentamicin, and tobramycin—are not well distributed to fatty tissue. Therefore, dosing based on actual body weight may lead to overdose and serious toxicity. In some cases, dosing must be based on lean body weight, which may be estimated from actuarial tables that give average weight range for height.

3. Metabolism and excretion (drug elimination)

Most drugs are metabolized in the liver and excreted by the kidneys. Hepatic diseases may affect one or more of the metabolic functions of the liver. Therefore, in patients with hepatic disease, the metabolism of a drug may be increased, decreased, or unchanged. Clearly, all patients with hepatic disease must be monitored closely for drug effect and toxicity. Some drugs (digoxin, gentamicin) are eliminated almost unchanged by the kidneys. For safe use of such drugs, renal function must be adequate or the drug will accumulate, producing toxic effects. Some drugs can alter the effect and excretion of other drugs. For example, they can stimulate hepatic metabolizing enzymes to speed up the rate of metabolism and change the drug effect. Or they can block or promote renal excretion of other drugs, causing them to accumulate and enhance their effects or causing them to be too rapidly excreted and so diminish their effects. Some slight elimination takes place by way of perspiration, saliva, breast milk, and so on. (Certain volatile anesthetics, however—halothane, for instance—are eliminated primarily by exhalation.)

The rate at which a drug is metabolized varies with the individual. In some patients, drugs are metabolized so quickly that their blood and tissue levels prove therapeutically inadequate. In others, the rate of metabolism is so slow that ordinary doses can produce toxic results.

Other modifying factors

An important factor that influences a drug's action and effect is its *binding to plasma proteins,* especially albumin, and other tissue components. Because only a free, unbound drug can act in the body, such binding greatly influences effectiveness and duration of effect.

The *patient's age* is another important factor. Elderly patients usually have decreased hepatic function, less muscle mass, and diminished renal function. Consequently, they need lower doses and sometimes longer dosage intervals to avoid toxicity. With similar consequences, neonates have underdeveloped metabolic enzyme systems and inadequate renal function. They need highly individualized dosage and careful monitoring.

Underlying disease can also markedly affect drug action and effect. For example, acidosis may cause insulin resistance. Genetic diseases, such as glucose-6-phosphate dehydrogenase (G6PD) deficiency and hepatic porphyria, may turn drugs into toxins with serious consequences. Patients with G6PD deficiency may develop hemolytic anemia when given sulfonamides or a number of other drugs. A genetically susceptible patient can develop an acute porphyria attack if given a barbiturate. Also, patients who have highly active hepatic enzyme systems (for example, rapid acetylators), when treated with isoniazid, can develop hepatitis from the rapid intrahepatic buildup of a toxic metabolite.

Things to consider about administration

1. Dosage forms do matter. Some tablets and capsules are too large to be readily swallowed by very ill patients. You may then request an oral solution or elixir of the same drug, but bear in mind that because a liquid is more easily and completely absorbed, it produces higher blood levels than a tablet. When a potentially toxic drug (such as digoxin) is given, the increased amount absorbed could cause toxicity. Sometimes a change in dosage form requires a change in dosage.

2. Routes of administration are not therapeutically interchangeable. For example, phenytoin (Dilantin) is readily absorbed orally but is slowly and erratically absorbed intramuscularly. On the other hand, carbenicillin must be given parenterally because oral administration yields inadequate blood levels to treat systemic infections. However, it can be given orally to treat urinary tract infections because it concentrates in the urine.

3. Improper storage can alter a drug's potency. Most drugs should be stored in tight containers protected from direct sunlight and extremes in temperature and humidity which can cause them to deteriorate. Some may require special storage conditions (such as refrigeration).

4. The timing of drug administration can be important. Sometimes giving an oral drug during or shortly after mealtime decreases the amount of drug absorbed. This is not clinically significant with most drugs and may in fact be desirable with irritating drugs such as aspirin or phenylbutazone. But penicillins and tetracyclines should not be scheduled for administration at mealtimes because certain foods can inactivate them. If in doubt about the effect of food on a certain drug, check with the pharmacist.

5. Consider the patient's age, height, and weight. The doctor will need this information when calculating the dose for many drugs. It should be accurately recorded on the patient's chart. This chart should also include current laboratory data, especially kidney and liver function studies, so the doctor can adapt dosage as needed.

6. Watch for metabolic changes. Monitor for any physiologic change that might alter drug effect. Examples: depressed respiratory function and the development of acidosis or alkalosis.

7. Know the patient's history. Whenever possible, obtain a comprehensive family history from the patient or his family. Ask about past reactions to drugs, possible genetic traits that might alter drug response, and the current use of other drugs. Multiple drug therapy can cause drug interactions that can dramatically change the effects of many drugs.

Drug interactions

When one drug administered in combination with or shortly after another drug alters the effect of one or both drugs, this is known as a drug interaction. Usually, the effect of one drug is increased or decreased. For instance, one drug may inhibit or stimulate the metabolism or excretion of the other; or it may release another from plasma protein-binding sites, freeing it for further action.

Combination therapy is based upon drug interaction. One drug, for example, may be given to potentiate another. Probenecid, which blocks the excretion of penicillin, is sometimes given with penicillin to maintain adequate blood levels of penicillin for a longer period. Often two drugs with similar action are given together precisely because of the additive effect that results. Aspirin and codeine, for instance, both analgesics, are often given in combination because together they provide greater relief from pain than either alone.

Drug interactions are sometimes used to prevent or antagonize certain adverse reactions. Hydrochlorothiazide and spironolactone, both diuretics, are often administered in combination, because the former is potassium-depleting, while the latter is potassium-sparing.

But not all drug interactions are beneficial. Multiple drugs can interact to produce effects that are often undesirable and sometimes hazardous. Harmful drug interactions decrease efficacy or increase toxicity. A hypertensive patient well controlled with guanethidine may see his blood pressure rise to its former high level if he takes the antidepressant amitriptyline (Elavil) at the same time. Such a drug effect is known as antagonism. Drug combinations that produce these effects should be avoided if possible. Another kind of inhibiting effect occurs when a tetracycline drug is administered with calcium- or magnesium-containing drugs or foods (such as antacids or milk). These combine with tetracycline in the GI tract and cause inadequate absorption of tetracycline.

Adverse reactions

Any drug effect other than what is therapeutically intended can be called an adverse reaction. It may be expected and benign, or unexpected and potentially harmful. Mild, but *predictable,* adverse reactions are sometimes called side effects. Drowsiness caused by antihistamines is an example of this. During hay fever season, a patient may have to contend with this drowsiness to get relief from hay fever symptoms. In such a case, the dosage may be adjusted up or down to balance therapeutic effects with side effects.

An adverse reaction may be tolerated for a necessary therapeutic effect, or it may be hazardous and unacceptable and require discontinuation of the drug. Some adverse reactions subside with continued use. As an example, the drowsiness associated with methyldopa (Aldomet) and the orthostatic hypotension associated with prazosin (Minipress) usually subside after several days, as the patient develops a tolerance to these effects. But many adverse reactions are dosage-related and lessen or disappear only if dosage is reduced. Although most adverse reactions are not therapeutically desirable, an occasional one can be put to clinical use. An outstanding example of this is the drowsiness associated with diphenhydramine (Benadryl), which makes it clinically useful as a mild hypnotic.

Hypersensitivity, a term sometimes used interchangeably with drug allergy, is the result of an antigen-antibody immune reaction that occurs in the body when a drug is given to a susceptible patient. One of the most dangerous of all drug hypersensitivities is penicillin allergy. In its severest form, penicillin anaphylaxis can rapidly become fatal.

Rarely, idiosyncratic reactions occur. These are highly unpredictable, individual, and unusual. Probably the best known idiosyncratic drug reaction is the aplastic anemia caused by the antibiotic chloramphenicol (Chloromycetin). This reaction appears in only 1 out of 40,000 patients, but when it does, it is often fatal. A more common idiosyncratic reaction is extreme sensitivity to very low doses of a drug, or insensitivity to higher-than-normal doses.

To deal with adverse reactions correctly, you need to be alert to even minor changes in the patient's clinical status. Such minor changes may be an early warning of pending toxicity. Listen to the patient's complaints about his reactions to a drug, and consider each complaint objectively. You may be able to reduce adverse reactions in several ways. Obviously, dosage reduction often helps. But often so does a simple rescheduling of the same dose. For example, pseudoephedrine (Sudafed) may produce stimulation that will be no problem if it's given early in the day; similarly, the drowsiness that occurs with antihistamines or tranquilizers can be totally harmless if the dose is given at bedtime. Most important, your patient needs to be told what adverse reactions to expect so he won't become worried or even stop taking the drug on his own. Of course, the patient should report any unusual or unexpected adverse reactions to the doctor.

Recognizing drug allergies or serious idiosyncratic reactions can sometimes be lifesaving. Ask each patient about drugs he is taking or has taken in the past and what, if any, unusual effects he experienced from taking them. If a patient claims to be allergic to a drug, ask him to tell you exactly what happens when he takes it. He may be calling a harmless side effect such as upset stomach an allergic reaction, or he may have a true tendency to anaphylaxis. In either case, you and the doctor need to know this. Of course, you must record and report any clinical changes throughout the patient's hospital stay. If you suspect a severe adverse reaction, withhold the drug until you can check with the pharmacist and the doctor.

Toxic reactions
Chronic drug toxicities are generally due to the cumulative effect and resulting buildup of the drug in the body. These effects may be extensions of the desired therapeutic effect. For example, guanethidine-induced norepinephrine depletion produces a desired antihypertensive effect, but in larger doses, this action often produces orthostatic hypotension.

Drug toxicities usually occur when drug blood levels rise due to impaired metabolism or excretion. For example, blood levels of theophylline rise when hepatic dysfunction impairs metabolism of the drug. Similarly, digoxin toxicity can follow impaired renal function because digoxin is eliminated from the body almost exclusively by the kidneys (via glomerular filtration). Of course, toxic blood levels also follow excessive dosage. Aspirin tinnitus (ringing in ears) is usually a sign that the safe dose has been exceeded.

Most drug toxicities are predictable and dosage-related; fortunately, most are also readily reversible upon dosage adjustment. So it's essential to monitor patients carefully for physiologic changes that might alter drug effect. Watch especially for impaired hepatic and renal function. Warn the patient about signs of pending toxicity, and tell him what to do if a toxic reaction occurs. Also, be sure to emphasize the importance of taking a drug exactly as prescribed. Warn the patient about serious problems that could arise if he changes the dosage or the schedule for taking it.

Drugs and pregnancy
Ever since the thalidomide tragedy of the late 1950s—when thousands of malformed infants were born after their mothers used this mild sedative-hypnotic during pregnancy—use of drugs during pregnancy has been a source of serious medical concern and controversy. To identify drugs that may cause such teratogenic effects, preclinical drug studies always include tests on pregnant laboratory animals. These tests point out gross teratogenicity but do not clearly establish safety. Because different species react to drugs in different ways, animal studies do not rule out possible teratogenic effects in humans. For example, the preliminary studies on thalidomide gave no warning of teratogenic effects, and it was subsequently

released for general use in Europe.

What about the placental barrier? Once thought to protect the fetus from drug effects, the placenta isn't actually much of a barrier at all. Except for drugs with exceptionally large molecular structure, almost every drug administered to a pregnant woman crosses the placenta and enters the fetal circulation. An example of such large molecular size is heparin, the injectable anticoagulant. Theoretically, then, heparin could be used in a pregnant woman without fear of harming the fetus—but even heparin carries a warning for cautious use in pregnancy. Conversely, just because a drug crosses the placenta doesn't necessarily mean it's harmful to the fetus.

Actually, only one factor—stage of fetal development—seems clearly related to exaggerated risk during pregnancy. During two stages of pregnancy—the first and the third trimesters—the fetus is especially vulnerable to damage from maternal use of drugs. During these times, *all* drugs should be given with extreme caution.

The most sensitive period for drug-induced fetal malformation is the first trimester, when fetal organs are differentiating (organogenesis). During this time, *all* drugs should be withheld unless doing so would jeopardize the mother's health. Theoretically, during this sensitive time, even aspirin could harm the fetus. So, strongly advise your patient to avoid *all* self-prescribed drugs during early pregnancy.

The other time of special fetal sensitivity to drugs is the last trimester. The reason? At birth, when separated from his mother, the newborn must rely on his own metabolism to eliminate any remaining drug. Because his detoxifying systems are not fully developed, any residual drug may take a long time to be metabolized—and thus may induce prolonged toxic reactions. Consequently, drugs should be

used only when absolutely necessary during the last 3 months of pregnancy.

Of course, in many circumstances, pregnant women must continue to take certain drugs. For example, a woman with a seizure disorder who is well controlled with an anticonvulsant should continue to take it even during pregnancy. Or a pregnant woman with a bacterial infection must receive antibiotics. In such cases, the potential risk to the fetus is overbalanced by the mother's need. The relative risk to the fetus is expressed by the drug's pregnancy risk category (see Chapter 1).

Following these general guidelines can prevent indiscriminate and potentially harmful use of drugs in pregnancy:
• Before a drug is prescribed for a woman of childbearing age, she should be asked the date of her last menstrual period and whether there is a possibility she is pregnant.
• Especially during the first and the third trimesters, a pregnant patient should avoid *all* drugs except those *essential* to maintain the pregnancy or maternal health.
• Topical drugs are not exempt from the warning against indiscriminate use during pregnancy. Many topically applied drugs can be absorbed in large enough amounts to be harmful to the fetus.
• When a pregnant patient needs *any* drug, the doctor should prescribe the *safest* possible drug in the *lowest* possible dose to minimize any harmful effect to the fetus.
• Every pregnant patient should check with her doctor before taking *any* drug.

Drugs and lactation
Most drugs a nursing mother takes appear in breast milk. Drug levels in breast milk tend to be high when blood levels are high—generally, shortly after taking each dose. Therefore, the mother should be advised to

breast-feed *before* taking medication, not *after*.

Nevertheless, with very few exceptions, a mother who wishes to breast-feed may continue to do so with her doctor's permission. However, breast-feeding should be temporarily interrupted and replaced with bottle-feeding when the mother must take:

- tetracyclines
- chloramphenicol
- sulfonamides (during first 2 weeks postpartum)
- oral anticoagulants
- iodine-containing drugs
- antineoplastics.

To protect her infant, a nursing mother should avoid taking drugs indiscriminately. If she needs to take a drug to maintain her own health, she should first check with her doctor to be sure of taking the safest drug at the safest dose.

What to teach patients about proper use of drugs

Store drugs in their original containers, at room temperature, in places that are not accessible to children or exposed to sunlight. Avoid storage in the bathroom medicine cabinet or the glove compartment or trunk of an automobile, where extremes of temperature and humidity will cause them to deteriorate. Never share prescription drugs with others.

Learn the trade name and generic name of any drug you are taking. Be sure to tell doctors, dentists, or other health care professionals you see regularly that you are taking it. Before taking any drug, be sure you have informed your doctor, nurse, or pharmacist about any unusual reactions you've had to drugs in the past and about your allergies to foods and other substances, any special medical problems, and any drugs you've taken over the last few weeks, including any nonprescription drugs.

Always take any drug exactly as prescribed, at the recommended dosage schedule and duration of treatment.

To avoid hazardous mistakes, always read the label before taking any drug. When using a drug prescribed for occasional or prolonged use, check the container for an expiration date (if available).

Never mix different drugs in a single container, and don't remove any drug from its original container or remove the label. Relying on your memory to identify a drug and specific directions for its use is extremely hazardous.

Discard any drugs that are outdated or no longer needed.

Before you have any surgery (including dental surgery), tell the doctor about all of the drugs that you have been taking.

Be sure to tell the doctor, nurse, or pharmacist about any side effects or unpleasant effects you've experienced while taking a drug. Such effects may require medical attention.

If you suspect that you or someone else has taken an overdose, call your doctor, poison control center, or pharmacist immediately. Keep syrup of ipecac in your home to induce vomiting, but induce vomiting only if one of these professionals has advised you to do so.

Drug therapy in children

A child's absorption, distribution, metabolism, and excretion processes undergo profound changes that affect drug dosage. To ensure optimal drug effect and minimal toxicity, consider these factors when administering drugs to a child.

Absorption

Drug absorption in children depends on the form of the drug; its physical properties; other drugs or substances, such as food, taken simultaneously; physiologic changes; and concurrent disease.

• The pH of neonatal gastric fluid is neutral or slightly acidic and becomes more acidic as the infant matures. This affects drug absorption. For example, nafcillin and penicillin G, erratically absorbed or malabsorbed in an adult due to degradation by gastric acid, are better absorbed in an infant due to low gastric acidity.

• Various infant formulas or milk products may increase gastric pH and impede absorption of acidic drugs. So, if possible, give a child oral medications when his stomach is empty.

• Gastric emptying time and transit time through the small intestine—which is longer in children than in adults—can affect absorption. Also, intestinal hypermotility (as in diarrhea) can diminish the drug's absorption.

• A child's comparatively thin epidermis allows increased absorption of topical drugs.

Distribution

As with absorption, changes in body weight and physiology during childhood can significantly influence a drug's distribution and effects. In a premature infant, body fluid makes up about 85% of total body weight; in a full-term infant, 55% to 70%; and in an adult, 50% to 55%. Extracellular fluid (mostly blood) constitutes 40% of a neonate's body weight, compared with 20% in an adult. Intracellular fluid remains fairly constant throughout life and has little effect on drug dosage.

Since most drugs travel through extracellular fluid to reach their receptors, however, extracellular fluid volume influences a water-soluble drug's concentration and effect. Children have a larger proportion of fluid to solid body weight, so their distribution area is proportionately greater.

Because the proportion of fat to lean body mass increases with age, the distribution of fat-soluble drugs is more limited in children than adults. As a result, a drug's lipid- or water-solubility affects the dosage for a child.

Binding to plasma proteins
As the result of a decrease in albumin concentration or intermolecular attraction between drug and plasma protein, many drugs are less bound to plasma proteins in infants than in adults.

Furthermore, preparations that bind plasma proteins may displace endogenous compounds, such as bilirubin or free fatty acids. Conversely, an endogenous compound may displace a weakly bound drug. For example, displacement of bound bilirubin can cause a rise in unbound bilirubin, which can lead to increased risk of kernicterus at normal bilirubin levels.

Since only an unbound, or free, drug has a pharmacologic effect, any alteration in ratio of a protein-bound to an unbound active drug can greatly influence its effect.

Several diseases and disorders, such as nephrotic syndrome and malnutrition, can also decrease plasma protein and increase the concentration of an unbound drug, intensifying the drug's effect or producing toxicity.

Metabolism
A newborn's ability to metabolize a drug depends on the integrity of his hepatic enzyme system, his intrauterine exposure to the drug, and the nature of the drug itself.

Certain metabolic mechanisms are underdeveloped in neonates. Glucuronidation, the mechanism that neutralizes drugs, for example, is insufficiently developed to permit full pediatric doses until the infant is 1 month old. Because of this, the use of chloramphenicol in a newborn may cause gray baby syndrome, illustrating the newborn's inability to metabolize the drug. Use of chloramphenicol in neonates, therefore, requires decreased dosage (25 mg/kg/day) and monitoring of blood levels.

Conversely, intrauterine exposure to drugs may induce precocious development of hepatic enzyme mechanisms, increasing the infant's capacity to metabolize potentially harmful substances.

Older children can metabolize some drugs (theophylline, for example) more rapidly than adults. This ability may be due to their increased hepatic metabolic activity. Larger doses than those recommended for adults may be required.

Also, preparations given concurrently to a child may alter hepatic metabolism and induce release of hepatic enzymes. Phenobarbital, for example, can induce hepatic enzyme production and accelerate metabolism of drugs given concurrently.

Excretion
Renal excretion of a drug is the net effect of glomerular filtration, active tubular secretion, and passive tubular reabsorption. Because so many drugs are excreted in the urine, the degree of renal development or presence of renal disease can profoundly affect a child's dosage requirements.

If a child is unable to excrete a drug renally, drug accumulation and possible toxicity may result unless dosage is reduced.

Physiologically, an infant's kidneys differ from an adult's in that they have:
• high resistance to blood flow and receive a smaller proportion of cardiac output
• incomplete glomerular and tubular development and short, incomplete loops of Henle (A child's glomerular filtration reaches adult values by age 2½ to 5 months; his tubular secretion may reach adult values by age 7 to 12 months.)
• low glomerular filtration rate (Penicillins are eliminated by this route.)
• decreased ability to concentrate urine or reabsorb various filtered compounds
• reduced ability by the proximal tubules to secrete organic acids.

Both children and adults have diurnal variations in urine pH that correlate with sleep-wake patterns.

Calculating and monitoring pediatric dosages
When calculating pediatric dosages, don't use formulas that modify adult dosages: a child is not a scaled-down

version of an adult. Pediatric dosages should be calculated on the basis of either body weight (mg/kg) or body surface area (mg/m²).

• Reevaluate dosages at regular intervals to ensure necessary adjustments as the child develops.

• Although useful for adults and older children, don't use dosages based on body surface area in premature or full-term infants. Use the body weight method instead.

• Don't exceed the maximum adult dosage when calculating amounts per kilogram of body weight (except with certain drugs, such as theophylline, if indicated).

• Obtain an accurate maternal drug history—prescription and nonprescription drugs, vitamins, and herbs or other health foods taken during pregnancy.

• Drugs passed through breast milk can also have adverse effects on the nursing infant. Before a drug is prescribed for a breast-feeding mother, the potential effects on the infant should be investigated. For example, sulfa drugs given to a breast-feeding mother for a urinary tract infection appear in breast milk and may cause kernicterus at lower-than-normal levels of unconjugated bilirubin. Also, high concentrations of isoniazid appear in breast milk. Since this drug is metabolized by the liver, an infant's immature hepatic enzyme mechanisms cannot metabolize the drug, and the infant may suffer central nervous system (CNS) toxicity.

Oral medications

• *When giving oral medication to an infant,* administer it in liquid form if possible. For accuracy, measure and give the preparation by syringe; never use a vial or cup.

• Lift the patient's head to prevent aspiration of the medication, and press down on his chin to prevent choking.

• You may also place the drug in a nipple and allow the infant to suck the contents.

• *If the patient is a toddler,* explain how you're going to give him the medication. If possible, have the parents enlist the child's cooperation.

• Don't mix medication with food or call it "candy" even if it has a pleasant taste.

• Let the child drink liquid medication from a calibrated medication cup rather than from a spoon: it's easier and more accurate. If the preparation is available only in tablet form, crush it and mix it with a compatible syrup. (Check with the pharmacist to make sure the tablet can be crushed without losing its effectiveness.)

• *If the patient's an older child* who can swallow a tablet or capsule by himself, have him place the medication on the back of his tongue and swallow it with water or fruit juice. Remember, milk or milk products may interfere with drug absorption.

Intravenous infusions

When administering I.V. infusions to children, note the following special considerations.

Protecting the insertion site
In infants, use a peripheral vein or a scalp vein in the temporal region for I.V. infusions. The scalp vein is safest in that the needle is not likely to be dislodged; however, the head must be shaved around the site. Disfigurement may also result from the needle and infiltrated fluids. For these reasons, the scalp veins are not used as frequently today as they were in the past.

The extremities are the most accessible insertion sites; however, since patients tend to move about, take these precautions:

• Protect the insertion site to prevent catheter or needle dislodgment.

• Use a padded arm board to minimize dislodgment. Remove the arm board during range-of-motion exercises.

• Place the clamp out of the child's reach; if extension tubing is used to allow the child greater mobility, securely tape the connection.

• Restrain the child only when necessary.

• To allay anxiety, give a simple explanation to the child who must be restrained while asleep.

Maintaining flow rate and fluid balance

While administering a continuous I.V. infusion to a child, monitor flow rate and check the patient's condition and insertion site at least hourly—more frequently when giving drug intermittently.

Adjust the flow rate only while the patient is composed; crying and emotional upset can constrict blood vessels. Flow rate may be retarded if a pump isn't used. Flow should be adequate because some drugs (calcium, for example) can be very irritating at low flow rates.

Making dilutions

Some drugs are hyperosmolar; in infants, these drugs must be diluted to prevent radical changes in fluid that might induce CNS hemorrhage. Sodium bicarbonate, for example, must be diluted to half-strength to lower osmolality and lessen the risk of CNS bleeding.

In general, however, use the minimum amount of compatible fluid over the shortest recommended period of time. Remember also to check the total daily fluid intake and the amount allotted to medication.

Intramuscular injections

Intramuscular injections are preferred when the drug cannot be given by other parenteral routes and rapid absorption is necessary.

• In children under 2 years, the vastus lateralis muscle is the preferred injection site; in older children, either the ventrogluteal area or the gluteus medius muscle can be used.

• To determine correct needle size, consider the patient's age, muscle mass, and nutritional status and the drug's viscosity; record and rotate injection sites.

• Explain to the patient that the injection will hurt, but that the medication will help him. Restrain him during the injection, and comfort him afterward.

Dermatomucosal medications

• Use eardrops warmed to room temperature; cold drops can cause considerable pain and possibly vertigo.

• To administer drops, turn the patient on his side, with the affected ear up. If he is younger than 3 years, pull the pinna down and back; if he is older than 3 years, pull the pinna up and back.

• Avoid using inhalants in very young children: obtaining their cooperation is difficult.

• Before attempting to administer medication through a metered-dose nebulizer to an older child, explain the inhaler to him. Then have him hold the nebulizer upside down and close his lips around the mouthpiece. Have him exhale; pinch his nostrils shut; and when he starts to inhale, release one dose of medication into his mouth. Tell the patient to continue inhaling until his lungs feel full.

• Most inhaled agents are not useful if taken orally; therefore, if you doubt the patient's ability to use the inhalant correctly, don't use it.

Parenteral nutrition

Intravenous nutrition is given to patients who can't or won't take adequate food orally and patients with hypermetabolic conditions who need I.V. supplementation. The latter group includes premature infants and children who have burns or other major trauma, intractable diarrhea, malabsorption syndromes, gastrointestinal abnormalities, emotional disorders (such as anorexia nervosa), and congenital abnormalities.

Before fat emulsions are administered to infants and children, however, potential benefits must be weighed against possible risks.

Fats—supplied as 10% or 20% emulsions—are administered both peripherally and centrally. Their use is limited by the child's ability to metabolize them. An infant or child with a diseased liver cannot efficiently metabolize fats, for example.

Some fats, however, must be supplied both to prevent essential fatty acid deficiency and to permit normal growth and development. A minimum of calories (2% to 4%) must be supplied as linoleic acid—an essential fatty acid found in lipids. In infants, fats are essential for normal neurologic development.

Nevertheless, fat solutions may decrease oxygen perfusion and may adversely affect children with pulmonary disease. This risk can be minimized by supplying only the minimum fat needed for essential fatty acid requirements and not the usual intake of 40% to 50% of the child's total calories.

Fatty acids can also displace bilirubin bound to serum albumin, causing a rise in free, unconjugated bilirubin and an increased risk of kernicterus. However, fat solutions may interfere with some bilirubin assays and cause falsely elevated levels. To avoid this complication, a blood sample should be drawn 4 hours after infusion of the lipid emulsion; or if the emulsion is introduced over 24 hours, the blood sample should be centrifuged before the assay is performed.

Drug therapy in elderly patients

If you're providing drug therapy for elderly patients, you'll want to understand physiologic and pharmacokinetic changes that may alter drug dosage, common adverse reactions, and compliance problems in elderly patients.

Physiologic changes affecting drug action

As a person ages, gradual physiologic changes occur. Some of these age-related changes may alter the therapeutic and toxic effects of medications.

Body composition
Proportions of fat, lean tissue, and water in the body change with age. Total body mass and lean body mass tend to decrease; the proportion of body fat tends to increase.

Varying from person to person, these changes in body composition affect the relationship between a drug's concentration and solubility in the body.

For example, a water-soluble drug, such as gentamicin, is not distributed to fat. Since there's relatively less lean tissue in an elderly person, more drug remains in the blood.

Gastrointestinal function
In elderly patients, decreases in gastric acid secretion and GI motility slow the emptying of stomach contents and the movement of intestinal contents through the entire tract. Furthermore, inconclusive research shows that elderly patients may have more difficulty absorbing medica-

tions. This is a particularly significant problem with drugs having a narrow therapeutic range, such as digoxin, in which any change in absorption can be crucial.

Hepatic function
The liver's ability to metabolize certain drugs decreases with age. This is due to diminished blood flow to the liver, which results from the age-related decrease in cardiac output and from the diminished activity of certain liver enzymes. When an elderly patient takes certain sleep medications, such as secobarbital, his liver's reduced ability to metabolize the drug may produce a hangover effect the next morning.

Decreased hepatic function may cause:
• more intense drug effects due to higher blood levels
• longer-lasting drug effects due to prolonged blood concentrations
• greater incidence of drug toxicity.

Renal function
Although an elderly person's renal function is usually sufficient to eliminate excess body fluid and waste, his ability to eliminate some medications may be reduced by 50% or more.

Many medications commonly used by elderly patients, such as digoxin, are excreted primarily through the kidneys. If the kidneys' ability to excrete the drug is decreased, high blood concentrations may result. Digoxin toxicity, therefore, is relatively common in elderly patients who are not receiving a reduced digoxin dosage to account for their decreased renal function.

Drug dosages can be modified to compensate for age-related decreases in renal function. Aided by laboratory tests, such as blood urea nitrogen and serum creatinine, clinical pharmacists and doctors can adjust medication dosages so the patient receives the expected therapeutic benefits without the risk of toxicity. Observe your patient for signs of toxicity. A patient taking digoxin, for example, may experience anorexia, nausea, vomiting, or confusion.

Adverse drug reactions
As compared with younger people, elderly patients experience twice as many adverse drug reactions relating to greater drug consumption, poor compliance, and physiologic changes.

Signs and symptoms of adverse drug reactions—confusion, weakness, and lethargy—are often mistakenly attributed to senility or disease. If the adverse reaction isn't identified, the patient may continue to receive the drug. Furthermore, he may receive unnecessary additional medication to treat complications caused by the original medication. This can sometimes result in the pattern of inappropriate and excessive medication use referred to as "polypharmacy."

Although any medication can cause adverse reactions, most of the serious reactions in the elderly are caused by relatively few medications. Be particularly alert for toxicities resulting from diuretics, antihypertensives, digoxin, corticosteroids, sleeping aids, and nonprescription drugs.

Diuretic toxicity
Because total body water content decreases with age, normal dosages of potassium-wasting diuretics, such as hydrochlorothiazide and furosemide, may result in fluid loss and even dehy-

dration in an elderly patient.

These diuretics may deplete serum potassium, causing weakness in the patient; and they may raise blood uric acid and glucose levels, complicating preexisting gout and diabetes mellitus.

Antihypertensive toxicity
Many elderly people experience lightheadedness or fainting when using antihypertensive medications. This is partially due to the fact that hypertension in elderly patients is partly a response to such changes as atherosclerosis and decreased elasticity of the blood vessels. Antihypertensive drugs lower blood pressure too rapidly, resulting in insufficient blood flow to the brain. This may cause dizziness, fainting, or even stroke.

Consequently, dosages of antihypertensive drugs must be carefully individualized for each patient. In elderly patients, overaggressive treatment of high blood pressure may clearly do more harm than good, so treatment goals should be reasonable. While it may be appropriate to bring blood pressure down to 120/85 mm Hg for a young hypertensive patient, a more reasonable goal for some elderly hypertensive patients would be 150/95 mm Hg.

Digoxin toxicity
As the body's renal function and rate of excretion decline, digoxin concentrations in the blood may build to toxic levels, causing nausea, vomiting, diarrhea, and—most serious—cardiac dysrhythmias. Try to prevent severe toxicity by observing your patient for early signs, such as appetite loss, confusion, or depression.

Corticosteroid toxicity
Elderly patients on corticosteroids may experience short-term effects, including fluid retention and psychological manifestations ranging from mild

euphoria to acute psychotic reactions. Long-term toxic effects, such as osteoporosis, can be especially severe in elderly patients who have been taking prednisone or related steroidal compounds for months or even years. To prevent serious toxicity, carefully monitor patients on long-term regimens. Observe them for subtle changes in appearance, mood, and mobility, as well as for signs of impaired healing and fluid and electrolyte disturbances.

Sleeping aid toxicity
Sedatives or sleeping aids, such as flurazepam, may cause excessive sedation or residual drowsiness.

Nonprescription drug toxicity
When aspirin and aspirin-containing analgesics are used in moderation, toxicity is minimal, but prolonged ingestion may cause GI irritation and gradual blood loss resulting in severe anemia. Although anemia from chronic aspirin consumption can affect all age-groups, elderly patients may be less able to compensate because of their already reduced iron stores.

Laxatives may cause diarrhea in elderly patients who are extremely sensitive to drugs such as bisacodyl. Chronic oral use of mineral oil as a lubricating laxative may result in lipid pneumonia due to aspiration of small residual oil droplets in the patient's mouth.

Patient noncompliance
Poor compliance is a problem with patients of all ages. However, in elderly patients, specific factors linked to aging—such as diminished visual acuity, hearing loss, forgetfulness, the common need for multiple drug therapy, and various socioeconomic factors—combine to make compliance a special problem. Approximately one-third of elderly patients fail to comply

with their prescribed drug therapy. They may fail to take prescribed doses or to follow the correct schedule; they may take medications prescribed for previous disorders, discontinue medications prematurely, or use p.r.n. medications indiscriminately.

Review your patient's medication regimen with him. Be sure he understands the medication amount and the time and frequency of doses. Also, explain how he should take each medication, that is, with food or water or by itself.

Give your patient whatever help you can to avoid drug therapy problems, and refer him to the doctor or pharmacist if he needs further information.

5

Drug therapy and the nursing process

The nursing process guides nursing decisions about drug administration to ensure the patient's safety and meet medical and legal standards. This process, in five steps, provides thorough assessment, appropriate nursing diagnosis, purposeful planning, appropriate interventions, and constant evaluation.

First step: Assessment
During assessment, the nurse focuses on direct data collection by:
• obtaining a drug history from the patient, parent, spouse, or significant other
• reviewing the patient's previous medical history
• performing a physical examination of the patient
• obtaining relevant laboratory or diagnostic test results.

Drug history
Data collection begins at admission to the hospital or in an outpatient setting with specific questions about the patient's background, including allergies, medical history, habits, socioeconomic status, life-style and beliefs, and sensory deficits. These aspects of the patient's background can have significant influence on drug therapy.

Allergies
The patient's allergy profile includes the patient's reactions to both drugs and food. Information about allergic reactions to drugs must specify the drug, when the allergic reaction oc-

curred, the situation and setting at the time of the reaction, a description of the reaction, and any contributing factors. Examples of contributing factors might include the concurrent use of alcohol or recreational drugs, or a significant change in nutritional patterns. Asking the patient to describe his allergic reaction is especially important to help determine whether the patient actually reacts adversely to a drug or simply dislikes taking it.

Allergies to foods can also affect a drug therapy. For example, allergies to shellfish can interfere with use of drugs that contain iodine or are byproducts of shellfish. Allergies to eggs are significant in patients who are to receive vaccines, which are commonly derived from chick embryos.

Prescription drugs
The patient's drug history should explore the following:
• the reason for using the drug
• the patient's knowledge of the appropriate dosage and schedule of administration
• the patient's knowedge about determining effectiveness of the drug (if appropriate), adverse effects the drug might cause, what to do about adverse effects, and when to contact the doctor
• route of administration
• the pattern of administration at home
• use of OTC drugs
• cognitive status.
  Note any special monitoring the pa-

tient must perform, such as blood glucose monitoring before insulin administration or checking radial pulse rate before taking digoxin. Make sure the patient is performing such procedures correctly and that the results are within acceptable limits.

Discuss the effects of drug therapy with the patient and determine if new symptoms or unpredicted adverse effects have developed. Noting the patient's pattern of administration may provide insight into why a particular drug regimen succeeds or fails.

Over-the-counter drugs
A comprehensive drug history should also list any OTC drugs the patient is taking. Many OTC drugs can inhibit or potentiate the effects of a prescribed drug. For example, aspirin potentiates the anticoagulant effects of warfarin.

OTC drugs include a wide range of products from common aspirin and nutritional supplements to various sprays and cleansing agents. The patient may not think of all of these products as drugs, so the nurse may have to suggest a general list of products to get an accurate response.

Dosage and frequency of use are just as important as the type of the OTC product the patient is using. One tablet of aspirin taken once a day may have no effect on concomitant drug therapy; however, a higher dosage (such as that used for arthritis) could influence it profoundly.

Medical history
In gathering the medical history, note any chronic diseases or disorders the patient may have and record the following information for each:
• date of diagnosis
• initial prescribed treatment
• current treatment
• the doctor in charge.

Careful attention to this part of the medical history can uncover one of the most important problems with drug therapy —conflicting and incompatible drug regimens. The patient who does not have a family physician to oversee and coordinate all care may seek the care of several specialists who may prescribe drug treatment without knowing what other drugs the patient is taking. A carefully detailed medical history can uncover such problems. The nurse who identifies such conflicting or overlapping drug therapy must call them to the appropriate doctor's attention and then teach the patient about the importance of informing all care-givers about all drugs he is taking.

Habits
Carefully consider dietary habits and the use of recreational drugs.

Certain foods can directly affect the effectiveness of many drugs. For example, a person who is taking the anticoagulant warfarin (Coumadin) should not increase his intake of green leafy vegetables because they contain significant levels of Vitamin K that can antagonize the drug's anticoagulant effect.

Recreational drugs can profoundly affect a patient's health and impair the effectiveness of a drug therapy. Consider the possible use of alcohol, tobacco, caffeine, and illicit drugs, such as marijuana, cocaine, and heroin. For example, if the patient uses alcohol, note the frequency of use, the amount, and the type of alcohol consumed. Carefully document the intake of stimulants, such as caffeine, because they significantly affect a patient's cardiovascular status and nervous system. Record the type of stimulant (coffee, tea, soda, or chocolate), the frequency of intake, and the amount consumed.

For the patient who smokes, document the following information:
• the length of time the patient has smoked

- what the patient smokes (cigarettes, cigar, or pipe)
- how many cigarettes or cigars the patient smokes per day
- the brand of cigarettes or cigars the patient smokes
- the brand of tobacco and how much he chews per day, if he chews it.

Defining the patient's use of illicit drugs may be difficult. However, the nurse who suspects such use should encourage the patient to discuss it honestly, emphasizing that these drugs have profound effects that may cause serious drug interactions. If the patient admits using illicit drugs, document the drug, the amount and frequency of use, and the route of administration.

Socioeconomic status
Note the patient's age, educational level, occupation, and insurance coverage. These factors may be significant to compliance and to an effective care plan. The patient's age, for example, can determine whom to include in the care plan (parents or other family members) and the level of information that is appropriate for teaching the patient.

Knowing the patient's educational background and occupation helps the nurse select interventions at an appropriate level, plan a drug regimen that fits the patient's daily routine, and encourage compliance. Knowing the patient's insurance status will help you anticipate probable length of stay based on the appropriate Diagnosis Related Group (DRG), and the patient's need for financial assistance and counseling. Remember that noncompliance frequently results from inability to afford costly medications.

Life-style and beliefs
Support systems, marital status, childbearing status, attitudes toward health and health care, use of the health care system, and daily patterns of activities all affect the plan of care and patient compliance. For example, an 18-year-old single parent, who is a high-school dropout on medical assistance and has no family support, will probably require more extensive teaching and support to gain a commitment and compliance to drug therapy than a 40-year-old affluent professional, with a lot of family support who can understand why she needs the drug and can readily pay for it.

Sensory deficits
Any sensory deficit can significantly shape an appropriate care plan. For example, impaired vision, paralysis of one or more extremities, loss of a limb, or loss of sensation in an extremity can impair the patient's ability to administer a subcutaneous injection, break a scored tablet, or open a medication container. Color blindness may cause difficulty in distinguishing between two medications. Hearing impairment can prevent effective patient instruction. Any sensory deficit requires careful consideration in any plan of prescribed drug therapy.

Clinical status
Two other factors can profoundly influence drug therapy: the patient's cognitive status and systemic effects of the prescribed drugs. A patient's intact cognitive abilities ensure that he can understand and implement the actions necessary for compliance. During the interview, note if the patient is alert and oriented, if he is able to interact appropriately with people, and if his conversation is appropriate to the subject being discussed. Consider whether the patient can think clearly, and express his thoughts coherently. Finally, check both short-term and long-term memory because the patient needs both to follow a specified drug regimen. If such evaluation identifies a cognitive deficit, de-

termine the probable cause, which can range from a transient drug-related effect to permanent neurologic impairment, and then determine whether or not the patient can carry out the prescribed drug regimen. If not, the nurse must find another way to ensure that the patient receives the prescribed therapy.

After completing the drug history, perform a physical examination to assess those body systems that may be affected by a particular drug the patient is taking or that may be prescribed. Every drug has a desired effect on a body system but it may have an undesired effect on another. For example, chemotherapeutic agents destroy cancerous cells but they also affect normal cells and often cause the patient to experience hair loss, diarrhea, or nausea. Therefore, examine the patient for expected drug effects; also closely monitor the patient for potentially harmful adverse effects.

Second step: Formulating a nursing diagnosis

Using information gathered during assessment, define any potential or actual drug-related problems by formulating each in a relevant nursing diagnosis. The most common problem statements related to drug therapy are "Knowledge deficit," "Noncompliance," and "Alteration in Health Maintenance."

Third step: Planning

Nursing diagnoses provide the framework for planning interventions and outcome criteria (patient goals).

Outcome criteria state the desired patient behaviors or responses that should result from nursing care. Outcome criteria should be measurable and objective, concise, realistic for the patient, and attainable by nursing management; they should express patient behavior in terms of expectations and specify a time frame. A typical outcome statement is "The patient verbalizes major adverse effects related to his chemotherapy drugs prior to discharge."

Fourth step: Intervention

After developing the outcome criteria, the nurse determines the interventions needed to help the patient reach the desired behavior or goals. Drug-related interventions may focus on patient teaching for a drug's action, adverse effects, scheduling, steps to avoid or treat a drug reaction, or drug administration techniques.

Appropriate interventions related to drug therapy will also include administration procedures, administration techniques, legal and ethical concerns, patient teaching, and any special concerns related to special groups of patients (geriatric, pediatric, and pregnant or breast-feeding patients). Such interventions may be independent nursing actions, such as turning a bedridden patient every 2 hours, or may be nursing actions that require a doctor's order.

Fifth step: Evaluation

The final component of the nursing process, evaluation, is a formal and systematic process for determining the effectiveness of nursing care. This process enables the nurse to determine whether outcome criteria were met, and thereby make informed decisions about subsequent interventions. For example, if the patient experienced relief of headache within 1 hour after the nurse administered a p.r.n. analgesic, the outcome criterion was met. If the headache was the same or worse, the outcome criterion was not met and requires reassessment, which may require replanning or may yield new data that invalidates the nursing diagnosis or suggests new nursing interventions that are more specific or more acceptable to the patient. Such reassessment could lead to a higher dosage, a different analgesic, or a re-evaluation of the cause.

Evaluation enables the nurse to design and implement a revised care plan, to continuously re-evaluate outcome criteria, and to replan until each nursing diagnosis is resolved.

Amebicides and trichomonacides

carbarsone
chloroquine hydrochloride
(See Chapter 9, ANTIMALARIALS.)
chloroquine phosphate
(See Chapter 9, ANTIMALARIALS.)
emetine hydrochloride
iodoquinol (diiodohydroxyquin)
metronidazole (systemic)
metronidazole hydrochloride
paromomycin sulfate

COMBINATION PRODUCTS
None.

---

carbarsone
Carbarsone Pulvules

Pregnancy Risk Category: D

MECHANISM OF ACTION
An organic arsenic derivative with amebicidal activity in the intestinal lumen, possibly due to inhibition of sulfhydryl enzymes.

INDICATIONS & DOSAGE
Intestinal amebiasis—
Adults: 250 mg P.O. b.i.d. or t.i.d. for 10 days. Rectal (as retention enema): 2 g dissolved in 200 ml warm 2% sodium bicarbonate solution, every other night for 5 doses. Solution should be retained overnight. Discontinue oral therapy when enema is given.
Children: average total dosage is 75 mg/kg P.O. daily in 3 divided doses over 10-day period. Recommended total dosage varies according to age— 2 to 4 years, 2 g total; 5 to 8 years, 3 g total; 9 to 12 years, 4 g total; and over 12 years, 5 g total.

ADVERSE REACTIONS
Blood: *agranulocytosis.*
CNS: neuritis, convulsions, *hemorrhagic encephalitis.*
EENT: sore throat, retinal edema, visual disturbances.
GI: epigastric pain and burning, irritation, *nausea, vomiting,* diarrhea, anorexia, constipation, increased motility, abdominal cramps.
GU: polyuria, albuminuria, kidney damage.
Hepatic: hepatomegaly, jaundice, hepatitis.
Skin: eruptions, *exfoliative dermatitis,* pruritus.
Other: edema of wrists, ankles, and knees; weight loss; splenomegaly.

INTERACTIONS
None significant.

NURSING CONSIDERATIONS
• Contraindicated as initial treatment in hepatic or renal disease; in patients with contracted visual or color fields; and in patients with known hypersensitivity or intolerance to any arsenical treatment.
• Don't exceed recommended dose; toxicity may result. If second treatment is needed, allow at least 10 days between courses.
• Monitor for signs of acute arsenic toxicity: sore throat; edema of wrists, ankles, and knees; nausea and vomiting. Acute toxicity may be treated with dimercaprol.
• Divide carbarsone capsule to obtain

required dose. Give in ½ glass orange juice or milk, in small amount of 1% sodium bicarbonate solution, or in jelly or other food.
• Discontinue upon first sign of intolerance or toxicity. Fatal exfoliative dermatitis has been reported.
• Tell patient to report any unusual symptoms, even post-treatment.
• Liver function tests should precede therapy. Careful inspection of skin, vision testing, and palpation of liver and spleen should be repeated regularly.
• Monitor intake/output. Record number, frequency, and character of stools.
• If ordered, give a cleansing enema of 2% sodium bicarbonate before giving carbarsone enema.
• All members of household may need to have stools examined.
• Deliver stool specimen to lab promptly; movements of parasites are seen only when stool is warm. Amebic cysts in stool indicate need for additional therapy. Stool specimen should be studied 1 week after stopping therapy and monthly for 1 year.
• To help prevent reinfestation, teach patient about the need for good personal hygiene, especially handwashing technique. Patient should refrain from preparing food until stools are negative.

---

emetine hydrochloride

Pregnancy Risk Category: X

MECHANISM OF ACTION
Kills *Entamoeba histolytica* by a mechanism related to the inhibition of protein synthesis.

INDICATIONS & DOSAGE
Acute fulminating amebic dysentery—
Adults: 1 mg/kg daily up to 60 mg daily (1 or 2 doses) deep S.C. or I.M. 3 to 5 days (only until symptoms are under control). Give another antiame-

bic drug simultaneously.
Children: 1 mg/kg daily in 2 doses I.M. for up to 5 days.
Amebic hepatitis and abscess—
Adults: 60 mg daily (1 or 2 doses) deep S.C. or I.M. for 10 days.

ADVERSE REACTIONS
CNS: dizziness, headache, mild sensory disturbances, central or peripheral nerve function changes, neuromuscular symptoms (weakness, aching, stiffness, tenderness, pain, tremors).
CV: *acute toxicity*—can occur at any dose (hypotension, tachycardia, precordial pain, dyspnea, *ECG abnormalities,* gallop rhythm, cardiac dilatation, severe acute degenerative myocarditis, pericarditis, congestive failure).
GI: *nausea, vomiting, diarrhea,* abdominal cramps, loss of sense of taste.
Metabolic: decreased serum potassium levels.
Skin: eczematous, urticarial purpuric lesions.
Local: skeletal muscle stiffness, aching, tenderness, *muscle weakness at injection site, cellulitis.*
Other: edema.

INTERACTIONS
None significant.

NURSING CONSIDERATIONS
• Contraindicated in cardiac or renal disease, except with amebic abscess or hepatitis not controlled by chloroquine or metronidazole; in patients who have received a course of emetine less than 6 to 8 weeks previously; in children, except for those with severe dysentery unresponsive to other amebicides; and in patients with polyneuropathy or muscle disease. Use with caution and in reduced dosage in elderly or debilitated patients, patients with hypotension, or those about to undergo surgery.

Italicized side effects are common or life-threatening.
*Liquid form contains alcohol.   **May contain tartrazine.

• Record pulse rate and blood pressure 2 to 3 times daily. Discontinue use if drug produces tachycardia, precipitous fall in blood pressure, neuromuscular symptoms, marked gastrointestinal effects, or considerable weakness. Weakness and muscle symptoms usually precede more serious symptoms and serve as a guide for avoiding toxicity.

• Because of potential for cardiovascular toxicity, don't exceed recommended dose or extend therapy beyond 10 days. Impose bed rest during treatment and for several days thereafter.

• Drug may alter ECG tracings for 6 weeks. ECG should be taken before therapy, after fifth dose, upon completion, and 1 week after therapy. Patterns can resemble those of myocardial infarction. First and most consistent change is T wave inversion.

• Deep S.C. administration is preferred; I.M. is acceptable, but I.V. route can be cardiotoxic and is contraindicated. Rotate sites and apply warm soaks.

• Record intake/output; odor and consistency of stools; and presence of mucus, blood, or other foreign matter. Send warm specimens to lab for analysis. Repeat fecal examinations at 3-month intervals to assure elimination of amebae. Patients with acute amebic dysentery often become asymptomatic carriers. Check family members and suspected contacts.

• Suspect emetine-induced reaction if stools increase in number following initial relief of diarrhea.

• To help prevent reinfestation, teach patient about the need for good personal hygiene, especially handwashing technique. Patient should refrain from preparing food until stools are negative.

• Drug is very irritating. Avoid contact with eyes and mucous membranes.

iodoquinol (diiodohydroxyquin)
Diodoquin♦♦, Diquinol, Yodoxin

Pregnancy Risk Category: C

MECHANISM OF ACTION
An iodine derivative with amebicidal activity in the intestinal lumen. Its precise mechanism of action is unknown.

INDICATIONS & DOSAGE
Intestinal amebiasis—
Adults: 630 to 650 mg P.O. t.i.d. for 20 days. Total daily dosage should not exceed 2 g.
Children: usual dosage 30 to 40 mg/kg of body weight daily in 2 to 3 divided doses for 20 days.

Additional courses of iodoquinol therapy should not be repeated before a resting interval of 2 to 3 weeks.

ADVERSE REACTIONS
Blood: *agranulocytosis.*
CNS: neurotoxicity (dose-related), dysesthesia, weakness, vertigo, malaise, headache, agitation, retrograde amnesia, ataxia, *peripheral neuropathy.*
EENT: *optic neuritis,* optic atrophy, loss of vision.
GI: anorexia, nausea, vomiting, abdominal cramps, diarrhea, increased motility, constipation, epigastric burning and pain, gastritis, anal irritation and itching.
Skin: pruritus, hives, papular and pustular eruptions, urticaria, discoloration of hair and nails.
Other: thyroid enlargement, fever, chills, generalized furunculosis, hair loss.

INTERACTIONS
None significant.

NURSING CONSIDERATIONS
• Contraindicated in patients with

---

known hypersensitivity to 8-hy-droxyquinoline derivatives or iodine-containing preparations. Diiodohy-droxyquin causes hepatic damage in such patients. Also contraindicated in hepatic or renal disease or preexisting optic neuropathy.

• Patient should have periodic ophthalmologic examinations during treatment.

• Give after meals. Crush tablets and mix with applesauce or chocolate syrup.

• Record intake/output and color and amount of stool. Send warm specimens to lab for analysis.

• Watch for diarrhea during the first 2 or 3 days of treatment. Notify doctor if it continues past 3 days.

• Advise patient not to discontinue the medication prematurely. Tell him to notify doctor if skin rash occurs.

• May interfere with thyroid function tests for up to 6 months after discontinuation of drug.

• To help prevent reinfestation, teach patient about the need for good personal hygiene, especially handwashing technique. Patient should refrain from preparing food until stools are negative.

---

metronidazole
Apo-Metronidazole◆◆, Flagyl◆, Metizol, Metric 21, Metryl, Neo-Metric◆◆, Novonidazol◆◆, PMS Metronidazole◆◆, Protostat

metronidazole hydrochloride
Flagyl I.V.◆, Flagyl I.V. RTU, Metro I.V., Novonidazol◆◆

Pregnancy Risk Category: B

MECHANISM OF ACTION
A direct-acting trichomonacide and amebicide that works at both intestinal and extraintestinal sites.

INDICATIONS & DOSAGE
Amebic hepatic abscess—
Adults: 500 to 750 mg P.O. t.i.d. for 5 to 10 days.
Children: 35 to 50 mg/kg daily (in 3 doses) for 10 days.
Intestinal amebiasis—
Adults: 750 mg P.O. t.i.d. for 5 to 10 days.
Children: 35 to 50 mg/kg daily (in 3 doses) for 10 days. Follow this therapy with oral iodoquinol.
Trichomoniasis—
Adults (both male and female): 250 mg P.O. t.i.d. for 7 days or 2 g P.O. in single dose; 4 to 6 weeks should elapse between courses of therapy.
Refractory trichomoniasis—
Women: 250 mg P.O. b.i.d. for 10 days.
Treatment of bacterial infections caused by anaerobic microorganisms—
Adults: Loading dose is 15 mg/kg I.V. infused over 1 hour (approximately 1 g for a 70-kg adult). Maintenance dose is 7.5 mg/kg I.V. or P.O. q 6 hours (approximately 500 mg for a 70-kg adult). The first maintenance dose should be administered 6 hours following the loading dose. Maximum dosage not to exceed 4 g daily.
Giardiasis—
Adults: 250 mg P.O. t.i.d. for 5 days.
Children: 5 mg/kg P.O. t.i.d. for 5 days.
Prevention of postoperative infection in contaminated or potentially contaminated colorectal surgery—
Adults: 15 mg/kg infused over 30 to 60 minutes and completed approximately 1 hour before surgery. Then, 7.5 mg/kg infused over 30 to 60 minutes at 6 and 12 hours after the initial dose.

ADVERSE REACTIONS
Blood: transient leukopenia, neutropenia.
CNS: vertigo, headache, ataxia, incoordination, confusion, irritability,

---

Italicized side effects are common or life-threatening.
*Liquid form contains alcohol.   **May contain tartrazine.

depression, restlessness, weakness, fatigue, drowsiness, insomnia, sensory neuropathy, paresthesias of extremities, psychic stimulation, neuromyopathy.
CV: ECG change (flattened T wave), edema (with I.V. R.T.U. preparation).
GI: abdominal cramping, stomatitis, *nausea, vomiting, anorexia,* diarrhea, constipation, proctitis, dry mouth.
GU: darkened urine, polyuria, dysuria, pyuria, incontinence, cystitis, decreased libido, dyspareunia, dryness of vagina and vulva, sense of pelvic pressure.
Skin: pruritus, flushing.
Local: *thrombophlebitis after I.V. infusion.*
Other: overgrowth of nonsusceptible organisms, especially *Candida* (glossitis, furry tongue), metallic taste, fever, gynecomastia.

INTERACTIONS
Alcohol: disulfiram-like reaction (nausea, vomiting, headache, cramps, flushing). Don't use together.
Disulfiram: acute psychoses and confusional states. Don't use together.

NURSING CONSIDERATIONS
Warning: This drug has been shown to be carcinogenic in mice and possibly rats. Unnecessary use should be avoided.
• If indicated during pregnancy for trichomoniasis, the 7-day regimen is preferred over the 2-g single-dose regimen.
• Use cautiously in patients with a history of blood dyscrasia or CNS disorder, and in patients with retinal or visual field changes. Use with caution in hepatic disease or alcoholism and in conjunction with known hepatotoxic drugs.
• Tell patient to avoid alcohol or alcohol-containing medications during therapy and for 48 hours after therapy is completed.
• Give oral form with meals to mini-

mize GI distress.
• Tell patient metallic taste and dark or red-brown urine may occur.
• Record number and character of stools when used in the treatment of amebiasis. Metronidazole should be used only after *Trichomonas vaginalis* has been confirmed by wet smear or culture or *Entamoeba histolytica* has been identified. Asymptomatic sexual partners of patients being treated for *T. vaginalis* infection should be treated simultaneously to avoid reinfection. Instruct patient in proper hygiene.
• The I.V. form should be administered by slow infusion only. Don't give I.V. push.
• Follow package instructions carefully when mixing the I.V. solution.
• Don't refrigerate Flagyl I.V. RTU
• Flagyl I.V. RTU may cause sodium retention. Observe carefully for edema, especially in patients also receiving corticosteroids.
• Topical metronidazole gel is available for the treatment of acne rosacea.

paromomycin sulfate
Humatin
Pregnancy Risk Category: C

MECHANISM OF ACTION
Acts as an amebicide in intestinal sites, effective in the presence or absence of bacteria. Its specific mechanism of action is unknown.

INDICATIONS & DOSAGE
Intestinal amebiasis, acute and chronic—
Adults and children: 25 to 35 mg/kg daily P.O. in 3 doses for 5 to 10 days after meals.
Tapeworms (fish, beef, pork, dog)—
Adults: 1 g P.O. q 15 minutes for 4 doses.
Children: 11 mg/kg P.O. q 15 minutes for 4 doses.

ADVERSE REACTIONS
Blood: eosinophilia.
CNS: headache, vertigo.
EENT: ototoxicity.
GI: anorexia, *nausea, vomiting, epigastric pain and burning, abdominal cramps,* diarrhea, constipation, increased motility, steatorrhea, pruritus ani, malabsorption syndrome.
GU: hematuria, nephrotoxicity.
Skin: rash, exanthema, pruritus.
Other: overgrowth of nonsusceptible organisms.

INTERACTIONS
None significant.

NURSING CONSIDERATIONS
• Contraindicated in patients with impaired renal function or intestinal obstruction. Use with caution in patients with ulcerative lesions of the bowel to avoid inadvertent absorption and resulting renal toxicity. Poorly absorbed orally, but will accumulate with renal impairment or ulcerative lesions.
• Ask about history of sensitivity to drug before giving first dose.
• Administer after meals.
• To help prevent reinfestation, teach patient about the need for good personal hygiene, especially handwashing technique. Patient should refrain from preparing food until stools are negative.
• Criterion of cure is absence of amebae in stools examined weekly for 6 weeks after treatment and thereafter at monthly intervals for 2 years. Examine feces of family members or suspected contacts.
• Avoid high doses or prolonged therapy.
• Watch for signs of superinfection (continued fever and other signs of new infections, especially monilial infections).

Italicized side effects are common or life-threatening.
*Liquid form contains alcohol.   **May contain tartrazine.

7

Anthelmintics

mebendazole
niclosamide
oxamniquine
piperazine adipate
piperazine citrate
praziquantel
pyrantel pamoate
quinacrine hydrochloride
(mepacrine hydrochloride)
thiabendazole

COMBINATION PRODUCTS
None.

---

mebendazole
Vermox♦

Pregnancy Risk Category: C

MECHANISM OF ACTION
Selectively and irreversibly inhibits
uptake of glucose and other nutrients
in susceptible helminths.

INDICATIONS & DOSAGE
Pinworm—
Adults and children over 2 years:
100 mg P.O. as a single dose. If infection persists 3 weeks later, repeat
treatment.
Roundworm, whipworm, hookworm—
Adults and children over 2 years:
100 mg P.O. b.i.d. for 3 days. If infection persists 3 weeks later, repeat
treatment.

ADVERSE REACTIONS
GI: occasional, transient abdominal
pain and diarrhea in massive infection
and expulsion of worms.

INTERACTIONS
None significant.

NURSING CONSIDERATIONS
• Tablets may be chewed, swallowed
whole, or crushed and mixed with
food.
• No dietary restrictions, laxatives, or
enemas are necessary.
• Treat all family members.
• Teach patient about the need for
good personal hygiene, especially
good handwashing technique. To
avoid reinfection, teach him to wash
perianal area daily. Change undergarments and bedclothes daily. Wash
hands and clean fingernails before
meals and after bowel movements.
Advise patient to refrain from preparing food during infestation.

---

niclosamide
Niclocide

Pregnancy Risk Category: B

MECHANISM OF ACTION
Inhibits the metabolic process of oxi-
dative phosphorylation in tapeworms.

INDICATIONS & DOSAGE
Tapeworms (fish and beef)—
Adults: 4 tablets (2 g) chewed thor-
oughly as a single dose.
Children (more than 34 kg): 3 tablets
(1.5 g) chewed thoroughly as a single
dose.
Children (11 to 34 kg): 2 tablets (1 g)
chewed thoroughly as a single dose.
Dwarf tapeworm—
Adults: 4 tablets chewed thoroughly

as a single daily dose for 7 days.
Children (more than 34 kg): 3 tablets chewed thoroughly on the first day, then 2 tablets for the next 6 days.
Children (11 to 34 kg): 2 tablets chewed thoroughly on the first day, then one tablet daily for the next 6 days.

ADVERSE REACTIONS
CNS: drowsiness, dizziness, headache.
EENT: oral irritation, bad taste in mouth.
GI: *nausea, vomiting, anorexia,* diarrhea.
Skin: rash, pruritus ani.

INTERACTIONS
None reported.

NURSING CONSIDERATIONS
• Instruct patient to chew tablets thoroughly and wash down with water; for smaller children, the tablets can be crushed and mixed with water or applesauce.
• Tablets should be taken as a single dose after breakfast.
• A mild laxative should be administered to cleanse the bowel prior to initiation of niclosamide therapy in patients who are constipated.
• When treating dwarf tapeworms, urge patient to drink fruit juices. This helps to eliminate the accumulated intestinal mucus under which they lodge.
• Teach patient about the need for good personal hygiene, especially good handwashing technique. Advise patient to refrain from preparing food during infestation.
• Patient is not considered cured until the stool has been negative for tapeworms for at least 3 months.

oxamniquine
Vansil

Pregnancy Risk Category: C

MECHANISM OF ACTION
Reduces the egg load of *Schistosoma mansoni,* but its exact mechanism of action is unknown.

INDICATIONS & DOSAGE
Treatment of schistosomiasis caused by Schistosoma mansoni—
Adults and children: 12 to 15 mg/kg given as a single oral dose.

ADVERSE REACTIONS
CNS: convulsions, *dizziness, drowsiness, headache.*
GI: nausea, vomiting, abdominal pain, anorexia.
Skin: urticaria.

INTERACTIONS
None significant.

NURSING CONSIDERATIONS
• Use cautiously in patients with a history of convulsive conditions. Epileptiform convulsions have rarely been observed within the first few hours after ingestion. Patients with a history of convulsions should be kept under medical supervision.
• Instruct patient to avoid driving and other hazardous activities if he's dizzy or drowsy.
• GI tolerance is improved if the drug is given after meals.
• Although *S. mansoni* infection is rare in the United States and Canada, travelers or immigrants from such areas as Puerto Rico, Latin America, and Africa may have contracted the infection from contaminated water.

---

piperazine adipate
Entacyl♦♦

piperazine citrate
Antepar, Bryrel, Pin-Tega Tabs,
Pipril, Ta-Verm, Veriga♦♦,
Vermazine, Vermirex♦♦

Pregnancy Risk Category: B

MECHANISM OF ACTION
Blocks neuromuscular action, paralyzing the worm and causing its expulsion by normal peristalsis.

INDICATIONS & DOSAGE
Pinworm—
Adults and children: 65 mg/kg P.O. daily 7 to 8 days. Maximum daily dosage is 2.5 g.
Roundworm—
Adults: 3.5 g P.O. in single doses for 2 consecutive days.
Children: 75 mg/kg P.O. daily in single doses for 2 consecutive days. Maximum daily dosage is 3.5 g.

ADVERSE REACTIONS
CNS: ataxia, tremors, choreiform movements, muscular weakness, myoclonus, hyporeflexia, paresthesias, convulsions, sense of detachment, EEG abnormalities, memory defect, *headache, vertigo.*
EENT: nystagmus, blurred vision, paralytic strabismus, cataracts with visual impairment, lacrimation, difficulty in focusing, rhinorrhea.
GI: *nausea, vomiting,* diarrhea, abdominal cramps.
Skin: urticaria, photodermatitis, *erythema multiforme,* purpura, eczematous skin reactions.
Other: arthralgia, fever, bronchospasm, hemolytic anemia.

INTERACTIONS
Pyrantel pamoate: Possible pharmacologic antagonism. Don't administer together.

NURSING CONSIDERATIONS
• Contraindicated in hepatic and/or renal impairment, or convulsive disorders. Use with caution in severe malnutrition or anemia.
• Discontinue if CNS or significant GI reactions occur.
• Because of potential neurotoxicity, avoid prolonged or repeated treatment, especially in children.
• No dietary restrictions, laxatives, or enemas are necessary.
• May be taken with food; but, for best absorption, tell patient to take on empty stomach.
• Mix powder for oral suspension in 57 ml. water, milk, or fruit juice.
• Treat all family members.
• Teach patient about the need for good personal hygiene, especially good handwashing technique. To avoid reinfection, teach him to wash perianal area, to change undergarments and bedclothes daily, and to wash hands and clean fingernails before meals and after bowel movements. Advise patient to refrain from preparing food during infestation.
• Mix powder for oral suspension in 57 ml water, milk, or fruit juice.

praziquantel
Biltricide

Pregnancy Risk Category: B

MECHANISM OF ACTION
Causes a contraction of schistosomes by a specific effect on the permeability of the cell membrane.

INDICATIONS & DOSAGE
Treatment of schistosomiasis caused by Schistosoma mekongi, S. japonicum, S. mansoni, *and* S. haematobium—
Adults and children 4 years and older: 20 mg/kg P.O. t.i.d. as a 1-day treatment. The interval between doses should be between 4 and 6 hours.

ADVERSE REACTIONS
CNS: *drowsiness, malaise,* headache, dizziness.
GI: abdominal discomfort, nausea.
Hepatic: minimal increase in liver enzymes.
Skin: urticaria.
Other: fever.

INTERACTIONS
None significant.

NURSING CONSIDERATIONS
• Contraindicated with ocular cysticercosis.
• May produce drowsiness. Tell patient to drive or operate machinery cautiously on the day of treatment and the day after treatment.
• Adverse effects may be more frequent or serious in patients with a heavy worm burden.
• In the event of overdose, give a fast-acting laxative.
• Advise patient to take the tablet during meals and to wash down the unchewed tablet with a liquid.
• Tablets taste very bitter. Keeping them in the mouth may cause gagging or vomiting.
• Praziquantel is effective for several different species of *Schistosoma*.
• May also be effective against liver flukes.

pyrantel pamoate
Antiminth, Combantrin♦♦

Pregnancy Risk Category: C

MECHANISM OF ACTION
Blocks neuromuscular action, paralyzing the worm and causing its expulsion by normal peristalsis.

INDICATIONS & DOSAGE
Roundworm and pinworm—
Adults and children over 2 years: single dosage of 11 mg/kg P.O. Maximum dosage 1 g. For pinworm, dosage should be repeated in 2 weeks.

ADVERSE REACTIONS
CNS: headache, dizziness, drowsiness, insomnia.
GI: anorexia, nausea, vomiting, gastralgia, cramps, diarrhea, tenesmus.
Hepatic: transient elevation of AST (SGOT).
Skin: rashes.
Other: fever, weakness.

INTERACTIONS
Piperazine salts: Possible pharmacologic antagonism. Don't administer together.

NURSING CONSIDERATIONS
• Use cautiously in severe malnutrition or anemia, or in hepatic dysfunction. Treat for anemia, dehydration, or malnutrition before giving drug.
• No dietary restrictions, laxatives, or enemas are necessary.
• May be taken with food, milk, or fruit juices. Shake well before pouring.
• Treat all family members.
• Teach patient about the need for good personal hygiene, especially good handwashing technique. To avoid reinfection, teach him to wash perianal area daily, to change undergarments and bedclothes daily, and to wash hands and clean fingernails before meals and after bowel movements. Advise patient to refrain from preparing food during infestation.
• Protect drug from light. Store below 30° C. (86° F.).
• Now available without a prescription. Urge patient to read the enclosed consumer information that tells how to identify and recognize pinworms.

quinacrine hydrochloride (mepacrine hydrochloride)
Atabrine♦

Pregnancy Risk Category: C

MECHANISM OF ACTION
Inhibits DNA metabolism in suscepti-

ble parasites.

INDICATIONS & DOSAGE
Treatment of giardiasis—
Adults: 300 mg P.O. in 3 divided doses for 5 to 7 days.
Children: 7 mg/kg/day P.O. given in 3 divided doses after meals for 5 days. Maximum 300 mg/day. If necessary, the dosage may be repeated in 2 weeks.
Tapeworms (beef, pork, and fish)—
Adults and children over 14 years: 4 doses of 200 mg given 10 minutes apart (800 mg total).
Children 11 to 14 years: 600 mg total dosage, administered in 3 or 4 divided doses, 10 minutes apart.
Children 5 to 10 years: 400 mg total dosage, administered in 3 or 4 divided doses, 10 minutes apart.

ADVERSE REACTIONS
CNS: *headache, dizziness, nervousness, vertigo, mood shifts, nightmares, seizures.*
GI: *diarrhea, anorexia, nausea, abdominal cramps,* vomiting.
GU: yellow urine.
Skin: pleomorphic skin eruptions, yellow discoloration.

INTERACTIONS
None significant.

NURSING CONSIDERATIONS
• Contraindicated if patient is taking primaquine since primaquine toxicity could be increased.
• Use with extreme caution in porphyria or psoriasis; may exacerbate these conditions.
• Use with caution in hepatic disease, alcoholism, severe renal or cardiac disease, psychosis, and G6PD deficiency, and in those over 60 years or under 1 year.
• Give after meals with large glass of water, tea, or fruit juice to reduce GI irritation. Bitter taste may be disguised by jam or honey.

• Nausea and vomiting after large doses may be lessened by taking sodium bicarbonate with each dose.
• Administer a saline cathartic 1 to 2 hours after drug is given, to expel the worm.
• Collect all of stool after treatment. Don't put toilet paper in bedpan. Look for the scolex (attachment organ), which will be stained yellow from drug.
• Warn patient about temporary yellow color of skin and urine—it is not jaundice.
• Patient should be on a bland, nonfat, semisolid diet for 24 hours, and should fast after the evening meal before treatment.

thiabendazole
Mintezol♦

Pregnancy Risk Category: C

MECHANISM OF ACTION
Unknown.

INDICATIONS & DOSAGE
Systemic infection with pinworm, roundworm, threadworm, whipworm, cutaneous larva migrans, and trichinosis—
Adults or children: 25 mg/kg P.O. in 2 doses daily for 2 successive days. Maximum dosage is 3 g daily.
Cutaneous infestations with larva migrans (creeping eruption)—
Adults and children: 25 mg/kg P.O. b.i.d. for 2 to 5 days. Maximum 3 g daily. If lesions persist after 2 days, repeat course.
Pinworm—2 doses daily for 1 day; repeat in 7 days.
Roundworm, threadworm, whipworm—2 doses daily for 2 successive days.
Trichinosis—2 doses daily for 2 to 4 successive days.

ADVERSE REACTIONS
CNS: impaired mental alertness, im-

paired physical coordination, *drowsiness, giddiness,* headache, dizziness.
GI: *anorexia, nausea, vomiting,* diarrhea, epigastric distress.
Skin: rash, pruritus, *erythema multiforme.*
Other: lymphadenopathy, fever, flushing, chills.

INTERACTIONS
None significant.

NURSING CONSIDERATIONS
• Use with caution in hepatic or renal dysfunction, severe malnutrition, and anemia, and in patients who are vomiting. Supportive therapy indicated for anemic, dehydrated, or malnourished patients. In children under 15 kg, weigh benefits of therapy against risks.
• Warn that medication may cause drowsiness and dizziness.
• Give after meals. Shake suspension before measuring; chew tablets before swallowing.
• No dietary restrictions, laxatives, or enemas are necessary.
• Treat all family members.
• Teach patient about the need for good personal hygiene, especially good handwashing technique. To avoid reinfection, teach him to wash perianal area daily, to change undergarments and bedclothes daily, and to wash hands and clean fingernails before meals and after bowel movements. Advise patient to refrain from preparing food during infestation.

Antifungals

amphotericin B
flucytosine (5-FC)
griseofulvin microsize
griseofulvin ultramicrosize
ketoconazole
miconazole
nystatin

COMBINATION PRODUCTS
None.

amphotericin B
Fungizone♦

Pregnancy Risk Category: B

MECHANISM OF ACTION
Probably acts by binding to sterols in
the fungal cell membrane, altering
cell permeability and allowing leakage of intracellular components.

INDICATIONS & DOSAGE
*Systemic fungal infections (histoplas-
mosis, coccidioidomycosis, blastomycosis, cryptococcosis, disseminated
moniliasis, aspergillosis, phycomy-
cosis), meningitis—*
Adults and children: initially, 1 mg
in 250 ml of dextrose 5% in water infused over 2 to 4 hours; or 0.25 mg/kg
daily by slow infusion over 6 hours.
Increase daily dosage gradually as patient tolerance develops to maximum
1 mg/kg daily. Therapy must not exceed 1.5 mg/kg. If drug is discontinued for 1 week or more, administration must resume with initial dose and
again increase gradually.
Topical (3% cream, lotion, ointment):
apply liberally and rub well into af-

fected area b.i.d. to q.i.d.
Intrathecal: 25 mcg/0.1 ml diluted
with 10 to 20 ml of cerebrospinal
fluid and administered by barbotage 2
or 3 times weekly. Initial dose should
not exceed 100 mcg.
Coccidioidal arthritis—
Adults: 5 to 15 mg into joint spaces.

ADVERSE REACTIONS
Blood: normochromic, normocytic
anemia.
CNS: headache, peripheral neuropathy; with intrathecal administration—
peripheral nerve pain, paresthesias.
CV: hypotension, *cardiac dysrhythmias, asystole.*
GI: *anorexia, weight loss, nausea,*
vomiting, dyspepsia, diarrhea, epigastric cramps.
GU: abnormal renal function with *hypokalemia, azotemia, hyposthenuria,*
renal tubular acidosis, nephrocalcino-
sis; with large doses—permanent
renal impairment, anuria, oliguria.
Local: burning, stinging, irritation,
tissue damage with extravasation,
thrombophlebitis, pain at site of injection.
Other: arthralgia, myalgia, muscle
weakness secondary to hypokalemia,
fever, chills, malaise, generalized
pain.

INTERACTIONS
Other nephrotoxic antibiotics: may
cause additive kidney toxicity. Administer very cautiously.

NURSING CONSIDERATIONS
• Use cautiously in patients with im-

paired renal function.
• Use parenterally only in hospitalized patients, under close supervision, when diagnosis of potentially fatal fungal infection has been confirmed.
• Monitor vital signs; fever and hypotension may appear 1 to 2 hours after start of I.V. infusion and should subside within 4 hours of discontinuation.
• Monitor intake/output; report change in urine appearance or volume. Renal damage usually reversible if drug is stopped at first sign of dysfunction.
• Obtain liver and renal function studies weekly. If BUN exceeds 40 mg/100 ml, or if serum creatinine exceeds 3 mg/100 ml, doctor may reduce or stop drug until renal function improves. Monitor CBC weekly. Stop drug if alkaline phosphatase or bilirubin levels become elevated.
• Monitor potassium levels closely. Report any signs of hypokalemia. Check calcium and magnesium levels twice weekly. Perform liver and renal function studies and monitor CBCs weekly.
• In the dry state, store at 2° to 8° C. (35.6° to 46.4° F.). Protect from light. Expires 2 years after date of manufacture. Reconstitute with 10 ml sterile water only. Mixing with solutions containing sodium chloride, other electrolytes, or bacteriostatic agents, such as benzyl alcohol, causes precipitation. Do not use if solution contains precipitate or foreign matter.
• Appears to be compatible with limited amounts of heparin sodium, hydrocortisone sodium succinate, and methylprednisolone sodium succinate.
• Reconstituted solution is stable for 1 week under refrigeration or 24 hours at room temperature. It has 24-hour stability in room light.
• An initial test dose may be prescribed: 1 mg is added to 50 to 250 ml of dextrose 5% in water and infused over 20 to 30 minutes and the patient's pulse, respiratory rate, temperature, and blood pressure are monitored for at least 4 hours. Some clinicians give this test dose more slowly (over a 4 hour period).
• Severity of some side effects can be reduced by premedication with aspirin, antihistamines, antiemetics, or small doses of corticosteroids; addition of phosphate buffer and heparin to the solution; and alternate-day dose schedule. For severe reactions, drug may have to be stopped for varying periods.
• For I.V. infusion, an in-line filter with mean pore diameter larger than 1 micron can be used. Infuse very slowly; rapid infusion may result in cardiovascular collapse. Warn patient of possible discomfort at infusion site and other potential side effects. Advise patient that several months of therapy may be needed to assure adequate response.
• Administer in distal veins. If veins become thrombosed, doctor can change to every-other-day regimen.
• Antibiotics should be given separately; don't mix or piggyback with amphotericin B.
• Topical preparations may stain clothing.

---

flucytosine (5-FC)
Ancobon, Ancotil♦♦

Pregnancy Risk Category: C

MECHANISM OF ACTION
Appears to penetrate fungal cells, where it is converted to fluorouracil, a known metabolic antagonist. Causes defective protein synthesis.

INDICATIONS & DOSAGE
For severe fungal infections caused by susceptible strains of Candida *(including septicemia, endocarditis, urinary tract and pulmonary infections) and* Cryptococcus *(meningitis, pulmonary*

infection, and possible urinary tract infections)—

Adults and children weighing more than 50 kg: 50 to 150 mg/kg daily q 6 hours P.O.

Adults and children weighing less than 50 kg: 1.5 to 4.5 g/m²/day in 4 divided doses P.O.

Severe infections, such as meningitis, may require doses up to 250 mg/kg.

ADVERSE REACTIONS
Blood: anemia, *leukopenia*, bone marrow suppression, *thrombocytopenia*.
CNS: dizziness, drowsiness, confusion, headache, vertigo.
GI: *nausea, vomiting, diarrhea,* abdominal bloating.
Hepatic: elevated AST (SGOT), ALT (SGPT).
Metabolic: elevated serum alkaline phosphatase, BUN, serum creatinine.
Skin: occasional rash.

INTERACTIONS
None significant.

NURSING CONSIDERATIONS
• Use with extreme caution in patients with impaired hepatic or renal function or bone marrow depression.
• Hematologic tests and renal and liver function studies should precede therapy and should be repeated at frequent intervals thereafter. Before treatment, susceptibility tests should establish that organism is flucytosine-sensitive. Tests should be repeated weekly to monitor drug resistance.
• GI side effects are reduced if capsules are given over a 15-minute period.
• Monitor intake/output; report any marked change.
• If possible, blood level assays of drug should be performed regularly to maintain flucytosine at therapeutic level (25 to 120 mcg/ml). Higher blood levels may be toxic.

• Drug is usually combined with amphotericin because they are synergistic.
• Inform patient that adequate therapeutic response may take weeks or months.

---

griseofulvin microsize
Fulvicin-U/F♦, Grifulvin V, Grisactin, Grisovin-FP♦♦

griseofulvin ultramicrosize
Fulvicin P/G♦, Grisactin Ultra, Gris-PEG

Pregnancy Risk Category: C

MECHANISM OF ACTION
Arrests fungal cell activity by disrupting its mitotic spindle structure.

INDICATIONS & DOSAGE
Ringworm infections of skin, hair, nails (tinea corporis, tinea pedis, tinea capitis) when caused by Trichophyton, Microsporum, *or* Epidermophyton—
Adults: 500 mg (microsize) P.O. daily in single or divided doses. Severe infections may require up to 1 g daily. Alternatively, may give 330 to 375 mg ultramicrosize in single or divided doses.
Tinea pedis and tinea unguium—
Adults: 0.75 to 1 g (microsize) P.O. daily. Alternatively, may give 660 to 750 mg ultramicrosize P.O. daily.
Children: 11 mg/kg/day (microsize) P.O. Alternatively, may give 7.3 mg/kg/day of the ultramicrosize.

ADVERSE REACTIONS
Blood: leukopenia, *granulocytopenia* (requires discontinuation of drug).
CNS: headaches (in early stages of treatment), transient decrease in hearing, fatigue with large doses, occasional mental confusion, impaired performance of routine activities, psychotic symptoms, dizziness, insomnia.

GI: nausea, vomiting, excessive thirst, flatulence, diarrhea.
Metabolic: porphyria.
Skin: rash, urticaria, photosensitivity (may aggravate lupus erythematosus).
Other: estrogen-like effects in children, oral thrush.

INTERACTIONS
Alcohol: may cause tachycardia, diaphoresis, and flushing. Avoid alcohol.
Barbiturates: decreased griseofulvin blood levels due to decreased absorption or increased metabolism. Avoid using together or administer griseofulvin t.i.d.
Coumarin anticoagulants: decreased effectiveness. Monitor prothrombin times when used concurrently.
Oral contraceptives: decreased effectiveness. Suggest alternate methods of contraception.

NURSING CONSIDERATIONS
• Contraindicated in porphyria or hepatocellular failure. Since griseofulvin is a penicillin derivative, cross-sensitivity is possible. Use cautiously in penicillin-sensitive patients. Use only when topical treatment fails to arrest mycotic disease.
• CBC should be repeated regularly.
• Advise patient that prolonged treatment may be needed to control infection and prevent relapse, even if symptoms abate in first few days of therapy. Tell patient to keep skin clean and dry and to maintain good hygiene. Caution him to avoid intense sunlight.
• Most effectively absorbed and causes least GI distress when given after high-fat meal.
• Effective treatment of tinea pedis may require concomitant use of topical agent.
• Diagnosis of infecting organism should be verified in lab. Continue drug until clinical and laboratory examinations confirm complete eradication.
• Because griseofulvin ultramicrosize is dispersed in polyethylene glycol (PEG), it is absorbed more rapidly and completely than microsize preparations and is effective at one half to two thirds the usual griseofulvin dose.
• Advise patient to avoid alcoholic beverages.

---

ketoconazole
Nizoral◆

Pregnancy Risk Category: C

MECHANISM OF ACTION
Inhibits purine transport and DNA, RNA, and protein synthesis; increases cell wall permeability, making the fungus more susceptible to osmotic pressure.

INDICATIONS & DOSAGE
Treatment of systemic candidiasis, chronic mucocandidiasis, oral thrush, candiduria, coccidioidomycosis, histoplasmosis, chromomycosis, and paracoccidioidomycosis; severe cutaneous dermatophyte infections resistant to therapy with topical or oral griseofulvin—
Adults and children over 40 kg: initially, 200 mg P.O. daily single dose. Dosage may be increased to 400 mg once daily in patients who don't respond to lower dosage.
Children less than 20 kg: 50 mg (¼ tablet) daily single dose.
Children 20 to 40 kg: 100 mg (½ tablet) daily single dose.

ADVERSE REACTIONS
CNS: headache, nervousness, dizziness.
GI: *nausea, vomiting,* abdominal pain, diarrhea, constipation.
Hepatic: elevated liver enzymes, *fatal hepatotoxicity.*
Skin: itching.
Other: gynecomastia with breast tenderness in males.

Italicized side effects are common or life-threatening.
*Liquid form contains alcohol.   **May contain tartrazine.

INTERACTIONS

Antacids, anticholinergics, H₂ blockers: decreased absorption of ketoconazole. Wait at least 2 hours after ketoconazole dose before administering these drugs.

Rifampin, isoniazid: increases ketoconazole metabolism. Monitor for decreased antifungal effect.

NURSING CONSIDERATIONS

• Ketoconazole is not effective in patients with achlorhydria because drug requires acidity for dissolution and absorption. Instruct such patients to dissolve each tablet in 4 ml aqueous solution of 0.2 N hydrochloric acid; and, to avoid contact with teeth, to sip the mixture through a straw (glass or plastic). Tell patient to follow with a glass of water.
• Make sure patient understands that treatment should be continued until all clinical and laboratory tests indicate that active fungal infection has subsided. If drug is discontinued too soon, infection will recur. Minimum treatment for candidiasis is 7 to 14 days. Minimum treatment for other systemic fungal infections is 6 months. Minimum treatment for resistant dermatophyte infections is at least 4 weeks.
• Reassure patient that, although nausea is common early in therapy, it will subside. To minimize nausea, you may, with doctor's permission, divide the daily dosage into 2 doses. Taking with meals also helps to decrease nausea.
• Also available as an oral suspension.
• Monitor for elevated liver enzymes and nausea that does not subside, as well as unusual fatigue, jaundice, dark urine, or pale stools. May be signs of hepatotoxicity.
• Much larger doses (up to 800 mg/day) can be used to effectively treat fungal meningitis and intracerebral fungal lesions.

• Ketoconazole is the most effective oral antifungal drug available.
• Because of the potential of serious liver toxicity, ketoconazole should not be prescribed or used for such less serious conditions as fungus infections of the skin or nails.

---

miconazole
Monistat I.V.♦

Pregnancy Risk Category: B

MECHANISM OF ACTION
Inhibits purine transport and DNA, RNA, and protein synthesis; increases cell wall permeability, making the fungus more susceptible to osmotic pressure.

INDICATIONS & DOSAGE
Treatment of systemic fungal infections (coccidioidomycosis, candidiasis, cryptococcosis, paracoccidioidomycosis), chronic mucocutaneous candidiasis—
Adults: 200 to 3,600 mg/day. Dosages may vary with diagnosis and with infective agent. May divide daily dosage over 3 infusions, 200 to 1,200 mg per infusion. Dilute in at least 200 ml of 0.9% sodium chloride. Repeated courses may be needed because of relapse or reinfection.
Children 1 year and older: 20 to 40 mg/kg/day. Do not exceed 15 mg/kg per infusion.
Fungal meningitis—
Adults: 20 mg intrathecally as an adjunct to intravenous administration, q 3 to 7 days.

ADVERSE REACTIONS
Blood: transient decreases in hematocrit, thrombocytopenia.
CNS: dizziness, drowsiness.
GI: *nausea, vomiting,* diarrhea.
Metabolic: *transient decrease in serum sodium.*
Skin: *pruritic rash.*
Local: *phlebitis at injection site.*

INTERACTIONS
None significant.

NURSING CONSIDERATIONS
• Rapid injection of undiluted miconazole may produce dysrhythmias. Dilute infusion with at least 200 ml of 0.9% sodium chloride and infuse over 30 to 60 minutes.
• Acute cardiorespiratory arrest has occurred with the first dose. The first dose should be given under continuous medical supervision with emergency resuscitative equipment immediately available.
• Premedication with antiemetic may lessen nausea and vomiting.
• Avoid administration at mealtime in order to lessen GI adverse reactions.
• Lesser incidence and severity of adverse reactions with this drug may offer a significant advantage over other antifungals.
• Pruritic rash may persist for weeks after drug is discontinued. Pruritus may be controlled with oral or I.V. diphenhydramine.
• In treatment of fungal meningitis and urinary bladder infections, must be supplemented with intrathecal administration and bladder irrigation, respectively.
• Inform patient that adequate therapeutic response may take weeks or months.
• Monitor levels of hemoglobin, hematocrit, electrolytes, and lipids regularly. Transient elevations in serum cholesterol and triglycerides may be due to castor oil vehicle.

---

nystatin
Mycostatin*♦, Nadostine♦♦,
Nilstat♦, Nystex*
Pregnancy Risk Category: B

MECHANISM OF ACTION
Probably acts by binding to sterols in the fungal cell membrane, altering cell permeability and allowing leakage of intracellular components.

INDICATIONS & DOSAGE
Gastrointestinal infections—
Adults: 500,000 to 1 million units as oral tablets, t.i.d.
Treatment of oral, vaginal, and intestinal infections caused by Candida albicans (Monilia) *and other* Candida *species—*
Adults: 400,000 to 600,000 units oral suspension q.i.d. for oral candidiasis.
Children and infants over 3 months: 250,000 to 500,000 units oral suspension q.i.d.
Newborn and premature infants: 100,000 units oral suspension q.i.d.
Vaginal infections—
Adults: 100,000 units, as vaginal tablets, inserted high into vagina, daily or b.i.d. for 14 days.

ADVERSE REACTIONS
GI: transient nausea, vomiting, diarrhea (usually with large oral dosage).

INTERACTIONS
None significant.

NURSING CONSIDERATIONS
• Nystatin is virtually nontoxic and nonsensitizing when used orally, vaginally, or topically, but advise patient to report redness, swelling, or irritation.
• Vaginal tablets can be used by pregnant women up to 6 weeks before term to prevent thrush in newborns.
• Continue therapy during menstruation.
• Instruct patient to wash applicator thoroughly after each use.
• Explain that use of antibiotics, oral contraceptives, and corticosteroids; diabetes; reinfection by sexual partner; and tight-fitting panty hose are predisposing factors of vaginal infection.
• For treatment of oral candidiasis (thrush): Be sure the mouth is clean of food debris before administering

---

Italicized side effects are common or life-threatening.
*Liquid form contains alcohol.   **May contain tartrazine.

drug, then tell patient to hold suspension in mouth for several minutes before swallowing. When treating infants, swab medication on oral mucosa. Instruct patient in good oral hygiene techniques. Tell patient overuse of mouthwash or poorly fitting dentures, especially in older patients, may alter flora and promote infection.

• Advise patient to continue medication for 1 to 2 weeks after symptomatic improvement to ensure against reinfection. Consult doctor for exact length of therapy.

• For treatment of oral candidiasis, immunosuppressed patients sometimes take vaginal tablets (100,000 units) by mouth since this provides prolonged contact with oral mucosa.

• Instruct patient in careful hygiene for affected areas.

• Not effective against systemic infections.

Antimalarials

chloroquine hydrochloride
chloroquine phosphate
hydroxychloroquine sulfate
primaquine phosphate
pyrimethamine
quinine sulfate

COMBINATION PRODUCTS
ARALEN PHOSPHATE WITH PRIMA-
QUINE PHOSPHATE: chloroquine phosphate 500 mg (300 mg base) and primaquine phosphate 79 mg (45 mg
base).
FANSIDAR: sulfadoxine 500 mg and
pyrimethamine 25 mg.
M-KYA, Q-VEL: quinine sulfate 64.8
mg and vitamin E 400 U (as d,l alpha-
tocopheryl acetate).

chloroquine hydrochloride
Aralen HCl♦

chloroquine phosphate
Aralen Phosphate♦

Pregnancy Risk Category: C

MECHANISM OF ACTION
As an antimalarial, may bind to and
alter the properties of DNA in susceptible parasites. As an amebicide,
mechanism of action is unknown.

INDICATIONS & DOSAGE
*Suppressive prophylaxis and treatment
of acute attacks of malaria due to*
Plasmodium vivax, P. malariae, P.
ovale, *and susceptible strains of* P.
falciparum—
Adults: initially, 600 mg (base) P.O.,
then 300 mg P.O. at 6, 24, and 48
hours. Or 160 to 200 mg (base) I.M.
initially; repeat in 6 hours if needed.
Switch to oral therapy as soon as possible.
Children: initially, 10 mg (base)/kg
P.O., then 5 mg (base)/kg dose P.O. at
6, 24, and 48 hours (do not exceed
adult dose). Or 5 mg (base)/kg I.M.
initially; repeat in 6 hours if needed.
Switch to oral therapy as soon as possible.
Malaria suppressive treatment—
Adults and children: 5 mg (base)/kg
P.O. (not to exceed 300 mg) weekly
on same day of the week (begin 2
weeks before entering endemic area
and continue for 8 weeks after leaving). If treatment begins after exposure, double the initial dose (600 mg
for adults, 10 mg/kg for children) in 2
divided doses P.O. 6 hours apart.
Extraintestinal amebiasis—
Adults: 160 to 200 mg chloroquine
(hydrochloride) base I.M. daily for no
more than 12 days. As soon as possible, substitute 1 g (600 mg base)
chloroquine phosphate P.O. daily for
2 days; then 500 mg (300 mg base)
daily for at least 2 to 3 weeks. Treatment is usually combined with an effective intestinal amebicide.
Children: 10 mg/kg of chloroquine
(hydrochloride) base for 2 to 3 weeks.
Maximum 300 mg daily.
*Rheumatoid arthritis and lupus ery-
thematosus—*
250 mg chloroquine phosphate daily
with evening meal.

ADVERSE REACTIONS
Blood: *agranulocytosis, aplastic ane-*

Italicized side effects are common or life-threatening.
*Liquid form contains alcohol.   **May contain tartrazine.

mia, hemolytic anemia, thrombocytopenia.
CNS: mild and transient headache, neuromyopathy, psychic stimulation, fatigue, irritability, nightmares, convulsions, dizziness.
CV: hypotension, ECG changes.
EENT: *visual disturbances* (blurred vision; difficulty in focusing; reversible corneal changes; generally irreversible, sometimes progressive or delayed, retinal changes, such as narrowing of arterioles; macular lesions; pallor of optic disk; optic atrophy; patchy retinal pigmentation, often leading to blindness); ototoxicity (nerve deafness, vertigo, tinnitus).
GI: anorexia, abdominal cramps, diarrhea, nausea, vomiting, stomatitis.
Skin: pruritus, lichen planus-like eruptions, skin and mucosal pigmentary changes, pleomorphic skin eruptions.

INTERACTIONS
Magnesium and aluminum salts, kaolin: Decreased GI absorption. Separate administration times.

NURSING CONSIDERATIONS
• Contraindicated in retinal or visual field changes or porphyria. Use with extreme caution in presence of severe GI, neurologic, or blood disorders. Drug concentrates in liver; use cautiously in patients with hepatic disease or alcoholism. Use with caution in patients with G6PD deficiency or psoriasis; drug may exacerbate these conditions.
• Complete blood cell counts and liver function studies should be made periodically during prolonged therapy; if severe blood disorder appears that is not attributable to disease under treatment, drug may need to be discontinued.
• Overdosage can quickly lead to toxic symptoms: headache, drowsiness, visual disturbances, cardiovascular collapse, and convulsions, followed by respiratory and cardiac arrest. Children are extremely susceptible to toxicity; avoid long-term treatment.
• Baseline and periodic ophthalmologic examinations needed. Tell patient to report blurred vision, increased sensitivity to light, or muscle weakness. Check periodically for ocular muscle weakness after long-term use. Audiometric examinations recommended before, during, and after therapy, especially if long term.
• Drug should be taken immediately before or after meals on same day each week.
• To avoid exacerbated drug-induced dermatoses, warn patient to avoid excessive exposure to sun.

---

hydroxychloroquine sulfate
Plaquenil♦

Pregnancy Risk Category: C

MECHANISM OF ACTION
May bind to and alter the properties of DNA.

INDICATIONS & DOSAGE
Suppressive prophylaxis of attacks of malaria due to Plasmodium vivax, P. malariae, P. ovale, *and susceptible strains of* P. falciparum—
Adults and children: for suppression: 5 mg (base)/kg body weight P.O. (not to exceed 310 mg) weekly on same day of the week (begin 2 weeks prior to entering and continue for 8 weeks after leaving endemic area). If not started prior to exposure, double initial dose (620 mg for adults, 10 mg/kg for children) in 2 divided doses P.O. 6 hours apart.
Treatment of acute malarial attacks—
Adults and children over 15 years: initially, 800 mg (sulfate) P.O., then 400 mg after 6 to 8 hours, then 400 mg daily for 2 days (total 2 g sulfate salt).

Children 11 to 15 years: 600 mg (sulfate) P.O. stat, then 200 mg 8 hours later, then 200 mg 24 hours later (total 1 g sulfate salt).

Children 6 to 10 years: 400 mg (sulfate) P.O. stat, then 2 doses of 200 mg at 8-hour intervals (total 800 mg sulfate salt).

Children 2 to 5 years: 400 mg (sulfate) P.O. stat, then 200 mg 8 hours later (total 600 mg sulfate salt).

Children under 1 year: 100 mg (sulfate) P.O. stat; then 3 doses of 100 mg 6 to 9 hours apart (total 400 mg sulfate salt).

Lupus erythematosus (chronic discoid and systemic)—
Adults: 400 mg P.O. daily or b.i.d., continued for several weeks or months, depending on response. Prolonged maintenance dosage—200 to 400 mg P.O. daily.

Rheumatoid arthritis—
Adults: initially, 400 to 600 mg P.O. daily. When good response occurs (usually in 4 to 12 weeks), cut dosage in half.

ADVERSE REACTIONS

Blood: *agranulocytosis, leukopenia,* thrombocytopenia, hemolysis in patients with G6PD deficiency, *aplastic anemia.*

CNS: irritability, nightmares, ataxia, convulsions, psychic stimulation, toxic psychosis, vertigo, tinnitus, nystagmus, lassitude, fatigue, dizziness, hypoactive deep tendon reflexes, skeletal muscle weakness.

EENT: visual disturbances (blurred vision; difficulty in focusing; reversible corneal changes; generally irreversible, sometimes progressive or delayed, retinal changes, e.g., narrowing of arterioles; macular lesions; pallor of optic disk; optic atrophy; visual field defects; patchy retinal pigmentation, often leading to blindness), ototoxicity (irreversible nerve deafness, tinnitus, labyrinthitis).

GI: anorexia, abdominal cramps, diarrhea, nausea, vomiting.

Skin: pruritus, lichen planus-like eruptions, skin and mucosal pigmentary changes, pleomorphic skin eruptions.

Other: weight loss, alopecia, bleaching of hair.

INTERACTIONS

Magnesium and aluminum salts, kaolin: Decreased GI absorption. Separate administration times.

NURSING CONSIDERATIONS

• Contraindicated in patients with retinal or visual field changes, or porphyria. Use with extreme caution in presence of severe GI, neurologic, or blood disorders. Drug concentrates in the liver; use cautiously in patients with hepatic disease or alcoholism. Use with caution in patients with G6PD deficiency or psoriasis; drug may exacerbate these conditions.

• Complete blood cell counts and liver function studies should be made periodically during prolonged therapy; if severe blood disorder appears that is not attributable to disease under treatment, consider discontinuing.

• Overdosage can quickly lead to toxic symptoms: headache, drowsiness, visual disturbances, cardiovascular collapse, and convulsions, followed by respiratory and cardiac arrest. Children are extremely susceptible to toxicity; avoid long-term treatment.

• Baseline and periodic ophthalmologic examinations needed. Tell patient to report blurred vision, increased sensitivity to light, or muscle weakness. Check periodically for ocular muscle weakness after long-term use. Audiometric examinations recommended before, during, and after therapy, especially if long term.

• Drug should be taken immediately before or after meals on same day of each week.

Italicized side effects are common or life-threatening.
*Liquid form contains alcohol.   **May contain tartrazine.

primaquine phosphate
Pregnancy Risk Category: C

MECHANISM OF ACTION
A gametocidal drug that destroys exo-erythrocytic forms and prevents delayed primary attack. Its precise mechanism of action is unknown.

INDICATIONS & DOSAGE
Radical cure of relapsing vivax malaria, eliminating symptoms and infection completely; prevention of relapse—
Adults: 15 mg (base) P.O. daily for 14 days. (26.3 mg tablet = 15 mg of base).

ADVERSE REACTIONS
Blood: leukopenia, hemolytic anemia in G6PD deficiency, methemoglobinemia in NADH methemoglobin reductase deficiency, leukocytosis, mild anemia, *granulocytopenia, agranulocytosis.*
CNS: headache.
EENT: disturbances of visual accommodation.
GI: nausea, vomiting, epigastric distress, abdominal cramps.
Skin: urticaria.

INTERACTIONS
Magnesium and aluminum salts: Decreased GI absorption. Separate administration times.

NURSING CONSIDERATIONS
• Contraindicated in lupus erythematosus and rheumatoid arthritis; in patients taking bone marrow suppressants and potentially hemolytic drugs.
• Use with a fast-acting antimalarial, such as chloroquine. Use full dose to reduce possibility of drug-resistant strains.
• Light-skinned patients taking more than 30 mg daily, dark-skinned patients taking more than 15 mg (base) daily, and patients with severe anemia or suspected sensitivity should have frequent blood studies and urine examinations. Sudden fall in hemoglobin concentration, erythrocyte or leukocyte count, or marked darkening of the urine suggests impending hemolytic reactions.
• Observe closely for tolerance in patients with previous idiosyncrasy (manifested by hemolytic anemia, methemoglobinemia, or leukopenia); family or personal history of favism; erythrocytic G6PD deficiency or NADH methemoglobin reductase deficiency.
• Administer drug with meals or with antacids.

pyrimethamine
Daraprim♦, Fansidar (with sulfadoxine)
Pregnancy Risk Category: C

MECHANISM OF ACTION
Inhibits the enzyme dihydrofolate reductase, thereby impeding reduction of folic acid.

INDICATIONS & DOSAGE
Malaria prophylaxis and transmission control (pyrimethamine)—
Adults and children over 10 years: 25 mg P.O. weekly.
Children 4 to 10 years: 12.5 mg P.O. weekly.
Children under 4 years: 6.25 mg P.O. weekly.
   Continue in all age groups at least 10 weeks after leaving endemic areas.
Acute attacks of malaria (Fansidar)—
Adults: 2 to 3 tablets as a single dose, either alone or in sequence with quinine or primaquine.
Children 9 to 14 years: 2 tablets.
Children 4 to 8 years: 1 tablet.
Children under 4 years: ½ tablet.
Malaria prophylaxis (Fansidar)—
Adults: 1 tablet weekly, or 2 tablets q 2 weeks.
Children 9 to 14 years: ¾ tablet

weekly, or 1½ tablets q 2 weeks.
Children 4 to 8 years: ½ tablet
weekly, or 1 tablet q 2 weeks.
Children under 4 years: ¼ tablet
weekly, or ½ tablet q 2 weeks.
*Acute attacks of malaria (pyrimeth-
amine)—*
Not recommended alone in nonim-
mune persons; use with faster-acting
antimalarials, such as chloroquine,
for 2 days to initiate transmission control and suppressive cure.
Adults and children over 15 years:
25 mg P.O. daily for 2 days.
Children under 15 years: 12.5 mg
P.O. daily for 2 days.
Toxoplasmosis (pyrimethamine)—
Adults: initially, 100 mg P.O., then
25 mg P.O. daily for 4 to 5 weeks;
during same time give 1 g sulfadiazine P.O. q 6 hours.
Children: initially, 1 mg/kg P.O.,
then 0.25 mg/kg daily for 4 to 5
weeks, along with 100 mg sulfadi-
azine/kg P.O. daily, divided q 6
hours.

ADVERSE REACTIONS
Blood: *agranulocytosis, aplastic anemia,* megaloblastic anemia, bone
marrow suppression, leukopenia,
thrombocytopenia, pancytopenia.
CNS: stimulation and convulsions
(acute toxicity).
GI: anorexia, vomiting, diarrhea,
atrophic glossitis.
Skin: rashes, *erythema multiforme
(Stevens-Johnson syndrome), toxic epidermal necrolysis.*

INTERACTIONS
*Folic acid and para-aminobenzoic
acid:* decreased antitoxoplasmic effects. May require dosage adjustment.
Sulfonamides, co-trimoxazole: increased adverse effects. Use together
cautiously.

NURSING CONSIDERATIONS
• Sulfadoxine, an ingredient in Fansidar, is a sulfonamide; therefore, this

combination is contraindicated in porphyria. Use cautiously in impaired hepatic or renal function, severe allergy
or bronchial asthma, or G6PD deficiency.
• Contraindicated in chloroquine-
resistant malaria. Use cautiously in
convulsive disorders; smaller doses
may be needed. Also use cautiously
following treatment with chloroquine.
• Warn patient taking Fansidar to
stop drug and notify doctor at first
sign of skin rash.
• Dosages required to treat toxoplasmosis approach toxic levels. Twice-
weekly blood counts, including platelets, are required. If signs of folic or
folinic acid deficiency develop, dosage should be reduced or discontinued while patient receives parenteral
folinic acid (leucovorin) until blood
counts become normal.
• Give with meals to minimize GI
distress.
• The first dose of Fansidar, when
taken prophylactically, should be
taken 1 to 2 days before traveling to an
endemic area.
• Because of the possibility of severe
skin reactions, Fansidar should be
used only in regions where chloroquine-resistant malaria is prevalent
and only when the traveler plans to
stay in the region longer than 3 weeks.

quinine sulfate
Legatrin, Novoquinine♦♦,
Quinamm, Quindan, Quine-200,
Quine-300, Quiphile, Strema
Pregnancy Risk Category: X

MECHANISM OF ACTION
Mechanism of antiprotozoal action is
unknown, but the drug is often referred to as a generalized proto-
plasmic poison. As a muscle relaxant,
quinine appears to have a direct effect
on muscle fibers that decreases their
response to repetitive stimulation.

INDICATIONS & DOSAGE

Malaria due to Plasmodium falciparum *(chloroquine-resistant)*—
Adults: 650 mg P.O. q 8 hours for 10 days, with 25 mg pyrimethamine q 12 hours for 3 days, and with 500 mg sulfadiazine q.i.d. for 5 days.
Nocturnal leg cramps—
Adults: 260 to 300 mg P.O. at bedtime or after the evening meal.

ADVERSE REACTIONS

Blood: hemolytic anemia, thrombocytopenia, *agranulocytosis,* hypoprothrombinemia.
CNS: severe headache, apprehension, excitement, confusion, delirium, syncope, hypothermia, convulsions (with toxic doses).
CV: hypotension, *cardiovascular collapse* with overdosage or rapid I.V. administration.
EENT: altered color perception, photophobia, blurred vision, night blindness, amblyopia, scotoma, diplopia, mydriasis, optic atrophy, tinnitus, impaired hearing.
GI: epigastric distress, diarrhea, nausea, vomiting.
GU: renal tubular damage, anuria.
Skin: rashes, pruritus.
Local: thrombosis at infusion site.
Other: asthma, flushing.

INTERACTIONS

Sodium bicarbonate: elevates quinine levels by decreasing quinine excretion. Use together cautiously.

NURSING CONSIDERATIONS

• Contraindicated in G6PD deficiency. Use with caution in cardiovascular conditions.
• Discontinue if any signs of idiosyncrasy or toxicity occur.
• Quinine is no longer used for acute attacks of malaria due to *Plasmodium vivax* or for suppression of malaria due to organism resistance.
• Administer after meals to minimize GI distress. Do not crush tablets, as the drug is irritating to gastric mucosa.
• When parenteral therapy is necessary or when oral therapy is not feasible, quinine dihydrochloride may be obtained from the Centers for Disease Control. Administer by slow infusion (over at least 1 hour).

10

Antituberculars and antileprotics

capreomycin sulfate
clofazimine
cycloserine
dapsone
ethambutol hydrochloride
ethionamide
isoniazid (INH)
pyrazinamide
rifampin
streptomycin sulfate
   (See Chapter 11, AMINOGLYCOSIDES.)

COMBINATION PRODUCTS
P-I-N FORTE: isoniazid 100 mg and pyridoxine HCl 5 mg.
RIFAMATE: isoniazid 150 mg and rifampin 300 mg.
RIMACTANE/INH DUAL PACK: Thirty 300-mg isoniazid tablets and sixty 300-mg rifampin capsules.

---

capreomycin sulfate
Capastat

Pregnancy Risk Category: C

MECHANISM OF ACTION
Unknown (bactericidal).

INDICATIONS & DOSAGE
Adjunctive treatment in pulmonary tuberculosis—
Adults: 15 mg/kg/day up to 1 g I.M. daily injected deeply into large muscle mass for 60 to 120 days; then 1 g 2 to 3 times weekly for a period of 18 to 24 months. Maximum dosage should not exceed 20 mg/kg daily. Must be given in conjunction with another antitubercular drug.

ADVERSE REACTIONS
Blood: eosinophilia, leukocytosis, leukopenia.
CNS: headache.
EENT: *ototoxicity* (tinnitus, vertigo, hearing loss).
GU: *nephrotoxicity* (elevated BUN and nonprotein nitrogen, casts, red blood cells, leukocytes; tubular necrosis; proteinuria; decreased creatinine clearance).
Local: pain, induration, excessive bleeding and sterile abscesses at injection site.
Metabolic: hypokalemia, alkalosis, hepatotoxicity.
Other: neuromuscular blockade

INTERACTIONS
None significant.

NURSING CONSIDERATIONS
• Contraindicated in patients receiving other ototoxic or nephrotoxic drugs. Use cautiously in patients with impaired renal function, history of allergies, or hearing impairment.
• Considered a "second-line" drug in the treatment of tuberculosis.
• Drug is never given I.V. Intravenous use may cause neuromuscular blockade.
• Administer deep into large muscle mass to minimize local reactions. If approved by the doctor, reconstitute I.M. dose with 0.5% lidocaine hydrochloride without epinephrine. Apply ice to injection site p.r.n. for pain.
• Evaluate patient's hearing before and every 1 to 2 weeks during therapy. Notify doctor if patient com-

---

Italicized side effects are common or life-threatening.
*Liquid form contains alcohol.   **May contain tartrazine.

plains of tinnitus, vertigo, or hearing impairment.
• Monitor renal function (output, specific gravity, urinalysis, BUN, and serum creatinine) before and during therapy; notify doctor of decreasing renal function. Dose must be reduced in renal impairment.
• Straw- or dark-colored solution does not indicate a loss in potency. Do not administer solutions that contain a precipitate.

clofazimine
Lamprene

Pregnancy Risk Category: C

MECHANISM OF ACTION
Inhibits mycobacterial growth by binding preferentially to mycobacterial DNA. Also has anti-inflammatory effects that suppress skin reactions of erythema nodosum leprosum.

INDICATIONS & DOSAGE
Treatment of dapsone-resistant leprosy—
Adults: 100 mg P.O. daily in combination with other antileprotics for 3 years. Then, clofazimine *alone*, 100 mg daily.
Erythema nodosum leprosum—
Adults: 100 to 200 mg P.O. daily for up to 3 months. Taper dosage to 100 mg daily as soon as possible. Dosages above 200 mg daily are not recommended.

ADVERSE REACTIONS
EENT: conjunctival and corneal pigmentation.
GI: *epigastric pain, diarrhea, nausea, vomiting, GI intolerance, bowel obstruction, GI bleeding.*
Skin: *Pink to brownish black pigmentation, ichthyosis and dryness,* rash, itching.
Other: *Splenic infarction,* discolored body fluids and excrement.

INTERACTIONS
None significant.

NURSING CONSIDERATIONS
• Use cautiously in GI dysfunction, such as abdominal pain and diarrhea.
• Advise patient to take the drug with meals.
• Doses that exceed 100 mg daily should be given for as short a period as possible and only under close medical supervision.
• If patient complains of colicky or burning abdominal pain or of any other GI symptom, report this to the doctor, who may reduce the dose or increase the interval between doses.
• Warn patient that clofazimine may discolor skin, body fluids, and excrement. The color ranges from red to brownish black. Reassure patient that the unsightly skin discoloration is reversible but may not disappear until several months or years after drug treatment ends.
• Recommend application of skin oil or cream to help reverse skin dryness or ichthyosis.

cycloserine
Seromycin

Pregnancy Risk Category: C

MECHANISM OF ACTION
Inhibits cell wall biosynthesis by inhibiting the utilization of amino acids (bacteriostatic).

INDICATIONS & DOSAGE
Adjunctive treatment in pulmonary or extrapulmonary tuberculosis—
Adults: initially, 250 mg P.O. q 12 hours for 2 weeks; then, if blood levels are below 25 to 30 mcg/ml and there are no clinical signs of toxicity, dosage is increased to 250 mg P.O. q 8 hours for 2 weeks. If optimum blood levels are still not achieved, and there are no signs of clinical toxicity, then dosage is increased to 250 mg P.O. q

6 hours. Maximum dosage is 1 g/day. If CNS toxicity occurs, drug is discontinued for 1 week, then resumed at 250 mg daily for 2 weeks. If no serious toxic effects occur, dosage is increased by 250-mg increments q 10 days until blood level of 25 to 30 mcg/ml is obtained.

ADVERSE REACTIONS
CNS: drowsiness, headache, tremor, dysarthria, vertigo, confusion, loss of memory, *possible suicidal tendencies and other psychotic symptoms, nervousness, hallucinations, depression,* hyperirritability, paresthesias, paresis, hyperreflexia.
Other: hypersensitivity (allergic dermatitis).

INTERACTIONS
Isoniazid: monitor for CNS toxicity (dizziness or drowsiness).
Ethanol or ethionamide: increased risk of CNS toxicity (seizures).

NURSING CONSIDERATIONS
• Contraindicated in seizure disorders, depression or severe anxiety, severe renal insufficiency, or chronic alcoholism. Use cautiously in impaired renal function; reduced dosage required.
• Considered a "second-line" drug in the treatment of tuberculosis.
• Obtain specimen for culture and sensitivity tests before therapy begins and periodically thereafter to detect possible resistance.
• Serious neurologic effects can be precipitated by ingestion of alcohol; warn patient to avoid alcohol.
• Toxic reactions may occur with blood levels above 30 mcg/ml.
• Pyridoxine, anticonvulsants, tranquilizers, or sedatives may help to relieve adverse reactions.
• Observe for psychiatric symptoms.
• Monitor hematologic tests and renal and liver function studies.
• Instruct patient to take drug exactly as prescribed; warn against discontinuing use without doctor's approval.

dapsone
Avlosulfon♦♦
Pregnancy Risk Category: A

MECHANISM OF ACTION
Inhibits folic acid biosynthesis in susceptible organisms (bactericidal).

INDICATIONS & DOSAGE
All forms of leprosy (Hansen's disease)—
Adults: 100 mg P.O. daily for indefinite period, plus rifampin 600 mg daily for 6 months.
Children: 1.4 mg/kg P.O. daily.
Prophylaxis for leprosy patient's close contacts—
Adults: 50 mg P.O. daily.
Children age 6 to 12: 25 mg P.O. daily.
Children age 2 to 5: 25 mg P.O. three times weekly.
Infants age 6 to 23 months: 12 mg P.O. three times weekly.
Children under age 6 months: 6 mg P.O. three times weekly.
Dermatitis herpetiformis—
Adults: 50 mg. P.O. daily; may increase to 400 mg. daily.
Malaria suppression or prophylaxis due to chloroquine-resistant Plasmodium falciparum *when other agents aren't available—*
Adults: 100 mg. P.O. weekly; usually given with pyrimethimine 12.5 mg. P.O. weekly.
Children: 2 mg/kg P.O. weekly, with pyrimethamine 0.25 mg/kg weekly.
  Continue prophylaxis during exposure and for 6 months after exposure.
Treatment of Pneumocystis carinii *pneumonia in patients with AIDS—*
Adults: 100 mg P.O. daily in conjunction with trimethoprim 20 mg/kg P.O. daily (usually divided q.i.d.).

ADVERSE REACTIONS
Blood: *aplastic anemia, agranulocytosis, hemolytic anemia;* methemoglobinemia; possible leukopenia.
CNS: psychosis, headache, dizziness, lethargy, severe malaise, paresthesias.
EENT: tinnitus, allergic rhinitis.
GI: anorexia, abdominal pain, nausea, vomiting.
Hepatic: hepatitis, cholestatic jaundice.
Skin: allergic dermatitis (generalized or fixed maculopapular rash).

INTERACTIONS
Probenecid: elevates levels of dapsone. Use together with extreme caution.

NURSING CONSIDERATIONS
• Use cautiously in chronic renal, hepatic, or cardiovascular disease or refractory types of anemia.
• Use cautiously in G6PD deficiency.
• Therapy should be interrupted if generalized, diffuse dermatitis occurs.
• Dapsone dosage should be reduced or temporarily discontinued if hemoglobin falls below 9 g/dl; if leukocyte count falls below 5,000/mm³; if erythrocyte count falls below 2.5 million/mm³ or remains low.
• Antihistamines may help to combat dapsone-induced allergic dermatitis.
• Erythema nodosum type of lepra reaction may occur during therapy as a result of *Mycobacterium leprae* bacilli (malaise, fever, painful inflammatory induration in the skin and mucosa, iritis, and neuritis). In severe cases, therapy should be stopped and glucocorticoids given cautiously.
• Obtain CBC before treatment and monitor frequently throughout therapy (weekly for the first month, monthly for 6 months, and semiannually thereafter).
• Also used to treat relapsing polychondritis and as prophylaxis against malaria. Has been used investigationally to treat rheumatoid arthritis, allergic vasculitis, relapsing polychondritis, and postular and inflammatory dermatoses.
• Instruct nursing mothers to report cyanosis in infants, as this indicates high sulfone level.

ethambutol hydrochloride
Etibi♦♦, Myambutol♦

Pregnancy Risk Category: B

MECHANISM OF ACTION
Interferes with the synthesis of RNA, thus inhibiting protein metabolism (bacteriostatic).

INDICATIONS & DOSAGE
Adjunctive treatment in pulmonary tuberculosis—
Adults and children over 13 years: initial treatment for patients who have not received previous antitubercular therapy is 15 mg/kg P.O. daily single dose.
Re-treatment: 25 mg/kg P.O. daily single dose for 60 days with at least one other antitubercular drug; then decrease to 15 mg/kg P.O. daily single dose.

ADVERSE REACTIONS
CNS: headache, dizziness, mental confusion, possible hallucinations, peripheral neuritis (numbness and tingling of extremities).
EENT: optic neuritis (vision loss and loss of color discrimination, especially red and green).
GI: anorexia, nausea, vomiting, abdominal pain.
Metabolic: *elevated uric acid.*
Other: anaphylactoid reactions, fever, malaise, bloody sputum.

INTERACTIONS
None significant.

NURSING CONSIDERATIONS
• Contraindicated in optic neuritis and in children under 13 years. Use cautiously in impaired renal function, cataracts, recurrent eye inflammations, gout, and diabetic retinopathy.
• Dose must be reduced in renal impairment.
• Perform visual acuity and color discrimination tests before and during therapy.
• Always monitor serum uric acid; observe patient for symptoms of gout.
• Reassure patient that visual disturbances will disappear several weeks to months after drug is stopped.

ethionamide
Trecator-SC

Pregnancy Risk Category: D

MECHANISM OF ACTION
Unknown (bacteriostatic).

INDICATIONS & DOSAGE
Adjunctive treatment in pulmonary or extrapulmonary tuberculosis (when primary therapy with streptomycin or isoniazid cannot be used or has failed)—
Adults: 500 mg to 1 g P.O. daily in divided doses. Concomitant administration of other effective antitubercular drugs and pyridoxine recommended.
Children: 12 to 15 mg/kg P.O. daily in 3 to 4 doses. Maximum dosage is 750 mg.

ADVERSE REACTIONS
Blood: thrombocytopenia.
CNS: *peripheral neuritis,* psychic disturbances (especially mental depression).
CV: postural hypotension.
GI: *anorexia,* metallic taste in mouth, nausea, vomiting, sialorrhea, *epigastric distress,* diarrhea, stomatitis, weight loss.
Hepatic: jaundice, hepatitis, elevated

AST (SGOT) and ALT (SGPT).
Skin: rash, *exfoliative dermatitis.*

INTERACTIONS
None significant.

NURSING CONSIDERATIONS
• Contraindicated in severe hepatic damage. Use cautiously in diabetes mellitus.
• Culture and sensitivity tests should be performed before starting therapy. Stop drug if skin rash occurs; may progress to exfoliative dermatitis.
• Monitor hepatic function every 2 to 4 weeks.
• Give with meals or antacids to minimize GI effects. Patient may require antiemetic.
• Pyridoxine may be ordered to prevent neuropathy.
• Instruct patient to take this drug exactly as prescribed; warn against discontinuing drug without doctor's consent.
• Warn patient to avoid excess alcohol ingestion because it may make him more vulnerable to liver damage.

isoniazid (INH)
DOW-Isoniazid, Isotamine♦♦, Laniazid, Nydrazid**, PMS-Isoniazid♦♦

Pregnancy Risk Category: C

MECHANISM OF ACTION
Inhibits cell wall biosynthesis by interfering with lipid and DNA synthesis (bactericidal).

INDICATIONS & DOSAGE
Primary treatment against actively growing tubercle bacilli—
Adults: 5 mg/kg P.O. or I.M. daily single dose, up to 300 mg/day, continued for 6 months to 2 years.
Infants and children: 10 to 20 mg/kg P.O. or I.M. daily single dose, up to 300 to 500 mg/day, continued for 18 months to 2 years. Concomitant ad-

ministration of at least one other effective antitubercular drug is recommended.

Preventive therapy against tubercle bacilli of those closely exposed or those with positive skin test whose chest X-rays and bacteriologic studies are consistent with nonprogressive tuberculous disease—

Adults: 300 mg P.O. daily single dose, continued for 1 year.

Infants and children: 10 mg/kg P.O. daily single dose, up to 300 mg/day, continued for 1 year.

ADVERSE REACTIONS

Blood: *agranulocytosis,* hemolytic anemia, *aplastic anemia,* eosinophilia, leukopenia, neutropenia, thrombocytopenia, methemoglobinemia, pyridoxine-responsive hypochromic anemia.

CNS: *peripheral neuropathy* (especially in the malnourished, alcoholics, diabetics, and slow acetylators), usually preceded by paresthesias of hands and feet, psychosis.

GI: nausea, vomiting, epigastric distress, constipation, dryness of the mouth.

Hepatic: *hepatitis, occasionally severe and sometimes fatal, especially in elderly patients.*

Metabolic: hyperglycemia, metabolic acidosis.

Local: irritation at injection site.

Other: rheumatic syndrome and systemic lupus erythematosus–like syndrome; hypersensitivity (fever, rash, lymphadenopathy, vasculitis).

INTERACTIONS

Aluminum-containing antacids and laxatives: may decrease the rate and amount of isoniazid absorbed. Give isoniazid at least 1 hour before antacid or laxative.

Disulfiram: neurologic symptoms, including changes in behavior and coordination, may develop with concomitant isoniazid use. Avoid concomitant use.

Carbamazepine: increased risk of isoniazid hepatotoxicity. Use together very cautiously.

Corticosteroids: may decrease therapeutic effectiveness. Monitor need for larger isoniazid dose.

NURSING CONSIDERATIONS

• Contraindicated in acute hepatic disease or isoniazid-associated hepatic damage. Use cautiously in chronic non-isoniazid-associated hepatic disease, seizure disorders (especially those taking phenytoin), severe renal impairment, chronic alcoholism; and in elderly patients.

• Isoniazid pharmacokinetics may vary among patients, since its metabolism occurs in the liver by genetically controlled acetylation. Fast acetylators metabolize the drug up to five times as fast as slow acetylators. About 50% of blacks and whites are slow acetylators; over 80% of Chinese, Japanese, and Eskimos are fast acetylators.

• Monitor hepatic function. Tell patient to notify doctor immediately if symptoms of hepatic impairment occur (loss of appetite, fatigue, malaise, jaundice, dark urine).

• Alcohol may be associated with increased incidence of isoniazid-related hepatitis. Advise against use.

• Pyridoxine should be given to prevent peripheral neuropathy, especially in malnourished patients.

• Instruct patient to take this drug exactly as prescribed; warn against discontinuing drug without doctor's consent.

• Encourage patient to fully comply with treatment, which may take months or years.

• Advise patient to take with food if GI irritation occurs.

• Reportedly effective when used investigationally to treat arthritis and action tremor in multiple sclerosis.

pyrazinamide
PMS Pyrazinamide♦♦, Tebrazid♦♦

Pregnancy Risk Category: C

MECHANISM OF ACTION
Unknown (bactericidal).

INDICATIONS & DOSAGE
Adjunctive treatment of tuberculosis (when primary and secondary antitubercular drugs cannot be used or have failed)—
Adults: 20 to 35 mg/kg P.O. daily, divided in 3 to 4 doses. Maximum dosage is 3 g daily.

ADVERSE REACTIONS
Blood: sideroblastic anemia, possible bleeding tendency due to thrombocytopenia.
GI: anorexia, nausea, vomiting.
GU: dysuria.
Hepatic: hepatitis.
Metabolic: interference with control in diabetes mellitus, *hyperuricemia*.
Other: malaise, fever, arthralgia.

INTERACTIONS
None significant.

NURSING CONSIDERATIONS
• Contraindicated in severe hepatic disease. Use cautiously in diabetes mellitus or gout.
• Nearly 100% excreted in urine; reduced dose needed in patients with renal impairment.
• Perform liver function studies and examination for jaundice, liver tenderness, or enlargement before and frequently during therapy.
• Watch closely for signs of gout and of hepatic impairment (loss of appetite, fatigue, malaise, jaundice, dark urine, and liver tenderness). Notify doctor at once.
• Question doses that exceed 35 mg/kg, as they may cause liver damage.
• Monitor hematopoietic studies and serum uric acid.

• When used with surgical management of tuberculosis, start pyrazinamide 1 to 2 weeks before surgery and continue for 4 to 6 weeks postoperatively.

rifampin
Rifadin♦, Rimactane♦, Rofact♦♦

Pregnancy Risk Category: C

MECHANISM OF ACTION
Inhibits DNA-dependent RNA polymerase, thus impairing RNA synthesis (bactericidal).

INDICATIONS & DOSAGE
Primary treatment in pulmonary tuberculosis—
Adults: 600 mg P.O. daily single dose 1 hour before or 2 hours after meals.
Children over 5 years: 10 to 20 mg/kg P.O. daily single dose 1 hour before or 2 hours after meals. Maximum dosage is 600 mg daily. Concomitant administration of other effective antitubercular drugs is recommended.
Meningococcal carriers—
Adults: 600 mg P.O. b.i.d. for 2 days.
Children 1 to 12 years: 10 mg/kg P.O. b.i.d. or 2 days, not to exceed 600 mg/dose.
Infants 3 months to 1 year: 5 mg/kg P.O. b.i.d. for 2 days.
Prophylaxis of Hemophilus influenza type b—
Adults and children: 20 mg/kg P.O. once daily for 4 days. Do not exceed 600 mg/day.

ADVERSE REACTIONS
Blood: thrombocytopenia, transient leukopenia, hemolytic anemia.
CNS: headache, fatigue, *drowsiness*, ataxia, dizziness, mental confusion, generalized numbness.
GI: epigastric distress, anorexia, nausea, vomiting, abdominal pain, diarrhea, flatulence, sore mouth and tongue.
Metabolic: hyperuricemia.

Italicized side effects are common or life-threatening.
*Liquid form contains alcohol.   **May contain tartrazine.

Hepatic: *serious hepatotoxicity as well as transient abnormalities in liver function tests.*
Skin: pruritus, urticaria, rash.
Other: flu-like syndrome, discoloration of body fluids.

INTERACTIONS
Para-aminosalicylate sodium, ketoconazole: may interfere with absorption of rifampin. Give these drugs 8 to 12 hours apart.
Probenecid: may increase rifampin levels. Use cautiously.
Alcohol: may increase risk of hepatotoxicity.

NURSING CONSIDERATIONS
• Contraindicated in clinically active hepatitis.
• Use cautiously in hepatic disease or in those receiving other hepatotoxic drugs.
• Monitor hepatic function, hematopoietic studies, and serum uric acid.
• Watch closely for signs of hepatic impairment (loss of appetite, fatigue, malaise, jaundice, dark urine, liver tenderness). Notify doctor if these occur.
• Warn patient about drowsiness and the possibility of red-orange discoloration of urine, feces, saliva, sweat, sputum, and tears. Soft contact lenses may be permanently stained.
• Rifampin is not considered a teratogen. However, it may cause hemorrhaging in the newborns of rifampin-treated mothers.
• Advise patient to avoid alcoholic beverages while taking this drug. May increase risk of hepatotoxicity.
• Give 1 hour before or 2 hours after meals for optimal absorption; however, if GI irritation occurs, patient may take rifampin with meals.
• Increases enzyme activity of liver; may require increased doses of warfarin, corticosteroids, oral contraceptives, and oral hypoglycemics. See each drug entry for specific drug interactions.
• Concomitant treatment with at least one other antitubercular drug is recommended.

11

Aminoglycosides

amikacin sulfate
gentamicin sulfate
kanamycin sulfate
neomycin sulfate
netilmicin sulfate
streptomycin sulfate
tobramycin sulfate

COMBINATION PRODUCTS
NEOSPORIN G.U. IRRIGANT: 40 mg
neomycin sulfate and 200,000 units
polymixin B sulfate/ml.

---

amikacin sulfate
Amikin♦

Pregnancy Risk Category: C

MECHANISM OF ACTION
Inhibits protein synthesis by binding
directly to the 30S ribosomal subunit.
Generally bactericidal.

INDICATIONS & DOSAGE
Serious infections caused by sensitive
Pseudomonas aeruginosa, Escherichia coli, Proteus, Klebsiella, Serratia, Enterobacter, Acinetobacter,
Providencia, Citrobacter, Staphylococcus—
**Adults and children with normal
renal function:** 15 mg/kg/day divided q 8 to 12 hours I.M. or I.V. infusion (in 100 to 200 ml dextrose 5%
in water run in over 30 to 60 minutes). May be given by direct I.V.
push if necessary.
**Neonates with normal renal func-
tion:** initially, 10 mg/kg I.M. or I.V.
infusion (in dextrose 5% in water run
in over 1 to 2 hours), then 7.5 mg/kg
q 12 hours I.M. or I.V. infusion.
Meningitis—
Adults: systemic therapy as above;
may also use up to 20 mg intrathecally or intraventricularly daily.
Children: systemic therapy as above;
may also use 1 to 2 mg intrathecally
daily.
*Uncomplicated urinary tract infec-
tions—*
Adults: 250 mg I.M. or I.V. b.i.d.
**Adults with impaired renal func-
tion:** initially, 7.5 mg/kg. Subsequent
doses and frequency determined by
blood amikacin levels and renal function studies.

ADVERSE REACTIONS
CNS: headache, lethargy, *neuromuscular blockade.*
EENT: *ototoxicity (tinnitus, vertigo,
hearing loss).*
GU: *nephrotoxicity (cells or casts in
urine, oliguria, proteinuria, decreased creatinine clearance, increased BUN and serum creatinine
levels).*

INTERACTIONS
Cephalothin: increased nephrotoxicity. Use together cautiously.
Dimenhydrinate: may mask symptoms of ototoxicity. Use with caution.
I.V. loop diuretics (e.g. furosemide):
increase ototoxicity. Use cautiously.
*Other aminoglycosides, amphotericin
B, cisplatin, methoxyflurane:* increases nephrotoxicity. Use together
cautiously.
Parenteral penicillins (e.g. carbenicillin, ticarcillin): amikacin inactivation

---

in vitro. Don't mix together in I.V.

NURSING CONSIDERATIONS
• Use cautiously in impaired renal function, in neonates and infants, and in elderly patients.
• Obtain specimen for culture and sensitivity tests before first dose. Therapy may begin pending test results.
• Weigh patient and obtain baseline renal function studies before therapy begins.
• Monitor renal function (output, specific gravity, urinalysis, BUN and creatinine levels, and creatinine clearance). Notify doctor of signs of decreasing renal function.
• Patient should be well hydrated while taking drug to minimize chemical irritation of the renal tubules.
• Evaluate patient's hearing before and during therapy. Notify doctor if patient complains of tinnitus, vertigo, or hearing loss.
• Watch for superinfection (continued fever and other signs of new infections, especially of upper respiratory tract).
• Usual duration of therapy is 7 to 10 days. If no response after 3 to 5 days, therapy may be stopped and new specimens obtained for culture and sensitivity.
• Peak blood levels that are above 35 mcg/ml and trough levels that are above 10 mcg/ml may be associated with higher incidence of toxicity.
• After I.V. infusion, flush line with normal saline solution or dextrose 5% in water.
• Draw blood for peak amikacin level 1 hour after I.M. injection and 30 minutes to 1 hour after infusion ends; for trough levels, draw blood just before next dose. Don't collect blood in a heparinized tube because heparin is incompatible with aminoglycosides.
• Potency of drug is not affected if solution turns light yellow.

gentamicin sulfate
Cidomycin◆◆, Garamycin◆, Gentafair, Jenamicin

Pregnancy Risk Category: C

MECHANISM OF ACTION
Inhibits protein synthesis by binding directly to the 30S ribosomal subunit. Generally bactericidal.

INDICATIONS & DOSAGE
Serious infections caused by sensitive Pseudomonas aeruginosa, Escherichia coli, Proteus, Klebsiella, Serratia, Enterobacter, Citrobacter, Staphylococcus—
Adults with normal renal function: 3 mg/kg daily in divided doses q 8 hours I.M. or I.V. infusion (in 50 to 200 ml of normal saline solution or dextrose 5% in water infused over 30 minutes to 2 hours). May be given by direct I.V. push if necessary. For life-threatening infections, patient may receive up to 5 mg/kg daily in 3 to 4 divided doses.
Children with normal renal function: 2 to 2.5 mg/kg I.M. or I.V. infusion q 8 hours.
Infants and neonates over 1 week with normal renal function: 2.5 mg/kg q 8 hours I.M. or I.V. infusion.
Neonates under 1 week: 2.5 mg/kg I.V. q 12 hours. For I.V. infusion, dilute in normal saline solution or dextrose 5% in water and infuse over 30 minutes to 2 hours.
Meningitis—
Adults: systemic therapy as above; may also use 4 to 8 mg intrathecally daily.
Children: systemic therapy as above; may also use 1 to 2 mg intrathecally daily.
Endocarditis prophylaxis for GI or GU procedure or surgery—
Adults: 1.5 mg/kg I.M. or I.V. 30 to 60 minutes before procedure or surgery and q 8 hours after, for 2 doses. Given with aqueous penicillin G or

ampicillin.
Children: 2.5 mg/kg I.M. or I.V. 30 to 60 minutes before procedure or surgery and q 8 hours after, for 2 doses. Given with aqueous penicillin G or ampicillin.
Patients with impaired renal function: initial dose is same as for those with normal renal function. Subsequent doses and frequency determined by renal function studies and serum concentrations of gentamicin. *Posthemodialysis to maintain therapeutic blood levels—*
Adults: 1 to 1.7 mg/kg I.M. or I.V. infusion after each dialysis.
Children: 2 mg/kg I.M. or I.V. infusion after each dialysis.

ADVERSE REACTIONS
CNS: headache, lethargy, *neuromuscular blockade*.
EENT: *ototoxicity (tinnitus, vertigo, hearing loss)*.
GU: *nephrotoxicity (cells or casts in the urine; oliguria; proteinuria; decreased creatinine clearance; increased BUN, nonprotein nitrogen, and serum creatinine levels)*.

INTERACTIONS
Cephalothin: increases nephrotoxicity. Use together cautiously.
Dimenhydrinate: may mask symptoms of ototoxicity. Use with caution.
I.V. loop diuretics (e.g. furosemide): increase ototoxicity. Use cautiously.
Other aminoglycosides, methoxyflurane: increase ototoxicity and nephrotoxicity. Use together cautiously.
Parenteral penicillins (e.g. carbenicillin and ticarcillin): gentamicin inactivation in vitro. Don't mix together in I.V.

NURSING CONSIDERATIONS
• Use cautiously in impaired renal function, and in neonates, infants, and elderly patients.
• Obtain specimen for culture and sensitivity tests before first dose.

Therapy may begin pending test results.
• Weigh patient and obtain baseline renal function studies before therapy begins.
• Monitor renal function (output, specific gravity, urinalysis, BUN and creatinine levels, and creatinine clearance). Notify doctor of signs of decreasing renal function.
• Patient should be well hydrated while taking drug to minimize chemical irritation of the renal tubules.
• After completing I.V. infusion, flush the line with normal saline solution or dextrose 5% in water.
• Evaluate patient's hearing before and during therapy. Notify doctor if patient complains of tinnitus, vertigo, or hearing loss.
• Watch for superinfection (continued fever and other signs of new infections, especially of upper respiratory tract).
• Usual duration of therapy is 7 to 10 days. If no response in 3 to 5 days, therapy may be stopped and new specimens obtained for culture and sensitivity.
• Peak blood levels above 12 mcg/ml and trough levels (those drawn just before next dose) above 2 mcg/ml may be associated with higher incidence of toxicity.
• Draw blood for peak gentamicin level 1 hour after I.M. injection and 30 minutes to 1 hour after infusion ends; for trough levels, draw blood just before next dose. Don't collect blood in a heparinized tube because heparin is incompatible with aminoglycosides.
• Hemodialysis (8 hours) removes up to 50% of drug from blood.
• Intrathecal form (without preservatives) should be used when intrathecal administration is indicated.

Italicized side effects are common or life-threatening.
*Liquid form contains alcohol.   **May contain tartrazine.

kanamycin sulfate
Kantrex, Klebcil

Pregnancy Risk Category: D

MECHANISM OF ACTION
Inhibits protein synthesis by binding directly to the 30S ribosomal subunit. Generally bactericidal.

INDICATIONS & DOSAGE
Serious infections caused by sensitive Escherichia coli, Proteus, Enterobacter aerogenes, Klebsiella pneumoniae, Serratia marcescens, Acinetobacter—
Adults and children with normal renal function: 15 mg/kg daily divided q 8 to 12 hours deep I.M. into upper outer quadrant of buttocks or I.V. infusion (diluted 500 mg/200 ml of normal saline solution or dextrose 5% in water infused at 60 to 80 drops/minute). Maximum daily dosage is 1.5 g.
Neonates: 15 mg/kg daily I.M. or I.V. divided q 12 hours.
Adjunctive treatment in hepatic coma—
Adults: 8 to 12 g daily P.O. in divided doses.
Preoperative bowel sterilization—
Adults: 1 g P.O. q 1 hour for 4 doses, then q 4 hours for 4 doses; or 1 g P.O. q 1 hour for 4 doses, then q 6 hours for 36 to 72 hours.
Intraperitoneal irrigation—
500 mg in 20 ml sterile distilled water instilled via catheter into wound after patient is fully recovered from anesthesia and neuromuscular blocking agent effects.
Wound irrigation—
Up to 2.5 mg/ml in normal saline solution irrigant.

ADVERSE REACTIONS
CNS: headache, lethargy, *neuromuscular blockade.*
EENT: o*totoxicity (tinnitus, vertigo, hearing loss).*
GU: *nephrotoxicity (cells or casts in the urine, oliguria, proteinuria, decreased creatinine clearance, increased BUN and serum creatinine levels).*

INTERACTIONS
Cephalothin: increases nephrotoxicity. Use together cautiously.
Dimenhydrinate: may mask symptoms of ototoxicity. Use with caution.
I.V. loop diuretics (e.g., furosemide): increase ototoxicity. Use cautiously.
Other aminoglycosides, amphotericin B, cisplatin, methoxyflurane: increases nephrotoxicity. Don't use together.
Parenteral penicillins (e.g., carbenicillin, ticarcillin): kanamycin inactivation in vitro. Don't mix together in I.V.

NURSING CONSIDERATIONS
• Oral use contraindicated in intestinal obstruction and treatment of systemic infection. Use cautiously in patients with impaired renal function and in the elderly.
• Obtain specimen for culture and sensitivity tests before first dose. Therapy may begin pending test results.
• Weigh patient and obtain baseline renal function studies before therapy begins.
• Monitor renal function (output, specific gravity, urinalysis, BUN and creatinine levels, and creatinine clearance). Notify doctor of signs of decreasing renal function.
• Patient should be well hydrated while taking drug to minimize chemical irritation of the renal tubules.
• Evaluate patient's hearing before and during therapy. Notify doctor if patient complains of tinnitus, vertigo, or hearing loss.
• Watch for superinfection (continued fever and other signs of new infection, especially of upper respiratory tract).
• If no response in 3 to 5 days, ther-

apy may be stopped and new specimens obtained for culture and sensitivity.

• Peak blood levels over 30 mcg/ml and trough levels over 10 mcg/ml may be associated with increased incidence of toxicity.

neomycin sulfate
Mycifradin

Pregnancy Risk Category: C

MECHANISM OF ACTION
Inhibits protein synthesis by binding directly to the 30S ribosomal subunit. Generally bactericidal.

INDICATIONS & DOSAGE
Infectious diarrhea caused by enteropathogenic Escherichia coli—
Adults: 50 mg/kg daily P.O. in 4 divided doses for 2 to 3 days.
Children: 50 to 100 mg/kg daily P.O. divided q 4 to 6 hours for 2 to 3 days.
Suppression of intestinal bacteria preoperatively—
Adults: 1 g P.O. q 1 hour for 4 doses, then 1 g q 4 hours for the balance of the 24 hours. A saline cathartic should precede therapy.
Children: 40 to 100 mg/kg daily P.O. divided q 4 to 6 hours. First dose should be preceded by saline cathartic.
Adjunctive treatment in hepatic coma—
Adults: 1 to 3 g P.O. q.i.d. for 5 to 6 days; or 200 ml of 1% or 100 ml of 2% solution as enema retained for 20 to 60 minutes q 6 hours.

ADVERSE REACTIONS
CNS: headache, lethargy.
EENT: *ototoxicity (tinnitus, vertigo, hearing loss).*
GI: nausea, vomiting.
GU: *nephrotoxicity (cells or casts in the urine, oliguria, proteinuria, decreased creatinine clearance, increased BUN and serum creatinine*

levels).
Skin: rash, urticaria.

INTERACTIONS
Cephalothin: Increases nephrotoxicity. Use together cautiously.
Dimenhydrinate: may mask symptoms of ototoxicity. Use with caution.
I.V. loop diuretics (e.g. furosemide): increase ototoxicity. Use cautiously.
Other aminoglycosides, amphotericin B, cisplatin, methoxyflurane: increases nephrotoxicity. Use together cautiously.

NURSING CONSIDERATIONS
• Contraindicated in intestinal obstruction. Use cautiously in impaired renal function, ulcerative bowel lesions, and in elderly patients.
• The ototoxic and nephrotoxic properties of neomycin limit its usefulness. Limited absorption prevents substantial systemic effects.
• Nonabsorbable at recommended dosage. However, more than 4 g/day may be systemically absorbed and lead to nephrotoxicity.
• Weigh patient and obtain baseline renal function studies before therapy begins.
• Obtain specimen for culture and sensitivity tests before first dose. Therapy may begin pending test results.
• Watch for superinfection (fever or other signs of new infection).
• Monitor renal function (output, specific gravity, urinalysis, BUN and creatinine levels, and creatinine clearance). Notify doctor of signs of decreasing renal function.
• Patient should be well hydrated while taking drug to minimize chemical irritation of the renal tubules.
• Watch for respiratory depression in patients with renal disease, hypocalcemia, or neuromuscular diseases, such as myasthenia gravis.
• Evaluate hearing of patient with hepatic or renal disease before and dur-

---

Italicized side effects are common or life-threatening.
*Liquid form contains alcohol.   **May contain tartrazine.

ing prolonged therapy. Notify doctor if patient complains of tinnitus, vertigo, or hearing loss. Onset of deafness may occur several weeks after drug is stopped.
• An adjunctive treatment of hepatic coma, neomycin is used to decrease ammonia-producing flora in the GI tract. During such treatment, decrease patient's dietary protein and assess neurologic status frequently.
• For preoperative disinfection, provide a low-residue diet and a cathartic immediately before oral administration of neomycin.
• Available in combination with polymyxin B as a urinary bladder irrigant.

netilmicin sulfate
Netromycin♦

Pregnancy Risk Category: C

MECHANISM OF ACTION
Inhibits protein synthesis by binding directly to the 30S ribosomal subunit. Generally bactericidal.

INDICATIONS & DOSAGE
Serious infections caused by sensitive Pseudomonas aeruginosa, Escherichia coli, Proteus, Klebsiella, Serratia, Enterobacter, Citrobacter, Staphylococcus—
Adults and children over 12 years: 3 to 6.5 mg/kg/day by I.M. injection or I.V. infusion. May be given q 12 hours to treat serious urinary tract infections and q 8 to 12 hours to treat serious systemic infections.
Infants and children 6 weeks to 12 years: 5.5 to 8 mg/kg/day by I.M. injection or I.V. infusion given either as 1.8 to 2.7 mg/kg q 8 hours or as 2.7 to 4 mg/kg q 12 hours.
Neonates under 6 weeks: 4 to 6.5 mg/kg/day by I.M. injection or I.V. infusion given as 2 to 3.25 mg/kg q 12 hours.
Patients with impaired renal function: Initial dose is the same as for patients with normal renal function. Subsequent doses and frequency are determined by renal function studies and serum concentration of netilmicin.

ADVERSE REACTIONS
CNS: headache, lethargy, *neuromuscular blockade*.
EENT: *ototoxicity (tinnitus, vertigo, hearing loss)*.
GU: *nephrotoxicity (cells or casts in the urine; oliguria; proteinuria; decreased creatinine clearance; increased BUN, nonprotein nitrogen, and serum creatinine levels)*.

INTERACTIONS
Cephalothin: increases nephrotoxicity. Use together cautiously.
Dimenhydrinate: may mask symptoms of ototoxicity. Use with caution.
I.V. loop diuretics (e.g. furosemide): increase ototoxicity. Use cautiously.
Other aminoglycosides, amphotericin B, cisplatin, methoxyflurane: increases nephrotoxicity. Use together cautiously.
Parenteral penicillins (e.g., carbenicillin, ticarcillin): netilmicin inactivation. Don't mix together in I.V.

NURSING CONSIDERATIONS
• Use cautiously in impaired renal function and in neonates, infants, and elderly patients.
• Obtain specimen for culture and sensitivity tests before first dose. Therapy may begin pending test results.
• Weigh patient and obtain baseline renal function studies before therapy begins.
• Monitor renal function (output, specific gravity, urinalysis, BUN and creatinine levels, and creatinine clearance). Notify doctor of signs of decreasing renal function.
• Patient should be well hydrated while taking drug to minimize chemical irritation of the renal tubules.

- After completing I.V. infusion, flush the line with normal saline solution or dextrose 5% in water.
- Evaluate patient's hearing before and during therapy. Notify doctor if patient complains of tinnitus, vertigo, or hearing loss.
- Watch for superinfection (continued fever and other signs of new infections, especially of upper respiratory tract).
- Usual duration of therapy is 7 to 10 days. If no response in 3 to 5 days, therapy may be stopped and new specimens obtained for culture and sensitivity.
- Peak blood levels above 16 mcg/ml and trough levels (those drawn just before next dose) above 4 mcg/ml may be associated with higher incidence of toxicity.
- Draw blood for peak netilmicin level 1 hour after I.M. injection and 30 minutes to 1 hour after infusion ends; for trough levels, draw blood just before next dose. Don't draw blood in a heparinized tube because heparin is incompatible with aminoglycosides.
- Netromycin is the newest aminoglycoside. Some studies show that this drug is less ototoxic than other drugs in its class.

streptomycin sulfate
Pregnancy Risk Category: D

MECHANISM OF ACTION
Inhibits protein synthesis by binding directly to the 30S ribosomal subunit. Generally bactericidal.

INDICATIONS & DOSAGE
Streptococcal endocarditis—
Adults: 10 mg/kg I.M. (maximum 0.5 g) q 12 hours for 2 weeks with penicillin.
Primary and adjunctive treatment in tuberculosis—
Adults: with normal renal function, 1

g I.M. daily for 2 to 3 months, then 1 g 2 or 3 times a week. Inject deeply into upper outer quadrant of buttocks.
Children: with normal renal function, 20 mg/kg daily in divided doses injected deeply into large muscle mass. Give concurrently with other antitubercular agents, but *not* with capreomycin, and continue until sputum specimen becomes negative.
Patients with impaired renal function: initial dose is same as for those with normal renal function. Subsequent doses and frequency determined by renal function study results.
Enterococcal endocarditis—
Adults: 1 g I.M. q 12 hours for 2 weeks, then 500 mg I.M. q 12 hours for 4 weeks with penicillin.
Tularemia—
Adults: 1 to 2 g I.M. daily in divided doses injected deep into upper outer quadrant of buttocks. Continue until patient is afebrile for 5 to 7 days.

ADVERSE REACTIONS
EENT: *ototoxicity (tinnitus, vertigo, hearing loss).*
GU: some nephrotoxicity (not nearly as frequent as with other aminoglycosides).
Local: pain, irritation, and sterile abscesses at injection site.
Skin: *exfoliative dermatitis.*
Other: *hypersensitivity* (rash, fever, urticaria, and angioneurotic edema).

INTERACTIONS
Cephalothin: increases nephrotoxicity. Use together cautiously.
Dimenhydrinate: may mask symptoms of streptomycin-induced ototoxicity. Use together cautiously.
I.V. loop diuretics (e.g. furosemide): increase ototoxicity. Use cautiously.

NURSING CONSIDERATIONS
- Contraindicated in labyrinthine disease. Use cautiously in impaired renal function and in the elderly.
- Obtain specimen for culture and

sensitivity tests before first dose except when treating tuberculosis. Therapy may begin pending test results.
• Patient should be well hydrated while taking drug to minimize chemical irritation of the renal tubules.
• Evaluate patient's hearing before, during, and 6 months after therapy. Notify doctor if patient complains of hearing loss, roaring noises, or fullness in ears.
• Watch for superinfection (continued fever and other signs of new infections).
• Protect hands when preparing. Drug is irritating.
• Endocarditis prophylaxis is recommended for all patients with rheumatic or congenital heart disease or with prosthetic heart valve. Patients should receive prophylactic antibiotics during GI or GU procedures or surgery.
• In primary treatment of tuberculosis, streptomycin is discontinued when sputum becomes negative.
• Draw blood for peak streptomycin level 1 to 2 hours after I.M. injection; for trough levels, draw blood just before next dose. Don't use a heparinized tube because heparin is incompatible with aminoglycosides.

tobramycin sulfate
Nebcin♦

Pregnancy Risk Category: D

MECHANISM OF ACTION
Inhibits protein synthesis by binding directly to the 30S ribosomal subunit. Generally bactericidal.

INDICATIONS & DOSAGE
Serious infections caused by sensitive strains of Escherichia coli, Proteus, Klebsiella, Enterobacter, Serratia, Staphylococcus aureus, Pseudomonas, Citrobacter, Providencia—
Adults and children with normal renal function: 3 mg/kg I.M. or I.V. daily divided q 8 hours. Up to 5 mg/kg I.M. or I.V. daily divided q 6 to 8 hours for life-threatening infections.
Neonates under 1 week: up to 4 mg/kg I.M. or I.V. daily divided q 12 hours. For I.V. use, dilute in 50 to 100 ml normal saline solution or dextrose 5% in water for adults and in less volume for children. Infuse over 20 to 60 minutes.
Patients with impaired renal function: initial dose is same as for those with normal renal function. Subsequent doses and frequency determined by renal function study results and serum concentrations of tobramycin.

ADVERSE REACTIONS
CNS: headache, lethargy, *neuromuscular blockade.*
EENT: *ototoxicity (tinnitus, vertigo, hearing loss).*
GU: *nephrotoxicity (cells or casts in the urine, oliguria, proteinuria, decreased creatinine clearance, increased BUN and serum creatinine levels).*

INTERACTIONS
Cephalothin: increase nephrotoxicity. Use together cautiously.
Dimenhydrinate: may mask symptoms of ototoxicity. Use with caution.
I.V. loop diuretics (e.g., furosemide): increase ototoxicity. Use cautiously.
Other aminoglycosides, amphotericin B, cisplatin, methoxyflurane: increases nephrotoxicity. Use together cautiously.
Parenteral penicillins (e.g., carbenicillin and ticarcillin): tobramycin inactivation in vitro. Don't mix together in I.V.

NURSING CONSIDERATIONS
• Use cautiously in impaired renal function and in the elderly.
• Obtain specimen for culture and sensitivity tests before first dose. Therapy may begin pending test re-

sults.
• Weigh patient and obtain baseline renal function studies before starting therapy.
• Usual duration of therapy is 7 to 10 days.
• Monitor renal function (output, specific gravity, urinalysis, BUN and creatinine levels, and creatinine clearance). Notify doctor of signs of decreasing renal function.
• Patient should be well hydrated while taking drug to minimize chemical irritation of the renal tubules.
• Evaluate patient's hearing before and during therapy. Notify doctor if patient complains of tinnitus, vertigo, or hearing loss.
• Watch for superinfection (continued fever and other signs of new infections).
• Peak blood levels over 12 mcg/ml and trough levels above 2 mcg/ml may be associated with increased incidence of toxicity.
• Draw blood for peak tobramycin level 1 hour after I.M. injection and 30 minutes to 1 hour after infusion ends; draw blood for trough level just before next dose. Don't collect blood in a heparinized tube because heparin is incompatible with aminoglycosides.
• After I.V. infusion, flush line with normal saline solution or dextrose 5% in water.

12

Penicillins

amdinocillin
amoxicillin/clavulanate
  potassium
amoxicillin trihydrate
ampicillin
ampicillin sodium
ampicillin sodium/sulbactam
  sodium
ampicillin trihydrate
azlocillin sodium
bacampicillin hydrochloride
carbenicillin disodium
carbenicillin indanyl sodium
cloxacillin sodium
cyclacillin
dicloxacillin sodium
methicillin sodium
mezlocillin sodium
nafcillin sodium
oxacillin sodium
penicillin G benzathine
penicillin G potassium
penicillin G procaine
penicillin G sodium
penicillin V
penicillin V potassium
piperacillin sodium
ticarcillin disodium
ticarcillin disodium/clavulanate
  potassium

COMBINATION PRODUCTS
AUGMENTIN, CLAVULIN ♦ ♦: amoxicillin 250 mg and clavulanate potassium 125 mg per tablet; amoxicillin 500 mg and clavulanate potassium 125 mg per tablet; amoxicillin 125 mg and potassium clavulanate 31.5 mg per 5 ml oral suspension; amoxicillin 250 mg and potassium clavulanate 31.5 mg per 5 ml oral suspension; amoxicillin 125 mg and potassium clavulanate 31.5 mg per chewable tablet; amoxicillin 250 mg and potassium clavulanate 31.5 mg per chewable tablet.
POLYCILLIN-PRB: ampicillin trihydrate 3.5g and probenecid 1g per bottle.
PRINCIPEN WITH PROBENECID: ampicillin trihydrate 3.5g and probenecid 1g per 9-capsule regimen.
TIMENTIN INJECTION: ticarcillin disodium 3 g and clavulanate potassium 100 mg per vial.
UNASYN INJECTION: ampicillin sodium 1 g and sulbactam sodium 500 mg per vial; ampicillin sodium 2 g and sulbactam sodium 1 g per vial.

---

amdinocillin
Coactin

Pregnancy Risk Category: B

MECHANISM OF ACTION
Although classified as a penicillin, amdinocillin differs structurally and in mechanism of action. It binds to a minor penicillin-binding protein (PPB 2) and prevents the bacterial cell from elongating. Generally considered bacteriostatic.

INDICATIONS & DOSAGE
Treatment of complicated and uncomplicated urinary tract infections due to susceptible strains of Escherichia coli, Klebsiella, *and* Enterobacter—
Adults: 10 mg/kg I.M. or I.V. q 4 to 6 hours.

ADVERSE REACTIONS
Blood: *eosinophilia; thrombocytosis.*
CNS: dizziness.
GI: diarrhea, nausea, vomiting.
Local: thrombophlebitis.
Other: *hypersensitivity (erythematous maculopapular rash, urticaria, anaphylaxis),* overgrowth of nonsusceptible organisms.

INTERACTIONS
Probenecid: increases blood levels of amdinocillin and other penicillins. Probenecid may be used for this purpose.

NURSING CONSIDERATIONS
• Use cautiously in patients with other drug allergies, especially to cephalosporins (possible cross-allergenicity).
• Obtain specimen for culture and sensitivity tests before first dose. Therapy may begin pending test results.
• Watch for superinfection (fever or other signs of new infection).
• Before giving amdinocillin, ask patient about any allergic reactions to penicillin. However, a negative history doesn't rule out future penicillin allergy.
• Amdinocillin may act synergistically with other penicillins and cephalosporins and is frequently prescribed in combination with these drugs. May be a less toxic alternative to aminoglycosides.
• Dosage should be decreased in patients with moderate-to-severe renal failure.

---

amoxicillin/clavulanate potassium
Augmentin, Clavulin♦♦

Pregnancy Risk Category: B

MECHANISM OF ACTION
An aminopenicillin that acts by preventing bacterial cell wall synthesis during active replication. Clavulanic acid increases amoxicillin effectiveness by inactivating beta lactamases, which destroy amoxicillin.

INDICATIONS & DOSAGE
Lower respiratory infections, otitis media, sinusitis, skin and skin structure infections, and urinary tract infections caused by susceptible strains of gram-positive and gram-negative organisms—
Adults: 250 mg (based on the amoxicillin component) P.O. q 8 hours. For more severe infections, 500 mg q 8 hours.
Children: 20 to 40 mg/kg/day (based on the amoxicillin component) given in divided doses q 8 hours.

ADVERSE REACTIONS
Blood: anemia, thrombocytopenia, thrombocytopenic purpura, eosinophilia, leukopenia.
GI: *nausea,* vomiting, *diarrhea.*
Other: *hypersensitivity (erythematous maculopapular rash, urticaria, anaphylaxis),* overgrowth of nonsusceptible organisms.

INTERACTIONS
Probenecid: increases blood levels of amoxicillin and other penicillins. Probenecid may be used for this purpose.

NURSING CONSIDERATIONS
• Use cautiously in patients with other drug allergies, especially to cephalosporins (possible cross-allergenicity), and in mononucleosis (high incidence of maculopapular rash). Before giving, ask patient about any allergic reactions to penicillin. However, a negative history doesn't rule out future penicillin allergy.
• Obtain specimen for culture and sensitivity tests before first dose. Therapy may begin pending test results.
• Watch for superinfection (fever or other signs of new infection).

Italicized side effects are common or life-threatening.
*Liquid form contains alcohol.   **May contain tartrazine.

- Tell patient to take drug exactly as prescribed, even after he feels better. Patient should take entire quantity prescribed.
- Give with food to prevent GI distress.
- Incidence of diarrhea is greater than with amoxicillin alone.
- Large doses may cause increased yeast growth. Report symptoms to doctor.
- With prolonged therapy, bacterial and fungal superinfection may occur, especially in elderly, debilitated, or immunosuppressed patients. Close observation is essential.
- Both the "250" and "500" tablets contain the same amount of clavulanic acid (125 mg). Therefore, two "250" tablets are not equivalent to one "500" tablet.
- Particularly useful in clinical settings with high prevalence of amoxicillin-resistant organisms.
- Give amoxicillin/potassium clavulanate least 1 hour before bacteriostatic antibiotics.

---

amoxicillin trihydrate

Amoxil♦, Apo-Amoxi♦♦, Axicillin♦♦, Novamoxin♦♦, Polymox♦, Trimox, Utimox, Wymox

Pregnancy Risk Category: B

MECHANISM OF ACTION

An aminopenicillin that is bactericidal against microorganisms by inhibiting cell wall synthesis during active multiplication. Bacteria resist amoxicillin by producing penicillinases—enzymes that hydrolyze amoxicillin.

INDICATIONS & DOSAGE

Systemic infections, acute and chronic urinary tract infections caused by susceptible strains of gram-positive and gram-negative organisms—
Adults: 750 mg to 1.5 g P.O. daily in divided doses given q 8 hours.

Children: 20 to 40 mg/kg P.O. daily in divided doses given q 8 hours.
Uncomplicated gonorrhea—
Adults: 3 g P.O. with 1 g probenecid given as a single dose.
Uncomplicated urinary tract infections caused by susceptible organisms—
Adults: 3 g P.O. given as a single dose.

ADVERSE REACTIONS

Blood: anemia, thrombocytopenia, thrombocytopenic purpura, eosinophilia, leukopenia.
GI: *nausea,* vomiting, *diarrhea.*
Other: *hypersensitivity (erythematous maculopapular rash, urticaria, anaphylaxis),* overgrowth of nonsusceptible organisms.

INTERACTIONS

Probenecid: increases blood levels of amoxicillin and other penicillins. Probenecid may be used for this purpose.

NURSING CONSIDERATIONS

- Use cautiously in patients with other drug allergies, especially to cephalosporins (possible cross-allergenicity), and in mononucleosis—high incidence of maculopapular rash in those receiving amoxicillin.
- Obtain specimen for culture and sensitivity tests before first dose. Therapy may begin pending test results.
- Watch for superinfection (fever or other signs of new infection).
- Before giving amoxicillin, ask patient if he's had any allergic reactions to penicillin. However, a negative history of penicillin allergy is no guarantee against a future allergic reaction.
- Tell patient to take medication exactly as prescribed, even after he feels better. Entire quantity prescribed should be taken.
- Give with food to prevent GI distress.
- Large doses may cause increased

---

yeast growths. Report symptoms to doctor.
• With prolonged therapy, bacterial and fungal superinfection may occur, especially in the elderly, debilitated, or those with low resistance to infection due to immunosuppressives or irradiation. Close observation essential.
• Warn patient never to use leftover amoxicillin for a new illness or to share it with family and friends.
• Trimox oral suspension may be stored at room temperature for up to 2 weeks. Be sure to check individual product labels for storage information.
• Tell patient to call the doctor if rash, fever, or chills develop. A rash is the most common allergic reaction. The rash is most common if the patient is also taking allopurinol.
• Amoxicillin and ampicillin have similar clinical applications.
• Urine glucose determinations may be false-positive with copper sulfate tests (Clinitest); glucose enzymatic tests (Clinistix, Tes-Tape) are not affected.
• Give amoxicillin at least 1 hour before bacteriostatic antibiotics.

ampicillin
Amcill, Ampicin♦♦, Ampilean♦♦, Apo-Ampi♦♦, Novo Ampicillin♦♦, Omnipen, Penbritin♦♦, Principen

ampicillin sodium
Omnipen-N♦, Polycillin-N, Totacillin-N

ampicillin trihydrate
Amcill, D-Amp, Omnipen, Penamp-250, Penamp-500, Polycillin, Principen-250, Principen-500, Totacillin

Pregnancy Risk Category: B

MECHANISM OF ACTION
An aminopenicillin that is bactericidal against microorganisms by inhibiting cell wall synthesis during active multiplication. Bacteria resist ampicillin by producing penicillinases—enzymes that hydrolyze ampicillin.

INDICATIONS & DOSAGE
Systemic infections, acute and chronic urinary tract infections caused by susceptible strains of gram-positive and gram-negative organisms—
Adults: 1 to 4 g P.O. daily, divided into doses given q 6 hours; 2 to 12 g I.M. or I.V. daily, divided into doses given q 4 to 6 hours.
Children: 50 to 100 mg/kg P.O. daily, divided into doses given q 6 hours; or 100 to 200 mg/kg I.M. or I.V. daily, divided into doses given q 6 hours.
Meningitis—
Adults: 8 to 14 g I.V. daily for 3 days, then I.M. divided q 3 to 4 hours.
Children: up to 300 mg/kg I.V. daily for 3 days, then I.M. divided q 4 hours.
Uncomplicated gonorrhea—
Adults: 3.5 g P.O. with 1 g probenecid given as a single dose.

ADVERSE REACTIONS
Blood: anemia, thrombocytopenia, thrombocytopenic purpura, eosinophilia, leukopenia.
GI: *nausea,* vomiting, *diarrhea,* glossitis, stomatitis.
Local: pain at injection site, vein irritation, thrombophlebitis.
Other: *hypersensitivity (erythematous maculopapular rash, urticaria, anaphylaxis), overgrowth of nonsusceptible organisms.*

INTERACTIONS
Probenecid: increases blood levels of ampicillin and other penicillins. Probenecid may be used for this purpose.

NURSING CONSIDERATIONS
• Use cautiously in patients with other drug allergies, especially to

---

Italicized side effects are common or life-threatening.
*Liquid form contains alcohol.   **May contain tartrazine.

cephalosporins (possible cross-allergenicity), and in mononucleosis—high incidence of maculopapular rash in those receiving ampicillin.
• Obtain specimen for culture and sensitivity tests before first dose. Therapy may begin pending test results.
• Watch for superinfection (fever or other signs of new infection).
• Before giving ampicillin, ask patient if he's had any allergic reactions to penicillin. However, a negative history of penicillin allergy is no guarantee against a future allergic reaction.
• Tell patient to take medication exactly as prescribed, even after he feels better. Entire quantity prescribed should be taken.
• Tell the patient to call the doctor if rash, fever, or chills develop. A rash is the most common allergic reaction. Rash is most common if the patient is also taking allopurinol.
• When given orally, drug may cause GI disturbances. Food may interfere with absorption, so give 1 to 2 hours before meals or 2 to 3 hours after.
• Don't give I.M. or I.V. unless infection is severe or patient can't take oral dose.
• Dosage should be altered in patients with impaired renal functions.
• When giving I.V., mix with dextrose 5% in water or a saline solution. Don't mix with other drugs or solutions: they might be incompatible.
• Give I.V. intermittently to prevent vein irritation. Change site every 48 hours.
• With large doses or prolonged therapy, bacterial or fungal superinfection may occur, especially in patients who are elderly, debilitated, or have low resistance to infection resulting from treatment with immunosuppressive agents or radiation. Close observation is essential.
• Warn patient never to use leftover ampicillin for a new illness or to share it with family and friends.

• Intitial dilution in vial is stable for 1 hour. Follow manufacturer's direction for stability data when ampicillin is further diluted for I.V. infusion.
• In pediatric meningitis, may be given concurrently with parenteral chloramphenicol for 24 hours pending cultures.
• Urine glucose determinations may be false-positive with copper sulfate tests (Clinitest); glucose enzymatic tests (Clinistix, Tes-Tape) are not affected.
• Give ampicillin at least 1 hour before bacteriostatic antibiotics.

ampicillin sodium/ sulbactam sodium
Unasyn
Pregnancy Risk Category: C

MECHANISM OF ACTION
Ampicillin (an aminopenicillin) inhibits cell wall synthesis during active multiplication. Sulbactam inactivates bacterial beta-lactamase, the enzyme that inactivates ampicillin and provides bacterial resistance to it.

INDICATIONS & DOSAGE
Intraabdominal, gynecologic, and integumentary infections caused by susceptible strains of bacteria—
Adults: dosage expressed as total drug (each 1.5-g vial contains 1 g ampicillin sodium and 0.5 g sulbactam sodium): 1.5 to 3 g I.M. or I.V. q 6 hours. Maximum daily dose is 4 g sulbactam (12 g of the combined drugs).

ADVERSE REACTIONS
CNS: fatigue, malaise, headache, chills.
CV: edema, erythema.
GI: diarrhea, nausea, vomiting, flatulence, abdominal distention.
GU: dysuria, urine retention.
Local: pain at injection site, thrombophlebitis.
Other: rash, itching, candidiasis,

anaphylaxis.

INTERACTIONS
Probenecid: increased levels of ampicillin. Probenecid may be used for this purpose.

NURSING CONSIDERATIONS
• Use cautiously in patients with other drug allergies, especially to cephalosporins (possible cross-allergenicity), and in mononucleosis—high incidence of maculopapular rash in those receiving ampicillin.
• Obtain specimen for culture and sensitivity tests before first dose. Therapy may begin pending test results.
• Watch for superinfection (fever or other signs of new infection).
• Before giving ampicillin, ask patient if he's had any allergic reactions to penicillin. However, a negative history of penicillin allergy is no guarantee against a future allergic reaction.
• When preparing I.V. injection, reconstitute powder with any of the following diluents: normal saline solution, dextrose 5% in water, lactated Ringer's injection, ⅙ M sodium lactate, dextrose 5% and 0.45% saline injection, and 10% invert sugar. Stability varies with diluent, temperature, and concentration of solution.
• After reconstitution, allow vials to stand for a few minutes to allow foam to dissipate. This will permit visual inspection of contents for particles.
• Give I.V. dose by slow injection (over 10 to 15 minutes), or dilute in 50 to 100 ml of a compatible diluent and infuse over 15 to 30 minutes.
• When administering I.M., give by deep injection. Drug may be reconstituted with sterile water for injection, or 0.5% or 2% lidocaine hydrochloride injection. Add 3.2 ml to a 1.5-g vial (or 6.4 ml to a 3-g vial) to yield a concentration of 375 mg/ml.
• Tell the patient to call the doctor if rash, fever, or chills develop. A rash

is the most common allergic reaction.
• Dosage should be altered in patients with impaired renal functions.
• When giving I.V., mix with dextrose 5% in water or saline solution. Don't mix with other drugs or solutions: they might be incompatible.
• Give I.V. intermittently to prevent vein irritation. Change site every 48 hours.
• Large doses may cause increased yeast growths. Report symptoms to doctor.
• With prolonged therapy, bacterial and fungal superinfections may occur, especially in patients who are elderly, debilitated, or who have low resistance to infection because of treatment with immunosuppressive agents or radiation. Close observation is essential.
• Urine glucose determinations may be false-positive with copper sulfate tests (Clinitest); glucose enzymatic tests (Clinistix, Tes-Tape) are not affected.
• Give ampicillin/sulbactam at least 1 hour before bacteriostatic antibiotics.

azlocillin sodium
Azlin

Pregnancy Risk Category: B

MECHANISM OF ACTION
An extended-spectrum penicillin that is bactericidal against microorganisms by inhibiting cell wall synthesis during active multiplication. Bacteria resist azlocillin by producing penicillinases—enzymes that hydrolyze azlocillin.

INDICATIONS & DOSAGE
Serious infections caused by susceptible strains of gram-negative organisms, including Pseudomonas aeruginosa—
Adults: 200 to 350 mg/kg daily I.V. given in four to six divided doses. Usual dose is 3 g q 4 hours (18 g

daily). Maximum daily dosage is 24 g. May be administered by I.V. intermittent infusion or by direct slow I.V. injection.

Children with acute exacerbation of cystic fibrosis: 75 mg/kg q 4 hours (450 mg/kg daily). Maximum daily dosage is 24 g.

Azlocillin should not be used in neonates.

ADVERSE REACTIONS
Blood: *bleeding with high doses,* neutropenia, eosinophilia, leukopenia, *thrombocytopenia.*
CNS: neuromuscular irritability, headache, dizziness.
GI: nausea, diarrhea.
Local: pain at injection site, vein irritation, phlebitis.
Metabolic: *hypokalemia.*
Other: *hypersensitivity (edema, fever, chills, rash, pruritus, urticaria, anaphylaxis), overgrowth of nonsusceptible organisms.*

INTERACTIONS
Aminoglycoside antibiotics (e.g., gentamicin, tobramycin): chemically incompatible. Don't mix together in I.V. solution.

NURSING CONSIDERATIONS
• Use cautiously in patients hypersensitive to drugs, especially to cephalosporins (possible cross-allergenicity), and in bleeding tendencies, uremia, or hypokalemia.
• Obtain specimen for culture and sensitivity tests before first dose. Therapy may begin pending test results.
• Watch for superinfection (fever or other signs of new infection).
• Before giving azlocillin, ask patient if he's had allergic reactions to penicillin. A negative history of penicillin allergy, however, is no guarantee against future allergic reactions.
• Dosage should be altered in patients with impaired renal functions.

• Check CBC and platelets frequently. Drug may cause thrombocytopenia.
• Monitor serum potassium level.
• Patient with high serum level of azlocillin may have seizures. Institute seizure precautions.
• When giving I.V., mix with dextrose 5% in water or other suitable I.V. fluids.
• Give I.V. intermittently to prevent vein irritation. Change site every 48 hours.
• Rapid administration may cause chest discomfort. Don't infuse over a period of less than 5 minutes.
• Almost always used with another antibiotic, such as gentamicin.
• With prolonged therapy, superinfections may occur, especially in the elderly or debilitated, or in those patients with low resistance to infection due to immunosuppressors or irradiation. Monitor patient closely.
• Azlocillin is less likely to cause hypokalemia than similar antibiotics, such as carbenicillin and ticarcillin.
• Drug may be better suited to patients on salt-free diets than carbenicillin and ticarcillin (contains 2.17 mEq Na^+/g of azlocillin).
• Give azlocillin at least 1 hour before bacteriostatic antibiotics.

---

bacampicillin hydrochloride
Penglobe♦♦, Spectrobid
Pregnancy Risk Category: B

MECHANISM OF ACTION
An aminopenicillin that is converted to ampicillin in vivo, each mg of bacampicillin yields 623 to 727 mcg ampicillin. It is bactericidal against microorganisms by inhibiting cell wall synthesis during active multiplication. Bacteria resist bacampicillin by producing penicillinases—enzymes that hydrolyze its active form (ampicillin).

INDICATIONS & DOSAGE

Upper and lower respiratory tract infections due to streptococci, pneumococci, staphylococci, and Hemophilus influenzae; urinary tract infections due to Escherichia coli, Proteus mirabilis, and Streptococcus faecalis; skin infections due to streptococci and susceptible staphylococci—
Adults and children weighing more than 25 kg: 400 to 800 mg P.O. q 12 hours.
Gonorrhea—
Usual dosage is 1.6 g plus 1 g probenecid given as a single dose.

Not recommended for children under 25 kg.

ADVERSE REACTIONS

Blood: anemia, thrombocytopenia, thrombocytopenic purpura, eosinophilia, leukopenia.
GI: *nausea,* vomiting, *diarrhea,* glossitis, stomatitis.
Other: *hypersensitivity (erythematous maculopapular rash, urticaria, anaphylaxis),* overgrowth of nonsusceptible organisms.

INTERACTIONS

Probenecid: increases blood levels of bacampicillin or other penicillins. Probenecid may be used for this purpose.

NURSING CONSIDERATIONS

• Use cautiously in patients with other drug allergies, especially to cephalosporins (possible cross-allergenicity), and in mononucleosis. This drug, like ampicillin, is linked to a high incidence of maculopapular rash.
• Obtain specimen for culture and sensitivity tests before first dose. Therapy may begin pending test results.
• Watch for superinfection (fever or other signs of new infection).
• Before giving bacampicillin, ask patient if he's had any previous allergic reactions to penicillin. However, a negative history of penicillin allergy is no guarantee against a future allergic reaction.
• Bacampicillin is especially formulated to produce high blood levels of antibiotic when administered twice daily.
• Diarrhea may occur less frequently with bacampicillin than with ampicillin.
• Tell patient to take medication even after he feels better. Entire quantity prescribed should be taken.
• Tell patient to call the doctor if rash, fever, or chills develop. A rash is the most common allergic reaction.
• With prolonged therapy, bacterial or fungal superinfection may occur, especially in the elderly or the debilitated, and in those with low resistance to infection due to immunosuppressors or irradiation. Close observation is essential.
• Warn patient never to use leftover bacampicillin for a new illness or to share it with family and friends.
• Unlike ampicillin, bacampicillin tablets may be taken with meals without fear of diminished drug absorption. Give with food to prevent GI distress. However, bacampicillin suspension should be taken on an empty stomach.
• Administer bacampicillin at least 1 hour before bacteriostatic antibiotics.

carbenicillin disodium
Geopen, Pyopen♦

Pregnancy Risk Category: B

MECHANISM OF ACTION

Bactericidal against microorganisms by inhibiting cell wall synthesis during active multiplication. Bacteria resist carbenicillin by producing penicillinases—enzymes that hydrolyze its active form.

INDICATIONS & DOSAGE

Systemic infections caused by suscepti-

Italicized side effects are common or life-threatening.
*Liquid form contains alcohol.   **May contain tartrazine.

ble strains of gram-positive and especially gram-negative organisms (including Proteus, Pseudomonas aeruginosa)—
Adults: 30 to 40 g daily I.V. infusion, divided into doses given q 4 to 6 hours.
Children: 300 to 500 mg/kg daily I.V. infusion, divided into doses given q 4 to 6 hours.
Urinary tract infections—
Adults: 200 mg/kg daily I.M. or I.V. infusion, divided into doses given q 4 to 6 hours.
Children: 50 to 200 mg/kg daily I.M. or I.V. infusion, divided into doses given q 4 to 6 hours.

ADVERSE REACTIONS
Blood: *bleeding with high doses,* neutropenia, eosinophilia, leukopenia, *thrombocytopenia.*
CNS: neuromuscular irritability.
GI: nausea.
Local: pain at injection site, vein irritation, phlebitis.
Metabolic: *hypokalemia.*
Other: *hypersensitivity (edema, fever, chills, rash, pruritus, urticaria, anaphylaxis),* overgrowth of nonsusceptible organisms.

INTERACTIONS
Aminoglycoside antibiotics (e.g., gentamicin, tobramycin): chemically incompatible. Don't mix together in I.V.
Probenecid: increases blood levels of carbenicillin and other penicillins. Probenecid may be used for this purpose.

NURSING CONSIDERATIONS
• Use cautiously in patients with other drug allergies, especially to cephalosporins (possible cross-allergenicity), and in bleeding tendencies, uremia, and hypokalemia. Use cautiously in patients on sodium-restricted diets; contains 4.7 mEq sodium/g.
• Obtain specimen for culture and sensitivity tests before first dose. Therapy may begin pending test results.
• Watch for superinfection (fever or other signs of new infection).
• Before giving carbenicillin, ask patient if he's had any allergic reactions to penicillin. However, a negative history of penicillin allergy is no guarantee against a future allergic reaction.
• Dosage should be altered in patients with impaired renal function. Patients with impaired renal function are susceptible to nephrotoxicity. Monitor intake/output.
• Check CBC and platelets frequently. Drug may cause thrombocytopenia.
• Monitor serum potassium level. Patients may develop hypokalemia due to large amount of sodium in the preparation.
• If patient has high blood level of this drug, he may have seizures. Institute seizure precautions.
• When giving I.V., mix with dextrose 5% in water or other suitable I.V. fluids.
• Give I.V. intermittently to prevent vein irritation. Change site every 48 hours.
• Almost always used with another antibiotic, such as gentamicin.
• Large doses may cause increased yeast growths. Report symptoms to doctor.
• With prolonged therapy, other superinfections may occur, especially in the elderly, debilitated, or those with low resistance to infection due to immunosuppressives or irradiation. Close observation is essential.
• Give carbenicillin at least 1 hour before bacteriostatic antibiotics.

carbenicillin indanyl sodium
Geocillin, Geopen Oral♦♦

Pregnancy Risk Category: B

MECHANISM OF ACTION
Bactericidal against microorganisms by inhibiting cell wall synthesis during active multiplication. Bacteria resist carbenicillin by producing penicillinases—enzymes that hydrolyze its active form.

INDICATIONS & DOSAGE
Urinary tract infection and prostatitis caused by susceptible strains of gram-negative organisms—
Adults: 382 to 764 mg P.O. q.i.d.
  Not recommended for children.

ADVERSE REACTIONS
Blood: leukopenia, neutropenia, eosinophilia, anemia, thrombocytopenia.
GI: *nausea,* vomiting, *diarrhea, flatulence, abdominal cramps, unpleasant taste.*
Other: *hypersensitivity (rash, chills, fever, urticaria, pruritus, anaphylaxis),* overgrowth of nonsusceptible organisms.

INTERACTIONS
None significant.

NURSING CONSIDERATIONS
• Use cautiously in patients with other drug allergies, especially to cephalosporins (possible cross-allergenicity).
• Obtain specimen for culture and sensitivity tests before first dose. Therapy may begin pending test results.
• Watch for superinfection (fever or other signs of new infection).
• Before giving carbenicillin, ask patient if he's had any allergic reactions to penicillin. However, a negative history of penicillin allergy is no guaran-

tee against a future allergic reaction.
• Tell patient to take medication exactly as prescribed, even after he feels better. Entire quantity prescribed should be taken.
• Tell patient to call the doctor if he develops rash, fever, or chills. A rash is the most common allergic reaction.
• When given orally, drug may cause GI disturbances. Food may interfere with absorption, so give 1 to 2 hours before meals or 2 to 3 hours after.
• With large doses or prolonged therapy, bacterial or fungal superinfections may occur, especially in patients who are elderly, debilitated, or have low resistance to infection because of treatment with immunosuppressive agents or radiation. Close observation is essential.
• Warn patient never to use leftover carbenicillin for a new illness or to share it with family and friends.
• Use only in patients whose creatinine clearance is 10 ml/minute or more.
• Excellent treatment for *Pseudomonas* urinary tract infections in ambulatory patients.
• May be useful in treatment of cystitis, but not pyelonephritis.
• Not effective for any systemic infection because blood levels are nil.

cloxacillin sodium
Apo-Cloxi♦♦, Bactopen♦♦, Cloxapen, Novocloxin♦♦, Orbenin♦♦, Tegopen♦

Pregnancy Risk Category: B

MECHANISM OF ACTION
Bactericidal against microorganisms by inhibiting cell wall synthesis during active multiplication. Bacteria resist penicillins by producing penicillinases—enzymes that convert penicillins to inactive penicilloic acis. Cloxacillin resists these enzymes.

INDICATIONS & DOSAGE

Systemic infections caused by penicillinase-producing staphylococci—
Adults: 2 to 4 g P.O. daily, divided into doses given q 6 hours.
Children: 50 to 100 mg/kg P.O. daily, divided into doses given q 6 hours.

ADVERSE REACTIONS

Blood: eosinophilia.
GI: *nausea,* vomiting, *epigastric distress, diarrhea.*
Other: *hypersensitivity (rash, urticaria, chills, fever, sneezing, wheezing, anaphylaxis),* overgrowth of nonsusceptible organisms.

INTERACTIONS

Probenecid: increases blood levels of cloxacillin and other penicillins. Probenecid may be used for this purpose.

NURSING CONSIDERATIONS

• Use with caution in patients with other drug allergies, especially to cephalosporins (possible cross-allergenicity).
• Obtain specimen for culture and sensitivity tests before first dose. Therapy may begin pending test results.
• Watch for superinfection (fever or other signs of new infection).
• Before giving cloxacillin, ask patient if he's had any allergic reactions to penicillin. However, a negative history of penicillin allergy is no guarantee against a future allergic reaction.
• Tell patient to take medication exactly as prescribed, even if he feels better. Entire quantity prescribed should be taken.
• Tell patient to call the doctor if rash, fever, or chills develop. A rash is the most common allergic reaction.
• When given orally, drug may cause GI disturbances. Food may interfere with absorption, so give 1 to 2 hours before meals or 2 to 3 hours after.
• Patient should take each dose with a full glass of water, not fruit juice or carbonated beverage, because acid will inactivate the drug.
• With prolonged therapy, other superinfections may occur, especially in the elderly, debilitated, or those with low resistance to infection due to immunosuppressives or irradiation. Close observation is essential.
• Warn patient never to use leftover cloxacillin for a new illness or to share it with family and friends.
• Give cloxacillin at least 1 hour before bacteriostatic antibiotics.

---

cyclacillin
Cyclapen-W
Pregnancy Risk Category: B

MECHANISM OF ACTION

Bactericidal against microorganisms by inhibiting cell wall synthesis during active multiplication. Bacteria resist cyclacillin by producing penicillinases—enzymes that hydrolyze cyclacillin to an inactive form.

INDICATIONS & DOSAGE

Systemic and urinary tract infections caused by susceptible strains of gram-positive and gram-negative organisms—
Adults: 250 to 500 mg P.O. q.i.d. in equally spaced doses.
Children: 50 to 100 mg/kg daily t.i.d. in equally divided doses.

ADVERSE REACTIONS

Blood: anemia, thrombocytopenia, thrombocytopenic purpura, leukopenia, neutropenia, eosinophilia.
GI: *nausea,* vomiting, diarrhea.
Other: *hypersensitivity (edema, fever, chills, rash, pruritus, urticaria, anaphylaxis),* overgrowth of nonsusceptible organisms.

INTERACTIONS

Probenecid: increases blood levels of cyclacillin. Probenecid may be used

---

for this purpose.

NURSING CONSIDERATIONS
• Contraindicated in patients allergic to other penicillins.
• Obtain specimen for culture and sensitivity tests before first dose. Therapy may begin pending test results.
• Watch for superinfection (fever or other signs of new infection).
• Before giving cyclacillin, ask patient if he's had any allergic reactions to penicillin. However, a negative history of penicillin allergy is no guarantee against a future allergic reaction.
• Tell patient he must take all medication exactly as prescribed, for as long as ordered, even after he feels better.
• Patients with renal insufficiency should receive less drug in accordance with their creatinine clearance level.
• Large doses of cyclacillin may cause increased yeast growths. Watch for signs and symptoms, and report to doctor.
• With prolonged therapy, bacterial and fungal superinfection may occur, especially in the elderly, debilitated, or those with low resistance to infection due to immunosuppressives or irradiation. Close observation is essential.
• Warn patient never to use leftover cyclacillin for a new illness or to share it with family and friends.
• Tell patient to call the doctor if he develops rash, fever, or chills. A rash is the most common allergic reaction.
• Studies show that cyclacillin is as effective as amoxicillin in treating acute otitis media and causes less diarrhea.
• Give cyclacillin at least 1 hour before bacteriostatic antibiotics.

dicloxacillin sodium
Dycill, Dynapen♦, Pathocil
Pregnancy Risk Category: B

MECHANISM OF ACTION
Bactericidal against microorganisms by inhibiting cell wall synthesis during active multiplication. Bacteria resist penicillins by producing penicillinases—enzymes that convert penicillins to inactive penicilloic acid. Dicloxacillin resists these enzymes.

INDICATIONS & DOSAGE
Systemic infections caused by penicillinase-producing staphylococci—
Adults: 1 to 2 g daily P.O., divided into doses given q 6 hours.
Children: 25 to 50 mg/kg P.O. daily, divided into doses given q 6 hours.

ADVERSE REACTIONS
Blood: eosinophilia.
GI: *nausea,* vomiting, *epigastric distress,* flatulence, *diarrhea.*
Other: *hypersensitivity (pruritus, urticaria, rash, anaphylaxis),* overgrowth of nonsusceptible organisms.

INTERACTIONS
Probenecid: increases blood levels of dicloxacillin and other penicillins. Probenecid may be used for this purpose.

NURSING CONSIDERATIONS
• Use cautiously in patients allergic to cephalosporins (possible cross-allergenicity).
• Obtain specimen for culture and sensitivity tests before first dose. Therapy may begin pending test results.
• Watch for superinfection (fever or other signs of new infection).
• Before giving dicloxacillin, ask patient if he's had any allergic reactions to penicillin. However, a negative history of penicillin allergy is no guarantee against a future allergic reaction.

- Tell patient to take medication exactly as prescribed, even if he feels better. Entire quantity prescribed should be taken.
- Tell patient to call the doctor if rash, fever, or chills develop. A rash is the most common allergic reaction.
- Drug may cause GI disturbances. Food may interfere with absorption, so give 1 to 2 hours before meals or 2 to 3 hours after.
- With prolonged therapy, other superinfections may occur, especially in the elderly, debilitated, or those with low resistance to infection due to immunosuppressives or irradiation. Close observation is essential.
- Periodic assessments of renal, hepatic, and hematopoietic function should be made when therapy is prolonged.
- Warn patient never to use leftover dicloxacillin for a new illness or to share it with family and friends.
- Give dicloxacillin at least 1 hour before bacteriostatic antibiotics.

methicillin sodium
Staphcillin

Pregnancy Risk Category: B

MECHANISM OF ACTION
Bactericidal against microorganisms by inhibiting cell wall synthesis during active multiplication. Bacteria resist penicillins by producing penicillinases—enzymes that convert penicillins to inactive penicilloic acids. Methicillin resists these enzymes.

INDICATIONS & DOSAGE
Systemic infections caused by penicillinase-producing staphylococci—
Adults: 4 to 12 g I.M. or I.V. daily, divided into doses given q 4 to 6 hours.
Children: 100 to 200 mg/kg I.M. or I.V. daily, divided into doses given q 4 to 6 hours.

ADVERSE REACTIONS
Blood: *eosinophilia,* hemolytic anemia, transient neutropenia.
CNS: neuropathy, seizures with high doses.
GI: glossitis, stomatitis.
GU: interstitial nephritis.
Local: *vein irritation, thrombophlebitis.*
Other: *hypersensitivity (chills, fever, edema, rash, urticaria, anaphylaxis),* overgrowth of nonsusceptible organisms.

INTERACTIONS
Probenecid: increases blood levels of methicillin and other penicillins. Probenecid may be used for this purpose.

NURSING CONSIDERATIONS
- Use cautiously in patients with other drug allergies, especially to cephalosporins (possible cross-allergenicity), and in infants.
- Obtain specimen for culture and sensitivity tests before first dose. Therapy may begin pending test results.
- Watch for superinfection (fever or other signs of new infection).
- Methicillin-resistant strains of Staphylococci should be treated with vancomycin.
- Before giving methicillin, ask patient if he's had any allergic reactions to penicillin. However, a negative history of penicillin allergy is no guarantee against a future allergic reaction.
- If ordered 4 times a day, be sure to give every 6 hours—even during the night.
- Closely monitor renal function. Urinalysis should be done frequently to detect interstitial nephritis.
- If patient has high blood level of this drug, he may have seizures. Institute seizure precautions.
- When giving I.V., mix with a normal saline solution. Don't mix with others because methicillin may be inactivated. Initial dilution must be

---

made with sterile water for injection.
• Give I.V. intermittently to prevent vein irritation. Change site every 48 hours.
• With prolonged therapy, other superinfections may occur, especially in the elderly, debilitated, or those with low resistance to infection due to immunosuppressives or irradiation. Close observation is essential.
• Periodic assessment of hepatic, renal, and hematopoietic function is required during prolonged therapy.
• Give methicillin at least 1 hour before bacteriostatic antibiotics.

mezlocillin sodium
Mezlin

Pregnancy Risk Category: B

MECHANISM OF ACTION
Bactericidal against microorganisms by inhibiting cell wall synthesis during active multiplication. Bacteria resist mezlocillin by producing penicillinases—enzymes that hydrolyze mezlocillin.

INDICATIONS & DOSAGE
Systemic infections caused by susceptible strains of gram-positive and especially gram-negative organisms (including Proteus, Pseudomonas aeruginosa)—
Adults: 200 to 300 mg/kg daily I.V. or I.M. given in 4 to 6 divided doses. Usual dose is 3 g q 4 hours or 4 g q 6 hours. For very serious infections, up to 24 g daily may be administered.
Children to age 12: 50 mg/kg q 4 hours by I.V. infusion or direct I.V. injection.

ADVERSE REACTIONS
Blood: *bleeding with high doses,* neutropenia, eosinophilia, leukopenia, *thrombocytopenia.*
CNS: neuromuscular irritability.
GI: nausea, diarrhea.
Local: pain at injection site, vein irri-

tation, phlebitis.
Metabolic: *hypokalemia.*
Other: *hypersensitivity (edema, fever, chills, rash, pruritus, urticaria, anaphylaxis), overgrowth of nonsusceptible organisms.*

INTERACTIONS
Aminoglycoside antibiotics (e.g., gentamicin, tobramycin): chemically incompatible. Don't mix together in I.V. solution. Give 1 hour apart, especially in patients with renal insufficiency.

NURSING CONSIDERATIONS
• Use cautiously in patients hypersensitive to drugs, especially to cephalosporins (possible cross-hypersensitivity), and in bleeding tendencies, uremia, and hypokalemia.
• Obtain specimen for culture and sensitivity tests before first dose. Therapy may begin pending test results.
• Watch for superinfection (fever or other signs of new infection).
• Before giving mezlocillin, ask patient if he's had allergic reactions to penicillin. A negative history of penicillin allergy, however, is no guarantee against future allergic reaction.
• Dosage should be altered in patients with impaired renal function.
• Check CBC and platelets frequently. Drug may cause thrombocytopenia.
• Monitor serum potassium level.
• Patient with high serum level of this drug may have seizures. Institute seizure precautions.
• When giving I.V., mix with dextrose 5% in water or other suitable I.V. fluids.
• Give I.V. intermittently to prevent vein irritation. Change site every 48 hours.
• Almost always used with another antibiotic, such as gentamicin.
• With prolonged therapy, superinfections may occur, especially in the elderly or debilitated, or those with

---

Italicized side effects are common or life-threatening.
*Liquid form contains alcohol.   **May contain tartrazine.

low resistance to infection due to immunosuppressors or irradiation. Monitor patient closely.
• Compared with similar antibiotics, such as carbenicillin and ticarcillin, mezlocillin is less likely to cause hypokalemia.
• Drug may be better suited to patients on salt-free diets than carbenicillin and ticarcillin (contains 1.85 mEq Na/g of mezlocillin).
• Give mezlocillin at least 1 hour before bacteriostatic antibiotics.

nafcillin sodium
Nafcil, Nallpen, Unipen♦

Pregnancy Risk Category: B

MECHANISM OF ACTION
Bactericidal against microorganisms by inhibiting cell wall synthesis during active multiplication. Bacteria resist nafcillin by producing penicillinases—enzymes that hydrolyze nafcillin.

INDICATIONS & DOSAGE
Systemic infections caused by penicillinase-producing staphylococci—
Adults: 2 to 4 g P.O. daily, divided into doses given q 6 hours; 2 to 12 g I.M. or I.V. daily, divided into doses given q 4 to 6 hours.
Children: 50 to 100 mg/kg P.O. daily, divided into doses given q 4 to 6 hours; or 100 to 200 mg/kg I.M. or I.V. daily, divided into doses given q 4 to 6 hours.

ADVERSE REACTIONS
Blood: transient leukopenia, neutropenia, granulocytopenia, thrombocytopenia with high doses.
GI: *nausea,* vomiting, diarrhea.
Local: *vein irritation, thrombophlebitis.*
Other: *hypersensitivity (chills, fever, rash, pruritus, urticaria, anaphylaxis).*

INTERACTIONS
Probenecid: increases blood levels of nafcillin and other penicillins. Probenecid may be used for this purpose.

NURSING CONSIDERATIONS
• Use cautiously in patients with other drug allergies, especially to cephalosporins (possible cross-allergenicity), and in GI distress.
• Obtain specimen for culture and sensitivity tests before first dose. Therapy may begin pending test results.
• Watch for superinfection (fever or other signs of new infection).
• Before giving nafcillin, ask patient if he's had any allergic reactions to penicillin. However, a negative history of penicillin allergy is no guarantee against a future allergic reaction.
• Tell patient to take medication exactly as prescribed, even if he feels better. Entire quantity prescribed should be taken.
• Tell patient to call the doctor if rash, fever, or chills develop. A rash is the most common allergic reaction.
• When given orally, drug may cause GI disturbances. Food may interfere with absorption, so give 1 to 2 hours before meals or 2 to 3 hours after.
• When giving I.V., mix with dextrose 5% in water or a saline solution.
• Give I.V. intermittently to prevent vein irritation. Change site every 48 hours.
• With prolonged therapy, other superinfections may occur, especially in the elderly, debilitated, or those with low resistance to infection due to immunosuppressives or irradiation. Close observation is essential.
• Give nafcillin at least 1 hour before bacteriostatic antibiotics.

oxacillin sodium
Bactocill, Prostaphlin
Pregnancy Risk Category: B

MECHANISM OF ACTION
Bactericidal against microorganisms by inhibiting cell wall synthesis during active multiplication. Bacteria resist penicillins by producing penicillinases—enzymes that convert penicillins to inactive penicilloic acids. Oxacillin resists these enzymes.

INDICATIONS & DOSAGE
Systemic infections caused by penicillinase-producing staphylococci—
Adults: 2 to 4 g P.O. daily, divided into doses given q 6 hours; 2 to 12 g I.M. or I.V. daily, divided into doses given q 4 to 6 hours.
Children: 50 to 100 mg/kg P.O. daily, divided into doses given q 6 hours; 100 to 200 mg/kg I.M. or I.V. daily, divided into doses given q 4 to 6 hours.

ADVERSE REACTIONS
Blood: granulocytopenia, thrombocytopenia, eosinophilia, hemolytic anemia, transient neutropenia.
CNS: neuropathy.
GI: oral lesions.
GU: interstitial nephritis, transient hematuria, proteinuria.
Hepatic: hepatitis, elevated enzymes.
Local: *thrombophlebitis.*
Other: *hypersensitivity (fever, chills, rash, urticaria, anaphylaxis),* overgrowth of nonsusceptible organisms.

INTERACTIONS
Probenecid: increases blood levels of oxacillin and other penicillins. Probenecid may be used for this purpose.

NURSING CONSIDERATIONS
• Use cautiously in patients with other drug allergies, especially to cephalosporins (possible cross-allergenicity), in premature newborns, and in infants.
• Obtain specimen for culture and sensitivity tests before first dose. Therapy may begin pending test results.
• Watch for superinfection (fever or other signs of new infection).
• Before giving oxacillin, ask patient if he's had any allergic reactions to penicillin. However, a negative history of penicillin allergy is no guarantee against a future allergic reaction.
• Tell the patient to take medication exactly as prescribed, even if he feels better. The entire quantity prescribed should be taken.
• Tell patient to call the doctor if rash, fever, or chills develop. A rash is the most common allergic reaction.
• When given orally, drug may cause GI disturbances. Food may interfere with absorption, so give 1 to 2 hours before meals or 2 to 3 hours after.
• Don't give I.M. or I.V. unless infection is severe or patient can't take oral dose.
• Periodic liver function studies are indicated; watch for elevated AST (SGOT) and ALT (SGPT).
• When giving I.V., mix with dextrose 5% in water or a saline solution.
• Give I.V. intermittently to prevent vein irritation. Change site every 48 hours.
• With prolonged therapy, other superinfections may occur, especially in the elderly, debilitated, or those with low resistance to infection due to immunosuppressives or irradiation. Close observation is essential.
• Give oxacillin at least 1 hour before bacteriostatic antibiotics.

penicillin G benzathine
Bicillin L-A♦, Megacillin
Pregnancy Risk Category: B

MECHANISM OF ACTION
Bactericidal against microorganisms by inhibiting cell wall synthesis dur-

---

ing active multiplication. Bacteria resist penicillin by producing penicillinases—enzymes that convert penicillin to inactive penicilloic acid.

INDICATIONS & DOSAGE
Congenital syphilis—
Children under age 2: 50,000 units/kg I.M. as a single dose.
Group A streptococcal upper respiratory infections—
Adults: 1.2 million units I.M. in a single injection.
Children over 27 kg: 900,000 units I.M. in a single injection.
Children under 27 kg: 300,000 to 600,000 units I.M. in a single injection.
Prophylaxis of poststreptococcal rheumatic fever—
Adults and children: 1.2 million units I.M. once a month or 600,000 units twice a month.
Syphilis of less than 1 year's duration—
Adults: 2.4 million units I.M. in a single dose.
Syphilis of more than 1 year's duration—
Adults: 2.4 million units I.M. weekly for 3 successive weeks.

ADVERSE REACTIONS
Blood: eosinophilia, hemolytic anemia, thrombocytopenia, leukopenia.
CNS: neuropathy, seizures with high doses.
Local: pain and sterile abscess at injection site.
Other: *hypersensitivity (maculopapular and exfoliative dermatitis, chills, fever, edema, anaphylaxis).*

INTERACTIONS
Probenecid: increases blood levels of penicillin. Probenecid may be used for this purpose.

NURSING CONSIDERATIONS
• Use cautiously in patients with other drug allergies, especially to cephalosporins (possible cross-allergenicity).
• Obtain specimen for culture and sensitivity tests before first dose. Therapy may begin pending test results.
• Watch for superinfection (fever or other signs of new infection).
• Before giving penicillin, ask patient if he's had any allergic reactions to this drug. However, a negative history of penicillin allergy is no guarantee against a future allergic reaction.
• Tell patient to call the doctor if rash, fever, or chills develop. Fever and eosinophilia are the most common allergic reactions.
• Shake medication well before injection.
• Never give I.V.—inadvertent I.V. administration has caused cardiac arrest and death.
• Very slow absorption time makes allergic reactions difficult to treat.
• Inject deeply into upper outer quadrant of buttocks in adults; in midlateral thigh in infants and small children.
• Give penicillin G benzathine at least 1 hour before bacteriostatic antibiotics.

penicillin G potassium
Megacillin♦♦, NovoPen-G♦♦, P-50♦♦, Pentids**, Pfizerpen

Pregnancy Risk Category: B

MECHANISM OF ACTION
Bactericidal against microorganisms by inhibiting cell wall synthesis during active multiplication. Bacteria resist penicillin by producing penicillinases—enzymes that convert penicillin to inactive penicilloic acid.

INDICATIONS & DOSAGE
Moderate to severe systemic infections—
Adults: 1.6 to 3.2 million units P.O. daily in divided doses given q 6 hours

(1 mg = 1,600 units); 1.2 to 24 million units I.M. or I.V. daily in divided doses given q 4 hours.

Children: 25,000 to 100,000 units/kg P.O. daily in divided doses given q 6 hours; or 25,000 to 300,000 units/kg I.M. or I.V. daily in divided doses given q 4 hours.

ADVERSE REACTIONS

Blood: hemolytic anemia, leukopenia, thrombocytopenia.
CNS: neuropathy, seizures with high doses.
Metabolic: possible severe potassium poisoning with high doses (hyperreflexia, seizures, coma).
Local: *thrombophlebitis, pain at injection site.*
Other: *hypersensitivity (rash, urticaria, maculopapular eruptions, exfoliative dermatitis, chills, fever, edema, anaphylaxis),* overgrowth of nonsusceptible organisms.

INTERACTIONS

Probenecid: increases blood levels of penicillin. Probenecid may be used for this purpose.

NURSING CONSIDERATIONS

• Use cautiously in patients with other drug allergies, especially to cephalosporins (possible cross-allergenicity).
• Obtain specimen for culture and sensitivity tests before first dose. Therapy may begin pending test results.
• Watch for superinfection (fever or other signs of new infection).
• Before giving penicillin, ask patient if he's had any allergic reactions to this drug. However, a negative history of penicillin allergy is no guarantee against a future allergic reaction.
• Tell patient to take medication exactly as prescribed, even if he feels better, and to take entire amount prescribed.
• Tell patient to call the doctor if

rash, fever, or chills develop. A rash is the most common allergic reaction.
• When given orally, drug may cause GI disturbances. Food may interfere with absorption, so give 1 to 2 hours before meals or 2 to 3 hours after.
• Extremely painful when given I.M. Inject deep into large muscle.
• Patients with poor renal function are predisposed to high blood levels. Monitor renal function closely.
• If patient has high blood level of this drug, he may have seizures. Institute seizure precautions.
• When giving I.V., mix with dextrose 5% in water or a saline solution.
• Give I.V. intermittently to prevent vein irritation. Change site every 48 hours.
• With prolonged therapy, other superinfections may occur, especially in elderly or debilitated patients or those with low resistance to infection because of treatment with immunosuppressive agents or radiation. Close observation is essential.
• Warn patient never to use leftover penicillin for a new illness or to share penicillin with family and friends.
• Give penicillin G potassium at least 1 hour before bacteriostatic antibiotics.

---

penicillin G procaine

Ayercillin♦♦, Crysticillin A.S., Duracillin A.S., Pfizerpen-AS, Wycillin♦

Pregnancy Risk Category: B

MECHANISM OF ACTION

Bactericidal against microorganisms by inhibiting cell wall synthesis during active multiplication. Bacteria resist penicillin by producing penicillinases—enzymes that convert penicillin to inactive penicilloic acid.

INDICATIONS & DOSAGE

Moderate to severe systemic infections—
Adults: 600,000 to 1.2 million units

I.M. daily given as a single dose.
Children: 300,000 units I.M. daily
given as a single dose.
Uncomplicated gonorrhea—
Adults and children over 12 years:
give 1 g probenecid; then 30 minutes
later give 4.8 million units of penicillin G procaine I.M., divided into two
injection sites.
Pneumococcal pneumonia—
Adults and children over 12 years:
300,000 to 600,000 units I.M. daily q
6 to 12 hours.

ADVERSE REACTIONS
Blood: thrombocytopenia, hemolytic
anemia, leukopenia.
CNS: arthralgia, seizures.
Other: *hypersensitivity (rash, urticaria, chills, fever, edema, prostra-
tion, anaphylaxis),* overgrowth of
nonsusceptible organisms.

INTERACTIONS
Probenecid: increases blood levels of
penicillin. Probenecid may be used
for this purpose.

NURSING CONSIDERATIONS
• Contraindicated in patients with hypersensitivity to procaine. Use cautiously in patients with other drug allergies, especially to cephalosporins
(possible cross-allergenicity).
• Obtain specimen for culture and
sensitivity tests before first dose.
Therapy may begin pending test results.
• Watch for superinfection (fever or
other signs of new infection).
• Before giving penicillin, ask patient
if he's had any allergic reactions to
this drug. However, a negative history
of penicillin allergy is no guarantee
against a future allergic reaction.
• Tell patient to call doctor if rash, fever, or chills develop. A rash is the
most common allergic reaction.
• Give deep I.M. in upper outer
quadrant of buttocks in adults; in midlateral thigh in small children. Do not

give subcutaneously. Don't massage
injection site.
• Never give I.V.—inadvertent I.V.
administration has caused death, due
to CNS toxicity from procaine.
• Due to slow absorption rate, allergic reactions are hard to treat.
• With prolonged therapy, other superinfections may occur, especially in
the elderly, debilitated, or those with
low resistance to infection due to immunosuppressives or irradiation.
Close observation is essential.
• Periodic evaluations of renal and
hematopoietic function are recommended.
• Give penicillin G procaine at least 1
hour before bacteriostatic antibiotics.

penicillin G sodium
Crystapen♦♦

Pregnancy Risk Category: B

MECHANISM OF ACTION
Bactericidal against microorganisms
by inhibiting cell wall synthesis during active multiplication. Bacteria resist penicillin by producing penicillinases—enzymes that convert penicillin to inactive penicilloic acid.

INDICATIONS & DOSAGE
*Moderate to severe systemic infec-
tions—*
Adults: 1.2 to 24 million units daily
I.M. or I.V., divided into doses given
q 4 hours.
Children: 25,000 to 300,000 units/kg
daily I.M. or I.V., divided into doses
given q 4 hours.
*Endocarditis prophylaxis for dental
surgery—*
Adults: 2 million units I.V. or I.M. 30
to 60 minutes before procedure, then
1 million units 6 hours later.

ADVERSE REACTIONS
Blood: hemolytic anemia, leuko-
penia, thrombocytopenia.
CNS: arthralgia, neuropathy, sei-

zures.
CV: *congestive heart failure with high doses.*
Local: *vein irritation, pain at injection site, thrombophlebitis.*
Other: *hypersensitivity (chills, fever, edema, maculopapular rash, exfoliative dermatitis, urticaria, anaphylaxis),* overgrowth of nonsusceptible organisms.

INTERACTIONS
Probenecid: increases blood levels of penicillin. Probenecid may be used for this purpose.

NURSING CONSIDERATIONS
• Contraindicated in patients on sodium restriction. Use cautiously in patients with other drug allergies, especially to cephalosporins (possible cross-allergenicity).
• Obtain specimen for culture and sensitivity tests before first dose. Therapy may begin pending test results.
• Watch for superinfection (fever or other signs of new infection).
• Before giving penicillin, ask patient if he's had any allergic reactions to this drug. However, a negative history of penicillin allergy is no guarantee against a future allergic reaction.
• If patient has high blood level of this drug, he may have seizures. Institute seizure precautions.
• Give I.V. intermittently to prevent vein irritation. Change site every 48 hours.
• With prolonged therapy, bacterial or fungal superinfections may occur, especially in patients who are elderly, debilitated, or who have low resistance to infection because of treatment with immunosuppressive agents or radiation.
• Give penicillin G sodium at least 1 hour before bacteriostatic antibiotics.

penicillin V

penicillin V potassium
Apo-Pen-VK♦♦, Beepen-VK, Betapen-VK, Ledercillin VK♦, Nadopen-V♦♦, NovoPen-VK♦♦, Penapar VK, Pen Vee K♦, PVF K♦♦, Robicillin VK, V-Cillin K♦, VC-K, Veetids**

Pregnancy Risk Category: B

MECHANISM OF ACTION
Bactericidal against microorganisms by inhibiting cell wall synthesis during active multiplication. Bacteria resist penicillin by producing penicillinases—enzymes that convert penicillin to inactive penicilloic acid.

INDICATIONS & DOSAGE
Mild to moderate systemic infections—
Adults: 250 to 500 mg (400,000 to 800,000 units) P.O. q 6 hours.
Children: 15 to 50 mg/kg (25,000 to 90,000 units/kg) P.O. daily, divided into doses given q 6 to 8 hours.
Endocarditis prophylaxis for dental surgery—
Adults: 2 g P.O. 30 to 60 minutes before procedure, then 1 g 6 hours after.
Children under 30 kg: half of the adult dose.

ADVERSE REACTIONS
Blood: eosinophilia, hemolytic anemia, leukopenia, thrombocytopenia.
CNS: neuropathy.
GI: *epigastric distress,* vomiting, diarrhea, *nausea.*
Other: *hypersensitivity (rash, urticaria, chills, fever, edema, anaphylaxis),* overgrowth of nonsusceptible organisms.

INTERACTIONS
Neomycin: decreases absorption of penicillin. Give penicillin by injection.
Probenecid: increases blood levels of penicillin. Probenecid may be used

---

Italicized side effects are common or life-threatening.
*Liquid form contains alcohol.   **May contain tartrazine.

for this purpose.

NURSING CONSIDERATIONS
• Use cautiously in patients with other drug allergies, especially to cephalosporins (possible cross-allergenicity), and in GI disturbances.
• Obtain specimen for culture and sensitivity tests before first dose. Therapy may begin pending test results.
• Watch for superinfection (fever or other signs of new infection).
• Before giving penicillin, ask patient if he's had any allergic reactions to this drug. However, a negative history of penicillin allergy is no guarantee against a future allergic reaction.
• Tell patient to take medication exactly as prescribed, even if he feels better. Entire quantity prescribed should be taken.
• Tell patient to call the doctor if rash, fever, or chills develop. A rash is the most common allergic reaction.
• May cause GI disturbances. Food may interfere with absorption, so give 1 to 2 hours before meals or 2 to 3 hours after.
• Patient should take each dose with a full glass of water, not fruit juice or a carbonated beverage, because acid will inactivate the drug.
• Patients being treated for streptococcal infections should take the drug until the full 10-day course is completed.
• With prolonged therapy, bacterial and fungal superinfections may occur, especially in patients who are elderly, debilitated, or who have low resistance to infection because of treatment with immunosuppressive agents or radiation. Close observation is essential.
• Periodic renal and hematopoietic function studies are recommended in patients receiving prolonged therapy.
• Warn patient never to use leftover penicillin for a new illness or to share penicillin with family and friends.

• Give penicillin V at least 1 hour before bacteriostatic antibiotics.

piperacillin sodium
Pipracil♦

Pregnancy Risk Category: B

MECHANISM OF ACTION
Bactericidal against microorganisms by inhibiting cell wall synthesis during active multiplication. Bacteria resist penicillin by producing penicillinases—enzymes that convert penicillin to inactive penicilloic acid.

INDICATIONS & DOSAGE
Systemic infections caused by susceptible strains of gram-positive and especially gram-negative organisms (including Proteus, Pseudomonas aeruginosa*)—*
Adults and children over 12 years: 100 to 300 mg/kg daily divided q 4 to 6 hours I.V. or I.M. Doses for children under 12 years not established.
Prophylaxis of surgical infections—
Adults: 2 g I.V., given 30 to 60 minutes before surgery. Depending on type of surgery, dose may be repeated during surgery, and once or twice more after surgery.

ADVERSE REACTIONS
Blood: *bleeding with high doses,* neutropenia, eosinophilia, leukopenia, *thrombocytopenia.*
CNS: neuromuscular irritability, headache, dizziness.
GI: nausea, diarrhea.
Local: pain at injection site, vein irritation, phlebitis.
Metabolic: *hypokalemia.*
Other: *hypersensitivity (edema, fever, chills, rash, pruritus, urticaria, anaphylaxis),* overgrowth of nonsusceptible organisms.

INTERACTIONS
Aminoglycoside antibiotics (e.g., gentamicin, tobramycin): chemically in-

compatible.

NURSING CONSIDERATIONS
• Use cautiously in patients hypersensitive to drugs, especially to cephalosporins (possible cross-hypersensitivity), and in bleeding tendencies, uremia, and hypokalemia.
• Cystic fibrosis patients tend to be most susceptible to fever or rash.
• Obtain specimen for culture and sensitivity tests before first dose. Therapy may begin pending test results.
• Watch for superinfection (fever or other signs of new infection).
• Before giving piperacillin, ask patient if he's had allergic reactions to penicillin. A negative history of penicillin allergy, however, is no guarantee against future allergic reaction.
• Dosage should be altered in patients with impaired renal function.
• Check CBC and platelets frequently. Drug may cause thrombocytopenia.
• Monitor serum potassium level.
• Patient with high serum level of this drug may have seizures. Institute seizure precautions.
• Give I.V. intermittently to prevent vein irritation. Change site every 48 hours.
• Almost always used with another antibiotic, such as gentamicin.
• With prolonged therapy, bacterial and fungal superinfections may occur, especially in patients who are elderly, debilitated, who have low resistance to infection because of treatment with immunosuppressive agents or radiation. Monitor patient closely.
• Drug may be better suited to patients on salt-free diets than carbenicillin and ticarcillin (contains 1.98 mEq Na/g of piperacillin).
• Piperacillin has shown greater activity against *Pseudomonas aeruginosa* than carbenicillin, ticarcillin, or mezlocillin.
• Give piperacillin at least 1 hour before bacteriostatic antibiotics.

---

ticarcillin disodium
Ticar♦

Pregnancy Risk Category: B

MECHANISM OF ACTION
Bactericidal against microorganisms by inhibiting cell wall synthesis during active multiplication. Bacteria resist penicillin by producing penicillinases—enzymes that convert penicillin to inactive penicilloic acid.

INDICATIONS & DOSAGE
Severe systemic infections caused by susceptible strains of gram-positive and especially gram-negative organisms (including Pseudomonas, *Proteus)—*
Adults: 18 g I.V. or I.M. daily, divided into doses given q 4 to 6 hours.
Children: 200 to 300 mg/kg I.V. or I.M. daily, divided into doses given q 4 to 6 hours.

ADVERSE REACTIONS
Blood: leukopenia, neutropenia, eosinophilia, *thrombocytopenia,* hemolytic anemia.
CNS: seizures, neuromuscular excitability.
GI: nausea, diarrhea.
Metabolic: *hypokalemia.*
Local: pain at injection site, vein irritation, phlebitis.
Other: *hypersensitivity (rash, pruritus, urticaria, chills, fever, edema, anaphylaxis),* overgrowth of nonsusceptible organisms.

INTERACTIONS
Aminoglycoside antibiotics (e.g., gentamicin, tobramycin): chemically incompatible. Don't mix together in I.V.
Probenecid: increases blood levels of ticarcillin and other penicillins. Probenecid may be used for this purpose.

Italicized side effects are common or life-threatening.
*Liquid form contains alcohol.   **May contain tartrazine.

NURSING CONSIDERATIONS

• Use cautiously in other drug allergies, especially to cephalosporins (possible cross-allergenicity), and in impaired renal function, hemorrhagic conditions, hypokalemia, or sodium restrictions (contains 5.2 mEq Na/g).

• Obtain specimen for culture and sensitivity tests before first dose. Therapy may begin pending test results.

• Watch for superinfection (fever or other signs of new infection).

• Before giving ticarcillin, ask patient if he's had any allergic reactions to penicillin. However, a negative history of penicillin allergy is no guarantee against a future allergic reaction.

• Dosage should be decreased in patients with impaired renal functions.

• Check CBC and platelets frequently. Drug may cause thrombocytopenia.

• If patient has high blood level of this drug, he may develop seizures. Institute seizure precautions.

• When giving I.V., mix with dextrose 5% in water or other suitable I.V. fluids.

• Give I.V. intermittently to prevent vein irritation. Change site every 48 hours.

• Administer deep I.M. into large muscle.

• Almost always used with another antibiotic, such as gentamicin.

• With prolonged therapy, bacterial and fungal superinfections may occur, especially in patients who are elderly, debilitated, who have low resistance to infection because of treatment with immunosuppressive agents or radiation. Close observation is essential.

• Monitor serum potassium.

• Give ticarcillin at least 1 hour before bacteriostatic antibiotics.

ticarcillin disodium/ clavulanate potassium
Timentin

Pregnancy Risk Category: B

MECHANISM OF ACTION
Clavulanic acid increases ticarcillin's effectiveness by inactivating beta lactamases, which destroy ticarcillin.

INDICATIONS & DOSAGE
Treatment of infections of the lower respiratory tract, urinary tract, bones and joints, skin and skin structure, and septicemia when caused by beta-lactamase–producing strains of bacteria or by ticarcillin-susceptible organisms—
Adults: 3.1-g vial (contains ticarcillin 3 g and clavulanate potassium 0.1 g) administered by I.V. infusion q 4 to 6 hours.

ADVERSE REACTIONS
Blood: leukopenia, neutropenia, eosinophilia, *thrombocytopenia*, hemolytic anemia.
CNS: seizures, neuromuscular excitability.
GI: nausea, diarrhea.
Metabolic: *hypokalemia.*
Local: pain at injection site, vein irritation, phlebitis.
Other: *hypersensitivity (rash, pruritus, urticaria, chills, fever, edema, anaphylaxis),* overgrowth of nonsusceptible organisms.

INTERACTIONS
Probenecid: increases blood levels of ticarcillin. Probenecid may be used for this purpose.
Aminoglycoside antibiotics (e.g., gentamicin, tobramycin): chemically incompatible. Don't mix together in I.V.

NURSING CONSIDERATIONS
• Use cautiously in patients with other drug allergies, especially to cephalosporins (possible cross-aller-

genicity), and in impaired renal function, hemorrhagic conditions, hypokalemia, or sodium restrictions.

• Obtain specimen for culture and sensitivity tests before first dose. Therapy may begin pending test results.

• Watch for superinfection (fever or other signs of new infection).

• Before giving Timentin, ask patient if he's had any allergic reactions to penicillin. However, a negative history of penicillin allergy is no guarantee against a future allergic reaction.

• Dosage should be decreased in patients with impaired renal functions.

• Check CBC and platelets frequently. Drug may cause thrombocytopenia.

• Monitor serum potassium.

• Administer by I.V. infusion over 30 minutes. Don't give by I.V. push or I.M.

• Particularly useful in clinical settings with a high prevalence of ticarcillin-resistant organisms.

• Give ticarcillin disodium/clavulanate potassium at least 1 hour before bacteriostatic antibiotics.

13

Cephalosporins

cefaclor
cefadroxil monohydrate
cefamandole nafate
cefazolin sodium
cefonicid sodium
cefoperazone sodium
ceforanide
cefotaxime sodium
cefotetan disodium
cefoxitin sodium
ceftazidime
ceftizoxime sodium
ceftriaxone sodium
cefuroxime axetil
cefuroxime sodium
cephalexin monohydrate
cephalothin sodium
cephapirin sodium
cephradine
moxalactam disodium

COMBINATION PRODUCTS
None.

---

cefaclor
Ceclor♦

Pregnancy Risk Category: B

MECHANISM OF ACTION
Inhibits cell wall synthesis, promoting osmotic instability. Usually bactericidal.

INDICATIONS & DOSAGE
Treatment of infections of respiratory or urinary tracts, skin, and soft tissue; and otitis media due to Hemophilus influenzae, Streptococcus pneumoniae, S. pyogenes, Escherichia coli, Proteus mirabilis, Klebsiella *species, and staphylococci—*
Adults: 250 to 500 mg P.O. q 8 hours. Total daily dose should not exceed 4 g.
Children: 20 mg/kg daily P.O. in divided doses q 8 hours. In more serious infections, 40 mg/kg daily are recommended, not to exceed 1 g per day.

ADVERSE REACTIONS
Blood: transient leukopenia, lymphocytosis, anemia, eosinophilia.
CNS: dizziness, headache, somnolence.
GI: *nausea,* vomiting, *diarrhea,* anorexia, *pseudomembranous colitis.*
GU: red and white cells in urine, vaginal moniliasis, vaginitis.
Skin: *maculopapular rash,* dermatitis.
Other: hypersensitivity, fever.

INTERACTIONS
Probenecid: may inhibit excretion and increase blood levels of cefaclor.

NURSING CONSIDERATIONS
• Contraindicated in hypersensitivity to other cephalosporins. Use cautiously in impaired renal function and in those with history of sensitivity to penicillin. Ask patient if he's had any reaction to previous cephalosporin or penicillin therapy before administering first dose.
• Obtain specimen for culture and sensitivity tests before first dose. Therapy may begin pending test results.
• Major clinical use appears to be in

---

treating otitis media caused by *H. influenzae* when resistant to ampicillin or amoxicillin. Drug is a second-generation cephalosporin.
• Tell patient to take medication exactly as prescribed, even after he feels better, and to take entire amount prescribed.
• Call doctor if skin rash develops.
• Prolonged use may result in overgrowth of nonsusceptible organisms. Careful observation of patient for superinfection is essential.
• Store reconstituted suspension in refrigerator. Stable for 14 days if refrigerated. Shake well before using.
• Drug may be taken with meals.
• Cefaclor is a relatively expensive antibiotic and should be used only when the organism is resistant to other agents.
• If ordered, total daily dose of cefaclor may be administered twice daily rather than 3 times daily with similar therapeutic results.
• Urine glucose determinations may be false-positive with copper sulfate tests (Clinitest); glucose enzymatic tests (Clinistix, Tes-Tape) are not affected.

---

cefadroxil monohydrate
Duricef♦, Ultracef

Pregnancy Risk Category: B

MECHANISM OF ACTION
Inhibits cell wall synthesis, promoting osmotic instability. Usually bactericidal.

INDICATIONS & DOSAGE
Treatment of urinary tract infections caused by Escherichia coli, Proteus mirabilis, *and* Klebsiella *species; infections of skin and soft tissue; and streptococcal pharyngitis—*
Adults: 500 mg to 2 g P.O. per day, depending on the infection being treated. Usually given in once-daily or b.i.d. dosage.

Children: 30 mg/kg daily in 2 divided doses.

ADVERSE REACTIONS
Blood: transient neutropenia, eosinophilia, leukopenia, anemia.
CNS: dizziness, headache, malaise, paresthesias.
GI: *pseudomembranous colitis, nausea,* anorexia, vomiting, *diarrhea,* glossitis, *dyspepsia,* abdominal cramps, anal pruritus, tenesmus, oral candidiasis (thrush).
GU: genital pruritus, moniliasis.
Skin: *maculopapular and erythematous rashes.*
Other: dyspnea.

INTERACTIONS
Probenecid: may inhibit excretion and increase blood levels of cefadroxil.

NURSING CONSIDERATIONS
• Contraindicated in patients with hypersensitivity to other cephalosporins. Use cautiously in impaired renal function and in those with history of sensitivity to penicillin. Ask patient if he's had any reaction to previous cephalosporin or penicillin therapy before administering first dose.
• Obtain specimen for culture and sensitivity tests before first dose. Therapy may begin pending test results.
• If creatinine clearance is below 50 ml/minute, dosage interval should be lengthened so drug doesn't accumulate.
• Tell patient to take medication exactly as prescribed, even after he feels better, and to take entire amount prescribed.
• Call doctor if skin rash develops.
• Since absorption not delayed by presence of food, tell the patient to take with food or milk to lessen GI discomfort.
• Longer half-life permits once- or twice-daily dosing.
• Urine glucose determinations may

---

be false-positive with copper sulfate tests (Clinitest); glucose enzymatic tests (Clinistix, Tes-Tape) are not affected.

• Prolonged use may result in overgrowth of nonsusceptible organisms. Careful observation of patient for superinfection is essential.

cefamandole nafate
Mandol♦

Pregnancy Risk Category: B

MECHANISM OF ACTION
Inhibits cell wall synthesis, promoting osmotic instability. Usually bactericidal.

INDICATIONS & DOSAGE
Treatment of serious infections of respiratory and genitourinary tracts, skin and soft-tissue infections, bone and joint infections, septicemia, and peritonitis due to Escherichia coli *and other coliform bacteria,* S. aureus *(penicillinase- and nonpenicillinase-producing),* S. epidermidis, *group A beta-hemolytic streptococci,* Klebsiella, Hemophilus influenzae, Proteus mirabilis, *and* Enterobacter—
Adults: 500 mg to 1 g q 4 to 8 hours. In life-threatening infections, up to 2 g q 4 hours may be needed.
Infants and children: 50 to 100 mg/kg daily in equally divided doses q 4 to 8 hours. May be increased to total daily dose of 150 mg/kg (not to exceed maximum adult dose) for severe infections.

Total daily dosage is same for I.M. or I.V. administration and depends on susceptibility of organism and severity of infection. In patients with impaired renal function, doses or frequency of administration must be modified according to degree of renal impairment, severity of infection, and susceptibility of organism. Should be injected deep I.M. into a large muscle mass, such as gluteus or lateral aspect of thigh.

ADVERSE REACTIONS
Blood: transient neutropenia, eosinophilia, hemolytic anemia, *hypoprothrombinemia,* bleeding.
CNS: headache, malaise, paresthesias, dizziness.
GI: *pseudomembranous colitis,* nausea, anorexia, vomiting, *diarrhea,* glossitis, dyspepsia, abdominal cramps, tenesmus, anal pruritus, oral candidiasis (thrush).
GU: genital pruritus and moniliasis.
Skin: *maculopapular and erythematous rashes, urticaria.*
Local: *at injection site—pain, induration, sterile abscesses,* temperature elevation, tissue sloughing; *phlebitis and thrombophlebitis with I.V. injection.*
Other: *hypersensitivity,* dyspnea.

INTERACTIONS
Ethyl alcohol: may cause a disulfiram-like reaction. Warn patients not to drink alcohol for several days after discontinuing cefamandole.
Probenecid: may inhibit excretion and increase blood levels of cefamandole.

NURSING CONSIDERATIONS
• Contraindicated in patients with hypersensitivity to other cephalosporins. Use cautiously in impaired renal function and in those with history of sensitivity to penicillin. Ask patient if he's had any reaction to previous cephalosporin or penicillin therapy before administering first dose.
• Obtain specimen for culture and sensitivity tests before first dose. Therapy may begin pending test results.
• Not as effective as cefoxitin in treating anaerobic infections.
• For most cephalosporin-sensitive organisms, cefamandole offers little advantage over previously available agents.
• For I.V. use, reconstitute 1 g with

10 ml of sterile water for injection, dextrose 5% or 0.9% sodium chloride for injection.
• Don't mix with I.V. infusions containing magnesium or calcium ions; chemically incompatible.
• I.M. cefamandole is not as painful as cefoxitin. Does not require addition of lidocaine.
• After reconstitution, drug remains stable for 24 hours at room temperature or 96 hours under refrigeration.
• The chemical structure of this drug includes the methylthiotetrazole (MTT) side chain that has been associated with bleeding disorders. If bleeding occurs, it can be promptly reversed with administration of vitamin K.
• Prolonged use may result in overgrowth of nonsusceptible organisms. Careful observation of patient for superinfection is essential.
• Urine glucose determinations may be false-positive with copper sulfate tests (Clinitest); glucose enzymatic tests (Clinistix, Tes-Tape) are not affected.

cefazolin sodium
Ancef♦, Kefzol♦
Pregnancy Risk Category: B

MECHANISM OF ACTION
Inhibits cell wall synthesis, promoting osmotic instability. Usually bactericidal.

INDICATIONS & DOSAGE
Treatment of serious infections of respiratory and genitourinary tracts, skin and soft-tissue infections, bone and joint infections, septicemia, and endocarditis due to Escherichia coli, *Enterobacteriaceae, gonococci,* Hemophilus influenzae, Klebsiella, Proteus mirabilis, Staphylococcus aureus, Streptococcus pneumoniae, *and group A beta-hemolytic streptococci; and perioperative prophylaxis—*

Adults: 250 mg I.M. or I.V. q 8 hours to 1 g q 6 hours. Maximun 12g/day in life-threatening situations.
Children over 1 month: 8 to 16 mg/kg I.M. or I.V. q 8 hours, or 6 to 12 mg/kg q 6 hours.
   Total daily dosage is same for I.M. or I.V. administration and depends on susceptibility of organism and severity of infection. In patients with impaired renal function, doses or frequency of administration must be modified according to degree of renal impairment, severity of infection, and susceptibility of organism. Should be injected deep I.M. into a large muscle mass, such as gluteus or lateral aspect of thigh.

ADVERSE REACTIONS
Blood: transient neutropenia, leukopenia, eosinophilia, anemia.
CNS: dizziness, headache, malaise, paresthesias.
GI: *pseudomembranous colitis,* nausea, anorexia, vomiting, *diarrhea,* glossitis, dyspepsia, abdominal cramps, anal pruritus, tenesmus, oral candidiasis (thrush).
GU: genital pruritus and moniliasis, vaginitis.
Skin: *maculopapular and erythematous rashes, urticaria.*
Local: *at injection site—pain, induration, sterile abscesses, tissue sloughing; phlebitis and thrombophlebitis with I.V. injection.*
Other: *hypersensitivity,* dyspnea.

INTERACTIONS
Probenecid: may inhibit excretion and increase blood levels of cefazolin.

NURSING CONSIDERATIONS
• Use cautiously in impaired renal function and in those with history of sensitivity to penicillin. Ask patient if he's ever had any reaction to cephalosporin or penicillin therapy before administering first dose.
• Avoid doses greater than 4 g daily

in patients with severe renal impairment.

• Obtain specimen for culture and sensitivity tests before first dose. Therapy may begin pending test results.

• Because of long duration of effect, most infections can be treated with a dose q 8 hours.

• For I.M. administration, reconstitute with sterile water, bacteriostatic water, or 0.9% sodium chloride solution as follows: 2 ml to 250-mg vial; 2 ml to 500-mg vial; 2.5 ml to 1-g vial. Shake well until dissolved. Resultant concentration: 125 mg/ml, 225 mg/ml, 330 mg/ml, respectively.

• Not as painful as other cephalosporins when given I.M.

• Alternate injection sites if I.V. therapy lasts longer than 3 days. Use of small I.V. needles in the larger available veins may be preferable.

• Reconstituted cefazolin sodium is stable for 24 hours at room temperature or 96 hours under refrigeration.

• About 40% to 75% of patients receiving cephalosporins show a false-positive direct Coombs' test; only a few of these indicate hemolytic anemia.

• Prolonged use may result in overgrowth of nonsusceptible organisms. Monitor carefully for superinfection.

• Considered the first-generation cephalosporin of choice by most authorities.

• Urine glucose determinations may be false-positive with copper sulfate tests (Clinitest); glucose enzymatic tests (Clinistix, Tes-Tape) are not affected.

---

cefonicid sodium
Monocid

Pregnancy Risk Category: B

MECHANISM OF ACTION
Inhibits cell wall synthesis, promoting osmotic instability. Usually bactericidal.

INDICATIONS & DOSAGE
Treatment of serious infections of the lower respiratory and urinary tract; skin and skin structure infections; septicemia; and bone and joint infections. Susceptible microorganisms include Streptococcus pneumoniae, Klebsiella pneumoniae, Escherichia coli, Hemophilus influenzae, Proteus mirabilis, Staphyloccus aureus and epidermidis, and Streptococcus pyogenes—

Adults: Usual dosage is 1 g I.V. or I.M. q 24 hours. In life-threatening infections, 2 g q 24 hours.

Total daily dosage is same for I.M. or I.V. administration and depends on susceptibility of organism and severity of infection. In patients with impaired renal function, doses or frequency of administration must be modified according to degree of renal impairment, severity of infection, and susceptibility of organism. Should be injected deep I.M. into a large muscle mass, such as gluteus or lateral aspect of thigh.

ADVERSE REACTIONS
Blood: transient neutropenia, leukopenia, eosinophilia, anemia.
CNS: dizziness, headache, malaise, paresthesias.
GI: *pseudomembranous colitis,* nausea, anorexia, vomiting, diarrhea, glossitis, dyspepsia, abdominal cramps, anal pruritus, tenesmus, oral candidiasis (thrush).
GU: genital pruritus and moniliasis, vaginitis.
Skin: *maculopapular and erythematous rashes, urticaria.*
Local: *at injection site—pain, induration, sterile abscesses, tissue sloughing; phlebitis and thrombophlebitis with I.V. injection.*
Other: hypersensitivity, dyspnea.

INTERACTIONS
Probenecid: may inhibit excretion and increase blood levels of cefonicid.

NURSING CONSIDERATIONS
• Contraindicated in patients with hypersensitivity to other cephalosporins. Use cautiously in impaired renal function and in those with history of sensitivity to penicillin. Ask patient if he's had any reaction to previous cephalosporin or penicillin therapy before administering first dose.
• Obtain specimen for culture and sensitivity tests before first dose. Therapy may begin pending test results.
• When administering 2-g I.M. doses once daily, one-half the dose should be administered in different large muscle masses.
• Prolonged use may result in overgrowth of nonsusceptible organisms. Observe patient carefully for superinfection.
• Has been promoted as a cost-effective agent for surgical prophylaxis.

---

cefoperazone sodium
Cefobid♦

Pregnancy Risk Category: B

MECHANISM OF ACTION
Inhibits cell wall synthesis, promoting osmotic instability. Usually bactericidal.

INDICATIONS & DOSAGE
Treatment of serious infections of the respiratory tract; intraabdominal, gynecologic, and skin infections; bacteremia, septicemia. Susceptible microorganisms include Streptococcus pneumoniae *and* pyogenes; Staphylococcus aureus *(penicillinase and nonpenicillinase-producing)* and epidermidis; enterococcus; *Escherichia coli;* Klebsiella; Hemophilus influenzae; Enterobacter; Citrobacter; Proteus; *some* Pseudomonas, *including* Pseudomonas aeruginosa; *and* Bacteroides fragilis—
Adults: Usual dosage is 1 to 2 g q 12 hours I.M. or I.V. In severe infections, or infections caused by less sensitive organisms, the total daily dosage or frequency may be increased up to 16 g/day in certain situations.

No dosage adjustment is usually necessary in patients with renal impairment. However, doses of 4 g/day should be given very cautiously in patients with hepatic disease. Should be injected deep I.M. into a large muscle mass, such as gluteus or lateral aspect of the thigh.

ADVERSE REACTIONS
Blood: transient neutropenia, eosinophilia, hemolytic anemia, *hypoprothrombinemia, bleeding.*
CNS: headache, malaise, paresthesias, dizziness.
GI: *pseudomembranous colitis,* nausea, anorexia, vomiting, *diarrhea,* glossitis, dyspepsia, abdominal cramps, tenesmus, anal pruritus, oral candidiasis (thrush).
Hepatic: mildly elevated liver enzymes.
GU: genital pruritus and moniliasis.
Skin: *maculopapular and erythematous rashes, urticaria.*
Local: *at injection site—pain, induration, sterile abscesses, temperature elevation, tissue sloughing; phlebitis and thrombophlebitis with I.V. injection.*
Other: hypersensitivity, dyspnea.

INTERACTIONS
Probenecid: may inhibit excretion and increase blood levels of cefoperazone.
Ethyl alcohol: may cause a disulfiram-like reaction. Warn patients not to drink alcohol for several days after discontinuing cefoperazone.

NURSING CONSIDERATIONS
• Contraindicated in patients with hypersensitivity to other cephalosporins.

Italicized side effects are common or life-threatening.
*Liquid form contains alcohol.   **May contain tartrazine.

Use cautiously in impaired renal function and in those with history of sensitivity to penicillin. Ask patient if he's had any reaction to previous cephalosporin or penicillin therapy before administering first dose.

• Obtain specimen for culture and sensitivity tests before first dose. Therapy may begin pending test results.

• Cefoperazone is one of the third-generation cephalosporins. It has greater activity than first-generation cephalosporins against gram-negative organisms, but less activity against gram-positive organisms.

• Because of high degree of biliary excretion, may cause more diarrhea than other cephalosporins.

• The chemical structure of this drug includes the methylthiotetrazole (MTT) side chain that has been associated with bleeding disorders. If bleeding occurs, it can be promptly reversed with administration of vitamin K. Monitor prothrombin time regularly.

• Prolonged use may result in overgrowth of nonsusceptible organisms. Careful observation of patient for superinfection is essential.

• Urine glucose determinations may be false-positive with copper sulfate tests (Clinitest); glucose enzymatic tests (Clinistix, Tes-Tape) are not affected.

ceforanide
Precef

Pregnancy Risk Category: B

MECHANISM OF ACTION
Inhibits cell wall synthesis, promoting osmotic instability. Usually bactericidal.

INDICATIONS & DOSAGE
Treatment of serious infections of the lower respiratory and urinary tract, skin and skin structure infections, en-docarditis, septicemia, and bone and joint infections. Susceptible microorganisms include Streptococcus pneumoniae and pyogenes, Klebsiella pneumoniae, Escherichia coli, Hemophilus influenzae, Proteus mirabilis, and Staphylococcus aureus *and* epidermidis—

Adults: 0.5 to 1 g I.V. or I.M. q 12 hours.
Children: 20 to 40 mg/kg/day in equally divided doses q 12 hours.
Prophylaxis of surgical infections— 0.5 to 1 g I.M. or I.V. 1 hour prior to surgery.

Total daily dosage is same for I.M. or I.V. administration and depends on susceptibility of organism and severity of infection. In patients with impaired renal function, doses or frequency of administration must be modified according to degree of renal impairment, severity of infection, and susceptibility of organism. Should be injected deep I.M. into a large muscle mass, such as gluteus or lateral aspect of thigh.

ADVERSE REACTIONS
Blood: transient neutropenia, leukopenia, eosinophilia, thrombocytopenia.
CNS: confusion, headache, lethargy.
GI: *pseudomembranous colitis,* nausea, anorexia, vomiting, diarrhea, glossitis, dyspepsia, abdominal cramps, oral candidiasis (thrush).
GU: genital pruritus and moniliasis, vaginitis.
Hepatic: transient elevation in liver enzymes.
Skin: *maculopapular and erythematous rashes, urticaria.*
Local: *at injection site—pain, induration, sterile abscesses, tissue sloughing; phlebitis and thrombophlebitis with I.V. injection.*
Other: hypersensitivity, dyspnea.

INTERACTIONS
Probenecid: may inhibit excretion and

increase blood levels of ceforanide.

NURSING CONSIDERATIONS
• Contraindicated in patients with hypersensitivity to other cephalosporins. Use cautiously in impaired renal function and in those with history of sensitivity to penicillin. Ask patient if he's had a previous reaction to cephalosporin or penicillin therapy before administering first dose.
• Obtain specimen for culture and sensitivity tests before first dose. Therapy may begin pending test results.
• Upon reconstitution, ceforanide injection may appear cloudy. Let stand briefly to allow solution to deaerate and clarify.
• Prolonged use may result in overgrowth of nonsusceptible organisms. Observe patient carefully for superinfection.
• Ceforanide is a second-generation cephalosporin which may be administered twice daily.

---

cefotaxime sodium
Claforan♦

Pregnancy Risk Category: B

MECHANISM OF ACTION
Inhibits cell wall synthesis, promoting osmotic instability. Usually bactericidal.

INDICATIONS & DOSAGE
Treatment of serious infections of the lower respiratory and urinary tracts, CNS infections, gynecologic infections, bacteremia, septicemia, and skin infections. Among susceptible microorganisms are streptococci, including Streptococcus pneumoniae *and* pyogenes; Staphylococcus aureus *(penicillinase- and nonpenicillinase-producing)* and epidermidis; Escherichia coli; Klebsiella; Hemophilus influenzae; Enterobacter; Proteus; *and* Peptostreptococcus—

Adults: usual dose is 1 g I.V. or I.M. q 6 to 8 hours. Up to 12 g daily can be administered in life-threatening infections.

Total daily dosage is same for I.M. or I.V. administration and depends on susceptibility of organism and severity of infection. In patients with impaired renal function, doses or frequency of administration must be modified according to degree of renal impairment, severity of infection, and susceptibility of organism. Should be injected deep I.M. into a large muscle mass, such as gluteus or lateral aspect of thigh.

ADVERSE REACTIONS
Blood: transient neutropenia, eosinophilia, hemolytic anemia.
CNS: headache, malaise, paresthesias, dizziness.
GI: *pseudomembranous colitis,* nausea, anorexia, vomiting, *diarrhea,* glossitis, dyspepsia, abdominal cramps, tenesmus, anal pruritus, oral candidiasis (thrush).
GU: genital pruritus and moniliasis.
Skin: *maculopapular and erythematous rashes, urticaria.*
Local: *at injection site—pain, induration, sterile abscesses, temperature elevation, tissue sloughing; phlebitis and thrombophlebitis with I.V. injection.*
Other: hypersensitivity, dyspnea, elevated temperature.

INTERACTIONS
Probenecid: may inhibit excretion and increase blood levels of cefotaxime. Use together cautiously.

NURSING CONSIDERATIONS
• Contraindicated in patients with hypersensitivity to other cephalosporins. Use cautiously in impaired renal function and in those with history of sensitivity to penicillin. Ask patient if he's had any reaction to previous cephalosporin or penicillin therapy before ad-

---

Italicized side effects are common or life-threatening.
*Liquid form contains alcohol.   **May contain tartrazine.

ministering first dose.
• Obtain specimen for culture and sensitivity tests before first dose. Therapy may begin pending test results.
• Prolonged use may result in overgrowth of nonsusceptible organisms. Careful observation of patient for superinfection is essential.
• Cefotaxime was the first of the so-called third-generation cephalosporins. It has increased antibacterial activity against gram-negative microorganisms.
• Some doctors may prescribe cefotaxime in clinical situations in which they formerly prescribed aminoglycosides. However, this drug is usually not effective against infections caused by *Pseudomonas* organisms.
• Urine glucose determinations may be false-positive with copper sulfate tests (Clinitest); glucose enzymatic tests (Clinistix, Tes-Tape) are not affected.

---

cefotetan disodium
Cefotan

Pregnancy Risk Category: B

MECHANISM OF ACTION
Inhibits cell wall synthesis, promoting osmotic instability. Usually bactericidal.

INDICATIONS & DOSAGE
Treatment of serious infections of the urinary and lower respiratory tracts, and gynecologic, skin and skin structure, intraabdominal, and bone and joint infections. Among susceptible microorganisms are streptococci, Staphylococcus aureus *(penicillinase-and nonpenicillinase-producing)* and epidermidis, Escherichia coli, Klebsiella, Enterobacter, Proteus, Hemophilus influenzae, Neisseria gonorrhoeae, *and* Bacteroides, including B. fragilis.
Adults: 1 to 2 g I.V. or I.M. q 12

hours for 5 to 10 days. Up to 6 g daily in life-threatening infections.
Total daily dosage is same for I.M. or I.V. administration and depends on susceptibility of organism and severity of infection. In patients with impaired renal function, doses or frequency of administration must be modified according to degree of renal impairment, severity of infection, and susceptibility of organism. Should be injected deep I.M. into a large muscle mass, such as gluteus or lateral aspect of thigh.

ADVERSE REACTIONS
Blood: transient neutropenia, eosinophilia, hemolytic anemia.
CNS: headache, malaise, paresthesias, dizziness.
GI: *pseudomembranous colitis,* nausea, anorexia, vomiting, *diarrhea,* glossitis, dyspepsia, abdominal cramps, tenesmus, anal pruritus.
GU: genital pruritus and moniliasis.
Skin: *maculopapular and erythematous rashes, urticaria.*
Local: *at injection site—pain, induration, sterile abscesses, tissue sloughing; phlebitis and thrombophlebitis with I.V. injection.*
Other: *hypersensitivity,* dyspnea, elevated temperature.

INTERACTIONS
Ethyl alcohol: may cause a disulfiram-like reaction. Warn patients not to drink alcohol for several days after discontinuing cefotetan.
Probenecid: may inhibit excretion and increase blood levels of cefotetan.

NURSING CONSIDERATIONS
• Contraindicated in patients with hypersensitivity to other cephalosporins. Use cautiously in impaired renal status and in those with history of sensitivity to penicillin. Ask patient if he's had any reaction to previous cephalosporin or penicillin therapy before administering first dose.

• Obtain specimen for culture and sensitivity tests before first dose. Therapy may begin pending test results.
• For I.V. use, reconstitute with sterile water for injection. Then, may be mixed with 50 to 100 ml of dextrose 5% in water or 0.9% sodium chloride solution.
• I.M. injection may be reconstituted with sterile water or bacteriostatic water for injection, normal saline, 0.5% or 1% lidocaine hydrochloride. Shake to dissolve and let stand until clear.
• Reconstituted solution remains stable for 24 hours at room temperature or 96 hours when refrigerated.
• The chemical structure of this drug includes the methylthiotetrazole (MTT) side chain that has been associated with bleeding disorders. However, such bleeding has not been reported with this drug.
• Prolonged use may result in overgrowth of nonsusceptible organisms. Monitor patient for superinfection.
• Cefotetan is similar to cefoxitin in that it's particularly useful in intraabdominal and gynecologic infection (highly active against *B. fragilis*).

cefoxitin sodium
Mefoxin♦
Pregnancy Risk Category: B

MECHANISM OF ACTION
Inhibits cell wall synthesis, promoting osmotic instability. Usually bactericidal.

INDICATIONS & DOSAGE
Treatment of serious infection of respiratory and genitourinary tracts, skin and soft-tissue infections, bone and joint infections, bloodstream and intra-abdominal infections caused by Escherichia coli *and other coliform bacteria,* Staphylcoccus aureus *(penicillinase- and nonpenicillinase-*

producing) and epidermidis, *strepto-cocci,* Klebsiella, Hemophilus influenzae, *and* Bacteroides, *including* B. fragilis—
Adults: 1 to 2 g q 6 to 8 hours for uncomplicated forms of infection. Up to 12 g daily in life-threatening infections.
Children: 80 to 160 mg/kg daily given in 4 to 6 equally divided doses.
Total daily dosage is same for I.M. or I.V. administration and depends on susceptibility of organism and severity of infection. In patients with impaired renal function, doses or frequency of administration must be modified according to degree of renal impairment, severity of infection, and susceptibility of organism. Should be injected deep I.M. into a large muscle mass, such as gluteus or lateral aspect of thigh.

ADVERSE REACTIONS
Blood: transient neutropenia, eosinophilia, hemolytic anemia.
CNS: headache, malaise, paresthesias, dizziness.
GI: *pseudomembranous colitis,* nausea, anorexia, vomiting, *diarrhea,* glossitis, dyspepsia, abdominal cramps, tenesmus, anal pruritus, oral candidiasis (thrush).
GU: genital pruritus and moniliasis.
Skin: *maculopapular and erythematous rashes, urticaria.*
Local: *at injection site—pain, induration, sterile abscesses, tissue sloughing; phlebitis and thrombophlebitis with I.V. injection.*
Other: *hypersensitivity,* dyspnea, elevated temperature.

INTERACTIONS
Probenecid: may inhibit excretion and increase blood levels of cefoxitin.

NURSING CONSIDERATIONS
• Contraindicated in patients with hypersensitivity to other cephalosporins. Use cautiously in impaired renal sta-

tus and in those with history of sensitivity to penicillin. Ask patient if he's had any reaction to previous cephalosporin or penicillin therapy before administering first dose.

• Obtain specimen for culture and sensitivity tests before first dose. Therapy may begin pending test results.

• A very useful cephalosporin when anaerobic or mixed aerobic-anaerobic infection is suspected, especially *B. fragilis.*

• Associated with development of thrombophlebitis. Assess I.V. site frequently.

• For I.V. use, reconstitute 1 g with at least 10 ml of sterile water for injection, and 2 g with 10 to 20 ml. Solutions of dextrose 5% and 0.9% sodium chloride for injection can also be used.

• I.M. injection can be reconstituted with 0.5% or 1% lidocaine HCl (without epinephrine) to minimize pain.

• After reconstitution, remains stable for 24 hours at room temperature or 1 week under refrigeration.

• Prolonged use may result in overgrowth of nonsusceptible organisms. Monitor patient for superinfection.

• Urine glucose determinations may be false-positive with copper sulfate tests (Clinitest); glucose enzymatic tests (Clinistix, Tes-Tape) are not affected.

ceftazidime
Fortaz♦,Magnacef♦♦, Tazicef, Tazidime

Pregnancy Risk Category: B

MECHANISM OF ACTION
Inhibits cell wall synthesis, promoting osmotic instability. Usually bactericidal.

INDICATIONS & DOSAGE
Treatment of serious infections of the lower respiratory and urinary tracts, gynecologic infections, bacteremia, septicemia, intraabdominal infections, CNS infections, and skin infections. Among susceptible microorganisms are streptococci, including Streptococcus pneumoniae *and* pyogenes; Staphylococcus aureus *(penicillinase- and nonpenicillinase-producing);* Escherichia coli; Klebsiella; Proteus; Enterobacter; Hemophilus influenzae; Pseudomonas; and some strains of Bacteroides—

Adults: 1 g I.V. or I.M. q 8 to 12 hours; up to 6 g daily in life-threatening infections.

Children 1 month to 12 years: 30 to 50 mg/kg I.V. q 8 hours.

Neonates 0 to 4 weeks: 30 mg/kg I.V. q 12 hours.

Total daily dosage is same for I.M. or I.V. administration and depends on susceptibility of organism and severity of infection. In patients with impaired renal function, doses or frequency of administration must be modified according to degree of renal impairment, severity of infection, and susceptibility of organism. Should be injected deep I.M. into a large muscle mass, such as gluteus or lateral aspect of thigh.

ADVERSE REACTIONS
Blood: *eosinophilia; thrombocytosis,* leukopenia.
CNS: headache, dizziness.
GI: *pseudomembranous enterocolitis,* nausea, vomiting, diarrhea, dysgeusia, abdominal cramps.
GU: genital pruritus and moniliasis.
Hepatic: transient elevation in liver enzymes.
Skin: *maculopapular and erythematous rashes,* urticaria.
Local: *at injection site—pain, induration, sterile abscesses, tissue sloughing; phlebitis and thrombophlebitis with I.V. injection.*
Other: *hypersensitivity,* dyspnea, elevated temperature.

INTERACTIONS
Sodium bicarbonate–containing solutions: make ceftazidime unstable. Don't mix together.

NURSING CONSIDERATIONS
• Contraindicated in patients with hypersensitivity to other cephalosporins. Use cautiously in patients with history of sensitivity to penicillin. Ask patient if he's had any previous reaction to cephalosporin or penicillin therapy before administering first dose.
• Obtain specimen for culture and sensitivity tests before first dose. Therapy may begin pending test results.
• The vials of ceftazidime are supplied under reduced pressure. When the antibiotic is dissolved, carbon dioxide is released and a positive pressure develops. Each brand of ceftazidime includes specific instructions for reconstitution. Read and follow these instructions carefully.
• This third-generation cephalosporin has excellent activity against infections caused by *Pseudomonas aeruginosa.* May be prescribed for these infections, especially when aminoglycosides are potentially too dangerous.
• Prolonged use may result in overgrowth of nonsusceptible organisms. Monitor carefully for superinfection.

---

ceftizoxime sodium
Cefizox

Pregnancy Risk Category: B

MECHANISM OF ACTION
Inhibits cell wall synthesis, promoting osmotic instability. Usually bactericidal.

INDICATIONS & DOSAGE
*Treatment of serious infections of the lower respiratory and urinary tracts, gynecological infections, bacteremia, septicemia, meningitis, intraabdominal infections, bone and joint infec-*tions, and skin infections. Among susceptible microorganisms are streptococci, including Streptococcus pneumoniae *and* pyogenes; Staphylococcus saureus *(penicillinase- and nonpenicillinase-producing)* and epidermidis; Escherichia coli; Klebsiella; Hemophilus influenzae; Enterobacter; Proteus; *some* Pseudomonas; and Peptostreptococcus—
Adults: Usual dosage is 1 to 2 g I.V. or I.M. q 8 to 12 hours. In life-threatening infections, up to 2 g q 4 hours.

Total daily dosage is same for I.M. or I.V. administration and depends on susceptibility of organism and severity of infection. In patients with impaired renal function, doses or frequency of administration must be modified according to degree of renal impairment, severity of infection, and susceptibility of organism. Should be injected deep I.M. into a large muscle mass, such as gluteus or lateral aspect of thigh.

ADVERSE REACTIONS
Blood: transient neutropenia, eosinophilia, hemolytic anemia.
CNS: headache, malaise, paresthesias, dizziness.
GI: *pseudomembranous colitis,* nausea, anorexia, vomiting, *diarrhea,* glossitis, dyspepsia, abdominal cramps, tenesmus, anal pruritus.
GU: genital pruritus and moniliasis.
Skin: *maculopapular and erythematous rashes, urticaria.*
Local: *at injection site—pain, induration, sterile abscesses, tissue sloughing; phlebitis and thrombophlebitis with I.V. injection.*
Other: hypersensitivity, dyspnea, elevated temperature.

INTERACTIONS
Probenecid: may inhibit excretion and increase blood levels of ceftizoxime.

NURSING CONSIDERATIONS
• Contraindicated in patients with hy-

persensitivity to other cephalosporins. Use cautiously in impaired renal function and in those with history of sensitivity to penicillin. Ask patient if he's had any reaction to previous cephalosporin or penicillin therapy before administering first dose.
• Obtain specimen for culture and sensitivity tests before first dose. Therapy may begin pending test results.
• Prolonged use may result in overgrowth of nonsusceptible organisms. Monitor carefully for superinfection.
• Ceftizoxime is a third-generation cephalosporin, which is comparable in activity to cefotaxime, moxalactam, ceftriaxone and cefoperazone. No significant degree of bleeding or disulfiram-type reaction has been reported with its use.

ceftriaxone sodium
Rocephin♦

Pregnancy Risk Category: B

MECHANISM OF ACTION
Inhibits cell wall synthesis, promoting osmotic instability. Usually bactericidal.

INDICATIONS & DOSAGE
Treatment of serious infections of the lower respiratory and urinary tracts, gynecological infections, bacteremia, septicemia, intraabdominal infections, and skin infections. Susceptible microorganisms are streptococci, including Streptococcus pneumoniae *and* pyogenes; Staphylococcus aureus *(penicillinase- and nonpenicillinase-producing)* and epidermidis; Escherichia coli; Klebsiella; Hemophilus influenzae; Enterobacter; Proteus; Pseudomonas; *and* Peptostreptococcus—
Adults: 1 to 2 g I.M. or I.V. once daily or in equally divided doses twice daily. Total daily dose should not exceed 4 g.

Children: 50 to 75 mg/kg, given in divided doses q 12 hours.
Treatment of meningitis—
Adults and children: 100 mg/kg given in divided doses q 12 hours. May give loading dose of 75 mg/kg.
    Total daily dose is same for I.M. or I.V. administration and depends on susceptibility of organism and severity of infection. Should be injected deep I.M. into a large muscle mass, such as gluteus or lateral aspect of thigh.

ADVERSE REACTIONS
Blood: *eosinophilia; thrombocytosis,* leukopenia.
CNS: headache, dizziness.
GI: *pseudomembranous enterocolitis,* nausea, vomiting, diarrhea, dysgeusia, abdominal cramps.
GU: genital pruritus and moniliasis.
Hepatic: transient elevation in liver enzymes.
Skin: *maculopapular and erythematous rashes, urticaria.*
Local: *at injection site—pain, induration, sterile abscesses, tissue sloughing; phlebitis and thrombophlebitis with I.V. injection.*
Other: hypersensitivity, dyspnea, elevated temperature.

INTERACTIONS
Probenecid: may inhibit excretion and increase blood levels of ceftriaxone.

NURSING CONSIDERATIONS
• Contraindicated in patients with hypersensitivity to other cephalosporins. Use cautiously in history of sensitivity to penicillin. Ask patient if he's had any previous reaction to cephalosporin or penicillin therapy before administering first dose.
• Obtain specimen for culture and sensitivity tests before first dose. Therapy may begin pending test results.
• A third-generation cephalosporin with the longest half-life of any avail-

---

able cephalosporin. Allows once-daily dose regimen.
• Dosage adjustment generally not needed in patients with renal insufficiency.
• Commonly used in home antibiotic programs for outpatient treatment of serious infections, such as osteomyelitis.
• Prolonged use may result in overgrowth of nonsusceptible organisms. Monitor carefully for superinfection.

cefuroxime axetil
Ceftin

cefuroxime sodium
Kefurox, Zinacef♦

Pregnancy Risk Category: B

MECHANISM OF ACTION
Inhibits cell wall synthesis, promoting osmotic instability. Usually bactericidal.

INDICATIONS & DOSAGE
Treatment of serious infections of the lower respiratory and urinary tract; skin and skin structure infections; septicemia, meningitis, and gonorrhea. Among susceptible organisms are Streptococcus pneumoniae and pyogenes, Hemophilus influenzae, Klebsiella, Staphylococcus aureus, Escherichia coli, Enterobacter, and Neisseria gonorrhoeae—
Adults: Usual dosage of cefuroxime sodium is 750 mg to 1.5 g I.M. or I.V. q 8 hours, usually for 5 to 10 days. For life-threatening infections and infections caused by less susceptible organisms, 1.5 g I.M. or I.V. q 6 hours; for bacterial meningitis, up to 3 g I.V. q 6 hours.
Alternatively, administer cefuroxime axetil 250 mg P.O. q 12 hours. For severe infections or less susceptible organisms, dosage may be increased to 500 mg P.O. q 12 hours.
Children and infants over 3

months: 50 to 100 mg/kg/day cefuroxime sodium I.M. or I.V. Higher doses are administered when treating meningitis. Alternatively, give cefuroxime axetil 125 mg P.O. q 12 hours.
Uncomplicated urinary tract infections—
Adults: 125 to 250 mg P.O. q 12 hours.
Otitis media—
Children under age 2: 125 mg P.O. q 12 hours.
Children age 2 and over: 250 mg P.O. q 12 hours.

ADVERSE REACTIONS
Blood: transient neutropenia, eosinophilia, hemolytic anemia, decrease in hemoglobin and hematocrit.
CNS: headache, malaise, paresthesias, dizziness.
GI: *pseudomembranous colitis,* nausea, anorexia, vomiting, *diarrhea,* glossitis, dyspepsia, abdominal cramps, tenesmus, anal pruritus.
GU: genital pruritus and moniliasis.
Skin: *maculopapular and erythematous rashes, urticaria.*
Local: *at injection site—pain, induration, sterile abscesses, temperature elevation, tissue sloughing; phlebitis and thrombophlebitis with I.V. injection.*
Other: hypersensitivity, dyspnea.

INTERACTIONS
Probenecid: may inhibit excretion and increase blood levels of cefuroxime.

NURSING CONSIDERATIONS
• Contraindicated in hypersensitivity to other cephalosporins. Use cautiously in patients with impaired renal function and in those with history of sensitivity to penicillin. Ask patient if he's had any reaction to previous cephalosporin or penicillin therapy before administering first dose.
• Total daily dosage is same for I.M. or I.V. administration and depends on susceptibility of organism and sever-

Italicized side effects are common or life-threatening.
*Liquid form contains alcohol.   **May contain tartrazine.

ity of infection. In patients with impaired renal function, doses or frequency of administration must be modified according to degree of renal impairment, severity of infection, and susceptibility of organism. Should be injected deep I.M. into a large muscle mass, such as gluteus or lateral aspect of thigh.
• Absorption of cefuroxime axetil is enhanced by food.
• Cefuroxime axetil is available only in tablet form, which may be crushed for patients who cannot swallow tablets. However, it has a bitter taste that is difficult to mask, even with food. Alternative therapy may be necessary.
• Obtain specimen for culture and sensitivity tests before first dose. Therapy may begin pending test results.
• Prolonged use may result in overgrowth of nonsusceptible organisms. Monitor patient carefully for superinfection.
• Cefuroxime is a second-generation cephalosporin similar to cefamandole. However, cefuroxime has not been associated with prothrombin deficiency and bleeding as are some of the other cephalosporins. Advantage over some other cephalosporins is that cefuroxime is useful in treating meningitis.

cephalexin monohydrate
Ceporex♦♦, Keflet, Keflex♦, Keftab, Novolexin♦♦

Pregnancy Risk Category: B

MECHANISM OF ACTION
Inhibits cell wall synthesis, promoting osmotic instability. Usually bactericidal.

INDICATIONS & DOSAGE
Treatment of infections of respiratory or genitourinary tract, skin and soft-tissue infections, bone and joint infections, and otitis media due to Esche-

richia coli *and other coliform bacteria, group A beta-hemolytic streptococci,* Hemophilus influenzae, Klebsiella, Proteus mirabilis, Streptococcus pneumoniae, *and staphylococci—*
Adults: 250 mg to 1 g P.O. q 6 hours.
Children: 6 to 12 mg/kg P.O. q 6 hours. Maximum 25 mg/kg q 6 hours.

ADVERSE REACTIONS
Blood: transient neutropenia, eosinophilia, anemia.
CNS: dizziness, headache, malaise, paresthesias.
GI: *pseudomembranous colitis, nausea, anorexia,* vomiting, *diarrhea,* glossitis, dyspepsia, abdominal cramps, anal pruritus, tenesmus, oral candidiasis (thrush).
GU: genital pruritus and moniliasis, vaginitis.
Skin: *maculopapular and erythematous rashes, urticaria.*
Other: *hypersensitivity,* dyspnea.

INTERACTIONS
Probenecid: may increase blood levels of cephalosporins.

NURSING CONSIDERATIONS
• Use cautiously in impaired renal function and in those with history of sensitivity to penicillin. Ask patient if he's had any reaction to previous cephalosporin or penicillin therapy before administering first dose.
• Obtain specimen for culture and sensitivity tests before first dose. Therapy may begin pending test results.
• Tell patient to take medication exactly as prescribed, even after he feels better. Group A beta-hemolytic streptococcal infections should be treated for a minimum of 10 days.
• Tell patient to take with food or milk to lessen GI discomfort.
• Call doctor if skin rash develops.
• Preparation of oral suspension: add required amount of water to powder in two portions. Shake well after each

addition. After mixing, store in refrigerator. Stable for 14 days without significant loss of potency. Keep tightly closed and shake well before using.

• Prolonged use may result in overgrowth of nonsusceptible organisms. Monitor closely for superinfection.

• About 40% to 75% of patients receiving cephalosporins show a false-positive direct Coombs' test, but only a few of these indicate hemolytic anemia.

• Urine glucose determinations may be false-positive with copper sulfate tests (Clinitest); glucose enzymatic tests (Clinistix, Tes-Tape) are not affected.

---

cephalothin sodium
Ceporacin◆◆, Keflin◆

Pregnancy Risk Category: B

MECHANISM OF ACTION
Inhibits cell wall synthesis, promoting osmotic instability. Usually bactericidal.

INDICATIONS & DOSAGE
Treatment of serious infections of respiratory, genitourinary, or gastrointestinal tract; skin and soft-tissue infections (including peritonitis); bone and joint infections; septicemia; endocarditis; and meningitis due to Escherichia coli *and other coliform bacteria,* Enterobacteriaceae, enterococci, gonococci, group A beta-hemolytic streptococci, Hemophilus influenzae, Klebsiella, Proteus mirabilis, Salmonella, Staphylococcus aureus, Shigella, Streptococcus pneumoniae and viridans, *and* staphylococci—
Adults: 500 mg to 1 g I.M. or I.V. (or intraperitoneally) q 4 to 6 hours; in life-threatening infections, up to 2 g q 4 hours.
Children: 14 to 27 mg/kg I.V. q 4 hours, or 20 to 40 mg/kg q 6 hours; dose should be proportionately less in accordance with age, weight, and severity of infection.

Dosage schedule is determined by degree of renal impairment, severity of infection, and susceptibility of causative organism. Should be injected deep I.M. into a large muscle mass, such as gluteus or lateral aspect of thigh. I.V. route is preferable in severe or life-threatening infections.

ADVERSE REACTIONS
Blood: transient neutropenia, eosinophilia, hemolytic anemia.
CNS: headache, malaise, paresthesias, dizziness.
GI: *pseudomembranous colitis,* nausea, anorexia, vomiting, *diarrhea,* glossitis, dyspepsia, abdominal cramps, tenesmus, anal pruritus, oral candidiasis (thrush).
GU: *nephrotoxicity,* genital pruritus and moniliasis.
Skin: *maculopapular and erythematous rashes, urticaria.*
Local: *at injection site—pain, induration, sterile abscesses, tissue sloughing; phlebitis and thrombophlebitis with I.V. injection.*
Other: *hypersensitivity,* dyspnea, fever.

INTERACTIONS
Probenecid: may increase blood levels of cephalosporins. Use together cautiously.
Aminoglycosides: increased nephrotoxicity. Monitor kidney function tests carefully.

NURSING CONSIDERATIONS
• Use cautiously in impaired renal function and in those with history of sensitivity to penicillin. Ask patient if he's had any reaction to previous cephalosporin or penicillin therapy before administering first dose.
• Obtain specimen for culture and sensitivity tests before first dose. Therapy may begin pending test results.

Italicized side effects are common or life-threatening.
*Liquid form contains alcohol.   **May contain tartrazine.

- Drug causes severe pain when administered I.M.; avoid this route if possible.
- When giving this drug I.V., check frequently for vein irritation and phlebitis. Alternate injection sites if I.V. therapy lasts longer than 3 days. Use of small I.V. needle in the larger available veins may be preferable. Addition of a small concentration of heparin (100 units) or hydrocortisone (10 to 25 mg) may reduce incidence of phlebitis.
- For I.M. administration, reconstitute each gram of cephalothin sodium with 4 ml of sterile water for injection, providing 500 mg in each 2.2 ml. If vial contents do not dissolve completely, add an additional 0.2 to 0.4 ml diluent, and warm contents slightly.
- For I.V. administration, dilute contents of 4-g vial with at least 20 ml of sterile water for injection, dextrose 5% injection, or 0.9% sodium chloride injection and add to one of following I.V. solutions: acetated Ringer's injection, dextrose 5% injection, dextrose 5% in lactated Ringer's injection, Ionosol B in dextrose 5% in water, lactated Ringer's injection, Normosol-N in dextrose 5% in water, Plasma-Lyte injection, Plasma-Lyte-N injection in dextrose 5%, Ringer's injection, or 0.9% sodium chloride injection. Choose solution and fluid volume according to patient's fluid and electrolyte status.
- Prolonged use may result in overgrowth of nonsusceptible organisms. Monitor for superinfection.
- About 40% to 75% of patients receiving cephalosporins show a false-positive direct Coombs' test; only a few of these indicate hemolytic anemia.
- Urine glucose determinations may be false-positive with copper sulfate tests (Clinitest); glucose enzymatic tests (Clinistix, Tes-Tape) are not affected.

cephapirin sodium
Cefadyl♦

Pregnancy Risk Category: B

MECHANISM OF ACTION
Inhibits cell wall synthesis, promoting osmotic instability. Usually bactericidal.

INDICATIONS & DOSAGE
Serious infections of respiratory, genitourinary, or gastrointestinal tract; skin and soft-tissue infections; bone and joint infections (including osteomyelitis); septicemia; endocarditis due to Streptococcus pneumoniae, Escherichia coli, *group A beta-hemolytic streptococci,* Hemophilus influenzae, Klebsiella, Proteus mirabilis, Staphylococcus aureus, *and* Streptococcus viridans—
Adults: 500 mg to 1 g I.V. or I.M. q 4 to 6 hours up to 12 g daily.
Children over 3 months: 10 to 20 mg/kg I.V. or I.M. q 6 hours; dose depends on age, weight, and severity of infection.

Should be injected deep I.M. into a large muscle mass, such as gluteus or lateral aspect of thigh. Depending on causative organism and severity of infection, patients with reduced renal function may be treated adequately with a lower dose (7.5 to 15 mg/kg q 12 hours). Patients with severely reduced renal function and who are to be dialyzed should receive same dose just before dialysis and q 12 hours thereafter.

ADVERSE REACTIONS
Blood: transient neutropenia, eosinophilia, anemia.
CNS: dizziness, headache, malaise, paresthesias.
GI: *pseudomembranous colitis,* nausea, anorexia, vomiting, *diarrhea,* glossitis, dyspepsia, abdominal cramps, tenesmus, anal pruritus, oral candidiasis (thrush).

GU: *genital pruritus and moniliasis,* vaginitis.

Skin: *maculopapular and erythematous rashes, urticaria.*

Local: *at injection site—pain, induration, sterile abscesses, tissue sloughing; phlebitis and thrombophlebitis with I.V. injection.*

Other: *hypersensitivity,* dyspnea.

INTERACTIONS
Probenecid: may increase blood levels of cephalosporins.

NURSING CONSIDERATIONS
• Use cautiously in impaired renal function and in those with a history of sensitivity to penicillin. Ask patient if he's had any reaction to previous cephalosporin or penicillin therapy before administering first dose.
• Obtain specimen for culture and sensitivity tests before first dose. Therapy may begin pending test results.
• For I.M. administration, reconstitute 1-g vial with 2 ml sterile water for injection or bacteriostatic water for injection so that 1.2 ml contains 500 mg of cephapirin. I.M. injection is painful; prepare patient for this.
• When giving this drug I.V., check frequently for vein irritation and phlebitis. Alternate injection sites if I.V. therapy lasts longer than 3 days. Use of small I.V. needles in the larger available veins may be preferable.
• Prepare I.V. infusion using dextrose injection, sodium chloride injection, or bacteriostatic water for injection as diluent: 20 ml yields 1 g per 10 ml; 50 ml yields 1 g per 25 ml; 100 ml yields 1 g per 50 ml.
• I.V. infusion with Y-tubing: during infusion of cephapirin solution, it is desirable to stop other solution. Check volume of cephapirin solution carefully so that calculated dose is infused. When Y-tubing is used, dilute 4-g vial with 40 ml of diluent.
• Reconstituted cephapirin is stable

and compatible for 10 days under refrigeration and for 24 hours at room temperature.
• Prolonged use may result in overgrowth of nonsusceptible organisms. Monitor for superinfection.
• About 40% to 75% of patients receiving cephalosporins show a false-positive direct Coombs' test, but only a few indicate hemolytic anemia.
• Urine glucose determinations may be false-positive with copper sulfate tests (Clinitest); glucose enzymatic tests (Clinistix, Tes-Tape) are not affected.

---

cephradine
Anspor, Velosef♦**

Pregnancy Risk Category: B

MECHANISM OF ACTION
Inhibits cell wall synthesis, promoting osmotic instability. Usually bactericidal.

INDICATIONS & DOSAGE
Serious infection of respiratory, genitourinary, or gastrointestinal tract; skin and soft-tissue infections; bone and joint infections; septicemia; endocarditis; and otitis media due to Escherichia coli *and other coliform bacteria,* group A beta-hemolytic streptococci, Hemophilus influenzae, Klebsiella, Proteus mirabilis, Staphylococcus aureus, Streptococcus pneumoniae and viridans, *and staphylococci*—
Adults: 500 mg to 1 g I.M. or I.V. 2 to 4 times daily; do not exceed 8 g daily. Or 250 to 500 mg P.O. q 6 hours. Severe or chronic infections may require larger and/or more frequent doses (up to 1 g P.O. q 6 hours).
Children over 1 year: 6 to 12 mg/kg P.O. q 6 hours. 12 to 25 mg/kg I.M. or I.V. q 6 hours.
Otitis media—19 to 25 mg/kg P.O. q 6 hours. Do not exceed 4 g daily.
   All patients, regardless of age and weight: larger doses (up to 1 g q.i.d.)

Italicized side effects are common or life-threatening.
*Liquid form contains alcohol.   **May contain tartrazine.

may be given for severe or chronic infections. Parenteral therapy may be followed by oral. Injections should be given deep I.M. into a large muscle mass, such as gluteus or lateral aspect of thigh.

ADVERSE REACTIONS
Blood: transient neutropenia, eosinophilia.
CNS: dizziness, headache, malaise, paresthesias.
GI: *pseudomembranous colitis, nausea, anorexia,* vomiting, heartburn, glossitis, dyspepsia, abdominal cramping, *diarrhea,* tenesmus, anal pruritus, oral candidiasis (thrush).
GU: genital pruritus and moniliasis, vaginitis.
Skin: *maculopapular and erythematous rashes, urticaria.*
Local: *at injection site—pain, induration, sterile abscesses, tissue sloughing; phlebitis and thrombophlebitis with I.V. injection.*
Other: *hypersensitivity,* dyspnea.

INTERACTIONS
Probenecid: may increase blood levels of cephalosporins.

NURSING CONSIDERATIONS
• Contraindicated in patients with hypersensitivity to other cephalosporins.
• Use cautiously in impaired renal function and in those with a history of sensitivity to penicillin. Ask patient if he's had any reaction to previous cephalosporin or penicillin therapy before administering first dose.
• Obtain specimen for culture and sensitivity tests before first dose. Therapy may begin pending test results.
• When giving this drug I.V., check frequently for vein irritation and phlebitis. Alternate injection sites if I.V. therapy lasts longer than 3 days. Use of small I.V. needle in the larger available veins may be preferable.
• Tell patient to take medication ex-

actly as prescribed, even after he feels better. Group A beta-hemolytic streptococcal infections should be treated for a minimum of 10 days.
• Tell patient to take the oral dosage form with food or milk to lessen GI discomfort.
• I.M. injection is painful.
• For I.M. administration, reconstitute with sterile water for injection or with bacteriostatic water for injection as follows: 1.2 ml to 250-mg vial; 2 ml to 500-mg vial; 4 ml to 1-g vial. I.M. solutions must be used within 2 hours if kept at room temperature and within 24 hours if refrigerated. Solutions may vary in color from light straw to yellow without affecting potency.
• When preparing cephradine for intravenous administration, when available, use preparation specifically supplied for infusion. Follow specific product directions carefully when reconstituting.
• Prolonged use may result in overgrowth of nonsusceptible organisms. Monitor for superinfection.
• About 40% to 75% of patients receiving cephalosporins show a false-positive direct Coombs' test, but only a few indicate hemolytic anemia.
• Urine glucose determinations may be false-positive with copper sulfate tests (Clinitest); glucose enzymatic tests (Clinistix, Tes-Tape) are not affected.
• Cephradine is the only cephalosporin available in both oral and injectable forms.

moxalactam disodium
Moxam♦

Pregnancy Risk Category: C

MECHANISM OF ACTION
Inhibits cell wall synthesis, promoting osmotic instability. Usually bactericidal.

INDICATIONS & DOSAGE

Treatment of serious infections of lower respiratory and urinary tract, CNS infections, intraabdominal infections, gynecologic infections, bacteremia, septicemia, and skin infections. Susceptible microorganisms include Streptococcus pneumoniae *and* pyogenes; Staphylococcus aureus *(penicillinase- and nonpenicillinase-producing)* and epidermidis; Escherichia coli; Klebsiella; Hemophilus influenzae; Enterobacter; Proteus; *some* Pseudomonas; *and* Peptostreptococcus—

Adults: Usual daily dose is 2 to 6 g I.M. or I.V. administered in divided doses q 8 hours for 5 to 10 days, or up to 14 days. Up to 12 g daily may be needed in life-threatening infections or in infections due to less susceptible organisms.

Children: 50 mg/kg I.M. or I.V. q 6 to 8 hours.

Neonates: 50 mg/kg I.M. or I.V. q 8 to 12 hours.

Total daily dosage is same for I.M. or I.V. administration and depends on susceptibility of organism and severity of infection. In patients with impaired renal function, doses or frequency of administration must be modified according to degree of impairment, severity of infection, and susceptibility of organism. Should be injected deep I.M. into the gluteus or lateral aspect of thigh.

ADVERSE REACTIONS

Blood: transient neutropenia, eosinophilia, hemolytic anemia, *hypoprothrombinemia, bleeding.*
CNS: headache, malaise, paresthesias, dizziness.
GI: *pseudomembranous colitis,* nausea, anorexia, vomiting, *diarrhea,* glossitis, dyspepsia, abdominal cramps, tenesmus, pruritus ani, oral candidiasis (thrush).
GU: genital moniliasis.
Skin: *maculopapular and erythematous rashes, urticaria.*
Local: *pain at injection site, induration, sterile abscesses, tissue sloughing; phlebitis and thrombophlebitis with I.V. injection.*
Other: *hypersensitivity,* dyspnea, elevated temperature.

INTERACTIONS

Ethyl alcohol: may cause a disulfiram-like reaction. Warn patients not to drink alcohol for several days after discontinuing moxalactam.

NURSING CONSIDERATIONS

• Contraindicated in patients with hypersensitivity to other cephalosporins. Use cautiously in impaired renal function and in those with history of sensitivity to penicillin. Before giving first dose, ask patient if he's had any reaction to penicillin.
• Obtain specimen for culture and sensitivity tests before first dose. Therapy may begin pending test results.
• For direct intermittent I.V. administration, add 10 ml of sterile water for injection, dextrose 5% injection, or 0.9% NaCl injection/g of moxalactam.
• Prolonged use may result in overgrowth of nonsusceptible organisms. Monitor closely for superinfection.
• Bleeding associated with hypoprothrombinemia can be prevented with vitamin K. Doctor may order 10 mg vitamin K per week to be given prophylactically.
• The chemical structure of this drug includes the methylthiotetrazole (MTT) side chain that has been associated with bleeding disorders. If bleeding occurs, it can be promptly reversed with the administration of vitamin K. Monitor prothrombin times regularly.
• Moxalactam does not interefere with urine glucose determinations.
• Moxalactam is a third-generation cephalosporin.

Italicized side effects are common or life-threatening.
*Liquid form contains alcohol.   **May contain tartrazine.

14

Tetracyclines

demeclocycline hydrochloride
doxycycline hyclate
minocycline hydrochloride
oxytetracycline hydrochloride
tetracycline hydrochloride

COMBINATION PRODUCTS
None.

demeclocycline hydrochloride
Declomycin♦

Pregnancy Risk Category: D

MECHANISM OF ACTION
Exerts bacteriostatic effect by binding to the 30S ribosomal subunit of microorganisms, thus inhibiting protein synthesis.

INDICATIONS & DOSAGE
Infections caused by susceptible gram-negative and gram-positive organisms, trachoma, rickettsiae—
Adults: 150 mg P.O. q 6 hours or 300 mg P.O. q 12 hours.
Children over 8 years: 6 to 12 mg/kg P.O. daily, divided q 6 to 12 hours.
Gonorrhea—
Adults: 600 mg P.O. initially, then 300 mg P.O. q 12 hours for 4 days (total 3 g).
Uncomplicated urethral, endocervical, or rectal infection caused by Chlamydia trachomatis—
Adults: 300 mg P.O. q.i.d. for at least 7 days.
Syndrome of inappropriate antidiuretic hormone (a hyposmolar state)—
Adults: 600 to 1,200 mg P.O. daily in divided doses.

ADVERSE REACTIONS
Blood: neutropenia, eosinophilia.
CV: pericarditis.
EENT: dysphagia, glossitis.
GI: anorexia, *nausea, vomiting, diarrhea,* enterocolitis, anogenital inflammation.
Metabolic: *increased BUN,* diabetes insipidus syndrome (polyuria, polydipsia, weakness).
Skin: *maculopapular and erythematous rashes, photosensitivity, increased pigmentation, urticaria.*
Other: hypersensitivity.

INTERACTIONS
Antacids (including sodium bicarbonate) and laxatives containing aluminum, magnesium, or calcium; food, milk, or other dairy products: decrease antibiotic absorption. Give antibiotic 1 hour before or 2 hours after any of the above.
Ferrous sulfate and other iron products, zinc: decrease antibiotic absorption. Give demeclocycline 3 hours after or 2 hours before iron administration.
Methoxyflurane: may cause nephrotoxicity with tetracyclines. Monitor carefully.

NURSING CONSIDERATIONS
• Use with extreme caution in impaired renal or hepatic function. Use of these drugs during last half of pregnancy and in children under 8 years may cause permanent discoloration of teeth, enamel defects, and retardation

---

of bone growth.
- Obtain specimen for culture and sensitivity tests before first dose. Therapy may begin pending test results.
- Check expiration date. Outdated or deteriorated demeclocycline has been associated with nephrotoxicity.
- Do not expose these drugs to light or heat; store in tight container.
- Monitor for overgrowth of nonsusceptible organisms. Check patient's tongue for signs of monilia infection. Stress good oral hygiene. If superinfection occurs, drug should be discontinued.
- Observe patient for diarrhea, which may result from local irritation or superinfection.
- Warn patient to avoid direct sunlight and ultraviolet light. A sunscreen may help prevent photosensitivity reactions. Photosensitivity persists for some time after discontinuation of drug.
- Effectiveness is reduced when taken with milk or other dairy products, food, antacids, or iron products. Explain this to patient. Tell patient to take each dose with a full glass of water on an empty stomach, at least 1 hour before meals or 2 hours afterward. Give at least 1 hour before bedtime to prevent esophagitis.
- Instruct patient to take medication for as long as prescribed, exactly as prescribed, even after he feels better, and to take entire amount prescribed.
- May cause false-negative reading of Clinistix or Tes-Tape.

doxycycline hyclate
Doxy-100, Doxy-200, Doxy-Caps, Doxychel, Doxy-Lemmon, Doxy-Tabs, Vibramycin•, Vibra-Tabs

Pregnancy Risk Category: D

MECHANISM OF ACTION
Exerts bacteriostatic effect by binding to the 30S ribosomal subunit of microorganisms, thus inhibiting protein synthesis.

INDICATIONS & DOSAGE
Infections caused by sensitive gram-negative and gram-positive organisms, trachoma, rickettsiae, Mycoplasma, *and* Chlamydia—
Adults: 100 mg P.O. q 12 hours on first day, then 100 mg P.O. daily; or 200 mg I.V. on first day in 1 or 2 infusions, then 100 to 200 mg I.V. daily.
Children over 8 years (under 45 kg): 4.4 mg/kg P.O. or I.V. daily, divided q 12 hours first day, then 2.2 to 4.4 mg/kg daily. For children over 45 kg, dosage is same as adults.
 Give I.V. infusion slowly (minimum 1 hour). Infusion must be completed within 12 hours (within 6 hours in lactated Ringer's solution or dextrose 5% in lactated Ringer's solution).
Gonorrhea in patients allergic to penicillin—
Adults: 200 mg P.O. initially, followed by 100 mg P.O. at bedtime, and 100 mg P.O. b.i.d. for 3 days; or 300 mg P.O. initially and repeat dose in 1 hour.
Primary or secondary syphilis in patients allergic to penicillin—
Adults: 300 mg P.O. daily in divided doses for 10 days.
Uncomplicated urethral, endocervical or rectal infections caused by Chlamydia trachomatis *or* Ureaplasma urealyticum—
Adults: 100 mg P.O. b.i.d. for at least 7 days.
To prevent "traveler's diarrhea" commonly caused by enterotoxigenic Escherichia coli—
Adults: 100 mg P.O. daily.

ADVERSE REACTIONS
Blood: neutropenia, eosinophilia.
CNS: intracranial hypertension.
CV: pericarditis.
EENT: sore throat, glossitis, dysphagia.

Italicized side effects are common or life-threatening.
*Liquid form contains alcohol.   **May contain tartrazine.

GI: anorexia, *epigastric distress, nausea,* vomiting, *diarrhea,* enterocolitis, anogenital inflammation.
Skin: *maculopapular and erythematous rashes, photosensitivity, increased pigmentation, urticaria.*
Local: thrombophlebitis.
Other: hypersensitivity.

INTERACTIONS

Antacids (including sodium bicarbonate) and laxatives containing aluminum, magnesium, or calcium: decrease antibiotic absorption. Give antibiotic 1 hour before or 2 hours after any of the above.
Ferrous sulfate and other iron products, zinc: decrease antibiotic absorption. Give doxycycline 3 hours after or 2 hours before iron administration.
Phenobarbital, carbamazepine, alcohol: decrease antibiotic effect. Avoid if possible.

NURSING CONSIDERATIONS

• Use of these drugs during last half of pregnancy and in children under 8 years may cause permanent discoloration of teeth, enamel defects, and retardation of bone growth.
• Patient may develop thrombophlebitis with I.V. administration.
• Obtain specimen for culture and sensitivity tests before first dose. Therapy may begin pending test results.
• Don't expose drug to light or heat. Protect from sunlight during infusion.
• Monitor for overgrowth of nonsusceptible organisms. Check patient's tongue for signs of monilia infection. Stress good oral hygiene. If superinfection occurs, drug should be discontinued.
• Observe patient for diarrhea, which may result from local irritation or superinfection.
• May be taken with milk or food if GI adverse effects develop.
• Do not give with antacids.
• Tell patient to take medication ex-

actly as prescribed, even after he feels better, and to take entire amount prescribed.
• Reconstitute powder for injection with sterile water for injection. Use 10 ml in 100-mg vial and 20 ml in 200-mg vial. Dilute solution to 100 to 1,000 ml for I.V. infusion. Do not infuse solutions more concentrated than 1 mg/ml.
• Reconstituted solution is stable for 72 hours refrigerated.
• Doxycycline may be used in patients with renal impairment; does not accumulate or cause a significant rise in BUN.
• Parenteral form may cause false-positive reading of Clinitest. All forms may cause false-negative reading of Clinistix or Tes-Tape.
• Should not be taken within 1 hour of bedtime because of increased incidence of dysphagia.

---

minocycline hydrochloride
Minocin♦*
Pregnancy Risk Category: D

MECHANISM OF ACTION
Exerts bacteriostatic effect by binding to the 30S ribosomal subunit of microorganisms, thus inhibiting protein synthesis.

INDICATIONS & DOSAGE
Infections caused by sensitive gram-negative and gram-positive organisms, trachoma, amebiasis—
Adults: initially, 200 mg P.O., I.V.; then 100 mg q 12 hours or 50 mg P.O. q 6 hours.
Children over 8 years: initially, 4 mg/kg P.O., I.V.; then 4 mg/kg P.O. daily, divided q 12 hours. Give I.V. in 500 to 1,000 ml solution without calcium, over 6 hours.
Gonorrhea in patients sensitive to penicillin—
Adults: initially, 200 mg, then 100 mg q 12 hours for 4 days.

Syphilis in patients sensitive to penicillin—
Adults: initially, 200 mg, then 100 mg q 12 hours for 10 to 15 days.
Meningococcal carrier state—
100 mg P.O. q 12 hours for 5 days.
Uncomplicated urethral, endocervical, or rectal infection caused by Chlamydia trachomatis *or* Ureaplasma urealyticam—
Adults: 100 mg b.i.d. for at least 7 days.
Uncomplicated gonoccocal urethritis in men—
Adults: 100 mg b.i.d. for 5 days.

ADVERSE REACTIONS
Blood: neutropenia, eosinophilia.
CNS: *light-headedness, dizziness from vestibular toxicity.*
CV: pericarditis.
EENT: dysphagia, glossitis.
GI: *anorexia,* epigastric distress, *nausea,* vomiting, *diarrhea,* enterocolitis, inflammatory lesions in anogenital region.
Metabolic: increased BUN.
Skin: *maculopapular and erythematous rashes, photosensitivity, increased pigmentation, urticaria.*
Local: *thrombophlebitis.*
Other: hypersensitivity.

INTERACTIONS
Antacids (including sodium bicarbonate) and laxatives containing aluminum, magnesium, or calcium: decrease antibiotic absorption. Give antibiotic 1 hour before or 2 hours after any of the above.
Ferrous sulfate and other iron products, zinc: decrease antibiotic absorption. Tetracyclines should be given 3 hours after or 2 hours before iron administration.
Methoxyflurane: may cause severe nephrotoxicity with tetracyclines. Monitor carefully.

NURSING CONSIDERATIONS
• Use with extreme caution in im-

paired renal or hepatic function. Use during last half of pregnancy and in children under 8 years may cause permanent discoloration of teeth, enamel defects, and retardation of bone growth.
• Patient may develop thrombophlebitis with I.V. administration of this drug. Avoid extravasation.
• Obtain specimen for culture and sensitivity tests before first dose. Therapy may begin pending test results.
• Do not expose these drugs to light or heat. Keep cap tightly closed.
• Monitor for overgrowth of nonsusceptible organisms. Check patient's tongue for signs of monilia infection. Stress good oral hygiene. If superinfection occurs, drug should be discontinued.
• Observe patient for diarrhea, which may result from local irritation or superinfection.
• May be taken with food. Tell patient to take medication exactly as prescribed, even after he feels better, and to take entire amount prescribed.
• May cause tooth discoloration in young adults. Observe for brown pigmentation and inform doctor if it occurs.
• Reconstitute 100 mg powder with 5 ml sterile water for injection, with further dilution of 500 to 1,000 ml for I.V. infusion. Stable for 24 hours at room temperature.
• Parenteral form may cause false-positive reading of Clinitest. All forms may cause false-negative reading of Clinistix or Tes-Tape.

oxytetracycline hydrochloride
E.P. Mycin, Terramycin♦
Pregnancy Risk Category: D

MECHANISM OF ACTION
Exerts bacteriostatic effect by binding to the 30S ribosomal subunit of mi-

croorganisms, thus inhibiting protein synthesis.

INDICATIONS & DOSAGE

Infections caused by sensitive gram-negative and gram-positive organisms, trachoma, rickettsiae—
Adults: 250 mg P.O. q 6 hours; 100 mg I.M. q 8 to 12 hours; 250 mg I.M. as a single dose.
Children over 8 years: 25 to 50 mg/kg P.O. daily, divided q 6 hours; 15 to 25 mg/kg I.M. daily, divided q 8 to 12 hours
Brucellosis—
Adults: 500 mg P.O. q.i.d. for 3 weeks with streptomycin 1 g I.M. q 12 hours first week, once daily second week.
Syphilis in patients sensitive to penicillin—
Adults: 30 to 40 g total dosage P.O., divided equally over 10 to 15 days.
Gonorrhea in patients sensitive to penicillin—
Adults: initially, 1.5 g P.O. followed by 0.5 g q.i.d. for a total of 9 g.

ADVERSE REACTIONS

Blood: neutropenia, eosinophilia.
CNS: intracranial hypertension.
CV: pericarditis.
EENT: dysphagia, glossitis.
GI: *anorexia, nausea,* vomiting, *diarrhea,* enterocolitis, anogenital inflammation.
Metabolic: *increased BUN.*
Skin: *maculopapular and erythematous rashes, urticaria, photosensitivity, increased pigmentation.*
Local: *irritation after I.M. injection, thrombophlebitis.*
Other: hypersensitivity.

INTERACTIONS

Antacids (including sodium bicarbonate) and laxatives containing aluminum, magnesium, or calcium; food, milk, or other dairy products: decrease antibiotic absorption. Give antibiotic 1 hour before or 2 hours after.

Ferrous sulfate and other iron products, zinc: decrease antibiotic absorption. Give tetracyclines 3 hours after or 2 hours before iron administration.
Methoxyflurane: may cause severe nephrotoxicity with tetracyclines.

NURSING CONSIDERATIONS

• Use with extreme caution in impaired renal or hepatic function. Use during last half of pregnancy and in children under 8 years may cause permanent discoloration of teeth, enamel defects, and retardation of bone growth.
• Obtain specimen for culture and sensitivity tests before first dose. Therapy may begin pending test results.
• Check expiration date. Outdated or deteriorated oxytetracycline has been associated with nephrotoxicity.
• Do not expose these drugs to light or heat.
• Inject I.M. dose deeply. Warn that it may be painful. Rotate sites. I.M. preparations contain a local anesthetic; ask patient about hypersensitivity to local anesthetics.
• Monitor for overgrowth of nonsusceptible organisms. Check patient's tongue for signs of monilia infection. Stress good oral hygiene. If superinfection occurs, drug should be discontinued.
• Observe patient for diarrhea, which may result from local irritation or superinfection.
• Warn patient to avoid direct sunlight and ultraviolet light. A sunscreen may help prevent photosensitivity reactions. Photosensitivity persists for considerable time after discontinuation of drug.
• Effectiveness is reduced when taken with milk or other dairy products, food, antacids, or iron products. Explain this to patient. Tell patient to take each dose with a full glass of water on an empty stomach, at least 1 hour before meals or 2 hours after-

ward. Give at least 1 hour before bedtime to prevent esophagitis.
• Tell patient to take medication exactly as prescribed, even after he feels better, and to take entire amount prescribed.
• For I.V. use, reconstitute 250 mg and 500 mg powder for injection with 10 ml sterile water.
• Dilute to at least 100 ml in dextrose 5% in water, normal saline solution, or Ringer's solution. Do not mix with any other drug.
• Store reconstituted solutions in refrigerator. Stable for 48 hours.
• Parenteral form may cause false-positive reading of Clinitest. All forms may cause false-negative reading of Clinistix or Tes-Tape.

---

tetracycline hydrochloride

Achromycin♦, Achromycin V♦,
Apo-Tetra♦♦, Bristacycline,
Cyclopar, Kesso-tetra, Nor-Tet,
Novotetra♦♦, Panmycin**, Robitet,
Sarocycline, Sumycin, Tetracap,
Tetracyn♦, Tetralan, Tetralean♦♦

Pregnancy Risk Category: D

MECHANISM OF ACTION
Exerts bacteriostatic effect by binding to the 30S ribosomal subunit of microorganisms, thus inhibiting protein synthesis.

INDICATIONS & DOSAGE
Infections caused by sensitive gram-negative and gram-positive organisms, trachoma, rickettsiae, Mycoplasma, *and* Chlamydia—
Adults: 250 to 500 mg P.O. q 6 hours; 250 mg I.M. daily or 150 mg I.M. q 12 hours; or 250 to 500 mg I.V. q 8 to 12 hours (I.M. and I.V. hydrochloride salt only).
Children over 8 years: 25 to 50 mg/ kg P.O. daily, divided q 6 hours; 15 to 25 mg/kg daily (maximum 250 mg) I.M. single dose or divided q 8 to 12 hours; or 10 to 20 mg/kg I.V. daily,

divided q 12 hours.
Uncomplicated urethral, endocervical, or rectal infection caused by Chlamydia trachomatis—
Adults: 500 mg P.O. q.i.d. for at least 7 days.
Brucellosis—
Adults: 500 mg P.O. q 6 hours for 3 weeks with streptomycin 1 g I.M. q 12 hours week 1 and daily week 2.
Gonorrhea in patients sensitive to penicillin—
Adults: initially, 1.5 g P.O., then 500 mg q 6 hours for 7 days.
Syphilis in patients sensitive to penicillin—
Adults: 30 to 40 g total in equally divided doses over 10 to 15 days.
Acne—
Adults and adolescents: initially, 250 mg P.O. q 6 hours, then 125 to 500 mg P.O. daily or every other day.
Shigellosis—
Adults: 2.5 g P.O. in 1 dose.

ADVERSE REACTIONS
Blood: neutropenia, eosinophilia.
CNS: dizziness, headache, intracranial hypertension.
CV: pericarditis.
EENT: sore throat, glossitis, dysphagia.
GI: anorexia, *epigastric distress, nausea,* vomiting, *diarrhea,* stomatitis, enterocolitis, inflammatory lesions in anogenital region.
Hepatic: hepatotoxicity with large doses given I.V.
Metabolic: *increased BUN.*
Skin: *maculopapular and erythematous rashes, urticaria, photosensitivity, increased pigmentation.*
Local: *irritation after I.M. injection, thrombophlebitis.*

INTERACTIONS
Antacids (including sodium bicarbonate) and laxatives containing aluminum, magnesium, or calcium; food, milk, or other dairy products: decrease antibiotic absorption. Give an-

---

Italicized side effects are common or life-threatening.
*Liquid form contains alcohol.   **May contain tartrazine.

tibiotic 1 hour before or 2 hours after any of the above.

Ferrous sulfate and other iron products, zinc: decrease antibiotic absorption. Give tetracyclines 3 hours after or 2 hours before iron administration.

Methoxyflurane: may cause severe nephrotoxicity with tetracyclines.

NURSING CONSIDERATIONS

• Use with extreme caution in impaired renal or hepatic function. Use during last half of pregnancy and in children under 8 years may cause permanent discoloration of teeth, enamel defects, and retardation of bone growth.

• Obtain specimen for culture and sensitivity tests before first dose. Therapy may begin pending test results.

• Effectiveness reduced when taken with milk or other dairy products, food, antacids, or iron products. Explain this to patient. Tell patient to take each dose with a full glass of water on an empty stomach, at least 1 hour before meals or 2 hours afterward. Give at least 1 hour before bedtime to prevent esophagitis.

• Patient may develop thrombophlebitis with I.V. administration. Avoid extravasation.

• Check expiration date. Outdated or deteriorated tetracycline has been associated with nephrotoxicity.

• Discard I.M. solutions after 24 hours because they deteriorate. Exception: discard Achromycin solution in 12 hours.

• Do not expose to light or heat.

• Inject I.M. dose deeply. Warn patient that it may be painful. Rotate sites. I.M. preparations often contain a local anesthetic; ask patient about hypersensitivity to local anesthetics.

• Monitor for overgrowth of nonsusceptible organisms. Check patient's tongue for signs of monilia infection. Stress good oral hygiene. Stop drug if superinfection occurs.

• Observe patient for diarrhea, which may result from local irritation or superinfection.

• Warn patient to avoid direct sunlight and ultraviolet light. A sunscreen may help prevent photosensitivity reactions. Photosensitivity persists after discontinuation of drug.

• Tell patient to take drug exactly as prescribed, even after he feels better, and to take entire amount prescribed.

• For I.V. use, reconstitute 100 mg and 250 mg powder for injection with 5 ml sterile water; with 10 ml for 500 mg. Further dilute in 100 to 1,000 ml volume of dextrose 5% in 0.9% saline solution. Refrigerate diluted solution for I.V. use and use within 24 hours. Exception: use Achromycin solution immediately.

• Do not mix tetracycline solution with any other I.V. additive.

• For I.M. use, reconstitute 100 mg powder for injection with 2 ml sterile water for injection. Concentration will be 50 mg/ml. Amount of diluent for 250-mg injection varies according to brand. Check with pharmacy or follow manufacturer's instructions.

• Parenteral form may cause false-positive reading of Clinitest. All forms may cause false-negative reading of Clinistix or Tes-Tape.

• Tetracycline may be used as a pleural sclerosing agent in malignant pleural effusions. Instilled through chest tube.

15

Sulfonamides

co-trimoxazole
  (sulfamethoxazole-
  trimethoprim)
sulfadiazine
  (sulfafurazole)
sulfamethoxazole
sulfasalazine
sulfisoxazole

COMBINATION PRODUCTS
AZO SULFAMETHOXAZOLE♦♦, URO
GANTANOL♦♦

AZO GANTANOL: sulfamethoxazole
500 mg and phenazopyridine hydrochloride 100 mg.

AZO GANTRISIN: sulfisoxazole 500
mg and phenazopyridine hydrochloride 50 mg.

NEOTRIZINE: sulfadiazine 167 mg,
sulfamerazine 167 mg, and sulfa-
methazine 167 mg.

PEDIAZOLE♦: sulfisoxazole 600 mg
and erythromycin ethylsuccinate 200
mg per 5 ml.

TERFONYL: sulfadiazine 167 mg, sulfamerazine 167 mg, and sulfametha-
zine 167 mg.

THIOSULFIL-A: sulfamethizole 250
mg and phenazopyridine hydrochloride 50 mg.

TRIPLE SULFA: sulfadiazine 167 mg,
sulfamerazine 167 mg, and sulfa-
methazine 167 mg.

UROBIOTIC-250: sulfamethizole 250
mg, oxytetracycline (as the hydrochloride) 250 mg, and phenazopyridine hydrochloride 50 mg.

co-trimoxazole (sulfamethoxazole-trimethoprim)
Apo-Sulfatrim♦♦, Apo-Sulfatrim
DS♦♦, Bactrim♦*, Bactrim DS,
Bactrim I.V. Infusion, Cotrim, Cotrim
D.S., Novotrimel♦♦, Novotrimel
DS♦♦, Protrin♦♦, Protrin DF♦♦,
Roubac♦♦, Roubac DS♦♦,
Septra♦*, Septra DS, Septra I.V.
Infusion, SMZ-TMP,
Sulfamethoprim, Sulfamethoprim
DS, Sulmeprim, Uroplus DS,
Uroplus SS

Pregnancy Risk Category: C (D if near term)

MECHANISM OF ACTION
The sulfamethoxazole component inhibits the formation of dihydrofolic
acid from para-aminobenzoic acid
(PABA). The trimethoprim component inhibits dihydrofolate reductase.
Both decrease bacterial folic acid synthesis.

INDICATIONS & DOSAGE
*Urinary tract infections and shigel-
losis—*

Adults: 160 mg trimethoprim/800 mg
sulfa (double strength tablet) P.O. q
12 hours for 10 to 14 days in urinary
tract infections and for 5 days in shigellosis. For simple cystitis or acute
urethral syndrome, may give one to
three double strength tablets as a single dose.

Children: 8 mg/kg trimethoprim/40
mg/kg sulfa P.O. per 24 hours, in two
divided doses q 12 hours (10 days for

urinary tract infections; for 5 days in shigellosis).

Otitis media—
Children: 8 mg/kg trimethoprim/40 mg/kg sulfa P.O. per 24 hours, in two divided doses q 12 hours for 10 days.

Pneumocystis carinii *pneumonitis—*
Adults and children: 20 mg/kg trimethoprim/ 100 mg/kg sulfa P.O. per 24 hours, in equally divided doses q 6 hours for 14 days.

Chronic bronchitis—
Adults: 160 mg trimethoprim/800 mg sulfa P.O. q 12 hours for 10 to 14 days. Not recommended for infants under 2 months old.

ADVERSE REACTIONS

Blood: *agranulocytosis, aplastic anemia,* megaloblastic anemia, thrombocytopenia, leukopenia, hemolytic anemia.
CNS: headache, mental depression, seizures, hallucinations.
GI: *nausea, vomiting, diarrhea,* abdominal pain, anorexia, stomatitis.
GU: toxic nephrosis with oliguria and anuria, crystalluria, hematuria.
Hepatic: jaundice.
Skin: *erythema multiforme (Stevens-Johnson syndrome), generalized skin eruption, epidermal necrolysis, exfoliative dermatitis,* photosensitivity, urticaria, pruritus.
Other: *hypersensitivity, serum sickness, drug fever, anaphylaxis.*

INTERACTIONS

Ammonium chloride, ascorbic acid: doses sufficient to acidify urine may cause precipitation of sulfonamide and crystalluria. Don't use together.

NURSING CONSIDERATIONS

• Contraindicated in porphyria. Use cautiously and in reduced dosages in impaired hepatic or renal function and in those with severe allergy or bronchial asthma, G6PD deficiency, and blood dyscrasias.
• Adverse reactions, especially hypersensitivity reactions, occur much more frequently in AIDS patients.
• I.V. infusion must be diluted in dextrose 5% in water prior to administration. Don't mix with other drugs or solutions.
• I.V. infusion must be infused slowly over 60 to 90 minutes. Don't give by rapid infusion or bolus injection. Must be used within 2 hours of mixing. Do not refrigerate.
• This combination is often used in extremely ill immunosuppressed patients when prescribed for treatment of *Pneumocystis carinii* pneumonia.
• Oral suspension available.
• Note that the "DS" or "DF" product means "double strength."
• Promptly report skin rash, sore throat, fever, or mouth sores—early signs of blood dyscrasias.
• Watch for superinfection (fever or other signs of new infection).
• Obtain specimen for culture and sensitivity tests before first dose. Therapy may begin pending test results.
• Tell patient to take medication exactly as prescribed, even if he feels better, and to take entire amount prescribed.
• Used effectively for treatment of chronic bacterial prostatitis.
• Used prophylactically for recurrent urinary tract infections in women and for "traveler's diarrhea."

sulfadiazine
Microsulfon

Pregnancy Risk Category: B (D if near term)

MECHANISM OF ACTION
Inhibits formation of dihydrofolic acid from para-aminobenzoic acid (PABA), decreasing bacterial folic acid synthesis.

INDICATIONS & DOSAGE
Urinary tract infection—

Unmarked trade names available in the United States only.
♦Also available in Canada.   ♦♦Available in Canada only.   ◊Also available OTC.

Adults: initially, 2 to 4 g P.O., then 500 mg to 1 g P.O. q 6 hours.
Children: initially, 75 mg/kg or 2 g/m² P.O., then 150 mg/kg or 4 g/m² P.O. in 4 to 6 divided doses daily. Maximum daily dosage is 6 g.
Rheumatic fever prophylaxis, as an alternative to penicillin—
Children over 30 kg: 1 g P.O. daily.
Children under 30 kg: 500 mg P.O. daily.
Adjunctive treatment in toxoplasmosis—
Adults: 4 g P.O. in divided doses q 6 hours for 3 to 4 weeks, discontinued for 1 week; given with pyrimethamine 25 mg P.O. daily for 3 to 4 weeks.
Children: 100 mg/kg P.O. in divided doses q 6 hours for 3 to 4 weeks; given with pyrimethamine 2 mg/kg daily for 3 days, then 1 mg/kg daily for 3 to 4 weeks.

ADVERSE REACTIONS
Blood: *agranulocytosis, aplastic anemia,* megaloblastic anemia, thrombocytopenia, leukopenia, hemolytic anemia.
CNS: headache, mental depression, convulsions, hallucinations.
GI: *nausea, vomiting, diarrhea,* abdominal pain, anorexia, stomatitis.
GU: toxic nephrosis with oliguria and anuria, crystalluria, hematuria.
Hepatic: jaundice.
Skin: *erythema multiforme (Stevens-Johnson syndrome), generalized skin eruption, epidermal necrolysis, exfoliative dermatitis,* photosensitivity, urticaria, pruritus.
Local: irritation, extravasation.
Other: *hypersensitivity, serum sickness, drug fever, anaphylaxis.*

INTERACTIONS
Ammonium chloride, ascorbic acid: doses sufficient to acidify urine may cause precipitation of sulfonamide and crystalluria. Don't use together.
PABA-containing drugs: inhibit antibacterial action. Don't use together.

NURSING CONSIDERATIONS
• Contraindicated in porphyria or in infants under 2 months (except in congenital toxoplasmosis). Use cautiously in reduced doses in impaired hepatic or renal function, bronchial asthma, history of multiple allergies, G6PD deficiency, and blood dyscrasias.
• Tell patient to drink a full glass of water with each dose and to drink plenty of water throughout the day to prevent crystalluria. Monitor input/output. Intake should be sufficient to produce output of 1,500 ml daily (between 3,000 and 4,000 ml daily for adults). To aid in prevention of crystalluria, sodium bicarbonate may be administered to alkalinize urine. Monitor urine pH daily.
• Watch for superinfection (fever or other signs of new infection).
• Obtain specimen for culture and sensitivity tests before first dose. Therapy may begin pending test results.
• Tell patient to take medication exactly as prescribed, even if he feels better, and to take entire amount prescribed.
• Warn patient to avoid direct sunlight and ultraviolet light to prevent photosensitivity reaction.
• Give drug on schedule to maintain constant blood level.
• Monitor for signs of blood dyscrasias (purpura, ecchymosis, sore throat, fever, and pallor). Report them immediately.
• Monitor urine cultures, CBCs, and urinalyses before and during therapy.
• Folic or folinic acid may be used during rest periods in toxoplasmosis therapy to reverse hematopoietic depression and/or anemia associated with pyrimethamine and sulfadiazine.
• Protect drug from light.

Italicized side effects are common or life-threatening.
*Liquid form contains alcohol.   **May contain tartrazine.

sulfamethoxazole
Apo-Sulfamethoxazole♦♦,
Gantanol♦, Gantanol DS

Pregnancy Risk Category: B (D if near term)

MECHANISM OF ACTION
Inhibits formation of dihydrofolic acid from para-aminobenzoic acid (PABA), decreasing bacterial folic acid synthesis.

INDICATIONS & DOSAGE
Urinary tract and systemic infections—
Adults: initially, 2 g P.O., then 1 g P.O. b.i.d. up to t.i.d. for severe infections.
Children and infants over 2 months: initially, 50 to 60 mg/kg P.O., then 25 to 30 mg/kg b.i.d. Maximum dosage should not exceed 75 mg/kg daily.
Lymphogranuloma venereum (genital, inguinal, or anorectal infection)—
Adults: 1 g P.O. daily for at least 2 weeks.

ADVERSE REACTIONS
Blood: *agranulocytosis, aplastic anemia,* megaloblastic anemia, thrombocytopenia, leukopenia, hemolytic anemia.
CNS: headache, mental depression, seizures, hallucinations.
GI: *nausea, vomiting, diarrhea,* abdominal pain, anorexia, stomatitis.
GU: toxic nephrosis with oliguria and anuria, crystalluria, hematuria.
Hepatic: jaundice.
Skin: *erythema multiforme (Stevens-Johnson syndrome), generalized skin eruption, epidermal necrolysis, exfoliative dermatitis,* photosensitivity, urticaria, pruritus.
Other: *hypersensitivity, serum sickness, drug fever, anaphylaxis.*

INTERACTIONS
Ammonium chloride, ascorbic acid: doses sufficient to acidify urine may cause precipitation of sulfonamide and crystalluria. Don't use together.
PABA-containing drugs: inhibit antibacterial action. Don't use together.

NURSING CONSIDERATIONS
• Contraindicated in porphyria or in infants under 2 months (except in congenital toxoplasmosis). Use cautiously and in reduced dosages in impaired hepatic or renal function and in those with severe allergy or bronchial asthma, G6PD deficiency, and blood dyscrasias.
• Tell patient to drink a full glass of water with each dose and to drink plenty of water during the day to prevent crystalluria. Monitor fluid intake/output. Intake should be sufficient to produce output of 1,500 ml daily (between 3,000 and 4,000 ml daily for adults). To aid in prevention of crystalluria, sodium bicarbonate may be administered to alkalinize urine. Monitor urine pH daily.
• Watch for superinfection (fever or other signs of new infection).
• Obtain specimen for culture and sensitivity tests before first dose. Therapy may begin pending test results.
• Tell patient to take medication exactly as prescribed, even if he feels better, and to take entire amount prescribed.
• Warn patient to avoid direct sunlight and ultraviolet light to prevent photosensitivity reaction.
• Monitor urine cultures, CBCs, and urinalyses before and during therapy.
• Sulfamethoxazole is also used in adjunctive therapy for treatment of toxoplasmosis.
• Instruct patient to report early signs of blood dyscrasias (sore throat, fever, and pallor) to doctor immediately.

sulfasalazine (salazosulfapyridine)
Azulfidine, Azulfidine EN-Tabs, PMS Sulfasalazine E.C.♦♦, Salazopyrin♦♦, Salazopyrin EN-Tabs♦♦, S.A.S.♦, S.A.S.-Enteric

Pregnancy Risk Category: B (D if near term)

MECHANISM OF ACTION
Inhibits formation of dihydrofolic acid from para-aminobenzoic acid (PABA), decreasing bacterial folic acid synthesis.

INDICATIONS & DOSAGE
Mild to moderate ulcerative colitis, adjunctive therapy in severe ulcerative colitis—
Adults: initially, 3 to 4 g P.O. daily in evenly divided doses; usual maintenance dosage is 1.5 to 2 g P.O. daily in divided doses q 6 hours. May need to start with 1 to 2 g initially, with a gradual increase in dosage to minimize adverse effects.
Children over 2 years: initially, 40 to 60 mg/kg P.O. daily, divided into 3 to 6 doses; then 30 mg/kg daily in 4 doses. May need to start at lower dose if GI intolerance occurs.

ADVERSE REACTIONS
Blood: *agranulocytosis, aplastic anemia,* megaloblastic anemia, thrombocytopenia, leukopenia, hemolytic anemia.
CNS: headache, mental depression, seizures, hallucinations.
GI: *nausea, vomiting, diarrhea,* abdominal pain, anorexia, stomatitis.
GU: toxic nephrosis with oliguria and anuria, crystalluria, hematuria.
Hepatic: jaundice, hepatoxicity.
Skin: *erythema multiforme (Stevens-Johnson syndrome), generalized skin eruption, epidermal necrolysis, exfoliative dermatitis,* photosensitivity, urticaria, pruritus.
Other: *hypersensitivity, serum sick-*

ness, drug fever, anaphylaxis, oligospermia, infertility.

INTERACTIONS
None significant.

NURSING CONSIDERATIONS
• Contraindicated in porphyria. Use cautiously and in reduced dosages in impaired hepatic or renal function and in those with severe allergy, bronchial asthma, and G6PD deficiency. Also contraindicated in intestinal and urinary obstruction, and in patients allergic to salicylates.
• Watch for superinfection (fever or other signs of new infection).
• Obtain specimen for culture and sensitivity tests before first dose. Therapy may begin pending test results.
• Tell patient to take medication exactly as prescribed, even if he feels better, and to take entire amount prescribed.
• Warn patient to avoid direct sunlight and ultraviolet light to prevent photosensitivity reaction.
• Colors alkaline urine orange-yellow.
• Adverse reactions are usually those affecting GI tract. Minimize symptoms by spacing doses evenly and administering after food intake.
• Also available as an oral suspension.

sulfisoxazole (sulfafurazole)
Azo-Sulfisoxazole♦♦, Gantrisin♦, Lipo Gantrisin, Novosoxazole♦♦

Pregnancy Risk Category: B (D if near term)

MECHANISM OF ACTION
Inhibits formation of dihydrofolic acid from para-aminobenzoic acid (PABA), decreasing bacterial folic acid synthesis.

Italicized side effects are common or life-threatening.
*Liquid form contains alcohol.   **May contain tartrazine.

INDICATIONS & DOSAGE
Urinary tract and systemic infections—

Adults: initially, 2 to 4 g P.O., then 1 to 2 g P.O. q.i.d.; extended-release suspension 4 to 5 g P.O. q 12 hours.
Children over 2 months: initially, 75 mg/kg P.O. daily or 2 g/m² P.O. daily in divided doses q 6 hours, then 150 mg/kg or 4 g/m² P.O. daily in divided doses q 6 hours; extended-release suspension 60 to 70 mg/kg P.O. q 12 hours.

ADVERSE REACTIONS
Blood: *agranulocytosis, aplastic anemia,* megaloblastic anemia, thrombocytopenia, leukopenia, hemolytic anemia.
CNS: headache, mental depression, seizures, hallucinations.
GI: *nausea, vomiting, diarrhea,* abdominal pain, anorexia, stomatitis.
GU: toxic nephrosis with oliguria and anuria, crystalluria, hematuria.
Hepatic: jaundice.
Skin: *erythema multiforme (Stevens-Johnson syndrome), generalized skin eruption, epidermal necrolysis, exfoliative dermatitis,* photosensitivity, urticaria, pruritus.
Other: *hypersensitivity, serum sickness, drug fever, anaphylaxis.*

INTERACTIONS
Ammonium chloride, ascorbic acid: doses sufficient to acidify urine may cause crystalluria and precipitation of sulfonamide. Don't use together.
PABA-containing drugs: inhibit antibacterial action. Don't use together.

NURSING CONSIDERATIONS
• Contraindicated in porphyria and in infants under 2 months (except in congenital toxoplasmosis). Use cautiously in impaired hepatic or renal function, severe allergy or bronchial asthma, and G6PD deficiency.
• Tell patient to drink a full glass of water with each dose and to drink plenty of water throughout the day to prevent crystalluria. Monitor intake/output. Intake should be sufficient to produce output of 1,500 ml daily (between 3,000 and 4,000 ml daily for adults). To aid in prevention of crystalluria, sodium bicarbonate may be administered to alkalinize urine. Monitor urine pH daily.
• Watch for superinfection (fever or other signs of new infection).
• Obtain specimen for culture and sensitivity tests before first dose. Therapy may begin pending test results.
• Tell patient to take medication exactly as prescribed, even if he feels better, and to take entire amount prescribed.
• Warn patient to avoid direct sunlight and ultraviolet light to prevent photosensitivity reaction.
• Monitor urine cultures, CBCs, prothrombin time, and urinalyses before and during therapy.
• Gantrisin suspension and Lipo Gantrisin suspension cannot be interchanged, since the latter is an extended-release preparation.
• Sulfisoxazole-pyrimethamine combination is used to treat toxoplasmosis.
• Tell patient to report early signs of blood dyscrasias (sore throat, fever, and pallor) immediately to doctor.
• When given preoperatively, the patient should receive a low-residue diet and a minimal number of enemas and cathartics.
• Although often given, initial loading dose is not necessary.

16

Urinary tract antiseptics

cinoxacin
methenamine hippurate
methenamine mandelate
methylene blue
nalidixic acid
nitrofurantoin
nitrofurantoin macrocrystals
norfloxacin

COMBINATION PRODUCTS
AZO GANTANOL: sulfamethoxazole 500 mg and phenazopyridine HCl 100 mg.
AZO GANTRISIN: sulfisoxazole 500 mg and phenazopyridine HCl 50 mg.
CYSTEX: methenamine 165 mg, salicylamide 65 mg, sodium salicylate 97 mg, and benzoic acid 32 mg.
HEXALOL: methenamine 40.8 mg, phenyl salicylate 18.1 mg, atropine sulfate 0.03 mg, hyoscyamine 0.03 mg, benzoic acid 4.5 mg, and methylene blue 5.4 mg.
THIOSULFIL-A: sulfamethizole 250 mg and phenazopyridine HCl 50 mg.
URO-PHOSPHATE: methenamine 300 mg and sodium acid phosphate 500 mg. Sugar coated.
UROQUID-ACID: methenamine mandelate 350 mg and sodium acid phosphate 200 mg.
UROQUID-ACID NO. 2: methenamine mandelate 500 mg and sodium acid phosphate 500 mg.

cinoxacin
Cinobac

Pregnancy Risk Category: B

MECHANISM OF ACTION
Inhibits microbial DNA synthesis.

INDICATIONS & DOSAGE
Treatment of initial and recurrent urinary tract infections caused by susceptible strains of Escherichia coli, Klebsiella, Enterobacter, Proteus mirabilis, Proteus vulgaris, *and* Proteus morgani, Serratia, *and* Citrobacter—

Adults and children over 12 years: 1 g P.O. daily, in two to four divided doses for 7 to 14 days.

Not recommended for children under 12 years.

ADVERSE REACTIONS
CNS: *dizziness, headache,* drowsiness, insomnia, seizures.
EENT: photosensitivity.
GI: *nausea, vomiting, abdominal pain,* diarrhea.
Skin: rash, urticaria, pruritus, photosensitivity.

INTERACTIONS
Probenecid: may decrease urine levels of cinoxacin by inhibiting renal tubular secretion. Monitor for increased toxicity and reduced antibacterial effectiveness.

NURSING CONSIDERATIONS
• Contraindicated in patients with hypersensitivity to nalidixic acid. Use

Italicized side effects are common or life-threatening.
*Liquid form contains alcohol.   **May contain tartrazine.

cautiously in patients with impaired renal and hepatic function.
• Not effective against *Pseudomonas*, enterococci, or staphylococci.
• Obtain clean-catch urine specimen for culture and sensitivity before starting therapy and repeat p.r.n. Therapy may begin pending test results.
• Remind patient to continue taking this drug, even when he feels better, and to take entire amount prescribed.
• High urine levels permit twice-daily dosing.
• Report CNS adverse effects to doctor immediately. They indicate serious toxicity and usually mean that administration of drug should be stopped.
• Cinoxacin should be taken with meals to help decrease GI side effects.
• Warn patient about photosensitizing effects of the drug, and advise him to avoid very bright sunlight and use sunblock.

methenamine hippurate
Hiprex**, Hip-Rex♦♦, Urex

methenamine mandelate
Mandameth, Mandelamine♦, Sterine♦♦

Pregnancy Risk Category: C

MECHANISM OF ACTION
In acid urine, methenamines are hydrolyzed to ammonia and to formaldehyde, which is responsible for antibacterial action against gram-positive and gram-negative organisms. Mandelic and hippuric acids, with which methenamines are combined, are also antibacterial by unknown mechanisms.

INDICATIONS & DOSAGE
Long-term prophylaxis or suppression of chronic urinary tract infections—
Adults and children over 12 years: 1 g (hippurate) P.O. q 12 hours.

Children 6 to 12 years: 500 mg to 1 g (hippurate) P.O. q 12 hours.
Urinary tract infections, infected residual urine in patients with neurogenic bladder—
Adults: 1 g (mandelate) P.O. q.i.d. after meals.
Children 6 to 12 years: 500 mg (mandelate) P.O. q.i.d. after meals.
Children under 6 years: 50 mg/kg (mandelate) divided in 4 doses after meals.

ADVERSE REACTIONS
GI: nausea, vomiting, diarrhea.
GU: with high doses, urinary tract irritation, dysuria, frequency, albuminuria, hematuria.
Hepatic: elevated liver enzymes.
Skin: rashes.

INTERACTIONS
Acetazolamide: antagonizes methenamine effect. Use together cautiously.
Alkalinizing agents: inhibit methenamine action. Don't use together.

NURSING CONSIDERATIONS
• Contraindicated in renal insufficiency, severe hepatic disease, or severe dehydration.
• Ineffective against *Candida* infection.
• Oral suspension contains vegetable oil. Administer cautiously to elderly or debilitated patients, because aspiration could cause lipid pneumonia.
• Monitor intake/output. Intake should be at least 1,500 to 2,000 ml daily.
• Obtain a clean-catch urine specimen for culture and sensitivity tests before starting therapy, and repeat p.r.n. Therapy may begin pending test results.
• Limit intake of alkaline foods, such as vegetables, milk, and peanuts. May drink cranberry, plum, and prune juices. These juices or ascorbic acid may be used to acidify urine.
• Warn patient not to take antacids,

including Alka-Seltzer and sodium bicarbonate.
• For best results, maintain urine pH at 5.5 or below. Use Nitrazine paper to check pH. Large doses of ascorbic acid (12 g/day) may be necessary to effectively acidify urine.
• *Proteus* and *Pseudomonas* tend to raise urine pH; urine acidifiers are usually necessary when treating these infections.
• Obtain liver function studies periodically during long-term therapy.
• Administer after meals to minimize GI upset.
• If rash appears, withhold dose and contact doctor.

methylene blue
Urolene Blue

Pregnancy Risk Category: C (D if injected intra-amniotically)

MECHANISM OF ACTION
Methylene blue is a mildly antiseptic dye. High concentrations convert the ferrous iron of reduced hemoglobin to ferric iron to form methemoglobin. This mechanism is the basis for its use as an antidote in cyanide poisoning. Low concentrations of methylene blue can hasten conversion of methemoglobin to hemoglobin.

INDICATIONS & DOSAGE
Cystitis, urethritis—
Adults: 65 mg P.O. b.i.d. or t.i.d. after meals with glass of water.
Methemoglobinemia and cyanide poisoning—
Adults and children: 1 to 2 mg/kg of 1% sterile solution slow I.V.

ADVERSE REACTIONS
Blood: anemia (long-term use).
GI: nausea, vomiting, diarrhea, blue-green stool.
GU: dysuria, bladder irritation, blue-green urine.
Other: fever (large doses).

INTERACTIONS
None significant.

NURSING CONSIDERATIONS
• Contraindicated in renal insufficiency.
• Monitor intake/output carefully. Intake should be at least 2,000 ml daily.
• Monitor hemoglobin; possibility of anemia from accelerated destruction of erythrocytes.
• Turns urine and stool blue-green.
• Seldom used as urinary tract antiseptic.
• I.V. form has been used to treat nitrite intoxication.
• Use caution when handling injectable form, since the liquid can stain the skin. Avoid extravasation. S.C. injection can cause necrotic abcess formation.

nalidixic acid
NegGram♦

Pregnancy Risk Category: B

MECHANISM OF ACTION
Inhibits microbial DNA synthesis.

INDICATIONS & DOSAGE
Acute and chronic urinary tract infections caused by susceptible gram-negative organisms (Proteus, Klebsiella, Enterobacter, *and* Escherichia coli)—
Adults: 1 g P.O. q.i.d. for 7 to 14 days; 2 g daily for long-term use.
Children over 3 months: 55 mg/kg P.O. daily divided q.i.d. for 7 to 14 days; 33 mg/kg daily for long-term use.

ADVERSE REACTIONS
Blood: eosinophilia.
CNS: drowsiness, weakness, headache, dizziness, vertigo, seizures in epileptics, confusion, hallucinations.
EENT: sensitivity to light, change in color perception, diplopia, blurred vision.

GI: *abdominal pain, nausea, vomiting,* diarrhea.
Skin: pruritus, photosensitivity, urticaria, rash.
Other: angioedema, fever, chills, increased intracranial pressure and bulging fontanelles in infants and children.

INTERACTIONS
None significant.

NURSING CONSIDERATIONS
• Contraindicated in convulsive disorders. Use with caution in impaired hepatic or renal function, or severe cerebral arteriosclerosis. Should be used very cautiously in prepubertal children; erosion of cartilage of immature animals has been reported.
• Not effective against *Pseudomonas* or infections outside of the urinary tract.
• Tell the patient to report visual disturbances; these usually disappear with reduced dose.
• Obtain specimen for culture and sensitivity tests before starting therapy and repeat p.r.n. Therapy may begin pending test results.
• Obtain CBC, renal and liver function studies during long-term therapy.
• Resistant bacteria may emerge within the first 48 hours of therapy.
• May cause a false-positive Clinitest reaction. Use Clinistix or Tes-Tape to monitor urine glucose. Also gives false elevations in urine vanillylmandelic acid (VMA) and 17-ketosteroids. Repeat tests after therapy is completed.
• Avoid undue exposure to sunlight due to photosensitivity. Patient may continue to be photosensitive for as long as 3 months after drug is discontinued.

nitrofurantoin
Apo-Nitrofurantoin♦♦, Furadantin, Furalan, Furan, Furanite, Macrodantin, Nephronex♦♦, Nitrofan, Novofuran♦♦

nitrofurantoin macrocrystals
Macrodantin♦
Pregnancy Risk Category: B

MECHANISM OF ACTION
Bacteriostatic in low concentration and possibly bactericidal in high concentration. Interferes with bacterial enzyme systems.

INDICATIONS & DOSAGE
Pyelonephritis, pyelitis, and cystitis due to susceptible Escherichia coli, Staphylococcus aureus, *enterococci; certain strains of* Klebsiella, Proteus, *and* Enterobacter—
Adults and children over 12 years: 50 to 100 mg P.O. q.i.d. with milk or meals.
Children 1 month to 12 years: 5 to 7 mg/kg P.O. daily, divided q.i.d.
Long-term suppression therapy—
Adults: 50 to 100 mg P.O. daily at bedtime.
Children: 1 to 2 mg/kg P.O. daily at bedtime.

ADVERSE REACTIONS
Blood: hemolysis in patients with G6PD deficiency (reversed after stopping drug), *agranulocytosis,* thrombocytopenia.
CNS: peripheral neuropathy, headache, dizziness, drowsiness, *ascending polyneuropathy with high doses or renal impairment.*
GI: *anorexia, nausea, vomiting,* abdominal pain, *diarrhea.*
Hepatic: hepatitis.
Skin: maculopapular, erythematous, or eczematous eruption; pruritus; urticaria; *exfoliative dermatitis; Stevens-Johnson syndrome.*

Unmarked trade names available in the United States only.
♦Also available in Canada.   ♦♦Available in Canada only.   ◊Also available OTC.

Other: asthmatic attacks in patients with history of asthma; *anaphylaxis;* hypersensitivity; transient alopecia; drug fever; overgrowth of nonsusceptible organisms in the urinary tract; *pulmonary sensitivity reactions (cough, chest pains, fever, chills, dyspnea).*

INTERACTIONS

Magnesium-containing antacids: decreased nitrofurantoin absorption. Separate administration times by 1 hour.
Nalidixic acid, norfloxacin: possible decreased effectiveness. Avoid using together.
Probenecid, sulfinpyrazone: increased blood levels and decreased urine levels. May result in increased toxicity and lack of therapeutic effect. Don't use together.

NURSING CONSIDERATIONS

• Contraindicated in moderate to severe renal impairment, anuria, oliguria, or creatinine clearance under 40 ml/minute; use cautiously in G6PD deficiency.
• Hypersensitivity may develop when used for long-term therapy.
• Obtain specimen for culture and sensitivity tests before starting therapy and repeat p.r.n. Therapy may begin pending test results.
• Monitor CBC regularly.
• Give with food or milk to minimize GI distress.
• Some patients may experience fewer GI adverse effects with nitrofurantoin macrocrystals.
• Monitor intake/output carefully. May turn urine brown or darker.
• Store in amber container. Keep away from metals other than stainless steel or aluminum to avoid precipitate formation. Warn patients not to use pillboxes made of these materials.
• Continue treatment for 3 days after sterile urine specimens have been obtained.

• Monitor pulmonary status.
• Has no effect in blood or tissue outside the urinary tract.
• Monitor for superinfection. Use of nitrofurantoin may result in growth of nonsusceptible organisms, especially *Pseudomonas.*
• May cause false-positive results with urine sugar test using copper sulfate reduction method (Clinitest) but not with glucose oxidase tests (Tes-Tape, Diastix, Clinistix).

norfloxacin
Noroxin♦

Pregnancy Risk Category: C

MECHANISM OF ACTION
Inhibits bacterial DNA synthesis, mainly by inhibiting DNA gyrase. Bactericidal.

INDICATIONS & DOSAGE
Treatment of complicated or uncomplicated urinary tract infections caused by susceptible strains of Escherichia coli, Klebsiella, Enterobacter, Proteus, Pseudomonas aeruginosa, Citrobacter, Staphylococcus aureus *(and* epidermidis*), and group D streptococci—*
Adults: For uncomplicated infections, 400 mg P.O. b.i.d. for 7 to 10 days. For complicated infections, 400 mg b.i.d. for 10 to 21 days.

ADVERSE REACTIONS
CNS: fatigue, somnolence, headache, dizziness.
GI: nausea, constipation, flatulence, heartburn.
Hepatic: transient elevations of AST (SGOT) and ALT (SGPT).
Skin: rash.

INTERACTIONS
Antacids: may hinder absorption.
Nitrofurantoin: decreases norfloxacin's effectiveness. Don't use together.

Italicized side effects are common or life-threatening.
*Liquid form contains alcohol.   **May contain tartrazine.

NURSING CONSIDERATIONS

• Contraindicated in patients with hypersensitivity to nalidixic acid and cinoxacin.

• Warn patients not to exceed the recommended dosages. Advise them to drink several glasses of water throughout the day to maintain hydration and adequate urine output.

• Advise patients to take the drug 1 hour before or 2 hours after meals since the presence of food may hinder absorption.

• Because norfloxacin may cause dizziness, patients should avoid hazardous activities that require alertness and good coordination until the CNS effects of the drug are known.

♦ Also available in Canada.   ♦ ♦ Available in Canada only.   ◊ Also available OTC.

17

Antivirals

acyclovir sodium
amantadine hydrochloride
ribavirin
vidarabine monohydrate
    (adenine arabinoside, ara-A)
zidovudine (azidothymidine,
    AZT)

COMBINATION PRODUCTS
None.

---

acyclovir sodium
Zovirax♦

Pregnancy Risk Category: C

MECHANISM OF ACTION
Becomes incorporated into viral DNA
and inhibits viral multiplication.

INDICATIONS & DOSAGE
*Treatment of initial and recurrent epi-
sodes of mucocutaneous herpes simplex virus (HSV-1 and HSV-2) infections in immunocompromised patients;
severe initial episodes of herpes genitalis in patients who are not immunocompromised—*
Adults and children over 11 years: 5
mg/kg, given at a constant rate over a
period of 1 hour by I.V. infusion q 8
hours for 7 days (5 days for herpes
genitalis).
Children under 12 years: 250 mg/
m², given at a constant rate over a period of 1 hour by I.V. infusion q 8
hours for 7 days (5 days for herpes
genitalis).
Treatment of initial genital herpes—
Adults: 200 mg P.O. q 4 hours while
awake (a total of 5 capsules daily).

Treatment should continue for 10
days.
*Intermittent therapy for recurrent gen-
ital herpes—*
Adults: 200 mg P.O. q 4 hours while
awake (a total of 5 capsules daily).
Treatment should continue for 5 days.
Initiate therapy at the first sign of recurrence.
*Chronic suppressive therapy for recur-
rent genital herpes—*
Adults: 200 mg P.O. t.i.d. for up to 6
months.

ADVERSE REACTIONS
CNS: (associated with I.V. dosage):
*headache, encephalopathic changes
(lethargy, obtundation, tremors, confusion, hallucinations, agitation, seizures, coma).*
CV: hypotension.
GI: (associated with P.O. dosage):
nausea, vomiting, diarrhea.
GU: *transient elevations of serum creatinine,* hematuria.
Local: *inflammation, vesicular eruptions and phlebitis at injection site.*
Skin: rash, itching.

INTERACTIONS
Probenecid: increased acyclovir blood
levels. Monitor for possible toxicity.

NURSING CONSIDERATIONS
For I.V. form:
● Don't administer topically, intra-
muscularly, orally, subcutaneously, or
ophthalmically.
● Don't give by bolus injection.
● Infusion must be administered over
at least 1 hour to prevent renal tubular

Italicized side effects are common or life-threatening.
*Liquid form contains alcohol.   **May contain tartrazine.

damage. Bolus injection, dehydration (decreased urine output), preexisting renal disease, and the concomitant use of other nephrotoxic drugs increase the risk of renal toxicity.

• Notify doctor if serum creatinine level does not return to normal within a few days. He may increase hydration, adjust dose, or discontinue acyclovir.

• Encephalopathic changes are more likely in patients with neurologic disorders or in those who have had neurologic reactions to cytotoxic drugs.

• Patient must be adequately hydrated during acyclovir infusion.

For P.O. form:

• Teach patient that drug is effective in managing the disease but does not eliminate or cure it.

• Instruct patient that acyclovir will not prevent spread of infection to others.

• Urge patient to recognize the early symptoms of infection (such as tingling, itching, or pain) so he can take acyclovir before the infection fully develops.

amantadine hydrochloride
Symadine, Symmetrel♦

Pregnancy Risk Category: C

MECHANISM OF ACTION
Interferes with influenza A virus penetration into susceptible cells. Its action in the treatment of parkinsonism is unknown.

INDICATIONS & DOSAGE
Prophylaxis or symptomatic treatment of influenza type A virus, respiratory tract illnesses—
Adults to age 64 and children age 10 and over: 200 mg P.O. daily in a single dose or divided b.i.d.
Children 1 to 9 years: 4.4 to 8.8 mg/kg P.O. daily, divided b.i.d. or t.i.d. Don't exceed 150 mg daily.
Adults over age 64: 100 mg P.O.

once daily.
Treatment should continue for 24 to 48 hours after symptoms disappear. Prophylaxis should start as soon as possible after initial exposure and continue for at least 10 days after exposure. May continue prophylactic treatment up to 90 days for repeated or suspected exposures if influenza vaccine unavailable. If used with influenza vaccine, continue dose for 2 to 3 weeks until protection from vaccine develops.
To treat drug-induced extrapyramidal reactions—
Adults: 100 mg P.O. b.i.d., up to 300 mg daily in divided doses. Patient may benefit from as much as 400 mg daily, but dosages over 200 mg must be closely supervised.
To treat idiopathic parkinsonism, parkinsonian syndrome—
Adults: 100 mg P.O. b.i.d.; in patients who are seriously ill or receiving other antiparkinsonism drugs, 100 mg daily for at least 1 week, then 100 mg b.i.d., p.r.n.

ADVERSE REACTIONS
CNS: depression, fatigue, confusion, dizziness, psychosis, hallucinations, anxiety, *irritability*, ataxia, *insomnia*, weakness, headache, light-headedness, difficulty concentrating.
CV: peripheral edema, orthostatic hypotension, CHF.
GI: anorexia, nausea, constipation, vomiting, dry mouth.
GU: urine retention.
Skin: *livedo reticularis* (with prolonged use).

INTERACTIONS
None significant.

NURSING CONSIDERATIONS
• Use cautiously in epilepsy, congestive heart failure, peripheral edema, hepatic disease, mental illness, eczematoid rash, renal impairment, orthostatic hypotension, and cardiovascular

disease, and in elderly patients.
• For best absorption, drug should be taken after meals.
• Instruct patient to report adverse reactions to the doctor, especially dizziness, depression, anxiety, nausea, and urine retention.
• Elderly patients are more susceptible to neurological adverse effects. Taking the drug in two daily doses rather than single dose may reduce their incidence.
• If orthostatic hypotension occurs, instruct patient not to stand or change positions too quickly.
• If insomnia occurs, dose should be taken several hours before bedtime.
• When prescribed for parkinsonism, warn patient against discontinuing drug abruptly since this might precipitate a parkinsonian crisis.

ribavirin
Virazole♦

Pregnancy Risk Category: X

MECHANISM OF ACTION
Inhibits viral activity by an unknown mechanism. Thought to inhibit RNA and DNA synthesis by depleting intracellular nucleotide pools.

INDICATIONS & DOSAGE
Treatment of hospitalized infants and young children infected by respiratory syncytial virus (RSV)—
Infants and young children: Solution in concentration of 20 mg/ml delivered via the Viratek Small Particle Aerosol Generator (SPAG-2). Treatment is carried out for 12 to 18 hours/day for at least 3, and no more than 7, days.

ADVERSE REACTIONS
Blood: anemia, reticulocytosis.
EENT: conjunctivitis.
Other: rash or erythema of eyelids.

INTERACTIONS
None significant.

NURSING CONSIDERATIONS
• Contraindicated in females who are or may become pregnant during treatment with drug.
• Ribavirin aerosol is indicated only for severe lower respiratory tract infection due to respiratory syncytial virus (RSV). Although treatment may be started while awaiting diagnostic test results, existence of RSV infection must be eventually documented.
• Most infants and children with RSV infection don't require treatment because the disease is often mild and self-limiting. Infants with underlying conditions, such as prematurity or cardiopulmonary disease get RSV in its severest form, and benefit most from treatment with ribavirin aerosol.
• This treatment must be accompanied by, and does not replace, supportive respiratory and fluid management.
• Ribavirin aerosol *must* be administered by the Viratek Small Particle Aerosol Generator (SPAG-2). Don't use any other aerosol generating device.
• Ribavarin may precipitate in ventilator apparatus which may result in equipment malfunction with serious consequences. The use of ribavirin in ventilator dependant patients is not recommended.
• The water used to reconstitute this drug must not contain any antimicrobial agent. Use sterile USP water for injection, *not* bacteriostatic water.
• Discard solutions placed in the SPAG-2 unit at least every 24 hours before adding newly reconstituted solution.
• Store reconstituted solutions at room temperature for 24 hours.

---

vidarabine monohydrate (adenine arabinoside, ara-A)
Vira-A♦

Pregnancy Risk Category: C

MECHANISM OF ACTION
Becomes incorporated into viral DNA and inhibits viral multiplication.

INDICATIONS & DOSAGE
Herpes simplex virus encephalitis—
Adults and children (including neonates): 15 mg/kg I.V. daily for 10 days. Slowly infuse the total daily dose by I.V. infusion at a constant rate over 12-to 24-hour period. Avoid rapid or bolus injection.

ADVERSE REACTIONS
Blood: anemia, neutropenia, thrombocytopenia.
CNS: tremor, dizziness, hallucinations, confusion, psychosis, ataxia.
GI: *anorexia, nausea,* vomiting, diarrhea.
Hepatic: elevated AST (SGOT), bilirubin.
Skin: pruritus, rash.
Local: pain at injection site.
Other: weight loss.

INTERACTIONS
Allopurinol: concurrent therapy increases risk of CNS adverse effects.

NURSING CONSIDERATIONS
• Will reduce mortality caused by herpes simplex virus encephalitis from 70% to 28%. No evidence that vidarabine is effective in encephalitis due to other viruses.
• Don't give I.M. or subcutaneously because of low solubility and poor absorption.
• Monitor hematologic tests, such as hemoglobin, hematocrit, WBC, and platelets during therapy. Also monitor renal and liver function studies.
• Patient with impaired renal function may need dosage adjustment.
• Once in solution, vidarabine is stable at room temperature for at least 2 weeks.
• Use with an I.V. filter of 0.45 μm or smaller.
• Must be diluted to a concentration of less than 0.5 mg/ml.
• Any I.V. solution is suitable as a diluent.

zidovudine (azidothymidine, AZT)
Retrovir

Pregnancy Risk Category: C

MECHANISM OF ACTION
Prevents replication of the human immunodeficiency virus (HIV) by inhibiting the enzyme reverse transcriptase.

INDICATIONS & DOSAGE
Patients with AIDS or advanced AIDS-related complex who have confirmed Pneumocystis carinii *pneumonia or a* T_4 *lymphocyte count below 200—*
Adults: 200 mg P.O. q 4 hours around the clock.

ADVERSE REACTIONS
Blood: *Severe bone marrow depression (resulting in anemia), granulocytopenia, thrombocytopenia.*
CNS: *headache,* agitation, restlessness, insomnia, confusion, anxiety.
Skin: rash, itching.

INTERACTIONS
Acyclovir: possible lethargy and fatigue. Use together cautiously.
Co-trimoxazole, acetaminophen: may impair hepatic metabolism of zidovudine, increasing the drug's toxicity.
Other cytotoxic drugs: additive adverse effects on the bone marrow.

NURSING CONSIDERATIONS
• Zidovudine frequently causes a low red blood cell count by suppressing

the bone marrow. Advise patients that they may need blood transfusions during treatment with zidovudine.

• Remind patients that they *must* comply with the every-4-hour dosage schedule. Suggest ways to avoid missing doses, such as the use of alarm clocks.

• Warn patients not to take any other drugs for AIDS (especially from the "street") unless their doctors have approved them. Some purported AIDS "cures" may interfere with zidovudine's effectiveness.

• The drug has been shown to temporarily decrease morbidity and mortality in certain patients with AIDS or AIDS-related complex.

• The optimum duration of treatment, as well as the dosage for optimum effectiveness and minimum toxicity, is not yet known.

Italicized side effects are common or life-threatening.
*Liquid form contains alcohol.   **May contain tartrazine.

18

Miscellaneous anti-infectives

aztreonam
bacitracin
chloramphenicol
chloramphenicol palmitate
chloramphenicol sodium
  succinate
ciprofloxacin
clindamycin hydrochloride
clindamycin palmitate
  hydrochloride
clindamycin phosphate
erythromycin base
erythromycin estolate
erythromycin ethylsuccinate
erythromycin gluceptate
erythromycin lactobionate
erythromycin stearate
imipenem/cilastatin sodium
lincomycin hydrochloride
pentamidine isethionate
polymyxin B sulfate
spectinomycin dihydrochloride
trimethoprim
vancomycin hydrochloride

COMBINATION PRODUCTS
None.

---

aztreonam
Azactam

Pregnancy Risk Category: B

MECHANISM OF ACTION
Inhibits bacterial cell wall synthesis,
ultimately causing cell wall destruction. Bactericidal.

INDICATIONS & DOSAGE
*Treatment of urinary tract infections,
lower respiratory tract infections, sep-*
*ticemia, skin and skin structure infec-
tions, intraabdominal infections, and
gynecologic infections caused by various gram-negative organisms—*
Adults: 500 mg to 2 g I.V. or I.M. q 8
to 12 hours. For severe systemic or
life-threatening infections, 2 g q 6 to
8 hours may be given. Maximum dosage is 8 g daily.

ADVERSE REACTIONS
GI: diarrhea, nausea, vomiting.
Hepatic: transient elevations of AST
(SGOT) and ALT (SGPT).
Local: thrombophlebitis at I.V. site,
discomfort and swelling at I.M. injec-
tion site.

INTERACTIONS
None significant.

NURSING CONSIDERATIONS
• Use cautiously in elderly patients
and in impaired renal function.
• Aztreonam is a narrow-spectrum
antibiotic, effective solely against
gram-negative organisms. Because it
is ineffective against gram-positive
and anaerobic organisms, aztreonam
must be used with other antibiotics
for immediate treatment of life-
threatening illnesses.
• Patients who are allergic to penicillins or cephalosporins may not be allergic to aztreonam since there is no
cross-allergenicity.
• To administer a bolus of aztreonam,
inject it slowly (over 3 to 5 minutes)
directly into a vein or I.V. tubing.
• I.M. injections should be given
deep into a large muscle mass, such as

the upper outer quadrant of the gluteus maximus or the lateral part of the thigh.
• Obtain specimen for culture and sensitivity tests before first dose. Therapy may begin pending test results.
• Watch for superinfection (fever or other signs of new infection).
• Aztreonam is the first commercially available member of a new antibiotic family, the monobactams. Its effectiveness against gram-negative organisms is comparable to that of the aminoglycoside antibiotics, without the ototoxicity or nephrotoxicity usually associated with the aminoglycosides.

bacitracin

Pregnancy Risk Category: C

MECHANISM OF ACTION
Hinders bacterial cell wall synthesis, damaging the bacterial plasma membrane and making the cell more vulnerable to osmotic pressure.

INDICATIONS & DOSAGE
Pneumonia or empyema caused by susceptible staphylococci—
Infants over 2.5 kg: 1,000 units/kg I.M. daily, divided q 8 to 12 hours.
Infants under 2.5 kg: 900 units/kg I.M. daily, divided q 8 to 12 hours.
   Although the FDA approves the use of bacitracin in infants only, adults with susceptible staphylococcal infections may receive 10,000 to 25,000 units I.M. q 6 hours (maximum 25,000 units/dose, 100,000 units daily).

ADVERSE REACTIONS
Blood: blood dyscrasias, eosinophilia.
GI: nausea, vomiting, anorexia, diarrhea, rectal itching or burning.
GU: *nephrotoxicity (albuminuria,* cylindruria, oliguria, anuria, increased

BUN, tubular and glomerular necrosis).
Skin: urticaria, rash.
Local: *pain at injection site.*
Other: superinfection, fever, *anaphylaxis,* neuromuscular blockade.

INTERACTIONS
None significant.

NURSING CONSIDERATIONS
• Contraindicated in impaired renal function. Use cautiously in myasthenia gravis and neuromuscular disease.
• Obtain specimen for culture and sensitivity tests before first dose. Therapy may begin pending test results.
• For I.M. administration only. Give deep I.M.; injection may be painful; dilute in solution containing sodium chloride and 2% procaine hydrochloride (if hospital policy permits). Do not dilute in procaine hydrochloride if patient is sensitive to procaine or PABA derivatives.
• Maintain adequate fluid intake, and monitor urine output closely. If intake or output decreases, notify the doctor.
• Obtain baseline renal function studies before starting therapy. Monitor daily during therapy. Notify doctor of any change.
• Concentration of bacitracin should be between 5,000 and 10,000 units/ml. Store in refrigerator. Drug is inactivated if stored at room temperature.
• Report adverse effects to the doctor immediately.
• May be used with neomycin as a bowel preparation, or in solution as a wound irrigating agent.
• Urine pH should be kept above 6.0 to reduce the risk of nephrotoxicity.
• Prolonged therapy may result in overgrowth of nonsusceptible organisms, especially *Candida albicans.*
• Don't administer by I.V. route; drug is irritating to vein and predisposes patient to severe thrombophlebitis.

Italicized side effects are common or life-threatening.
*Liquid form contains alcohol.   **May contain tartrazine.

chloramphenicol
Chloromycetin, Novochlorocap♦♦

chloramphenicol palmitate
Chloromycetin Palmitate

chloramphenicol sodium succinate
Chloromycetin, Pentamycetin♦♦,
Sodium Succinate♦

Pregnancy Risk Category: C

MECHANISM OF ACTION
Inhibits bacterial protein synthesis by binding to the 50S subunit of the ribosome.

INDICATIONS & DOSAGE
Hemophilus influenzae *meningitis, acute* Salmonella typhi *infection, and meningitis, bacteremia, or other severe infections caused by sensitive* Salmonella *species,* Rickettsia, *lymphogranuloma, psittacosis, or various sensitive gram-negative organisms—*
Adults and children: 50 to 100 mg/kg P.O. or I.V. daily, divided q 6 hours. Maximum dosage is 100 mg/kg daily.
Premature infants and neonates 2 weeks or younger: 25 mg/kg P.O. or I.V. daily, divided q 6 hours. I.V. route must be used to treat meningitis.

ADVERSE REACTIONS
Blood: *aplastic anemia,* hypoplastic anemia, *granulocytopenia,* thrombocytopenia.
CNS: headache, mild depression, confusion, delirium, peripheral neuropathy with prolonged therapy.
EENT: optic neuritis (in patients with cystic fibrosis), glossitis, decreased visual acuity.
GI: nausea, vomiting, stomatitis, diarrhea, enterocolitis.
Other: infections by nonsusceptible organisms, hypersensitivity reaction (fever, rash, urticaria, *anaphylaxis*), *gray baby syndrome in premature and newborn infants (abdominal distention, gray cyanosis, vasomotor collapse, respiratory distress, death within a few hours of onset of symptoms).*

INTERACTIONS
Acetaminophen: elevates chloramphenicol levels. Monitor for chloramphenicol toxicity.

NURSING CONSIDERATIONS
• Use cautiously in impaired hepatic or renal function, and with other drugs causing bone marrow depression or blood disorders. *Don't use for infections caused by organisms susceptible to other agents or for trivial infections; use only when clearly indicated for severe infection.*
• Obtain specimen for culture and sensitivity tests before first dose. Therapy may begin pending test results.
• Monitor CBC, platelets, serum iron, and reticulocytes before and every 2 days during therapy. Stop drug immediately if anemia, reticulocytopenia, leukopenia, or thrombocytopenia develops.
• Instruct patient to report adverse reactions to the doctor, especially nausea, vomiting, diarrhea, fever, confusion, sore throat, or mouth sores.
• Tell patient to take medication for as long as prescribed, exactly as directed, even after he feels better.
• Give I.V. slowly over 1 minute. Check injection site daily for phlebitis and irritation.
• Reconstitute 1-g vial of powder for injection with 10 ml sterile water for injection. Concentration will be 100 mg/ml. Stable for 30 days at room temperature, but refrigeration recommended. Do not use cloudy solutions.
• Monitor for evidence of superinfection by nonsusceptible organisms.
• Therapeutic plasma concentrations are 5 to 25 mcg/ml.

ciprofloxacin
Cipro

Pregnancy Risk Category: C

MECHANISM OF ACTION
A broad-spectrum quinolone antibiotic. Exact mechanism is unknown, but bactericidal effects may result from drug's ability to inhibit bacterial DNA gyrase and to prevent DNA replication in susceptible bacteria.

INDICATIONS & DOSAGE
Mild to moderate urinary tract infections—
Adults: 250 mg P.O. q 12 hours.
Severe or complicated urinary tract infections; mild to moderate bone and joint infections; mild to moderate respiratory tract infections; mild to moderate skin and skin structure infections; infectious diarrhea—
Adults: 500 mg P.O. q 12 hours.
Severe or complicated bone or joint infections; severe respiratory tract infections; severe skin and skin structure infection—
Adults: 750 mg P.O. q 12 hours.

ADVERSE REACTIONS
CNS: headache, restlessness, tremor, light-headedness, confusion, hallucinations, *seizures.*
GI: nausea, diarrhea, vomiting, abdominal pain or discomfort, oral candidiasis.
GU: crystalluria.
Other: rash.

INTERACTIONS
Antacids containing magnesium hydroxide or aluminum hydroxide: decreased ciprofloxacin absorption. Separate administration by at least 2 hours.
Probenecid: may elevate serum level of ciprofloxacin.
Theophylline: increased plasma theophylline concentrations and prolonged theophylline half-life.

NURSING CONSIDERATIONS
• Contraindicated in patients sensitive to quinolone antibiotics, in pregnant or breast-feeding women, and in children. Quinolone antibiotics have been shown to produce arthropathy in young laboratory animals.
• Obtain specimen for culture and sensitivity tests before first dose. Therapy may begin pending test results.
• The preferred time for dosing is 2 hours after a meal. Food does not affect absorption but may delay peak serum levels.
• May cause CNS stimulation. Use with caution in CNS disorders, such as severe cerebral arteriosclerosis or epilepsy, and in other patients who are at an increased risk of seizures.
• May cause dizziness or light-headedness. Warn patient to avoid hazardous tasks that require alertness, such as driving, until CNS effects of the drug are known.
• Advise patient to drink plenty of fluids to reduce the risk of crystalluria.
• Dosage adjustments may be necessary in patients with renal dysfunction.
• Prolonged use may result in overgrowth of organisms that are resistant to ciprofloxacin.

clindamycin hydrochloride
Cleocin HCl, Dalacin C♦♦

clindamycin palmitate hydrochloride
Cleocin Pediatric, Dalacin C palmitate♦♦

clindamycin phosphate
Cleocin, Cleocin phosphate♦♦, Dalacin C♦♦, Dalacin C phosphate

Pregnancy Risk Category: B

MECHANISM OF ACTION
Inhibits bacterial protein synthesis by

binding to the 50S subunit of the ribosome.

INDICATIONS & DOSAGE

Infections caused by sensitive staphylococci, streptococci, pneumococci, Bacteroides, Fusobacterium, Clostridium perfringens, *and other sensitive aerobic and anaerobic organisms—*

Adults: 150 to 450 mg P.O. q 6 hours; or 300 mg I.M. or I.V. q 6, 8, or 12 hours. Up to 2,700 mg I.M. or I.V. daily, divided q 6, 8, or 12 hours.

May be used for severe infections.
Children over 1 month: 8 to 25 mg/kg P.O. daily, divided q 6 to 8 hours; or 15 to 40 mg/kg I.M. or I.V. daily, divided q 6 hours.

ADVERSE REACTIONS

Blood: transient leukopenia, eosinophilia, thrombocytopenia.
GI: *nausea,* vomiting, abdominal pain, *diarrhea, pseudomembranous enterocolitis,* esophagitis, flatulence, anorexia, *bloody or tarry stools, dysphagia.*
Hepatic: elevated AST (SGOT), alkaline phosphatase, bilirubin.
Skin: maculopapular rash, urticaria.
Local: *pain,* induration, *sterile abscess with I.M. injection;* thrombophlebitis, erythema, and pain after I.V. administration.
Other: unpleasant or bitter taste, *anaphylaxis.*

INTERACTIONS

Erythromycin: antagonist that may block access of clindamycin to its site of action; don't use together.

NURSING CONSIDERATIONS

• Contraindicated in patients with known hypersensitivity to the antibiotic congener lincomycin; also in patients with history of GI disease, especially colitis. Use cautiously in newborns and patients with renal or hepatic disease, asthma, or significant allergies.
• Monitor renal, hepatic, and hematopoietic functions during prolonged therapy.
• Obtain specimen for culture and sensitivity tests before first dose. Therapy may begin pending test results.
• Don't use in meningitis. Drug does not penetrate blood/brain barrier.
• Don't refrigerate reconstituted oral solution, as it will thicken. Drug is stable for 2 weeks at room temperature.
• Instruct patient to report adverse reactions to the doctor, especially diarrhea. Warn patient not to treat such diarrhea himself.
• Advise patients taking the capsule form to take with a full glass of water to prevent dysphagia.
• Don't give diphenoxylate compound (Lomotil) to treat drug-induced diarrhea. May prolong and worsen diarrhea.
• Give deep I.M. Rotate sites. Warn that I.M. injection may be painful. Doses greater than 600 mg per injection are not recommended.
• When giving I.V., check site daily for phlebitis and irritation. For I.V. infusion, dilute each 300 mg in 50 ml solution, and give no faster than 30 mg/minute.
• Watch for superinfection (fever or other signs of new infection).
• I.M. injection may cause creatinine phospokinase level to rise due to muscle irritation.
• Topical form available to treat acne.

erythromycin base
Apo-Erythro base♦♦, E-Mycin♦,
Eryc♦, Eryc Sprinkle, Ery-Tab,
Erythromid♦♦, Ilotycin♦,
Novorythro♦♦, PCE Dispersatabs,
Robimycin

erythromycin estolate
Ilosone♦, Novorythro♦♦

erythromycin
ethylsuccinate
Apo-Erythro-ES♦♦, E.E.S.,
E-Mycin E, EryPed, Erythrocin♦,
Pediamycin, Wyamycin E

erythromycin gluceptate
Ilotycin♦

erythromycin lactobionate
Erythrocin♦

erythromycin stearate
Apo-Erythro-S♦♦, Erypar,
Erythrocin♦, Novorythro♦♦,
Wyamycin S

Pregnancy Risk Category: B

MECHANISM OF ACTION
Inhibits bacterial protein synthesis by
binding to the 50S subunit of the ribosome.

INDICATIONS & DOSAGE
*Acute pelvic inflammatory disease
caused by* Neisseria gonorrhoeae—
Women: 500 mg I.V. (erythromycin
gluceptate, lactobionate) q 6 hours for
3 days, then 250 mg (erythromycin
base, estolate, stearate) or 400 mg
(erythromycin ethylsuccinate) P.O. q
6 hours for 7 days.
*Endocarditis prophylaxis for dental
procedures in patients allergic to penicillin—*
Adults: 1 g (erythromycin base, estolate, stearate) P.O. 1 hour before procedure, then 500 mg P.O. 6 hours
later.
Intestinal amebiasis—

Adults: 250 mg (erythromycin base,
estolate, stearate) P.O. q 6 hours for
10 to 14 days.
Children: 30 to 50 mg/kg (erythromycin base, estolate, stearate) P.O.
daily, divided q 6 hours for 10 to 14
days.
*Mild-to-moderately severe respiratory
tract, skin, and soft tissue infections
caused by sensitive group A beta-
hemolytic streptococci,* Diplococcus
pneumoniae, Mycoplasma pneumoniae, Corynebacterium diphtheriae,
Bordetella pertussis, Listeria mono-
cytogenes—
Adults: 250 to 500 mg (erythromycin
base, estolate, stearate) P.O. q 6
hours; or 400 to 800 mg (erythromycin ethylsuccinate) P.O. q 6 hours; or
15 to 20 mg/kg I.V. daily, as continuous infusion or divided q 6 hours.
Children: 30 mg/kg to 50 mg/kg (oral
erythromycin salts) P.O. daily, divided q 6 hours; or 15 to 20 mg/kg
I.V. daily, divided q 4 to 6 hours.
Syphilis—
Adults: 500 mg (erythromycin base,
estolate, stearate) P.O. q.i.d. for 15
days.
Legionnaire's Disease—
Adults: 500 mg to 1 g I.V. or P.O. q 6
hours for 21 days.
*Uncomplicated urethral, endocervi-
cal, or rectal infections where tetracyclines are contraindicated—*
Adults: 500 mg P.O. q.i.d. for at least
7 days.
Urogenital Chlamydia trachomatis *infections during pregnancy—*
Adults: 500 mg P.O. q.i.d. for at least
7 days or 250 mg P.O. q.i.d. for at
least 14 days.
Conjunctivitis caused by Chlamydia
trachomatis *in newborns—*
Newborns: 50 mg/kg/day in 4 divided
doses for at least 2 weeks.
Pneumonia of infancy due to Chlamydia trachomatis—
Infants: 50 mg/kg/day in 4 divided
doses for at least 3 weeks.

Italicized side effects are common or life-threatening.
*Liquid form contains alcohol.   **May contain tartrazine.

ADVERSE REACTIONS
EENT: hearing loss with high I.V. doses.
GI: *abdominal pain and cramping, nausea, vomiting, diarrhea.*
Hepatic: cholestatic jaundice (with erythromycin estolate).
Skin: urticaria, rashes.
Local: *venous irritation, thrombophlebitis following I.V. injection.*
Other: overgrowth of nonsusceptible bacteria or fungi; *anaphylaxis;* fever.

INTERACTIONS
Clindamycin, lincomycin: may be antagonistic. Don't use together.
Theophylline: decreased erythromycin blood level and increased theophylline toxicity. Use together cautiously.

NURSING CONSIDERATIONS
• Erythromycin estolate contraindicated in hepatic disease. Use other erythromycin salts cautiously in impaired hepatic function.
• Obtain specimen for culture and sensitivity tests before first dose. Therapy may begin pending test results.
• For best absorption, instruct patient to take oral form of drug with a full glass of water 1 hour before or 2 hours after meals. If tablets are coated, they may be taken with meals. Tell patient not to drink fruit juice with medication. Chewable erythromycin tablets should not be swallowed whole.
• Coated forms of erythromycin are associated with lower incidence of GI problems. May be more tolerable in patients who cannot easily tolerate erythromycin.
• When administering suspension, be sure to note the concentration.
• May cause overgrowth of nonsusceptible bacteria or fungi. Monitor for signs and symptoms of superinfection.
• Tell patient to take medication for as long as prescribed, exactly as directed, even after he feels better, and to take entire amount prescribed. Treat streptococcal infections for 10 days.
• Report adverse effects, especially nausea, abdominal pain, and fever.
• Erythromycin estolate may cause serious hepatotoxicity in adults (reversible cholestatic jaundice). Monitor hepatic function (increased levels of bilirubin, AST [SGOT], ALT [SGPT], and alkaline phosphatase may occur). Other erythromycin salts cause hepatotoxicity to a lesser degree. Patients who develop hepatotoxicity from estolate may react similarly to treatment with any erythromycin preparation.
• I.V. dose should be administered over 60 minutes. Reconstitute according to manufacturer's directions and dilute each 250 mg in at least 100 ml 0.9% normal saline solution.
• Erythromycin lactobionate should not be administered with other drugs.
• Topical form available to treat acne.

imipenem/cilastatin sodium
Primaxin♦
Pregnancy Risk Category: C

MECHANISM OF ACTION
Imipenem is bactericidal and inhibits bacterial cell wall synthesis. Cilastatin inhibits the enzymatic breakdown of imipenem in the kidney, making it effective in the urinary tract.

INDICATIONS & DOSAGE
Treatment of serious infections of the lower respiratory and urinary tracts, intraabdominal and gynecologic infections, bacterial septicemia, bone and joint infections, skin and soft tissue infections, and endocarditis. Most known microorganisms susceptible: Staphylococcus, Streptococcus, Escherichia coli, Klebsiella, Proteus, Enterobacter, Pseudomonas aeruginosa, *and* Bacteroides, *including* B. fra-

gilis—
Adults: 250 mg to 1 g by I.V. infusion q 6 to 8 hours. Maximum daily dosage is 50 mg/kg/day or 4 g/day, whichever is less.

ADVERSE REACTIONS
CNS: *seizures*, dizziness.
CV: hypotension.
GI: nausea, vomiting, diarrhea, *pseudomembranous colitis*.
Skin: rash, urticaria, pruritus.
Local: *thrombophlebitis, pain at injection site*.
Other: *hypersensitivity*.

INTERACTIONS
None significant.

NURSING CONSIDERATIONS
• Use cautiously in patients allergic to penicillins or cephalosporins because this drug is chemically similar. Ask patient if he's had a hypersensitivity reaction to either of these drugs before administering first dose of imipenem.
• Use cautiously in patients who have a history of seizure disorders, especially if they also have compromised renal function. If patient develops seizures that persist despite anticonvulsant therapy, notify doctor. The drug should then be discontinued.
• Don't administer by direct I.V. bolus injection. Each 250- or 500-mg dose should be given by I.V. infusion over 20 to 30 minutes. Each 1-g dose should be infused over 40 to 60 minutes. If nausea occurs, the infusion may be slowed.
• When reconstituting powder, shake until the solution is clear. Solutions may range from colorless to yellow and variations of color within this range don't affect the drug's potency. After reconstitution, solution is stable for 10 hours at room temperature and for 48 hours when refrigerated.
• Imipenem/cilastatin has the broadest antibacterial spectrum of any available antibiotic. The drug is most valuable for empiric treatment of infections and for mixed infections that would otherwise require a combination of antibiotics, often including an aminoglycoside.
• Patients with impaired renal function may need lower dosage or longer intervals between doses.
• Obtain specimen for culture and sensitivity tests before first dose. Therapy may begin pending test results.
• Monitor patient for bacterial or fungal superinfections and resistant infections during and after therapy.

lincomycin hydrochloride
Lincocin♦

Pregnancy Risk Category: B

MECHANISM OF ACTION
Inhibits bacterial protein synthesis by binding to the 50S subunit of the ribosome.

INDICATIONS & DOSAGE
Respiratory tract, skin and soft tissue, and urinary tract infections; osteomyelitis, septicemia caused by sensitive group A beta-hemolytic streptococci, pneumococci, and staphylococci—
Adults: 500 mg P.O. q 6 to 8 hours (not to exceed 8 g daily); or 600 mg I.M. daily or q 12 hours; or 600 mg to 1 g I.V. q 8 to 12 hours (not to exceed 8 g daily).
Children over 1 month: 30 to 60 mg/kg P.O. daily, divided q 6 to 8 hours; or 10 mg/kg I.M. daily or divided q 12 hours; or 10 to 20 mg/kg I.V. daily, divided q 6 to 8 hours. For I.V. infusion, dilute to 100 ml; infuse over 1 hour to avoid hypotension.

ADVERSE REACTIONS
Blood: *neutropenia, leukopenia*, thrombocytopenia, purpura.
CNS: dizziness, headache.
CV: hypotension with rapid I.V. infu-

sion.
EENT: glossitis, tinnitus.
GI: nausea, vomiting, *pseudomembranous colitis, persistent diarrhea,* abdominal cramps, stomatitis, pruritus ani.
GU: vaginitis.
Hepatic: cholestatic jaundice.
Skin: rashes, urticaria.
Local: pain at injection site.
Other: hypersensitivity, angioedema.

INTERACTIONS
Antidiarrheal medication (kaolin, pectin, attapulgite): reduce oral absorption of lincomycin by as much as 90%. Antidiarrheals should be avoided or given at least 2 hours before lincomycin.

NURSING CONSIDERATIONS
• Contraindicated in patients with hypersensitivity to clindamycin. Use cautiously in GI disorders (especially colitis), asthma or significant allergies, hepatic or renal disease, and endocrine or metabolic disorders.
• Obtain specimen for culture and sensitivity tests before first dose. Therapy may begin pending test results.
• For best absorption, instruct patient to take drug with a full glass of water 1 hour before or 2 hours after meals.
• Tell patient to take medication exactly as directed, even after he feels better, and to take entire amount prescribed.
• Tell patient to report adverse reactions to doctor, especially diarrhea. Warn him not to treat diarrhea himself because it may reflect the onset of antibiotic associated pseudomembraneous colitis.
• Monitor for signs of bacterial and fungal superinfection, especially when therapy exceeds 10 days.
• Give deep I.M. Rotate sites. Warn that I.M. injection may be painful.
• When giving I.V., check site daily for phlebitis and irritation. Rotate infusion sites regularly.
• Rapid I.V. infusion may cause hypotension and syncope. Monitor blood pressure in patients receiving the drug parenterally.
• Monitor hepatic function (increased levels of alkaline phosphatase, AST (SGOT), ALT (SGPT), bilirubin may occur).
• Monitor CBC and platelets. Stop drug immediately if neutropenia, leukopenia, or other blood disorders develop.

pentamidine isethionate
Pentam 300
Pregnancy Risk Category: C

MECHANISM OF ACTION
Interferes with biosynthesis of DNA, RNA, phospholipids, and proteins in susceptible organisms.

INDICATIONS & DOSAGE
Treatment of pneumonia due to Pneumocystis carinii—
Adults and children: 4 mg/kg I.V. or I.M. once a day for 14 days.
Prevention of Pneumocystis carinii *pneumonia in high-risk individuals—*
Adults: 300 mg by inhalation (using a Respirgard II nebulizer) once every 4 weeks.

ADVERSE REACTIONS
Blood: *leukopenia,* thrombocytopenia, anemia.
CNS: confusion, hallucinations.
CV: *hypotension,* tachycardia.
Endocrine: *hypoglycemia,* hyperglycemia, hypocalcemia.
GI: nausea, anorexia, metallic taste.
GU: *elevated serum creatinine,* renal toxicity.
Hepatic: elevated liver enzymes.
Local: *sterile abscess, pain or induration at injection site.*
Skin: rash, facial flushing, pruritus.
Other: fever.

INTERACTIONS
None significant.

NURSING CONSIDERATIONS
• Once the diagnosis of *Pneumocystis carinii* pneumonia has been firmly established, there are no absolute contraindications to pentamidine therapy.
• Use cautiously in hypertension, hypotension, hypoglycemia, hypocalcemia, leukopenia, thrombocytopenia, anemia, and hepatic or renal dysfunction.
• Patient should be lying down when receiving the drug because sudden, severe hypotension may develop. Monitor blood pressure during administration and several times thereafter until blood pressure is stable.
• When administering I.V., infuse over 60 minutes to minimize risk of hypotension.
• Monitor blood glucose, serum creatinine, and BUN daily. After parenteral administration, blood glucose may decrease initially; hypoglycemia may be severe in 5% to 10% of patients. This may be followed by hyperglycemia and insulin-dependant diabetes mellitus (which may be permanent).
• Pain and induration occur universally with I.M. injection. Administer by deep I.M. injection.
• In patients with AIDS, pentamidine may produce less severe adverse reactions than the alternative treatment co-trimoxazole.Therefore, in some AIDS patients, pentamidine is considered the treatment of choice.

---

polymyxin B sulfate
Aerosporin♦

Pregnancy Risk Category: B

MECHANISM OF ACTION
Hinders bacterial cell wall synthesis, damaging the bacterial plasma membrane and making the cell more vulnerable to osmotic pressure.

INDICATIONS & DOSAGE
Acute urinary tract infections or septicemia caused by sensitive Pseudomonas aeruginosa, *or when other antibiotics are ineffective or contraindicated; bacteremia caused by sensitive* Enterobacter aerogenes *and* Klebsiella pneumoniae, *or acute urinary tract infections caused by* Escherichia coli—
Adults and children: 15,000 to 25,000 units/kg daily I.V. infusion, divided q 12 hours; or 25,000 to 30,000 units/kg daily, divided q 4 to 8 hours. I.M. not advised due to severe pain at injection site.
Meningitis caused by sensitive P. aeruginosa *or* Hemophilus influenzae *when other antibiotics ineffective or contraindicated—*
Adults and children over 2 years: 50,000 units intrathecally once daily for 3 to 4 days, then 50,000 units every other day for at least 2 weeks after cerebrospinal fluid tests are negative and cerebrospinal fluid sugar is normal.
Children under 2 years: 20,000 units intrathecally once daily for 3 to 4 days, then 25,000 units every other day for at least 2 weeks after cerebrospinal fluid tests are negative and cerebrospinal fluid sugar is normal.

ADVERSE REACTIONS
CNS: irritability, drowsiness, facial flushing, weakness, ataxia, respiratory paralysis, headache and meningeal irritation with intrathecal administration, peripheral and perioral paresthesias, seizures, *coma.*
EENT: blurred vision.
GU: *nephrotoxicity* (albuminuria, cylindruria, hematuria, proteinuria, decreased urine output, increased BUN).
Skin: urticaria.
Local: *pain at I.M. injection site.*
Other: hypersensitivity reactions with fever, *anaphylaxis.*

Italicized side effects are common or life-threatening.
*Liquid form contains alcohol.   **May contain tartrazine.

INTERACTIONS
None significant.

NURSING CONSIDERATIONS
• Use cautiously in impaired renal function or myasthenia gravis.
• Give only to hospitalized patients under constant medical supervision.
• For meningitis, must give intrathecally to achieve adequate cerebrospinal fluid levels.
• Give deep I.M. Warn that injection may be painful. If patient isn't allergic to procaine, use 1% procaine (if hospital policy permits) as diluent to decrease pain. Rotate sites.
• Don't give solution containing local anesthetics I.V. or intrathecally.
• When giving I.V., check site daily for phlebitis and irritation. Dilute each 500,000 units in 300 to 500 ml dextrose 5% in water; infuse over 60 to 90 minutes. Rotate I.V. sites regularly.
• Parenteral solutions should be refrigerated and used within 72 hours.
• Monitor renal function (BUN, serum creatinine, creatinine clearance, urine output) before and during therapy. Intake should be sufficient to maintain output at 1,500 ml/day (between 3,000 and 4,000 ml/day for adults).
• Obtain specimen for culture and sensitivity tests before first dose. Therapy may begin pending test results.
• Notify doctor immediately if patient develops fever, CNS adverse effects, rash, or symptoms of nephrotoxicity.
• If patient is scheduled for surgery, notify anesthesiologist of preoperative treatment with this drug since it may prolong neuromuscular blockade.

spectinomycin dihydrochloride
Trobicin♦

Pregnancy Risk Category: B

MECHANISM OF ACTION
Inhibits protein synthesis by binding to the 30S subunit of the ribosome.

INDICATIONS & DOSAGE
Gonorrhea—
Adults: 2 to 4 g I.M. single dose injected deeply into the upper outer quadrant of the buttock.

ADVERSE REACTIONS
CNS: insomnia, dizziness.
GI: nausea.
GU: decreased urine output.
Skin: urticaria.
Local: pain at injection site.
Other: fever, chills (may mask or delay symptoms of incubating syphilis).

INTERACTIONS
None significant.

NURSING CONSIDERATIONS
• Not effective in the treatment of syphilis.
• Serologic test for syphilis should be done before treatment dose and 3 months after.
• Use 20G needle to administer drug. The 4-g dose (10 ml) should be divided into two 5-ml injections—one in each buttock.
• Shake vial vigorously after reconstitution and before withdrawing dose. Store at room temperature after reconstitution and use within 24 hours.
• Should be reserved for penicillin-resistant strains of gonorrhea.

trimethoprim
Proloprim♦, Trimpex

Pregnancy Risk Category: C

MECHANISM OF ACTION
Interferes with the action of dihydrofolate reductase, inhibiting bacterial synthesis of folic acid.

INDICATIONS & DOSAGE
Treatment of uncomplicated urinary tract infections caused by susceptible strains of Escherichia coli, Proteus mirabilis, Klebsiella, *and* Enterobacter—
Adults: 100 mg P.O. every 12 hours for 10 days.
Not recommended for children under 12 years.

ADVERSE REACTIONS
Blood: thrombocytopenia, leukopenia, megaloblastic anemia, methemoglobinemia.
GI: *epigastric distress, nausea, vomiting,* glossitis.
Skin: *rash, pruritus, exfoliative dermatitis.*
Other: fever.

INTERACTIONS
None significant.

NURSING CONSIDERATIONS
• Contraindicated in documented megaloblastic anemia due to folate deficiency.
• Clinical signs such as sore throat, fever, pallor, or purpura may be early indications of serious blood disorders. Complete blood counts should be done routinely. Prolonged use of trimethoprim at high doses may cause bone marrow suppression.
• Dosage should be decreased in patients with severely impaired renal function. Give cautiously to patients with impaired hepatic function.
• Obtain specimen for culture and sensitivity tests before first dose.

Therapy may begin pending test results.
• Instruct patient to continue taking the drug, even if he feels better, and to take entire amount prescribed.

vancomycin hydrochloride
Vancocin♦

Pregnancy Risk Category: C

MECHANISM OF ACTION
Hinders bacterial cell wall synthesis, damaging the bacterial plasma membrane and making the cell more vulnerable to osmotic pressure.

INDICATIONS & DOSAGE
Severe staphylococcal infections when other antibiotics ineffective or contraindicated—
Adults: 500 mg I.V. q 6 hours, or l g q 12 hours.
Children: 44 mg/kg I.V. daily, divided q 6 hours.
Neonates: 10 mg/kg I.V. daily, divided q 6 to 12 hours.
Antibiotic-associated pseudomembranous and staphylococcal enterocolitis—
Adults: 125 to 500 mg P.O. q 6 hours for 7 to 10 days.
Children: 44 mg/kg P.O. daily, divided q 6 hours.
Endocarditis prophylaxis for dental procedures—
Adults: 1 g I.V. slowly over 1 hour, starting 1 hour before procedure. No repeat dose is necessary.

ADVERSE REACTIONS
Blood: transient eosinophilia, leukopenia.
EENT: tinnitus, ototoxicity (deafness).
GI: nausea.
Skin: "red-neck" syndrome (maculopapular rash on face, neck, trunk, and extremities).
Local: pain or thrombophlebitis with I.V. administration, necrosis.

Italicized side effects are common or life-threatening.
*Liquid form contains alcohol.   **May contain tartrazine.

Other: chills, fever, *anaphylaxis,* overgrowth of nonsusceptible organisms.

INTERACTIONS
None significant.

NURSING CONSIDERATIONS
• Use cautiously in patients receiving other neurotoxic, nephrotoxic, or ototoxic drugs. Use cautiously in impaired hepatic or renal function; also in those with preexisting hearing loss; in patients over 60 years; and in patients with allergies to other antibiotics. Patients with renal dysfunction require adjustment of dosage or dosing interval.
• Obtain specimen for culture and sensitivity tests before first dose. Therapy may begin pending test results.
• Tell patient to take medication exactly as directed, even after he feels better, and to take entire amount prescribed. Treat staphylococcal endocarditis for at least 4 weeks.
• Patients should receive auditory function tests before and during prolonged therapy.
• Tell patient to report adverse reactions at once, especially fullness or ringing in ears. Stop drug immediately if these occur.
• Do not give drug I.M.
• For I.V. infusion, dilute in 200 ml sodium chloride injection or 5% glucose solution and infuse over 60 minutes. Check site daily for phlebitis and irritation. Report pain at infusion site. Avoid extravasation. Severe irritation and necrosis can result.
• Monitor patient carefully for "redneck" syndrome. Stop infusion and notify doctor promptly if you see this reaction.
• Refrigerate I.V. solution after reconstitution and use within 96 hours.
• Monitor renal function (BUN, serum creatinine, urinalysis, creatinine clearance, and urine output) before and during therapy. Also monitor for signs of superinfection.
• Oral preparation stable for 2 weeks if refrigerated.

19

Cardiac glycosides, glycoside neutralizer, and amrinone

amrinone lactate
deslanoside
digitoxin
digoxin
digoxin immune FAB (ovine)

COMBINATION PRODUCTS
None.

---

amrinone lactate
Inocor♦

Pregnancy Risk Category: C

MECHANISM OF ACTION
Produces inotropic action by increasing cellular levels of cyclic adenosine monophosphate. Produces vasodilation through a direct relaxant effect on vascular smooth muscle.

INDICATIONS & DOSAGE
Short-term management of CHF—
Adults: initially, 0.75 mg/kg I.V. bolus over 2 to 3 minutes. Then begin maintenance infusion of 5 to 10 mcg/kg/minute. Additional bolus of 0.75 mg/kg may be given 30 minutes after start of therapy. Total daily dosage should not exceed 10 mg/kg.

ADVERSE REACTIONS
Blood: *thrombocytopenia* (dose dependent).
CV: *dysrhythmias,* hypotension.
GI: nausea, vomiting, cramps, dyspepsia, diarrhea.
Hepatic: elevated enzymes, possible hepatotoxicity.

Local: burning at site of injection.
Other: hypersensitivity.

INTERACTIONS
Digitalis glycosides: Enhanced inotropic effect. Beneficial drug interaction.
Disopyramide: excessive hypotension. Don't administer concurrently.

NURSING CONSIDERATIONS
• Don't use in severe aortic or pulmonic valvular disease. Use cautiously in idiopathic hypertrophic subaortic stenosis. Not recommended during acute phase of myocardial infarction.
• Dosage should be based on clinical response, including assessment of pulmonary artery pressures and cardiac output. Cardiovascular effects begin within 2 to 5 minutes after starting infusion, and may last for 30 minutes to 2 hours after infusion is discontinued.
• Amrinone may be added to digitalis glycoside therapy in atrial fibrillation and flutter since it enhances AV conduction and increases ventricular response rate.
• Amrinone should be administered with a continuous infusion pump.
• Monitor blood pressure and heart rate throughout the infusion. Slow or stop infusion and notify doctor if patient's blood pressure falls.
• Monitor platelet count. Platelet count below 150,000 mm^3 usually requires a decreased dosage.
• Administer amrinone as supplied, or dilute in normal or half-strength

---

Italicized side effects are common or life-threatening.
*Liquid form contains alcohol.   **May contain tartrazine.

normal saline solution to a concentration of 1 to 3 mg/ml. Use diluted solution within 24 hours. Don't mix other drugs into this solution.
• Furosemide will form a precipitate with amrinone solutions. Don't mix together.
• Don't dilute with solutions containing dextrose because a slow chemical reaction occurs over 24 hours. However, amrinone can be injected into running dextrose infusions through a Y connector or directly into the tubing.
• Amrinone is primarily prescribed for patients who have not responded to therapy with digitalis, diuretics, and vasodilators.

deslanoside
Cedilanid♦♦, Cedilanid-D

Pregnancy Risk Category: C

MECHANISM OF ACTION
Promotes movement of calcium from extracellular to intracellular cytoplasm and inhibits sodium-potassium activated adenosine triphosphatase. These actions strengthen myocardial contraction.

INDICATIONS & DOSAGE
CHF, paroxysmal atrial tachycardia, atrial fibrillation and flutter—
Adults: loading dose is 1.2 to 1.6 mg I.M. or slow I.V. in two divided doses over 24 hours; for maintenance, use another glycoside. Not recommended for children.

ADVERSE REACTIONS
The following are signs of toxicity that may occur with all cardiac glycosides:
CNS: *fatigue, generalized muscle weakness, agitation,* hallucinations, headache, malaise, dizziness, vertigo, stupor, paresthesias.
CV: *increased severity of CHF, dysrhythmias (most commonly conduction disturbances with or without AV block,*
premature ventricular contractions, and supraventricular dysrhythmias), hypotension.
   Toxic effects on heart may be life-threatening and require immediate attention.
EENT: *yellow-green halos around visual images, blurred vision,* light flashes, photophobia, diplopia.
GI: *anorexia, nausea,* vomiting, diarrhea.

INTERACTIONS
Amphotericin B, carbenicillin, ticarcillin, corticosteroids, and diuretics (including loop diuretics, chlorthalidone, metolazone, and thiazides): hypokalemia, predisposing patient to digitalis toxicity. Monitor serum potassium.
Parenteral calcium, thiazides: hypercalcemia and hypomagnesemia, predisposing patient to digitalis toxicity. Monitor serum calcium and serum magnesium.

NURSING CONSIDERATIONS
• Contraindicated in presence of any digitalis-induced toxicity; ventricular fibrillation; ventricular tachycardia unless caused by CHF. Administering calcium salts to digitalized patient is contraindicated. Calcium affects cardiac contractility and excitability in much the same way as glycosides and may lead to serious dysrhythmias in digitalized patient. Use with extreme caution in elderly patients, and in those with acute myocardial infarction, incomplete AV block, chronic constrictive pericarditis, idiopathic hypertrophic subaortic stenosis, renal insufficiency, severe pulmonary disease, or hypothyroidism.
• Use only for rapid digitilization, not maintenance therapy. Deslanoside has a low therapeutic index, and its dosage should be based upon patient response.
• Maintenance therapy with an oral digitalis glycoside is usually initiated

within 12 to 24 hours.
• Hypothyroid patients are sensitive to effects of glycosides; hyperthyroid patients may need larger doses.
• Obtain baseline data (heart rate and rhythm, blood pressure, and electrolytes) before giving first dose. Monitor ECG continuously.
• Question patient about recent use of cardiac glycosides (within the previous 2 to 3 weeks) before administering a loading dose. Always divide loading dose over first 24 hours unless clinical situation indicates otherwise.
• Dosage is adjusted to patient's clinical condition and is monitored by serum levels of cardiac glycoside, calcium, potassium, magnesium, and by ECG.
• Take apical-radial pulse for a full minute. Record and report to doctor any significant changes (sudden increase or decrease in rate, pulse deficit, irregular beats, and particularly regularization of a previously irregular rhythm). Check blood pressure and obtain 12-lead ECG with these changes.
• Excessive slowing of the pulse rate (60 beats/minute or less) may be a sign of digitalis toxicity. Withhold drug and notify doctor.
• Observe eating patterns. Ask patient about nausea, vomiting, anorexia, visual disturbances, and other symptoms of toxicity.
• I.M. injection is painful; give I.V. if possible. I.V. administration also provides for a more rapid effect.
• Monitor serum potassium carefully. Take corrective action *before* hypokalemia occurs.

digitoxin
Crystodigin
Pregnancy Risk Category: C

MECHANISM OF ACTION
Promotes movement of calcium from extracellular to intracellular cytoplasm and inhibits sodium-potassium activated adenosine triphosphatase. These actions strengthen myocardial contraction.

INDICATIONS & DOSAGE
CHF, paroxysmal atrial tachycardia, atrial fibrillation and flutter—
Adults: loading dose is 1.2 to 1.6 mg I.V. or P.O. in divided doses over 24 hours; average maintenance dosage is 0.15 mg daily (range: 0.05 to 0.3 mg daily).
Children 2 to 12 years: loading dose is 0.03 mg/kg or 0.75 mg/m² I.M., I.V., or P.O. in divided doses over 24 hours; maintenance dosage is one-tenth of loading dose or 0.003 mg/kg or 0.075 mg/m² daily. Monitor closely for toxicity.
Children 1 to 2 years: loading dose is 0.04 mg/kg over 24 hours in divided doses; maintenance dosage is 0.004 mg/kg daily. Monitor closely for toxicity.
Children 2 weeks to 1 year: loading dose is 0.045 mg/kg I.M., I.V., or P.O. in divided doses over 24 hours; maintenance dosage is 0.0045 mg/kg daily. Monitor closely for toxicity.
Premature infants, neonates, severely ill older infants: loading dose is 0.022 mg/kg I.M., I.V., or P.O. in divided doses over 24 hours; maintenance dosage is 0.0022 mg/kg daily. Monitor closely for toxicity.

ADVERSE REACTIONS
The following are signs of toxicity that may occur with all cardiac glycosides:
CNS: *fatigue, generalized muscle weakness, agitation, hallucinations,* headache, malaise, dizziness, vertigo, stupor, paresthesias.
CV: *increased severity of CHF, dysrhythmias (most commonly conduction disturbances with or without AV block, premature ventricular contractions, and supraventricular dysrhythmias),* hypotension.
Toxic effects on heart may be life-

threatening and require immediate attention.
EENT: *yellow-green halos around visual images, blurred vision,* light flashes, photophobia, diplopia.
GI: *anorexia, nausea,* vomiting, diarrhea.

INTERACTIONS

Antacids, kaolin-pectin: decreased absorption of oral digitoxin. Schedule doses as far as possible from oral digitoxin administration.
Cholestyramine, colestipol, metoclopramide: decreased absorption of oral digitoxin. Monitor for decreased effect and low blood levels. Dosage may have to be increased.
Amphotericin B, carbenicillin, ticarcillin, corticosteroids, and diuretics (including loop diuretics, chlorthalidone, metolazone, and thiazides): hypokalemia, predisposing patient to digitalis toxicity. Monitor serum potassium.
Parenteral calcium, thiazides: hypercalcemia and hypomagnesemia, predisposing patient to digitalis toxicity. Monitor serum calcium and serum magnesium.
Phenylbutazone, phenobarbital, phenytoin, rifampin: faster metabolism and shorter duration of digitoxin. Observe for underdigitalization.
Cimetidine: decreased digitoxin metabolism. Monitor for digitoxin toxicity.
Quinidine, verapamil: Possible increased serum digitoxin levels. Monitor patient closely.

NURSING CONSIDERATIONS

• Contraindicated in presence of any digitalis-induced toxicity; ventricular fibrillation; ventricular tachycardia unless caused by CHF. Administering calcium salts to digitalized patient is contraindicated. Calcium affects cardiac contractility and excitability in much the same way as glycosides and may lead to serious dysrhythmias in digitalized patient. Use with extreme caution in acute myocardial infarction, incomplete AV block, chronic constrictive pericarditis, idiopathic hypertrophic subaortic stenosis, severe pulmonary disease, and hypothyroidism; and in elderly patients.
• Hypothyroid patients are very sensitive to glycosides; hyperthyroid patients may need larger doses.
• Obtain baseline data (heart rate and rhythm, blood pressure, and electrolytes) and question patient about recent use of cardiac glycosides (within the previous 2 to 3 weeks) before administering a loading dose. Always divide loading dose over first 24 hours unless clinical situation indicates otherwise.
• Dosage is adjusted to patient's clinical condition and is monitored by serum levels of cardiac glycoside, calcium, potassium, magnesium, and by ECG.
• Take apical-radial pulse for a full minute. Record and report to doctor any significant changes (sudden increase or decrease in rate, pulse deficit, irregular beats, and particularly regularization of a previously irregular rhythm). Check blood pressure and obtain 12-lead ECG with these changes.
• Excessive slowing of the pulse rate (60 beats/minute or less) may be a sign of digitalis toxicity. Withhold drug and notify doctor.
• Monitor serum potassium carefully. Take corrective action *before* hypokalemia occurs.
• Encourage the patient to eat potassium-rich foods.
• I.M. injection is painful and poorly absorbed; give I.V. if parenteral route is necessary.
• Digitoxin is a long-acting drug; watch for cumulative effects and signs of toxicity, especially in children and elderly patients. Ask patient about nausea, vomiting, anorexia, visual disturbances, and other symptoms of

toxicity.
- Protect solution from light.
- Instruct patient and responsible family member about drug action, dosage regimen, how to take pulse, reportable signs, and follow-up plans.
- Don't substitute one brand for another.
- Therapeutic blood levels of digitoxin range from 25 to 35 ng/ml.
- Digitoxin toxicity may be treated by administering agents that bind the drug in the intestine (for example, colestipol and cholestyramine). Dysrhythmias may be treated with phenytoin I.V. Potentially life-threatening toxicity may be treated by specific antigen-binding fragments (such as digoxin immune FAB).

---

digoxin
Lanoxicaps, Lanoxin♦*,
Novodigoxin♦♦

Pregnancy Risk Category: C

MECHANISM OF ACTION
Promotes movement of calcium from extracellular to intracellular cytoplasm and inhibits sodium-potassium activated adenosine triphosphatase. These actions strengthen myocardial contraction.

INDICATIONS & DOSAGE
CHF, paroxysmal atrial tachycardia, atrial fibrillation and flutter—
Adults: loading dose is 0.5 to 1 mg I.V. or P.O. in divided doses over 24 hours; maintenance dosage is 0.125 to 0.5 mg I.V. or P.O. daily (average 0.25 mg). Larger doses are often needed for treatment of dysrhythmias, depending on patient response. Smaller loading and maintenance doses should be given in patients with impaired renal function.
Adults over 65 years: 0.125 mg P.O. daily as maintenance dose. Frail or underweight elderly patients may require only 0.0625 mg daily or 0.125

mg every other day.
Children over 2 years: loading dose is 0.02 to 0.04 mg/kg P.O. divided q 8 hours over 24 hours; I.V. loading dose is 0.015 to 0.035 mg/kg; maintenance dosage is 0.012 mg/kg P.O. daily divided q 12 hours.
Children 1 month to 2 years: loading dose is 0.035 to 0.060 mg/kg P.O. in three divided doses over 24 hours; I.V. loading dose is 0.03 to 0.05 mg/kg; maintenance dosage is 0.01 to 0.02 mg/kg P.O. daily divided q 12 hours.
Neonates under 1 month: loading dose is 0.035 mg/kg P.O. divided q 8 hours over 24 hours; I.V. loading dose is 0.02 to 0.03 mg/kg; maintenance dosage is 0.01 mg/kg P.O. daily divided q 12 hours.
Premature infants: loading dose is 0.025 mg/kg I.V. in three divided doses over 24 hours; maintenance dosage is 0.01 mg/kg I.V. daily divided q 12 hours.

ADVERSE REACTIONS
The following are signs of toxicity that may occur with all cardiac glycosides:
CNS: *fatigue, generalized muscle weakness, agitation, hallucinations,* headache, malaise, dizziness, vertigo, stupor, paresthesias.
CV: *increased severity of CHF, dysrhythmias (most commonly conduction disturbances with or without AV block, premature ventricular contractions, and supraventricular dysrhythmias),* hypotension.
  Toxic effects on heart may be lifethreatening and require immediate attention.
EENT: *yellow-green halos around visual images, blurred vision,* light flashes, photophobia, diplopia.
GI: *anorexia, nausea,* vomiting, diarrhea.

INTERACTIONS
Antacids, kaolin-pectin: decreased absorption of oral digoxin. Schedule

---

Italicized side effects are common or life-threatening.
*Liquid form contains alcohol.   **May contain tartrazine.

doses as far as possible from oral digoxin administration.

Cholestyramine, colestipol, metoclopramide: decreased absorption of oral digoxin. Monitor for decreased effect and low blood levels. Dosage may have to be increased.

Quinidine, diltiazem, amiodarone, nifedipine, verapamil: increased digoxin blood levels. Monitor for toxicity.

Amphotericin B, carbenicillin, ticarcillin, corticosteroids, and diuretics (including loop diuretics, chlorthalidone, metolazone, and thiazides): hypokalemia, predisposing patient to digitalis toxicity. Monitor serum potassium.

Parenteral calcium, thiazides: hypercalcemia and hypomagnesemia, predisposing patient to digitalis toxicity. Monitor serum calcium and serum magnesium.

Anticholinergics: may increase digoxin absorption of oral tablets. Monitor blood levels and observe for toxicity.

Amiloride: inhibits and increases digoxin excretion. Monitor for altered digoxin effect.

NURSING CONSIDERATIONS

• Contraindicated in presence of any digitalis-induced toxicity; ventricular fibrillation; ventricular tachycardia unless caused by CHF. Administering calcium salts to digitalized patient is contraindicated. Calcium affects cardiac contractility and excitability in much the same way as glycosides and may lead to serious dysrhythmias in digitalized patient. Use with extreme caution in elderly patients, and in those with acute myocardial infarction, incomplete AV block, chronic constrictive pericarditis, idiopathic hypertrophic subaortic stenosis, renal insufficiency, severe pulmonary disease, or hypothyroidism. Dosage must be reduced in renal impairment.

• Infuse I.V. dose slowly over at least 5 minutes.

• Hypothyroid patients are very sensitive to glycosides; hyperthyroid patients may need larger doses.

• Obtain baseline data (heart rate and rhythm, blood pressure, and electrolytes) before giving first dose.

• Question patient about recent use of cardiac glycosides (within the previous 2 to 3 weeks) before administering a loading dose. Always divide loading dose over first 24 hours unless clinical situation indicates otherwise.

• Dose is adjusted to patient's clinical condition and is monitored by serum levels of cardiac glycoside, calcium, potassium, magnesium, and by ECG. Obtain blood for digoxin levels 8 hours after last P.O. dose.

• Take apical-radial pulse for a full minute. Record and report to doctor any significant changes (sudden increase or decrease in rate, pulse deficit, irregular beats, and particularly regularization of a previously irregular rhythm). Check blood pressure and obtain 12-lead ECG with these changes.

• Excessive slowing of the pulse rate (60 beats/minute or less) may be a sign of digitalis toxicity. Withhold drug and notify doctor.

• Observe eating patterns. Ask patient about nausea, vomiting, anorexia, visual disturbances, and other symptoms of toxicity.

• Monitor serum potassium carefully. Take corrective action *before* hypokalemia occurs. Encourage patient to eat potassium-rich foods.

• Withhold drug for 1 to 2 days before elective electrocardioversion. Adjust dose after cardioversion.

• Instruct patient and responsible family member about drug action, dosage regimen, how to take pulse, reportable signs, and follow-up plans.

• Don't substitute one brand for another.

• When changing from oral tablets or elixir to parenteral therapy, dosage should be reduced by 20% to 25%.

When changing from liquid-filled capsules to parenteral therapy, dosage is about equivalent because absorption is best using liquid-filled capsules. Therefore, when changing from oral tablets or elixir to liquid-filled capsules, reduce dose by 20% to 25%.
• Therapeutic blood levels of digoxin range from 0.5 to 2.0 ng/ml.

digoxin immune FAB (ovine)
Digibind

Pregnancy Risk Category: C

MECHANISM OF ACTION
Binds molecules of digoxin and digitoxin, making them unavailable for binding at site of action on cells in the body.

INDICATIONS & DOSAGE
Treatment of potentially life-threatening digoxin or digitoxin intoxication—
Adults and children: administered I.V. over 30 minutes or as a bolus if cardiac arrest is imminent. The dosage varies according to the amount of digoxin or digitoxin to be neutralized. Average dosage is 10 vials (400 mg). However, if the toxicity resulted from acute digoxin ingestion, and neither a serum digoxin level nor an estimated ingestion amount is known, 20 vials (800 mg) should be administered. See package insert for complete, specific dosage instructions.

ADVERSE REACTIONS
CV: CHF, rapid ventricular rate (both caused by reversal of the cardiac glycoside's therapeutic effects).
Metabolic: hypokalemia.
Other: *hypersensitivity*.

INTERACTIONS
None reported.

NURSING CONSIDERATIONS
• Since digoxin immune FAB is de-

rived from digoxin-specific antibody fragments obtained from immunized sheep, use cautiously in persons known to be allergic to ovine proteins. In these high-risk patients, skin testing is recommended. A limited supply of this drug is available at major medical centers or from the manufacturer (call 1-800-334-4828 or, in North Carolina, 1-800-672-7223).
• This antidote should be used only for life-threatening overdose in patients in shock or cardiac arrest; with ventricular dysrhythmias, such as ventricular tachycardia or fibrillation; with progressive bradycardia, such as severe sinus bradycardia; or with second- or third-degree AV block not responsive to atropine.
• Monitor potassium closely.
• In most patients, signs of digitalis toxicity disappear within a few hours.
• Best to infuse this drug through a 0.22-mcm membrane filter. However, give by bolus injection if cardiac arrest is considered imminent.
• Refrigerate powder for reconstitution. Reconstituted product should be used immediately, but it may be stored for up to 4 hours in the refrigerator.
• Digoxin immune FAB will interfere with digitalis immunoassay measurements, so standard serum digoxin levels will be misleading until the drug is cleared from the body (about 2 days).
• Total serum digoxin levels may rise after administration of this drug, but this reflects FAB-bound (inactive) digoxin.

Italicized side effects are common or life-threatening.
*Liquid form contains alcohol.   **May contain tartrazine.

20

Antiarrhythmics

amiodarone hydrochloride
atropine sulfate
bretylium tosylate
disopyramide
disopyramide phosphate
encainide hydrochloride
esmolol hydrochloride
flecainide acetate
lidocaine hydrochloride
  (lignocaine hydrochloride)
mexiletine hydrochloride
phenytoin
  (See Chapter 30, ANTICONVULSANTS.)
phenytoin sodium
  (See Chapter 30, ANTICONVULSANTS.)
procainamide hydrochloride
propranolol hydrochloride
  (See Chapter 21, ANTIANGINALS.)
quinidine gluconate
quinidine polygalacturonate
quinidine sulfate
tocainide hydrochloride

COMBINATION PRODUCTS
None.

---

amiodarone hydrochloride
Cordarone ♦

Pregnancy Risk Category: C

MECHANISM OF ACTION
A Group III antiarrhythmic that prolongs the refractory period and action
potential duration and decreases repolarization.

INDICATIONS & DOSAGE
*Ventricular and supraventricular dys-
rhythmias, including recurrent supraventricular tachycardia (Wolff-Parkin-*
*son-White syndrome), atrial fibrilla-
tion and flutter, and ventricular tachycardia refractory to other antiarrhythmics—*
Adults: loading dose is 5 to 10 mg/kg
by I.V. infusion via central line, followed by I.V. infusion of 10 mg/kg/
day for 3 to 5 days. (*Note:* I.V. use of
amiodarone is investigational.) Or,
give loading dose of 800 to 1,600 mg
P.O. daily for 1 to 3 weeks until initial
therapeutic response occurs. Maintenance dosage is 200 to 600 mg P.O.
daily.

ADVERSE REACTIONS
CNS: peripheral neuropathy, extrapy-
ramidal symptoms, headache, *mal-
aise, fatigue.*
CV: bradycardia, hypotension, *dys-
rhythmias, CHF.*
EENT: *corneal microdeposits,* visual
disturbances.
Endocrine: hypothyroidism, hyper-
thyroidism, gynecomastia.
GI: *nausea, vomiting,* constipation.
Hepatic: *altered liver enzymes,* he-
patic dysfunction.
Respiratory: *severe pulmonary toxic-
ity (pneumonitis/alveolitis).*
Skin: *photosensitivity,* blue-gray skin
pigmentation.
Other: muscle weakness.

INTERACTIONS
Antihypertensives: increased hypotensive effect. Use together cautiously.
*Beta blockers, calcium channel block-
ers:* increased cardiac depressant effects. Use together cautiously.
Warfarin: increased anticoagulant ef-

---

fect. Monitor patient closely.

NURSING CONSIDERATIONS
• Use cautiously in preexisting brady-cardia or sinus node disease; conduction disturbances; severely depressed ventricular function; and marked cardiomegaly. Use cautiously (if at all) in patients receiving Class I antiarrhythmics.
• Amiodarone is often effective for treatment of dysrhythmias resistant to other drug therapy. However, large incidence of side effects limits its use.
• Most patients treated show corneal microdeposits upon slit-lamp ophthalmologic examination. Onset of this effect from 1 to 4 months after beginning amiodarone therapy. However, only 2% to 3% have actual visual disturbances. To minimize this complication, recommend instillation of methylcellulose ophthalmic solution during amiodarone therapy.
• Monitor carefully for pulmonary toxicity, which can be fatal. Incidence increases in patients receiving more than 400 mg/day.
• Monitor for symptoms of pneumonitis—exertional dyspnea, nonproductive cough, and pleuritic chest pain. Monitor pulmonary function tests and chest X-ray.
• Monitor blood pressure and heart rate and rhythm frequently. Continuous ECG monitoring should be performed during initiation and alteration of dosage. Notify doctor of any significant change.
• Monitor hepatic and thyroid function tests. Monitor serum electrolytes, particularly potassium and magnesium levels.
• Divide oral loading dose into three equal doses and give with meals to decrease GI intolerance. Maintenance dosage may be given once daily, but may be divided into two doses taken with meals if GI intolerance occurs.
• Advise patient to use a sunscreen to prevent photosensitivity. Monitor for

burning or tingling skin followed by erythema and possible skin blistering.
• Amiodarone's adverse effects are more prevalent at high doses but are generally reversible when drug therapy is stopped. Resolution of adverse reactions may take up to 4 months.

---

atropine sulfate
Pregnancy Risk Category: C

MECHANISM OF ACTION
An anticholinergic, it inhibits acetylcholine at the parasympathetic neuroeffector junction, blocking vagal effects on the sinoatrial node; this enhances conduction through the AV node and speeds heart rate.

INDICATIONS & DOSAGE
Symptomatic bradycardia, bradydysrhythmia (junctional or escape rhythm)—
Adults: usually 0.5 to 1 mg I.V. push; repeat q 5 minutes, to maximum of 2 mg. Lower doses (less than 0.5 mg) can cause bradycardia.
Children: 0.01 mg/kg dose up to maximum of 0.4 mg; or 0.3 mg/m² dose; may repeat q 4 to 6 hours.
Antidote for anticholinesterase insecticide poisoning—
Adults and children: 2 mg I.M. or I.V. repeated hourly until muscarinic symptoms disappear. Severe cases may require up to 6 mg I.M. or I.V. q 1 hour.
Preoperatively for diminishing secretions and blocking cardiac vagal reflexes—
Adults: 0.4 to 0.6 mg I.M. 45 to 60 minutes before anesthesia.
Children: 0.01 mg/kg I.M. up to a maximum dose of 0.4 mg 45 to 60 minutes before anesthesia.

ADVERSE REACTIONS
Blood: leukocytosis.
CNS: *headache, restlessness,* ataxia, disorientation, hallucinations, delir-

ium, coma, *insomnia, dizziness;* excitement, agitation, and confusion (especially in elderly patients).
CV: 1 to 2 mg—*tachycardia, palpitations; greater than 2 mg—extreme tachycardia, angina.*
EENT: 1 mg—*slight mydriasis,* photophobia; 2 mg—*blurred vision, mydriasis.*
GI: *dry mouth (common even at low doses),* thirst, *constipation,* nausea, vomiting.
GU: urine retention.
Skin: hot, flushed skin.

INTERACTIONS
Methotrimeprazine: may produce extrapyramidal symptoms. Monitor patient carefully.

NURSING CONSIDERATIONS
• Contraindicated in narrow-angle glaucoma, obstructive uropathy, obstructive disease of GI tract, myasthenia gravis, paralytic ileus, intestinal atony, unstable cardiovascular status in acute hemorrhage, and toxic megacolon.
• Adverse reactions vary considerably with dose. Most common is dry mouth.
• Many of the adverse effects (such as dry mouth and constipation) are an extension of the drug's pharmacologic activity and may be expected.
• Watch for tachycardia in cardiac patients.
• Antidote for atropine overdose is physostigmine salicylate.
• Other anticholinergic drugs may increase vagal blockage.
• When given I.V., may cause paradoxical initial bradycardia. Usually disappears within 2 minutes.
• Monitor intake/output. Drug causes urine retention and urinary hesitancy; have patient void before receiving the drug.
• Monitor closely for urine retention in elderly men with benign prostatic hypertrophy.

bretylium tosylate
Bretylate♦♦, Bretylol
Pregnancy Risk Category: C

MECHANISM OF ACTION
A Group III antiarrhythmic that initially exerts transient adrenergic stimulation through release of norepinephrine. Subsequent depletion of norepinephrine causes adrenergic blocking actions to predominate. Repolarization is prolonged; duration of action potential and effective refractory period are increased.

INDICATIONS & DOSAGE
Ventricular fibrillation—
Adults: 5 mg/kg by I.V. push over 1 minute. If necessary, increase dose to 10 mg/kg and repeat q 15 to 30 minutes until 30 mg/kg have been given.
Other ventricular dysrhythmias—
Adults: initially, 500 mg diluted to 50 ml with dextrose 5% in water or normal saline solution and infused I.V. over more than 8 minutes at 5 to 10 mg/kg. Dose may be repeated in 1 to 2 hours. Thereafter, repeat q 6 to 8 hours.
I.V. maintenance—
Adults: infused in diluted solution of 500 ml dextrose 5% in water or normal saline solution at 1 to 2 mg/minute.
I.M. injection—
Adults: 5 to 10 mg/kg undiluted. Repeat in 1 to 2 hours if needed. Thereafter, repeat q 6 to 8 hours.
  Not recommended for children.

ADVERSE REACTIONS
CNS: *vertigo, dizziness, lightheadedness, syncope* (usually secondary to hypotension).
CV: *severe hypotension (especially orthostatic), bradycardia,* anginal pain, transient dysrhythmias.
GI: severe nausea, vomiting (with rapid infusion).

INTERACTIONS

All antihypertensives: may potentiate hypotension. Monitor blood pressure. *Other antiarrhythmics:* additive or antagonistic antiarrhythmic effects. Monitor for additive toxicity.

NURSING CONSIDERATIONS

• There are no contraindications to the use of bretylium in the treatment of ventricular fibrillation or life-threatening dysrhythmias; however, patients who are hypersensitive to corn or corn products should not receive the commercially available preparation mixed in dextrose 5% in water.

• Use cautiously in patients with fixed cardiac output, aortic stenosis, and pulmonary hypertension to avoid severe and sudden drop in blood pressure.

• Avoid initiating bretylium therapy concomitantly with digitalis glycoside therapy. Do not use in digitalized patients unless the dysrhythmia is life-threatening, not caused by digitalis, and is unresponsive to other drugs.

• Monitor blood pressure and heart rate and rhythm continuously. Notify doctor immediately of any significant change. If supine systolic blood pressure falls below 75 mm Hg, notify doctor; he may order norepinephrine, dopamine, or volume expanders to raise blood pressure.

• The initial release of norepinephrine caused by bretylium may induce transient hypertension and dysrhythmias. Monitor patient closely.

• Keep patient in the supine position until tolerance to hypotension develops. Tell patient to avoid sudden postural changes.

• Follow dosage directions carefully to avoid nausea and vomiting.

• Rotate I.M. injection sites to prevent tissue damage, and don't exceed 3-ml volume in any one site.

• To be used with other cardiopulmonary resuscitative measures, such as CPR, countershock, epinephrine, sodium bicarbonate, and lidocaine.

• Avoid subtherapeutic doses (less than 5 mg/kg), because such doses may cause hypotension.

• Ventricular tachycardia and other ventricular dysrhythmias respond less rapidly to treatment than ventricular fibrillation.

• Dosage should be decreased in renal impairment.

• Monitor carefully if pressor amines (sympathomimetics) are given to correct hypotension, because bretylium potentiates pressor amines.

• Ineffective treatment for atrial dysrhythmias.

• Has been used investigationally to treat hypertension.

• Observe for increased anginal pain in susceptible patients.

• Observe patient for adverse reactions and notify doctor if any occur.

---

disopyramide
Rythmodan♦♦

disopyramide phosphate
Norpace♦, Norpace CR♦

Pregnancy Risk Category: C

MECHANISM OF ACTION

A Class Ia antiarrhythmic that depresses phase O. It prolongs the action potential. All Class I drugs have membrane stabilizing effects.

INDICATIONS & DOSAGE

Premature ventricular contractions (unifocal, multifocal, or coupled); ventricular tachycardia not severe enough to require electrocardioversion—

Adults: Usual maintenance dosage 150 to 200 mg P.O. q 6 hours; for patients who weigh less than 50 kg or those with renal, hepatic, or cardiac impairment—100 mg P.O. q 6 hours. May give sustained-release capsule q 12 hours. Recommended dosages in

---

Italicized side effects are common or life-threatening.
*Liquid form contains alcohol.   **May contain tartrazine.

advanced renal insufficiency: creatinine clearance 15 to 40 ml/minute—100 mg q 10 hours; creatinine clearance 5 to 15 ml/minute—100 mg q 20 hours; creatinine clearance 1 to 5 ml/minute—100 mg q 30 hours.
Children 12 to 18 years: 6 to 15 mg/kg daily.
Children 4 to 12 years: 10 to 15 mg/kg daily.
Children 1 to 4 years: 10 to 20 mg/kg daily.
Children less than 1 year: 10 to 30 mg/kg daily.

All children's dosages should be divided into equal amounts and given q 6 hours.

ADVERSE REACTIONS
CNS: dizziness, agitation, depression, fatigue, muscle weakness, syncope.
CV: *hypotension, CHF, heart block, edema, weight gain, dysrhythmias.*
EENT: *blurred vision, dry eyes, dry nose.*
GI: nausea, vomiting, anorexia, bloating, abdominal pain, *constipation, dry mouth.*
GU: urine retention and urinary hesitancy.
Hepatic: cholestatic jaundice.
Metabolic: hypoglycemia.
Skin: rash in 1% to 3% of patients.

INTERACTIONS
Phenytoin: increases disopyramide's metabolism. Monitor for decreased antiarrhythmic effect.

NURSING CONSIDERATIONS
• Contraindicated in cardiogenic shock or second- or third-degree heart block with no pacemaker. Use very cautiously, and avoid, if possible, in CHF. Use cautiously in underlying conduction abnormalities, urinary tract diseases (especially prostatic hypertrophy), hepatic or renal impairment, myasthenia gravis, or narrow-angle glaucoma. Adjust dosage in renal insufficiency.
• Don't give sustained-release capsule for rapid control of ventricular dysrhythmias; when therapeutic blood levels must be rapidly attained; in cardiomyopathy or possible cardiac decompensation; or in severe renal impairment.
• When transferring patient from immediate-release to sustained-release capsules, advise him to begin a sustained-release capsule 6 hours after the last immediate-release capsule was taken.
• Discontinue if heart block develops, if QRS complex widens by more than 25%, or if Q-T interval lengthens by more than 25% above baseline.
• Correct any underlying electrolyte abnormalities before use.
• Watch for recurrence of dysrhythmias and check for adverse reactions; notify doctor if any occur.
• Check apical pulse before administering drug. Notify doctor if pulse rate is slower than 60 beats/minute or faster than 120 beats/minute.
• Teach patient the importance of taking drug on time, exactly as prescribed. To do this, he may have to use an alarm clock for night doses.
• Relieve discomfort of dry mouth by chewing gum or hard candy.
• Manage constipation with proper diet or bulk laxatives.
• Use of disopyramide with other antiarrhythmics may cause further myocardial depression.
• Most doctors prefer to prescribe disopyramide for patients not in heart failure who can't tolerate quinidine or procainamide.
• Pharmacist may prepare disopyramide suspension from 100-mg capsules using cherry syrup. Protect suspension from light. It should be dispensed in amber glass bottles. May be best for young children.

encainide hydrochloride
Enkaid

Pregnancy Risk Category: C

MECHANISM OF ACTION
A Class Ic antiarrhythmic that depresses phase O and fast sodium channel activity. Unlike Class Ia and Ib agents, it does not prolong or shorten the action potential. All Class I drugs have membrane-stabilizing effects.

INDICATIONS & DOSAGE
Treatment of life-threatening ventricular dysrhythmias, such as sustained ventricular tachycardia—
Adults: initially, 25 mg P.O. t.i.d. at approximately 8-hour intervals. After 3 to 5 days, dosage may be increased to 35 mg t.i.d. if necessary. After an additional 3 to 5 days, dosage may be increased to 50 mg t.i.d. Maximum daily dosage is 75 mg q.i.d.

ADVERSE REACTIONS
CNS: *dizziness, blurred vision, insomnia, headache,* tremor.
CV: *new or worsened dysrhythmias,* palpitations, edema, *chest pains, cardiac arrest.*
GI: dry mouth, constipation, nausea, vomiting.
Other: dyspnea, weakness.

INTERACTIONS
Cimetidine: may increase encainide blood levels. Use together cautiously.

NURSING CONSIDERATIONS
• Contraindicated in preexisting second- or third-degree AV block or right bundle branch block when associated with a left hemiblock, unless a pacemaker is present; in cardiogenic shock and severe hypokalemia.
• Findings from the Cardiac Arrhythmia Suppression Trial (CAST) include a greater-than-twofold increase in the number of deaths and nonfatal cardiac arrest in patients treated with encain-
ide. Therefore, it should be used only in immediately life-threatening dysrhythmias.
• Patients with a history of sustained ventricular tachycardia or fibrillation taking more than 200 mg daily may be at a higher risk of developing new or worsened dysrhythmias, especially during the first week of therapy.
• Use cautiously in cardiomyopathy or sick sinus syndrome.
• Patients who receive encainide dosage of 200 mg/day or more should be hospitalized.
• Encainide may induce several ECG changes, including prolonged PR and QRS intervals; however, ECG changes are not good predictors of effectiveness, overdose, or toxicity.
• Allowing at least 3 days to adjust to the dosage before increasing it significantly reduces the risk of proarrhythmia. Warn patient of the risk of increasing his own encainide dosage.
• Some patients who are well controlled on 50 mg t.i.d. or less may be treated as effectively with a 12-hour dosage schedule to ease compliance. Discuss this possibility with the doctor.

esmolol hydrochloride
Brevibloc

Pregnancy Risk Category: C

MECHANISM OF ACTION
Ultrashort-acting beta-adrenergic blocking agent. Decreases heart rate and blood pressure.

INDICATIONS & DOSAGE
Supraventricular tachycardia—
Adults: loading dose is 500 mcg/kg/minute by I.V. infusion over 1 minute, followed by a 4-minute maintenance infusion of 50 mcg/kg/minute. If adequate response does not occur within 5 minutes, repeat the loading dose followed by a maintenance infusion of 100 mcg/kg/minute. Maximum main-

tenance infusion is 200 mcg/kg/min-ute.

ADVERSE REACTIONS
CNS: dizziness, somnolence, head-ache, agitation, fatigue.
CV: *hypotension* (sometimes with diaphoresis).
GI: *nausea,* vomiting.
Local: inflammation and induration at infusion site.
Other: bronchospasm.

INTERACTIONS
Morphine: may increase esmolol blood levels. Titrate esmolol care-fully.
Reserpine (and other catecholamine-depleting drugs): may cause additive bradycardia and hypotension. Titrate esmolol carefully.

NURSING CONSIDERATIONS
• Contraindicated in sinus bradycar-dia, heart block greater than first de-gree, cardiogenic shock, or overt heart failure.
• Use cautiously in impaired renal function, diabetes, or bronchospasm.
• Monitor continuous ECG and blood pressure during infusion. Up to 50% of all patients treated with esmolol develop hypotension. Monitor closely, especially if patient's pretreatment blood pressure was low.
• Hypotension can usually be re-versed within 30 minutes by decreas-ing the dose or, if necessary, by stop-ping the infusion.
• Esmolol is recommended only for short-term use, no longer than 48 hours.
• If a local reaction develops at the infusion site, change to another site. Avoid butterfly needles.
• Don't give esmolol by I.V. push; use a controlled infusion device. Drug must be diluted before infusion.
• Esmolol solutions are incompatible with diazepam, furosemide, sodium bicarbonate, and thiopental sodium.

• When patient's heart rate becomes stable, esmolol will be replaced by al-ternative (longer-acting) antiarrhyth-mics, such as propranolol, digoxin, or verapamil. As the replacement drug is started, the esmolol infusion should be gradually reduced over 1 hour.
• Esmolol has an ultrashort duration of action and can be accurately ti-trated. Therefore, it has advantages over other beta blockers in treating cardiac dysrhythmias.

flecainide acetate
Tambocor◆

Pregnancy Risk Category: C

MECHANISM OF ACTION
A Class Ic antiarrhythmic that de-presses phase O. Unlike Class Ia and Ib agents, however, it does not pro-long or shorten the action potential. All Class I drugs have membrane sta-bilizing effects.

INDICATIONS & DOSAGE
Treatment of life-threatening ventricu-lar dysrhythmias, such as sustained ventricular tachycardia—
Adults: 100 mg P.O. q 12 hours. May be increased in increments of 50 mg b.i.d. q 4 days until efficacy is achieved. Maximum dosage is 400 mg daily for most patients.

ADVERSE REACTIONS
CNS: *dizziness, headache,* fatigue, tremor.
CV: *new or worsened dysrhythmias,* chest pain, *CHF, cardiac arrest.*
EENT: *blurred vision and other vi-sual disturbances.*
GI: nausea, constipation, abdominal pain.
Other: *dyspnea,* edema.

INTERACTIONS
Amiodarone, cimetidine, digoxin, propranolol: altered pharmacokinet-ics. Monitor for toxicity.

NURSING CONSIDERATIONS

• Contraindicated in preexisting second- or third-degree AV block or right bundle branch block when associated with a left hemiblock, unless a pacemaker is present; contraindicated in cardiogenic shock.

• Findings from the Cardiac Arrhythmia Suppression Trial (CAST) include a greater-than-twofold increase in the number of deaths and nonfatal cardiac arrest in patients treated with flecainide. Therefore, it should be used only in immediately life-threatening dysrhythmias, such as sustained ventricular tachycardia.

• Flecainide can alter endocardial pacing thresholds. Determine pacing threshold 1 week before and after initiating therapy in patients with pacemakers.

• Use cautiously in preexisting CHF, cardiomyopathy, severe renal or hepatic disease, prolonged Q-T interval, sick sinus syndrome, or blood dyscrasias.

• Hypokalemia or hyperkalemia may alter the effect of flecainide and should be corrected before this drug is given.

• Incidence of adverse effects increases when trough blood levels exceed 1 mcg/ml. Periodically monitor blood levels, especially in patients with renal failure or CHF.

• Most patients can be adequately maintained on an every-12-hour dosage schedule, but some need to receive flecainide every 8 hours.

• Full therapeutic effect of flecainide may take 3 to 5 days. The doctor may order I.V. lidocaine while awaiting full effect.

• Loading doses may aggravate dysrhythmias and are therefore not recommended.

• Twice-daily dosing for flecainide aids patient compliance.

• Therapeutic serum levels of flecainide range from 0.2 to 1 mcg/ml.

lidocaine hydrochloride (lignocaine hydrochloride)

Lido Pen Auto-Injector, Xylocaine♦, Xylocard♦♦

Pregnancy Risk Category: B

MECHANISM OF ACTION

A Class Ib antiarrhythmic that depresses phase O. It shortens the action potential. All Class I drugs have membrane stabilizing effects.

INDICATIONS & DOSAGE

Ventricular dysrhythmias from myocardial infarction, cardiac manipulation, or cardiac glycosides; ventricular tachycardia—

Adults: 50 to 100 mg (1 to 1.5 mg/kg) I.V. bolus at 25 to 50 mg/minute. Give half this amount to elderly patients or patients under 50 kg, and to those with CHF or hepatic disease. Repeat bolus q 3 to 5 minutes until dysrhythmias subside or adverse reactions develop. Don't exceed 300-mg total bolus during a 1-hour period. Simultaneously, begin constant infusion of 1 to 4 mg/minute. If single bolus has been given, repeat smaller bolus 15 to 20 minutes after start of infusion to maintain therapeutic serum level. After 24 hours of continuous infusion, decrease rate by half.

I.M. administration: 200 to 300 mg in deltoid muscle only.

Children: 1mg/kg by I.V. bolus, followed by infusion of 30 mcg/kg/minute.

ADVERSE REACTIONS

CNS: *confusion, tremors,* lethargy, somnolence, *stupor, restlessness,* slurred speech, euphoria, depression, *light-headedness,* paresthesias, muscle twitching, *convulsions.*

CV: *hypotension,* bradycardia, further dysrhythmias.

EENT: *tinnitus, blurred or double vision.*

Other: *anaphylaxis,* soreness at in-

---

jection site, sensations of cold, diaphoresis.

INTERACTIONS
Cimetidine, beta blockers: decreased metabolism of lidocaine. Monitor for toxicity.
Phenytoin: additive cardiac depressant effects. Monitor carefully.

NURSING CONSIDERATIONS
• Contraindicated in patients who are allergic to related local anesthetics of the amide type, such as Nupercaine.
• Use cautiously in complete or second-degree heart block. Use of lidocaine with epinephrine (for local anesthesia) to treat dysrhythmias is contraindicated. Use with caution in elderly patients, those with CHF, renal or hepatic disease, or those who weigh less than 50 kg. Such patients will need a reduced dose.
• In many severely ill patients, seizures may be the first clinically apparent sign of toxicity. However, severe reactions usually are preceded by somnolence, confusion, and paresthesias.
• If toxic signs (such as dizziness) occur, stop drug at once and notify doctor. Continued infusion could lead to seizures and coma. Give oxygen via nasal cannula, if not contraindicated. Keep oxygen and CPR equipment readily available.
• Patients receiving infusions must be attended *at all times,* and be on a cardiac monitor. Use a continuous infusion pump for administering infusion precisely. Do not exceed an infusion rate of 4 mg/minute. A faster rate greatly increases risk of toxicity.
• Monitor patient's response, especially blood pressure and serum electrolytes, BUN, and creatinine. Notify doctor promptly if abnormalities develop.
• Discontinue infusion and notify doctor if dysrhythmias worsen or ECG changes, such as widening QRS

complex or substantially prolonged PR interval, are evident.
• A bolus dose not followed by infusion will have a short-lived effect.
• A patient who has received lidocaine I.M. will show a sevenfold increase in serum creatinine phosphokinase (CPK) level. Such CPK originates in the skeletal muscle, not the heart. Test isoenzymes if using I.M. route.
• Used investigationally to treat refractory status epilepticus.
• Therapeutic serum levels are 2 to 5 mcg/ml.

---

mexiletine hydrochloride
Mexitil♦

Pregnancy Risk Category: C

MECHANISM OF ACTION
A Class Ib antiarrhythmic that depresses phase O. It shortens the action potential. All Group I drugs have membrane stabilizing effects.

INDICATIONS & DOSAGE
Treatment of refractory ventricular dysrhythmias, including ventricular tachycardia and premature ventricular contractions—
Adults: 200 to 400 mg P.O. followed by 200 mg q 8 hours. May increase dose to 400 mg q 8 hours if satisfactory control is not obtained. Some patients may respond well to an every-12-hour schedule. May give up to 450 mg q 12 hours.

ADVERSE REACTIONS
CNS: *tremor, dizziness,* blurred vision, ataxia, diplopia, confusion, nystagmus, nervousness, headache.
CV: hypotension, bradycardia, widened QRS complex, dysrhythmias.
GI: nausea, vomiting.
Skin: rash.

INTERACTIONS
Phenytoin, rifampin, phenobarbital:

decreased mexiletine blood levels. Monitor carefully.
Cimetidine: increased mexiletine blood levels. Monitor carefully.

NURSING CONSIDERATIONS
• Contraindicated in cardiogenic shock or preexisting second- or third-degree AV block (if pacemaker is not present).
• Early sign of mexiletine toxicity is tremor, usually a fine tremor of the hands. This progresses to dizziness and later to ataxia and nystagmus as the drug's blood level increases. Question your patient about these symptoms.
• When changing from lidocaine to mexiletine, stop the infusion when the first mexiletine dose is given. Keep the infusion line open, however, until the dysrhythmia appears to be satisfactorily controlled.
• May administer oral dose with meals to lessen GI distress.
• Therapeutic levels range from 0.75 to 2 mcg/ml.
• Monitor blood pressure and heart rate and rhythm frequently. Notify doctor of any significant change.
• Patients who respond well to mexiletine can often be maintained on a q 12 hour schedule. Notify doctor if you feel the patient is a good candidate for q 12 hour therapy. Twice-daily dosage eases compliance.

---

procainamide hydrochloride
Procan SR♦, Promine, Pronestyl♦**, Pronestyl-SR♦, Rhythmin

Pregnancy Risk Category: C

MECHANISM OF ACTION
A Class Ia antiarrhythmic that depresses phase O. It prolongs the action potential. All Class I drugs have membrane stabilizing effects.

INDICATIONS & DOSAGE
Premature ventricular contractions, ventricular tachycardia, atrial dysrhythmias unresponsive to quinidine, paroxysmal atrial tachycardia—
Adults: 100 mg q 5 minutes slow I.V. push, no faster than 25 to 50 mg/minute until dysrhythmias disappear, adverse reactions develop, or 1 g has been given. When dysrhythmias disappear, give continuous infusion of 2 to 6 mg/minute. Usual effective dose is 500 to 600 mg. If dysrhythmias recur, repeat bolus as above and increase infusion rate; 0.5 to 1 g I.M. q 4 to 8 hours until oral therapy begins.
Loading dose for atrial fibrillation or paroxysmal atrial tachycardia—
Adults: 1 to 1.25 g P.O. If dysrhythmias persist after 1 hour, give additional 750 mg. If no change occurs, give 500 mg to 1 g q 2 hours until dysrhythmias disappear or adverse reactions occur.
Loading dose for ventricular tachycardia—
Adults: 1 g P.O. Maintenance dosage is 50 mg/kg daily q 3 hours; average is 250 to 500 mg q 3 hours.
Note: Sustained-release tablet may be used for maintenance dosing when treating ventricular tachycardia, atrial fibrillation, and paroxysmal atrial tachycardia. Dose is 500 mg to 1 g q 6 hours.

ADVERSE REACTIONS
Blood: thrombocytopenia, *neutropenia* (especially with sustained-release forms), *agranulocytosis,* hemolytic anemia, *increased antinuclear antibodies titer.*
CNS: hallucinations, confusion, seizures, depression.
CV: *severe hypotension, bradycardia,* AV block, ventricular fibrillation (after parenteral use).
GI: *nausea, vomiting, anorexia, diarrhea, bitter taste.*
Skin: *maculopapular rash.*
Other: *fever, lupus erythematosus*

Italicized side effects are common or life-threatening.
*Liquid form contains alcohol.   **May contain tartrazine.

syndrome (especially after prolonged administration), myalgia.

INTERACTIONS

Cimetidine: may increase procaina-mide blood levels. Monitor for toxic-ity.

Amiodarone: increased procainamide levels and possible drug toxicity.

Neuromuscular blocking agents: increased skeletal muscle relaxant effects. Monitor patient closely.

NURSING CONSIDERATIONS

• Contraindicated in patients with hypersensitivity to procaine and related drugs; with complete, second-, or third-degree heart block unassisted by electrical pacemaker; or with myasthenia gravis. Use with caution in CHF or other conduction disturbances, such as bundle branch block or cardiac glycoside intoxication, or with hepatic or renal insufficiency.

• Patients receiving infusions must be *attended at all times.* Use a continuous infusion pump to administer the infusion precisely.

• Monitor serum electrolytes, especially potassium level. Hypokalemia predisposes patients to dysrhythmias.

• Monitor blood pressure and ECG continuously during I.V. administration. Watch for prolonged Q-T and QRS intervals, heart block, or increased dysrhythmias. If these occur, withhold drug, obtain rhythm strip, and notify doctor immediately.

• Keep patient supine for I.V. administration if hypotension occurs.

• If procainamide is administered too rapidly, I.V. hypotension can occur. Watch closely for adverse reactions and notify doctor if they occur. Instruct patient to report fever, rash, muscle pain, diarrhea, bleeding, bruises, or pleuritic chest pain.

• Procainamide solution for injection may become discolored. If so, check with pharmacy and prepare to discard.

• Monitor CBC frequently during first 3 months of therapy, particularly in patients taking sustained-release dosage forms.

• Decrease dose in hepatic and renal dysfunction, and give over 6 hours. Half-life of procainamide is increased as much as threefold in these states.

• N-acetylprocainamide (NAPA), an active metabolite, may accumulate when renal function is decreased. This may add to toxicity.

• Patient with CHF has a lower volume of distribution and can be treated with lower doses.

• Positive antinuclear antibody titer is common in about 60% of patients who don't have symptoms of lupus erythematosus syndrome. This response seems related to prolonged use, not dosage.

• After prolonged atrial fibrillation, restoration of normal rhythm may result in thromboembolism, due to dislodgment of thrombi from atrial wall. Anticoagulation usually advised before restoration of normal sinus rhythm.

• Stress importance of taking drug exactly as prescribed. Patient may have to set an alarm clock for night doses.

• Reassure patients who are taking the extended-release form of procainamide that a wax matrix 'ghost' from the tablet may be passed in the stool. The drug is completely absorbed before this occurs.

• Elderly patients may be more likely to develop hypotension. Monitor blood pressure carefully.

quinidine gluconate
(62% quinidine base)
Duraquin, Quinaglute Dura-Tabs♦,
Quinalan, Quinate♦♦

quinidine polygalacturonate
(60.5% quinidine base)
Cardioquin♦

quinidine sulfate
(83% quinidine base)
Apo-Quinidine♦♦, CinQuin,
Novoquindin♦♦, Quine, Quinidex
Extentabs♦, Quinora

Pregnancy Risk Category: C

MECHANISM OF ACTION
A Class Ia antiarrhythmic that depresses phase O. It prolongs the action potential. All Class I drugs have membrane stabilizing effects.

INDICATIONS & DOSAGE
Atrial flutter or fibrillation—
Adults: 200 mg quinidine sulfate or equivalent base P.O. q 2 to 3 hours for 5 to 8 doses with subsequent daily increases until sinus rhythm is restored or toxic effects develop. Administer quinidine only after digitalization to avoid increasing AV conduction. Maximum dosage is 3 to 4 g daily.
Paroxysmal supraventricular tachycardia—
Adults: 400 to 600 mg I.M. gluconate q 2 to 3 hours until toxic side effects develop or dysrhythmia subsides.
Premature atrial and ventricular contractions; paroxysmal atrioventricular junctional rhythm; paroxysmal atrial tachycardia; paroxysmal ventricular tachycardia; maintenance after cardioversion of atrial fibrillation or flutter—
Adults: test dose is 50 to 200 mg P.O., then monitor vital signs before beginning therapy. Quinidine sulfate or equivalent base 200 to 400 mg P.O. q 4 to 6 hours; or initially, quinidine gluconate 600 mg I.M., then up to 400 mg q 2 hours, p.r.n.; or quinidine gluconate 800 mg (10 ml of the commercially available solution) added to 40 ml dextrose 5% in water, infused I.V. at 16 mg (1 ml)/minute.
Children: test dose is 2 mg/kg; 3 to 6 mg/kg q 2 to 3 hours for 5 doses P.O. daily.

ADVERSE REACTIONS
Blood: *hemolytic anemia, thrombocytopenia, agranulocytosis.*
CNS: *vertigo, headache, lightheadedness,* confusion, restlessness, cold sweat, pallor, fainting, dementia.
CV: *premature ventricular contractions; severe hypotension; SA and AV block; ventricular fibrillation, tachycardia; aggravated CHF; ECG changes (particularly widening of QRS complex, notched P waves, widened Q-T interval, ST segment depression).*
EENT: *tinnitus,* excessive salivation, blurred vision.
GI: *diarrhea, nausea, vomiting,* anorexia, abdominal pains.
Hepatic: hepatotoxicity including granulomatous hepatitis.
Skin: rash, petechial hemorrhage of buccal mucosa, pruritus.
Other: angioedema, acute asthmatic attack, respiratory arrest, *fever, cinchonism.*

INTERACTIONS
Acetazolamide, antacids, sodium bicarbonate: may increase quinidine blood levels due to alkaline urine. Monitor for increased effect.
Barbiturates, phenytoin, rifampin: may antagonize quinidine activity. Monitor for decreased quinidine effect.
Cimetidine: increased serum quinidine levels. Monitor for increased effect.
Digoxin: increased serum digoxin levels after initiating quinidine therapy. Monitor closely.

Italicized side effects are common or life-threatening.
*Liquid form contains alcohol.   **May contain tartrazine.

Nifedipine: may decrease quinidine blood levels. Monitor carefully.
Verapamil: may result in hypotension. Monitor blood pressure.
Warfarin: increased anticoagulant effect. Monitor closely.

NURSING CONSIDERATIONS

• Contraindicated in cardiac glycoside toxicity when AV conduction is grossly impaired and in complete AV block with AV nodal or idioventricular pacemaker. Use with caution in myasthenia gravis. Anticholinesterase drug doses may have to be increased.
• May increase toxicity of digitalis derivatives. Use with caution in patients previously digitalized. Monitor digoxin levels.
• Monitor liver function tests during the first 4 to 8 weeks of therapy.
• The I.V. route should only be used to treat acute dysrhythmias. For maintenance, give only by oral or I.M. route.
• Dosage varies—some patients may require drug q 4 hours; others, q 6 hours. Titrate dose by both clinical response and blood levels.
• When changing route of administration, alter dosage to compensate for variations in quinidine base content.
• Dosage should be decreased in CHF and hepatic disease.
• Check apical pulse rate and blood pressure before starting therapy. If you detect extremes in pulse rate, withhold drug and notify doctor at once.
• Lidocaine may be effective in treating quinidine-induced dysrhythmias, because it increases AV conduction.
• GI adverse reactions, especially diarrhea, are signs of toxicity. Notify doctor. Check quinidine blood levels, which are toxic when greater than 8 mcg/ml. GI symptoms may be decreased by giving with meals. Monitor patient response carefully.
• Instruct patient to notify doctor if skin rash, fever, unusual bleeding, bruising, ringing in ears, or visual disturbance occurs.
• After long-standing atrial fibrillation, restoration of normal sinus rhythm may result in thromboembolism due to dislodgment of thrombi from atrial wall. Anticoagulation often advised before restoration of normal atrial rhythm.
• Never use discolored (brownish) quinidine solution.
• Store away from heat and direct light.
• The Centers for Disease Control (CDC) is investigating the use of quinidine gluconate for the treatment of severe *Plasmodium falciparum* malaria when quinine dihydrochloride is unavailable. Contact the CDC malaria branch for further information.

---

tocainide hydrochloride
Tonocard♦

Pregnancy Risk Category: C

MECHANISM OF ACTION
A Class Ib antiarrhythmic that depresses phase O. It shortens the action potential. All Class I drugs have membrane stabilizing effects.

INDICATIONS & DOSAGE
Suppression of symptomatic ventricular dysrhythmias, including frequent premature ventricular contractions and ventricular tachycardia—
Adults: initially, 400 mg P.O. q 8 hours. Usual dosage is between 1,200 and 1,800 mg daily in three divided doses.

ADVERSE REACTIONS
Blood: aplastic anemia.
CNS: *light-headedness, tremors,* restlessness, paresthesias, confusion, dizziness.
CV: hypotension, dysrhythmias, *CHF.*
EENT: blurred vision.
GI: *nausea, vomiting, epigastric*

---

pain, constipation, diarrhea, anorexia.
Hepatic: hepatitis.
Skin: skin rash.

INTERACTIONS
Beta blockers: decreased myocardial contractility; increased CNS toxicity.

NURSING CONSIDERATIONS
• Contraindicated in patients who are hypersensitive to lidocaine or other amide-type local anesthetics and in patients with second- or third-degree AV block in the absence of a ventricular pacemaker.
• Use cautiously in CHF or diminished cardiac reserve.
• Use cautiously in hepatic or renal impairment. These patients may often be treated effectively with a lower dose.
• Therapeutic blood levels range from 4 to 10 mcg/ml.
• Adverse reactions are generally mild, transient, and reversible by reducing dosage. GI reactions can be minimized by taking the drug with food.
• Dizziness and falling are more likely to occur in elderly patients.
• Monitor patient for tremor. This may indicate the approaching of maximum dose.
• Considered by cardiologists as an "oral lidocaine." May ease transition from I.V. lidocaine to oral antiarrhythmic therapy. Monitor patient carefully during this transition period.

Italicized side effects are common or life-threatening.
*Liquid form contains alcohol.   **May contain tartrazine.

21

Antianginals

diltiazem hydrochloride
erythrityl tetranitrate
isosorbide dinitrate
nadolol
nicardipine
nifedipine
nitroglycerin (glyceryl trinitrate)
pentaerythritol tetranitrate
propranolol hydrochloride
verapamil hydrochloride

COMBINATION PRODUCTS

ANGIJEN NO. 1: pentaerythritol tetranitrate 20 mg and phenobarbital sodium 15 mg.
ARCOTRATE NO. 3: pentaerythritol tetranitrate 20 mg and phenobarbital sodium 8 mg.
BITRATE: pentaerythritol tetranitrate 15 mg and phenobarbital sodium 20 mg.
DIMYCOR: pentaerythritol tetranitrate 10 mg and phenobarbital sodium 15 mg.
NITROTYM-PLUS: nitroglycerin 2.5 mg and butabarbital sodium 48 mg.
PERBUZEM: pentaerythritol tetranitrate 10 mg and butabarbital sodium 15 mg.

---

diltiazem hydrochloride
Cardizem♦, Cardizem SR

Pregnancy Risk Category: C

MECHANISM OF ACTION
Inhibits calcium ion influx across cardiac and smooth muscle cells, decreasing myocardial contractility and oxygen demand, and dilates coronary arteries and peripheral arterioles.

INDICATIONS & DOSAGE
Management of vasospastic (also called Prinzmetal's or variant) angina and classic chronic stable angina pectoris—
Adults: 30 mg P.O. t.i.d. or q.i.d. before meals and at bedtime. Dosage may be gradually increased to a maximum of 360 mg/day, in divided doses.
Hypertension—
Adults: 90 mg P.O. b.i.d. (sustained release capsule). Titrate dosage to effect. Maximum recommended dosage is 360 mg/day.

ADVERSE REACTIONS
CNS: *headache, fatigue, drowsiness,* dizziness, nervousness, depression, insomnia, confusion.
CV: *edema, dysrhythmias,* flushing, bradycardia, hypotension, conduction abnormalities.
GI: *nausea,* vomiting, diarrhea.
GU: nocturia, polyuria.
Hepatic: transient elevation of liver enzymes.
Skin: *rash,* pruritus.
Other: photosensitivity.

INTERACTIONS
Cimetidine: may inhibit diltiazem metabolism. Monitor for toxicity.
Digoxin: diltiazem may increase serum levels of digoxin. Monitor for toxicity.
Propranolol (and other beta blockers): may prolong cardiac conduction time. Use together cautiously.

NURSING CONSIDERATIONS
• Contraindicated in sick sinus syn-

Unmarked trade names available in the United States only.
♦ Also available in Canada.   ♦ ♦ Available in Canada only.   ◊ Also available OTC.

drome, unless a functioning ventricular pacemaker is present; hypotension when systolic blood pressure is less than 90 mm Hg; and second- or third-degree AV block.

• Use cautiously in elderly patients because duration of action may be prolonged.

• Use cautiously in impaired ventricular function or conduction abnormalities.

• Use cautiously in impaired hepatic or renal function.

• Monitor blood pressure during initiation of therapy and dosage adjustments. Assist patients with ambulation during initiation of diltiazem therapy because dizziness may occur.

• If systolic pressure is less than 90 mm Hg, or heart rate is less than 60 beats/minute, withhold dose and notify doctor.

• If nitrate therapy is prescribed during titration of diltiazem dosage, urge patient to continue compliance. Sublingual nitroglycerin, especially, may be taken concomitantly as needed when anginal symptoms are acute.

• Of the available calcium antagonists, diltiazem may offer the lowest risk of adverse effects.

• Used investigationally to treat supraventricular tachycardia.

• May be useful as migraine prophylaxis in some patients. However, diltiazem itself may cause headaches.

---

erythrityl tetranitrate
Cardilate♦

Pregnancy Risk Category: C

MECHANISM OF ACTION
Reduces cardiac oxygen demand by decreasing left ventricular end-diastolic pressure (preload) and, to a lesser extent, systemic vascular resistance (afterload). Also increases blood flow through the collateral coronary vessels.

INDICATIONS & DOSAGE
Prophylaxis and long-term management of frequent or recurrent anginal pain, reduced exercise tolerance associated with angina pectoris—
Adults: 5 mg orally, sublingually, or buccally t.i.d., increasing in 2 to 3 days if needed.

ADVERSE REACTIONS
CNS: *headache, sometimes with throbbing; dizziness;* weakness.
CV: *orthostatic hypotension, tachycardia, flushing, palpitations,* fainting.
GI: nausea, vomiting.
Local: sublingual burning.
Skin: cutaneous vasodilation.
Other: hypersensitivity reactions.

INTERACTIONS
None significant.

NURSING CONSIDERATIONS
• Contraindicated in hypersensitivity to nitrites, head trauma, cerebral hemorrhage, or severe anemia. Use with caution in hypotension.

• Monitor blood pressure and intensity and duration of response to drug.

• May cause headaches, especially at first. Treat headache with aspirin or acetaminophen. Dosage may need to be reduced temporarily, but tolerance usually develops.

• Tell patient to take medication regularly, even long-term, if ordered, and to keep it easily accessible at all times. Physiologically necessary but not habit-forming.

• Additional dose may be taken before anticipated stress or at bedtime if angina is nocturnal.

• Advise patient to avoid alcoholic beverages; may produce increased hypotension.

• May cause orthostatic hypotension. To minimize it, patient should change to upright position slowly. He should go up and down stairs carefully, and lie down at the first sign of dizziness.

Italicized side effects are common or life-threatening.
*Liquid form contains alcohol.   **May contain tartrazine.

• Teach patient to take sublingual tablet at first sign of attack. He should wet the tablet with saliva, place it under the tongue until completely absorbed, and sit down and rest. Dose may be repeated every 10 to 15 minutes for a maximum of three doses. If no relief, patient should call doctor or go to hospital emergency room. If patient complains of tingling sensation with drug placed sublingually, he may try holding tablet in buccal pouch.

• Teach patient to take oral tablet on empty stomach, either half an hour before or 1 to 2 hours after meals, and to swallow oral tablets whole.

• Drug should not be discontinued abruptly—coronary vasospasm may occur.

• Store drug in cool place, in a tightly closed container, away from light. To ensure freshness, replace supply every 3 months. Remove cotton from container, since it absorbs drug.

---

isosorbide dinitrate

Apo-ISDN♦♦, Cedocard-SR♦♦, Coronex♦♦, Dilatrate-SR, Iso-Bid, Isonate, Isorbid Isordil♦, Isotrate, Novosorbide♦♦, Sorbitrate, Sorbitrate SA

Pregnancy Risk Category: C

MECHANISM OF ACTION

Reduces cardiac oxygen demand by decreasing left ventricular end-diastolic pressure (preload) and, to a lesser extent, systemic vascular resistance (afterload). Also increases blood flow through the collateral coronary vessels.

INDICATIONS & DOSAGE

Treatment of acute anginal attacks (sublingual and chewable tablets only); prophylaxis in situations likely to cause anginal attacks; treatment of chronic ischemic heart disease (by preload reduction)—
Adults: *Sublingual form—*2.5 to 10

mg under the tongue for prompt relief of anginal pain, repeated q 2 to 3 hours during acute phase, or q 4 to 6 hours for prophylaxis.
*Chewable form—*5 to 10 mg, p.r.n., for acute attack or q 2 to 3 hours for prophylaxis but only after initial test dose of 5 mg to determine risk of severe hypotension.
*Oral form—*5 to 30 mg P.O. q.i.d. for prophylaxis only (use smallest effective dose); sustained-release forms 40 mg P.O. q 6 to 12 hours.
Adjunct with other vasodilators, such as hydralazine and prazosin, in treatment of severe chronic CHF—
Adults: *Oral or chewable form—*20 to 40 mg q 4 hours.

ADVERSE REACTIONS

CNS: *headache, sometimes with throbbing; dizziness;* weakness.
CV: *orthostatic hypotension, tachycardia, palpitations, ankle edema,* fainting.
GI: nausea, vomiting.
Local: sublingual burning.
Skin: cutaneous vasodilation, *flushing.*
Other: hypersensitivity reactions.

INTERACTIONS

Antihypertensives: possibly increased hypotensive effects. Monitor closely during initial therapy.

NURSING CONSIDERATIONS

• Contraindicated in hypersensitivity to nitrites, head trauma, cerebral hemorrhage, or severe anemia. Use with caution in hypotension.

• Monitor blood pressure and intensity and duration of response to drug.

• May cause headaches, especially at first. Treat headache with aspirin or acetaminophen. Dosage may need to be reduced temporarily, but tolerance usually develops.

• Tell patient to take medication regularly, even long-term, if ordered, and

---

to keep it easily accessible at all times. Physiologically necessary but not habit-forming.
• Additional dose may be taken before anticipated stress or at bedtime if angina is nocturnal.
• Advise patient to avoid alcoholic beverages; they may produce increased hypotension.
• May cause orthostatic hypotension. To minimize it, patient should change to upright position slowly. He should go up and down stairs carefully, and lie down at the first sign of dizziness.
• Teach patient to take sublingual tablet at first sign of attack. He should wet the tablet with saliva, place it under the tongue until completely absorbed, and sit down and rest. Dose may be repeated every 10 to 15 minutes for a maximum of three doses. If no relief, patient should call doctor or go to hospital emergency room. If patient complains of tingling sensation with drug placed sublingually, he may try holding tablet in buccal pouch.
• Warn patient not to confuse sublingual with oral form.
• Teach patient to take oral tablet on empty stomach, either half an hour before or 1 to 2 hours after meals; to swallow oral tablets whole; and to chew chewable tablets thoroughly before swallowing.
• Drug should not be discontinued abruptly—coronary vasospasm may occur.
• Store in cool place, in tightly closed container, away from light.
• Has been used investigationally in treatment of congestive heart failure and diffuse esophageal spasms.

---

nadolol
Corgard♦

Pregnancy Risk Category: C

MECHANISM OF ACTION
A beta-adrenergic blocker that reduces cardiac oxygen demand by blocking catecholamine-induced increases in heart rate, blood pressure, and force of myocardial contraction. Depresses renin secretion.

INDICATIONS & DOSAGE
Management of angina pectoris—
Adults: 40 mg P.O. once daily, initially. Dosage may be increased in 40- to 80-mg increments until optimum response occurs. Usual maintenance dosage range is 80 to 240 mg once daily.
Treatment of hypertension—
Adults: 40 mg P.O. once daily, initially. Dosage may be increased in 40- to 80-mg increments until optimum response occurs. Usual maintenance dosage is 80 to 320 mg once daily. Doses of 640 mg may be necessary in rare cases.

ADVERSE REACTIONS
CNS: fatigue, lethargy.
CV: *bradycardia, hypotension, CHF,* peripheral vascular disease.
GI: nausea, vomiting, diarrhea.
Metabolic: hypoglycemia without tachycardia.
Skin: rash.
Other: *increased airway resistance,* fever.

INTERACTIONS
Cardiac glycosides: excessive bradycardia and increased depressant effect on myocardium. Use together cautiously.
Epinephrine: severe vasoconstriction and reflex bradycardia. Monitor blood pressure and observe patient carefully.
Indomethacin: decreased antihypertensive effect. Monitor blood pressure and adjust dosage.
Insulin, hypoglycemic drugs (oral): can alter dosage requirements in previously stabilized diabetics. Observe patient carefully.

Italicized side effects are common or life-threatening.
*Liquid form contains alcohol. **May contain tartrazine.

NURSING CONSIDERATIONS
• Contraindicated in bronchial asthma, sinus bradycardia and greater than first-degree conduction block, and cardiogenic shock.
• Elderly patients may experience enhanced adverse reactions. Dose may need to be adjusted.
• Use cautiously in patients with heart failure, chronic bronchitis, renal or hepatic insufficiency, or emphysema.
• Always check patient's apical pulse before giving this drug. If slower than 60 beats/minute, withhold drug and call doctor.
• Monitor blood pressure frequently. If patient develops severe hypotension, administer a vasopressor as ordered.
• Don't discontinue abruptly; can exacerbate angina and myocardial infarction. Gradually reduce dosage over 1 to 2 weeks.
• Teach patient about his disease and therapy. Explain the importance of taking this drug as prescribed, even when he's feeling well. Tell outpatient not to discontinue drug suddenly, but to call doctor if unpleasant adverse reactions occur.
• Has been used in a limited number of patients with atrial flutter or fibrillation. Also has been used for a few patients in the treatment of migraine headaches.
• This drug masks common signs of shock, hyperthyroidism, and hypoglycemia.
• May be given without regard to meals.

nicardipine
Cardene

Pregnancy Risk Category: C

MECHANISM OF ACTION
Inhibits calcium ion influx across cardiac and smooth muscle cells, thus decreasing myocardial contractility and oxygen demand, and dilates coronary arteries and arterioles.

INDICATIONS AND DOSAGE
Chronic stable angina (used alone or in combination with beta blockers)—
Adults: Initially 20 mg P.O. t.i.d. Titrate dosage according to patient response. Usual dosage range is 20 to 40 mg P.O. t.i.d.
Hypertension—
Adults: Initially 20 to 40 mg P.O. t.i.d. Increase dosage according to patient response.

ADVERSE REACTIONS
CNS: dizziness or light-headedness, headache, paresthesias, drowsiness, asthenia.
CV: peripheral edema, palpitations, angina, tachycardia.
GI: nausea, abdominal discomfort, dry mouth.
Skin: rash, flushing.

INTERACTIONS
Beta-adrenergic blocking agents: may increase cardiac depressant effects. Monitor patient closely.
Cimetidine: may decrease metabolism of calcium channel blocking agents. Monitor for increased pharmacologic effect.
Cyclosporine: nicardipine may increase plasma levels of cyclosporine. Monitor for toxicity.
Theophylline: pharmacologic effects of theophylline may be enhanced. Monitor for toxicity.

NURSING CONSIDERATIONS
• Contraindicated in patients with hypersensitivity to nicardipine, and in advanced aortic stenosis. Use cautiously in cardiac conduction disturbances, hypotension, and CHF.
• Some patients may experience increased frequency, severity, or duration of chest pain at beginning of therapy or during dosage adjustments. The mechanism for this adverse effect

is not known. Advise patient to report chest pain immediately.
• Allow at least 3 days between dosage adjustments to achieve steady plasma levels.
• Measure blood pressure frequently during initial therapy. Maximum blood pressure response occurs about 1 hour after dosing. Check for potential orthostatic hypotension 1 to 2 hours after first dose. Because large swings in blood pressure may occur depending upon blood level of drug, assess adequacy of antihypertensive effect 8 hours after dosing.
• Patients with renal impairment should be titrated slowly to optimal response. Begin therapy with 20 mg P.O. t.i.d.
• Patients with hepatic impairment should receive lower initial doses (20 mg P.O. b.i.d.) and be carefully titrated to optimal response.

nifedipine
Adalat♦, Adalat P.A.♦♦, Apo-Nifed♦, Novo-Nifedin♦, Procardia
Pregnancy Risk Category: C

MECHANISM OF ACTION
Inhibits calcium ion influx across cardiac and smooth muscle cells, decreasing myocardial contractility and oxygen demand, and dilates coronary arteries and arterioles.

INDICATIONS & DOSAGE
Management of vasospastic (also called Prinzmetal's or variant) angina and classic chronic stable angina pectoris; treatment of hypertension and Raynaud's disease—
Adults: Starting dose is 10 mg P.O. t.i.d. Usual effective dose range is 10 to 20 mg t.i.d. Some patients may require up to 30 mg q.i.d. Maximum daily dosage is 180 mg.

ADVERSE REACTIONS
CNS: *dizziness, light-headedness,* *flushing, headache,* weakness, syncope.
CV: peripheral edema, hypotension, palpitations.
EENT: nasal congestion.
GI: *nausea, heartburn,* diarrhea.
Metabolic: hypokalemia.
Other: muscle cramps, dyspnea.

INTERACTIONS
Propranolol (and other beta blockers): may cause hypotension and heart failure. Use together cautiously.
Cimetidine, ranitidine: decreased nifedipine metabolism.

NURSING CONSIDERATIONS
• Use cautiously in CHF or hypotension.
• Monitor blood pressure regularly, especially in patients who are also taking beta blockers or antihypertensives.
• Use cautiously in elderly patients because duration of action may be prolonged.
• Monitor serum potassium level regularly.
• Patient may briefly develop anginal exacerbation when beginning drug therapy or when dosage is increased. Reassure him that this symptom is temporary.
• Although rebound effect hasn't been observed when drug is stopped, dosage should still be reduced slowly under doctor's supervision.
• If patient is kept on nitrate therapy while drug dosage is being titrated, urge him to continue his compliance. Sublingual nitroglycerin, especially, may be taken as needed when anginal symptoms are acute.
• Instruct patient to swallow the capsule whole without breaking, crushing, or chewing it.
• There's no sublingual form of nifedipine available. However, the liquid in the oral capsule can be withdrawn by puncturing the capsule with a needle. Instill the drug into the buccal pouch.

Italicized side effects are common or life-threatening.
*Liquid form contains alcohol.   **May contain tartrazine.

• Sublingual nifedipine may be useful in decreasing blood pressure during hypertensive emergencies. Continuous blood pressure and ECG monitoring is recommended.

• Protect capsules from direct light and moisture and store at room temperature.

---

nitroglycerin (glyceryl trinitrate)

Deponit, Klavikordal, Niong, Nitro-Bid♦, Nitro-Bid I.V.♦, Nitrocap, Nitrocap T.D., Nitrocine, Nitrodisc, Nitro-Dur, Nitro-Dur II, Nitrogard, Nitrogard SR, Nitrol♦, Nitrolin, Nitrolingual♦, Nitrol TSAR, Nitronet, Nitrong♦, Nitrong S.R.♦Nitrospan, Nitrostat♦, Nitrostat I.V.♦, NTS, Transderm-Nitro, Tridil♦

Pregnancy Risk Category: C

MECHANISM OF ACTION
Reduces cardiac oxygen demand by decreasing left ventricular end-diastolic pressure (preload) and, to a lesser extent, systemic vascular resistance (afterload). Also increases blood flow through the collateral coronary vessels.

INDICATIONS & DOSAGE
Prophylaxis against chronic anginal attacks—
Adults: 1 sustained-release capsule q 8 to 12 hours; or 2% ointment: Start with ½″ ointment, increasing by ½″ increments until headache occurs, then decreasing to previous dose. Range of dosage with ointment is 2″ to 5″. Usual dose is 1″ to 2″. Alternatively, transdermal disc or pad (Nitrodisc, Nitro-Dur, or Transderm-Nitro) may be applied to hairless site once daily.
Relief of acute angina pectoris, prophylaxis to prevent or minimize anginal attacks when taken immediately before stressful events—
Adults: 1 sublingual tablet (gr ¹⁄₄₀₀,

¹⁄₂₀₀, ¹⁄₁₅₀, ¹⁄₁₀₀) dissolved under the tongue or in the buccal pouch immediately upon indication of anginal attack. May repeat q 5 minutes for 15 minutes. Or, using Nitrolingual spray, spray one or two doses into mouth, preferably onto or under the tongue. May repeat q 3 to 5 minutes to a maximum of 3 doses within a 15-minute period. Or, transmucosally, 1 to 3 mg q 3 to 5 hours during waking hours.
To control hypertension associated with surgery; to treat CHF associated with myocardial infarction; to relieve angina pectoris in acute situations; to produce controlled hypotension during surgery (by I.V. infusion)—
Adults: initial infusion rate is 5 mcg/minute. May be increased by 5 mcg/minute q 3 to 5 minutes until a response is noted. If a 20 mcg/minute rate doesn't produce a response, dosage may be increased by as much as 20 mcg/minute q 3 to 5 minutes.

ADVERSE REACTIONS
CNS: *headache, sometimes with throbbing; dizziness;* weakness.
CV: *orthostatic hypotension, tachycardia, flushing, palpitations,* fainting.
GI: nausea, vomiting.
Skin: cutaneous vasodilation.
Local: sublingual burning.
Other: hypersensitivity reactions.

INTERACTIONS
Antihypertensives: possibly enhanced hypotensive effect. Monitor closely.

NURSING CONSIDERATIONS
• Contraindicated in hypersensitivity to nitrites, head trauma, cerebral hemorrhage, hypertrophic cardiomyopathy, or severe anemia. Use with caution in hypotension.
• Monitor blood pressure and intensity and duration of response to drug.
• May cause headaches, especially at first. Treat headache with aspirin or acetaminophen. Dosage may need to

---

be reduced temporarily, but tolerance usually develops.
• Tell patient to take medication regularly, even long-term, if ordered, and to keep it easily accessible at all times. Physiologically necessary but not habit-forming.
• Additional dose may be taken before anticipated stress or at bedtime if angina is nocturnal.
• Advise patient to avoid alcoholic beverages; may produce increased hypotension.
• May cause orthostatic hypotension. To minimize it, patient should change to upright position slowly. He should go up and down stairs carefully, and lie down at the first sign of dizziness.
• Teach patient to take sublingual tablet at first sign of attack. He should wet the tablet with saliva, place it under the tongue until completely absorbed, and sit down and rest. Dose may be repeated every 10 to 15 minutes for a maximum of three doses. If no relief, patient should call doctor or go to hospital emergency room. If patient complains of tingling sensation with drug placed sublingually, he may try holding tablet in buccal pouch.
• Although a burning sensation used to be an indication of tablet potency, today many brands don't produce this sensation.
• Store drug in cool, dark place in a tightly closed container. To ensure freshness, replace supply of sublingual tablets every 3 months. Remove cotton from container, since it absorbs drug.
• Tell patient to store nitroglycerin sublingual tablets in original container or other container specifically approved for this use.
• Advise patient not to carry bottle close to body. Patient should carry it in jacket pocket or purse.
• Teach patient to take oral tablet on empty stomach, either half an hour before or 1 to 2 hours after meals; to swallow oral tablets whole; and to

chew chewable tablets thoroughly before swallowing.
• To apply ointment, spread uniform, thin layer on any nonhairy area. Do not rub in. Cover with plastic film to aid absorption and to protect clothing. If using Tape-Surrounded Appli-Ruler (TSAR) system, keep the TSAR on skin to protect patient's clothing and to ensure that ointment remains in place.
• Be sure to remove all excess ointment from previous site before applying the next dose.
• Avoid getting ointment on fingers.
• Transdermal dosage forms can be applied to any hairless part of the skin except distal parts of the arms or legs, because absorption will not be maximal at these sites.
• Be sure to remove transdermal patch before defibrillation. Because of its aluminum backing, the electric current may cause the patch to explode.
• When terminating transdermal treatment of angina, gradually reduce the dosage and frequency of application over 4 to 6 weeks.
• Instruct patient to use caution when wearing transdermal patch near microwave oven. Leaking radiation may heat patch's metallic backing and cause burns.
• The various brands of transdermal nitroglycerin products can be interchanged to achieve the prescribed dose. Now, standardized labels specify the amount of nitroglycerin released over 24 hours.
• If nitroglycerin lingual aerosol (Nitrolingual) has been prescribed for patient, instruct him how to use this device correctly. Remind him he should *not* inhale the spray, but should release the spray onto or under the tongue. Also tell him not to swallow immediately after administering the spray—wait about 10 seconds or so before swallowing.
• The transmucosal dosage form may

Italicized side effects are common or life-threatening.
*Liquid form contains alcohol.   **May contain tartrazine.

be used to provide relief from an acute anginal attack as well as for prophylaxis.

• Tell patient to place the transmucosal tablet between lip and gum above the incisors, or between cheek and gum. Tell him not to swallow or chew tablet; this will make it ineffective.

• When administering as an I.V. infusion, be sure to use the special nonabsorbing tubing supplied by the manufacturer, because up to 80% of the drug can be absorbed by regular plastic tubing. Also, be sure to prepare in a glass bottle or container, and use a controlled infusion pump.

• Closely monitor vital signs during infusion.

---

pentaerythritol tetranitrate
Dilar, Duotrate, Naptrate, Pentritol, Pentylan, Peritrate♦, Peritrate Forte♦♦, Peritrate SA♦, PETN

Pregnancy Risk Category: C

MECHANISM OF ACTION
Reduces cardiac oxygen demand by decreasing left ventricular end-diastolic pressure (preload) and, to a lesser extent, systemic vascular resistance (afterload). Also increases blood flow through the collateral coronary vessels.

INDICATIONS & DOSAGE
Prophylaxis against angina pectoris—
Adults: 10 to 20 mg P.O. q.i.d.; may be titrated upward to 40 mg P.O. q.i.d. half an hour before or 1 hour after meals and h.s.; 80 mg sustained-release preparations P.O. b.i.d.

ADVERSE REACTIONS
CNS: *headache, sometimes with throbbing; dizziness;* weakness.
CV: *orthostatic hypotension, tachycardia, flushing, palpitations,* fainting.
GI: nausea, vomiting.

Skin: cutaneous vasodilation.
Other: hypersensitivity reactions.

INTERACTIONS
None significant.

NURSING CONSIDERATIONS
• Contraindicated in head trauma, cerebral hemorrhage, or severe anemia. Use with caution in hypotension and glaucoma.

• Monitor blood pressure and intensity and duration of response to drug.

• May cause headaches, especially at first. Treat with aspirin or acetaminophen. Dosage may need to be reduced temporarily, but tolerance usually develops.

• Medication should be taken regularly, even long-term, if ordered. Physiologically necessary but not habit-forming.

• Additional doses may be taken before anticipated stress or at bedtime for nocturnal angina.

• Not to be used for relief of acute anginal attacks.

• May cause orthostatic hypotension. To minimize it, patient should change to upright position slowly. He should go up and down stairs carefully, and lie down at the first sign of dizziness.

• Advise patient to avoid alcoholic beverages; may exacerbate hypotension.

• Drug should not be discontinued abruptly—coronary vasospasm may occur.

• Store in cool place, in a tightly covered container away from light.

---

propranolol hydrochloride
Apo-Propranolol♦♦, Detensol♦♦, Inderal♦, Inderal LA♦, Novo-pranol♦♦, pms-Propranolol♦♦

Pregnancy Risk Category: C

MECHANISM OF ACTION
A beta-adrenergic blocker that reduces cardiac oxygen demand by

---

blocking catecholamine-induced increases in heart rate, blood pressure, and force of myocardial contraction. Depresses renin secretion. Also prevents vasodilation of the cerebral arteries.

INDICATIONS & DOSAGE

Management of angina pectoris—
Adults: 10 to 20 mg t.i.d. or q.i.d. Or, one 80-mg sustained-release capsule daily. Dosage may be increased at 7- to 10-day intervals. The average optimum dosage is 160 mg daily.
To reduce mortality following myocardial infarction—
Adults: 180 to 240 mg P.O. daily in divided doses. Usually administered t.i.d. to q.i.d.
Supraventricular, ventricular, and atrial dysrhythmias; tachydysrhythmias caused by excessive catecholamine action during anesthesia, hyperthyroidism, and pheochromocytoma—
Adults: 1 to 3 mg I.V. diluted in 50 ml dextrose 5% in water or normal saline solution infused slowly, not to exceed 1 mg/minute. After 3 mg have been infused, another dose may be given in 2 minutes; subsequent doses no sooner than q 4 hours. Usual maintenance dosage is 10 to 80 mg P.O. t.i.d. or q.i.d.
Hypertension—
Adults: initial treatment of hypertension: 80 mg P.O. daily in two to four divided doses or the sustained-release form once daily. Increase at 3- to 7-day intervals to maximum daily dosage of 640 mg. Usual maintenance dosage for hypertension is 160 to 480 mg daily.
Prevention of frequent, severe, uncontrollable, or disabling migraine or vascular headache—
Adults: initially, 80 mg daily in divided doses or one sustained-release capsule daily. Usual maintenance dosage is 160 to 240 mg daily, divided t.i.d. or q.i.d.

ADVERSE REACTIONS

CNS: *fatigue, lethargy,* vivid dreams, hallucinations.
CV: *bradycardia, hypotension, CHF,* peripheral vascular disease.
GI: nausea, vomiting, diarrhea.
Metabolic: hypoglycemia without tachycardia.
Skin: rash.
Other: *increased airway resistance,* fever, arthralgia.

INTERACTIONS

Aminophylline: antagonized beta-blocking effects of propranolol. Use together cautiously.
Cardiac glycosides, verapamil: excessive bradycardia and increased depressant effect on myocardium. Use together cautiously.
Cimetidine: inhibits propranolol's metabolism. Monitor for greater beta-blocking effect.
Epinephrine: severe vasoconstriction. Monitor blood pressure and observe patient carefully.
Insulin, hypoglycemic drugs (oral): can alter requirements for these drugs in previously stabilized diabetics. Monitor for hypoglycemia.
Isoproterenol, glucagon: antagonized propranolol effect. May be used therapeutically and in emergencies.

NURSING CONSIDERATIONS

• Contraindicated in diabetes mellitus, asthma, or allergic rhinitis; during ethyl ether anesthesia; with sinus bradycardia and in heart block greater than first degree; in cardiogenic shock; and with right ventricular failure secondary to pulmonary hypertension. Use with caution in patients with CHF or respiratory disease, and in patients taking other antihypertensive drugs.
• Elderly patients may experience enhanced adverse reactions. Dosage may need to be adjusted.
• Always check patient's apical pulse before giving this drug. If you detect

Italicized side effects are common or life-threatening.
*Liquid form contains alcohol.   **May contain tartrazine.

extremes in pulse rates, withhold drug and call the doctor immediately.
• Monitor blood pressure, ECG, and heart rate and rhythm frequently, especially during I.V. administration. If patient develops severe hypotension, notify doctor. He may prescribe a vasopressor.
• After prolonged atrial fibrillation, restoration of normal sinus rhythm may result in thromboembolism due to dislodgment of thrombi from atrial wall. Anticoagulation often advised before restoration of normal atrial rhythm.
• Teach patient about his disease and therapy. Explain the importance of taking this drug as prescribed, even when he's feeling well. Tell outpatient not to discontinue his drug suddenly; abrupt discontinuation can exacerbate angina and myocardial infarction. Tell patient to call doctor if unpleasant adverse reactions occur.
• This drug masks common signs of shock and hypoglycemia.
• Food may increase the absorption of propranolol. Give consistently with meals.
• Compliance may be improved by administering this drug twice daily, or by sustained-release capsule. Check with doctor.
• Has also been used to treat aggression and rage, stage fright, recurrent GI bleeding, and menopausal symptoms.
• *Don't discontinue before surgery for pheochromocytoma.* Before any surgical procedure, notify anesthesiologist that patient is receiving propranolol.
• Double-check dose and route. I.V. doses are much smaller than P.O.
• Glucagon may be prescribed to reverse propranolol overdose.

verapamil hydrochloride
Calan, Calan SR, Isoptin♦, Isoptin SR♦

Pregnancy Risk Category: C

MECHANISM OF ACTION
Inhibits calcium ion influx across cardiac and smooth muscle cells, thus decreasing myocardial contractility and oxygen demand, and dilates coronary arteries and arterioles.

INDICATIONS & DOSAGE
Management of vasospastic (also called Prinzmetal's or variant) angina and classic chronic, stable angina pectoris—
Adults: starting dose is 80 mg P.O. t.i.d. or q.i.d. Dosage may be increased at weekly intervals. Some patients may require up to 480 mg daily.
Treatment of atrial dysrhythmias—
Adults: 0.075 to 0.15 mg/kg (5 to 10 mg) I.V. push over 2 minutes with ECG and blood pressure monitoring. Repeat dose in 30 minutes if no response. Follow bolus injection with maintenance infusion of 0.005 mg/kg/minute.
Children 1 to 15 years: 0.1 to 0.3 mg/kg and I.V. bolus over 2 minutes.
Children less than 1 year: 0.1 to 0.2 mg/kg as I.V. bolus over 2 minutes under continuous ECG monitoring.
  Dose can be repeated in 30 minutes if no response.
Migraine headache prophylaxis—
Adults: 80 mg P.O. q.i.d.
Treatment of hypertension—
Adults: 240-mg sustained-release tablet once daily in the morning. If response is not adequate, may give an additional half tablet in the evening or one tablet q 12 hours. Alternatively, may give 80-mg immediate-release tablet t.i.d. or q.i.d.

ADVERSE REACTIONS
CNS: dizziness, headache, fatigue.
CV: *transient hypotension, CHF,* bra-

dycardia, AV block, ventricular asystole, peripheral edema.
GI: *constipation,* nausea (primarily from oral form).
Hepatic: elevated liver enzymes.

INTERACTIONS

Carbamazepine, digitalis glycosides: verapamil may increase the serum levels of these drugs. Monitor patient for toxicity.
Lithium: verapamil may decrease serum lithium levels. Monitor patient closely.
Propranolol (and other beta blockers, including ophthalmic timolol), disopyramide: may cause heart failure. Use together cautiously.
Quinidine, antihypertensives: may result in hypotension. Monitor blood pressure.
Rifampin: may decrease oral bioavailability of verapamil. Monitor patient for lack of effect.

NURSING CONSIDERATIONS

• Contraindicated in advanced heart failure, AV block, severe left ventricular dysfunction, cardiogenic shock, sinus node disease, and severe hypotension.
• Use cautiously in elderly patients because duration of action may be prolonged. Administer I.V. doses over at least 3 minutes to minimize the risk of adverse effects.
• Use cautiously in myocardial infarction followed by coronary occlusion, sick sinus syndrome, impaired AV conduction, or heart failure with atrial tachydysrhythmia; and in hepatic or renal disease.
• All patients receiving I.V. verapamil should be monitored electrocardiographically. Monitor the R-R interval.
• Liver function tests should be done periodically.
• Patients with severely compromised cardiac function or those receiving beta blockers should receive lower doses of verapamil. Monitor these patients closely. Do not administer I.V. beta blockers at the same time as I.V. verapamil.
• Notify doctor if such signs of CHF as swelling of hands and feet or shortness of breath occur.
• If patient is kept on nitrate therapy while drug dosage of oral verapamil is being titrated, urge him to continue his compliance. Sublingual nitroglycerin, especially, may be taken as needed when anginal symptoms are acute.
• Taking extended-release tablets with food may decrease rate and extent of absorption, but allows smaller fluctuations of peak and trough blood levels.
• Preliminary studies show verapamil to be highly effective in the prophylaxis of migraine headache.

22

Antihypertensives

acebutolol
atenolol
captopril
clonidine hydrochloride
deserpidine
diazoxide
diltiazem hydrochloride
(See Chapter 21, ANTIANGINALS.)
enalapril maleate
guanabenz acetate
guanadrel sulfate
guanethidine sulfate
guanfacine hydrochloride
hydralazine hydrochloride
labetalol
lisinopril
mecamylamine hydrochloride
methyldopa
metoprolol tartrate
metyrosine
minoxidil
nadolol
(See Chapter 21, ANTIANGINALS.)
nitroprusside sodium
pargyline hydrochloride
penbutolol sulfate
phenoxybenzamine
  hydrochloride
phentolamine mesylate
pindolol
prazosin hydrochloride
propranolol hydrochloride
(See Chapter 21, ANTIANGINALS.)
rauwolfia serpentina
rescinnamine
reserpine
terazocin hydrochloride
timolol maleate
trimethaphan camsylate
verapamil hydrochloride
(See Chapter 21, ANTIANGINALS.)

COMBINATION PRODUCTS
ALDOCLOR-150: chlorothiazide 150 mg and methyldopa 250 mg.
ALDOCLOR-250: chlorothiazide 250 mg and methyldopa 250 mg.
ALDORIL-15♦: hydrochlorothiazide 15 mg and methyldopa 250 mg.
ALDORIL-25♦: hydrochlorothiazide 25 mg and methyldopa 250 mg.
ALDORIL D30: hydrochlorothiazide 30 mg and methyldopa 500 mg.
ALDORIL D50: hydrochlorothiazide 50 mg and methyldopa 500 mg.
APRESAZIDE 25/25: hydrochlorothiazide 25 mg and hydralazine HCl 25 mg.
APRESAZIDE 50/50: hydrochlorothiazide 50 mg and hydralazine HCl 50 mg.
APRESAZIDE 100/50: hydrochlorothiazide 50 mg and hydralazine HCl 100 mg.
APRESODEX: hydrochlorothiazide 15 mg and hydralazine HCl 25 mg.
APRESOLINE-ESIDRIX: hydrochlorothiazide 15 mg and hydralazine HCl 25 mg.
CAM-AP-ES: hydrochlorothiazide 15 mg, hydralazine HCl 25 mg, and reserpine 0.1 mg.
CAPOZIDE 50/25: hydrochlorothiazide 25 mg and captopril 50 mg.
CAPOZIDE 50/15: hydrochlorothiazide 15 mg and captopril 50 mg.
CAPOZIDE 25/25: hydrochlorothiazide 25 mg and captopril 25 mg.
CAPOZIDE 25/15: hydrochlorothiazide 15 mg and captopril 25 mg.
CHERAPAS: hydrochlorothiazide 15 mg, hydralazine HCl 25 mg, and reserpine 0.1 mg.

Unmarked trade names available in the United States only.
♦ Also available in Canada.   ♦♦ Available in Canada only.   ◇ Also available OTC.

COMBIPRES 0.1♦: chlorthalidone 15 mg and clonidine HCl 0.1 mg.

COMBIPRES 0.2: chlorthalidone 15 mg and clonidine HCl 0.2 mg.

CORZIDE: nadolol 40 mg or 80 mg and bendroflumethiazide 5 mg.

DEMI-REGROTON: chlorthalidone 25 mg and reserpine 0.125 mg.

DIUPRES-250: chlorothiazide 250 mg and reserpine 0.125 mg.

DIUPRES-500: chlorothiazide 500 mg and reserpine 0.125 mg.

DIURESE-R: trichlormethiazide 4 mg and reserpine 0.1 mg.

DIURIGEN WITH RESERPINE: chlorothiazide 250 mg and reserpine 0.125 mg.

DIUTENSEN: methyclothiazide 2.5 mg and cryptenamine 2 mg (as tannate).

DIUTENSEN-R: methyclothiazide 2.5 mg and reserpine 0.1 mg.

ENDURONYL: methyclothiazide 5 mg and deserpidine 0.25 mg.

ENDURONYL-FORTE: methyclothiazide 5 mg and deserpidine 0.5 mg.

ESIMIL: hydrochlorothiazide 25 mg and guanethidine monosulfate 10 mg.

EUTRON FILMTABS: methyclothiazide 5 mg and pargyline HCl 25 mg.

EXNA-R TABLETS: benzthiazide 50 mg and reserpine 0.125 mg.

H.H.R.: hydrochlorothiazide 15 mg, hydralazine HCl 25 mg, and reserpine 0.1 mg.

HYDROMOX-R: quinethazone 50 mg and reserpine 0.125 mg.

HYDROPINE: hydroflumethiazide 25 mg and reserpine 0.125 mg.

HYDROPINE HP: hydroflumethiazide 50 mg and reserpine 0.125 mg.

HYDROPRES-25♦: hydrochlorothiazide 25 mg and reserpine 0.125 mg.

HYDRO-RESERP: hydrochlorothiazide 25 or 50 mg and reserpine 0.125 mg.

HYDRO-SERP: hydrochlorothiazide 25 or 50 mg and reserpine 0.125 mg.

HYDROSERPINE: hydrochlorothiazide 25 or 50 mg and reserpine 0.125 mg.

HYDROTENSIN-25 TABLETS: hydrochlorothiazide 25 mg and reserpine 0.125 mg.

INDERIDE 40/25: propranolol HCl 40 mg and hydrochlorothiazide 25 mg.

INDERIDE 80/25: propranolol HCl 80 mg and hydrochlorothiazide 25 mg.

INDERIDE LA 80/50: propranolol HCl 80 mg and hydrochlorothiazide 50 mg.

LOPRESSOR HCT 50/25: metoprolol tartrate 50 mg and hydrochlorothiazide 25 mg.

LOPRESSOR HCT 100/25: metoprolol tartrate 100 mg and hydrochlorothiazide 25 mg.

MAXZIDE: triamterene 75 mg and hydrochlorothiazide 50 mg.

METATENSIN TABLETS #2 or #4: trichlormethiazide 2 or 4 mg and reserpine 0.1 mg.

MINIZIDE 1: polythiazide 0.5 mg and prazosin 1 mg.

MINIZIDE 2: polythiazide 0.5 mg and prazosin 2 mg.

MINIZIDE 5: polythiazide 0.5 mg and prazosin 5 mg.

NAQUIVAL: trichlormethiazide 4 mg and reserpine 0.1 mg.

NATURETIN W/K 2.5 mg♦: bendroflumethiazide 2.5 mg and potassium chloride 500 mg.

NATURETIN W/K 5 mg♦: bendroflumethiazide 5 mg and potassium chloride 500 mg.

NORMOZIDE 100/25: labetalol 100 mg and hydrochlorothiazide 25 mg.

NORMOZIDE 200/25: labetalol 200 mg and hydrochlorothiazide 25 mg.

NORMOZIDE 300/25: labetalol 300 mg and hydrochlorothiazide 25 mg.

ORETICYL 25: hydrochlorothiazide 25 mg and deserpidine 0.125 mg.

ORETICYL 50: hydrochlorothiazide 50 mg and deserpidine 0.125 mg.

ORETICYL FORTE: hydrochlorothiazide 25 mg and deserpidine 0.25 mg.

RAUZIDE**: bendroflumethiazide 4 mg and powdered rauwolfia serpentina 50 mg.

REGROTON: chlorthalidone 50 mg and reserpine 0.25 mg.

RENESE-R: polythiazide 2 mg and reserpine 0.25 mg.

Italicized side effects are common or life-threatening.
*Liquid form contains alcohol.   **May contain tartrazine.

REZIDE: hydrochlorothiazide 15 mg, hydralazine HCl 25 mg, and reserpine 0.1 mg.

R-HCTZ-H: hydrochlorothiazide 15 mg, hydralazine HCl 25 mg, and reserpine 0.1 mg.

SALUTENSIN♦: hydroflumethiazide 50 mg and reserpine 0.125 mg.

SALUTENSIN DEMI: hydroflumethiazide 25 mg and reserpine 0.125 mg.

SER-A-GEN: hydrochlorothiazide 15 mg, hydralazine HCl 25 mg, and reserpine 0.1 mg.

SERALAZIDE: hydrochlorothiazide 15 mg, hydralazine HCl 25 mg, and reserpine 0.1 mg.

SER-AP-ES♦: hydrochlorothiazide 15 mg, reserpine 0.1 mg, and hydralazine HCl 25 mg.

SERPASIL-APRESOLINE #1**: reserpine 0.1 mg and hydralazine HCl 25 mg.

SERPASIL-APRESOLINE #2♦: reserpine 0.2 mg and hydralazine HCl 50 mg.

SERPASIL-ESIDRIX #1♦: hydrochlorothiazide 25 mg and reserpine 0.1 mg (called Serpasil-Esidrix 25 in Canada).

SERPASIL ESIDRIX #2: hydrochlorothiazide 50 mg and reserpine 0.1 mg.

SERPAZIDE: hydrochlorothiazide 15 mg, hydralazine HCl 25 mg, and reserpine 0.1 mg.

TENORETIC 50: atenolol 50 mg and chlorthalidone 25 mg.

TENORETIC 100: atenolol 100 mg and chlorthalidone 25 mg.

TIMOLIDE 10/25: timolol maleate 10 mg and hydrochlorothiazide 25 mg.

TRI-HYDROSERPINE: hydrochlorothiazide 15 mg, hydralazine HCl 25 mg, and reserpine 0.1 mg.

UNIPRES: hydrochlorothiazide 15 mg, reserpine 0.1 mg, and hydralazine HCl 25 mg.

VASERETIC: enalapril maleate 10 mg and hydrochlorothiazide 25 mg.

acebutolol
Monitan♦♦, Sectral♦

Pregnancy Risk Category: B

MECHANISM OF ACTION
A beta-selective blocking agent, acebutolol decreases myocardial contractility and decreases heart rate. It has mild intrinsic sympathomimetic activity.

INDICATIONS & DOSAGE
Treatment of hypertension—
Adults: 400 mg P.O. either as a single daily dosage or divided b.i.d. Patients may receive as much as 1,200 mg daily.
Ventricular dysrhythmias—
Adults: 400 mg P.O. daily divided b.i.d. Dosage is then increased to provide an adequate clinical response. Usual dosage is 600 to 1,200 mg daily.

ADVERSE REACTIONS
CNS: *fatigue,* headache, dizziness, insomnia.
CV: chest pain, edema, bradycardia, CHF, *hypotension.*
GI: nausea, constipation, diarrhea, dyspepsia.
Metabolic: hypoglycemia without tachycardia.
Skin: rash.
Other: fever.

INTERACTIONS
Insulin, hypoglycemic drugs (oral): can alter dosage requirements in previously stabilized diabetics. Observe patient carefully.
Cardiac glycosides: excessive bradycardia and increased depressant effect on myocardium. Use together cautiously.
Indomethacin: decreased antihypertensive effect. Monitor blood pressure and adjust dosage.

Unmarked trade names available in the United States only.
♦ Also available in Canada.   ♦♦ Available in Canada only.   ◊ Also available OTC.

NURSING CONSIDERATIONS
- Contraindicated in persistently severe bradycardia, second- and third-degree heart block, overt cardiac failure, and cardiogenic shock.
- Use cautiously in patients with cardiac failure.
- Similar to metoprolol, acebutolol is a cardioselective beta blocker. This drug should be used with caution in patients with bronchospastic diseases such as asthma and emphysema.
- Dosage should be reduced in patients with decreased renal function.
- Elderly patients may require lower acebutolol doses. For such patients, dosage should not exceed 800 mg daily.
- Always check patient's apical pulse before giving this drug; if slower than 60 beats/minute, hold drug and call doctor.
- Acebutolol may mask the signs of hyperthyroidism and hyperglycemia, and potentiate insulin-induced hypoglycemia.
- Before surgery, notify anesthesiologist if patient is receiving this drug.
- Do not discontinue abruptly; can exacerbate angina and myocardial infarction.
- Teach patient about his disease and therapy. Explain the importance of taking this drug as prescribed, even when he's feeling well. Tell patient not to discontinue drug suddenly, but to call the doctor if unpleasant adverse effects occur.
- Instruct patient to check with doctor or pharmacist before taking OTC medications.

---

atenolol
Tenormin♦

Pregnancy Risk Category: C

MECHANISM OF ACTION
Blocks response to beta stimulation and depresses renin secretion.

INDICATIONS & DOSAGE
Treatment of hypertension—
Adults: initially, 50 mg P.O. daily as a single dose. Dosage may be increased to 100 mg once daily after 7 to 14 days. Dosages greater than 100 mg are unlikely to produce further benefit. Dosage adjustment is necessary in patients with creatinine clearance below 35 ml/minute.
Angina pectoris—
Adults: 50 mg P.O. once daily. May increase to 100 mg daily after 7 days for optimal effect. May give as much as 200 mg daily.

ADVERSE REACTIONS
CNS: fatigue, lethargy.
CV: *bradycardia, hypotension, congestive heart failure,* peripheral vascular disease.
GI: nausea, vomiting, diarrhea.
Skin: rash.
Other: fever.

INTERACTIONS
Antihypertensives: enhanced hypotensive effect. Use together cautiously.
Cardiac glycosides: excessive bradycardia and increased depressant effect on myocardium. Use together cautiously.
Indomethacin: decrease in antihypertensive effect. Monitor blood pressure and adjust dosage.
Insulin, hypoglycemic drugs (oral): can alter dosage requirements in previously stabilized diabetics. Observe patient carefully.

NURSING CONSIDERATIONS
- Contraindicated in sinus bradycardia and greater than first-degree conduction block, and cardiogenic shock.
- Use cautiously in cardiac failure.
- Similar to metoprolol, atenolol is a cardioselective beta blocker. Although atenolol can be used in patients with bronchospastic diseases such as asthma and emphysema, the drug should still be used cautiously in

---

such patients—especially when 100 mg are given. Twice-daily dosing may help minimize this risk.
- Dosage should be reduced if patient has renal insufficiency.
- Once-a-day dosage encourages patient compliance. Counsel your patient to take the drug at a regular time every day. Drug can be dispensed in a 28-day calendar pack.
- Full antihypertensive effect may not appear for 1 to 2 weeks after initiating therapy.
- Always check patient's apical pulse before giving this drug; if slower than 60 beats/minute, hold drug and call doctor.
- Monitor blood pressure frequently.
- Don't discontinue abruptly; can exacerbate angina and myocardial infarction. Drug should be withdrawn gradually over a 2-week period.
- Teach patient about his disease and therapy. Explain the importance of taking this drug as prescribed, even when he's feeling well. Tell patient not to discontinue drug suddenly, but to call the doctor if unpleasant adverse effects occur.
- Instruct patient to check with doctor or pharmacist before taking OTC medications.
- This drug masks common signs of shock and hypoglycemia. However, atenolol doesn't potentiate insulin-induced hypoglycemia or delay recovery of blood glucose to normal levels.
- Has been prescribed effectively in the treatment of angina pectoris and in patients with alcohol withdrawal syndrome.
- Atenolol and other beta blockers are being prescribed to decrease mortality after myocardial infarction.

captopril
Capoten♦

Pregnancy Risk Category: C

MECHANISM OF ACTION
By inhibiting angiotensin-converting enzyme, prevents pulmonary conversion of angiotensin I to angiotensin II.

INDICATIONS & DOSAGE
Hypertension—
Adults: 25 mg P.O. b.i.d. or t.i.d. initially. If blood pressure isn't satisfactorily controlled in 1 to 2 weeks, dosage may be increased to 50 mg t.i.d. If not satisfactorily controlled after another 1 to 2 weeks, a diuretic should be added to regimen. If further blood pressure reduction is necessary, dosage may be raised to as high as 150 mg t.i.d. while continuing the diuretic. Maximum dosage is 450 mg daily. Daily dose may also be administered b.i.d.
Congestive heart failure—
Adults: 6.25 to 12.5 mg P.O. t.i.d. initially. May be gradually increased to 50 mg t.i.d. Maximum dosage is 450 mg daily.

ADVERSE REACTIONS
Blood: *leukopenia, agranulocytosis, pancytopenia.*
CNS: dizziness, fainting.
CV: *tachycardia, hypotension,* angina pectoris, CHF, pericarditis.
EENT: *loss of taste (dysgeusia), persistant cough.*
GU: *proteinuria, nephrotic syndrome, membranous glomerulopathy, renal failure,* urinary frequency.
GI: anorexia.
Metabolic: hyperkalemia.
Skin: *urticarial rash, maculopapular rash,* pruritus.
Other: fever, angioedema of face and extremities, transient increases in liver enzymes, persistent cough.

INTERACTIONS
NSAIDs: may reduce antihypertensive effect. Monitor blood pressure.
Potassium supplements: increased risk of hyperkalemia. Avoid these supplements unless hypokalemic blood levels are confirmed.
Antacids: decreased captopril effect. Separate administration times.

NURSING CONSIDERATIONS
• Use cautiously in impaired renal function or serious autoimmune disease (particularly systemic lupus erythematosus), or in patients who have been exposed to other drugs known to affect white cell counts or immune response.
• Proteinuria and nephrotic syndrome may occur in patients who are on captopril therapy. Those who develop persistent proteinuria or proteinuria that exceeds 1 g daily should have their captopril therapy reevaluated.
• Monitor patient's blood pressure and pulse rate frequently.
• Perform WBC and differential counts before starting treatment, every 2 weeks for the first 3 months of therapy, and periodically thereafter.
• Advise patients to report any sign of infection (sore throat, fever).
• Although captopril can be used alone, its beneficial effects are increased when a thiazide diuretic is added.
• May cause dizziness or fainting, especially during initiation of therapy. Advise patient to avoid sudden postural changes.
• Teach patient about his disease and therapy. Explain the importance of taking this drug as prescribed, even when he's feeling well. Tell outpatient not to discontinue drug suddenly, but to call the doctor if unpleasant adverse effects occur.
• Instruct patient to check with doctor or pharmacist before taking OTC medications.
• Elderly patients may be more sensitive to the drug's hypotensive effects.
• Should be taken 1 hour before meals since food in the GI tract may reduce absorption.
• Has been prescribed to treat rheumatoid arthritis.

clonidine hydrochloride
Catapres♦, Catapres-TTS, Dixarit♦♦

Pregnancy Risk Category: C

MECHANISM OF ACTION
Inhibits the central vasomotor centers, thereby decreasing sympathetic outflow.

INDICATIONS & DOSAGE
Essential, renal, and malignant hypertension—
Adults: initially, 0.1 mg P.O. b.i.d. Then increase by 0.1 to 0.2 mg daily on a weekly basis. Usual dosage range is 0.2 to 0.8 mg daily in divided doses; infrequently, dosages as high as 2.4 mg daily. No dosing recommendations for children.
Or, apply transdermal patch to a hairless area of intact skin on the upper arm or torso, once every 7 days.
To suppress abstinence symptoms during narcotics withdrawal—
Adults: 0.1 mg P.O. t.i.d.

ADVERSE REACTIONS
CNS: *drowsiness,* dizziness, fatigue, sedation, nervousness, headache, vivid dreams.
CV: orthostatic hypotension, bradycardia, *severe rebound hypertension.*
EENT: *dry mouth.*
GI: *constipation.*
GU: urine retention, impotence.
Metabolic: transient glucose intolerance (after large doses).
Skin: *pruritus, dermatitis* (from transdermal patch).

INTERACTIONS
CNS depressants: enhanced CNS de-

Italicized side effects are common or life-threatening.
*Liquid form contains alcohol.   **May contain tartrazine.

pression. Use together cautiously.
Propranolol and other beta blockers:
paradoxical hypertensive response.
Monitor carefully.
Tricyclic antidepressants and MAO inhibitors: may decrease antihypertensive effect. Use together cautiously.

NURSING CONSIDERATIONS

• Use cautiously in patients with severe coronary insufficiency, diabetes, myocardial infarction, cerebral vascular disease, chronic renal failure, or history of depression, or in those taking other antihypertensives.
• Monitor blood pressure and pulse rate frequently. Dosage is usually adjusted to patient's blood pressure and tolerance.
• May be given to rapidly lower blood pressure in some hypertensive emergency situations.
• Discontinuing clonidine for surgery is not recommended.
• Reduce dosage gradually over 2 to 4 days. If discontinued abruptly, this drug may cause severe hypertension.
• In patients receiving both clonidine and a beta blocker, the beta blocker should be gradually withdrawn before clonidine to minimize adverse effects.
• Teach patient about his disease and therapy. Explain the importance of taking this drug exactly as prescribed, even when he's feeling well. Tell outpatient not to discontinue this drug suddenly because this can cause severe rebound hypertension, but to call the doctor if unpleasant adverse effects occur. Warn that this drug can cause drowsiness, but that tolerance to this side effect will develop.
• Instruct patient to check with doctor or pharmacist before taking OTC medications.
• Observe for tolerance to the drug's therapeutic effects that may require an increased dosage.
• Inform patient that orthostatic hypotension can be minimized by rising slowly and avoiding sudden position

changes.
• Periodic eye examinations are recommended.
• Elderly patients may be more sensitive to hypotensive effects.
• Last dose should be taken immediately before retiring.
• Transdermal patch provides antihypertensive activity for up to 7 days. Available in three strengths: TTS-1 contains 2.5 mg; TTS-2 contains 5 mg; TTS contains 7.5 mg of clonidine.
• Transdermal patch usually adheres despite showering and other routine daily activities. An adhesive "overlay" is available to provide additional skin adherence if necessary. Instruct the patient to place the patch at a different site each week.
• Antihypertensive effects of transdermal clonidine may take 2 to 3 days to become apparent. Oral antihypertensive therapy may have to be continued in the interim.
• Remove patch before defibrillation to prevent arcing.
• Has been used investigationally for migraine headache prophylaxis and treatment of dysmenorrhea. May also suppress craving for nicotine in nicotine addiction.

---

deserpidine
Harmonyl

Pregnancy Risk Category: C

MECHANISM OF ACTION
Acts peripherally, inhibiting norepinephrine release and depleting norepinephrine stores in adrenergic nerve endings.

INDICATIONS & DOSAGE
Mild essential hypertension—
Adults: 0.25 mg P.O. once daily. No dosing recommendations for children.

ADVERSE REACTIONS
CNS: mental confusion, *depression,*

drowsiness, nervousness, paradoxical anxiety, nightmares, *sedation, extrapyramidal symptoms.*
CV: *bradycardia.*
EENT: *dry mouth, nasal stuffiness,* glaucoma.
GI: *hypersecretion of gastric acid, nausea, vomiting,* GI bleeding.
Skin: pruritus, rash.
Other: *impotence, weight gain.*

INTERACTIONS
MAO inhibitors: may cause excitability and hypertension. Avoid if possible.

NURSING CONSIDERATIONS
• Contraindicated in mental depression. Use cautiously in severe cardiac or cerebrovascular disease, peptic ulcer, ulcerative colitis, gallstones, or mental depressive disorders; in patients undergoing surgery; and in patients taking other antihypertensives or anticonvulsants.
• Monitor patient's blood pressure and pulse rate frequently.
• Teach patient about his disease and therapy. Explain the importance of taking this drug as prescribed, even when he's feeling well. Tell outpatient not to discontinue this drug suddenly, but to call the doctor if unpleasant adverse effects, such as mental depression, insomnia, or loss of appetite, occur. Warn that drug can cause drowsiness.
• Instruct patient to check with doctor or pharmacist before taking OTC medications.
• Advise patients to have periodic eye examinations.
• Watch patient closely for signs of mental depression. Warn him to notify doctor promptly if he experiences nightmares.
• Tell patient to avoid alcohol and to follow prescribed diet.
• Dry mouth can be relieved with chewing gum, sour hard candy, or ice chips. Tell patient to contact doctor if

relief is needed for nasal stuffiness.
• Give this drug with meals to increase absorption.
• Patient should weigh himself daily and notify doctor of any weight gain.

diazoxide
Hyperstat♦ (I.V. only)
Pregnancy Risk Category: C

MECHANISM OF ACTION
Directly relaxes arteriolar smooth muscle.

INDICATIONS & DOSAGE
Hypertensive crisis—
Adults and children: 1 to 3 mg/kg I.V. (up to a maximum of 150 mg) q 5 to 15 minutes until adequate response is seen. Repeat at intervals q 4 to 24 hours p.r.n.

ADVERSE REACTIONS
CNS: *headaches,* dizziness, lightheadedness, euphoria.
CV: *sodium and water retention, orthostatic hypotension,* sweating, flushing, warmth, angina, myocardial ischemia, dysrhythmias, ECG changes.
GI: *nausea, vomiting,* abdominal discomfort.
Metabolic: *hyperglycemia,* hyperuricemia.
Local: inflammation and pain from extravasation.

INTERACTIONS
Hydralazine: may cause severe hypotension. Use together cautiously.
Thiazide diuretics: may increase the effects of diazoxide. Use together cautiously.

NURSING CONSIDERATIONS
• Use cautiously in patients with impaired cerebral or cardiac function, diabetes, or uremia, or in those taking other antihypertensives.
• Monitor blood pressure and ECG

---

continuously. Patient should be supine or in Trendelenberg's position during and for 1 hour after infusion. Notify doctor immediately if severe hypotension develops. Keep norepinephrine available.
• Monitor patient's intake/output carefully. If fluid or sodium retention develops, doctor may want to order diuretics.
• Check patient's standing blood pressure before discontinuing close monitoring for hypotension.
• Take care to avoid extravasation.
• This drug may alter requirements for insulin, diet, or oral hypoglycemic drugs in previously controlled diabetics. Monitor blood glucose daily.
• Weigh patient daily. Notify doctor of any weight increase.
• Watch diabetics closely for signs of severe hyperglycemia or hyperosmolar nonketotic coma. Insulin may be needed.
• Check patient's uric acid levels frequently. Report abnormalities to doctor.
• Inform patient that orthostatic hypotension can be minimized by rising slowly and avoiding sudden position changes. Instruct patient to remain supine for 30 minutes after injection.
• Infusion of diazoxide has been shown to be as effective as a bolus in some patients.
• Protect I.V. solutions from light. Darkened I.V. solutions of diazoxide are subpotent and should not be used.

---

enalapril maleate
Vasotec♦

Pregnancy Risk Category: C

MECHANISM OF ACTION
By inhibiting angiotensin-converting enzyme, prevents pulmonary conversion of angiotensin I to angiotensin II.

INDICATIONS & DOSAGE
Treatment of hypertension—

Adults: Initially, 5 mg P.O. once daily, then adjust according to response. Usual dosage range is 10 to 40 mg daily as a single dose or two divided doses.

ADVERSE REACTIONS
Blood: neutropenia, *agranulocytosis.*
CNS: *headache, dizziness, fatigue,* insomnia.
CV: *hypotension.*
GI: diarrhea, nausea.
Skin: rash.
Other: persistent cough, *angioedema.*

INTERACTIONS
Lithium: lithium toxicity can occur. Monitor lithium levels.

NURSING CONSIDERATIONS
• Use cautiously in preexisting renal impairment or collagen vascular disease. Diabetic patients, patients with impaired renal function or CHF, and patients receiving drugs that can increase serum potassium may develop hyperkalemia. Monitor potassium intake and serum potassium level.
• If patient is taking a diuretic, it should be discontinued 2 to 3 days before beginning enalapril therapy. This will reduce the risk of hypotension. Then, if enalapril does not control blood pressure, diuretic therapy may be added.
• Teach patient about his disease and therapy. Explain the importance of taking this drug as prescribed, even when he's feeling well. Tell outpatient not to discontinue drug suddenly, but to call the doctor if unpleasant adverse effects occur.
• Instruct patient to check with doctor or pharmacist before taking OTC medications.
• Angioedema (including laryngeal edema) may occur, especially after the first enalapril dose. Advise patient to report any signs or symptoms such as swelling of face, eyes, lips, tongue,

---

Unmarked trade names available in the United States only.
♦ Also available in Canada.   ♦♦ Available in Canada only.   ◊ Also available OTC.

or breathing difficulty.
• Advise patient to report light-headedness, especially during the first few days of therapy, when it's most likely to occur.
• Advise patient to report any sign of infection.
• Enalapril is similar to captopril, the other angiotensin-converting enzyme inhibitor, but has a longer duration of action. Many patients may get satisfactory therapeutic results by taking enalapril once daily.

guanabenz acetate
Wytensin

Pregnancy Risk Category: C

MECHANISM OF ACTION
Inhibits the central vasomotor centers, thereby decreasing sympathetic outflow.

INDICATIONS & DOSAGE
Treatment of hypertension—
Adults: initially, 4 mg P.O. b.i.d. Dosage may be increased in increments of 4 to 8 mg/day q 1 to 2 weeks. Maximum dosage is 32 mg b.i.d. To ensure adequate overnight blood pressure control, give last dose h.s.

ADVERSE REACTIONS
CNS: *drowsiness, sedation, dizziness, weakness,* headache, ataxia, depression.
CV: *severe rebound hypertension.*
EENT: *dry mouth.*
GU: sexual dysfunction.

INTERACTIONS
CNS depressants: may cause increased sedation. Use together cautiously.

NURSING CONSIDERATIONS
• Use cautiously in vascular insufficiency, coronary insufficiency, recent myocardial infarction, cerebrovascular disease, or severe hepatic or renal failure.
• Don't stop guanabenz therapy abruptly. Rebound hypertension may occur.
• Advise patient to drive a car or operate machinery very cautiously until the CNS effects of the drug are known.
• Elderly patients may be more sensitive to hypotensive effects.
• Warn patient that his tolerance to alcohol or other CNS depressants may be diminished.
• Guanabenz can be used alone or in combination with a thiazide diuretic.
• Teach patient about his disease and therapy. Explain the importance of taking this drug as prescribed, even when he's feeling well. Tell outpatient not to discontinue drug suddenly, but to call the doctor if unpleasant adverse effects occur.
• Instruct patient to check with doctor or pharmacist before taking OTC medications.
• To relieve dry mouth, tell patient to chew sugarless gum or dissolve ice chips in the mouth.
• Has been used investigationally as an adjunct in the treatment of opiate withdrawal (4 mg P.O. b.i.d.).

guanadrel sulfate
Hylorel

Pregnancy Risk Category: B

MECHANISM OF ACTION
Acts peripherally, inhibiting norepinephrine release and depleting norepinephrine stores in adrenergic nerve endings.

INDICATIONS & DOSAGE
Treatment of hypertension—
Adults: initially, 5 mg P.O. b.i.d. Dosage can be adjusted until blood pressure is controlled. Most patients require doses of 20 to 75 mg/day, usually given b.i.d.

ADVERSE REACTIONS

CNS: *fatigue, dizziness,* drowsiness, faintness.
CV: *orthostatic hypotension,* edema.
GI: diarrhea.
Other: impotence, ejaculation disturbances.

INTERACTIONS

MAO inhibitors, ephedrine, norepinephrine, methylphenidate, tricyclic antidepressants, amphetamines, phenothiazines: may inhibit the antihypertensive effect of guanadrel. Adjust dose accordingly.

NURSING CONSIDERATIONS

• Contraindicated in known or suspected pheochromocytoma or frank CHF.
• Use cautiously in known regional vascular disease, asthma, and history of peptic ulcer disease.
• Guanadrel should be discontinued 48 to 72 hours before surgery to minimize the risk of vascular collapse during anesthesia.
• Don't give concurrently or within 1 week of therapy with an MAO inhibitor.
• Patient response varies widely with this drug and dosage must be individualized. Monitor both supine and standing blood pressure, especially during the period of dosage adjustment.
• Teach patient about his disease and therapy. Explain the importance of taking this drug as prescribed, even when he's feeling well. Tell patient not to discontinue this drug suddenly, but to call the doctor if unpleasant adverse effects occur.
• Instruct patient to check with doctor or pharmacist before taking OTC medications.
• Tell outpatient to avoid strenuous exercise, and warn that hot showers may cause hypotensive reaction.
• Inform patient that orthostatic hypotension can be minimized by rising slowly from a supine position and by avoiding sudden position changes.
• Elderly patients may be more sensitive to hypotensive effects.

guanethidine sulfate
Apo-Guanethidine♦♦, Ismelin♦
Pregnancy Risk Category: C

MECHANISM OF ACTION

Acts peripherally, inhibiting norepinephrine release and depleting norepinephrine stores in adrenergic nerve endings.

INDICATIONS & DOSAGE

For moderate to severe hypertension; usually used in combination with other antihypertensives—
Adults: initially, 10 mg P.O. daily. Increase by 10 mg at weekly to monthly intervals, p.r.n. Usual dose is 25 to 50 mg daily. Some patients may require up to 300 mg.
Children: initially, 200 mcg/kg P.O. daily. Increase gradually q 1 to 3 weeks to maximum of 8 times initial dose.

ADVERSE REACTIONS

CNS: *dizziness, weakness, syncope.*
CV: *orthostatic hypotension, bradycardia,* CHF, dysrhythmias.
EENT: *nasal stuffiness*
GI: *diarrhea.*
Other: *edema, weight gain, inhibition of ejaculation.*

INTERACTIONS

Levodopa, alcohol: may increase hypotensive effect of guanethidine. Use together cautiously.
MAO inhibitors, ephedrine, norepinephrine, methylphenidate, tricyclic antidepressants, amphetamines, phenothiazines: may inhibit the antihypertensive effect of guanethidine. Adjust dose accordingly.

NURSING CONSIDERATIONS
• Contraindicated in pheochromocytoma. Use cautiously in severe cardiac disease, recent myocardial infarction, cerebrovascular disease, peptic ulcer, impaired renal function, or bronchial asthma, or in patients taking other antihypertensives.
• Full antihypertensive effect may not appear for 1 to 3 weeks.
• Discontinue drug 2 to 3 weeks before elective surgery to reduce the possibility of vascular collapse and cardiac arrest during anesthesia.
• Teach patient about his disease and therapy. Explain the importance of taking this drug as prescribed, even when he's feeling well. Tell patient not to discontinue this drug suddenly, but to call the doctor if unpleasant adverse effects occur.
• Instruct patient to check with doctor or pharmacist before taking OTC medications.
• Tell outpatient to avoid strenuous exercise, and warn that hot showers may cause hypotensive reaction.
• Patient should receive instruction on low-sodium diet. Monitor for possible weight gain and edema.
• A hot environment may also potentiate the hypotensive effects of guanethidine.
• Inform patient that orthostatic hypotension can be minimized by rising slowly and avoiding sudden position changes. Dry mouth can be relieved with sugarless chewing gum, sour hard candy, or ice chips.
• Elderly patients may be more sensitive to hypotensive effects.
• If patient develops diarrhea, doctor may prescribe atropine or paregoric.

guanfacine hydrochloride
Tenex

Pregnancy Risk Category: B

MECHANISM OF ACTION
Inhibits the central vasomotor center,
thereby decreasing sympathetic outflow.

INDICATIONS & DOSAGE
Treatment of mild to moderate hypertension—
Adults: initially, 0.5 to 1 mg P.O. daily, h.s. Average dose is 1 to 3 mg daily.

ADVERSE REACTIONS
CNS: *drowsiness, dizziness,* fatigue, headache, insomnia.
CV: bradycardia, orthostatic hypotension, rebound hypertension.
EENT: dry mouth.
GI: *constipation,* diarrhea, nausea.
Skin: dermatitis, pruritus.

INTERACTIONS
None significant.

NURSING CONSIDERATIONS
• Use cautiously in severe coronary insufficiency, recent myocardial infarction, cerebrovascular disease, or chronic renal or hepatic insufficiency.
• Warn patients not to discontinue therapy abruptly. Rebound hypertension is less common than with similar drugs, such as clonidine, but may occur.
• Guanfacine reportedly has no adverse effect on blood lipids.
• May be used alone or with a diuretic.
• The incidence and severity of adverse reactions increase with higher dosages.
• Teach patient about his disease and therapy. Explain the importance of taking this drug as prescribed, even when he's feeling well. Tell outpatient not to discontinue drug suddenly, but to call the doctor if unpleasant adverse effects occur.
• Instruct patient to check with doctor or pharmacist before taking OTC medications.
• Because guanfacine causes drowsiness, advise patient to avoid activities

that require alertness until response to the drug is established.

• Guanfacine appears to be as effective as methyldopa and clonidine; long half-life permits once-daily dosing.

---

hydralazine hydrochloride
Apresoline♦**, Novo-Hylazin♦♦
Pregnancy Risk Category: C

MECHANISM OF ACTION
Directly relaxes arteriolar smooth muscle.

INDICATIONS & DOSAGE
Essential hypertension (oral, alone or in combination with other antihypertensives); to reduce afterload in severe CHF (with nitrates); and severe essential hypertension (parenteral to lower blood pressure quickly)—
Adults: initially, 10 mg P.O. q.i.d.; gradually increased to 50 mg q.i.d. Maximum recommended dosage is 200 mg daily, but some patients may require 300 to 400 mg daily. Can be given b.i.d. for CHF.
I.V.—10 to 20 mg given slowly and repeated as necessary, generally q 4 to 6 hours. Switch to oral antihypertensives as soon as possible.
I.M.—20 to 40 mg repeated as necessary, generally q 4 to 6 hours. Switch to oral antihypertensives as soon as possible.
Children: initially, 0.75 mg/kg P.O. daily in four divided doses (25 mg/m² daily). May increase gradually to 10 times this dosage, if necessary.
I.V.—give slowly 1.7 to 3.5 mg/kg daily or 50 to 100 mg/m² daily in four to six divided doses.
I.M.—1.7 to 3.5 mg/kg daily or 50 to 100 mg/m² daily in four to six divided doses.

ADVERSE REACTIONS
Blood: neutropenia, leukopenia.
CNS: peripheral neuritis, *headache*,

dizziness.
CV: orthostatic hypotension, *tachycardia*, dysrhythmias, *angina, palpitations, sodium retention*.
GI: *nausea, vomiting, diarrhea, anorexia*.
Skin: rash.
Other: *lupus erythematosus-like syndrome (especially with high doses), weight gain*.

INTERACTIONS
Diazoxide: may cause severe hypotension. Use together cautiously.

NURSING CONSIDERATIONS
• Use cautiously in cardiac disease, CVA, or severe renal impairment, and in those taking other antihypertensives.
• Monitor patient's blood pressure, pulse rate, and body weight frequently. Some clinicians combine hydralazine therapy with diuretics and beta-adrenergic blocking agents to decrease sodium retention and tachycardia, and to prevent anginal attacks.
• Watch patient closely for signs of lupus erythematosus-like syndrome (sore throat, fever, muscle and joint aches, skin rash). Call doctor immediately if any of these develop.
• Teach patient about his disease and therapy. Explain the importance of taking this drug as prescribed, even when he's feeling well. Tell outpatient not to discontinue this drug suddenly, but to call the doctor if unpleasant adverse effects occur.
• Instruct patient to check with doctor or pharmacist before taking OTC medications.
• Inform patient that orthostatic hypotension can be minimized by rising slowly and avoiding sudden position changes.
• Elderly patients may be more sensitive to hypotensive effects.
• Give this drug with meals to increase absorption.
• Compliance may be improved by

---

administering this drug b.i.d. Check with doctor.

• CBC, LE cell preparation, and antinuclear antibody titer determinations should be done before therapy and periodically during long-term therapy.

• Has been prescribed during pregnancy for treatment of eclampsia. Administered I.V.

labetalol

Normodyne, Trandate♦

Pregnancy Risk Category: C

MECHANISM OF ACTION
Blocks response to alpha and beta stimulation and depresses renin secretion.

INDICATIONS & DOSAGE
Treatment of hypertension—
Adults: 100 mg P.O. b.i.d. with or without a diuretic. Dose may be increased to 200 mg b.i.d. after 2 days. Further dose increases may be made q 1 to 3 days until optimum response is reached. Usual maintenance dosage is 200 to 400 mg b.i.d.
For severe hypertension and hypertensive emergencies—
Adults: Dilute 200 mg to 200 ml with dextrose 5% in water. Infuse at 2 mg/minute until satisfactory response is obtained. Then stop the infusion. May repeat q 6 to 8 hours.

Alternatively, administer by repeated I.V. injection: Initially, give 20 mg I.V. slowly over 2 minutes. May repeat injections of 40 to 80 mg q 10 minutes until maximum dose of 300 mg is reached.

ADVERSE REACTIONS
CNS: vivid dreams, fatigue, headache.
CV: *orthostatic hypotension and dizziness,* peripheral vascular disease, bradycardia.
EENT: nasal stuffiness.

Endocrine: hypoglycemia without tachycardia.
GI: nausea, vomiting, diarrhea.
GU: sexual dysfunction, urine retention.
Skin: rash.
Other: increased airway resistance, transient scalp tingling.

INTERACTIONS
Cimetidine: may enhance labetalol's effect. Give together cautiously.
Insulin, hypoglycemic drugs (oral): can alter dosage requirements in previously stabilized diabetics. Observe patient carefully.

NURSING CONSIDERATIONS
• Contraindicated in bronchial asthma.
• Use cautiously in CHF, hepatic failure, chronic bronchitis, emphysema, preexisting peripheral vascular disease, and pheochromocytoma.
• Monitor blood pressure frequently.
• Teach patient about his disease and therapy. Explain the importance of taking this drug as prescribed, even when he's feeling well. Tell outpatient not to discontinue this drug suddenly; abrupt discontinuation can exacerbate angina and myocardial infarction. Tell patient to call the doctor if unpleasant adverse effects occur.
• Instruct patient to check with doctor or pharmacist before taking OTC medications.
• This drug masks common signs of shock and hypoglycemia.
• Labetalol is a beta-adrenergic blocker which also has unique alpha-adrenergic blocking effects.
• Unlike other beta blockers, labetalol does not decrease heart rate or cardiac output.
• Dizziness is the most troublesome adverse reaction and tends to occur in early stages of treatment, in patients also receiving diuretics, and in patients receiving higher dosages. Inform patient that this can be mini-

---

Italicized side effects are common or life-threatening.
*Liquid form contains alcohol.   **May contain tartrazine.

mized by rising slowly and avoiding sudden position changes. Taking a dose at bedtime or taking smaller doses t.i.d. will also help minimize this adverse reaction. Discuss changes in medication schedule with doctor.
• Transient scalp tingling occurs occasionally at the beginning of labetalol therapy. This usually subsides quickly.
• When administered I.V. for hypertensive emergencies, labetalol produces a rapid, predictable fall in blood pressure within 5 to 10 minutes. Labetolol injection should be administered with a controlled infusion pump. Monitor blood pressure closely: q 5 minutes for 30 minutes, then q 30 minutes for 2 hours, then hourly for 6 hours. Patient should remain supine for 3 hours after infusion.

lisinopril
Prinivil, Zestril

Pregnancy Risk Category: C

MECHANISM OF ACTION
Lisinopril inhibits angiotensin converting enzyme (ACE), preventing pulmonary conversion of angiotensin I to angiotensin II, a potent vasoconstrictor. This decreases peripheral arterial resistance and aldosterone secretion, thereby reducing sodium and water retention and blood pressure.

INDICATIONS & DOSAGE
Mild to severe hypertension—
Adults: initially, 10 mg P.O. daily. Most patients are well controlled on 20 to 40 mg daily as a single dose.

ADVERSE REACTIONS
Blood: neutropenia.
CNS: *dizziness, headache, fatigue,* depression, somnolence, paresthesia.
CV: hypotension, *orthostasis,* chest pain.

EENT: *nasal congestion.*
GI: *diarrhea,* nausea, dyspepsia, dysgeusia.
GU: impotence.
Metabolic: hyperkalemia.
Skin: rash.
Other: *upper respiratory symptoms, cough, muscle cramps, angiodema,* decreased libido.

INTERACTIONS
Diuretics: excessive hypotension.
Indomethacin: attenuated hypotensive effect.
Potassium-sparing diuretics, potassium supplements, potassium-containing salt substitutes: possible hyperkalemia.

NURSING CONSIDERATIONS
• Lisinopril absorption is unaffected by food.
• Lisinopril attenuates potassium loss of thiazide diuretics. If patient is taking a diuretic, the diuretic should be discontinued 2 to 3 days before lisinopril therapy, or lisinopril dosage should be reduced to 5 mg once daily.
• If drug does not adequately control blood pressure, diuretics may be added.
• Teach patient about his disease and therapy. Explain the importance of taking this drug as prescribed, even when he's feeling well. Tell outpatient not to discontinue drug suddenly, but to call the doctor if unpleasant adverse effects occur.
• Instruct patient to check with doctor or pharmacist before taking OTC medications.
• Review WBC and differential counts before treatment every 2 weeks for 3 months, and periodically thereafter.
• Lower dosage is necessary in patients with impaired renal function.
• Beneficial effects of lisinopril may require several weeks of therapy.
• Tell patient to report light-headedness, especially in first few days of

treatment, so dose can be adjusted; signs of infection such as sore throat or fever, because drugs may decrease WBC count; facial swelling or difficulty breathing, because drug may cause angioedema; and loss of taste, which may necessitate discontinuation of drug.

• Advise patient to avoid sudden postural changes to minimize orthostatic hypotension.

mecamylamine hydrochloride
Inversine

Pregnancy Risk Category: C

MECHANISM OF ACTION
A ganglionic blocker; competes with acetylcholine for ganglionic cholinergic receptors.

INDICATIONS & DOSAGE
For moderate to severe essential hypertension and uncomplicated malignant hypertension—
Adults: initially, 2.5 mg P.O. b.i.d. Increase by 2.5 mg daily q 2 days. Average daily dose is 25 mg given in three divided doses. No dosing recommendations for children.

ADVERSE REACTIONS
CNS: *paresthesia,* sedation, *fatigue, tremor, choreiform movements,* seizures, psychic changes, dizziness, *weakness, headaches.*
CV: *orthostatic hypotension.*
EENT: *dry mouth,* glossitis, dilated pupils, *blurred vision.*
GI: *anorexia, nausea, vomiting, constipation, adynamic ileus, diarrhea.*
GU: urine retention, impotence.
Other: decreased libido.

INTERACTIONS
Alcohol, bethanecol: excessive hypotension. Don't use together.
Sodium bicarbonate, acetazolamide: may increase effect of mecamylamine. Use together cautiously. Watch for increased hypotensive effects and toxicity.

NURSING CONSIDERATIONS
• Contraindicated in recent myocardial infarction, uremia, or chronic pyelonephritis. Use cautiously in lower urinary tract pathology, renal insufficiency, glaucoma, pyloric stenosis, coronary insufficiency, or in patients taking other antihypertensives. Mecamylamine is usually reserved for moderate to severe hypertension that is refractory to other drugs.
• Effects of this drug are increased by high environmental temperature, fever, stress, or severe illness.
• Don't withdraw this drug suddenly; rebound hypertension may occur.
• Frequently monitor patient's standing blood pressure.
• Give with meals for more gradual absorption. Schedule the administration consistently with meals. Don't restrict sodium intake.
• If patient develops constipation from this drug, the doctor may want him to take milk of magnesia. Instruct patient to avoid bulk laxatives.
• Teach the patient about his disease and therapy. Explain the importance of taking this drug as prescribed, even when he's feeling well. Tell outpatient to call the doctor if unpleasant adverse reactions develop. Warn him against discontinuing the drug suddenly because this may cause severe rebound hypertension.
• Instruct patient to check with doctor or pharmacist before taking OTC medications.
• Inform patient that orthostatic hypotension can be minimized by rising slowly and avoiding sudden position changes. Dry mouth can be relieved with sugarless chewing gum, sour hard candy, or ice chips.

Italicized side effects are common or life-threatening.
*Liquid form contains alcohol.   **May contain tartrazine.

methyldopa
Aldomet♦, Apo-Methyldopa♦♦,
Dopamet♦♦, Novomedopa♦♦

Pregnancy Risk Category: B

MECHANISM OF ACTION
Inhibits the central vasomotor centers, thereby decreasing sympathetic outflow.

INDICATIONS & DOSAGE
For sustained mild to severe hypertension; should not be used for acute treatment of hypertensive emergencies—
Adults: initially, 250 mg P.O. b.i.d. to t.i.d. in first 48 hours. Then increase as needed q 2 days. May give entire daily dosage in the evening or h.s. Dosages may need adjustment if other antihypertensive drugs are added to or deleted from therapy. Maintenance dosage is 500 mg to 2 g daily in two to four divided doses. Maximum recommended daily dosage is 3 g.
I.V.—500 mg to 1 g q 6 hours, diluted in dextrose 5% in water, and administered over 30 to 60 minutes. Switch to oral antihypertensives as soon as possible.
Children: initially, 10 mg/kg P.O. daily in two to three divided doses; or 20 to 40 mg/kg I.V. daily in four divided doses. Increase dose daily until desired response occurs. Maximum daily dose is 65 mg/kg.

ADVERSE REACTIONS
Blood: *hemolytic anemia,* reversible granulocytopenia, thrombocytopenia.
CNS: *sedation,* headache, asthenia, weakness, dizziness, *decreased mental acuity,* involuntary choreoathetotic movements, psychic disturbances, depression, nightmares.
CV: bradycardia, *orthostatic hypotension,* aggravated angina, myocarditis, *edema, and weight gain.*
EENT: *dry mouth, nasal stuffiness.*

GI: diarrhea, pancreatitis.
Hepatic: *hepatic necrosis.*
Other: gynecomastia, lactation, skin rash, *drug-induced fever,* impotence.

INTERACTIONS
Norepinephrine, phenothiazines, tricyclic antidepressants, amphetamines: possible hypertensive effects. Monitor carefully.

NURSING CONSIDERATIONS
• Use cautiously in patients receiving other antihypertensives or MAO inhibitors and in patients with impaired hepatic function. Monitor blood pressure and pulse rate frequently.
• Methyldopa is frequently used to treat hypertension in pregnant women, apparently without ill effects to the fetus if the patient is closely monitored. Some clinicians recommend that therapy not begin between 16 and 20 weeks' gestation, if possible.
• Observe for involuntary choreoathetoid movements. Report to doctor; he may discontinue drug.
• Observe patient for side effects, particularly unexplained fever. Report adverse reactions to doctor.
• After dialysis, monitor patient for hypertension. Patient may need an extra dose of methyldopa.
• If patient requires blood transfusion, make sure he gets direct and indirect Coombs' tests to avoid crossmatching problems.
• Monitor blood studies (CBC) before and during therapy. Monitor hepatic function periodically, especially during the first 6 to 12 weeks of therapy.
• If patient has received this drug for several months, positive reaction to direct Coombs' test indicates hemolytic anemia.
• Weigh patient daily. Notify doctor of any weight increase. Salt and water retention may occur but can be relieved with diuretics.

• Teach patient about his disease and therapy. Explain the importance of taking this drug as prescribed, even when he's feeling well. Tell outpatient not to stop this drug suddenly, but to call the doctor if unpleasant adverse effects occur. Check dosage schedule with doctor.
• Warn patient that this drug may impair ability to perform tasks that require mental alertness, particularly at start of therapy. Once-daily dosage given at bedtime will minimize daytime drowsiness.
• Instruct patient to check with doctor or pharmacist before taking OTC medications.
• Inform patient that orthostatic hypotension can be minimized by rising slowly and avoiding sudden position changes. Dry mouth can be relieved with sugarless chewing gum, sour hard candy, or ice chips.
• Tell patient that urine may turn dark in toilet bowls treated with bleach.
• Elderly patients are more likely to experience sedation and hypotension.

metoprolol tartrate
Apo-Metoprolol♦♦, Betaloc♦♦,
Betaloc Durules♦♦, Lopresor♦♦,
Lopresor SR♦♦, Lopressor,
Novometoprol♦♦

Pregnancy Risk Category: B

MECHANISM OF ACTION
Blocks cardiac beta receptors and depresses renin secretion.

INDICATIONS & DOSAGE
For hypertension; may be used alone or in combination with other antihypertensives—
Adults: 50 mg b.i.d. or 100 mg once daily P.O. initially. Up to 200 to 400 mg daily in two to three divided doses. No dosage recommendations for children.
Early intervention in acute myocardial infarction—

Adults: Three injections of 5-mg I.V. boluses q 2 minutes. Then, 15 minutes after last dose, administer 50 mg P.O. q 6 hours for 48 hours. Maintenance dosage is 100 mg P.O. b.i.d.

ADVERSE REACTIONS
CNS: fatigue, lethargy, dizziness.
CV: *bradycardia, hypotension, CHF,* peripheral vascular disease.
GI: nausea, vomiting, diarrhea.
Skin: rash.
Other: fever, arthralgias.

INTERACTIONS
Barbiturates, rifampin: increased metabolism of metoprolol. Monitor for decreased effect.
Cardiac glycosides: excessive bradycardia and increased depressant effect on myocardium. Use together cautiously.
Chlorpromazine, cimetidine, verapamil: decreased hepatic clearance. Monitor for greater beta-blocking effect.
Indomethacin: decrease in antihypertensive effect. Monitor blood pressure and adjust dosage.
Insulin, hypoglycemic drugs (oral): can alter dosage requirements in previously stabilized diabetics. Observe patient carefully.

NURSING CONSIDERATIONS
• Use cautiously in heart failure, diabetes, respiratory or hepatic disease, or in patients taking other antihypertensives. Always check patient's apical pulse rate before giving this drug. If it's slower than 60 beats/minute, hold drug and call doctor immediately.
• Although most patients with asthma and bronchitis can take this drug without fear of worsening their condition, doses over 100 mg daily should be used cautiously.
• Monitor blood pressure frequently.
• Teach patient about his disease and therapy. Explain the importance of

taking this drug as prescribed, even when he's feeling well. Tell outpatient not to discontinue this drug suddenly; abrupt discontinuation can exacerbate angina and myocardial infarction. Instruct patient to call the doctor if unpleasant adverse effects occur.
• Instruct patient to check with doctor or pharmacist before taking OTC medications.
• This drug masks common signs of shock and hypoglycemia. However, metoprolol doesn't potentiate insulin-induced hypoglycemia or delay recovery of blood glucose to normal levels.
• Food may increase absorption of metoprolol. Give consistently with meals.
• Patient should have periodic eye examinations while taking drug.

metyrosine
Demser

Pregnancy Risk Category: C

MECHANISM OF ACTION
Inhibits the enzyme tyrosine hydroxylase, thus inhibiting endogenous catecholamine synthesis.

INDICATIONS & DOSAGE
Preoperative preparation of patients with pheochromocytoma; management of such patients when surgery is contraindicated; to control or prevent hypertension before or during pheochromocytomectomy—
Adults and children over 12 years: 250 mg P.O. q.i.d. May be increased by 250 to 500 mg q day to a maximum of 4 g daily in divided doses. When used for preoperative preparation, optimally effective dosage should be given for at least 5 to 7 days. In normotensive patients, doses are adjusted to produce a 50% reduction in urinary metanephrines and vanillylmandelic acid.

ADVERSE REACTIONS
CNS: *sedation,* extrapyramidal symptoms, such as speech difficulty and tremors, disorientation.
GI: *diarrhea,* nausea, vomiting, abdominal pain.
GU: *crystalluria,* hematuria.
Other: impotence, hypersensitivity.

INTERACTIONS
Phenothiazines and haloperidol: increased inhibition of catecholamine synthesis may result in extrapyramidal symptoms. Use cautiously.

NURSING CONSIDERATIONS
• During surgery, monitor blood pressure and ECG continuously. If a serious dysrhythmia occurs during anesthesia and surgery, treatment with a beta-blocking drug or lidocaine may be necessary.
• Warn patient that sedation almost always occurs in those treated with metyrosine. Sedation usually subsides after several days' treatment.
• Instruct patient to increase daily fluid intake to prevent crystalluria. Daily urine volume should be 2,000 ml or more.
• Insomnia may occur when metyrosine is stopped.
• If patient's hypertension is not adequately controlled by metyrosine, an alpha-adrenergic blocking agent, such as phenoxybenzamine, should be added to the regimen.

minoxidil
Loniten◆, Minodyl

Pregnancy Risk Category: C

MECHANISM OF ACTION
Produces direct arteriolar vasodilation.

INDICATIONS & DOSAGE
Treatment of severe hypertension—
Adults: 5 mg P.O. initially as a single dose. Effective dosage range is usu-

ally 10 to 40 mg daily. Maximum dosage is 100 mg daily.

Children under 12 years: 0.2 mg/kg as a single daily dose. Effective dosage range usually is 0.25 to 1 mg/kg daily. Maximum dosage is 50 mg.

ADVERSE REACTIONS

CV: *edema, tachycardia, pericardial effusion and tamponade, CHF,* ECG changes.

Skin: rash, *Stevens-Johnson syndrome.*

Other: *hypertrichosis* (elongation, thickening, and enhanced pigmentation of fine body hair), breast tenderness.

INTERACTIONS

Guanethidine: severe orthostatic hypotension. Advise patient to stand up slowly.

NURSING CONSIDERATIONS

• Contraindicated in pheochromocytoma. Patients with malignant hypertension should be hospitalized during initial therapy.

• A potent vasodilator: use only when other antihypertensives have failed.

• Instruct patient to take his own pulse. Patient should report an increase greater than 20 beats/minute to the doctor.

• Closely monitor blood pressure and pulse at beginning of therapy.

• Monitor intake/output and check for weight gain and edema. Tell outpatients to weigh themselves at least weekly and report substantial weight gain (more than 5 lb per week).

• Elderly patients may be more sensitive to hypotensive effects.

• About 8 out of 10 patients will experience hypertrichosis within 3 to 6 weeks of beginning treatment. Unwanted hair can be controlled with a depilatory or shaving. Assure patient that extra hair will disappear within 1 to 6 months of stopping minoxidil. Advise patient, however, not to dis-

continue drug without doctor's approval.

• Drug is usually prescribed with a beta-blocking drug to control tachycardia and a diuretic to counteract fluid retention. Make sure patient complies with total treatment regimen.

• Teach patient about his disease and therapy. Explain the importance of taking this drug as prescribed, even when he's feeling well. Tell outpatient not to discontinue drug suddenly, but to call the doctor if unpleasant adverse effects occur.

• A patient package insert has been prepared by the manufacturer of minoxidil, describing in layman's terms the drug and its adverse reactions. Be sure your patient receives this insert and reads it thoroughly. Provide an oral explanation also.

• Instruct patient to check with doctor or pharmacist before taking OTC medications.

• Prescribed in various topical forms for treatment of some types of male pattern baldness.

• Minoxidil is removed by hemodialysis. Be sure to administer dose after dialysis.

---

nitroprusside sodium
Nipride♦, Nitropress

Pregnancy Risk Category: C

MECHANISM OF ACTION
Relaxes both arteriolar and venous smooth muscle.

INDICATIONS & DOSAGE
To lower blood pressure quickly in hypertensive emergencies; to control hypotension during anesthesia; to reduce preload and afterload in cardiac pump failure or cardiogenic shock; may be used with or without dopamine—
Adults: 50-mg vial diluted with 2 to 3 ml of dextrose 5% in water I.V. and then added to 250, 500, or 1,000 ml

dextrose 5% in water. Infuse at 0.5 to 10 mcg/kg/minute. Average dose is 3 mcg/kg/minute. Maximum infusion rate is 10 mcg/kg/minute.

Patients taking other antihypertensive drugs along with nitroprusside are very sensitive to this drug. Adjust dosage accordingly.

ADVERSE REACTIONS
The following adverse reactions usually indicate overdosage:
CNS: *headache, dizziness,* ataxia, loss of consciousness, coma, weak pulse, absent reflexes, widely dilated pupils, *restlessness, muscle twitching, diaphoresis.*
CV: distant heart sounds, palpitations, dyspnea, shallow breathing.
GI: *vomiting, nausea, abdominal pain.*
Metabolic: acidosis.
Skin: pink color.

INTERACTIONS
None significant.

NURSING CONSIDERATIONS
• Use cautiously in hypothyroidism or hepatic or renal disease, or in patients receiving other antihypertensives. Keep patient supine when initiating or titrating nitroprusside therapy.
• Because of light sensitivity, wrap I.V. solution in foil. It's not necessary to wrap the tubing in foil. Fresh solution should have faint brownish tint. Discard after 24 hours.
• Obtain baseline vital signs before giving this drug, and find out what parameters the doctor wants to achieve.
• Check blood pressure every 5 minutes at start of infusion and every 15 minutes thereafter. If severe hypotension occurs, turn off I.V. nitroprusside—effects of drug quickly reverse. Notify doctor. If possible, an arterial pressure line should be started. Regulate drug flow to specified level.
• Don't use bacteriostatic water for

injection or sterile saline solution for reconstitution.
• Infuse with a continuous infusion pump.
• This drug is best run piggyback through a peripheral line with no other medication. Don't adjust rate of main I.V. line while drug is running. Even small bolus of nitroprusside can cause severe hypotension.
• Excessive doses or rapid infusion (>15 mcg/kg/minute) of this drug can cause cyanide toxicity, so check serum thiocyanate levels every 72 hours. Thiocyanate levels of greater than 100 mcg/ml are associated with toxicity. Watch for signs of thiocyanate toxicity: profound hypotension, metabolic acidosis, dyspnea, headache, loss of consciousness, ataxia, vomiting. If these occur, discontinue drug immediately and notify doctor.

pargyline hydrochloride
Eutonyl

Pregnancy Risk Category: C

MECHANISM OF ACTION
Inhibits the enzyme MAO.

INDICATIONS & DOSAGE
For moderate to severe hypertension, usually given in combination with other drugs—
Adults: initially, 25 to 50 mg P.O. once daily, if not receiving any other antihypertensive drugs. Then increase dosage by 10 mg daily at weekly intervals. Maximum daily dosage is 200 mg. Usual daily dosage for elderly patients or those who've had sympathectomy is 10 to 25 mg. When used in combination with other drugs, total daily dosage of pargyline should not exceed 25 mg. No dosage recommendations for children.

ADVERSE REACTIONS
CNS: *tremors,* convulsions, choreiform movements, psychic changes,

nightmares, hyperexcitability, sweating, dizziness, fainting, drowsiness.
CV: palpitations, orthostatic hypotension, fluid retention.
EENT: dry mouth, optic damage.
GI: nausea, vomiting, increased appetite, constipation.
Other: impotence.

INTERACTIONS
Amphetamines, ephedrine, levodopa, metaraminol, methotrimeprazine, methylphenidate, phenylephrine, phenylpropanolamine, pseudoephedrine: enhanced pressor effects. Use together cautiously.
Alcohol, barbiturates, and other sedatives; tranquilizers; narcotics; dextromethorphan; tricyclic antidepressants: unpredictable interactions. Should be used with caution and in reduced dosage.

NURSING CONSIDERATIONS
• Contraindicated in advanced renal failure, pheochromocytoma, hyperthyroidism, or Parkinson's disease; in hyperactive and hyperexcitable patients. Use cautiously in patients who are receiving other antihypertensives or who have hepatic disease. Pargyline should not be used to treat malignant hypertension.
• Discontinue this drug at least 2 weeks before elective surgery.
• Hypotensive effects of this drug are increased by high environmental temperatures, fever, stress, or severe illness. If patient develops severe hypotension, counteract with ephedrine or phenylephrine.
• Monitor blood pressure and pulse rate frequently. Take blood pressure while patient is standing.
• Patient should have periodic eye examinations during therapy.
• If patient is scheduled for surgery and has been taking this drug, be sure narcotic dosages are reduced.
• This drug may require up to several weeks to reach optimal effect. Toler-

ance to its hypotensive actions may develop, and other drugs may be necessary.
• Advise patient to take drug in the morning to avoid insomnia.
• Warn patient not to take any other medications, including over-the-counter cold remedies, without first getting medical approval.
• This drug is an MAO inhibitor. Tell patient not to eat foods with high tyramine content: for example, aged cheese, chianti wine, sour cream, canned figs, raisins, chicken livers, yeast extract, and pickled herring.
• Teach patient about his disease and therapy. Explain the importance of taking this drug as prescribed, even when he's feeling well. Tell outpatient not to discontinue this drug suddenly, but to call the doctor if unpleasant adverse effects occur.
• Instruct patient to check with doctor or pharmacist before taking OTC medications.
• Inform patient that orthostatic hypotension can be minimized by rising slowly and avoiding sudden position changes. Dry mouth can be relieved with sugarless chewing gum, sour hard candy, or ice chips.

penbutolol sulfate
Levatol

Pregnancy Risk Category: C

MECHANISM OF ACTION
Blocks both beta$_1$- and beta$_2$-adrenergic receptors.

INDICATIONS AND DOSAGE
Treatment of mild to moderate hypertension—
Adults: 20 mg P.O. once daily. Usually given with other antihypertensive agents, such as thiazide diuretics.

ADVERSE REACTIONS
CNS: syncope, dizziness, vertigo, headache, fatigue, mental depression,

paresthesias, hypoesthesia or hyperesthesia, lethargy, anxiety, nervousness, diminished concentration, sleep
disturbances, nightmares, bizarre or
frequent dreams, sedation, changes in
behavior, reversible mental depression, catatonia, hallucinations, alteration of time perception, memory
loss, emotional lability, light-headedness.
CV: *bradycardia,* chest pain, *CHF,*
asymptomatic hypotension, peripheral ischemia, worsening of angina or
arterial insufficiency, peripheral vascular insufficiency, claudication,
edema, *pulmonary edema,* vasodilation, symptomatic postural hypotension, tachycardia, palpitations, conduction disturbances, first-degree and
third-degree heart block, intensifica-
tion of AV block.
EENT: dry mouth.
GI: gastric pain, flatulence, nausea,
constipation, heartburn, vomiting,
taste alteration.
GU: impotence, nocturia, urine retention.
Metabolic: hyperglycemia, hypoglycemia.
Respiratory: pharyngitis, laryngospasm, respiratory distress, shortness
of breath.
Skin: pallor, flushing, rash.
Other: allergic reactions, eye discomfort, decreased libido.

INTERACTIONS
NSAIDs: possibly decreased antihypertensive effects.
Clonidine: may cause paradoxical hypertension when combined with beta-
adrenergic blocking agents. Also, beta
blockers may enhance rebound hypertension when clonidine is withdrawn.
*Beta-adrenergic blocking agents may
alter the hypoglycemic response to
these drugs. Monitor patient closely.*
Prazocin, terazocin: Beta blockers
may enhance the "first dose" orthostatic hypotension seen with these
drugs.

*Sympathomimetics, including isopro-
terenol, dopamine, dobutamine, or
norepinephrine:* decreased hypotensive response.
Theophylline: possibly decreased
bronchodilator effect.

NURSING CONSIDERATIONS
• Contraindicated in patients allergic
to penbutolol or other beta blockers.
Also contraindicated in sinus bradycardia, cardiogenic shock, CHF, overt
cardiac failure, and patients with
greater than first-degree heart block.
Beta-adrenergic blocking agents
should be avoided in patients with
pheochromocytoma unless alpha-adrenergic blocking agents are also
used. They should also be avoided in
patients with chronic airway disease,
such as chronic bronchitis or emphysema.
• Administer cautiously to patients
with a history of CHF controlled by
digitalis glycosides and diuretics.
• Advise patients not to discontinue
the drug abruptly, because sudden
withdrawal of other beta blockers has
precipitated angina and myocardial
infarction. However, clinical experience has shown that withdrawal of
beta blocker therapy in patients who
have had a myocardial infarction does
not present major problems.
• Administer with caution to patients
with a history of bronchospastic disease. Teach patient the signs and
symptoms of CHF (edema and pulmonary congestion). Advise them to contact the doctor if these symptoms occur.
• Always check patient's apical pulse
before giving this drug. If you detect
extremes in pulse rates, hold drug and
call doctor immediately.
• Monitor blood pressure, ECG, and
heart rate and rhythm frequently.
• Teach patient about his disease and
therapy. Explain the importance taking this drug, even when he's feeling
well. Tell patient to call doctor if un-

pleasant adverse effects occur.
• Advise patient to check with his doctor or pharmacist before taking OTC medications.

phenoxybenzamine hydrochloride
Dibenzyline

Pregnancy Risk Category: C

MECHANISM OF ACTION
An alpha-adrenergic blocker that noncompetitively blocks the effect of catecholamines on alpha-adrenergic receptors.

INDICATIONS & DOSAGE
To control hypertension and sweating secondary to pheochromocytoma; may be used in combination with propranolol to control excessive tachycardia—
Adults: initially, 10 mg P.O. daily. Increase by 10 mg daily q 4 days. Maintenance dosage is 20 to 60 mg daily.
Children: initially, 0.2 mg/kg or 6 mg/m² P.O. daily in a single dose. Maintenance dosage is 12 to 36 mg/m² daily as a single dose or in divided doses.
To control Raynaud's disease, frostbite, acrocyanosis—
Adults: initially, 10 mg P.O., then increase by 10 mg q 4 days to a maximum of 60 mg daily.

ADVERSE REACTIONS
CNS: lethargy, drowsiness.
CV: *orthostatic hypotension, tachycardia,* shock.
EENT: *nasal stuffiness, dry mouth, miosis.*
GI: vomiting, abdominal distress.
Other: *impotence, inhibition of ejaculation.*

INTERACTIONS
Antihypertensives: excessive hypotension. Use together cautiously.

NURSING CONSIDERATIONS
• Use cautiously in cerebrovascular or coronary insufficiency, advanced renal disease, or respiratory disease.
• Watch patient closely for side effects, and call doctor promptly if they occur. If severe hypotension develops, patient may require norepinephrine to counteract effect.
• Nasal congestion, inhibition of ejaculation, and impotence usually decrease with continued therapy.
• Patient with tachycardia may require concurrent propranolol therapy.
• Monitor patient's heart rate and blood pressure frequently.
• This drug may take several weeks to achieve optimal effect.
• Monitor respiratory status carefully. This drug may aggravate symptoms of pneumonia and asthma.
• Teach patient about his disease and therapy. Explain the importance of taking this drug as prescribed, even when he's feeling well. Tell outpatient not to discontinue this drug suddenly, but to call the doctor if unpleasant adverse effects occur.
• Instruct patient to check with doctor or pharmacist before taking OTC medications.
• Inform patient that orthostatic hypotension can be minimized by rising slowly and avoiding sudden position changes.
• Dry mouth can be relieved with sugarless chewing gum, sour hard candy, or ice chips. GI distress can be relieved by taking the drug in divided doses or with milk.
• Used investigationally to treat chronic urine retention.
• Small initial doses are increased gradually until desired effect is obtained. Patient should be observed after each dose for at least 4 days.

Italicized side effects are common or life-threatening.
*Liquid form contains alcohol.   **May contain tartrazine.

phentolamine mesylate
Regitine, Rogitine♦♦

Pregnancy Risk Category: C

MECHANISM OF ACTION
An alpha-adrenergic blocker that competitively blocks the effects of catecholamines on alpha-adrenergic receptors.

INDICATIONS & DOSAGE
To aid in diagnosis of pheochromocytoma; to control or prevent hypertension before or during pheochromocytomectomy—
Adults: I.V. diagnostic dose is 5 mg, with close monitoring of blood pressure.

Before surgical removal of tumor, give 2 to 5 mg I.M. or I.V. During surgery, patient may need small I.V. doses (1 mg) or small I.M. doses (3 mg).
Children: I.V. diagnostic dose is 0.1 mg/kg or 3 mg/m² as single dose, with close monitoring of blood pressure.

Before surgical removal of tumor, give 1 mg I.V. or 3 mg I.M. During surgery, patient may need small I.V. doses (1 mg).
To treat extravasation—
Adults and children: infiltrate area with 5 to 10 mg phentolamine in 10 ml normal saline solution. Must be done within 12 hours.

ADVERSE REACTIONS
CNS: *dizziness, weakness, flushing.*
CV: *hypotension,* shock, *dysrhythmias,* palpitations, *tachycardia,* angina pectoris.
GI: *diarrhea,* abdominal pain, *nausea, vomiting,* hyperperistalsis.
Other: *nasal stuffiness,* hypoglycemia.

INTERACTIONS
Epinephrine: excessive hypotension. Don't use together.

NURSING CONSIDERATIONS
• Contraindicated in angina, coronary artery disease, and history of myocardial infarction. Use cautiously in gastritis or peptic ulcer and in patients receiving other antihypertensives.
• Don't administer epinephrine to treat phentolamine-induced hypotension. May cause additional fall in blood pressure ("epinephrine reversal"). Use norepinephrine instead.
• When this drug is given as a diagnostic test for pheochromocytoma, check patient's blood pressure first; check blood pressure frequently during administration.
• Test is positive for pheochromocytoma if I.V. test dose causes severe hypotension.
• Don't give sedatives or narcotics 24 hours before diagnostic test. Rauwolfia alkaloids should be withdrawn at least 4 weeks before such testing.
• Has been used experimentally, alone or with papaverine, to treat impotence. Patients are taught to self-administer this drug by intracavernosal injection.

pindolol
Visken♦

Pregnancy Risk Category: B

MECHANISM OF ACTION
Blocks response to beta stimulation.

INDICATIONS & DOSAGE
Treatment of hypertension—
Adults: initially, 5 mg P.O. b.i.d. Dosage may be increased by 10 mg/day q 2 to 3 weeks up to a maximum of 60 mg/day.

ADVERSE REACTIONS
CNS: *insomnia, fatigue, dizziness, nervousness,* vivid dreams, hallucinations, lethargy.
CV: *edema,* bradycardia, CHF, peripheral vascular disease, hypoten-

sion.
EENT: visual disturbances.
GI: *nausea,* vomiting, diarrhea.
Metabolic: hypoglycemia without tachycardia.
Skin: rash.
Other: *increased airway resistance, muscle pain, joint pain,* chest pain.

INTERACTIONS
Insulin, hypoglycemic drugs (oral): can alter requirements for these drugs in previously stabilized diabetics. Monitor for hypoglycemia.
Cardiac glycosides: excessive bradycardia and increased depressant effect on myocardium. Use together cautiously.
Cimetidine: inhibits pindolol metabolism. Monitor for greater beta-blocking effect.
Epinephrine: severe vasoconstriction. Monitor blood pressure and observe patient carefully.
Indomethacin: decreased antihypertensive effect. Monitor blood pressure and adjust dosage.

NURSING CONSIDERATIONS
• Contraindicated in diabetes mellitus, asthma, allergic rhinitis; during ethyl ether anesthesia; in sinus bradycardia and heart block greater than first degree; in cardiogenic shock; in right ventricular failure secondary to pulmonary hypertension. Use with caution in CHF or respiratory disease, and in patients taking other antihypertensive drugs.
• Always check patient's apical pulse rate before giving this drug. If you detect extremes in pulse rates, hold medication and call doctor immediately.
• Monitor blood pressure frequently. If patient develops severe hypotension, notify doctor. He may prescribe a vasopressor.
• Teach patient about his disease and therapy. Explain the importance of taking this drug as prescribed, even

when he's feeling well. Tell outpatient not to discontinue this drug suddenly; abrupt discontinuation can exacerbate angina and myocardial infarction. Tell patient to call doctor if unpleasant adverse effects occur.
• Instruct patient to check with doctor or pharmacist before taking OTC medications.
• This drug masks common signs of shock and hypoglycemia.
• Pindolol may be taken without any special regard for meals.
• Many patients respond favorably to a dose of 5 mg t.i.d.
• The first commercially available beta blocker with partial beta-*agonist* activity. In other words, pindolol also *stimulates* beta-adrenergic receptors as well as blocks them. Therefore, it decreases cardiac output less than other beta-adrenergic blockers.
• May be advantageous for patients who develop bradycardia with other beta blockers.
• Withdraw drug gradually (over 1 to 2 weeks) after long-term administration.

---

prazosin hydrochloride
Minipress♦

Pregnancy Risk Category: C

MECHANISM OF ACTION
Relaxes both arteriolar and venous smooth muscle probably by blocking postsynaptic alpha receptors.

INDICATIONS & DOSAGE
For mild to moderate hypertension; used alone or in combination with a diuretic or other antihypertensive drugs; also used to decrease afterload in severe chronic congestive heart failure—
Adults: P.O. test dose is 1 mg given before bedtime to prevent "first-dose syncope." Initial dose is 1 mg t.i.d. Increase dosage slowly. Maximum daily dosage is 20 mg. Maintenance

dosage is 3 to 20 mg daily in three divided doses. A few patients have required dosages larger than this (up to 40 mg daily). If other antihypertensive drugs or diuretics are added to this drug, decrease prazosin dosage to 1 to 2 mg t.i.d. and retitrate.

ADVERSE REACTIONS
CNS: *dizziness,* headache, drowsiness, weakness, *"first-dose syncope,"* depression.
CV: orthostatic hypotension, *palpitations.*
EENT: blurred vision, dry mouth.
GI: vomiting, diarrhea, abdominal cramps, constipation, *nausea.*
GU: priapism, impotence.

INTERACTIONS
Propranolol and other beta blockers: syncope with loss of consciousness may occur more frequently. Advise patient to sit or lie down if he feels dizzy.

NURSING CONSIDERATIONS
• Use cautiously in patients receiving other antihypertensive drugs.
• Monitor patient's blood pressure and pulse rate frequently.
• If initial dose is greater than 1 mg, patient may develop severe syncope with loss of consciousness (first-dose syncope). Increase dosage slowly. Instruct patient to sit or lie down if he experiences dizziness.
• Elderly patients may be more sensitive to hypotensive effects.
• Teach patient about his disease and therapy. Explain the importance of taking this drug as prescribed, even when he's feeling well. Tell outpatient not to discontinue this drug suddenly, but to call the doctor if unpleasant adverse effects occur.
• Instruct patient to check with doctor or pharmacist before taking OTC medications.
• Inform patient that orthostatic hypotension can be minimized by rising slowly and avoiding sudden position changes. Dry mouth can be relieved with sugarless chewing gum, sour hard candy, or ice chips.
• Compliance *may* be improved by giving this drug once a day. Check with doctor.
• Has been used to treat Raynaud's disease.

---

rauwolfia serpentina
Raudixin**, Rauval, Rauverid, Wolfina
Pregnancy Risk Category: D

MECHANISM OF ACTION
Acts peripherally, inhibiting norepinephrine release and depleting norepinephrine stores in adrenergic nerve endings.

INDICATIONS & DOSAGE
Mild to moderate hypertension—
Adults: initially and for 1 to 3 weeks thereafter, 200 to 400 mg P.O. daily as a single dose or in two divided doses.
Maintenance dosage is 50 to 300 mg daily. No dosing recommendations for children.

ADVERSE REACTIONS
CNS: mental confusion, *depression, drowsiness, nervousness, paradoxical anxiety,* nightmares, sedation, headache, extrapyramidal symptoms.
CV: orthostatic hypotension, bradycardia, syncope.
EENT: *dry mouth, nasal stuffiness,* glaucoma.
GI: *hypersecretion of gastric acid, nausea, vomiting,* GI bleeding.
Skin: pruritus, rash.
Other: impotence, weight gain.

INTERACTIONS
Digitalis glycosides: rauwolfia may predispose patients to digitalis-induced dysrhythmias. Use together cautiously.

MAO inhibitors: may cause excitability and hypertension. Use together cautiously.

NURSING CONSIDERATIONS
• Contraindicated in depression. Use cautiously in severe cardiac or cerebrovascular disease, impaired renal function, peptic ulcer, ulcerative colitis, gallstones; in those undergoing surgery; in elderly or debilitated patients; and in those taking other antihypertensives or tricyclic antidepressants.
• Monitor patient's blood pressure and pulse rate frequently.
• Teach patient about his disease and therapy. Explain the importance of taking this drug as prescribed, even when he's feeling well. Tell outpatient not to discontinue this drug suddenly, but to call the doctor if unpleasant adverse effects occur.
• Instruct patient to check with doctor or pharmacist before taking OTC medications.
• Warn that this drug can cause drowsiness. Patient should not drive or perform other activities that require alertness and good coordination until CNS effects are known.
• Watch patient closely for signs of mental depression. Warn him to notify doctor promptly if he experiences nightmares.
• Inform patient that orthostatic hypotension can be minimized by rising slowly and avoiding sudden position changes. Dry mouth can be relieved with sugarless chewing gum, sour hard candy, or ice chips. Tell patient to contact doctor if relief is needed for nasal stuffiness.
• Give this drug with meals.
• Patient should weigh himself daily and notify doctor of any weight gain.
• Effects of this drug may last for 10 days after it's discontinued.
• Advise patient to have periodic eye examinations.

rescinnamine
Anaprel, Moderil

Pregnancy Risk Category: D

MECHANISM OF ACTION
Acts peripherally, inhibiting norepinephrine release and depleting norepinephrine stores in adrenergic nerve endings.

INDICATIONS & DOSAGE
For mild to moderate hypertension; may be used alone or in combination with other antihypertensives—
Adults: initially, 0.5 mg b.i.d. Maintenance dosage is 0.25 to 0.5 mg daily. No dosing recommendations for children.

ADVERSE REACTIONS
CNS: mental confusion, *depression, drowsiness, nervousness, anxiety, nightmares,* sedation, parkinsonism.
CV: *orthostatic hypotension, bradycardia, syncope.*
EENT: *dry mouth, nasal stuffiness,* glaucoma.
GI: *hypersecretion of gastric acid, nausea, vomiting,* GI bleeding.
Skin: pruritus, rash.
Other: *impotence, weight gain.*

INTERACTIONS
MAO inhibitors: may cause excitability and hypertension. Use together cautiously.

NURSING CONSIDERATIONS
• Contraindicated in depression. Use cautiously in severe cardiac or cerebrovascular disease, peptic ulcer, ulcerative colitis, gallstones, or in patients undergoing surgery; and in elderly or debilitated patients. Also use cautiously in patients taking other antihypertensives.
• Monitor patient's blood pressure and pulse rate frequently.
• Teach patient about his disease and therapy. Explain the importance of

taking this drug as prescribed, even when he's feeling well. Tell outpatient not to discontinue this drug suddenly, but to call the doctor if unpleasant adverse reactions develop.

• Instruct patient to check with doctor or pharmacist before taking OTC medications.

• Warn that this drug can cause drowsiness. Patients should not drive or perform other tasks that require alertness and coordination until the adverse CNS effects of the drug are known.

• Watch patient closely for signs of mental depression. Warn him to notify doctor promptly if he experiences nightmares.

• Inform patient that orthostatic hypotension can be minimized by rising slowly and avoiding sudden position changes. Dry mouth can be relieved with sugarless chewing gum, sour hard candy, or ice chips. Tell patient to contact doctor if relief is needed for nasal stuffiness.

• Give this drug with meals.

• Patient should weigh himself daily and notify doctor of any weight gain.

• Effects of this drug may last for 10 days after it's discontinued.

• Advise patient to have periodic eye examinations.

reserpine
Novo-Reserpine♦♦, Reserfia♦♦, Serpalan, Serpasil♦*

Pregnancy Risk Category: C

MECHANISM OF ACTION
Acts peripherally, inhibiting norepinephrine release and depleting norepinephrine stores in adrenergic nerve endings.

INDICATIONS & DOSAGE
Mild to moderate essential hypertension—
Adults: 0.1 to 0.25 mg P.O. daily.
Children: 5 to 20 mcg/kg P.O. daily.

ADVERSE REACTIONS
CNS: mental confusion, *depression, drowsiness, nervousness, paradoxical anxiety, nightmares,* extrapyramidal symptoms, sedation.
CV: *orthostatic hypotension, bradycardia, syncope.*
EENT: *dry mouth, nasal stuffiness,* glaucoma.
GI: *hyperacidity, nausea, vomiting,* GI bleeding.
Skin: pruritus, rash.
Other: *impotence, weight gain.*

INTERACTIONS
MAO inhibitors: may cause excitability and hypertension. Use together cautiously.

NURSING CONSIDERATIONS
• Contraindicated in depression. Use cautiously in severe cardiac or cerebrovascular disease, history of seizures, peptic ulcer, ulcerative colitis, gallstones, or mental depressive disorders; in patients undergoing surgery; and in those taking other antihypertensive drugs.

• Monitor patient's blood pressure and pulse rate frequently.

• Teach patient about his disease and therapy. Explain the importance of taking this drug as prescribed, even when he's feeling well. Tell outpatient not to discontinue this drug suddenly, but to call doctor if unpleasant adverse effects occur.

• Instruct patient to check with doctor or pharmacist before taking OTC medications.

• Warn patient that this drug can cause drowsiness. Tell him to avoid hazardous activities that require alertness and coordination until CNS effects of the drug are known.

• Warn female patient to notify doctor if she becomes pregnant.

• Watch patient closely for signs of mental depression. Warn him to notify doctor promptly if he experiences nightmares.

• Inform patient that orthostatic hypotension can be minimized by rising slowly and avoiding sudden position changes. Dry mouth can be relieved with sugarless chewing gum, sour hard candy, or ice chips. Tell patient to contact doctor if relief is needed for nasal stuffiness.
• Give this drug with meals.
• Patient should weigh himself daily and notify doctor of any weight gain.
• Effects of this drug may last for 10 days after it's discontinued.
• Advise patient to have periodic eye examinations.

terazocin hydrochloride
Hytrin

Pregnancy Risk Category: C

MECHANISM OF ACTION
Decreases blood pressure by vasodilation produced in response to blockade of alpha$_1$ adrenergic receptors.

INDICATIONS & DOSAGE
Hypertension—
Adults: initial dose is 1 mg P.O. h.s., gradually increased according to patient response. Usual dosage range is 1 to 5 mg daily. Maximum recommended dosage is 20 mg/day.

ADVERSE REACTIONS
CNS: *dizziness,* nervousness, paresthesia, somnolence, decreased libido.
CV: *palpitations,* postural hypotension, tachycardia, *peripheral edema.*
EENT: *nasal congestion,* sinusitis, blurred vision.
GI: *nausea.*
Other: *asthenia, headache,* back pain, muscle pain, dyspnea, weight gain, impotence.

INTERACTIONS
Antihypertensives: excessive hypotension. Use together cautiously.

NURSING CONSIDERATIONS
• Do not exceed initial dose of 1 mg.
• Instruct patient to avoid hazardous activities that require mental alertness (such as driving or operating heavy machinery) for 12 hours after the first dose.
• If terazocin is discontinued for several days, patient will need to be retitrated using initial dosing regimen (1 mg P.O. at bedtime).
• Teach patient about his disease and therapy. Explain the importance of taking this drug as prescribed, even when he's feeling well. Tell outpatient not to discontinue drug suddenly, but to call the doctor if unpleasant adverse effects occur.
• Instruct patient to check with doctor or pharmacist before taking OTC medications.

timolol maleate
Apo-Timolol♦♦, Blocadren♦

Pregnancy Risk Category: C

MECHANISM OF ACTION
Blocks response to beta stimulation and depresses renin secretion.

INDICATIONS & DOSAGE
Hypertension—
Adults: initially 10 mg P.O. b.i.d. Usual daily maintenance dosage is 20 to 40 mg. Maximum daily dosage is 60 mg. Drug is used either alone or in combination with diuretics.
Myocardial infarction (long-term prophylaxis in patients who have survived acute phase)—
Adults: Recommended dosage for long-term prophylaxis in survivors of acute myocardial infarction is 10 mg P.O. b.i.d.

ADVERSE REACTIONS
CNS: fatigue, lethargy, vivid dreams.
CV: *bradycardia, hypotension, CHF,* peripheral vascular disease.
GI: nausea, vomiting, diarrhea.

Italicized side effects are common or life-threatening.
*Liquid form contains alcohol.   **May contain tartrazine.

Metabolic: hypoglycemia without tachycardia.
Skin: rash.
Other: *increased airway resistance,* fever.

INTERACTIONS
Cardiac glycosides: excessive bradycardia and increased depressant effect on myocardium. Use together cautiously.
Indomethacin: decrease in antihypertensive effect. Monitor blood pressure and adjust dosage.
Insulin, hypoglycemic drugs (oral): can alter requirements for these drugs in previously stabilized diabetics. Monitor for hypoglycemia.

NURSING CONSIDERATIONS
• Contraindicated in diabetes mellitus, asthma, allergic rhinitis; during ethyl ether anesthesia; in sinus bradycardia and heart block greater than first degree; in cardiogenic shock; in right ventricular failure secondary to pulmonary hypertension. Use with caution in CHF, hepatic, renal, or respiratory disease, and in patients taking other antihypertensives.
• Always check patient's apical pulse rate before giving this drug. If you detect extremes in pulse rates, withhold medication and call the doctor immediately.
• Monitor blood pressure frequently.
• Teach patient about his disease and therapy. Explain the importance of taking drug as prescribed, even when he's feeling well. Tell patient not to discontinue drug suddenly: abrupt discontinuation can exacerbate angina and myocardial infarction. Tell patient to call doctor if unpleasant adverse effects occur.
• Instruct patient to check with doctor or pharmacist before taking OTC medications.
• This drug masks common signs of shock and hypoglycemia.
• If patient is taking the drug for hy-

pertension, warn him not to increase the dosage without first consulting his doctor. At least 7 days should intervene between increases in dosage.
• Do not discontinue therapy abruptly. Reduce dosage gradually over 1 to 2 weeks.
• Timolol is the first beta blocker approved for use in post-myocardial infarction patients. Like other beta blockers, it prolongs survival of myocardial infarction patients.

---

trimethaphan camsylate
Arfonad♦

Pregnancy Risk Category: C

MECHANISM OF ACTION
A ganglionic blocker that stabilizes postsynaptic membranes.

INDICATIONS & DOSAGE
To lower blood pressure quickly in hypertensive emergencies; for controlled hypotension during surgery—
Adults: 500 mg (10 ml) diluted in 500 ml dextrose 5% in water to yield concentration of 1 mg/ml I.V. Start I.V. drip at 1 to 2 mg/minute and titrate to achieve desired hypotensive response. Range is 0.3 mg to 6 mg/minute.

ADVERSE REACTIONS
CNS: dilated pupils, *extreme weakness.*
CV: *severe orthostatic hypotension, tachycardia.*
GI: anorexia, *nausea, vomiting, dry mouth.*
GU: urine retention.
Other: respiratory depression.

INTERACTIONS
Anesthetics, diuretics, procainamide: Increased hypotensive effect. Monitor patient closely.

NURSING CONSIDERATIONS
• Contraindicated in anemia, respira-

tory insufficiency. Use cautiously in arteriosclerosis; cardiac, hepatic, or renal disease; degenerative CNS disorders; Addison's disease; diabetes. Also use cautiously in patients receiving glucocorticoids or other antihypertensives.

• Monitor patient's blood pressure and vital signs continuously.

• Patient should be supine during drug administration. May require elevation of the head of the bed for maximal effect to avoid cerebral anoxia. Do not elevate bed more than 30°.

• Large doses have caused apnea and respiratory arrest.

• If extreme hypotension occurs, discontinue drug and call doctor. Use phenylephrine or mephentermine to counteract hypotension.

• Watch closely for respiratory distress, especially if large doses are used.

• Patient should receive oxygen therapy during use of this agent.

• Use continuous infusion pump to administer this drug slowly and precisely.

• Discontinue drug before wound closure in surgery to allow blood pressure to return to normal.

23

Vasodilators

amyl nitrite
cyclandelate
dipyridamole
ethaverine hydrochloride
isoxsuprine hydrochloride
nicotinyl alcohol tartrate
nimodipine
nylidrin hydrochloride
papaverine hydrochloride
tolazoline hydrochloride

COMBINATION PRODUCTS
HYDERGINE: dihydroergocornine mesylate 0.167 mg, dihydroergocristine mesylate 0.167 mg, and dihydroergocryptine mesylate 0.167 mg.

amyl nitrite
Pregnancy Risk Category: C

MECHANISM OF ACTION
Reduces cardiac oxygen demand by decreasing left ventricular end-diastolic pressure (preload) and systemic vascular resistance (afterload). Also increases blood flow through the collateral coronary vessels. Converts hemoglobin to methemoglobin (which binds cyanide) to treat cyanide poisoning.

INDICATIONS & DOSAGE
Relief of angina pectoris—
Adults and children: 0.2 to 0.3 ml by inhalation (one glass ampule inhaler), p.r.n.
Antidote for cyanide poisoning—
0.2 or 0.3 ml by inhalation for 30 to 60 seconds q 5 minutes until conscious.

ADVERSE REACTIONS
Blood: methemoglobinemia.
CNS: *headache, sometimes with throbbing;* dizziness; weakness.
CV: *orthostatic hypotension, tachycardia,* flushing, palpitations, fainting.
GI: nausea, vomiting.
Skin: cutaneous vasodilation.
Other: hypersensitivity reactions.

INTERACTIONS
None significant.

NURSING CONSIDERATIONS
• Contraindicated in hypersensitivity to nitrites. Use with caution in cerebral hemorrhage, hypotension, head injury, or glaucoma.
• Watch for orthostatic hypotension. Have patient sit down and avoid rapid position changes while inhaling drug.
• Extinguish all cigarettes before use, or ampule may ignite.
• Wrap ampule in cloth and crush. Hold near patient's nose and mouth so vapor is inhaled.
• Effective within 30 seconds but has a short duration of action (3 to 5 minutes).
• Keeping the head low, deep breathing, and movement of extremities may help relieve dizziness, syncope, or weakness from postural hypotension.
• Drug is often abused. Claimed to have aphrodisiac benefits. Sometimes called "Amy."
• Seldom, if ever, used for treatment of angina because it is expensive, inconvenient, and frequently causes adverse reactions.

Unmarked trade names available in the United States only.
♦ Also available in Canada.   ♦♦ Available in Canada only.   ◊ Also available OTC.

- Sometimes used to induce changes in heart murmurs. Patient inhales the drug until reflex tachycardia is induced, then discontinues.
- Store away from light.

cyclandelate
Cyclospasmol♦
Pregnancy Risk Category: C

MECHANISM OF ACTION
Directly relaxes smooth muscle due to the inhibition of phosphodiesterase, resulting in increased concentrations of cyclic adenosine monophosphate.

INDICATIONS & DOSAGE
Adjunct in intermittent claudication, arteriosclerosis obliterans, vasospasm and muscular ischemia associated with thrombophlebitis, nocturnal leg cramps, Raynaud's phenomenon, selected cases of ischemic cerebral vascular disease—
Adults: initially, 200 mg P.O. q.i.d. (before meals and h.s.); maximum is 400 mg P.O. q.i.d. When clinical response is noted, decrease dosage gradually until maintenance dosage is reached. Maintenance dosage is 400 to 800 mg daily in divided doses.

ADVERSE REACTIONS
CNS: *headache, tingling of the extremities, dizziness.*
CV: *mild flushing,* tachycardia.
GI: pyrosis, eructation, nausea, heartburn.
Other: *sweating.*

INTERACTIONS
None significant.

NURSING CONSIDERATIONS
- Use with extreme caution in severe obliterative coronary artery or cerebrovascular disease, because circulation to these diseased areas may be compromised by vasodilatory effects of the drug elsewhere (coronary steal syndrome). Use with caution in glaucoma or hypotension.
- Give with food or antacids to lessen GI distress.
- Use in conjunction with, not as a substitute for, appropriate medical or surgical therapy for peripheral or cerebrovascular disease.
- Short-term therapy is of little benefit. Instruct patient to expect long-term treatment and to continue to take medication.
- Adverse reactions usually disappear after several weeks of therapy.

dipyridamole
Persantine♦**
Pregnancy Risk Category: C

MECHANISM OF ACTION
Inhibits platelet adhesion. Also inhibits the enzymes adenosine deaminase and phosphodiesterase.

INDICATIONS & DOSAGE
Inhibition of platelet adhesion in prosthetic heart valves, in combination with warfarin or aspirin—
Adults: 75 to 100 mg P.O. q.i.d.
Transient ischemic attack—
Adults: 400 to 800 mg P.O. daily in divided doses.

ADVERSE REACTIONS
CNS: *headache, dizziness,* weakness.
CV: flushing, fainting, *hypotension.*
GI: *nausea,* vomiting, diarrhea.
Skin: rash.

INTERACTIONS
None significant.

NURSING CONSIDERATIONS
- Use with caution in hypotension, and in patients receiving anticoagulant therapy.
- Observe for side effects, especially with large doses. Monitor blood pressure.
- Administer 1 hour before meals.

Italicized side effects are common or life-threatening.
*Liquid form contains alcohol.   **May contain tartrazine.

May administer with meals if patient develops GI distress.
• Watch for signs of bleeding, prolonged bleeding time (large doses, long-term).
• Dipyridamole should not be used alone for the prophylaxis of thromboembolism in postoperative prosthetic valve patients; it should be used with oral anticoagulants. Its value as part of an antithrombotic regimen is controversial and may not be significantly better than aspirin alone.

ethaverine hydrochloride
Circubid, Etalent, Ethaquin, Ethatab, Ethavex, Isovex, Pavaspan, Spasodil

Pregnancy Risk Category: C

MECHANISM OF ACTION
Directly relaxes smooth muscle due to the inhibition of phosphodiesterase, resulting in increased concentrations of cyclic adenosine monophosphate.

INDICATIONS & DOSAGE
Long-term treatment of peripheral and cerebrovascular insufficiency associated with arterial spasm; spastic conditions of GI and GU tracts—
Adults: 100 to 200 mg P.O. t.i.d. or 150 mg of sustained-release preparation P.O. q 12 hours.

ADVERSE REACTIONS
CNS: *headache,* drowsiness.
CV: *hypotension, flushing,* sweating, vertigo, cardiac depression, dysrhythmias.
GI: *nausea, anorexia, abdominal distress, dry throat,* constipation, diarrhea.
Hepatic: jaundice, altered liver function tests.
Skin: rash.
Other: respiratory depression, malaise, lassitude.

INTERACTIONS
None significant.

NURSING CONSIDERATIONS
• Contraindicated in complete AV dissociation and severe hepatic disease. Use with caution in women who are pregnant or of childbearing age, and in glaucoma or pulmonary embolus; may precipitate dysrhythmias.
• Withhold dose and call doctor if signs of hepatic hypersensitivity develop (GI symptoms, altered liver function tests, jaundice, and eosinophilia).
• The FDA has announced this drug may not be effective for disease states indicated.

isoxsuprine hydrochloride
Vasodilan♦, Vasoprine

Pregnancy Risk Category: C

MECHANISM OF ACTION
Stimulates beta receptors and may also be a direct-acting peripheral vasodilator.

INDICATIONS & DOSAGE
Adjunct for relief of symptoms associated with cerebrovascular insufficiency, peripheral vascular diseases (such as arteriosclerosis obliterans, thromboangiitis obliterans, Raynaud's disease)—
Adults: 10 to 20 mg P.O. t.i.d. or q.i.d.

ADVERSE REACTIONS
CV: tachycardia, hypotension.
GI: vomiting, abdominal distress, intestinal distention.
Skin: severe rash.

INTERACTIONS
None significant.

NURSING CONSIDERATIONS
• Contraindicated in immediate postpartum period and arterial bleeding.

Use with caution in cardiovascular or cerebrovascular disease.
• Safe use in pregnancy and lactation not established, although drug has been used to inhibit contractions in premature labor.
• Isoxsuprine has also been used to minimize cramping in patients with severe primary dysmenorrhea.
• Discontinue if rash develops.
• Instruct patient to avoid sudden position changes to minimize the risk of orthostasis.

nicotinyl alcohol tartrate
Roniacol♦, Ronigen, Rycotin

Pregnancy Risk Category: C

MECHANISM OF ACTION
Converted to nicotinic acid, which produces peripheral vasodilation by a direct effect on vascular smooth muscle.

INDICATIONS & DOSAGE
Treatment of conditions of deficient circulation, such as peripheral vascular disease, vascular spasm, varicose ulcers, decubital ulcers, Ménière's disease, vertigo—
Adults: 50 to 100 mg P.O. b.i.d. or t.i.d. (may increase to 150 to 200 mg P.O. t.i.d. or q.i.d.); or 150- to 300-mg sustained-release tablets P.O. b.i.d.; 5 to 10 ml of elixir P.O. t.i.d.

ADVERSE REACTIONS
CNS: paresthesias.
CV: *transient flushing, orthostatic hypotension.*
GI: *gastric irritation.*
Skin: minor rashes, tingling.
Other: allergic reactions.

INTERACTIONS
Clonidine: may inhibit vasodilation. Observe for lack of response.

NURSING CONSIDERATIONS
• Contraindicted in active peptic ul-

cer or gastritis.
• Instruct the patient to avoid sudden position changes to minimize risk of orthostatic hypotension.
• Tolerance to most side effects develops with continued therapy.

nimodipine
Nimotop

Pregnancy Risk Category: C

MECHANISM OF ACTION
Inhibits calcium ion influx across cardiac and smooth muscle cells, thus decreasing myocardial contractility and oxygen demand, and dilates coronary arteries and arterioles. Initially thought to relieve vasospasm in patients after subarachnoid hemorrhage, its mechanism of action is not fully known.

INDICATIONS AND DOSAGE
Improvement of neurologic deficits in patients after subarachnoid hemorrhage from ruptured congenital aneurysms—
Adults: 60 mg P.O. every 4 hours for 21 days. Therapy should begin within 96 hours after subarachnoid hemorrhage.

ADVERSE REACTIONS
CNS: headaches.
CV: decreased blood pressure, flushing, edema.

INTERACTIONS
Antihypertensives: Possible enhanced hypotensive effect.
Calcium channel blockers: Possible enhanced cardiovascular effects.

NURSING CONSIDERATIONS
• There are no known contraindications to nimodipine therapy, and the drug was relatively well tolerated in clinical trials. Nimodipine should be reserved for patients who are in good neurological condition post-ictus (for

---

Italicized side effects are common or life-threatening.
*Liquid form contains alcohol.   **May contain tartrazine.

example, Hunt and Hess grades I to III).
• Patients with hepatic failure should receive lower doses. Begin therapy at 30 mg P.O. every 4 hours, with close monitoring of blood pressure and heart rate.
• Monitor blood pressure and heart rate in all patients, especially at the initiation of therapy.

nylidrin hydrochloride
Arlidin♦, Arlidin Forte♦♦, PMS Nylidrin♦♦

Pregnancy Risk Category: C

MECHANISM OF ACTION
Stimulates beta receptors and may directly relax vascular smooth muscle.

INDICATIONS & DOSAGE
To increase blood supply in vasospastic disorders (arteriosclerosis obliterans, thromboangiitis obliterans, diabetic vascular disease, night leg cramps, Raynaud's phenomenon and disease, ischemic ulcer, frostbite, acrocyanosis, acroparesthesia, sequelae of thrombophlebitis) and in circulatory disturbances of the middle ear (primary cochlear ischemia, cochlear striae, vascular ischemia, macular or ampullar ischemia); other disturbances caused by labyrinth artery spasm or obstruction—
Adults: 3 to 12 mg P.O. t.i.d. or q.i.d.

ADVERSE REACTIONS
CNS: trembling, *nervousness, weakness, dizziness (not associated with labyrinth artery insufficiency).*
CV: *palpitations, hypotension,* flushing.
GI: nausea, vomiting.

INTERACTIONS
None significant.

NURSING CONSIDERATIONS
• Contraindicated in acute myocardial infarction, paroxysmal tachycardia, angina pectoris, or thyrotoxicosis. Use with caution in uncompensated heart disease or peptic ulcer.
• Advise patient to avoid tasks that require mental alertness (such as driving or operating heavy machinery) until CNS effects of the drug are known.
• Instruct patient to avoid sudden posture changes to minimize the risks of orthostasis.

papaverine hydrochloride
Cerespan, Genabid, Pavabid, Pavabid HP, Pavacap, Pavacen, Pavagen ,Pava-Par, Pavarine, Pavased, Pavatime, Pavatine, Paverolan

Pregnancy Risk Category: C

MECHANISM OF ACTION
Directly relaxes smooth muscle from the inhibition of phosphodiesterase, resulting in increased concentrations of cyclic adenosine monophosphate.

INDICATIONS & DOSAGE
Relief of cerebral and peripheral ischemia associated with arterial spasm and myocardial ischemia; treatment of smooth muscle spasm (coronary occlusion, angina pectoris, sequelae of peripheral and pulmonary embolism, certain cerebral angiospastic states) and visceral spasms (biliary, ureteral, or GI colic)—
Adults: 60 to 300 mg P.O. 1 to 5 times daily, or 150- to 300-mg sustained-release preparations q 8 to 12 hours; 30 to 120 mg I.M. or I.V. q 3 hours, as indicated.

ADVERSE REACTIONS
CNS: *headache.*
CV: *increased heart rate, increased blood pressure* (with parenteral use), depressed AV and intraventricular conduction, hypotension, dysrhyth-

mias.
GI: constipation, *nausea*.
Other: *sweating, flushing*, malaise, hepatic damage, increased depth of respiration.

INTERACTIONS
None significant.

NURSING CONSIDERATIONS
• Contraindicated for I.V. use in patients with Parkinson's disease or complete AV block. Use with caution in glaucoma.
• Monitor blood pressure and heart rate and rhythm, especially in cardiac disease. Withhold dose and notify doctor immediately if changes occur.
• Not often used parenterally, except when immediate effect is desired.
• Give I.V. slowly (over 1 to 2 minutes) to avoid serious adverse reactions.
• Most effective when given early in the course of a disorder.
• Tell patient to take medication regularly; long-term therapy is required.
• Monitor for adverse hepatic effects in patients receiving long-term therapy.
• Do not add lactated Ringer's injection to the injectable form; will precipitate.
• Advise patient to avoid tasks that require mental alertness (such as driving or operating heavy machinery) until CNS effects of the drug are known.
• Instruct patient to avoid sudden posture changes to minimize the risks of orthostatic hypotension.
• The FDA has announced this drug may not be effective for disease states indicated.
• Has been used experimentally, alone or with phenoxybenzamine, to treat impotence in males. Patients are taught to self-administer by intercavernosal injection.

tolazoline hydrochloride
Priscoline♦, Tazol, Toloxan, Tolzol
Pregnancy Risk Category: C

MECHANISM OF ACTION
Direct-acting vasodilator. May have some alpha receptor blocking effects.

INDICATIONS & DOSAGE
Persistent pulmonary hypertension of the newborn—
Neonates: initially, 1 to 2 mg/kg I.V. over 10 minutes, followed by infusion of 1 to 2 mg/kg/hour.
Peripheral vasospastic disorders—
Adults: 10 to 50 mg I.M. or I.V. q.i.d.

ADVERSE REACTIONS
CV: *dysrhythmias, anginal pain, hypertension, flushing,* transient postural vertigo, palpitations.
GI: *nausea, vomiting, diarrhea, epigastric discomfort, exacerbation of peptic ulcer.*
Local: burning at injection site.
Other: weakness, paradoxical response in seriously damaged limbs, increased pilomotor activity, tingling, chilliness, apprehension, pulmonary hemorrhage.

INTERACTIONS
Ethyl alcohol: possible disulfiram reaction from accumulation of acetaldehyde. Use together cautiously.
Vasopressors (epinephrine, norepinephrine): may cause a paradoxical fall in blood pressure.

NURSING CONSIDERATIONS
• Contraindicated in coronary artery disease or active peptic ulcer, or following CVA. Use with caution in patients with history of peptic ulcer disease, gastritis, or known or suspected mitral stenosis.
• Response to treatment of persistent pulmonary hypertension of the newborn should be evident within 30 min-

utes. There is little information regarding infusions lasting longer than 48 hours.

• Keep patient warm during parenteral administration to increase response.

• Patient should be supine during infusion.

• Appearance of flushing usually indicates maximum tolerable dose.

• Monitor vital signs. Watch especially for blood pressure changes and dysrhythmias.

• Instruct patient to avoid alcohol; chills and flushing may occur.

• Warn patient against exposure to cold, which can aggravate tissue damage.

• Often used to distinguish between functional (vasospastic) and organic (obstructive) forms of peripheral vascular disease.

24

Antilipemics

cholestyramine
clofibrate
colestipol hydrochloride
dextrothyroxine sodium
gemfibrozil
lovastatin
niacin◇
   (See Chapter 101, VITAMINS AND
   MINERALS.)
probucol

COMBINATION PRODUCTS
None.

---

cholestyramine
Cholybar, Questran♦**

Pregnancy Risk Category: C

MECHANISM OF ACTION
Combines with bile acid to form an insoluble compound that is excreted.

INDICATIONS & DOSAGE
Primary hyperlipidemia, pruritus, and diarrhea due to excess bile acid; as adjunctive therapy for the reduction of elevated serum cholesterol in patients with primary hypercholesterolemia; and to reduce the risks of atherosclerotic coronary artery disease and myocardial infarction—
Adults: 4 g before meals and h.s., not to exceed 32 g daily. Each scoop or packet of Questran contains 4 g cholestyramine. Also available as Cholybar, a chewable candy bar (raspberry or caramel flavored) containing 4 g cholestyramine.
Children: 240 mg/kg daily P.O. in three divided doses with beverage or food. Safe dosage not established for children under 6 years.

ADVERSE REACTIONS
GI: *constipation,* fecal impaction, hemorrhoids, *abdominal discomfort,* flatulence, *nausea,* vomiting, steatorrhea.
Skin: *rashes,* irritation of skin, tongue, and perianal area.
Other: *vitamin A, D, and K deficiency from decreased absorption;* hyperchloremic acidosis with long-term use or very high dosage.

INTERACTIONS
Acetaminophen, coumarin anticoagulants, beta-adrenergic blocking agents, corticosteroids, digitalis glycosides, fat soluble vitamins (A,D,E and K), iron preparations, thiazide diuretics, thyroid hormone: absorption may be substantially decreased by cholestyramine. Separate administration times by at least 2 hours.

NURSING CONSIDERATIONS
• Patients who are taking this drug to reduce the risks of atherosclerotic heart disease should be encouraged to be aware of other cardiac disease risk factors. Recommend weight control and stop smoking programs.
• Monitor serum cholesterol and triglyceride levels regularly during cholestyramine therapy. Teach the patient about proper dietary management (restricting total fat and cholesterol intake), weight control, and exercise. Explain their importance in controlling elevated serum lipids.

Italicized side effects are common or life-threatening.
*Liquid form contains alcohol.   **May contain tartrazine.

• To mix powder, sprinkle powder on surface of preferred beverage or wet food. Let stand a few minutes, then stir to obtain uniform suspension.

• Mixing with carbonated beverages may result in excess foaming. Use large glass and mix slowly.

• Administer all other medications at least 1 hour before or 4 to 6 hours after cholestyramine to avoid blocking their absorption.

• Monitor bowel habits; treat constipation as needed. Encourage a diet high in fiber and fluids. If severe constipation develops, decrease dosage, add a stool softener, or discontinue drug.

• Monitor cardiac glycosides in patients receiving both medications concurrently. Should cholestyramine therapy be discontinued, cardiac glycoside toxicity may result unless dosage is adjusted.

• Watch for signs of folic acid and vitamin A, D, E, and K deficiency.

• May bind many drugs and cause decreased absorption. Check drug interaction list of individual drugs.

clofibrate
Atromid-S♦, Claripex♦♦,
Novofibrate♦♦

Pregnancy Risk Category: C

MECHANISM OF ACTION
Seems to inhibit biosynthesis of cholesterol at an early stage, but the exact mechanism is unknown.

INDICATIONS & DOSAGE
Hyperlipidemia and xanthoma tuberosum; Type III hyperlipidemia that does not respond adequately to diet—
Adults: 2 g P.O. daily in four divided doses. Some patients may respond to lower doses as assessed by serum lipid monitoring.

Should not be used in children.

ADVERSE REACTIONS
Blood: leukopenia.
CNS: fatigue, weakness.
GI: *nausea, diarrhea, vomiting,* stomatitis, *dyspepsia,* flatulence.
Hepatic: gallstones, *transient and reversible elevations of liver function tests.*
Skin: rashes, urticaria, pruritus, dry skin and hair.
Other: myalgias and arthralgias, resembling a flu-like syndrome; *weight gain; polyphagia;* fever, decreased libido.

INTERACTIONS
Furosemide, sulfonylureas: clofibrate may potentiate the clinical effect of these agents. Monitor patient closely.
Oral contraceptives, rifampin: may antagonize clofibrate's lipid-lowering effect. Monitor serum lipids.
Oral anticoagulants: clofibrate may potentiate the anticoagulant effects of warfarin or dicoumarol. Decreased anticoagulant dosage is necessary.
Probenecid: increased clofibrate effect. Monitor for toxicity.

NURSING CONSIDERATIONS
• Contraindicated in severe renal or hepatic disease.

• Warn patient to report flu-like symptoms to doctor immediately.

• Monitor renal and hepatic function, blood counts, and serum electrolyte and blood sugar levels. If liver function tests show steady rise, clofibrate should be discontinued.

• Should not be used indiscriminately. May pose increased risk of gallstones, heart disease, and cancer.

• Monitor serum cholesterol and triglycerides regularly during clofibrate therapy.

• Teach patient about proper dietary management (restricting total fat and cholesterol intake), weight control, and exercise. Explain their importance in controlling elevated serum lipids.

- If significant lipid lowering is not achieved within 3 months, drug should be discontinued.
- Clofibrate has been used investigationally to treat diabetes insipidus at doses of 1.5 to 2 g daily.

colestipol hydrochloride
Colestid♦

Pregnancy Risk Category: C

MECHANISM OF ACTION
Combines with bile acid to form an insoluble compound that is excreted.

INDICATIONS & DOSAGE
Primary hypercholesterolemia and xanthomas—
Adults: 15 to 30 g P.O. daily in two to four divided doses.

ADVERSE REACTIONS
GI: *constipation (common, may require decreasing the dosage),* fecal impaction, hemorrhoids, abdominal discomfort, flatulence, nausea, vomiting, steatorrhea.
Skin: rashes, irritation of skin, tongue, and perianal area.
Other: vitamin A, D, and K deficiency from decreased absorption; hyperchloremic acidosis with long-term use or very high dosage.

INTERACTIONS
Oral hypoglycemics: may antagonize response to colestipol. Monitor serum lipids.

NURSING CONSIDERATIONS
- Administer all other medications at least 1 hour before or 4 to 6 hours after colestipol to avoid blocking their absorption.
- Monitor cardiac glycoside levels in patients receiving both medications concurrently. Should colestipol therapy be discontinued, cardiac glycoside toxicity may result unless dosage is adjusted.

- Watch for signs of vitamin A, D, and K deficiency.
- Lowering dosage, increasing dietary fiber, or adding stool softener may relieve constipation.
- May bind many drugs and cause decreased absorption. Check drug interaction list of individual drugs.
- Administer this drug in at least 3 oz (90 ml) of juice, milk, or water. After drinking this preparation, patient should swirl a small additional amount of liquid in the same glass and then drink it to ensure ingestion of the entire dose.
- Palatability may be enhanced if the next daily dose is mixed and refrigerated the previous evening.
- Teach patient about proper dietary management (restricting total fat and cholesterol intake), weight control, and exercise. Explain their importance in controlling elevated serum lipids.

dextrothyroxine sodium
Choloxin♦**

Pregnancy Risk Category: C

MECHANISM OF ACTION
Accelerates hepatic catabolism of cholesterol and increases bile secretion to lower cholesterol levels.

INDICATIONS & DOSAGE
Hyperlipidemia in euthyroid patients, especially when cholesterol and triglyceride levels are elevated—
Adults: initial dose 1 to 2 mg P.O. daily, increased by 1 to 2 mg daily at monthly intervals to a total of 4 to 8 mg daily.
Children: initial dose 0.05 mg/kg P.O. daily, increased by 0.05 mg/kg daily at monthly intervals to a total of 4 mg daily.

ADVERSE REACTIONS
CV: palpitations, angina pectoris, dysrhythmias, ischemic myocardial

changes on ECG, *myocardial infarction.*
EENT: visual disturbances, ptosis.
GI: nausea, vomiting, diarrhea, constipation, decreased appetite.
Metabolic: *insomnia, weight loss, sweating,* flushing, hyperthermia, hair loss, menstrual irregularities.

INTERACTIONS
Digitalis glycosides: dextrothyroxine may enhance clinical effect. Use together cautiously.

NURSING CONSIDERATIONS
• Contraindicated in hepatic or renal disease, or iodism. Patients with history of cardiac disease, including dysrhythmias, hypertension, or angina pectoris, should receive very small doses.
• May increase need for insulin, diet therapy, or oral hypoglycemics in patients with diabetes.
• If the use of anticoagulants is being considered, discontinue drug 2 weeks before surgery to avoid possible potentiation of anticoagulant effect.
• Observe patient for signs of hyperthyroidism, such as nervousness, insomnia, and weight loss. If these occur, dosage should be decreased or drug discontinued.
• Teach patient about proper dietary management (restricting total fat and cholesterol intake), weight control, and exercise. Explain their importance in controlling elevated serum lipids.

gemfibrozil
Lopid♦

Pregnancy Risk Category: B

MECHANISM OF ACTION
Inhibits peripheral lipolysis and also reduces triglyceride synthesis in the liver.

INDICATIONS & DOSAGE
Treatment of type IV hyperlipidemia (hypertriglyceridemia) and severe hypercholesterolemia unresponsive to diet and other drugs—
Adults: 1,200 mg P.O. administered in two divided doses. Usual dosage range is 900 to 1,500 mg daily. If no beneficial effect is seen after 3 months of therapy, drug should be discontinued.

ADVERSE REACTIONS
Blood: anemia, leukopenia.
CNS: blurred vision, headache, dizziness.
GI: *abdominal and epigastric pain, diarrhea, nausea,* vomiting, flatulence.
Hepatic: bile duct obstruction, elevated enzymes.
Skin: rash, dermatitis, pruritus.
Other: painful extremities.

INTERACTIONS
Oral anticoagulants: gemfibrozil may enhance the clinical effects of oral anticoagulants. Monitor patient closely.

NURSING CONSIDERATIONS
• Contraindicated in hepatic or severe renal dysfunction—including primary biliary cirrhosis—and preexisting gallbladder disease.
• CBC and liver function tests should be done periodically during the first 12 months of therapy.
• Gemfibrozil is very closely related to clofibrate both chemically and pharmacologically.
• Instruct patient to take drug half an hour before breakfast and dinner.
• Should not be used indiscriminately. May pose risk of gallstones, heart disease, and cancer.
• Observe bowel movements for evidence of steatorrhea or other signs of bile duct obstruction.
• Because of possible dizziness and blurred vision, patient should avoid driving or other hazardous activities

until CNS effects of the drug are known.
• Teach patient about proper dietary management (restricting total fat and cholesterol intake), weight control, and exercise. Explain their importance in controlling elevated serum lipids.

---

lovastatin
Mevacor

Pregnancy Risk Category: X

MECHANISM OF ACTION
Lovastatin inhibits 3-hydroxy-3-methylglutaryl-coenzyme A (HMG-CoA) reductase. This enzyme is an early (and rate-limiting) step in the synthetic pathway of cholesterol.

INDICATIONS & DOSAGE
Reduction of low-density lipoprotein and total cholesterol levels in patients with primary hypercholesterolemia (types IIa and IIb)—
Adults: initially, 20 mg P.O. once daily with the evening meal. For patients with severely elevated cholesterol levels (for example, over 300 mg/dl), the initial dose should be 40 mg. The recommended range is 20 to 80 mg in single or divided doses.

ADVERSE REACTIONS
CNS: headache, dizziness.
EENT: blurred vision, dysgeusia.
GI: constipation, diarrhea, dyspepsia, flatus, abdominal pain or cramps, heartburn, nausea.
Metabolic: elevated serum transaminase levels, abnormal liver test results.
Skin: rash, pruritus.
Other: peripheral neuropathy, muscle cramps, myalgia, myositis, *rhabdomyolysis*.

INTERACTIONS
Cholestyramine, clofibrate: enhanced lipid-reducing effects.

Immunosuppressive agents, gemfibrozil: possible increased risk of polymyositis and rhabdomyolysis. Maximum recommended lovastatin dosage is 20 mg daily; monitor patient closely.

NURSING CONSIDERATIONS
• Initiate lovastatin only after diet and other nonpharmacologic therapies have proven ineffective. Patient should be on a standard cholesterol-lowering diet during therapy.
• Give lovastatin with the evening meal; absorption is enhanced and cholesterol biosynthesis is greater in the evening.
• Therapeutic response occurs in about 2 weeks, with maximum effects in 4 to 6 weeks. Effects of long-term use are unknown.
• Watch for signs of myositis.
• Liver function tests should be performed frequently at start of therapy and periodically thereafter.
• Store tablets at room temperature in a light-resistant container.
• Advise patient to restrict alcohol intake.
• Tell patient to advise doctor of any adverse reactions, particularly muscle aches and pains.
• Advise patient to have periodic eye examinations.
• Teach patient about proper dietary management (restricting total fat and cholesterol intake), weight control, and exercise. Explain their importance in controlling elevated serum lipids.

---

probucol
Lorelco♦

Pregnancy Risk Category: B

MECHANISM OF ACTION
Inhibits cholesterol transport from the intestine and may also decrease cholesterol synthesis. Appears to be more effective in patients with mild cholesterol elevations than in those with se-

vere hypercholesterolemia.

INDICATIONS & DOSAGE
Primary hypercholesterolemia—
Adults: 2 tablets (500 mg total) P.O.
b.i.d. with morning and evening
meals. Not recommended for children.

ADVERSE REACTIONS
GI: *diarrhea, flatulence, abdominal
pain, nausea, vomiting.*
Other: *hyperhidrosis,* fetid sweat, angioneurotic edema.

INTERACTIONS
Clofibrate: additive pharmacologic effects.

NURSING CONSIDERATIONS
• Drug's effect is enhanced when
taken with food.
• Contraindicated in patients with
dysrhythmias. Drug should be
stopped in any patient whose ECG
shows prolonged Q-T interval. Monitor ECG periodically.
• Teach patient about proper dietary
management (restricting total fat and
cholesterol intake), weight control,
and exercise. Explain their importance in controlling elevated serum
lipids.
• If female patient wishes to become
pregnant, withdrawal of drug and effective contraception is recommended
for 6 months due to the persistence of
the drug in the body.

25

Nonnarcotic analgesics and antipyretics

Salicylates
aspirin (acetylsalicylic acid)◊
choline magnesium trisalicylate
choline salicylate
magnesium salicylate◊
salsalate
sodium salicylate◊
sodium thiosalicylate

Urinary tract analgesic
phenazopyridine hydrochloride

Miscellaneous
acetaminophen (paracetamol)◊
diflunisal
methotrimeprazine
(See Chapter 29, SEDATIVE-HYPNOTICS.)

COMBINATION PRODUCTS
AMAPHEN: acetaminophen 325 mg, caffeine 40 mg, and butalbital 50 mg.
ANOQUAN: acetaminophen 325 mg, caffeine 40 mg, and butalbital 50 mg.
ARTHRALGEN: acetaminophen 250 mg and salicylamide 250 mg.
AXOTAL: aspirin 650 mg and butalbital 50 mg.
BC POWDER: aspirin 650 mg, salicylamide 195 mg, and caffeine 32 mg.
BC TABLETS: aspirin 325 mg, salicylamide 95 mg, and caffeine 16 mg.
BUTAL: aspirin 325 mg, caffeine 40 mg, and butalbital 50 mg.
CAMA, ARTHRITIS STRENGTH: aspirin 500 mg, magnesium oxide 150 mg, and aluminum hydroxide 150 mg.
COPE◊: aspirin 421 mg, caffeine 32 mg, magnesium hydroxide 50 mg, and aluminum hydroxide 25 mg.
DURADYNE◊: acetaminophen 180 mg, aspirin 230 mg, and caffeine 15 mg.

ESGIC: acetaminophen 325 mg, caffeine 40 mg, and butalbital 50 mg.
EXCEDRIN P.M.◊: acetaminophen 500 mg and diphenhydramine citrate 38 mg.
EXCEDRIN TABLETS◊: aspirin 250 mg, acetaminophen 250 mg, caffeine 65 mg.
FEMCAPS◊: acetaminophen 324 mg, caffeine 32 mg, ephedrine sulfate 8 mg, and atropine sulfate 0.0325 mg.
FIORICET: acetaminophen 325 mg, butalbital 50 mg, and caffeine 40 mg
FIORINAL: aspirin 325 mg, caffeine 40 mg, and butalbital 50 mg.
G-1: acetaminophen 500 mg, caffeine 40 mg, and butalbital 50 mg.
GEMNISYN◊: aspirin 325 mg and acetaminophen 325 mg.
ISOLLYL: aspirin 325 mg, caffeine 40 mg, and butalbital 50 mg.
MIDOL◊: aspirin 454 mg, caffeine 32.4 mg, and cinnemedrine HCl 14.9 mg.
PAC NEW REVISED FORMULA◊: aspirin 400 mg and caffeine 32 mg.
PHRENILIN: acetaminophen 325 mg and butalbital 50 mg.
PHRENILIN FORTE: acetaminophen 650 mg and butalbital 50 mg.
SINUTAB◊: acetaminophen 325 mg, chlorpheniramine 2 mg, and pseudoephedrine HCl 30 mg.
SINUTAB II MAXIMUM STRENGTH◊: acetaminophen 500 mg and pseudoephedrine HCl 30 mg.
SYNALGOS◊: aspirin 356.4 mg and caffeine 30 mg.
TRIGESIC◊: acetaminophen 125 mg, aspirin 230 mg, and caffeine 30 mg.
TRILISATE: choline salicylate 293 mg

Italicized side effects are common or life-threatening.
*Liquid form contains alcohol.   **May contain tartrazine.

and magnesium salicylate 362 mg.
VANQUISH◇: aspirin 227 mg, acetaminophen 194 mg, caffeine 33 mg, aluminum hydroxide 25 mg, and magnesium hydroxide 50 mg.

---

acetaminophen (paracetamol)◇
Acephen, Aceta*, Ace-Tabs♦♦, Acetaminophen Unicerts, Actamin, Actamin Extra, Anacin-3, Anacin-3 Maximum Strength, Anuphen, Apacet, Apacet Extra Strength, Apacet Oral Solution, APAP, Apo-Acetaminophen♦♦, Atasol♦♦, Atasol Forte♦♦, Banesin, Campain♦♦, Children's Anacin-3, Children's Apacet, Children's Genapap, Children's Panadol, Children's Tylenol, Children's Ty-PAP, Children's Ty-Tabs, Dapa, Datril, Datril Extra Strength, Dolanex *, Exdol♦♦, Exdol Strong♦♦, Genapap, Genebs, Genebs Extra Strength, Gentabs, Halenol, Infant's Anacin-3, Infant's Apacet, Infant's Tylenol, Infant's Ty-PAP, Liquiprin, Meda Cap, Meda Tab, Myapap, Neopap, Oraphen-PD, Panadol, Panadol Junior Strength, Panex, Paraphen♦♦, Pedric *, Phenaphen, Robigesic♦♦, Rounox♦♦, Suppap, Tapanol, Tapanol Extra Strength, Tempra♦, Tenol, Ty Caplets, Ty Caps, Tylenol♦*, Tylenol Extra Strength, Ty Tabs, Valadol*, Valorin

Pregnancy Risk Category: B

MECHANISM OF ACTION
Produces analgesia by blocking generation of pain impulses. This action is probably caused by inhibition of prostaglandin synthesis; it may also be caused by inhibition of the synthesis or action of other substances that sensitize pain receptors to mechanical or chemical stimulation. It relieves fever by central action in the hypothalamic heat-regulating center.

INDICATIONS & DOSAGE
Mild pain or fever—
Adults and children over 11 years: 325 to 650 mg P.O. or rectally q 4 hours, p.r.n. Maximum dosage should not exceed 4 g daily. Dosage for long-term therapy should not exceed 2.6 g daily.
Children 11 years: 480 mg/dose.
Children 9 to 10 years: 400 mg/dose.
Children 6 to 8 years: 320 mg/dose.
Children 4 to 5 years: 240 mg/dose.
Children 2 to 3 years: 160 mg/dose.
Children 12 to 23 months: 120 mg/dose.
Children 4 to 11 months: 80 mg/dose.
Children up to 3 months: 40 mg/dose.

ADVERSE REACTIONS
Hepatic: *severe liver damage with toxic doses.*
Skin: rash, urticaria.

INTERACTIONS
Diflunisal: increases acetaminophen blood levels. Don't use together.

NURSING CONSIDERATIONS
• Repeated use is contraindicated in anemia, or renal or hepatic disease.
• Has no significant anti-inflammatory effect.
• Warn patient that high doses or unsupervised chronic use can cause hepatic damage. Excessive ingestion of alcoholic beverages may increase the risk of hepatotoxicity.
• Should not be used for self-medication of marked fever (greater than 103.1° F. [39.5° C.]), fever persisting longer than 3 days, or recurrent fever unless directed by doctor.
• May increase the hypoprothrombinemic activity of warfarin when taken chronically for pain.
• Many nonprescription products contain acetaminophen. Be aware of this when calculating total daily dosages.

Unmarked trade names available in the United States only.
♦ Also available in Canada.   ♦♦ Available in Canada only.   ◇ Also available OTC.

• Recommend the liquid form for children and for all patients who have difficulty swallowing.

aspirin (acetylsalicylic acid)○

Ancasal♦♦, Arthrinol♦♦, Artria SR, ASA, ASA Enseals, Aspergum, Astrin♦♦, Bayer Aspirin, Coryphen♦♦, Easprin, Ecotrin♦, Empirin, Entrophen♦♦, Measurin, Norwich Aspirin, Novasen♦♦, Riphen-10♦♦, Sal-Adult♦♦, Sal-Infant♦♦, Supasa♦♦, Triaphen-10♦♦, ZORprin

Pregnancy Risk Category: C (D in 3rd trimester)

MECHANISM OF ACTION
• Produces analgesia by an ill-defined effect on the hypothalamus (central action) and by blocking generation of pain impulses (peripheral action). The peripheral action may involve inhibition of prostaglandin synthesis.
• Exerts its anti-inflammatory effect by inhibiting prostaglandin synthesis, may also inhibit the synthesis or action of other mediators of the inflammatory response.
• Relieves fever by acting on the hypothalamic heat-regulating center to produce peripheral vasodilation. This increases peripheral blood supply and promotes sweating, which leads to loss of heat and to cooling by evaporation.
• Also appears to impede clotting by blocking prostaglandin synthesis, which prevents formation of the platelet-aggregating substance thromboxane A_2.

INDICATIONS & DOSAGE
Adults:
Arthritis—2.6 to 5.4 g P.O. daily in divided doses.
Mild pain or fever—325 to 650 mg P.O. or rectally q 4 hours, p.r.n.

Thromboembolic disorders—325 to 650 mg P.O. daily or b.i.d.
Transient ischemic attacks in men—650 mg P.O. b.i.d. or 325 mg q.i.d.
To reduce the risk of heart attack in patients with previous myocardial infarction or unstable angina—325 mg P.O. once daily.
Children:
Arthritis—90 to 130 mg/kg P.O. daily divided q 4 to 6 hours.
Fever—40 to 80 mg/kg P.O. or rectally daily divided q 6 hours, p.r.n.
Mild pain—65 to 100 mg/kg P.O. or rectally daily divided q 4 to 6 hours, p.r.n.

ADVERSE REACTIONS
Blood: *prolonged bleeding time.*
EENT: *tinnitus and hearing loss.*
GI: *nausea, vomiting, GI distress, occult bleeding.*
Hepatic: abnormal liver function studies, hepatitis.
Skin: *rash,* bruising.
Other: *hypersensitivity manifested by anaphylaxis and/or asthma.*

INTERACTIONS
Ammonium chloride (and other urine acidifiers): increased blood levels of aspirin products. Monitor for aspirin toxicity.
Antacids in high doses (and other urine alkalinizers): decreased levels of aspirin products. Monitor for decreased aspirin effect.
Corticosteroids: enhance salicylate elimination. Monitor for decreased salicylate effect.
Oral anticoagulants and heparin: increase risk of bleeding. Avoid using together if possible.

NURSING CONSIDERATIONS
• Contraindicated in GI ulcer, GI bleeding, or aspirin hypersensitivity. Use cautiously in patients with hypoprothrombinemia, vitamin K deficiency, bleeding disorders, and in asthmatics with nasal polyps (may

---

Italicized side effects are common or life-threatening.
*Liquid form contains alcohol.   **May contain tartrazine.

cause severe bronchospasm).
• Because of epidemiologic association with Reye's syndrome, the Centers for Disease Control recommends that children or teenagers with chicken pox or influenza-like illness should not be given salicylates.
• Febrile, dehydrated children can develop toxicity rapidly.
• Elderly patients may be more susceptible to aspirin's toxic effects.
• Give with food, milk, antacid, or large glass of water to reduce GI adverse effects.
• Because of the many possible drug interactions involving aspirin, warn patients taking prescription drugs to check with doctor or pharmacist before taking OTC combinations containing aspirin.
• Therapeutic blood salicylate level in arthritis is 10 to 30 mg/100 ml. Tinnitus may occur at plasma levels of 30 mg/100 ml and above, but this is not a reliable indicator of toxicity, especially in very young and elderly patients.
• Concomitant use with alcohol, steroids or other NSAIDs may increase risk of GI bleeding.
• May cause an increase in serum levels of AST (SGOT), ALT (SGPT), alkaline phosphatase, and bilirubin.
• Keep out of reach of children—aspirin is one of the leading causes of poisoning in children. Encourage use of child-resistant containers in households with children.
• Advise patients receiving large doses of aspirin for an extended period of time to watch for petechiae, bleeding gums, and signs of GI bleeding, and to maintain adequate fluid intake. Obtain hemoglobin and prothrombin tests periodically.
• Enteric-coated products are slowly absorbed and are not suitable for acute effects. They do cause less GI bleeding and may be more suited for long-term therapy, such as arthritic therapy.

• There's no evidence that aspirin is effective in reducing the incidence of transient ischemic attacks in women.
• There is some evidence that aspirin may prevent sunburn and treat sunburn pain by preventing cells from manufacturing prostaglandins.
• If possible, stop aspirin dosage 10 days before elective surgery.
• For patients with swallowing difficulties, aspirin can be crushed and combined with soft food or dissolved in liquid. After mixing it with a liquid, administer it immediately, because the drug doesn't stay in solution. Don't crush enteric-coated aspirin.

choline magnesium trisalicylate
Trilisate♦

Pregnancy Risk Category: C

MECHANISM OF ACTION
• Produces analgesia by an ill-defined effect on the hypothalamus (central action) and by blocking generation of pain impulses (peripheral action). The peripheral action may involve inhibition of prostaglandin synthesis.
• Exerts its anti-inflammatory effect by inhibiting prostaglandin synthesis.
• Relieves fever by acting on the hypothalamic heat-regulating center to produce peripheral vasodilation. This increases peripheral blood supply and promotes sweating, which leads to loss of heat and to cooling by evaporation.

INDICATIONS & DOSAGE
Arthritis, mild—
Adults: 1 to 2 teaspoonfuls or tablets P.O. b.i.d. Total daily dosage can also be given at one time (usually h.s.)
Rheumatoid arthritis and osteoarthritis—
Adults: Initially, 3 g P.O. daily either as a single dose h.s. or in divided

doses. Dosage is adjusted according to patient response. Dosage range is 1 to 4.5 g daily.
Juvenile rheumatoid arthritis—
Children (12 to 37 kg): 50 mg/kg/day P.O. in divided doses.
Children (more than 37 kg): 2,250 mg given in divided doses.
Mild to moderate pain and fever—
Adults: 2 to 3 g P.O. daily divided b.i.d.
Children (12 to 37 kg): 50 mg/kg/day in divided doses.

ADVERSE REACTIONS
EENT: tinnitus and hearing loss.
GI: GI distress.
Skin: rash.
Other: *hypersensitivity manifested by anaphylaxis (rare).*

INTERACTIONS
Alcohol, steroids, and other NSAIDs: enhanced risk of adverse GI effects.
Ammonium chloride (and other urine acidifiers): increased blood levels of salicylates. Monitor for salicylate toxicity.
Antacids in high doses (and other urine alkalinizers): decreased levels of salicylates. Monitor for decreased salicylate effect.
Corticosteroids: enhance salicylate elimination. Monitor for decreased salicylate effect.
Oral anticoagulants, heparin: enhanced risk of bleeding. Use together cautiously.

NURSING CONSIDERATIONS
• Use cautiously in chronic renal failure, peptic ulcer disease, gastritis, and in patients with a known allergy to salicylates.
• Each '500' tablet or teaspoonful is equal in salicylate content to 650 mg aspirin.
• Because of epidemiologic association with Reye's syndrome, the Centers for Disease Control recommends that children or teenagers with

chicken pox or influenza-like illness should not be given salicylates.
• Causes less GI distress than aspirin. If antacid is needed, give it 2 hours after meals and give choline magnesium trisalicylate before meals.
• Tell patient to take tablets with food or a full glass of water. Solution may be mixed with fruit juice, but not antacids.
• Febrile, dehydrated children can develop toxicity rapidly.
• Therapeutic blood salicylate level in arthritis is 10 to 30 mg/100 ml. Tinnitus may occur at plasma levels of 30 mg/100 ml and above, but this is not a reliable indicator of toxicity, especially in very young and elderly patients.
• Obtain hemoglobin and prothrombin tests periodically in patients receiving large doses over an extended period of time.

choline salicylate
Arthropan
Pregnancy Risk Category: C

MECHANISM OF ACTION
• Produces analgesia by an ill-defined effect on the hypothalamus (central action) and by blocking generation of pain impulses (peripheral action). The peripheral action may involve inhibition of prostaglandin synthesis.
• Exerts its anti-inflammatory effect by inhibiting prostaglandin synthesis.
• Relieves fever by acting on the hypothalamic heat-regulating center to produce peripheral vasodilation. This increases peripheral blood supply and promotes sweating, which leads to loss of heat and to cooling by evaporation.

INDICATIONS & DOSAGE
Rheumatoid arthritis, osteoarthritis, minor pain or fever—
Adults and children over age 12:

One teaspoonful (870 mg choline salicylate) P.O. every 3 to 4 hours p.r.n. If tolerated and needed, dosage may be increased to 2 teaspoonfuls. Do not exceed 6 teaspoons daily.

ADVERSE REACTIONS
EENT: tinnitus and hearing loss.
GI: nausea, vomiting, GI distress.
Skin: rash.
Other: *hypersensitivity manifested by anaphylaxis (rare).*

INTERACTIONS
Alcohol, steroids, and other NSAIDs: enhanced risk of adverse GI effects.
Ammonium chloride (and other urine acidifiers): increased blood levels of salicylates. Monitor for salicylate toxicity.
Antacids in high doses (and other urine alkalinizers): decreased levels of salicylates. Monitor for decreased salicylate effect.
Corticosteroids: enhance salicylate elimination. Monitor for decreased salicylate effect.

NURSING CONSIDERATIONS
• Use cautiously in chronic renal failure, peptic ulcer disease, gastritis, and in patients with a known allergy to salicylates.
• Because of epidemiologic association with Reye's syndrome, the Centers for Disease Control recommends that children or teenagers with chicken pox or influenza-like illness should not be given salicylates.
• Causes less GI distress than aspirin. If antacid is needed, give it 2 hours after meals and give choline salicylate before meals.
• May mix drug with water, fruit juice, or carbonated drinks, but not antacids.
• Febrile, dehydrated children can develop toxicity rapidly.
• Therapeutic blood salicylate level in arthritis is 10 to 30 mg/100 ml. Tinnitus may occur at plasma levels of

30 mg/100 ml and above, but this is not a reliable indicator of toxicity, especially in very young and elderly patients.
• Obtain hemoglobin and prothrombin tests periodically in patients receiving large dosages over an extended period of time.

diflunisal
Dolobid♦

Pregnancy Risk Category: C

MECHANISM OF ACTION
Mechanism of action is unknown, but it is probably related to inhibition of prostaglandin synthesis.

INDICATIONS & DOSAGE
Mild to moderate pain and osteoarthritis—
Adults: 500 to 1,000 mg P.O. daily in two divided doses, usually q 12 hours. Maximum dosage 1,500 mg daily.
Adults over 65: Start with one-half the usual adult dose.

ADVERSE REACTIONS
CNS: *dizziness,* somnolence, insomnia, *headache.*
EENT: *tinnitus, visual disturbances (rare).*
GI: *nausea, dyspepsia, gastrointestinal pain, diarrhea,* vomiting, constipation, flatulence.
Skin: *rash,* pruritus, sweating, dry mucous membranes, stomatitis.

INTERACTIONS
Aspirin, antacids: decreased diflunisal blood levels. Monitor for possible decreased therapeutic effect.
Oral anticoagulants, thrombolytic agents: diflunisal may enhance pharmacologic effects of these agents. Use together cautiously.
Sulindac: diflunisal decreases blood levels of sulindac's active metabolite. Monitor for decreased pharmacologic

effect.

NURSING CONSIDERATIONS
• Contraindicated for patients in whom acute asthmatic attacks, urticaria, or rhinitis are precipitated by aspirin or other nonsteroidal anti-inflammatory drugs.
• Use cautiously in patients with active GI bleeding or history of peptic ulcer disease, renal impairment, compromised cardiac function, or those taking anticoagulants.
• Similar to aspirin, diflunisal is a salicylic acid derivative but is metabolized differently and has less effect on platelet function.
• May be administered with water, milk, or meals.
• Avoid the use of diflunisal in children and teenagers with viral illnesses and flu because of possible association with Reye's syndrome.

---

magnesium salicylate◇
Doan's Pills, Magan, Mobidin
Pregnancy Risk Category: C

MECHANISM OF ACTION
• Produces analgesia by an ill-defined effect on the hypothalamus (central action) and by blocking generation of pain impulses (peripheral action). The peripheral action may involve inhibition of prostaglandin synthesis.
• Exerts its anti-inflammatory effect by inhibiting prostaglandin synthesis.
• Relieves fever by acting on the hypothalamic heat-regulating center to produce peripheral vasodilation. This increases peripheral blood supply and promotes sweating, which leads to loss of heat and to cooling by evaporation.

INDICATIONS & DOSAGE
Arthritis—
Adults: 545 mg to 1.2 g P.O. t.i.d. or q.i.d. not to exceed 9.6 g daily.

Mild pain or fever—
Adults: 300 to 600 mg P.O. q 4 hours, not to exceed 3.5 g/24 hours.

ADVERSE REACTIONS
EENT: *tinnitus and hearing loss.*
GI: *nausea, vomiting, GI distress, occult bleeding.*
Hepatic: abnormal liver function studies, hepatitis.
Skin: *rash,* bruising.
Other: *hypersensitivity manifested by anaphylaxis and/or asthma.*

INTERACTIONS
Ammonium chloride (and other urine acidifiers): increased blood levels of salicylates. Monitor for salicylate toxicity.
Antacids in high doses (and other urine alkalinizers): decreased levels of salicylates. Monitor for decreased salicylate effect.
Corticosteroids: enhance salicylate elimination. Monitor for decreased salicylate effect.
Oral anticoagulants and heparin: increase risk of bleeding. Avoid using together if possible.

NURSING CONSIDERATIONS
• Contraindicated in severe chronic renal insufficiency because of risk of magnesium toxicity; GI ulcer; GI bleeding; or aspirin hypersensitivity. Use cautiously in hypoprothrombinemia, vitamin K deficiency, and bleeding disorders.
• Because of epidemiologic association with Reye's syndrome, the Centers for Disease Control recommends that children or teenagers with chicken pox or influenza-like illness should not be given salicylates.
• Febrile, dehydrated children can develop toxicity rapidly.
• Give with food, milk, antacid, or large glass of water to reduce GI adverse effects.
• Therapeutic blood salicylate level in arthritis is 10 to 30 mg/100 ml.

Italicized side effects are common or life-threatening.
*Liquid form contains alcohol.   **May contain tartrazine.

Tinnitus may occur at plasma levels of 300 mg/100 ml and above, but this is not a reliable indicator of toxicity, expecially in very young and elderly patients.
• Concomitant use with alcohol, steroids, or other NSAIDs may increase risk of GI bleeding.
• May cause an increase in serum levels of AST (SGOT), ALT (SGPT), alkaline phosphatase, and bilirubin.
• Obtain hemoglobin and prothrombin tests periodically in patients receiving large doses over an extended period of time.

phenazopyridine hydrochloride
Azo-Standard, Baridium, Eridium, Geridium, Phenazo♦♦, Phenazodine, Pyrazodine, Pyridiate, Pyridin, Pyridium♦, Pyronium♦♦, Urodine, Urogesic, Viridium

Pregnancy Risk Category: B

MECHANISM OF ACTION
Exerts local anesthetic action on urinary mucosa through unknown mechanism.

INDICATIONS & DOSAGE
Pain with urinary tract irritation or infection—
Adults: 100 to 200 mg P.O. t.i.d.
Children: 100 mg P.O. t.i.d.

ADVERSE REACTIONS
CNS: headache, vertigo.
GI: nausea.
Skin: rash.

INTERACTIONS
None significant.

NURSING CONSIDERATIONS
• Contraindicated in renal and hepatic insufficiency.
• Colors urine red or orange. May stain fabrics.

• Use only as analgesic. Use with antibiotic to treat urinary tract infection.
• Drug may be stopped in 3 days if pain is relieved.
• May alter Clinistix or Tes-Tape results. Use Clinitest for accurate urine glucose test results.
• Stop drug if skin or sclera becomes yellow-tinged. May indicate accumulation caused by impaired renal excretion.

salsalate
Disalcid, Mono-Gesic, Salflex, Salgesic, Salsitab

Pregnancy Risk Category: C

MECHANISM OF ACTION
• The salicylic ester of salicylic acid, each molecule of salsalate is hydrolyzed to two molecules of salicylate in vivo.
• Produces analgesia by an ill-defined effect on the hypothalamus (central action) and by blocking generation of pain impulses (peripheral action). The peripheral action may involve inhibition of prostaglandin synthesis.
• Exerts its anti-inflammatory effect by inhibiting prostaglandin synthesis; may also inhibit the synthesis or action of other mediators of the inflammatory response.

INDICATIONS & DOSAGE
Arthritis—
Adults: 3 g P.O. daily, divided b.i.d. or t.i.d. Usual maintenance dose is 2 to 4 g daily.

ADVERSE REACTIONS
EENT: *tinnitus and hearing loss.*
GI: *nausea, vomiting, GI distress, occult bleeding.*
Hepatic: abnormal liver function studies, hepatitis.
Skin: *rash,* bruising.
Other: *hypersensitivity manifested by anaphylaxis and asthma.*

INTERACTIONS

Ammonium chloride (and other urine acidifiers): increased blood levels of salicylates. Monitor for salicylate toxicity.

Antacids in high doses (and other urine alkalinizers): decreased levels of salicylates. Monitor for decreased salicylate effect.

Corticosteroids: compete for binding sites. Monitor for decreased salicylate effect.

Oral anticoagulants and heparin: possible increased risk of bleeding. Avoid using together if possible.

NURSING CONSIDERATIONS

• Contraindicated in salsalate hypersensitivity. Use cautiously in GI bleeding, aspirin hypersensitivity, and renal insufficiency. Use cautiously in hypoprothrombinemia, vitamin K deficiency, and bleeding disorders.

• Because of epidemiologic association with Reye's syndrome, the Centers for Disease Control recommends that children or teenagers with chicken pox or influenza-like illness should not be given salicylates.

• Give with food, milk, antacid, or large glass of water to reduce possible GI adverse effects.

• Therapeutic blood salicylate level in arthritis is 10 to 30 mg/100 ml. Tinnitus may occur at plasma levels of 30 mg/100 ml and above, but this is not a reliable indicator of toxicity, especially in very young and elderly patients.

• Concomitant use with alcohol, steroids, or other NSAIDs may increase risk of GI bleeding.

• May cause an increase in serum levels of AST (SGOT), ALT (SGPT), alkaline phosphatase, and bilirubin.

• Advise patients receiving large doses for extended period of time to watch for petechiae, bleeding gums, and signs of GI bleeding, and to maintain adequate fluid intake. Obtain hemoglobin and prothrombin tests periodically.

sodium salicylate◇
Uracel

Pregnancy Risk Category: C

MECHANISM OF ACTION

• Produces analgesia by an ill-defined effect on the hypothalamus (central action) and by blocking generation of pain impulses (peripheral action). The peripheral action may involve inhibition of prostaglandin synthesis.

• Exerts its anti-inflammatory effect by inhibiting prostaglandin synthesis; may also inhibit the synthesis or action of other mediators of the inflammatory response.

• Relieves fever by acting on the hypothalamic heat-regulating center to produce peripheral vasodilation. This increases peripheral blood supply and promotes sweating, which leads to loss of heat and to cooling by evaporation.

INDICATIONS & DOSAGE

Minor pain or fever—
Adults: 325 to 650 mg P.O. q 4 to 6 hours, p.r.n., or 500 mg slow I.V. infusion over 4 to 8 hours. Maximum dosage is 1 g daily.

Arthritis—
Adults: 3.5 to 5.4 g P.O. daily in divided doses.

ADVERSE REACTIONS

EENT: *tinnitus, hearing loss.*
GI: *nausea, vomiting, GI distress, occult bleeding.*
Hepatic: abnormal liver function studies, hepatitis.
Skin: *rash,* bruising.
Other: *hypersensitivity manifested by anaphylaxis and/or asthma.*
Local: thrombophlebitis (from I.V.).

INTERACTIONS

Ammonium chloride (and other urine

acidifiers): increased blood levels of salicylates. Monitor for salicylate toxicity.
Antacids in large doses (and other urine alkalinizers): decreased levels of salicylates. Monitor for decreased salicylate effect.
Corticosteroids: enhance salicylate elimination. Monitor for decreased salicylate effect.
Oral anticoagulants and heparin: increase risk of bleeding. Avoid using together if possible.

NURSING CONSIDERATIONS
• Contraindicated in GI ulcer, GI bleeding, or aspirin hypersensitivity. Use cautiously in hypoprothrombinemia, vitamin K deficiency, bleeding disorders, and asthma with nasal polyps (may cause severe bronchospasm).
• Use cautiously in CHF and hypertension because of increased sodium load.
• Because of epidemiologic association with Reye's syndrome, the Centers for Disease Control recommends that children or teenagers with chicken pox or influenza-like illness should not be given salicylates.
• Febrile, dehydrated children can develop toxicity rapidly.
• Give with food, milk, antacid, or large glass of water to reduce GI adverse effects.
• Therapeutic salicylate level in arthritis is 10 to 30 mg/100 ml. Tinnitus may occur at plasma levels of 30 mg/100 ml and above, but this is not a reliable indicator of toxicity, especially in very young and elderly patients.
• Concomitant use with alcohol, steroids, or other NSAIDs may increase risk of GI bleeding.
• May cause an increase in serum levels of AST (SGOT), ALT (SGPT), alkaline phosphatase, and bilirubin.
• Advise patients receiving large doses for extended period of time to watch for petechiae, bleeding gums,

and signs of GI bleeding, and to maintain adequate fluid intake. Obtain hemoglobin and prothrombin tests periodically.

sodium thiosalicylate
Rexolate, Tusal
Pregnancy Risk Category: C

MECHANISM OF ACTION
• Produces analgesia by an ill-defined effect on the hypothalamus (central action) and by blocking generation of pain impulses (peripheral action). The peripheral action may involve inhibition of prostaglandin synthesis.
• Relieves fever by acting on the hypothalamic heat-regulating center to produce peripheral vasodilation. This increases peripheral blood supply and promotes sweating, which leads to loss of heat and to cooling by evaporation.

INDICATIONS & DOSAGE
Mild pain—
Adults: 50 to 100 mg daily or every other day, I.M. or slow I.V.
Arthritis—
Adults: 100 mg daily I.M. or slow I.V.
Rheumatic fever—
Adults: 100 to 150 mg I.M. or slowly I.V. q 4 to 6 hours for 3 days, followed by 100 mg b.i.d. until asymptomatic.

ADVERSE REACTIONS
EENT: *tinnitus and hearing loss.*
GI: *nausea, vomiting, GI distress, occult bleeding.*
Hepatic: abnormal liver function studies, hepatitis.
Skin: *rash,* bruising.
Other: *hypersensitivity manifested by anaphylaxis and/or asthma.*

INTERACTIONS
Ammonium chloride (and other urine acidifiers): increased blood levels of

salicylates. Monitor for salicylate toxicity.
*Antacids in large doses (and other
urine alkalinizers):* decreased levels
of salicylates. Monitor for decreased
salicylate effect.
Corticosteroids: enhance salicylate
elimination. Monitor for decreased
salicylate effects.
Oral anticoagulants and heparin: increase risk of bleeding. Avoid using
together if possible.

NURSING CONSIDERATIONS
• Contraindicated in GI ulcer, GI
bleeding, or aspirin sensitivity. Use
cautiously in hypoprothrombinemia,
vitamin K deficiency, bleeding disorders, and asthma with nasal polyps
(may cause severe bronchospasm).
• Because of epidemiologic association with Reye's syndrome, the Centers for Disease Control recommends
that children or teenagers with
chicken pox or influenza-like illness
should not be given salicylates.
• Tinnitus, headache, dizziness, confusion, fever, sweating, thirst, drowsiness, dim vision, hyperventilation,
and tachycardia are signs of mild toxicity.
• May cause an increase in serum levels of AST (SGOT), ALT (SGPT), alkaline phosphatase, and bilirubin.

26

Nonsteroidal anti-inflammatory drugs

carprofen
diclofenac sodium
fenoprofen calcium
flurbiprofen
ibuprofen◇
indomethacin
indomethacin sodium trihydrate
ketoprofen
meclofenamate
mefenamic acid
naproxen
naproxen sodium
oxyphenbutazone
phenylbutazone
piroxicam
sulindac
tolmetin sodium

COMBINATION PRODUCTS
None.

carprofen
Rimadyl

Pregnancy Risk Category: C

MECHANISM OF ACTION
A nonsteroidal anti-inflammatory
agent, carprofen inhibits prostaglandin synthesis.

INDICATIONS & DOSAGE
*Mild to moderate inflammation, acute
pain syndromes, arthritis—*
Adults: 150 to 600 mg P.O. daily, in
two or three divided doses.

ADVERSE REACTIONS
GI: *pain, nausea, heartburn, dyspep-
sia, peptic ulceration.*
GU: frequency, burning, dysuria, he-

maturia, nephritis, proteinuria, renal
failure.
Skin: *eczema, rash, urticaria, photosensitivity.*
Other: elevated hepatic enzymes.

INTERACTIONS
None significant.

NURSING CONSIDERATIONS
• Contraindicated in asthmatics with
nasal polyps. Use cautiously in GI
disorders, angioedema, hypersensitivity to other noncorticosteroid anti-
inflammatory drugs (including aspirin), hepatic or renal disease, cardiac
decompensation, or known intrinsic
coagulation defects.
• Use cautiously in history of peptic
ulcer disease.
• Tell patient that full therapeutic effect may be delayed for 2 to 4 weeks.
• Check renal and hepatic function
periodically in long-term therapy.
Stop drug if abnormalities occur.
• Teach patient signs and symptoms
of GI bleeding.
• Tell patient to report to doctor immediately any signs or symptoms of
GI bleeding, visual disturbances, skin
rashes, weight gain, and edema.
• Give with meals or milk to reduce
GI side effects.

diclofenac sodium
Voltaren

Pregnancy Risk Category: B

MECHANISM OF ACTION
Produces anti-inflammatory, analge-

Unmarked trade names available in the United States only.
♦ Also available in Canada.   ♦♦ Available in Canada only.   ◇ Also available OTC.

sic, and antipyretic effects, possibly through inhibition of prostaglandin synthesis.

INDICATIONS AND DOSAGE
Ankylosing spondylitis—
Adults: 25 mg P.O. q.i.d. and h.s.
Osteoarthritis—
Adults: 50 mg P.O. b.i.d. or t.i.d., or 75 mg P.O. b.i.d.

ADVERSE REACTIONS
CNS: anxiety, depression, drowsiness, insomnia, irritability.
CV: *CHF,* hypertension.
EENT: tinnitus, laryngeal edema, swelling of the lips and tongue.
GI: abdominal pain or cramps, constipation, diarrhea, indigestion, nausea, abdominal distention, flatulence, peptic ulceration, GI bleeding, melena, bloody diarrhea, appetite change, colitis.
GU: azotemia, proteinuria, acute renal failure, oliguria, interstitial nephritis, papillary necrosis, nephrotic syndrome.
Hepatic: elevated hepatic enzymes, jaundice, hepatitis, hepatotoxicity.
Respiratory: asthma.
Skin: rash, pruritus, urticaria, eczema, dermatitis, alopecia, photosensitivity, bullous eruption, *Stevens-Johnson syndrome,* allergic purpura.
Other: *anaphylaxis,* anaphylactoid reactions, angioedema.

INTERACTIONS
Anticoagulants (including warfarin): possible increased incidence of bleeding. Monitor patient closely.
Aspirin: concomitant use not recommended by manufacturer.
Cyclosporine, digoxin, lithium, methotrexate: diclofenac may reduce renal clearance of these drugs, and increase risk of toxicity. Monitor patient closely.
Diuretics: diclofenac may decrease the effectiveness of diuretics.
Insulin, oral hypoglycemic agents: di-
clofenac may alter requirements for hypoglycemic agents. Monitor patient closely.
Potassium-sparing diuretics: diclofenac may enhance potassium retention resulting in increased serum potassium levels.

NURSING CONSIDERATIONS
• Contraindicated in patients with hypersensitivity to diclofenac, aspirin, or other NSAIDs. Also contraindicated in patients with a history of asthma, urticaria, or other allergic reactions after taking these drugs.
• Use cautiously in patients with a history of peptic ulcer disease.
• Elevations of liver tests may occur during therapy. Measure serum transaminase, especially ALT (SGPT) periodically, in patients undergoing long-term therapy. The first serum transaminase measurement should be made no later than 8 weeks after initiation of therapy.
• Tell patient to take diclofenac with milk or meals to minimize G.I. distress.
• Peptic ulceration and GI bleeding have occurred in patients taking diclofenac despite the absence of GI symptoms. Teach patient the signs and symptoms of GI bleeding, and tell him to contact the doctor if these symptoms appear.
• Teach patient the signs and symptoms of hepatotoxicity, including nausea, fatigue, lethargy, pruritus, jaundice, right upper quadrant tenderness, and flulike symptoms. Tell him to contact doctor immediately if these symptoms appear.

fenoprofen calcium
Nalfon♦

Pregnancy Risk Category: B (D in 3rd trimester)

MECHANISM OF ACTION
Produces anti-inflammatory, analge-

sic, and antipyretic effects, possibly through inhibition of prostaglandin synthesis.

INDICATIONS & DOSAGE
Rheumatoid arthritis and osteoarthritis—
Adults: 300 to 600 mg P.O. q.i.d. Maximum dosage is 3.2 g daily.
Mild to moderate pain—
Adults: 200 mg P.O. q 4 to 6 hours, p.r.n.

ADVERSE REACTIONS
Blood: prolonged bleeding time, anemia.
CNS: *headache, drowsiness, dizziness.*
CV: peripheral edema.
GI: *epigastric distress, nausea, vomiting, occult blood loss, peptic ulceration,* constipation, anorexia.
GU: reversible renal failure.
Hepatic: elevated enzymes.
Skin: *pruritus,* rash, urticaria.

INTERACTIONS
Aspirin: decreases fenoprofen half-life.
Oral anticoagulants, sulfonylureas: fenoprofen enhances pharmacologic effects of these drugs. Use together cautiously.

NURSING CONSIDERATIONS
• Contraindicated in asthmatics with nasal polyps and in patients with hypersensitivity to aspirin. Use cautiously in elderly patients and patients with GI disorders, angioedema, cardiovascular disease, or hypersensitivity to other noncorticosteroid anti-inflammatory drugs.
• Use cautiously in patients with history of peptic ulcer disease.
• Chronic use may enhance the risk of GI ulceration and bleeding. Teach patient signs and symptoms of GI bleeding. Tell patient to report any signs or symptoms to doctor immediately.

• Concomitant use with aspirin, alcohol, or steroids may increase the risk of GI side effects.
• Tell patient that full therapeutic effect may be delayed for 2 to 4 weeks.
• Check renal, hepatic, and auditory function periodically in long-term therapy. Stop drug if abnormalities occur.
• Give dose 30 minutes before or 2 hours after meals. If GI side effects occur, give with milk or meals.
• Prothrombin time may be prolonged in patients receiving coumarin-type anticoagulants. Fenoprofen decreases platelet aggregation and may prolong bleeding time.

flurbiprofen
Ansaid♦

Pregnancy Risk Category: B

MECHANISM OF ACTION
An NSAID, flurbiprofen interferes with prostaglandin synthesis.

INDICATIONS AND DOSAGE
Rheumatoid arthritis and osteoarthritis—
Adults: 200 to 300 mg P.O. daily, divided b.i.d. or t.i.d.

ADVERSE REACTIONS
CNS: headache, anxiety, insomnia, increased reflexes, tremors, amnesia, asthenia, drowsiness, malaise, depression, dizziness.
CV: edema.
EENT: rhinitis, tinnitus, visual changes.
GI: dyspepsia, diarrhea, abdominal pain, nausea, constipation, *GI bleeding,* flatulence, vomiting.
GU: urinary tract infection.
Hepatic: elevated liver enzymes.
Skin: rash.
Other: weight changes.

INTERACTIONS
Aspirin: decreased flurbiprofen lev-

els. Concomitant use is not recommended.
Diuretics: possible decreased diuretic effect. Monitor patient closely.
Oral anticoagulants: increased bleeding tendencies.
Monitor patient closely.

NURSING CONSIDERATIONS
• Contraindicated in patients with hypersensitivity including asthma or urticaria to aspirin or NSAIDs.
• Serious GI toxicity can occur at any time with patients taking chronic NSAID therapy. Teach patient the signs and symptoms of GI bleeding, and tell him to discontinue the drug and call the doctor if these symptoms appear.
• Elderly or debilitated patients and patients with impaired hepatic or renal function should be closely monitored and probably should receive lower doses. These patients may be at risk for renal toxicity. Periodically monitor renal function.
• Patients receiving long-term therapy should have periodic liver function studies, eye examinations, and hematocrit determinations.
• Tell patient to take drug with food, milk, or antacid if GI upset occurs.
• Advise patient to avoid hazardous activities that require mental alertness until the CNS effects of the drug are known.
• Tell patient to call doctor immediately if edema, substantial weight gain, black stools, skin rash, itching, or visual disturbances occur.

ibuprofen◇
Advil, Amersol♦♦, Apo-Ibuprofen♦♦, Cap-Profen, Haltran, Ibuprin, Ifen, Medipren, Midol-200, Motrin♦, Novoprofen♦♦, Nuprin, Pamprin-IB, Paxofen, Rufen, Tab-Profen, Trendar

Pregnancy Risk Category: B (D in 3rd trimester)

MECHANISM OF ACTION
Produces anti-inflammatory, analgesic, and antipyretic effects, possibly through inhibition of prostaglandin synthesis.

INDICATIONS & DOSAGE
Mild to moderate pain, arthritis, primary dysmenorrhea, gout, postextraction dental pain—
Adults: 200 to 800 mg P.O. t.i.d. or q.i.d. not to exceed 3.2 g/day.

ADVERSE REACTIONS
Blood: prolonged bleeding time.
CNS: headache, drowsiness, dizziness, aseptic meningitis.
CV: peripheral edema.
EENT: visual disturbances, tinnitus.
GI: *epigastric distress, nausea, occult blood loss, peptic ulceration.*
GU: reversible renal failure.
Hepatic: elevated enzymes.
Skin: pruritus, rash, urticaria.
Other: bronchospasm, edema.

INTERACTIONS
Furosemide, thiazide diuretics: ibuprofen may decrease the effectiveness of diuretics.
Oral anticoagulants, lithium: ibuprofen may increase plasma levels or pharmacologic effects of these agents. Monitor for toxicity.

NURSING CONSIDERATIONS
• Contraindicated in asthmatics with nasal polyps. Use cautiously in GI disorders, angioedema, hypersensitivity to other noncorticosteroid anti-in-

Italicized side effects are common or life-threatening.
*Liquid form contains alcohol.   **May contain tartrazine.

flammatory drugs (including aspirin), hepatic or renal disease, cardiac decompensation, or known intrinsic coagulation defects.
• Use cautiously with history of peptic ulcer disease.
• Tell patient that full therapeutic effect may be delayed for 2 to 4 weeks.
• Check renal and hepatic function periodically in long-term therapy. Stop drug if abnormalities occur.
• Teach patient signs and symptoms of GI bleeding. Tell patient to report to doctor immediately any GI symptoms or signs of bleeding, visual disturbances, skin rashes, weight gain, and edema.
• Give with meals or milk to reduce GI adverse effects.
• Concomitant use with aspirin, alcohol, or steroids may increase the risk of GI side effects.
• Available as several brands without prescription in the 200-mg tablet strength. Instruct patient not to exceed 1.2 g/day, or self-medicate for extended periods without consulting doctor.

---

indomethacin
Apo-Indomethacin♦♦, Indameth, Indocid♦♦, Indocid SR ♦♦, Indocin, Indocin SR, Indomed, Novomethacin♦♦, Zendole

indomethacin sodium trihydrate
Apo-Indomethacin♦♦, Indocid♦♦, Indocin I.V., Indometh, Novomethacin

Pregnancy Risk Category: B (D in 3rd trimester)

MECHANISM OF ACTION
Produces anti-inflammatory, analgesic, and antipyretic effects, possibly through inhibition of prostaglandin synthesis.

INDICATIONS & DOSAGE
Moderate to severe arthritis, ankylosing spondylitis—
Adults: 25 mg P.O. or rectally b.i.d. or t.i.d. with food or antacids; may increase dosage by 25 mg daily q 7 days up to 200 mg daily. Alternatively, sustained-release capsules (75 mg) may be given: 75 mg to start, in the morning or h.s., followed, if necessary, by 75 mg b.i.d.
Acute gouty arthritis—
Adults: 50 mg P.O. t.i.d. Reduce dose as soon as possible, then stop. Sustained-release capsules shouldn't be used for this condition.
To close a hemodynamically significant patent ductus arteriosus in premature infants (I.V. form only)—
Neonates less than 48 hours: 0.2 mg/kg I.V. followed by 2 doses of 0.1 mg/kg at 12- to 24-hour intervals.
Neonates 2 to 7 days: 0.2 mg/kg I.V. followed by 2 doses of 0.2 mg/kg at 12- to 24-hour intervals.
Over 7 days: 0.2 mg/kg I.V. followed by 2 doses of 0.25 mg/kg at 12- to 24-hour intervals.

ADVERSE REACTIONS
Oral form:
Blood: *hemolytic anemia, aplastic anemia, agranulocytosis,* leukopenia, *thrombocytopenic purpura,* iron deficiency anemia.
CNS: *headache, dizziness,* depression, drowsiness, confusion, peripheral neuropathy, seizures, psychic disturbances, syncope, *vertigo.*
CV: hypertension, *edema.*
EENT: *blurred vision, corneal and retinal damage,* hearing loss, tinnitus.
GI: *nausea, vomiting,* anorexia, *diarrhea, peptic ulceration, severe GI bleeding.*
GU: hematuria, hyperkalemia, acute renal failure.
Hepatic: elevated enzymes.
Skin: pruritus, urticaria, *Stevens-Johnson syndrome.*
Other: hypersensitivity (shocklike

symptoms, rash, respiratory distress, angioedema).
I.V. form:
Blood: decreased platelet aggregation.
GI: *bleeding,* vomiting.
GU: *renal dysfunction.*
Metabolic: *hyponatremia, hyperkalemia,* hypoglycemia.

INTERACTIONS
Aspirin: decreased blood levels of indomethacin.
Diflunisal, probenecid: decreases indomethacin excretion; watch for increased incidence of indomethacin adverse reactions.
Lithium: increased plasma lithium levels. Monitor for toxicity.
Thiazide diuretics, furosemide: impaired response to both drugs. Avoid using together if possible.
Triamterene: possible nephrotoxicity. Don't use together.

NURSING CONSIDERATIONS
Oral form:
• Contraindicated in aspirin hypersensitivity and GI disorders. Use cautiously in epilepsy, parkinsonism, hepatic or renal disease, cardiovascular disease, infection, and history of mental illness, and in elderly patients.
• Severe headache may occur. Decrease dose if headache persists.
• Has an antipyretic effect.
• Tell patient to notify doctor immediately if any visual or hearing changes occur. Patients taking drug long-term should have regular eye examinations, hearing tests, CBC, and renal function tests to monitor for toxicity.
• Irritating to GI tract. Give with meals. Teach patient signs and symptoms of GI bleeding. Tell patient to notify doctor of any GI side effects.
• Concomitant use with aspirin, alcohol, or steroids may increase the risk of GI side effects.
• CNS side effects are more common

and serious in elderly patients.
• Monitor for bleeding in patients receiving anticoagulants.
• Causes sodium retention; monitor for weight gain and increased blood pressure in patients with hypertension.
• Used investigationally as prophylaxis for gout when colchicine is not well tolerated.
• Due to high incidence of side effects when used chronically, indomethacin should not be used routinely as an analgesic or antipyretic.
I.V. form:
• Contraindicated in infants with untreated infection, active bleeding, coagulation defects or thrombocytopenia, necrotizing enterocolitis, or impaired renal function.
• Don't administer second or third scheduled dose if anuria or marked oliguria is evident.
• If ductus arteriosus reopens, a second course of one to three doses may be given. If ineffective, surgery may be necessary.
• Monitor carefully for bleeding and for reduced urine output. Stop drug and notify doctor if either occurs.

ketoprofen
Orudis♦, Orudis E♦♦

Pregnancy Risk Category: B (D in 3rd trimester)

MECHANISM OF ACTION
Produces anti-inflammatory, analgesic, and antipyretic effects, possibly through inhibition of prostaglandin synthesis.

INDICATIONS & DOSAGE
Rheumatoid arthritis and osteoarthritis—
Adults: 150 to 300 mg P.O. in three or four divided doses. Usual dosage is 75 mg t.i.d. Maximum dosage is 300 mg/day.

Italicized side effects are common or life-threatening.
*Liquid form contains alcohol.   **May contain tartrazine.

ADVERSE REACTIONS
Blood: prolonged bleeding time.
CNS: *headache,* dizziness, *CNS inhibition or excitation.*
EENT: tinnitus, visual disturbances.
GI: *nausea, abdominal pain, diarrhea, constipation, flatulence, peptic ulceration,* anorexia, vomiting, stomatitis.
GU: nephrotoxicity, *elevated BUN.*
Hepatic: elevated enzymes.
Skin: rash.

INTERACTIONS
Probenecid, aspirin: decreased plasma levels of ketoprofen.

NURSING CONSIDERATIONS
• Contraindicated in patients who are hypersensitive to aspirin or other NSAIDs.
• Use cautiously in patients with history of peptic ulcer disease or renal dysfunction.
• Teach patient signs and symptoms of GI bleeding. Tell patient to report these symptoms to doctor immediately.
• Tell patient to report visual or auditory adverse effects immediately.
• Concomitant use with aspirin, alcohol, or steroids may increase the risk of GI side effects.
• Tell patient that full therapeutic effect may be delayed for 2 to 4 weeks.
• Check renal and hepatic function periodically during long-term therapy.
• Give dose 30 minutes before or 2 hours after meals. If GI side effects occur, give with milk or meals.

---

meclofenamate
Meclomen

Pregnancy Risk Category: B (D in 3rd trimester)

MECHANISM OF ACTION
Produces anti-inflammatory, analgesic, and antipyretic effects, possibly through inhibition of prostaglandin synthesis.

INDICATIONS & DOSAGE
Rheumatoid arthritis and osteoarthritis—
Adults: 200 to 400 mg/day P.O. in three or four equally divided doses.

ADVERSE REACTIONS
Blood: leukopenia, thrombocytopenia, *agranulocytosis, aplastic anemia.*
CNS: fatigue, malaise, insomnia, *dizziness,* nervousness, *headache.*
CV: edema.
EENT: blurred vision, eye irritation.
GI: *abdominal pain, flatulence, peptic ulceration,* nausea, vomiting, *diarrhea,* hemorrhage.
GU: dysuria, hematuria, nephrotoxicity.
Hepatic: hepatotoxicity.
Skin: rash, urticaria.

INTERACTIONS
Aspirin: decreased plasma levels of meclofenamate.
Oral anticoagulants: enhanced anticoagulant effect. Monitor for toxicity.

NURSING CONSIDERATIONS
• Contraindicated in GI ulceration or inflammation. Use cautiously in hepatic or renal disease, cardiovascular disease, blood dyscrasias, diabetes mellitus, and in asthmatics with nasal polyps.
• Use cautiously in history of peptic ulcer disease. Also use cautiously in elderly patients, who are more likely to experience adverse reactions.
• Teach patient signs and symptoms of GI bleeding. Tell patient to report any signs or symptoms to doctor immediately.
• Concomitant use with aspirin, alcohol, or steroids may increase the risk of GI side effects.
• Warn patient against activities that require alertness until CNS effects of drug are known.

Unmarked trade names available in the United States only.
♦ Also available in Canada.   ♦ ♦ Available in Canada only.   ◊ Also available OTC.

- Stop drug if rash, visual disturbances, or diarrhea develops.
- Administer with food to minimize GI side effects.
- Concomitant use with alcohol, steroids, or other NSAIDs may enhance risk of GI toxicity.
- Almost identical in chemical structure to mefenamic acid.
- False-positive reactions for urine bilirubin using the diazo tablet test have been reported.
- Patients taking drug long-term should receive periodic testing of CBC and renal and hepatic function.

mefenamic acid
Ponstan♦♦, Ponstel
Pregnancy Risk Category: C

MECHANISM OF ACTION
Produces anti-inflammatory, analgesic, and antipyretic effects, possibly through inhibition of prostaglandin synthesis.

INDICATIONS & DOSAGE
Mild to moderate pain, dysmenorrhea—
Adults and children over 14 years:
Initially 500 mg P.O., then 250 mg q 6 hours, p.r.n. Maximum therapy 1 week.

ADVERSE REACTIONS
Blood: leukopenia, thrombocytopenia, *agranulocytosis, aplastic anemia.*
CNS: *drowsiness, dizziness,* nervousness, headache.
CV: edema.
EENT: blurred vision, eye irritation.
GI: nausea, vomiting, *diarrhea, peptic ulceration,* hemorrhage.
GU: dysuria, hematuria, nephrotoxicity.
Hepatic: hepatotoxicity.
Skin: rash, urticaria.

INTERACTIONS
None significant.

NURSING CONSIDERATIONS
- Contraindicated in GI ulceration or inflammation. Use cautiously in hepatic or renal disease, cardiovascular disease, blood dyscrasias, diabetes mellitus, and in asthmatics with nasal polyps.
- Use cautiously in history of peptic ulcer disease.
- Teach patient signs and symptoms of GI bleeding. Tell patient to report any signs and symptoms to doctor immediately.
- Concomitant use with aspirin, alcohol, or steroids may increase the risk of GI side effects.
- Warn patient against hazardous activities that require alertness until CNS effects of the drug are known.
- Severe hemolytic anemia may occur with prolonged use. Monitor CBC periodically.
- Stop drug if rash, visual disturbances, or diarrhea develops.
- Should not be administered for more than 1 week at a time, because risk of toxicity increases.
- Administer with food to minimize GI side effects.
- False-positive reactions for urine bilirubin using the diazo tablet test have been reported.

naproxen
Apo-Naproxen♦♦, Naprosyn♦, Naxen♦♦, Novonaprox♦♦

naproxen sodium
Anaprox♦, Anaprox D.S.

Pregnancy Risk Category: B (D in 3rd trimester)

MECHANISM OF ACTION
Produces anti-inflammatory, analgesic, and antipyretic effects, possibly through inhibition of prostaglandin synthesis.

INDICATIONS & DOSAGE
Arthritis, primary dysmenorrhea (free base)—
Adults: 250 to 500 mg P.O. b.i.d. Maximum dosage is 1,000 mg daily.
Mild to moderate pain and for treatment of primary dysmenorrhea (naproxen sodium)—
Adults: 2 tablets (275 mg each tablet) P.O. to start, followed by 275 mg q 6 to 8 hours as needed. Maximum daily dosage should not exceed 1,375 mg.

ADVERSE REACTIONS
Blood: prolonged bleeding time, *agranulocytosis,* neutropenia.
CNS: *headache,* drowsiness, *dizziness,* tinnitus.
CV: peripheral edema, dyspnea.
EENT: visual disturbances.
GI: *epigastric distress, occult blood loss, nausea, peptic ulceration.*
GU: nephrotoxicity.
Hepatic: elevated enzymes.
Skin: *pruritus, rash,* urticaria.

INTERACTIONS
None significant.

NURSING CONSIDERATIONS
• Contraindicated in asthmatics with nasal polyps.
• Use cautiously in elderly patients and in patients with renal disease, cardiovascular disease, GI disorders, angioedema, and in those highly allergic to noncorticosteroid anti-inflammatory agents, including aspirin.
• Use cautiously in patients with history of peptic ulcer disease.
• Teach patient signs and symptoms of GI bleeding. Tell patient to report any signs and symptoms to doctor immediately.
• Concomitant use with aspirin, alcohol, or steroids may increase the risk of GI side effects.
• Monitor CBC and renal and hepatic function periodically during long-term therapy. Advise patient to have periodic eye examinations.

• Tell patient taking naproxen that full therapeutic effect may be delayed 2 to 4 weeks.
• Advise patient to take drug with food or milk to minimize GI upset.
• Warn patient against taking both naproxen and naproxen sodium at the same time because both circulate in the blood as the naproxen anion.
• 275 mg naproxen sodium is equivalent to 250 mg naproxen free base.

---

oxyphenbutazone
Pregnancy Risk Category: D

MECHANISM OF ACTION
Produces anti-inflammatory, analgesic, and antipyretic effects, possibly through inhibition of prostaglandin synthesis.

INDICATIONS & DOSAGE
Pain, inflammation in arthritis, bursitis, superficial venous thrombosis—
Adults: 100 to 200 mg P.O. with food or milk t.i.d. or q.i.d.
Acute gouty arthritis—
Adults: 400 mg initially as single dose, then 100 mg q 4 hours for 4 days or until relief is obtained. Do not continue therapy for longer than 1 week.

ADVERSE REACTIONS
Blood: *bone marrow suppression (fatal aplastic anemia, agranulocytosis, thrombocytopenia),* hemolytic anemia, leukopenia.
CNS: restlessness, confusion, lethargy.
CV: hypertension, pericarditis, myocarditis, *cardiac decompensation.*
EENT: optic neuritis, blurred vision, retinal hemorrhage or detachment, hearing loss.
GI: *nausea, vomiting, diarrhea, peptic ulceration, occult blood loss.*
GU: proteinuria, hematuria, glomerulonephritis, nephrotic syndrome, *renal failure.*

Hepatic: *hepatitis.*
Metabolic: toxic and nontoxic goiter, respiratory alkalosis, metabolic acidosis.
Skin: petechiae, pruritus, purpura, various dermatoses from rash to *toxic necrotizing epidermolysis.*

INTERACTIONS
Insulin, oral hypoglycemic agents: enhanced hypoglycemic effect. Monitor patient closely.
Oral anticoagulants: enhanced risk of bleeding. Monitor patient closely.
Phenytoin, lithium: increased plasma levels after oxyphenbutazone administration.

NURSING CONSIDERATIONS
• Contraindicated in children under 14 years and in patients with senility, GI ulcer, blood dyscrasias, and renal, hepatic, cardiac, and thyroid disease. Should not be used in patients receiving long-term anticoagulant therapy.
• Tell patient to stop drug and notify doctor immediately if fever, sore throat, mouth ulcers, GI discomfort, black or tarry stools, bleeding, bruising, rash, or weight gain occurs.
• Teach patient signs and symptoms of GI bleeding. Tell patient to report any signs and symptoms to doctor immediately.
• Give with food, milk, or antacids.
• Complete physical examination and laboratory evaluation are recommended before therapy. Warn patient to remain under close medical supervision and to keep all doctor and laboratory appointments.
• Monitor CBC every 2 weeks or weekly in elderly patients. Report any abnormality to doctor immediately.
• Record patient's weight and intake/output daily. May cause sodium retention and edema.
• Response should be seen in 2 or 3 days. Stop drug if no response seen within 1 week.
• Patients over 60 years should not

receive drug for longer than 1 week.
• Has antipyretic effect.

phenylbutazone
Apo-Phenylbutazone♦♦, Azolid, Butazolidin♦, Butazone, Intrabutazone♦♦, Novobutazone♦♦
Pregnancy Risk Category: D

MECHANISM OF ACTION
Produces anti-inflammatory, analgesic, and antipyretic effects, possibly through inhibition of prostaglandin synthesis.

INDICATIONS & DOSAGE
Pain, inflammation in arthritis, bursitis, acute superficial thrombophlebitis—
Adults: initially, 100 to 200 mg P.O. t.i.d. or q.i.d. Maximum dosage is 600 mg daily. When improvement is obtained, decrease dosage to 100 mg t.i.d. or q.i.d.
Acute, gouty arthritis—
Adults: 400 mg initially as single dose, then 100 mg q 4 hours for 4 days or until relief is obtained. Do not continue therapy for longer than 1 week.

ADVERSE REACTIONS
Blood: *bone marrow suppression (fatal aplastic anemia, agranulocytosis,* thrombocytopenia), hemolytic anemia, leukopenia.
CNS: agitation, confusion, lethargy.
CV: hypertension, edema, pericarditis, myocarditis, *cardiac decompensation.*
EENT: optic neuritis, blurred vision, retinal hemorrhage or detachment, hearing loss.
GI: *nausea, vomiting, diarrhea, peptic ulceration, occult blood loss.*
GU: proteinuria, hematuria, glomerulonephritis, nephrotic syndrome, *renal failure.*
Hepatic: *hepatitis.*
Metabolic: hyperglycemia, toxic and

Italicized side effects are common or life-threatening.
*Liquid form contains alcohol.   **May contain tartrazine.

nontoxic goiter, respiratory alkalosis, metabolic acidosis.
Skin: petechiae, pruritus, purpura, various dermatoses from rash to *toxic necrotizing epidermolysis*.

INTERACTIONS
Cholestyramine: may alter phenylbutazone absorption. Give 1 hour before cholestyramine.
Insulin, oral hypoglycemics: enhanced hypoglycemic effect. Monitor patient closely.
Oral anticoagulants: enhanced risk of bleeding. Monitor patient closely.
Phenytoin, lithium: increased plasma levels after oxyphenbutazone administration.

NURSING CONSIDERATIONS
• Contraindicated in children under 14 years and in patients with senility, GI ulcer, blood dyscrasias, and renal, hepatic, cardiac, and thyroid disease. Should not be used in patients receiving long-term anticoagulant therapy.
• Warn patient to stop drug and notify doctor immediately if fever, sore throat, mouth ulcers, GI discomfort, black or tarry stools, bleeding, bruising, rash, or weight gain occurs.
• Teach patient signs and symptoms of GI bleeding. Tell patient to report any signs or symptoms to doctor immediately.
• Give with food, milk, or antacids.
• Complete physical examination and laboratory evaluation are recommended before therapy. Patient should remain under close medical supervision and keep all doctor and laboratory appointments.
• Monitor CBC every 2 weeks or weekly in elderly patients. Report any abnormalities to doctor right away.
• Record patient's weight and intake/output daily. May cause sodium retention and edema.
• Response should be seen in 3 to 4 days. Stop drug if no response within 1 week.

• Patients over 60 years should not receive this drug for longer than 1 week.
• This drug has limited use because it produces adverse reactions in up to 45% of patients.

piroxicam
Apo-Piroxicam♦♦, Feldene♦, Novopirocam♦♦

Pregnancy Risk Category: C

MECHANISM OF ACTION
Produces anti-inflammatory, analgesic, and antipyretic effects, possibly through inhibition of prostaglandin synthesis.

INDICATIONS & DOSAGE
Osteoarthritis and rheumatoid arthritis—
Adults: 20 mg P.O. once daily. If desired, the dose may be divided.

ADVERSE REACTIONS
Blood: prolonged bleeding time, anemia.
CNS: headache, drowsiness, dizziness.
CV: peripheral edema.
GI: *epigastric distress, nausea, occult blood loss, peptic ulceration, severe GI bleeding*.
GU: nephrotoxicity.
Hepatic: elevated enzymes.
Skin: pruritus, rash, urticaria, *photosensitivity*.

INTERACTIONS
Aspirin: decreased plasma levels of piroxicam.
Lithium: increased plasma lithium levels.
Oral anticoagulants: enhanced risk of bleeding. Monitor patient closely.
Oral hypoglycemic agents: enhanced hypoglycemic effects. Monitor patient closely.

NURSING CONSIDERATIONS
• Contraindicated in asthmatics with nasal polyps. Use cautiously in elderly patients and patients with angioedema, GI disorders, history of renal or peptic ulcer disease, cardiac disease, or hypersensitivity to other nonsteroidal anti-inflammatory drugs.
• Teach patient signs and symptoms of GI bleeding. Tell patient to report any signs or symptoms to doctor immediately.
• Tell patient full therapeutic effect may be delayed for 2 to 4 weeks.
• Causes adverse skin reactions more often than other drugs in its class. Photosensitivity reactions are the most common.
• Check renal, hepatic, and auditory function periodically during prolonged therapy. Drug should be discontinued if abnormalities occur.
• If GI side effects occur, give with milk or meals.
• The first NSAID approved by the FDA for once-daily administration. Has a longer half-life and, hence, a longer duration of action than other similar drugs.

sulindac
Clinoril♦

Pregnancy Risk Category: B (D in 3rd trimester)

MECHANISM OF ACTION
Produces anti-inflammatory, analgesic, and antipyretic effects, possibly through inhibition of prostaglandin synthesis.

INDICATIONS & DOSAGE
Osteoarthritis, rheumatoid arthritis, ankylosing spondylitis—
Adults: 150 mg P.O. b.i.d. initially; may increase to 200 mg P.O. b.i.d.
Acute subacromial bursitis or supraspinatus tendinitis, acute gouty arthritis—
Adults: 200 mg P.O. b.i.d. for 7 to 14 days. Dose may be reduced as symptoms subside.

ADVERSE REACTIONS
Blood: prolonged bleeding time, *aplastic anemia.*
CNS: dizziness, headache, nervousness.
EENT: tinnitus, transient visual disturbances.
GI: *epigastric distress, peptic ulceration, occult blood loss, nausea.*
Hepatic: elevated enzymes.
Skin: rash, pruritus.
Other: edema.

INTERACTIONS
None significant.

NURSING CONSIDERATIONS
• Contraindicated in acute asthmatics whose conditions are precipitated by aspirin or other nonsteroidal anti-inflammatory agents; in patients who have active ulcers and GI bleeding. Use cautiously in patients with a history of ulcers and GI bleeding, renal dysfunction, compromised cardiac function, hypertension; or in those receiving oral anticoagulants or oral hypoglycemic agents.
• To reduce GI side effects, give with food, milk, or antacids.
• Teach patient signs and symptoms of GI bleeding. Tell patient to report any signs and symptoms to doctor immediately.
• Patient should notify doctor and have complete visual examination if any visual disturbances occur.
• Tell patient to notify doctor immediately if prolonged bleeding occurs.
• Drug causes sodium retention. Patient should report edema and have blood pressure checked periodically.

Italicized side effects are common or life-threatening.
*Liquid form contains alcohol.   **May contain tartrazine.

tolmetin sodium
Tolectin♦, Tolectin DS♦

Pregnancy Risk Category: B (D in 3rd trimester)

MECHANISM OF ACTION
Produces anti-inflammatory, analgesic, and antipyretic effects, possibly through inhibition of prostaglandin synthesis.

INDICATIONS & DOSAGE
Rheumatoid arthritis, osteoarthritis, gout, dysmenorrhea, juvenile rheumatoid arthritis—
Adults: 400 mg P.O. t.i.d. or q.i.d. Maximum dosage is 2 g daily.
Children 2 years or older: 15 to 30 mg/kg daily in divided doses.

ADVERSE REACTIONS
Blood: prolonged bleeding time.
CNS: headache, dizziness, drowsiness.
GI: *epigastric distress, peptic ulceration, occult blood loss, nausea.*
GU: nephrotoxicity, pseudoproteinuria.
Skin: rash, urticaria, pruritus.
Other: sodium retention, edema.

INTERACTIONS
Oral anticoagulants: increased risk of bleeding. Monitor patient closely.

NURSING CONSIDERATIONS
• Contraindicated in asthmatics with nasal polyps. Use cautiously in cardiac and renal disease, GI bleeding, and history of peptic ulcer disease.
• Teach patient signs and symptoms of GI bleeding. Tell patient to report any signs or symptoms to doctor immediately.
• Give with food, milk, or antacids to reduce GI adverse effects.
• Tell patient therapeutic effect should begin within 1 week, but full therapeutic effect may be delayed 2 to 4 weeks.
• Double-strength capsule (400 mg) is available.
• Prolonged therapy requires periodic eye examinations and liver and renal function studies.
• Only NSAID reported to falsely elevate urinary protein, causing pseudoproteinuria.

27

Narcotic and opioid analgesics

alfentanil hydrochloride
buprenorphine hydrochloride
butorphanol tartrate
codeine phosphate
codeine sulfate
fentanyl citrate
hydromorphone hydrochloride
levorphanol tartrate
meperidine hydrochloride
  (pethidine hydrochloride)
methadone hydrochloride
morphine hydrochloride
morphine sulfate
nalbuphine hydrochloride
oxycodone hydrochloride
oxymorphone hydrochloride
pentazocine hydrochloride
pentazocine lactate
propoxyphene hydrochloride
propoxyphene napsylate
sufentanil citrate

COMBINATION PRODUCTS
AMACODONE: hydrocodone bitartrate 5 mg and acetaminophen 500 mg.
BANCAP HC: hydrocodone bitartrate 5 mg and acetaminophen 500 mg.
BUFF-A-COMP NO. 3: codeine phosphate 30 mg, aspirin 325 mg, caffeine 40 mg, and butalbital 50 mg.
DARVOCET-N 50: propoxyphene napsylate 50 mg and acetaminophen 325 mg.
DARVOCET-N 100: propoxyphene napsylate 100 mg and acetaminophen 650 mg.
DARVON COMPOUND: propoxyphene HCl 32 mg, aspirin 389 mg, and caffeine 32.4 mg.
DARVON COMPOUND-65: propoxyphene HCl 65 mg, aspirin 389 mg, and caffeine 32.4 mg.
DARVON-N WITH ASA: propoxyphene napsylate 100 mg and aspirin 325 mg.
DARVON WITH ASA: propoxyphene HCl 65 mg and aspirin 325 mg.
DEMEROL APAP: meperidine HCl 50 mg and acetaminophen 300 mg.
DOLACET: propoxyphene HCl 65 mg and acetaminophen 650 mg.
DOLENE AP-65: propoxyphene HCl 65 mg and acetaminophen 650 mg.
DOLENE COMPOUND-65: propoxyphene HCl 65 mg, aspirin 389 mg, and caffeine 32.4 mg.
DOXAPHENE COMPOUND: propoxyphene HCl 65 mg, aspirin 389 mg, and caffeine 32.4 mg.
DURADYNE DHC: hydrocodone bitartrate 5 mg and acetaminophen 500 mg.
EMPIRIN WITH CODEINE NO. 2: aspirin 325 mg and codeine phosphate 15 mg.
EMPIRIN WITH CODEINE NO. 3: aspirin 325 mg and codeine phosphate 30 mg.
EMPIRIN WITH CODEINE NO. 4: aspirin 325 mg and codeine phosphate 60 mg.
EMPRACET WITH CODEINE NO. 3: codeine phosphate 30 mg and acetaminophen 300 mg.
EMPRACET WITH CODEINE NO. 4: codeine phosphate 60 mg and acetaminophen 300 mg.
FIORINAL WITH CODEINE NO. 1: codeine phosphate 7.5 mg, aspirin 325 mg, caffeine 40 mg, and butalbital 50 mg.
FIORINAL WITH CODEINE NO. 2♦: codeine phosphate 15 mg, aspirin 325

mg, caffeine 40 mg, and butalbital 50 mg.

FIORINAL WITH CODEINE NO. 3♦: codeine phosphate 30 mg, aspirin 325 mg, caffeine 40 mg, and butalbital 50 mg.

HYCODAPHEN: hydrocodone bitartrate 5 mg and acetaminophen 500 mg.

INNOVAR (INJECTION)♦: fentanyl (as the citrate) 0.05 mg and droperidol 2.5 mg per ml.

PANTOPON♦: hydrochlorides of opium alkaloids. 20 mg is therapeutically equivalent to 15 mg morphine.

PERCOCET-5: acetaminophen 325 mg and oxycodone hydrochloride 5 mg.

PERCODAN♦: oxycodone hydrochloride 4.5 mg, oxycodone terephthalate 0.38 mg, and aspirin 325 mg.

PERCODAN-DEMI♦: oxycodone hydrochloride 2.25 mg, oxycodone terephthalate 0.19 mg, and aspirin 325 mg.

PHENAPHEN-650 WITH CODEINE: codeine phosphate 30 mg and acetaminophen 650 mg.

PHENAPHEN WITH CODEINE NO. 3: codeine phosphate 30 mg and acetaminophen 325 mg.

PHENAPHEN WITH CODEINE NO. 4: codeine phosphate 60 mg and acetaminophen 325 mg.

PHRENILIN WITH CODEINE NO. 3: codeine phosphate 30 mg, acetaminophen 325 mg, and butalbital 50 mg.

PROVAL NO. 3: codeine phosphate 30 mg and acetaminophen 325 mg.

TALACEN: pentazocine hydrochloride 25 mg and acetaminophen 650 mg.

TALWIN COMPOUND: pentazocine HCl 12.5 mg and aspirin 325 mg.

TYLENOL WITH CODEINE NO 1: acetaminophen 300 mg and codeine phosphate 7.5 mg.

TYLENOL WITH CODEINE NO. 2: acetaminophen 300 mg and codeine phosphate 15 mg.

TYLENOL WITH CODEINE NO. 3: acetaminophen 300 mg and codeine phosphate 30 mg.

TYLENOL WITH CODEINE NO. 4: acet-

aminophen 300 mg and codeine phosphate 60 mg.

TYLOX: acetaminophen 500 mg and oxycodone hydrochloride 5 mg.

VICODIN: hydrocodone bitartrate 5 mg and acetaminophen 500 mg.

WYGESIC: propoxyphene HCl 65 mg and acetaminophen 650 mg.

ZYDONE: hydrocodone bitartrate 5 mg and acetaminophen 500 mg.

alfentanil hydrochloride
Alfenta♦
Controlled Substance Schedule II

Pregnancy Risk Category: B (D for prolonged use or use of high doses at term)

MECHANISM OF ACTION
Binds with opiate receptors at many sites in the CNS (brain, brain stem, and spinal cord), altering both perception of and emotional response to pain through an unknown mechanism.

INDICATIONS & DOSAGE
Adjunct to general anesthetic—
Adults: initially, 8 to 50 mcg/kg I.V., then give increments of 3 to 15 mcg/kg I.V.
As a primary anesthetic—
Adults: initially, 130 to 245 mcg/kg I.V., then give 0.5 to 1.5 mcg/kg/minute I.V.

ADVERSE REACTIONS
CV: hypotension, hypertension, bradycardia, tachycardia.
GI: nausea, vomiting.
Skin: itching.
Other: chest wall rigidity, intraoperative muscle movement, *respiratory depression*.

INTERACTIONS
Alcohol, CNS depressants: additive effects. Use together cautiously.

NURSING CONSIDERATIONS
• Use cautiously in patients with head

injury, pulmonary disease, or decreased respiratory reserve.
• Should be administered only by persons specifically trained in the use of I.V. anesthetics.
• As a primary anesthetic, alfentanil may be prescribed for induction of anesthesia for general surgery requiring endotracheal intubation and medical ventilation.
• Discontinue infusion at least 10 to 15 minutes before the end of surgery.
• To administer small volumes of alfentanil accurately, use a tuberculin syringe.
• Keep narcotic antagonist (naloxone) and resuscitative equipment available when giving drug I.V..
• Dose should be reduced in elderly and debilitated patients.
• Monitor postoperative vital signs and bladder function periodically.

buprenorphine hydrochloride
Buprenex
Controlled Substance Schedule V

Pregnancy Risk Category: C (D for prolonged use or use of high doses at term)

MECHANISM OF ACTION
Binds with opiate receptors at many sites in the CNS (brain, brain stem, and spinal cord), altering both perception of and emotional response to pain through an unknown mechanism.

INDICATIONS & DOSAGE
Moderate to severe pain—
Adults: 0.3 mg I.M. or slow I.V. q 6 hours, p.r.n. or around the clock. May administer up to 0.6 mg per dose if necessary.

ADVERSE REACTIONS
CNS: *dizziness, sedation, headache,* confusion, nervousness, euphoria.
CV: hypotension.
GI: *nausea,* vomiting, constipation.

Skin: pruritus.
Other: *respiratory depression,* hypoventilation.

INTERACTIONS
Alcohol, CNS depressants: additive effects. Use together cautiously.
Narcotic analgesics: avoid concomitant use. Possible decreased analgesic effect.

NURSING CONSIDERATIONS
• Use cautiously in head injury and increased intracranial pressure, severe liver and kidney impairment, CNS depression, thyroid irregularities, and prostatic hypertrophy.
• Naloxone will not completely reverse the respiratory depression caused by buprenorphine overdose. Therefore, an overdose may necessitate mechanical ventilation. Larger than customary doses of naloxone (more than 0.4 mg) and doxapram may also be ordered.
• Psychological and physical addiction may occur.
• If dependence occurs, withdrawal symptoms may appear up to 14 days after drug is stopped.
• Possesses narcotic antagonist properties. May precipitate abstinence syndrome in narcotic-dependent patients.
• S.C. administration not recommended.
• Buprenorphine 0.3 mg is equal to 10 mg morphine and 75 mg meperidine in analgesic potency. Has longer duration of action than morphine or meperidine.

butorphanol tartrate
Stadol♦

Pregnancy Risk Category: B (D for prolonged use or use of high doses at term)

MECHANISM OF ACTION
Binds with opiate receptors at many

sites in the CNS (brain, brain stem, and spinal cord), altering both perception of and emotional response to pain through an unknown mechanism.

INDICATIONS & DOSAGE
Moderate to severe pain—
Adults: 1 to 4 mg I.M. q 3 to 4 hours, p.r.n. or around the clock; or 0.5 to 2 mg I.V. q 3 to 4 hours, p.r.n. or around the clock.

ADVERSE REACTIONS
CNS: *sedation, headache, vertigo, floating sensation,* lethargy, confusion, nervousness, unusual dreams, agitation, euphoria, hallucinations, flushing.
CV: palpitations, fluctuation in blood pressure.
EENT: diplopia, blurred vision.
GI: *nausea,* vomiting, dry mouth, constipation.
Skin: rash, hives, *clamminess, excessive sweating.*
Other: respiratory depression.

INTERACTIONS
Alcohol, CNS depressants: additive effects. Use together cautiously.
Narcotic analgesics: avoid concomitant use. Possible decreased analgesic effect.

NURSING CONSIDERATIONS
• Contraindicated in narcotic addiction; may precipitate narcotic abstinence syndrome. Use cautiously in head injury, increased intracranial pressure, acute myocardial infarction, ventricular dysfunction, coronary insufficiency, respiratory disease or depression, and renal or hepatic dysfunction.
• Psychological and physical addiction may occur.
• Possesses narcotic antagonist properties. May precipitate abstinence syndrome in narcotic-dependent patients.
• Respiratory depression apparently

does not increase with increased dosage.
• S.C. route not recommended.
• Also used as a preoperative medication, as the analgesic component of balanced anesthesia, and for relief of postpartum pain.

---

codeine phosphate
Paveral••

codeine sulfate
Controlled Substance Schedule II
Pregnancy Risk Category: C (D for prolonged use or use of high doses at term)

MECHANISM OF ACTION
Binds with opiate receptors at many sites in the CNS (brain, brain stem, and spinal cord), altering both perception of and emotional response to pain through an unknown mechanism. Also supresses the cough reflex by direct action on the cough center in the medulla.

INDICATIONS & DOSAGE
Mild to moderate pain—
Adults: 15 to 60 mg P.O. or 15 to 60 mg (phosphate) S.C. or I.M. q 4 hours, p.r.n. or around the clock.
Children: 3 mg/kg daily divided q 4 hours, p.r.n. or around the clock.
Nonproductive cough—
Adults: 8 to 20 mg P.O. q 4 to 6 hours. Maximum dosage is 120 mg/24 hours.
Children: 1 to 1.5 mg/kg P.O. daily in four divided doses. Maximum dosage is 60 mg/24 hours.

ADVERSE REACTIONS
CNS: *sedation, clouded sensorium, euphoria,* dizziness, seizures with large doses.
CV: *hypotension,* bradycardia.
GI: *nausea, vomiting, constipation, dry mouth,* ileus.
GU: *urine retention.*

Skin: pruritus, flushing.
Other: *respiratory depression*, physical dependence.

INTERACTIONS
Alcohol, CNS depressants: additive effects. Use together cautiously.

NURSING CONSIDERATIONS
• Use with extreme caution in head injury, increased intracranial pressure, increased cerebrospinal fluid pressure, hepatic or renal disease, hypothyroidism, Addison's disease, acute alcoholism, seizures, severe CNS depression, bronchial asthma, chronic obstructive pulmonary disease, respiratory depression, and shock; and in elderly or debilitated patients.
• Warn ambulatory patient to avoid activities that require alertness.
• Monitor respiratory and circulatory status and bowel function.
• For full analgesic effect, give before patient has intense pain.
• Codeine and aspirin or acetaminophen are often prescribed together to provide enhanced pain relief.
• Do not administer discolored injection solution.
• If used with general anesthetics, other narcotic analgesics, tranquilizers, sedatives, hypnotics, alcohol, tricyclic antidepressants, or MAO inhibitors, CNS depression is increased. Use together with extreme caution. Monitor patient response.
• An antitussive; don't use when cough is a valuable diagnostic sign or beneficial (as after thoracic surgery).
• Monitor cough type and frequency.
• Constipating effect makes codeine useful in the treatment of diarrhea.
• The abuse potential is much less than that of morphine.

fentanyl citrate
Sublimaze♦
Controlled Substance Schedule II

Pregnancy Risk Category: B (D for prolonged use or use of high doses at term)

MECHANISM OF ACTION
Binds with opiate receptors at many sites in the CNS (brain, brain stem, and spinal cord), altering both perception of and emotional response to pain through an unknown mechanism.

INDICATIONS & DOSAGE
Adjunct to general anesthetic—
Adults: 0.05 to 0.1 mg I.V. repeated q 2 to 3 minutes, p.r.n. Dose should be reduced in elderly and high-risk patients.
Postoperatively—
Adults: 0.05 to 0.1 mg I.M. q 1 to 2 hours p.r.n.
Preoperatively—
Adults: 0.05 to 0.1 mg I.M. 30 to 60 minutes before surgery.
Children 2 to 12 years: 1.7 to 3.3 mcg/kg I.M.

ADVERSE REACTIONS
CNS: *sedation, somnolence, clouded sensorium, euphoria,* dizziness, seizures with large doses.
CV: *hypotension,* bradycardia.
GI: nausea, vomiting, *constipation,* ileus.
GU: *urine retention.*
Other: *respiratory depression,* muscle rigidity, physical dependence.

INTERACTIONS
Alcohol, CNS depressants: additive effects. Use together cautiously.

NURSING CONSIDERATIONS
• Contraindicated in patients who have received MAO inhibitors within 14 days and who have myasthenia gravis. Use cautiously in head injury, increased cerebrospinal fluid pres-

sure, asthma, chronic obstructive pulmonary disease, respiratory depression, seizures, hepatic or renal disease, hypothyroidism, Addison's disease, alcoholism, increased intracranial pressure, CNS depression, and shock; and in elderly or debilitated patients.
• Keep narcotic antagonist (naloxone) and resuscitative equipment available when giving drug I.V.
• Monitor respirations of newborns exposed to drug during labor.
• Use as postoperative analgesic only in recovery room. Make sure another analgesic is ordered for later use.
• Often used with droperidol (Innovar) to produce neuroleptanalgesia.
• Monitor circulatory and respiratory status carefully.
• Respiratory depression, hypotension, profound sedation, and coma may result if used with other narcotic analgesics, general anesthetics, tranquilizers, alcohol, sedatives, hypnotics, tricyclic antidepressants, or MAO inhibitors. Fentanyl citrate dose should be reduced by one-fourth to one-third. Also give above drugs in reduced dosages.
• For better analgesic effect, give before patient has intense pain.
• When used postoperatively, encourage turning, coughing, and deep breathing to avoid atelectasis.
• Monitor bladder function in postoperative patients.
• Epidural injection or infusion has been used for postoperative analgesia, chronic pain management, or postpartum pain control.
• When administered by epidural injection, monitor the patient closely for respiratory depression. Immediately report a respiratory rate below 12.
• High doses can produce muscle rigidity. This effect can be reversed by administration of neuromuscular blocking agents.

hydromorphone hydrochloride
Dilaudid♦**, Dilaudid HP♦
Controlled Substance Schedule II

Pregnancy Risk Category: B (D for prolonged use or use of high doses at term)

MECHANISM OF ACTION
Binds with opiate receptors at many sites in the CNS (brain, brain stem, and spinal cord), altering both perception of and emotional response to pain through an unknown mechanism. Also suppresses the cough reflex by direct action on the cough center in the medulla.

INDICATIONS & DOSAGE
Moderate to severe pain—
Adults: 1 to 6 mg P.O. q 4 to 6 hours, p.r.n. or around the clock; or 2 to 4 mg I.M., S.C., or I.V. q 4 to 6 hours, p.r.n., or q 6 to 8 hours around the clock (I.V. dose should be given over 3 to 5 minutes); or 3 mg rectal suppository h.s., p.r.n., or q 6 to 8 hours around the clock.
Cough—
Adults: 1 mg P.O. q 3 to 4 hours p.r.n.
Children 6 to 12 years: 0.5 mg P.O. q 3 to 4 hours p.r.n.

ADVERSE REACTIONS
CNS: *sedation, somnolence, clouded sensorium,* dizziness, *euphoria,* seizures with large doses.
CV: *hypotension,* bradycardia.
GI: *nausea, vomiting, constipation,* ileus.
GU: *urine retention.*
Local: induration with repeated S.C. injections.
Other: *respiratory depression,* physical dependence.

INTERACTIONS
Alcohol, CNS depressants: additive effects. Use together cautiously.

NURSING CONSIDERATIONS
• Contraindicated in increased intracranial pressure and status asthmaticus. Use with extreme caution in patients with increased cerebrospinal fluid pressure, respiratory depression, hepatic or renal disease, hypothyroidism, shock, Addison's disease, acute alcoholism, seizures, head injury, severe CNS depression, brain tumor, bronchial asthma, and chronic obstructive pulmonary disease; and in elderly or debilitated patients.
• Warn ambulatory patient to avoid activities that require alertness.
• Monitor respiratory and circulatory status and bowel function.
• Keep narcotic antagonist (naloxone) available.
• Respiratory depression and hypotension can occur with I.V. administration. Give very slowly and monitor constantly. Keep recusitative equipment available.
• Rotate injection sites to avoid induration with S.C. injection.
• Commonly abused narcotic.
• If used with general anesthetics, other narcotic analgesics, tranquilizers, sedatives, hypnotics, alcohol, tricyclic antidepressants, or MAO inhibitors, CNS depression is increased. Hydromorphone dose should be reduced. Use together with extreme caution. Monitor patient response.
• Oral dosage form is particularly convenient for patients with chronic pain because tablets are available in 1 mg, 2 mg, 3 mg, and 4 mg. This enables these patients to titrate their own dose.
• For better analgesic effect, give before patient has intense pain.
• When used postoperatively, encourage turning, coughing, and deep breathing to avoid atelectasis.
• May worsen or mask gallbladder pain.
• Dilaudid HP, a highly concentrated form (10 mg/ml), may be administered in smaller volumes, preventing the discomfort associated with large-volume I.M. or S.C. injections.

levorphanol tartrate
Levo-Dromoran♦
Controlled Substance Schedule II

Pregnancy Risk Category: B (D for prolonged use or use of high doses at term)

MECHANISM OF ACTION
Binds with opiate receptors at many sites in the CNS (brain, brain stem, and spinal cord), altering both perception of and emotional response to pain through an unknown mechanism.

INDICATIONS & DOSAGE
Moderate to severe pain—
Adults: 2 to 3 mg P.O. or S.C. q 6 to 8 hours, p.r.n. or around the clock.

ADVERSE REACTIONS
CNS: *sedation, somnolence, clouded sensorium,* dizziness, *euphoria,* seizures with large doses.
CV: *hypotension,* bradycardia.
GI: *nausea, vomiting, constipation,* ileus.
GU: urine retention.
Other: *respiratory depression,* physical dependence.

INTERACTIONS
Alcohol, CNS depressants: additive effects. Use together cautiously.

NURSING CONSIDERATIONS
• Contraindicated in acute alcoholism, bronchial asthma, increased intracranial pressure, respiratory depression, and anoxia. Use with extreme caution in hepatic or renal disease, hypothyroidism, Addison's disease, seizures, head injury, severe CNS depression, brain tumor, chronic obstructive pulmonary disease, and shock; and in elderly or debilitated patients.
• Warn ambulatory patient to avoid

Italicized side effects are common or life-threatening.
*Liquid form contains alcohol.   **May contain tartrazine.

activities that require alertness.
- Monitor circulatory and respiratory status and bowel function.
- Warn patient drug has bitter taste.
- Protect from light.
- Keep narcotic antagonist (naloxone) available.
- If used with general anesthetics, other narcotic analgesics, tranquilizers, sedatives, hypnotics, alcohol, tricyclic antidepressants, or MAO inhibitors, CNS depression is increased. Reduce levorphanol dose. Use together with extreme caution. Monitor patient response.
- For better analgesic effect, give before patient has intense pain.
- When used postoperatively, encourage turning, coughing, and deep breathing to avoid atelectasis.

---

meperidine hydrochloride (pethidine hydrochloride)
Demerol♦
Controlled Substance Schedule II

Pregnancy Risk Category: B (D for prolonged use or use of high doses at term)

MECHANISM OF ACTION
Binds with opiate receptors at many sites in the CNS (brain, brain stem, and spinal cord), altering both perception of and emotional response to pain through an unknown mechanism.

INDICATIONS & DOSAGE
Moderate to severe pain—
Adults: 50 to 150 mg P.O., I.M., or S.C. q 3 to 4 hours, p.r.n. or around the clock.
Children: 1 to 1.8 mg/kg P.O., I.M., or S.C. q 4 to 6 hours. Maximum dosage is 100 mg q 4 hours, p.r.n. or around the clock.
Preoperatively—
Adults: 50 to 100 mg I.M. or S.C. 30 to 90 minutes before surgery.
Children: 1 to 2.2 mg/kg I.M. or S.C. 30 to 90 minutes before surgery.

ADVERSE REACTIONS
CNS: *sedation, somnolence, clouded sensorium, euphoria,* paradoxical excitement, tremors, dizziness, seizures with large doses.
CV: *hypotension,* bradycardia, tachycardia.
GI: *nausea, vomiting, constipation,* ileus.
GU: *urine retention.*
Local: pain at injection site, local tissue irritation and induration after S.C. injection; phlebitis after I.V. injection.
Other: *respiratory depression,* physical dependence, muscle twitching.

INTERACTIONS
Alcohol, CNS depressants: additive effects. Use together cautiously.
MAO inhibitors, barbiturates, isoniazid: increased CNS excitation or depression can be severe or fatal. Don't use together.
Phenytoin: decreased blood levels of meperidine. Monitor for decreased analgesia.

NURSING CONSIDERATIONS
- Contraindicated in patients who have received MAO inhibitors within 14 days. Use with extreme caution in patients with increased intracranial pressure, increased cerebrospinal fluid pressure, shock, CNS depression, head injury, asthma, chronic obstructive pulmonary disease, respiratory depression, supraventricular tachycardias, seizures, acute abdominal conditions, hepatic or renal disease, hypothyroidism, Addison's disease, urethral stricture, prostatic hypertrophy, and alcoholism; in children under 12 years; and in elderly or debilitated patients.
- May be used in some patients allergic to morphine.
- Meperidine and active metabolite normeperidine accumulate. Monitor for increased toxic effect, especially in patients with impaired renal func-

tion.
• Because meperidine toxicity often appears after several days of treatment, this drug is not recommended for treatment of chronic pain.
• Meperidine may be given slow I.V., preferably as a diluted solution. S.C. injection is very painful.
• Keep narcotic antagonist (naloxone) available when giving this drug I.V.
• Warn ambulatory patient to avoid activities that require alertness.
• Monitor respirations of newborns exposed to drug during labor. Have resuscitation equipment and naloxone available.
• P.O. dose less than half as effective as parenteral dose. Give I.M. if possible. When changing from parenteral to P.O. route, dose should be increased.
• Syrup has local anesthetic effect. Give with full glass of water.
• Chemically incompatible with barbiturates. Don't mix together.
• Monitor respiratory and cardiovascular status carefully. Don't give if respirations are below 12/minute or if change in pupils is noted.
• Monitor bladder function in postoperative patients.
• Monitor bowel function. Patient may need a laxative or stool softener.
• Watch for withdrawal symptoms if stopped abruptly after long-term use.
• If used with other narcotic analgesics, general anesthetics, phenothiazines, sedatives, hypnotics, tricyclic antidepressants, or alcohol, respiratory depression, hypotension, profound sedation, or coma may occur. Reduce meperidine dose. Use together with extreme caution.
• For better analgesic effect, give before patient has intense pain. Initially, administration on a fixed schedule may result in better pain control with a smaller daily dose by reducing patient anxiety. Once good pain control has been achieved, adjust scheduling

per individual requirements.
• Alternating a centrally active narcotic with a more peripherally active nonnarcotic analgesic (aspirin, acetaminophen, or NSAID) may improve pain control while requiring lower narcotic doses.
• When used postoperatively, encourage turning, coughing, and deep breathing to avoid atelectasis.

methadone hydrochloride
Dolophine♦, Methadose
Controlled Substance Schedule II

Pregnancy Risk Category: B (D for prolonged use or use of high doses at term)

MECHANISM OF ACTION
Binds with opiate receptors at many sites in the CNS (brain, brain stem, and spinal cord), altering both perception of and emotional response to pain through an unknown mechanism.

INDICATIONS & DOSAGE
Severe pain—
Adults: 2.5 to 10 mg P.O., I.M., or S.C. q 6 to 8 hours, p.r.n. or around the clock.
Narcotic abstinence syndrome—
Adults: 15 to 40 mg P.O. daily (highly individualized). Maintenance dosage is 20 to 120 mg P.O. daily. Adjust dose as needed. Daily dosages greater than 120 mg require special state and federal approval.

ADVERSE REACTIONS
CNS: *sedation, somnolence, clouded sensorium, euphoria,* dizziness, seizures with large doses.
CV: *hypotension,* bradycardia.
GI: *nausea, vomiting, constipation,* ileus.
GU: *urine retention.*
Local: pain at injection site, tissue irritation, induration following S.C. injection.
Other: *respiratory depression,* de-

creased libido, sweating, physical dependence.

INTERACTIONS
Alcohol, CNS depressants: additive effects. Use together cautiously.
Ammonium chloride and other urine acidifiers, phenytoin: may reduce methadone effect. Monitor for decreased pain control.
Rifampin: withdrawal symptoms; reduced blood levels of methadone. Use together cautiously.

NURSING CONSIDERATIONS
• Use with extreme caution in elderly or debilitated patients, or in patients with acute abdominal conditions, severe hepatic or renal impairment, hypothyroidism, Addison's disease, prostatic hypertrophy, urethral stricture, head injury, increased intracranial pressure, asthma, chronic obstructive pulmonary disease, respiratory depression, and CNS depression.
• When used as an adjunct in the treatment of narcotic addiction ("maintenance"), withdrawal will usually be delayed and mild.
• Safe use as maintenance drug in adolescent addicts not established.
• Once-daily dosage is adequate for maintenance. No advantage to divided doses.
• Oral liquid form legally required in maintenance programs. Completely dissolve tablets in 120 ml of orange juice or powdered citrus drink.
• Oral dose is half as potent as injected dose.
• Rotate injection sites.
• Has cumulative effect; marked sedation can occur after repeated doses.
• Monitor circulatory and respiratory status and bladder and bowel function. Patient may need laxatives or stool softeners.
• Warn ambulatory patient to avoid activities that require alertness.
• Regimented scheduling (around the clock) beneficial in severe, chronic

pain. When used for severe, chronic pain, tolerance may develop with long-term use, requiring a higher dose to achieve the same degree of analgesia. This is *not* a sign of addiction.
• Patient treated for narcotic abstinence syndrome will usually require an additional analgesic if pain control is necessary.
• Use with general anesthetics, tranquilizers, sedatives, hypnotics, alcohol, tricyclic antidepressants, or MAO inhibitors may cause respiratory depression, hypotension, profound sedation, or coma. Use together with extreme caution. Monitor patient response.
• Liquid form available for patients who are unable to swallow tablets.

morphine hydrochloride
Morphine hydrochloride♦♦, Morphitec♦♦, M.O.S.♦♦, M.O.S.-S.R.♦♦

morphine sulfate
Astramorph, Astramorph P.F., Duramorph PF, Epimorph♦♦, Morphine H.P.♦♦, MS Contin♦, MSIR, RMS Uniserts, Roxanol, Roxanol SR, Statex♦♦
Controlled Substance Schedule II

Pregnancy Risk Category: B (D for prolonged use or use of high doses at term)

MECHANISM OF ACTION
Binds with opiate receptors at many sites in the CNS (brain, brain stem, and spinal cord), altering both perception of and emotional response to pain through an unknown mechanism.

INDICATIONS & DOSAGE
Severe pain—
Adults: 4 to 15 mg S.C. or I.M.; or 30 to 60 mg P.O. or rectally q 4 hours, p.r.n. or around the clock. May be injected slow I.V. (over 4 to 5 minutes) diluted in 4 to 5 ml water for injec-

tion. May also administer controlled-release tablets q 8 to 12 hours. As an epidural injection, 5 mg via an epidural catheter q 24 hours.
Children: 0.1 to 0.2 mg/kg dose S.C. Maximum dosage is 15 mg.

In some situations, morphine may be administered by continuous I.V. infusion or by intraspinal and intrathecal injection.

ADVERSE REACTIONS

CNS: *sedation, somnolence, clouded sensorium, euphoria,* seizures with large doses, dizziness, *nightmares* (with long-acting oral forms).
CV: *hypotension,* bradycardia.
GI: *nausea, vomiting, constipation,* ileus.
GU: *urine retention.*
Other: *respiratory depression, physical dependence, pruritus and skin flushing (with epidural administration).*

INTERACTIONS

Alcohol, CNS depressants: additional effects. Use together cautiously.

NURSING CONSIDERATIONS

• Use with extreme caution in head injury, increased intracranial pressure, seizures, asthma, chronic obstructive pulmonary disease, alcoholism, prostatic hypertrophy, severe hepatic or renal disease, acute abdominal conditions, hypothyroidism, Addison's disease, increased cerebrospinal fluid pressure, urethral stricture, cardiac dysrhythmias, reduced blood volume, and toxic psychosis; and in elderly or debilitated patients.
• Warn ambulatory patient to avoid activities that require alertness.
• Monitor circulatory and respiratory status and bladder and bowel function. Don't give if respirations are below 12/minute.
• Constipation often severe with maintenance. Make sure stool softener or other laxative is ordered.

• Drug of choice in relieving pain of myocardial infarction. May cause transient decrease in blood pressure.
• Keep narcotic antagonist (naloxone) and resuscitative equipment available.
• Respiratory depression, hypotension, profound sedation, or coma may occur if used with general anesthetics, tranquilizers, sedatives, hypnotics, alcohol, tricyclic antidepressants, or MAO inhibitors. Reduce morphine dose. Use together with extreme caution. Monitor patient response.
• Regimented scheduling (around the clock) beneficial in severe, chronic pain.
• When used postoperatively, encourage turning, coughing, and deep breathing to avoid atelectasis.
• Oral solutions of various concentrations are available, as well as an intensified oral solution (20 mg/ml). Be sure to note the strength you are administering.
• Sublingual administration may be ordered. Measure out oral solution with tuberculin syringe. Administer dose a few drops at a time to allow maximal sublingual absorption and to minimize swallowing.
• Rectal suppository available in 5-, 10-, and 20-mg dosages. Refrigeration is not necessary. Note that in some patients, rectal and oral absorption may not be equivalent.
• Preservative-free preparations now available for epidural and intrathecal administration. The popularity of the epidural route is constantly increasing.
• When given epidurally, monitor closely for respiratory depression up to 24 hours after the injection. Check respiratory rate and depth every 30 to 60 minutes for 24 hours.
• May worsen or mask gallbladder pain.

Italicized side effects are common or life-threatening.
*Liquid form contains alcohol.   **May contain tartrazine.

nalbuphine hydrochloride
Nubain♦

Pregnancy Risk Category: B (D for prolonged use or use of high doses at term)

MECHANISM OF ACTION
Binds with opiate receptors at many sites in the CNS (brain, brain stem, and spinal cord), altering both perception of and emotional response to pain through an unknown mechanism.

INDICATIONS & DOSAGE
Moderate to severe pain—
Adults: 10 to 20 mg S.C., I.M., or I.V. q 3 to 6 hours, p.r.n. or around the clock. Maximum daily dosage is 160 mg.

ADVERSE REACTIONS
CNS: *sedation,* dizziness, nervousness, depression, restlessness, crying, euphoria, hostility, unusual dreams, confusion, hallucinations, delusions.
GI: cramps, dyspepsia, bitter taste, *nausea, vomiting,* constipation.
GU: urinary urgency.
Skin: itching, burning, urticaria.
Other: *respiratory depression.*

INTERACTIONS
Alcohol, CNS depressants: additive effects. Use together cautiously.
Narcotic analgesics: avoid concomitant use. Possible decreased analgesic effect.

NURSING CONSIDERATIONS
• Contraindicated in emotional instability, drug abuse, head injury, or increased intracranial pressure. Use cautiously in hepatic and renal disease. These patients may overreact to customary doses.
• Causes respiratory depression, which at 10 mg is equal to the respiratory depression produced by 10 mg of morphine.
• Respiratory depression can be reversed with naloxone. Keep recusitative equipment available, particulary when administering I.V.
• Psychological and physical dependence may occur.
• Monitor circulatory and respiratory status and bladder and bowel function. Don't give if respirations are below 12/minute.
• Constipation often severe with maintenance. Make sure stool softener or other laxative is ordered.
• Also acts as a narcotic antagonist; may precipitate abstinence syndrome. When administering to patients who have chronically received opiates, administer 25% of the usual dose initially. Observe for signs of withdrawal.
• Warn patient to avoid hazardous activities that require alertness until CNS effects of the drug are known.

oxycodone hydrochloride
Roxicodone, Supeudol♦♦
Controlled Substance Schedule II

Pregnancy Risk Category: B (D for prolonged use or use of high doses at term)

MECHANISM OF ACTION
Binds with opiate receptors at many sites in the CNS (brain, brain stem, and spinal cord), altering both perception of and emotional response to pain through an unknown mechanism.

INDICATIONS & DOSAGE
Moderate to severe pain—
Adults: available in combination with other drugs, such as aspirin (Codoxy, Percodan, Percodan-Demi) or acetaminophen (Percocet, Tylox). One to 2 tablets P.O. q 6 hours, p.r.n. or around the clock. Or 5 mg (5 ml) of Oxycodone oral solution or tablets P.O. q 6 hours.
Adults: (Supeudol) 1 to 3 suppositories rectally daily, p.r.n. or around the clock.

Children: (Percodan-Demi) ¼ to ½ tablet P.O. q 6 hours, p.r.n. or around the clock.

ADVERSE REACTIONS
CNS: *sedation, somnolence, clouded sensorium, euphoria*, dizziness, seizures with large doses.
CV: *hypotension*, bradycardia.
GI: *nausea, vomiting, constipation*, ileus.
GU: *urine retention*.
Other: *respiratory depression*, physical dependence.

INTERACTIONS
Alcohol, CNS depressants: additive effects. Use together cautiously.
Anticoagulants: oxycodone hydrochloride products containing aspirin may increase anticoagulant effect. Monitor clotting times. Use together cautiously.

NURSING CONSIDERATIONS
• Use with extreme caution in head injury, increased intracranial pressure, increased cerebrospinal fluid pressure, seizures, asthma, chronic obstructive pulmonary disease, alcoholism, prostatic hypertrophy, severe hepatic or renal disease, acute abdominal conditions, urethral stricture, hypothyroidism, Addison's disease, cardiac dysrhythmias, reduced blood volume, and toxic psychosis; and in elderly or debilitated patients.
• Don't give to children, except for Percodan-Demi and Percocet-Demi.
• Warn ambulatory patient to avoid activities that require alertness.
• Monitor circulatory and respiratory status and bladder and bowel function. Do not give if respirations are below 12/minute.
• Patient may require laxative or stool softener.
• For full analgesic effect, give before patient has intense pain.
• Give after meals or with milk.
• If used with general anesthetics,

other narcotic analgesics, tranquilizers, sedatives, hypnotics, alcohol, tricyclic antidepressants, or MAO inhibitors, CNS depression is increased. Reduce oxycodone dose. Use together with extreme caution. Monitor patient's response.
• Single-agent oxycodone solution or tablets are especially good for patients who shouldn't take aspirin or acetaminophen.

---

oxymorphone hydrochloride
Numorphan♦
Controlled Substance Schedule II

Pregnancy Risk Category: B (D for prolonged use or use of high doses at term)

MECHANISM OF ACTION
Binds with opiate receptors at many sites in the CNS (brain, brain stem, and spinal cord), altering both perception of and emotional response to pain through an unknown mechanism.

INDICATIONS & DOSAGE
Moderate to severe pain—
Adults: 1 to 1.5 mg I.M. or S.C. q 4 to 6 hours, p.r.n. or around the clock; or 0.5 mg I.V. q 4 to 6 hours, p.r.n. or around the clock; or 2.5 to 5 mg rectally q 4 to 6 hours, p.r.n. or around the clock.

ADVERSE REACTIONS
CNS: *sedation, somnolence, clouded sensorium, euphoria*, dizziness, seizures with large doses.
CV: *hypotension*, bradycardia.
GI: *nausea, vomiting, constipation*, ileus.
GU: *urine retention*.
Other: *respiratory depression*, physical dependence.

INTERACTIONS
Alcohol, CNS depressants: additive effects. Use together cautiously.

Italicized side effects are common or life-threatening.
*Liquid form contains alcohol.   **May contain tartrazine.

NURSING CONSIDERATIONS

• Use with extreme caution in head injury, increased intracranial pressure, seizures, asthma, chronic obstructive pulmonary disease, alcoholism, increased cerebrospinal fluid pressure, acute abdominal conditions, prostatic hypertrophy, severe hepatic or renal disease, urethral stricture, CNS depression, respiratory depression, hypothyroidism, Addison's disease, cardiac dysrhythmias, reduced blood volume, and toxic psychosis; and in elderly or debilitated patients.

• Warn ambulatory patient to avoid activities that require alertness.

• Monitor cardiovascular and respiratory status and bladder and bowel function. Don't give if respirations are below 12/minute.

• Patient may need laxative or stool softener.

• Well absorbed rectally. Alternative to narcotics with more limited dosage forms.

• Keep narcotic antagonist (naloxone) and resuscitative equipment available.

• If used with general anesthetics, tranquilizers, sedatives, hypnotics, alcohol, tricyclic antidepressants, or MAO inhibitors, CNS depression is increased. Reduce oxymorphone dose. Use together with extreme caution. Monitor patient's response.

• For better analgesic effect, give before patient has intense pain.

• When used postoperatively, encourage turning, coughing, and deep breathing to avoid atelectasis.

• Not intended for mild to moderate pain. May worsen gallbladder pain.

pentazocine hydrochloride♦♦
Fortral♦♦, Talwin♦♦

pentazocine lactate
Talwin, Talwin-Nx
Controlled Substance Schedule IV

Pregnancy Risk Category: B (D for prolonged use or use of high doses at term)

MECHANISM OF ACTION
Binds with opiate receptors at many sites in the CNS (brain, brain stem, and spinal cord), altering both perception of and emotional response to pain through an unknown mechanism.

INDICATIONS & DOSAGE
Moderate to severe pain—
Adults: 50 to 100 mg P.O. q 3 to 4 hours, p.r.n. or around the clock. Maximum oral dosage is 600 mg daily. Alternatively, may give 30 mg I.M., I.V., or S.C. q 3 to 4 hours, p.r.n. or around the clock. Maximum parenteral dosage is 360 mg daily. Single doses above 30 mg I.V. or 60 mg I.M. or S.C. not recommended.

ADVERSE REACTIONS
CNS: *sedation,* visual disturbances, *hallucinations,* drowsiness, dizziness, light-headedness, confusion, euphoria, headache, *psychotomimetic effects.*
GI: nausea, vomiting, dry mouth.
GU: *urine retention.*
Local: induration, nodules, sloughing, and sclerosis of injection site.
Other: *respiratory depression,* physical and psychological dependence.

INTERACTIONS
Alcohol, CNS depressants: additive effects. Use together cautiously.
Narcotic analgesics: avoid concomitant use. Possible decreased analgesic effect.

NURSING CONSIDERATIONS
• Contraindicated in emotional insta-bility, drug abuse, head injury, and in-creased intracranial pressure. Use cautiously in hepatic or renal disease.
• Tablets not well absorbed.
• Possesses narcotic antagonist prop-erties. May precipitate abstinence syndrome in narcotic-dependent pa-tients.
• Psychological and physical depen-dence may occur.
• Respiratory depression can be re-versed with naloxone.
• Do not mix in same syringe with soluble barbiturates.
• Warn ambulatory patient to avoid activities that require alertness.
• Talwin-Nx, the oral pentazocine available in the U.S., contains the nar-cotic antagonist naloxone. This pre-vents illicit I.V. use.

---

propoxyphene hydrochloride
Darvon♦, Dolene, Doraphen, Doxaphene, Novopropoxyn♦♦, Profene♦♦, Pro-Pox, Propoxycon, 642♦♦

propoxyphene napsylate
Darvocet-N, Darvon-N♦
Controlled Substance Schedule IV

Pregnancy Risk Category: C (D for prolonged use)

MECHANISM OF ACTION
Binds with opiate receptors at many sites in the CNS (brain, brain stem, and spinal cord), altering both per-ception of and emotional response to pain through an unknown mechanism.

INDICATIONS & DOSAGE
Mild to moderate pain—
Adults: 65 mg (hydrochloride) P.O. q 4 hours p.r.n.
Mild to moderate pain—
Adults: 100 mg (napsylate) P.O. q 4 hours p.r.n.

ADVERSE REACTIONS
CNS: *dizziness,* headache, sedation, euphoria, paradoxical excitement, in-somnia.
GI: nausea, vomiting, constipation.
Other: psychological and physical de-pendence.

INTERACTIONS
Alcohol, CNS depressants: additive effects. Use together cautiously.

NURSING CONSIDERATIONS
• Not to be prescribed for mainte-nance purposes in narcotic addiction.
• Warn ambulatory patient to avoid activities that require alertness until CNS effects of the drug are known.
• Warn patient not to exceed recom-mended dosage.
• Do not use caffeine or amphet-amines to treat overdose; may cause fatal seizures. Use narcotic antagonist instead.
• May cause false decreases in uri-nary steroid excretion tests.
• 65 mg propoxyphene HCl equals 100 mg propoxyphene napsylate.
• Can be considered a mild narcotic analgesic, but pain relief is equivalent to aspirin. Often used with aspirin or acetaminophen to maximize analgesic effects.
• Advise patient to limit alcohol in-take when taking this drug.

---

sufentanil citrate
Sufenta♦
Controlled Substance Schedule II

Pregnancy Risk Category: C (D for prolonged use or use of high doses at term)

MECHANISM OF ACTION
Binds with opiate receptors at many sites in the CNS (brain, brain stem, and spinal cord), altering both per-ception of and emotional response to pain through an unknown mechanism.

Italicized side effects are common or life-threatening.
*Liquid form contains alcohol.   **May contain tartrazine.

INDICATIONS & DOSAGE
Adjunct to general anesthetic—
Adults: 1 to 8 mcg/kg I.V. administered with nitrous oxide/oxygen.
As a primary anesthetic—
Adults: 8 to 30 mcg/kg I.V. administered with 100% oxygen and a muscle relaxant.

ADVERSE REACTIONS
CNS: chills.
CV: *hypotension,* hypertension, bradycardia, tachycardia.
GI: nausea, vomiting.
Skin: itching.
Other: *chest wall rigidity,* intraoperative muscle movement, *respiratory depression.*

INTERACTIONS
Alcohol, CNS depressants: additive effects. Use together cautiously.

NURSING CONSIDERATIONS
• Use cautiously in head injury, pulmonary disease, or decreased respiratory reserve.
• Should only be administered by persons specifically trained in the use of I.V. anesthetics.
• When used at doses of greater than 8 mcg/kg, postoperative mechanical ventilation and observation are essential because of extended postoperative respiratory depression.
• Keep narcotic antagonist (naloxone) and resuscitative equipment available when giving drug.
• Dose should be reduced in elderly and debilitated patients.
• Monitor postoperative vital signs frequently.
• Compared to fentanyl, sufentanil has a more rapid onset and shorter duration of action.
• High doses can produce muscle rigidity. This effect can be reversed by administration of neuromuscular blocking agents.

28

Narcotic antagonists

naloxone hydrochloride
naltrexone hydrochloride

COMBINATION PRODUCTS
None.

---

naloxone hydrochloride
Narcan♦

Pregnancy Risk Category: B

MECHANISM OF ACTION
Displaces previously administered narcotic analgesics from their receptors (competitive antagonism). Has no pharmacologic activity of its own.

INDICATIONS & DOSAGE
Known or suspected narcotic-induced respiratory depression, including that caused by pentazocine and propoxyphene—
Adults: 0.4 to 2 mg I.V., S.C., or I.M. May repeat q 2 to 3 minutes, p.r.n. If no response is observed after 10 mg has been administered, the diagnosis of narcotic-induced toxicity should be questioned.
Postoperative narcotic depression—
Adults: 0.1 to 0.2 mg I.V. q 2 to 3 minutes, p.r.n. Adult concentration is 0.4 mg/ml.
Children: 0.01 mg/kg dose I.M., I.V., or S.C. May repeat q 2 to 3 minutes.
  Note: If initial dose of 0.01 mg/kg does not result in clinical improvement, up to 10 times this dose (0.1 mg/kg) may be needed to be effective.
Neonates (asphyxia neonatorum): 0.01 mg/kg I.V. into umbilical vein.

May repeat q 2 to 3 minutes for 3 doses. Neonatal concentration (for children also) is 0.02 mg/ml.

ADVERSE REACTIONS
With higher-than-recommended doses: nausea, vomiting, tachycardia, hypertension, tremors.
In narcotic-dependent patients: withdrawal symptoms.

INTERACTIONS
None significant.

NURSING CONSIDERATIONS
• Use cautiously in cardiac irritability and narcotic addiction.
• Safest drug to use when cause of respiratory depression is uncertain.
• Monitor respiratory depth and rate. Be prepared to provide oxygen, ventilation, and other resuscitative measures.
• Respiratory rate increases within 1 to 2 minutes. Effect lasts 1 to 4 hours.
• Duration of narcotic may exceed that of the naloxone. Patient may relapse into respiratory depression.
• May be administered by continuous I.V. infusion, which is often necessary to control the adverse effects of epidurally administered morphine.
• Can see "overshoot" effect—respiratory rate exceeds the rate before respiratory depression.
• Although generally believed to be ineffective in respiratory depression caused by nonnarcotics, recent reports indicate that it may reverse coma induced by alcohol intoxication.
• Does *not* reverse respiratory de-

Italicized side effects are common or life-threatening.
*Liquid form contains alcohol.   **May contain tartrazine.

pression secondary to diazepam.
• May dilute adult concentration (0.4 mg) by mixing 0.5 ml with 9.5 ml sterile water or saline solution for injection to make neonatal concentration (0.02 mg/ml).
• Now available in 1-ml prefilled disposable syringes, 1-ml ampules, and 10-ml vials.
• Naloxone has been successfully used investigationally to treat the senile dementia of Alzheimer's disease.
• Also has been shown to improve circulation in refractory shock.
• Used by some researchers to relieve certain kinds of chronic constipation.

naltrexone hydrochloride
Trexan

Pregnancy Risk Category: C

MECHANISM OF ACTION
Reversibly blocks the subjective effects of intravenously administered opioids by occupying opiate receptors in the brain.

INDICATIONS & DOSAGE
As an adjunct for maintenance of an opioid-free state in detoxified individuals—
Adults: initially, 25 mg P.O. If no withdrawal signs occur within 1 hour, give an additional 25 mg. Once patient has been started on 50 mg q 24 hours, flexible maintenance schedule may be used. From 50 to 150 mg may be given daily, depending on the schedule prescribed.

ADVERSE REACTIONS
CNS: *insomnia, anxiety,* nervousness, headache, depression.
GI: *nausea, vomiting,* anorexia, *abdominal pain.*
Hepatic: hepatotoxicity.
Other: *muscle and joint pain.*

INTERACTIONS
None significant.

NURSING CONSIDERATIONS
• Contraindicated in patients receiving opioid analgesics, opioid-dependent patients, patients in acute opioid withdrawal, and in those with positive urine screen for opioids or acute hepatitis or liver failure.
• Treatment shouldn't begin until patient receives Narcan challenge, a provocative test of opioid dependency. If signs of opioid withdrawal persist after Narcan challenge, don't administer naltrexone.
• Use cautiously in mild liver disease or history of recent liver disease.
• Patients must be completely free of opioids before taking naltrexone, or they may experience severe withdrawal symptoms. Those who have been addicted to short-acting opioids (such as heroin and meperidine) must wait at least 7 days after the last opioid dose before starting naltrexone. Those who have been addicted to longer-acting opioids (such as methadone) should wait at least 10 days.
• In an emergency that requires opioid analgesia, a patient receiving naltrexone can be given an opioid analgesic. However, the dose must be higher than usual to surmount naltrexone's effect. Monitor for respiratory depression from the opioid, which may be longer and deeper.
• Naltrexone should be used only as part of a comprehensive rehabilitation program.
• A suggested flexible maintenance dosage regimen: 100 mg on Monday and Wednesday; 150 mg on Friday. This schedule would be preferred for those expected to be poor compliers.
• Advise the patient to carry a medical identification card. Warn him to tell medical personnel that he is taking naltrexone, if he needs medical treatment.
• Give patient the names of nonopioid drugs that he can continue to take for pain, diarrhea, or cough.

29

Sedative-hypnotics

amobarbital
amobarbital sodium
aprobarbital
butabarbital sodium
chloral hydrate
ethchlorvynol
ethinamate
flurazepam hydrochloride
glutethimide
methotrimeprazine
  hydrochloride
methyprylon
midazolam hydrochloride
paraldehyde
  (See Chapter 30, ANTICONVULSANTS.)
pentobarbital
pentobarbital sodium
phenobarbital sodium
  (See Chapter 30, ANTICONVULSANTS.)
secobarbital sodium
talbutal
temazepam
triazolam

COMBINATION PRODUCTS
Barbiturates
TRI-BARBS CAPSULE: phenobarbital
32 mg, butabarbital sodium 32 mg,
and secobarbital sodium 32 mg.
TUINAL 50 MG PULVULES: amobarbital sodium 25 mg and secobarbital sodium 25 mg.
TUINAL 100 MG PULVULES♦: amobarbital sodium 50 mg and secobarbital sodium 50 mg.
TUINAL 200 MG PULVULES♦: amobarbital sodium 100 mg and secobarbital sodium 100 mg.

amobarbital
Amytal♦

amobarbital sodium
Amytal Sodium♦
Controlled Substance Schedule II

*Pregnancy Risk Category: B
(according to manufacturer)*

MECHANISM OF ACTION
Probably interferes with transmission
of impulses from the thalamus to the
cortex of the brain. A barbiturate.

INDICATIONS & DOSAGE
Sedation—
Adults: usually 30 to 50 mg P.O.
b.i.d. or t.i.d. but may range from 15
to 120 mg b.i.d. to q.i.d.
Children: 3 to 6 mg/kg P.O. daily in
four equally divided doses.
Insomnia—
Adults: 65 to 200 mg P.O. or deep
I.M. h.s.; I.M. injection not to exceed
5 ml in any one site. Maximum dosage is 500 mg.
Children: 3 to 5 mg/kg deep I.M.
h.s.; I.M. injection not to exceed 5 ml
in any one site.
Preanesthetic sedation—
Adults and children: 200 mg P.O. or
I.M. 1 to 2 hours before surgery.
Manic reactions, as an adjunct in psychotherapy, anticonvulsant—
Adults and children over 6 years: 65
to 500 mg slow I.V.; rate not to exceed
100 mg/minute. Maximum dosage is
1 g.
Children under 6 years: 3 to 5 mg/
kg slow I.V. or I.M.

Italicized side effects are common or life-threatening.
*Liquid form contains alcohol.   **May contain tartrazine.

ADVERSE REACTIONS
CNS: *drowsiness, lethargy, hangover*, paradoxical excitement in elderly patients.
GI: nausea, vomiting.
Skin: rash, urticaria.
Local: pain, irritation, sterile abscess at injection site.
Other: *Stevens-Johnson syndrome*, angioedema, exacerbation of porphyria.

INTERACTIONS
Alcohol or other CNS depressants, including narcotic analgesics: excessive CNS and respiratory depression. Use together cautiously.
Griseofulvin: decreased absorption of griseofulvin.
MAO inhibitors: inhibit metabolism of barbiturates; may cause prolonged CNS depression. Reduce barbiturate dosage.
Oral anticoagulants, estrogens and oral contraceptives, doxycycline, corticosteroids: amobarbital may enhance the metabolism of these drugs. Monitor for decreased effect.
Rifampin: may decrease barbiturate levels. Monitor for decreased effect.

NURSING CONSIDERATIONS
• Contraindicated in uncontrolled severe pain, respiratory disease with dyspnea or obstruction, hypersensitivity to barbiturates, previous addiction to sedatives, or porphyria. Use with caution in hepatic or renal impairment.
• Elderly patients are more sensitive to the drug's adverse CNS effects. Assess mental status before initiating therapy.
• Use injection solution within 30 minutes after opening container to minimize deterioration. Don't use cloudy or precipitated solution. Don't shake solution; mix with sterile water only.
• Reserve I.V. injection for emergency treatment. Give under close supervision. Be prepared to give artificial respiration. Administer slowly I.V.; do not exceed 100 mg/minute.
• Administer I.M. injection deeply. Superficial injection may cause pain, sterile abscess, and sloughing.
• Because barbiturates potentiate narcotics, reduce dose when giving during labor. Excessive dose may cause respiratory depression in neonate.
• Remove cigarettes of patient receiving hypnotic dose.
• Supervise walking; raise bed rails, especially for elderly patients.
• Long-term high dosage may cause drug dependence and severe withdrawal symptoms. Withdraw barbiturates gradually.
• Prevent hoarding or self-overdosing by patients who are depressed, suicidal, or drug-dependent, or who have a history of drug abuse.
• Watch for signs of barbiturate toxicity: coma, pupillary constriction, cyanosis, clammy skin, and hypotension. Overdose can be fatal.
• Morning "hangover" common after hypnotic dose. Hypnotic doses suppress REM sleep. When drug is discontinued, patient may experience increased dreaming.
• Used in psychiatric settings as an "Amytal interview" to elicit information that patient can't or won't offer when fully conscious.

---

aprobarbital
Alurate*
Controlled Substance Schedule III

Pregnancy Risk Category: D

MECHANISM OF ACTION
Probably interferes with transmission of impulses from the thalamus to the cortex of the brain. A barbiturate.

INDICATIONS & DOSAGE
Sedation—
Adults: 15 to 40 mg P.O. t.i.d. or q.i.d.; usual dose is 40 mg t.i.d.

Insomnia—
Adults: 40 to 160 mg P.O. h.s.

ADVERSE REACTIONS
CNS: *drowsiness, lethargy, hangover,* paradoxical excitement in elderly patients.
GI: nausea, vomiting.
Skin: rash, urticaria.
Other: *Stevens-Johnson syndrome,* angioedema, exacerbation of porphyria.

INTERACTIONS
Alcohol or other CNS depressants, including narcotic analgesics: excessive CNS and respiratory depression. Use together cautiously.
Griseofulvin: decreased absorption of griseofulvin.
MAO inhibitors: inhibit metabolism of barbiturates; may cause prolonged CNS depression. Reduce barbiturate dosage.
Oral anticoagulants, estrogens and oral contraceptives, doxycycline, corticosteroids: aprobarbital may enhance the metabolism of these drugs. Monitor for decreased effectiveness.
Rifampin: may decrease barbiturate levels. Monitor for decreased effect.

NURSING CONSIDERATIONS
• Contraindicated in uncontrolled severe pain, respiratory disease with dyspnea or obstruction, hypersensitivity to barbiturates, previous addiction to sedatives, or porphyria. Use with caution in hepatic or renal impairment.
• Remove cigarettes of patient receiving hypnotic dose.
• Supervise walking; raise bed rails, especially for elderly patients.
• Long-term high dosage may cause drug dependence and severe withdrawal symptoms. Withdraw barbiturates gradually.
• Prevent hoarding or self-overdosing by patients who are depressed, suicidal, or drug-dependent, or who have a history of drug abuse.
• Available as elixir only, with alcohol 20%.
• Watch for signs of barbiturate toxicity: coma, pupillary constriction, cyanosis, clammy skin, and hypotension. Overdose can be fatal.
• Morning "hangover" common after hypnotic dose.
• Hypnotic doses suppress REM sleep. When drug discontinued, patient may experience increased dreaming.
• Women who use oral contraceptives should consider alternate birth control methods when taking this drug because it may enhance contraceptive hormone metabolism and decrease its effect.

---

butabarbital sodium
Barbased, Butalan, Buticaps, Butisol♦, Day-Barb♦♦, Sarisol No. 2
Controlled Substance Schedule III

Pregnancy Risk Category: D

MECHANISM OF ACTION
Probably interferes with transmission of impulses from the thalamus to the cortex of the brain. A barbiturate.

INDICATIONS & DOSAGE
Sedation—
Adults: 15 to 30 mg P.O. t.i.d. or q.i.d.
Children: 6 mg/kg P.O. divided t.i.d. Dosage range 7.5 to 30 mg P.O. t.i.d.
Preoperatively—
Adults: 50 to 100 mg P.O. 60 to 90 minutes before surgery.
Insomnia—
Adults: 50 to 100 mg P.O. h.s.

ADVERSE REACTIONS
CNS: *drowsiness, lethargy, hangover,* paradoxical excitement in elderly patients.
GI: nausea, vomiting.
Skin: rash, urticaria.
Other: *Stevens-Johnson syndrome,*

---

angioedema, exacerbation of porphyria.

INTERACTIONS
Alcohol or other CNS depressants, including narcotic analgesics: excessive CNS and respiratory depression. Use together cautiously.
Griseofulvin: decreased absorption of griseofulvin.
MAO inhibitors: inhibit the metabolism of barbiturates; may cause prolonged CNS depression. Reduce barbiturate dosage.
Oral anticoagulants, estrogens and oral contraceptives, doxycycline, corticosteroids: butabarbital may enhance the metabolism of these drugs. Monitor for decreased effect.
Rifampin: may decrease barbiturate levels. Monitor for decreased effect.

NURSING CONSIDERATIONS
• Contraindicated in uncontrolled severe pain, respiratory disease with dyspnea or obstruction, hypersensitivity to barbiturates, previous addiction to sedatives, or porphyria. Use with caution in hepatic or renal impairment.
• Elderly patients are more sensitive to the drug's adverse CNS effects. Assess mental status before initiating therapy.
• Remove cigarettes of patient receiving hypnotic dose.
• Supervise walking; raise bed rails, especially for elderly patients.
• Long-term high dosage may cause drug dependence and severe withdrawal symptoms. Withdraw barbiturates gradually.
• Prevent hoarding or self-overdosing by patients who are depressed, suicidal, or drug-dependent, or who have a history of drug abuse.
• Butisol sodium elixir is sugar-free.
• Watch for signs of barbiturate toxicity: coma, pupillary constriction, cyanosis, clammy skin, and hypotension. Overdose can be fatal.

• Prolonged administration is not recommended: drug is not shown to be effective after 14 days. A drug-free interval of at least 1 week is advised.
• Morning "hangover" common after hypnotic dose.
• Hypnotic doses suppress REM sleep. When drug is discontinued, patient may experience increased dreaming.
• Women who use oral contraceptives should consider alternate birth control methods when taking this drug because it may enhance contraceptive hormone metabolism and decrease its effect.

chloral hydrate
Aquachloral Suprettes, Noctec♦, Novochlorhydrate♦♦
Controlled Substance Schedule IV
Pregnancy Risk Category: C

MECHANISM OF ACTION
Unknown. Sedative effects may be caused by its primary metabolite, trichloroethanol.

INDICATIONS & DOSAGE
Sedation—
Adults: 250 mg P.O. or rectally t.i.d. after meals.
Children: 8 mg/kg P.O. t.i.d. Maximum dosage is 500 mg t.i.d.
Insomnia—
Adults: 500 mg to 1 g P.O. or rectally 15 to 30 minutes before bedtime.
Children: 50 mg/kg single dose. Maximum dosage is 1 g.
Premedication for EEG—
Children: 25 mg/kg single dose. Maximum dosage is 1 g.

ADVERSE REACTIONS
Blood: eosinophilia.
CNS: *hangover, drowsiness,* nightmares, dizziness, ataxia, paradoxical excitement.
GI: *nausea,* vomiting, diarrhea, flatulence.

Skin: hypersensitivity reactions.

INTERACTIONS
Alcohol or other CNS depressants, including narcotic analgesics: excessive CNS depression or vasodilation reaction. Use together cautiously.
Furosemide I.V.: sweating, flushes, variable blood pressure, and uneasiness. Use together cautiously or use a different hypnotic drug.
Oral anticoagulants: increased risk of bleeding. Monitor patient closely.

NURSING CONSIDERATIONS
• Contraindicated in marked hepatic or renal impairment and hypersensitivity to chloral hydrate or triclofos. Oral administration contraindicated in gastric disorders. Use with caution in severe cardiac disease, mental depression, and suicidal tendencies.
• Dilute or administer with liquid to minimize unpleasant taste and stomach irritation. Administer after meals.
• Prevent hoarding or self-overdosing by patients who are depressed, suicidal, or drug-dependent, or who have a history of drug abuse.
• Remove cigarettes of patient receiving hypnotic dose.
• Supervise walking; raise bed rails, especially for elderly patients.
• Large dosage may raise BUN level.
• May interfere with fluorometric tests for urine catecholamines and Reddy, Jenkins, Thorn test for urine 17-hydroxycorticosteroids. Do not administer drug for 48 hours before fluorometric test.
• Aqueous solutions are incompatible with alkaline substances.
• Store in dark container; store suppositories in refrigerator.

ethchlorvynol
Placidyl♦**
Controlled Substance Schedule IV
Pregnancy Risk Category: C

MECHANISM OF ACTION
Unknown.

INDICATIONS & DOSAGE
Sedation—
Adults: 100 to 200 mg P.O. b.i.d. or t.i.d.
Insomnia—
Adults: 500 mg to 1 g P.O. h.s. May repeat 100 to 200 mg if awakened in early morning.

ADVERSE REACTIONS
Blood: thrombocytopenia.
CNS: facial numbness, drowsiness, fatigue, nightmares, dizziness, residual sedation, muscular weakness, syncope, ataxia.
CV: hypotension.
EENT: unpleasant aftertaste, blurred vision.
GI: distress, nausea, vomiting.
Skin: rashes, urticaria.

INTERACTIONS
Alcohol or other CNS depressants, including narcotic analgesics, tricyclic antidepressants, and MAO inhibitors: excessive CNS depression. Use together cautiously.
Oral anticoagulants: ethchlorvynol may enhance the metabolism of coumarin derivitives, decreasing their effectiveness. Monitor closely.

NURSING CONSIDERATIONS
• Contraindicated in uncontrolled pain and porphyria. Use cautiously in hepatic or renal impairment; in elderly or debilitated patients; in mental depression with suicidal tendencies; and if patient has previously overreacted to barbiturates or alcohol.
• Give with milk or food to minimize transient dizziness or ataxia caused by

SEDATIVE-HYPNOTICS   **273**

rapid absorption.
• May cause dependence and severe withdrawal symptoms. Withdraw gradually.
• Prevent hoarding or self-overdosing by patients who are depressed, suicidal, or drug-dependent, or who have a history of drug abuse. Overdosage very difficult to treat and has a high mortality.
• Watch for signs of toxicity, such as poor muscle coordination, confusion, hypothermia, speech or vision disturbances, tremors, and weakness.
• 750-mg strength contains tartrazine dye. May cause allergic reactions in susceptible patients.
• Remove cigarettes of patient receiving hypnotic dose.
• Supervise walking; raise bed rails, especially for elderly patients.
• Slight darkening of liquid from exposure to air and light doesn't affect safety or potency, but store in tight, light-resistant container to avoid possible deterioration.
• Drug is effective for short-term use only; treatment period should not exceed 1 week.

ethinamate
Valmid
Controlled Substance Schedule IV

Pregnancy Risk Category: C

MECHANISM OF ACTION
Unknown.

INDICATIONS & DOSAGE
Insomnia—
Adults: 500 mg to 1 g P.O. 20 minutes before bedtime. Starting dose may be 250 mg for elderly or debilitated patients.

ADVERSE REACTIONS
Blood: thrombocytic purpura.
GI: mild upset.
Skin: rashes.
Other: fever (allergic reaction).

INTERACTIONS
Alcohol, CNS depressants: increased CNS depression. Avoid concomitant use.

NURSING CONSIDERATIONS
• Contraindicated for uncontrolled pain. Use cautiously in mental depression, suicidal tendencies, or history of drug abuse.
• Not recommended for use in children under age 15; paradoxical excitement in children has been reported.
• Not usually given for daytime sedation because of short duration of effect.
• Long-term use may cause dependence and severe withdrawal symptoms. Withdraw gradually.
• Prevent hoarding or self-overdosing by patients who are depressed, suicidal, or drug-dependent, or who have a history of drug abuse.
• Abrupt withdrawal may cause blood pressure and pulse rate changes, sweating, and hallucinations.
• Remove cigarettes of patient receiving dose.
• Supervise walking; raise bed rails, especially for elderly patients.
• In overdosage, treat CNS and respiratory depression same as barbiturate intoxication; ethinamate is dialyzable.
• May cause falsely elevated urine 17-ketosteroid (modified Zimmermann reaction) and 17-hydroxycorticosteroid levels (Porter-Silber test).
• Prolonged therapy not recommended; drug is not effective for more than 7 days.

flurazepam hydrochloride
Apo-Flurazepam♦♦, Dalmane♦, Durapam, Novoflupam♦♦, SamPam♦♦
Controlled Substance Schedule IV

Pregnancy Risk Category: D

MECHANISM OF ACTION
Acts on the limbic system, thalamus,

and hypothalamus of the central nervous system to produce hypnotic effects. A benzodiazepine.

INDICATIONS & DOSAGE
Insomnia—
Adults: 15 to 30 mg P.O. h.s. May repeat dose once.
Adults over 65: 15 mg P.O. h.s.

ADVERSE REACTIONS
Blood: leukopenia, granulocytopenia.
CNS: *daytime sedation, dizziness, drowsiness, disturbed coordination,* lethargy, confusion, *headache.*
GI: nausea, vomiting, heartburn.
Metabolic: elevated liver enzymes.

INTERACTIONS
Alcohol or other CNS depressants, including narcotic analgesics: excessive CNS depression. Use together cautiously.
Cimetidine: increased sedation. Monitor carefully.

NURSING CONSIDERATIONS
• Use cautiously in impaired hepatic or renal function, mental depression, suicidal tendencies, or history of drug abuse.
• Elderly patients are more sensitive to the drug's adverse CNS effects. Assess mental status before initiating therapy.
• Prevent hoarding or self-overdosing by patients who are depressed, suicidal, or drug-dependent, or who have a history of drug abuse.
• Remove cigarettes of patient receiving drug.
• Supervise walking; raise bed rails, especially for elderly patients.
• Dependence is possible with long-term use.
• More effective on second, third, and fourth nights of use because active metabolite accumulates. Encourage patient to continue drug if it doesn't work the first night.

glutethimide
Doriden♦, Doriglute
Controlled Substance Schedule III
Pregnancy Risk Category: C

MECHANISM OF ACTION
Unknown.

INDICATIONS & DOSAGE
Insomnia—
Adults: 250 to 500 mg P.O. h.s. May be repeated, but not less than 4 hours before intended awakening. Total daily dosage should not exceed 1 g.

ADVERSE REACTIONS
CNS: *residual sedation, dizziness, ataxia,* paradoxical excitation, headache, vertigo.
EENT: dry mouth, blurred vision.
GI: irritation, nausea.
GU: bladder atony.
Skin: rash, urticaria.

INTERACTIONS
Alcohol or other CNS depressants, including narcotic analgesics: excessive CNS depression. Use together cautiously.
Oral anticoagulants: glutethimide enhances the metabolism of coumarin derivitives. Monitor for decreased effect.

NURSING CONSIDERATIONS
• Contraindicated in uncontrolled pain, severe renal impairment, or porphyria. Use cautiously in mental depression, suicidal tendencies, history of drug abuse, prostatic hypertrophy, stenosing peptic ulcer, pyloroduodenal or bladder-neck obstruction, narrow-angle glaucoma, and cardiac dysrhythmias.
• Drug is effective for short-term use only.
• Remove cigarettes of patient receiving drug.
• Supervise walking; raise bed rails, especially for elderly patients.

Italicized side effects are common or life-threatening.
*Liquid form contains alcohol.   **May contain tartrazine.

• Prevent hoarding or self-overdosing by patients who are depressed, suicidal, or drug-dependent, or who have a history of drug abuse.

• Abrupt withdrawal may produce nausea, vomiting, nervousness, tremors, chills, fever, nightmares, insomnia, tachycardia, delirium, numbness of extremities, hallucinations, dysphagia, and seizures. Withdraw gradually.

• Monitor prothrombin times carefully when patient on glutethimide starts or ends anticoagulant therapy. Anticoagulant dose may need to be adjusted.

• Suppresses REM sleep, as do barbiturates. When drug is discontinued, patient may experience increased dreaming.

---

methotrimeprazine hydrochloride
Levoprome, Nozinan♦♦

Pregnancy Risk Category: C

MECHANISM OF ACTION
Acts on the limbic system, thalamus, and hypothalamus of the central nervous system to produce hypnotic effects. A phenothiazine.

INDICATIONS & DOSAGE
Postoperative analgesia—
Adults and children over 12 years: initially, 2.5 to 7.5 mg I.M. q 4 to 6 hours, then adjust dose.
Preanesthetic medication—
Adults and children over 12 years: 2 to 20 mg I.M. 45 minutes to 3 hours before surgery.
Sedation, analgesia—
Adults and children over 12 years: 10 to 20 mg deep I.M. q 4 to 6 hours as required.
Adults over 65 years: 5 to 10 mg I.M. q 4 to 6 hours.

ADVERSE REACTIONS
Blood: *agranulocytosis* and other dyscrasias after long-term high dosage.
CNS: *fainting, weakness, dizziness,* drowsiness, excessive sedation, amnesia, disorientation, euphoria, headache, slurred speech.
CV: *orthostatic hypotension,* palpitations.
EENT: dry mouth, nasal congestion.
GI: nausea, vomiting, abdominal discomfort.
GU: difficulty urinating.
Local: *pain, inflammation, swelling at injection site.*

INTERACTIONS
All antihypertensive agents: increased orthostatic hypotension. Don't use together.

NURSING CONSIDERATIONS
• Contraindicated in patients receiving concurrent antihypertensive drug therapy, including MAO inhibitors; also, in history of convulsive disorders; hypersensitivity to phenothiazines; severe cardiac, hepatic, or renal disease; previous overdose of CNS depressant; or coma. Use with extreme caution in elderly or debilitated patients with cardiac disease or in any patient who may suffer serious consequences from a sudden drop in blood pressure.

• Use low initial dose in susceptible patients; increase gradually while frequently checking pulse rate, blood pressure, and circulation.

• Expect drop in blood pressure 10 to 20 minutes after I.M. injection.

• Keep patient in bed or closely supervised for 6 to 12 hours after each of the first several injections because orthostatic hypotension may occur. If hypotension is severe, combat with phenylephrine, methoxamine, or levarterenol. Don't use epinephrine because it may worsen hypotension.

• Don't use for longer than 30 days except in terminal illness or when narcotics are contraindicated.

• In prolonged use, monitor liver

function and blood studies periodically.
• Inject I.M. into large muscle masses. Rotate sites. Do not administer subcutaneously, as local irritation results. I.V. injection not recommended.
• May be mixed in same syringe with reduced dose of atropine and scopolamine. Do not mix with other drugs. Protect solution from light.
• Rarely may cause neuroleptic malignant syndrome, with fever, leukocytosis, and dystonic reaction. Can be fatal if untreated.

methyprylon
Noludar♦
Controlled Substance Schedule III

Pregnancy Risk Category: B

MECHANISM OF ACTION
Raises threshold of arousal centers in the brain stem.

INDICATIONS & DOSAGE
Insomnia—
Adults: 200 to 400 mg P.O. 15 minutes before bedtime.
Children over 3 months: 50 mg P.O. at bedtime, increased to 200 mg, if necessary. Maximum dosage is 400 mg daily.

ADVERSE REACTIONS
Blood: thrombocytopenic purpura, neutropenia, *aplastic anemia.*
CNS: *morning drowsiness, dizziness,* headache, paradoxical excitation.
CV: hypotension.
GI: nausea, vomiting, diarrhea, esophagitis.
Skin: rash, pruritus.

INTERACTIONS
Alcohol or other CNS depressants, including narcotic analgesics: excessive CNS and respiratory depression. Use together cautiously.

NURSING CONSIDERATIONS
• Contraindicated in intermittent porphyria. Use cautiously in renal or hepatic impairment.
• Periodic blood counts are advisable during repeated or long-term use.
• May cause drug dependence and severe life-threatening withdrawal symptoms. Withdrawal should be gradual and closely monitored.
• Prevent hoarding or self-overdosing by patients who are depressed, suicidal, or drug-dependent, or who have a history of drug abuse.
• Remove cigarettes of patient receiving drug.
• Supervise walking; raise bed rails, especially for elderly patients.
• Value of this drug as a sedative has not been established.
• Overdosage symptoms include somnolence, confusion, constricted pupils, respiratory depression, hypotension, and coma. Hemodialysis is useful in severe intoxication.
• Suppresses REM sleep, as do barbiturates. When drug is discontinued, patient may experience increased dreaming.

midazolam hydrochloride
Versed♦
Controlled Substance Schedule IV

Pregnancy Risk Category: D

MECHANISM OF ACTION
Depresses the CNS at the limbic and subcortical levels of the brain.

INDICATIONS & DOSAGE
Preoperative sedation (to induce sleepiness or drowsiness and relieve apprehension)—
Adults: 0.07 mg to 0.08 mg/kg I.M. approximately 1 hour before surgery. May be administered with atropine or scopolamine and reduced doses of narcotics.
Conscious sedation before short diagnostic or endoscopic procedures—

Adults: initially, 0.035 mg/kg slowly I.V.(not to exceed 2.5 mg). Dose is then titrated in small amounts to a total dosage of 0.1 mg/kg.
Induction of general anesthesia—
Adults: 0.3 to 0.35 mg/kg I.V. over 20 to 30 seconds. Additional increments of 25% of the initial dose may be needed to complete induction. Up to 0.6 mg/kg total dosage may be given.

ADVERSE REACTIONS
CNS: headache, oversedation, involuntary movements, combativeness.
CV: variations in blood pressure and pulse rate.
GI: nausea, vomiting, hiccups.
Local: pain and tenderness at injection site.
Other: *decreased respiratory rate, apnea.*

INTERACTIONS
CNS depressants: may increase the risk of apnea. Prepare to adjust drug dosage.

NURSING CONSIDERATIONS
• Contraindicated in acute narrow-angle glaucoma. Don't give to patients in shock, coma, or acute alcohol intoxication. Use cautiously in CHF, COPD, or renal disease, and in elderly or debilitated patients.
• Before administering I.V. midazolam, have oxygen and resuscitative equipment available in case of severe respiratory depression. Excessive dosage or rapid infusion has been associated with respiratory arrest, particularly in elderly or debilitated patients.
• Monitor blood pressure during procedure, especially in patients who have also been premedicated with narcotics.
• Midazolam has a beneficial amnestic effect, which diminishes patient's recall of perioperative events. This drug offers advantages over diazepam, hydrozyzine, and barbiturates,

which are also prescribed for similar indications.
• When injecting I.M., give deep into a large muscle mass.
• May be mixed in the same syringe with morphine sulfate, meperidine, atropine sulfate, or scopolamine.
• When administering I.V., take care to avoid extravasation.

---

pentobarbital
Nembutal**

pentobarbital sodium
Nembutal Sodium♦*,
Novopentobarb♦♦
Controlled Substance Schedule II
Pregnancy Risk Category: D

MECHANISM OF ACTION
Probably interferes with transmission of impulses from the thalamus to the cortex of the brain. A barbiturate.

INDICATIONS & DOSAGE
Sedation—
Adults: 20 to 40 mg P.O. b.i.d., t.i.d., or q.i.d.
Children: 6 mg/kg daily P.O. in divided doses.
Insomnia—
Adults: 100 to 200 mg P.O. h.s. or 150 to 200 mg deep I.M.; 100 mg initially, I.V., then additional doses up to 500 mg; 120 to 200 mg rectally.
Children: 3 to 5 mg/kg I.M. Maximum dosage is 100 mg. Rectal dosages are 2 months to 1 year, 30 mg; 1 to 4 years, 30 to 60 mg; 5 to 12 years, 60 mg; 12 to 14 years, 60 to 120 mg.
Preanesthetic medication—
Adults: 150 to 200 mg I.M. or P.O. in two divided doses.

ADVERSE REACTIONS
CNS: *drowsiness, lethargy, hangover,* paradoxical excitement in elderly patients.
GI: nausea, vomiting.
Skin: rash, urticaria.

Other: *Stevens-Johnson syndrome,* angioedema, exacerbation of porphyria.

INTERACTIONS
Alcohol or other CNS depressants, including narcotic analgesics: excessive CNS and respiratory depression. Use together cautiously.
Griseofulvin: decreased absorption of griseofulvin.
MAO inhibitors: inhibit metabolism of barbiturates; may cause prolonged CNS depression. Reduce barbiturate dosage.
Oral anticoagulants, estrogens and oral contraceptives, doxycycline, corticosteroids: pentobarbital may enhance the metabolism of these drugs. Monitor for decreased effect.
Rifampin: may decrease barbiturate levels. Monitor for decreased effect.

NURSING CONSIDERATIONS
• Contraindicated in uncontrolled severe pain, respiratory disease with dyspnea or obstruction, hypersensitivity to barbiturates, previous addiction to sedatives, or porphyria. Use with caution in hepatic or renal impairment.
• Elderly patients are more sensitive to the drug's adverse CNS effects. Assess mental status before initiating therapy.
• Use injection solution within 30 minutes after opening container to minimize deterioration. Don't use cloudy solution.
• Parenteral solution alkaline. Avoid extravasation; may cause tissue necrosis.
• I.V. injection should be reserved for emergency treatment and should be given under close supervision. Be prepared to give artificial respiration.
• Administer I.M. injection deeply. Superficial injection may cause pain, sterile abscess, and sloughing.
• Do not mix with other medications.
• Remove cigarettes of patient receiving hypnotic dose.
• Supervise walking; raise bed rails, especially for elderly patients.
• May cause drug dependence and severe withdrawal symptoms. Withdraw barbiturates gradually.
• Prevent hoarding or self-overdosing by patients who are depressed, suicidal, or drug-dependent, or who have a history of drug abuse.
• No analgesic effect. May cause restlessness or delirium in presence of pain.
• Watch for signs of barbiturate toxicity: coma, pupillary constriction, cyanosis, clammy skin, and hypotension. Overdose can be fatal.
• To ensure accurate dosage, don't divide suppositories.
• Morning "hangover" common after hypnotic dose.
• Hypnotic doses suppress REM sleep. When drug is discontinued, patient may experience increased dreaming.

secobarbital sodium
Novosecobarb♦♦, Seconal Sodium♦
Controlled Substance Schedule II
Pregnancy Risk Category: D

MECHANISM OF ACTION
Probably interferes with transmission of impulses from the thalamus to the cortex of the brain. A barbiturate.

INDICATIONS & DOSAGE
Sedation, preoperatively—
Adults: 200 to 300 mg P.O. 1 to 2 hours before surgery.
Children: 50 to 100 mg P.O. or 4 to 5 mg/kg rectally 1 to 2 hours before surgery.
Insomnia—
Adults: 100 to 200 mg P.O. or I.M.
Children: 3 to 5 mg/kg I.M., not to exceed 100 mg, with no more than 5 ml injected in any one site or 4 to 5 mg/kg rectally.

Acute tetanus convulsion—
Adults and children: 5.5 mg/kg I.M.
or slow I.V., repeated q 3 to 4 hours, if
needed; I.V. injection rate not to exceed 50 mg per 15 seconds.
Acute psychotic agitation—
Adults: 50 mg/minute I.V. up to 250
mg I.V. initially, additional doses
given cautiously after 5 minutes if desired response is not obtained. Not to
exceed 500 mg total.
Status epilepticus—
Adults and children: 250 to 350 mg
I.M. or I.V.

ADVERSE REACTIONS
CNS: *drowsiness, lethargy, hangover,*
paradoxical excitement in elderly patients.
GI: nausea, vomiting.
Skin: rash, urticaria.
Other: *Stevens-Johnson syndrome,*
angioedema, exacerbation of porphyria.

INTERACTIONS
*Alcohol or other CNS depressants, in-
cluding narcotic analgesics:* excessive
CNS and respiratory depression. Use
together cautiously.
Griseofulvin: decreased absorption of
griseofulvin.
MAO inhibitors: inhibit metabolism of
barbiturates; may cause prolonged
CNS depression. Reduce barbiturate
dosage.
*Oral anticoagulants, estrogens and
oral contraceptives, doxycycline, corticosteroids:* secobarbital may enhance the metabolism of these drugs.
Monitor for decreased effect.
Rifampin: may decrease barbiturate
levels. Monitor for decreased effect.

NURSING CONSIDERATIONS
• Contraindicated in uncontrolled severe pain, respiratory disease with
dyspnea or obstruction, hypersensitivity to barbiturates, previous addiction
to sedatives, or porphyria. Use with
caution in hepatic or renal impair-

ment; also, in pregnant women with
toxemia or history of bleeding.
• Elderly patients are more sensitive
to the drug's adverse CNS effects. Assess mental status before initiating
therapy.
• Use injection solution within 30
minutes after opening container to
minimize deterioration. Don't use
cloudy solution.
• I.V. injection should be reserved for
emergency treatment and should be
given under close supervision. Be prepared to give artificial respiration.
• Give I.M. injection deeply. Superficial injection may cause pain, sterile
abscess, and sloughing.
• Because barbiturates potentiate narcotics, reduce dose when giving during labor. Excessive dose may cause
respiratory depression in neonate.
• Remove cigarettes of patient receiving hypnotic dose.
• Supervise walking; raise bed rails,
especially for elderly patients.
• May cause drug dependence and severe withdrawal symptoms. Withdraw
barbiturates gradually.
• Prevent hoarding or self-overdosing
by patients who are depressed, suicidal, or drug-dependent, or who have
a history of drug abuse.
• In renal insufficiency, use sterile
drug reconstituted with sterile water
for injection. Avoid commercial solution containing polyethylene glycol; it
may irritate kidneys.
• Secobarbital in polyethylene glycol
must be refrigerated.
• Secobarbital sodium injection not
compatible with lactated Ringer's solution.
• Sterile secobarbital sodium compatible with Ringer's injection and normal saline solution. Don't mix with
acidic solutions.
• To reconstitute, rotate ampule. Do
not shake.
• Watch for signs of barbiturate toxicity: coma, pupillary construction,
cyanosis, clammy skin, and hypoten-

sion. Overdose can be fatal.
• Morning "hangover" common after hypnotic dose.
• Hypnotic doses suppress REM sleep. When drug is discontinued, patient may experience increased dreaming.

talbutal
Lotusate
Controlled Substance Schedule III

Pregnancy Risk Category: D

MECHANISM OF ACTION
Probably interferes with transmission of impulses from the thalamus to the cortex of the brain. A barbiturate.

INDICATIONS & DOSAGE
Insomnia—
Adults: 120 mg P.O. h.s.

ADVERSE REACTIONS
CNS: *drowsiness, lethargy, hangover,* paradoxical excitement in elderly patients.
GI: nausea, vomiting.
Skin: rash, urticaria.
Other: *Stevens-Johnson syndrome,* angioedema, exacerbation of porphyria.

INTERACTIONS
Alcohol or other CNS depressants, including narcotic analgesics: excessive CNS and respiratory depression. Use together cautiously.
Griseofulvin: decreased absorption of griseofulvin.
MAO inhibitors: inhibit the metabolism of barbiturates; may cause prolonged CNS depression. Reduce barbiturate dosage.
Oral anticoagulants, estrogens and oral contraceptives, doxycycline, corticosteroids: talbutal may enhance the metabolism of these drugs. Monitor for decreased effect.
Rifampin: may decrease barbiturate levels. Monitor for decreased effect.

NURSING CONSIDERATIONS
• Contraindicated in uncontrolled severe pain, respiratory disease with dyspnea or obstruction, hypersensitivity to barbiturates, previous addiction to sedatives, or porphyria. Use with caution in hepatic or renal impairment.
• Remove cigarettes of patient receiving hypnotic dose.
• Supervise walking; raise bed rails, especially for elderly patients.
• May cause drug dependence and severe withdrawal symptoms. Withdraw barbiturates gradually.
• Prevent hoarding or self-overdosing by patients who are depressed, suicidal, or drug-dependent, or who have a history of drug abuse.
• Watch for signs of barbiturate toxicity: coma, pupillary constriction, cyanosis, clammy skin, and hypotension. Overdose can be fatal.
• Morning "hangover" common after hypnotic dose.
• Hypnotic doses suppress REM sleep. When drug is discontinued, patient may experience increased dreaming.
• Indicated only for short-term management of insomnia. Tolerance to hypnotic effects may develop after approximately 2 weeks.

temazepam
Razepam, Restoril♦, Temaz
Controlled Substance Schedule IV

Pregnancy Risk Category: X

MECHANISM OF ACTION
Acts on the limbic system, thalamus, and hypothalamus of the central nervous system to produce hypnotic effects. A benzodiazepine.

INDICATIONS & DOSAGE
Insomnia—
Adults: 15 to 30 mg P.O. h.s.
Adults over 65 years: 15 mg P.O. h.s.

Italicized side effects are common or life-threatening.
*Liquid form contains alcohol.   **May contain tartrazine.

ADVERSE REACTIONS
CNS: *drowsiness, dizziness, lethargy,* disturbed coordination, daytime sedation, confusion.
GI: anorexia, diarrhea.

INTERACTIONS
Alcohol or CNS depressants, including narcotic analgesics: increased CNS depression. Use together cautiously.

NURSING CONSIDERATIONS
• Use cautiously in impaired hepatic or renal function, mental depression, suicidal tendencies, and history of drug abuse. Use caution and low end of dosage range for elderly or debilitated patients.
• Elderly patients are more sensitive to the drug's adverse CNS effects. Assess mental status before initiating therapy.
• Prevent hoarding or self-overdosing by patients who are depressed, suicidal, or drug-dependent, or who have a history of drug abuse. Warn about increased alcohol effects and against hazardous activity requiring alertness or skill.
• Remove cigarettes of patient receiving drug.
• Supervise walking; raise bed rails, especially for elderly patients.
• May have less residual sedative effects ("hangover") the next day than flurazepam and diazepam. Relatively short-acting.
• May take as long as 2 to 2½ hours for onset of action.

triazolam
Halcion♦
Controlled Substance Schedule IV
Pregnancy Risk Category: X

MECHANISM OF ACTION
Acts on the limbic system, thalamus, and hypothalamus of the central nervous system to produce hypnotic effects. A benzodiazepine.

INDICATIONS & DOSAGE
Insomnia—
Adults: 0.125 to 0.25 mg P.O. h.s.
Adults over 65: 0.125 mg P.O. h.s.
May give up to 0.25 mg.

ADVERSE REACTIONS
CNS: *drowsiness, dizziness, headache,* rebound insomnia, amnesia, light-headedness, lack of coordination, mental confusion.
GI: nausea, vomiting.

INTERACTIONS
Alcohol or other CNS depressants, including narcotic analgesics: excessive CNS depression. Use together cautiously.
Cimetidine, erythromycin: may cause prolonged triazolam blood levels. Monitor for increased sedation.

NURSING CONSIDERATIONS
• Use cautiously in impaired hepatic or renal function, mental depression, suicidal tendencies, or history of drug abuse.
• Elderly patients are more sensitive to the drug's adverse CNS effects. Assess mental status before initiating therapy.
• Prevent hoarding or self-overdosing by patients who are depressed, suicidal, or drug-dependent, or who have a history of drug abuse.
• Remove cigarettes of patient receiving drug.
• Supervise walking; raise bed rails, especially for elderly patients.
• Dependence is possible with long-term use.
• Triazolam is a benzodiazepine compound with similarities to flurazepam. However, it is very short-acting and therefore has less tendency to cause morning drowsiness.
• Faster acting than temazepam, another benzodiazepine derivative.
• Warn patient not to take more than the prescribed amount since overdosage can occur at a total daily dose of 2

mg (or four times the highest recommended amount).

• Tell patient that rebound insomnia may develop for one or two nights after stopping therapy.

Italicized side effects are common or life-threatening.
*Liquid form contains alcohol.   **May contain tartrazine.

30

Anticonvulsants

acetazolamide sodium
   (See Chapter 63, DIURETICS.)
carbamazepine
clonazepam
diazepam
   (See Chapter 32, ANTIANXIETY AGENTS.)
ethosuximide
ethotoin
magnesium sulfate
mephenytoin
mephobarbital
metharbital
methsuximide
paraldehyde
paramethadione
phenacemide
phenobarbital
phenobarbital sodium
phensuximide
phenytoin
phenytoin sodium
phenytoin sodium (extended)
phenytoin sodium (prompt)
primidone
trimethadione
valproate sodium
valproic acid
divalproex sodium

COMBINATION PRODUCTS
DILANTIN WITH PHENOBARBITAL♦:
phenytoin sodium 100 mg and phenobarbital 16 mg.
DILANTIN WITH PHENOBARBITAL♦:
phenytoin sodium 100 mg and phenobarbital 32 mg.

carbamazepine
Apo-Carbamazepine♦♦, Epitol,
Mazepine♦♦, Tegretol♦, Tegretol
CR♦♦

Pregnancy Risk Category: C

MECHANISM OF ACTION
Stabilizes neuronal membranes and
limits seizure activity by either increasing efflux or decreasing influx of
sodium ions across cell membranes in
the motor cortex during generation of
nerve impulses.

INDICATIONS & DOSAGE
*Generalized tonic-clonic (grand mal)
and complex-partial (psychomotor)
seizures, mixed seizure patterns—*
Adults and children over 12 years:
initially, 200 mg P.O. b.i.d. May increase by 200 mg P.O. daily, in divided doses at 6- to 8-hour intervals.
Adjust to minimum effective level
when control achieved.
Children under 12 years: 10 to 20
mg/kg P.O. daily in two to four divided doses.
Trigeminal neuralgia—
Adults: initially, 100 mg P.O. b.i.d.
with meals. Increase by 100 mg q 12
hours until pain is relieved. Don't exceed 1.2 g daily. Maintenance dose is
200 to 400 mg P.O. b.i.d.

ADVERSE REACTIONS
Blood: *aplastic anemia, agranulocytosis,* eosinophilia, leukocytosis,
thrombocytopenia.
CNS: dizziness, *vertigo, drowsiness,*
fatigue, *ataxia,* worsening of sei-

zures.
CV: CHF, hypertension, hypotension, aggravation of coronary artery disease.
EENT: conjunctivitis, dry mouth and pharynx, blurred vision, diplopia, nystagmus.
GI: *nausea,* vomiting, abdominal pain, diarrhea, anorexia, *stomatitis,* glossitis.
GU: urinary frequency, urine retention, impotence, albuminuria, glycosuria, elevated BUN.
Hepatic: abnormal liver function tests, hepatitis.
Metabolic: water intoxication.
Skin: *rash,* urticaria, erythema multiforme, *Stevens-Johnson syndrome.*
Other: diaphoresis, fever, chills, pulmonary hypersensitivity.

INTERACTIONS
Phenytoin, primidone, phenobarbital, nicotinic acid: may decrease carbamazepine levels. Monitor for decreased effect.
Phenytoin, warfarin, doxycycline, theophylline, haloperidol: carbamazepine may decrease blood levels of these drugs. Monitor for decreased effect.
Propoxyphene: may raise carbamazepine levels. Use another analgesic.
Troleandomycin, erythromycin, isoniazid: may increase carbamazepine blood levels. Use cautiously.

NURSING CONSIDERATIONS
• Contraindicated in bone marrow suppression, or hypersensitivity to carbamazepine or tricyclic antidepressants. Use cautiously in cardiac, renal, or hepatic damage and increased intraocular pressure.
• Warn patient to avoid activities that require alertness and good psychomotor coordination until CNS effects of the drug are known.
• May cause mild to moderate dizziness and drowsiness when first taken. Effect usually disappears within 3 to 4

days. Should be taken three times a day, when possible, to provide consistent blood levels.
• Observe for signs of anorexia or subtle appetite changes, which may indicate excessive blood levels.
• Never stop the drug suddenly when treating seizures or status epilepticus. Notify doctor immediately if side effects occur.
• Obtain CBC, platelet and reticulocyte counts, and serum iron levels weekly for first 3 months, then monthly. If bone marrow suppression develops, stop drug. Obtain urinalysis, BUN, and liver function tests every 3 months. Periodic eye examinations are recommended.
• Tell patient to notify doctor immediately if fever, sore throat, mouth ulcers, or easy bruising occurs.
• Therapeutic carbamazepine blood level is 3 to 9 mcg/ml.
• Monitor blood levels and effects closely. Ask patient when last dose of medication was taken to approximately evaluate blood levels.
• When used for trigeminal neuralgia, an attempt should be made every 3 months to decrease dosage or stop drug.
• Chewable tablets are available for children.
• Generally reserved for seizures unresponsive to other anticonvulsants.
• Adverse effects may be minimized by increasing dosage gradually.
• An alternative to lithium in treatment of some affective disorders.
• Patient may take with food to minimize GI distress.

clonazepam
Klonopin, Rivotril♦
Controlled Substance Schedule IV
Pregnancy Risk Category: C

MECHANISM OF ACTION
Appears to act on the limbic system, thalamus, and hypothalamus to pro-

duce anticonvulsant effects. A benzodiazepine.

INDICATIONS & DOSAGE
*Absence (petit mal) and atypical ab-
sence seizures; akinetic and myoclonic
seizures—*
Adults: initial dosage should not exceed 1.5 mg P.O. daily, in three divided doses. May be increased by 0.5
to 1 mg q 3 days until seizures are
controlled. Maximum recommended
daily dosage is 20 mg.
Children up to 10 years or 30 kg:
0.01 to 0.03 mg/kg P.O. daily (not to
exceed 0.05 mg/kg daily), divided q 8
hours. Increase dosage by 0.25 to 0.5
mg q third day to a maximum maintenance dosage of 0.1 to 0.2 mg/kg
daily.

ADVERSE REACTIONS
Blood: leukopenia, thrombocytopenia, eosinophilia.
CNS: *drowsiness, ataxia, behavioral
disturbances (especially in children),*
slurred speech, tremor, confusion.
EENT: *increased salivation,* diplopia, nystagmus, abnormal eye movements.
GI: constipation, gastritis, change in
appetite, nausea, abnormal thirst,
sore gums.
GU: dysuria, enuresis, nocturia, urinary retention.
Skin: rash.
Other: respiratory depression.

INTERACTIONS
Alcohol, CNS depressants: increased
CNS depression. Monitor closely.

NURSING CONSIDERATIONS
• Contraindicated in hepatic disease;
chlordiazepoxide, diazepam, or other
benzodiazepine sensitivity; or acute
narrow-angle glaucoma. Use with
caution in chronic respiratory disease,
impaired renal function, and open-
angle glaucoma.
• Elderly patients are more sensitive

to the drug's CNS effects.
• Warn patient to avoid activities that
require alertness and good psychomotor coordination until CNS effects of
the drug are known.
• Never withdraw drug suddenly. Call
doctor at once if adverse effects develop.
• Obtain periodic CBC and liver
function tests.
• Monitor patient for oversedation.
• Withdrawal symptoms similar to
those of barbiturates.

ethosuximide
Zarontin♦

Pregnancy Risk Category: C

MECHANISM OF ACTION
Increases seizure threshold. Reduces
the paroxysmal spike-and-wave pattern of absence seizures by depressing
nerve transmission in the motor cortex. A succinimide derivative.

INDICATIONS & DOSAGE
Absence (petit mal) seizure—
Adults and children over 6 years:
initially, 250 mg P.O. b.i.d. May increase by 250 mg q 4 to 7 days up to
1.5 g daily.
Children 3 to 6 years: 250 mg P.O.
daily or 125 mg P.O. b.i.d. May increase by 250 mg q 4 to 7 days up to
1.5 g daily.

ADVERSE REACTIONS
Blood: leukopenia, eosinophilia,
agranulocytosis, pancytopenia, *aplastic anemia.*
CNS: *drowsiness,* headache, *fatigue,
dizziness,* ataxia, irritability, hiccups,
euphoria, lethargy.
EENT: myopia.
GI: *nausea, vomiting,* diarrhea, gum
hypertrophy, weight loss, cramps,
tongue swelling, *anorexia, epigastric
and abdominal pain.*
GU: vaginal bleeding.
Skin: urticaria, pruritic and erythem-

atous rashes, hirsutism.

INTERACTIONS
None significant.

NURSING CONSIDERATIONS
• Contraindicated in hypersensitivity to succinimide derivatives. Use cautiously in hepatic or renal disease.
• Never withdraw drug suddenly. Abrupt withdrawal may precipitate absence seizures. Call doctor immediately if adverse effects develop.
• Warn patient to avoid activities that require alertness and good psychomotor coordination until CNS effects of the drug are known.
• Obtain CBC every 3 months.
• Therapeutic blood levels 40 to 80 mcg/ml.
• May increase frequency of generalized tonic-clonic seizures when used alone in patients who have mixed types of seizures.
• May cause positive direct Coombs' test.
• Currently the drug of choice for treating absence seizures.
• Patient may take with food to minimize GI distress.

---

ethotoin
Peganone

Pregnancy Risk Category: D

MECHANISM OF ACTION
Stabilizes neuronal membranes and limits seizure activity by either increasing efflux or decreasing influx of sodium ions across cell membranes in the motor cortex during generation of nerve impulses. Hydantoin derivative.

INDICATIONS & DOSAGE
Generalized tonic-clonic (grand mal) or complex-partial (psychomotor) seizures—
Adults: initially, 250 mg P.O. q.i.d. after meals. May increase slowly over several days to 3 g daily divided q.i.d.

Children: initially, 250 mg P.O. b.i.d. May increase up to 250 mg P.O. q.i.d.

ADVERSE REACTIONS
Blood: thrombocytopenia, leukopenia, *agranulocytosis*, pancytopenia, megaloblastic anemia.
CNS: fatigue, insomnia, dizziness, headache, numbness.
CV: chest pain.
EENT: diplopia, nystagmus.
GI: *nausea, vomiting, diarrhea*, gingival hyperplasia (rare).
Skin: rash.
Other: fever, lymphadenopathy.

INTERACTIONS
Alcohol, folic acid: monitor for decreased ethotoin activity.
Oral anticoagulants, antihistamines, chloramphenicol, cimetidine, diazepam, diazoxide, disulfiram, isoniazid, phenylbutazone, salicylates, sulfamethizole, valproate: monitor for increased ethotoin activity and toxicity.
Phenacemide: paranoia. Use together cautiously.

NURSING CONSIDERATIONS
• Contraindicated in hydantoin hypersensitivity or hepatic or hematologic disorders. Use cautiously in patients receiving other hydantoin derivatives.
• Never withdraw drug suddenly. Call doctor at once if adverse effects develop.
• Warn patient to avoid activities that require alertness and good psychomotor coordination until CNS effects of the drug are known.
• Obtain CBC and urinalysis when therapy starts and monthly thereafter. Periodically monitor liver function tests on long-term use.
• Give after meals. Schedule doses as evenly as possible over 24 hours.
• Discontinue drug if lymphadenopathy or lupus-like syndrome (fever, bruising, and sore throat) develops.

Italicized side effects are common or life-threatening.
*Liquid form contains alcohol.   **May contain tartrazine.

• Heavy use of alcohol may diminish benefits of drug.
• Hydantoin derivative of choice in young adults who are prone to gingival hyperplasia caused by phenytoin. Otherwise, infrequently used in the treatment of epilepsy.
• Ethotoin generally produces milder adverse effects than phenytoin; however, the large doses required to maintain its therapeutic effect frequently cause GI distress.

magnesium sulfate

Pregnancy Risk Category: B

MECHANISM OF ACTION

May decrease acetylcholine released by nerve impulse, but its anticonvulsant mechanism is unknown.

INDICATIONS & DOSAGE

Hypomagnesemic seizures—
Adults: 1 to 2 g (as 10% solution) I.V. over 15 minutes, then 1 g I.M. q 4 to 6 hours, based on patient response and blood magnesium levels.
Seizures secondary to hypomagnesemia in acute nephritis—
Children: 0.2 ml/kg of 50% solution I.M. q 4 to 6 hours, p.r.n. or 100 mg/kg of 10% solution I.V. very slowly. Titrate dosage according to blood magnesium levels and seizure response.
Prevention or control of seizures in preeclampsia or eclampsia—
Women: initially, 4 g I.V. in 250 ml dextrose 5% in water and 4 g deep I.M. each buttock; then 4 g deep I.M. into alternate buttock q 4 hours, p.r.n. Alternatively, 4 g I.V. loading dose followed by 1 to 4 g hourly as an I.V. infusion.

ADVERSE REACTIONS

CNS: *sweating,* drowsiness, *depressed reflexes,* flaccid paralysis, hypothermia.
CV: *hypotension, flushing, circula-*tory collapse, depressed cardiac function, *heart block.*
Other: *respiratory paralysis,* hypocalcemia.

INTERACTIONS

Neuromuscular blocking agents: may cause increased neuromuscular blockade. Use cautiously.

NURSING CONSIDERATIONS

• Use cautiously in impaired renal function, myocardial damage, and heart block, and in women in labor.
• Magnesium sulfate can decrease the frequency and force of uterine contractions.
• Keep I.V. calcium gluconate available to reverse magnesium intoxication; however, use cautiously in patients undergoing digitalization due to danger of dysrhythmias.
• Monitor vital signs every 15 minutes when giving drug I.V.
• Watch for respiratory depression and signs of heart block. Respirations should be approximately 16/minute before each dose given.
• Monitor intake/output. Urine output should be 100 ml or more in 4-hour period before each dose.
• Check blood magnesium levels after repeated doses. Disappearance of knee-jerk and patellar reflexes is a sign of pending magnesium toxicity.
• Maximum infusion rate is 150 mg/minute. Rapid drip will induce uncomfortable feeling of heat.
• Especially when given I.V. to toxemic mothers within 24 hours before delivery, observe neonates for signs of magnesium toxicity, including neuromuscular or respiratory depression.
• Signs of hypermagnesemia begin to appear at blood levels of 4 mEq/liter.
• Has been used as a tocolytic agent (suppresses uterine contractions) to inhibit premature labor.

---

mephenytoin
Mesantoin♦

Pregnancy Risk Category: C

MECHANISM OF ACTION
Stabilizes neuronal membranes and limits seizure activity by either increasing efflux or decreasing influx of sodium ions across cell membranes in the motor cortex during generation of nerve impulses. Hydantoin derivative.

INDICATIONS & DOSAGE
Generalized tonic-clonic (grand mal) or complex-partial (psychomotor) seizures—
Adults: 50 to 100 mg P.O. daily. May increase by 50 to 100 mg at weekly intervals up to 200 mg P.O. t.i.d.
Children: initially, 50 to 100 mg P.O. daily or 100 to 450 mg/m² P.O. daily in three divided doses. May increase slowly by 50 to 100 mg at weekly intervals up to 200 mg P.O. t.i.d., divided q 8 hours. Dosage must be adjusted individually.

ADVERSE REACTIONS
Blood: *leukopenia,* neutropenia, *agranulocytosis,* thrombocytopenia, pancytopenia, eosinophilia.
CNS: ataxia, *drowsiness,* fatigue, irritability, choreiform movements, depression, tremor, sleeplessness, dizziness (usually transient).
EENT: conjunctivitis, diplopia, nystagmus.
GI: gingival hyperplasia, nausea and vomiting (with prolonged use).
Skin: *rashes, exfoliative dermatitis.*
Other: hypertrichosis, edema, dysarthria, lymphadenopathy, polyarthropathy, pulmonary fibrosis, photosensitivity.

INTERACTIONS
Alcohol, folic acid: monitor for decreased mephenytoin activity.
Oral anticoagulants, antihistamines, chloramphenicol, cimetidine, diazepam, diazoxide, disulfiram, isoniazid, phenylbutazone, salicylates, sulfamethizole, valproate: monitor for increased mephenytoin activity and toxicity.

NURSING CONSIDERATIONS
• Contraindicated in hydantoin hypersensitivity. Use cautiously in patients receiving other hydantoin derivatives.
• Tell patient to notify doctor if fever, sore throat, bleeding, or rash occurs.
• Periodically monitor liver function studies with long-term use. Check CBC and platelet count initially and every 2 weeks thereafter, up to 2 weeks after full dose is attained; then monthly for first year and every 3 months thereafter. Discontinue drug if neutrophil count becomes less than 1,600/mm³.
• Never withdraw drug suddenly. Call doctor if adverse effects develop.
• Warn patient to avoid activities that require alertness and good psychomotor coordination until CNS effects of the drug are known.
• Therapeutic blood level of mephenytoin and its active metabolite is 25 to 40 mcg/ml.
• Heavy use of alcohol may diminish benefit of drug.
• Potentially life-threatening blood dyscrasias limit this drug's usefulness.

mephobarbital
Mebaral♦
Controlled Substance Schedule IV

Pregnancy Risk Category: D

MECHANISM OF ACTION
Depresses monosynaptic and polysynaptic transmission in the CNS and increases the threshold for seizure activity in the motor cortex. A barbiturate.

INDICATIONS & DOSAGE
Generalized tonic-clonic (grand mal)

or absence (petit mal) seizures—
Adults: 400 to 600 mg P.O. daily or in divided doses.
Children: 6 to 12 mg/kg P.O. daily, divided q 6 to 8 hours (smaller doses are given initially and increased over 4 to 5 days as needed).

ADVERSE REACTIONS
Blood: megaloblastic anemia, *agranulocytosis,* thrombocytopenia.
CNS: *dizziness,* headache, *hangover,* confusion, paradoxical excitation, exacerbation of existing pain, drowsiness.
CV: hypotension, bradycardia.
GI: nausea, vomiting, epigastric pain.
Skin: urticaria, morbilliform rash, blisters, purpura, erythema multiforme.
Other: allergic reactions (facial edema).

INTERACTIONS
Alcohol and other CNS depressants, including narcotic analgesics: excessive CNS depression. Use cautiously.
Griseofulvin: decreased absorption of griseofulvin.
MAO inhibitors: potentiated barbiturate effect. Monitor patient for increased CNS and respiratory depression.
Oral anticoagulants, estrogens and oral contraceptives, doxycycline, corticosteroids: mephobarbital may enhance the metabolism of these drugs. Monitor for decreased effect.
Rifampin: may decrease barbiturate levels. Monitor for decreased effect.

NURSING CONSIDERATIONS
• Contraindicated in barbiturate hypersensitivity, porphyria, or respiratory disease with dyspnea or obstruction. Use cautiously in hepatic, renal, cardiac, or respiratory function impairment; myasthenia gravis; and myxedema.
• Never withdraw drug suddenly. Call

doctor at once if adverse effects develop.
• Warn patient to avoid activities that require alertness and good psychomotor coordination until CNS effects of drug are known.
• Store in light-resistant container.
• In adults, give total or largest dose at night if seizures occur then.
• Three-quarters of drug is metabolized to phenobarbital; therapeutic blood levels as phenobarbital are 15 to 40 mcg/ml.
• Periodically monitor CBC, BUN, and creatinine.
• Women who use oral contraceptives should consider alternate birth control methods when receiving this drug because it may enhance contraceptive hormone metabolism and decrease its effectiveness.
• Suppresses REM sleep, as do other barbiturates. When drug is discontinued, patient may experience increased dreaming.

---

metharbital
Gemonil
Controlled Substance Schedule III
Pregnancy Risk Category: D

MECHANISM OF ACTION
Depresses monosynaptic and polysynaptic transmission in the CNS and increases the threshold for seizure activity in the motor cortex. A barbiturate.

INDICATIONS & DOSAGE
Generalized tonic-clonic (grand mal) or absence (petit mal) seizures; myoclonic or mixed seizures—
Adults: initially, 100 mg P.O. daily to t.i.d. May increase to 800 mg daily in divided doses.
Children: 5 to 15 mg/kg P.O. daily, divided t.i.d. May increase to 50 to 100 mg P.O. daily, b.i.d., or t.i.d.

ADVERSE REACTIONS
Blood: megaloblastic anemia, *agranulocytosis,* thrombocytopenia.
CNS: *dizziness,* irritability, *drowsiness,* headache, confusion, excitation.
CV: hypotension.
GI: nausea, vomiting, discomfort.
Skin: rash, urticaria, purpura, erythema multiforme.

INTERACTIONS
Alcohol and other CNS depressants, including narcotic analgesics: excessive CNS depression. Use cautiously.
Griseofulvin: decreased absorption of griseofulvin.
MAO inhibitors: potentiated barbiturate effect. Monitor patient for increased CNS and respiratory depression.
Oral anticoagulants, estrogens and oral contraceptives, doxycycline, corticosteroids: metharbital may enhance the metabolism of these drugs. Monitor for decreased effect.
Rifampin: may decrease barbiturate levels. Monitor for decreased effect.

NURSING CONSIDERATIONS
• Contraindicated in barbiturate hypersensitivity, manifest or latent porphyria, or respiratory disease with dyspnea or obstruction. Use cautiously in hepatic, cardiac, or renal impairment.
• Don't stop drug abruptly. Call doctor at once if adverse effects develop.
• Warn patient to avoid activities that require alertness and good psychomotor coordination until CNS effects of the drug are known.
• Periodically monitor CBC, BUN, and creatinine.
• Women who use oral contraceptives should consider alternate birth control methods when receiving this drug because it may enhance contraceptive hormone metabolism and decrease its effectiveness.
• Seldom-used anticonvulsant. More sedative effects than phenobarbital.

methsuximide
Celontin♦

Pregnancy Risk Category: C

MECHANISM OF ACTION
Increases seizure threshold. Reduces the paroxysmal spike-and-wave pattern of absence seizures by depressing nerve transmission in the motor cortex. A succinimide derivative.

INDICATIONS & DOSAGE
Refractory absence (petit mal) seizures—
Adults and children: initially, 300 mg P.O. daily. May increase by 300 mg weekly. Maximum daily dosage is 1.2 g in divided doses.

ADVERSE REACTIONS
Blood: eosinophilia, leukopenia, monocytosis, pancytopenia.
CNS: *drowsiness, ataxia, dizziness,* irritability, nervousness, headache, insomnia, confusion, depression, aggressiveness.
EENT: blurred vision, photophobia, periorbital edema.
GI: *nausea, vomiting, anorexia,* diarrhea, weight loss, abdominal or epigastric pain.
Skin: urticaria, pruritic and erythematous rashes.

INTERACTIONS
None significant.

NURSING CONSIDERATIONS
• Contraindicated in hypersensitivity to succinimide derivatives. Use cautiously in hepatic or renal dysfunction.
• Never change or withdraw drug suddenly. Abrupt withdrawal may precipitate petit mal seizures. Call doctor immediately if adverse effects develop.
• Warn patient to avoid activities that require alertness and good psychomotor coordination until CNS effects of

---

Italicized side effects are common or life-threatening.
*Liquid form contains alcohol.   **May contain tartrazine.

the drug are known.
- Obtain CBC every 3 months; urinalysis and liver function tests every 6 months.
- Tell patient to call doctor promptly if lupus-like syndrome develops.
- May color urine pink or brown.
- Not as popular an anticonvulsant as ethosuximide.

---

paraldehyde
Paral
Controlled Substance Schedule IV
Pregnancy Risk Category: C

MECHANISM OF ACTION
Unknown.

INDICATIONS & DOSAGE
Refractory generalized tonic-clonic (grand mal) seizures, status epilepticus—
Adults: 5 to 10 ml I.M. (divide 10 ml dose into 2 injections); 0.2 to 0.4 ml/kg in 0.9% saline injection I.V.
Children: 0.15 ml/kg dose deep I.M. q 4 to 6 hours, p.r.n.; or 0.3 ml/kg rectally in olive oil q 4 to 6 hours; or 1 ml per year of age not to exceed 5 ml, repeated in 1 hour, p.r.n.; or dilute 5 ml in 95 ml 0.9% saline injection for I.V. infusion and titrate dose beginning at 5 ml/hour.
Sedation—
Adults: 4 to 10 ml P.O. or rectally; or 5 ml deep I.M. in upper outer quadrant of buttock. 3 to 5 ml I.V. (in emergency only).
Children: 0.15 ml/kg P.O., rectally, or deep I.M.
Insomnia—
Adults: 10 to 30 ml P.O. or rectally; 10 ml I.M. or I.V.
Children: 0.3 ml/kg P.O., rectally, or deep I.M.
Alcohol withdrawal syndrome—
Adults: 5 to 10 ml P.O. or rectally; or 5 ml deep I.M. q 4 to 6 hours for the first 24 hours, not to exceed a total of 60 ml P.O. or 30 ml I.M.; then q 6

hours on following days, not to exceed 40 ml P.O. or 20 ml I.M. per 24 hours.
Tetanus—
Adults: 4 to 5 ml I.V. (well diluted) or 12 ml (diluted 1:10) via gastric tube q 4 hours, p.r.n.; 5 to 10 ml I.M., p.r.n. to control seizures.

ADVERSE REACTIONS
CNS: confusion, tremor, weakness, irritability, dizziness.
CV: *I.V. administration may cause pulmonary edema or hemorrhage,* dilatation of right side of heart, *circulatory collapse.*
GI: irritation, *foul breath odor.*
GU: nephrosis with prolonged use.
Skin: *erythematous rash.*
Local: *pain,* sterile abscesses, sloughing of skin, fat necrosis, muscular irritation, nerve damage (if injection is near nerve trunk) at I.M. injection site.
Other: respiratory depression.

INTERACTIONS
Alcohol: increased CNS depression. Use with caution.
Disulfiram: increased paraldehyde and acetaldehyde blood levels; possible toxic disulfiram reaction. Use together cautiously.

NURSING CONSIDERATIONS
- Contraindicated in gastroenteritis with ulceration. Use cautiously in impaired hepatic function and asthma or other pulmonary disease.
- Use fresh supply. Don't expose to air. Don't use if liquid is brown or has a vinegary odor, or if container has been open longer than 24 hours.
- Watch closely for respiratory depression, especially in repeated doses.
- Dilute paraldehyde in olive oil or cottonseed oil 1:2 for rectal administration. Give as retention enema. May also use 200 ml normal saline solution to prepare enema.
- Keep patient's room well ventilated

---

to remove exhaled paraldehyde.
• May cause drug dependence and severe withdrawal symptoms.
• Oral or rectal administration of decomposed paraldehyde may cause severe corrosion of stomach or rectum.
• Dilute oral dose with iced juice or milk to mask taste and odor and to reduce GI distress.
• Parenteral form may be difficult to obtain commercially. Check with pharmacy for availability.
• Paraldehyde is rarely given parenterally because of the availability of less toxic alternatives. I.V. administration is not advisable except in extreme emergencies.
• Drug reacts with plastic. Use glass syringe and bottle for parenteral dose. Prepare fresh I.V. solution every 4 hours. I.V. administration very hazardous.
• Give I.M. dose deeply, away from nerve trunks; massage injection site. Limit I.M. volume to a maximum of 5 ml at any one site.

paramethadione
Paradione♦* **

Pregnancy Risk Category: D

MECHANISM OF ACTION
Raises the threshold for cortical seizures but does not modify seizure pattern. Decreases projection of focal activity and reduces both repetitive spinal-cord transmission and spike-and-wave patterns of absence (petit mal) seizures.

INDICATIONS & DOSAGE
Refractory absence (petit mal) seizures—
Adults: initially, 300 mg P.O. t.i.d. May increase by 300 mg weekly, up to 600 mg q.i.d., if needed.
Children over 6 years: 0.9 g P.O. daily in divided doses t.i.d. or q.i.d.
Children 2 to 6 years: 0.6 g P.O. daily in divided doses t.i.d. or q.i.d.

Children under 2 years: 0.3 g P.O. daily in divided doses b.i.d.

ADVERSE REACTIONS
Blood: neutropenia, leukopenia, eosinophilia, thrombocytopenia, pancytopenia, *agranulocytosis, hypoplastic and aplastic anemia.*
CNS: *drowsiness,* fatigue, vertigo, headache, paresthesias, irritability.
CV: hypertension, hypotension.
EENT: hemeralopia, photophobia, diplopia, epistaxis, retinal hemorrhage.
GI: nausea, vomiting, abdominal pain, weight loss, bleeding gums.
GU: albuminuria, vaginal bleeding.
Hepatic: abnormal liver function tests.
Skin: acneiform or morbilliform rash, *exfoliative dermatitis,* erythema multiforme, petechiae, alopecia.
Other: lymphadenopathy, lupus erythematosus.

INTERACTIONS
None significant.

NURSING CONSIDERATIONS
• Contraindicated in renal and hepatic dysfunction or severe blood dyscrasias. Use cautiously in retinal or optic nerve diseases.
• Never withdraw drug suddenly. Call doctor at once if adverse effects develop.
• Discontinue drug if scotomata or signs of hepatitis, systemic lupus erythematosus, lymphadenopathy, skin rash, nephrosis, hair loss, or generalized tonic-clonic seizures appear.
• Tell patient to report sore throat, fever, malaise, bruises, petechiae, or epistaxis to doctor immediately. Advise patient to wear dark glasses if photosensitivity occurs. Warn him not to drive car or operate machinery until CNS effects of the drug are known.
• Obtain liver function studies and urinalysis before therapy; then monthly.

Italicized side effects are common or life-threatening.
*Liquid form contains alcohol.   **May contain tartrazine.

- Dilute oral solution with water before giving because it contains 65% alcohol.
- Give drug with food or milk to minimize GI upset.
- Monitor CBC. Discontinue drug if neutrophil count falls below 2,500/mm³.

---

phenacemide
Phenurone

Pregnancy Risk Category: D

MECHANISM OF ACTION
Stabilizes neuronal membranes and limits seizure activity by either increasing efflux or decreasing influx of sodium ions across cell membranes in the motor cortex during generation of nerve impulses. Hydantoin derivative.

INDICATIONS & DOSAGE
Refractory, complex-partial (psychomotor), generalized tonic-clonic (grand mal), absence (petit mal), and atypical absence seizures—
Adults: 500 mg P.O. t.i.d. May increase by 500 mg weekly up to 5 g daily, p.r.n.
Children 5 to 10 years: 250 mg P.O. t.i.d. May increase by 250 mg weekly, up to 1.5 g daily, p.r.n.

ADVERSE REACTIONS
Blood: *aplastic anemia, agranulocytosis,* leukopenia.
CNS: drowsiness, dizziness, insomnia, headaches, paresthesias, *depression, suicidal tendencies,* aggressiveness.
GI: anorexia, weight loss.
GU: nephritis with marked albuminuria.
Hepatic: hepatitis, jaundice.
Skin: rashes.

INTERACTIONS
Anticonvulsants: enhanced risk of toxicity.
Ethotoin: paranoia. Use together cautiously.

NURSING CONSIDERATIONS
- Contraindicated in patients with preexisting personality disturbances or in patients achieving satisfactory seizure control with other anticonvulsants. Use with caution in patients with hepatic dysfunction or history of allergy, and when a hydantoin derivative is used concomitantly.
- Extremely toxic. Use drug only when other anticonvulsants are ineffective.
- Obtain liver function tests, CBCs, and urinalyses before and at monthly intervals during therapy.
- Tell patient to report sore throat or fever to doctor immediately.
- Warn patient to avoid activities that require alertness or good psychomotor coordination until CNS effects of the drug are known.
- Never withdraw drug suddenly. Call doctor at once if adverse effects develop.
- Tell patient's family to watch for personality or psychological changes and report them to doctor at once.
- When phenacemide replaces another anticonvulsant, phenacemide dosage should be increased slowly while the dosage of the drug being discontinued is decreased slowly to maintain adequate seizure control.
- Notify doctor if patient develops jaundice or other signs of hepatitis, abnormal urinary findings, or WBC count below 4,000/mm³.

phenobarbital
Barbita, Gardenal◆◆, Luminal◆◆, Solfoton

phenobarbital sodium
Luminal Sodium◆◆
Controlled Substance Schedule IV

Pregnancy Risk Category: D

MECHANISM OF ACTION
Depresses monosynaptic and polysynaptic transmission in the CNS and increases the threshold for seizure activity in the motor cortex. As a sedative, probably interferes with transmission of impulses from the thalamus to the cortex of the brain. A barbiturate.

INDICATIONS & DOSAGE
All forms of epilepsy, febrile seizures in children—
Adults: 100 to 200 mg P.O. daily, divided t.i.d. or given as single dosage at bedtime.
Children: 4 to 6 mg/kg P.O. daily, usually divided q 12 hours. It can, however, be administered once daily.
Status epilepticus—
Adults: 10 mg/kg as I.V. infusion no faster than 50 mg/minute. May give up to 20 mg/kg total. Administer in acute care or emergency area only.
Children: 5 to 10 mg/kg I.V. May repeat q 10 to 15 minutes up to total of 20 mg/kg. I.V. injection rate should not exceed 50 mg/minute.
Sedation—
Adults: 30 to 120 mg P.O. daily in two or three divided doses.
Children: 6 mg/kg P.O. divided t.i.d.
Insomnia—
Adults: 100 to 320 mg P.O. or I.M.
Children: 3 to 6 mg/kg.
Preoperative sedation—
Adults: 100 to 200 mg I.M. 60 to 90 minutes before surgery.
Children: 16 to 100 mg I.M. 60 to 90 minutes before surgery.
Hyperbilirubinemia—

Neonates: 7 mg/kg daily P.O. from first to fifth day of life; or 5 mg/kg daily I.M. on first day, repeated P.O. on second to seventh days.
Chronic cholestasis—
Adults: 90 to 180 mg P.O. daily in two or three divided doses.
Children under 12 years: 3 to 12 mg/kg daily P.O. in two or three divided doses.

ADVERSE REACTIONS
CNS: *drowsiness, lethargy, hangover,* paradoxical excitement in elderly patients.
GI: nausea, vomiting.
Skin: rash, *Stevens-Johnson syndrome,* urticaria.
Local: pain, swelling, thrombophlebitis, necrosis, nerve injury.
Other: angioedema.

INTERACTIONS
Alcohol and other CNS depressants, including narcotic analgesics: excessive CNS depression. Use cautiously.
Diazepam: increased effects of both drugs. Use together cautiously.
Griseofulvin: decreased absorption of griseofulvin.
MAO inhibitors: potentiated barbiturate effect. Monitor for increased CNS and respiratory depression.
Oral anticoagulants, estrogens and oral contraceptives, doxycycline, corticosteroids: may enhance the metabolism of these drugs. Monitor for decreased effect.
Primidone: monitor for excessive phenobarbital blood levels.
Rifampin: may decrease barbiturate levels. Monitor for decreased effect.
Valproic acid: increased phenobarbital levels. Monitor for toxicity.

NURSING CONSIDERATIONS
• Contraindicated in barbiturate hypersensitivity, porphyria, hepatic dysfunction, respiratory disease with dyspnea or obstruction, nephritis, and in lactating women. Use cautiously in

---

Italicized side effects are common or life-threatening.
*Liquid form contains alcohol.   **May contain tartrazine.

hyperthyroidism, diabetes mellitus, anemia, and in elderly or debilitated patients.

• Elderly patients are more sensitive to the drug's effects.

• I.V. injection should be reserved for emergency treatment and should be given slowly under close supervision. Monitor respirations closely.

• When administering I.V., do not give more than 60 mg/minute. Have recusitative equipment readily available.

• Give I.M. injection deeply. Superficial injection may cause pain, sterile abscess, and tissue sloughing.

• Do not use injectable solution if it contains a precipitate.

• Do not mix parenteral form with acidic solutions; precipitation may result.

• Watch for signs of barbiturate toxicity: coma, asthmatic breathing, cyanosis, clammy skin, and hypotension. Overdose can be fatal.

• Warn patient to avoid activities that require alertness and good psychomotor coordination until CNS effects of the drug are known.

• Don't stop drug abruptly. Call doctor immediately if adverse effects develop.

• Full therapeutic effects not seen for 2 to 3 weeks, except when loading dose is used.

• Therapeutic blood levels are 15 to 40 mcg/ml.

• Make sure patient is aware that phenobarbital is available in different milligram strengths and sizes.

phensuximide
Milontin♦

Pregnancy Risk Category: D

MECHANISM OF ACTION
Increases seizure threshold. Reduces the paroxysmal spike-and-wave pattern of absence seizures by depressing nerve transmission in the motor cor-

tex. A succinimide derivative.

INDICATIONS & DOSAGE
Absence (petit mal) seizures—
Adults and children: 500 mg to 1 g P.O. b.i.d. to t.i.d.

ADVERSE REACTIONS
Blood: transient leukopenia, pancytopenia, *agranulocytosis.*
CNS: muscular weakness, *drowsiness,* dizziness, ataxia, headache.
GI: nausea, vomiting, anorexia.
GU: urinary frequency, renal damage, hematuria.
Skin: pruritus, eruptions, erythema.
Other: lupus-like syndrome.

INTERACTIONS
None significant.

NURSING CONSIDERATIONS
• Contraindicated in hypersensitivity to succinimide derivatives. Use cautiously in patients with hepatic or renal disease.

• Never withdraw drug suddenly. Abrupt withdrawal may precipitate absence seizures. Call doctor immediately if adverse effects develop.

• Warn patient to avoid hazardous activities that require alertness and good coordination until CNS effects of the drug are known.

• Obtain CBCs every 3 months; urinalyses and liver function tests every 6 months.

• Tell patient to report lupus-like symptoms immediately.

• May color urine pink or red to reddish brown.

• Therapeutic blood level 40 to 80 mcg/ml.

• May increase incidence of generalized tonic-clonic seizures if used alone to treat patients with mixed seizure types.

---

phenytoin
Dilantin

phenytoin sodium
Dilantin♦

phenytoin sodium (extended)
Dilantin Kapseals♦

phenytoin sodium (prompt)
Diphenylan

Pregnancy Risk Category: D

MECHANISM OF ACTION
Stabilizes neuronal membranes and limits seizure activity by either increasing efflux or decreasing influx of sodium ions across cell membranes in the motor cortex during generation of nerve impulses. Produces antiarrhythmic effect by normalizing sodium influx to Purkinje's fibers when used to treat digitalis-induced dysrhythmias. A hydantoin derivative.

INDICATIONS & DOSAGE
Generalized tonic-clonic (grand mal) seizures, status epilepticus, nonepileptic seizures (post-head trauma, Reye's syndrome)—
Adults: loading dose is 900 mg to 1.5 g I.V. at 50 mg/minute or P.O. divided t.i.d., then start maintenance dosage of 300 mg P.O. daily (extended only) or divided t.i.d. (extended or prompt).
Children: loading dose is 15 mg/kg I.V. at 50 mg/minute or P.O. divided q 8 to 12 hours, then start maintenance dosage of 5 to 7 mg/kg P.O. or I.V. daily, divided q 12 hours.
If patient has not received phenytoin previously or has no detectable blood level, use loading dose—
Adults: 900 mg to 1.5 g I.V. divided into t.i.d. at 50 mg/minute. Do not exceed 500 mg each dose.
Children: 15 mg/kg I.V. at 50 mg/minute.
If patient has been receiving phenytoin but has missed one or more doses and has subtherapeutic levels—
Adults: 100 to 300 mg I.V. at 50 mg/minute.
Children: 5 to 7 mg/kg I.V. at 50 mg/minute. May repeat lower dose in 30 minutes if needed.
Neuritic pain (migraine, trigeminal neuralgia, Bell's palsy)—
Adults: 200 to 400 mg P.O. daily.
Ventricular dysrhythmias unresponsive to lidocaine or procainamide; supraventricular and ventricular dysrhythmias induced by cardiac glycosides—
Adults: loading dose is 1 g P.O. divided over first 24 hours, followed by 500 mg daily for 2 days, then maintenance dose of 300 mg P.O. daily; 250 mg I.V. over 5 minutes until dysrhythmias subside, adverse effects develop, or 1 g has been given. Infusion rate should never exceed 50 mg/minute (slow I.V. push).
Alternate method: 100 mg I.V. q 15 minutes until adverse effects develop, dysrhythmias are controlled, or 1 g has been given. May also administer entire loading dose of 1 g I.V. slowly at 25 mg/minute. Can be diluted in normal saline solution. I.M. dose not recommended because of pain and erratic absorption.
Children: 3 to 8 mg/kg P.O. or slow I.V. daily or 250 mg/m² daily given as single dose or in two divided doses.

ADVERSE REACTIONS
Blood: thrombocytopenia, leukopenia, *agranulocytosis*, pancytopenia, macrocytosis, megaloblastic anemia.
CNS: *ataxia, slurred speech, confusion,* dizziness, insomnia, nervousness, twitching, headache.
CV: hypotension, *ventricular fibrillation.*
EENT: *nystagmus, diplopia,* blurred vision.
GI: *nausea, vomiting, gingival hyperplasia (especially children).*

Italicized side effects are common or life-threatening.
*Liquid form contains alcohol.   **May contain tartrazine.

Hepatic: toxic hepatitis.

Skin: scarlatiniform or morbilliform rash; bullous, *exfoliative,* or purpuric *dermatitis; Stevens-Johnson syndrome;* lupus erythematosus; *hirsutism; toxic epidermal necrolysis;* photosensitivity.

Local: pain, necrosis, and inflammation at injection site; purple glove syndrome.

Other: periarteritis nodosa, lymphadenopathy, hyperglycemia, osteomalacia, hypertrichosis.

INTERACTIONS

Alcohol, dexamethasone, folic acid: monitor for decreased phenytoin activity.

Oral anticoagulants, antihistamines, amiodarone, chloramphenicol, cimetidine, cycloserine, diazepam, diazoxide, disulfiram, influenza vaccine, isoniazid, phenylbutazone, salicylates, sulfamethizole, valproate: monitor for increased phenytoin activity and toxicity.

Oral tube feedings with Osmolite or Isocal: may interfere with absorption of oral phenytoin. Schedule feedings as far as possible from drug administration.

NURSING CONSIDERATIONS

• Contraindicated in phenacemide or hydantoin hypersensitivity, bradycardia, SA and AV block, or Stokes-Adams syndrome. Use cautiously in hepatic or renal dysfunction, hypotension, myocardial insufficiency, and respiratory depression; in elderly or debilitated patients; and in patients receiving other hydantoin derivatives.

• Elderly patients tend to metabolize phenytoin slowly. Therefore, they may require lower dosages.

• Phenytoin requirements usually increase during pregnancy. Monitor serum levels closely.

• Don't withdraw drug suddenly. Call doctor at once if adverse effects develop.

• Warn patient to avoid activities that require alertness and good psychomotor coordination until CNS effects of the drug are known.

• Don't mix drug with dextrose 5% in water because it will precipitate. Clear I.V. tubing first with normal saline solution. Never use cloudy solution. May mix with normal saline solution if necessary and give as an infusion. Administer infusion over 30 to 60 minutes, when possible. Infusion must begin within 1 hour after preparation and should run through an in-line filter. Discard 4 hours after preparation. Preferably, administer slowly (50 mg/minute) as an I.V. bolus.

• Do not give I.M. unless dosage adjustments are made. Drug may precipitate at injection site, cause pain, and be erratically absorbed.

• Obtain CBC and serum calcium levels every 6 months, and periodically monitor hepatic function. Doctor may order folic acid and vitamin B_{12} if megaloblastic anemia is evident.

• Drug may color urine pink, red, or reddish-brown.

• Tell patient to carry identification stating that he's taking phenytoin.

• Stress importance of good oral hygiene and regular dental examinations. Gingivectomy may be necessary periodically.

• Drug should be stopped if rash appears. If rash is scarlet or measles-like, drug may be resumed after rash clears. If rash reappears, therapy should be stopped. If rash is exfoliative, purpuric, or bullous, don't resume drug.

• Use only clear solution for injection. Slight yellow color acceptable. Don't refrigerate.

• Avoid administering I.V. push phenytoin injections into veins in the back of the hand. Inject into larger veins to avoid discoloration known as purple glove syndrome.

• Divided doses given with or after meals may decrease GI adverse ef-

fects.
• Available as suspension. Shake well before each dose. Use solid forms (tablets or capsules) if possible.
• Therapeutic phenytoin blood level is 10 to 20 mcg/ml.
• Heavy use of alcohol may diminish benefits of drug.
• Phenytoin levels may be decreased in mononucleosis. Monitor for increased seizure activity.
• Dilantin brand and Bolar generic capsules are the only oral forms that can be given once daily. Toxic levels may result if any other brand is given once daily. Dilantin brand tablets and oral suspension should not be taken once daily.
• Advise patient not to change brands or dosage forms once stabilized on therapy.
• Suspension available as 30 mg/5 ml or 125 mg/5 ml. Read label carefully.
• The drug was formerly known as diphenylhydantoin.
• Also used to treat neuralgia and migraine headache.

primidone
Apo-Primidone♦♦, Myidone, Mysoline♦, Sertan♦♦
Pregnancy Risk Category: D

MECHANISM OF ACTION
Unknown, but some activity may be caused by phenobarbital, which is an active metabolite.

INDICATIONS & DOSAGE
Generalized tonic-clonic (grand mal) seizures, complex-partial (psychomotor) seizures—
Adults and children over 8 years: 250 mg P.O. daily. Increase by 250 mg weekly, up to maximum of 2 g daily, divided q.i.d.
Children under 8 years: 125 mg P.O. daily. Increase by 125 mg weekly, up to maximum of 1 g daily, divided q.i.d.

ADVERSE REACTIONS
Blood: leukopenia, eosinophilia.
CNS: *drowsiness, ataxia,* emotional disturbances, vertigo, hyperirritability, fatigue.
EENT: *diplopia,* nystagmus, edema of the eyelids.
GI: anorexia, *nausea, vomiting.*
GU: impotence, polyuria.
Skin: morbilliform rash, alopecia.
Other: edema, thirst.

INTERACTIONS
Carbamezepine: increased primidone levels. Observe for toxicity.
Phenytoin: stimulated conversion of primidone to phenobarbital. Observe for increased phenobarbital effect.

NURSING CONSIDERATIONS
• Contraindicated in phenobarbital hypersensitivity or porphyria.
• Don't withdraw drug suddenly. Call doctor at once if adverse effects develop.
• Warn patient to avoid hazardous activities that require alertness and good psychomotor coordination until CNS effects of the drug are known. Full therapeutic response may take 2 weeks or more.
• Therapeutic blood level of primidone is 5 to 12 mcg/ml. Therapeutic blood level of phenobarbital is 15 to 40 mcg/ml.
• CBC and routine blood chemistry should be done every 6 months.
• Partially converted to phenobarbital; use cautiously with phenobarbital.
• Shake liquid suspension well.

trimethadione
Tridione
Pregnancy Risk Category: D

MECHANISM OF ACTION
Raises the threshold for cortical seizure but does not modify seizure pattern. Decreases projection of focal activity and reduces both repetitive

spinal-cord transmission and spike-and-wave patterns of absence (petit mal) seizures. An oxazolidinedione derivative.

INDICATIONS & DOSAGE
Refractory absence (petit mal) seizures—
Adults: initially, 300 mg P.O. t.i.d. May increase by 300 mg weekly up to 600 mg P.O. q.i.d.
Children: 13 mg/kg P.O. t.i.d. or 335 mg/m² P.O. t.i.d.; alternatively
Children under 2 years: 100 mg P.O. t.i.d.
Children 2 to 6 years: 200 mg P.O. t.i.d.
Children 6 to 13 years: 300 mg P.O. t.i.d.
Children over 13 years: 400 mg P.O. t.i.d

ADVERSE REACTIONS
Blood: neutropenia, leukopenia, eosinophilia, thrombocytopenia, pancytopenia, *agranulocytosis, hypoplastic and aplastic anemia.*
CNS: *drowsiness,* fatigue, *malaise,* insomnia, dizziness, headache, paresthesias, irritability.
CV: hypertension, hypotension.
EENT: *hemeralopia,* diplopia, photophobia, epistaxis, retinal hemorrhage.
GI: nausea, vomiting, anorexia, abdominal pain, bleeding gums.
GU: nephrosis, albuminuria, vaginal bleeding.
Hepatic: abnormal liver function tests.
Skin: acneiform and morbilliform rash, *exfoliative dermatitis,* erythema multiforme, petechiae, alopecia.
Other: lymphadenopathy, systemic lupus-like syndrome, myasthenia-like syndrome.

INTERACTIONS
None significant.

NURSING CONSIDERATIONS
• Contraindicated in paramethadione and trimethadione hypersensitivity, severe blood dyscrasias, or hepatic dysfunction. Use with extreme caution in retinal and optic nerve diseases.
• Don't withdraw drug suddenly. Abrupt withdrawal may precipitate absence seizures. Call doctor immediately if adverse effects develop.
• Check CBC, hepatic function, and urinalysis before starting therapy and monthly thereafter. Drug should be stopped if neutrophil count falls below 2,500/mm³.
• Watch for impending toxicity; may precipitate tonic-clonic seizure.
• Warn patient to report skin rash, alopecia, sore throat, fever, bruises, or epistaxis to doctor immediately.
• Warn patient to avoid activities requiring alertness and good psychomotor coordination until CNS effects of the drug are known.
• Suggest sunglasses if vision blurs in bright light. Notify doctor.
• If scotomata or rash develops, drug should be discontinued.
• May increase risk of tonic-clonic seizures if used alone to treat patients who have mixed types of seizures.
• Has been largely replaced by succinimide derivatives.

---

valproate sodium
Depakene Syrup♦, Myproic Acid Syrup

valproic acid
Dalpro, Depa, Depakene♦, Myproic Acid

divalproex sodium
Depakote♦, Epival♦♦
Pregnancy Risk Category: D

MECHANISM OF ACTION
Increases brain levels of gamma-aminobutyric acid, which transmits in-

---

hibitory nerve impulses in the CNS.

INDICATIONS & DOSAGE
Simple and complex absence seizures (including petit mal), mixed seizure types (including absence seizures), investigationally in major motor (grand mal, tonic-clonic) seizures—
Adults and children: initially, 15 mg/kg P.O. daily divided b.i.d. or t.i.d.; then may increase by 5 to 10 mg/kg daily at weekly intervals up to maximum of 60 mg/kg daily, divided b.i.d. or t.i.d.

ADVERSE REACTIONS
Because drug usually used in combination with other anticonvulsants, adverse effects reported may not be caused by valproic acid alone.
Blood: *inhibited platelet aggregation, thrombocytopenia, increased bleeding time.*
CNS: *sedation,* emotional upset, depression, psychosis, aggression, hyperactivity, behavioral deterioration, muscle weakness, tremor.
EENT: stomatitis.
GI: *nausea, vomiting,* indigestion, diarrhea, abdominal cramps, constipation, increased appetite and weight gain, *anorexia,* pancreatitis. (*Note:* lower incidence of GI effects with divalproex.)
Hepatic: *elevated enzymes, toxic hepatitis.*
Metabolic: *elevated serum ammonia.*
Other: alopecia.

INTERACTIONS
Antacids, aspirin: May cause valproic acid toxicity. Use together cautiously and monitor blood levels.
Phenobarbital: increased phenobarbital levels.
Phenytoin: increased or decreased phenytoin levels.

NURSING CONSIDERATIONS
• Contraindicated in hepatic dysfunction. Use cautiously in children under 2 years; in children with congenital metabolic disorders or mental retardation; in patients with organic brain disease; and those taking multiple anticonvulsants.
• Tell patient not to disontinue the drug suddenly. Call doctor at once if adverse reactions develop.
• Obtain liver function studies, platelet counts, and prothrombin time before starting drug and every month thereafter, especially during the first 6 months of therapy.
• Serious or fatal hepatotoxicity may follow nonspecific symptoms, such as malaise, fever, and lethargy.
• Warn patient to avoid activities that require alertness and good psychomotor coordination until CNS effects of the drug are known.
• May give drug with food or milk to reduce GI adverse effects. Advise against chewing capsules; causes irritation of mouth and throat.
• May need to reduce dosage if tremors occur.
• May produce false-positive test results for ketones in urine.
• Available as tasty red syrup. Keep out of reach of children.
• Syrup is more rapidly absorbed. Peak effect within 15 minutes.
• Syrup shouldn't be mixed with carbonated beverages; may be irritating to mouth and throat.
• Don't administer syrup to patients who need sodium restriction. Check with doctor.
• Divalproex, a combination of valproic acid and valproate sodium, is available as an enteric-coated tablet. Divalproex minimizes GI intolerance.
• Valproic acid has been used investigationally to prevent recurrent febrile seizures in children.

31

Antidepressants

Monoamine oxidase inhibitors
isocarboxazid
phenelzine sulfate
tranylcypromine sulfate

Tricyclic antidepressants
amitriptyline hydrochloride
amoxapine
desipramine hydrochloride
doxepin hydrochloride
fluoxetine hydrochloride
imipramine hydrochloride
imipramine pamoate
maprotiline hydrochloride
nortriptyline hydrochloride
protriptyline hydrochloride
trimipramine maleate

Miscellaneous
trazodone hydrochloride

COMBINATION PRODUCTS
ETRAFON 2-10♦: perphenazine 2 mg and amitriptyline HCl 10 mg.
ETRAFON: perphenazine 2 mg and amitriptyline HCl 25 mg.
ETRAFON-A: perphenazine 4 mg and amitriptyline 10 mg.
ETRAFON-FORTE: perphenazine 4 mg and amitriptyline 25 mg.
LIMBITROL 10-25: chlordiazepoxide 10 mg and amitriptyline (as HCl) 25 mg.
LIMBITROL 5-12.5: chlordiazepoxide 5 mg and amitriptyline (as HCl) 12.5 mg.
TRIAVIL 2-10, TRIAVIL 4-10, TRIAVIL 2-25, TRIAVIL 4-25 are products identical to the Etrafon products listed above. Triavil is also available as TRIAVIL 4-50 (perphenazine 4 mg and

amitriptyline HCl 50 mg).

---

amitriptyline hydrochloride
Apo-Amitriptylene♦♦, Elavil♦, Emitrip, Endep, Enovil, Levate♦♦, Meravil♦♦, Novo-Triptyn♦♦, Rolavil
Pregnancy Risk Category: D

MECHANISM OF ACTION
Increases the amount of norepinephrine or serotonin, or both, in the CNS by blocking their reuptake by the presynaptic neurons. This action allows these neurotransmitters to accumulate.

INDICATIONS & DOSAGE
Treatment of depression—
Adults: 50 to 100 mg P.O. h.s., increasing to 200 mg daily; maximum dosage is 300 mg daily if needed; or 20 to 30 mg I.M. q.i.d. Alternatively, the entire dosage can be given at bedtime.
Elderly patients and adolescents: 30 mg P.O. daily in divided doses. May be increased to 150 mg.

ADVERSE REACTIONS
CNS: *drowsiness, dizziness,* excitation, tremors, weakness, confusion, headache, nervousness.
CV: *orthostatic hypotension, tachycardia, ECG changes,* hypertension.
EENT: *blurred vision,* tinnitus, mydriasis.
GI: *dry mouth, constipation,* nausea, vomiting, anorexia, paralytic ileus.
GU: *urine retention.*
Skin: rash, urticaria.

Unmarked trade names available in the United States only.
♦Also available in Canada.   ♦♦Available in Canada only.   ◊Also available OTC.

Other: *sweating,* allergy.
After abrupt withdrawal of long-term therapy: nausea, headache, malaise. (Does not indicate addiction.)

INTERACTIONS
Barbiturates: decrease tricyclic antidepressant (TCA) blood levels. Monitor for decreased antidepressant effect.
Cimetidine, methylphenidate: increases TCA blood levels. Monitor for enhanced antidepressant effect.
Epinephrine, norepinephrine: increase hypertensive effect. Use with caution.
MAO inhibitors: may cause severe excitation, hyperpyrexia, or seizures, usually with high dosage. Use together cautiously.

NURSING CONSIDERATIONS
• Contraindicated during acute recovery phase of myocardial infarction, in patients with history of seizure disorders, and in prostatic hypertrophy. Use with caution in patients who are suicide risks; in patients with urine retention, narrow-angle glaucoma, increased intraocular pressure, cardiovascular disease, impaired hepatic function, or hyperthyroidism; and in patients receiving thyroid medications, electroshock therapy, or elective surgery.
• Reduce dosage in elderly or debilitated persons and adolescents.
• Do not withdraw drug abruptly.
• If psychotic signs increase, dosage should be reduced. Record mood changes. Watch for suicidal tendencies. Allow minimum supply of tablets to lessen suicide risk.
• Check for urine retention and constipation. Increase fluids to lessen constipation. Suggest stool softener or high-fiber diet, if needed.
• Warn patient to avoid activities that require alertness and good psychomotor coordination until CNS effects of

the drug are known. Drowsiness and dizziness usually subside after first few weeks.
• Has strong anticholinergic effects; one of the most sedating tricyclic antidepressants. Avoid combining with alcohol or other depressants.
• Expect delay of 2 weeks or more before noticeable effect. Full effect may take 4 weeks or more.
• Dry mouth may be relieved with sugarless hard candy or gum. Saliva substitutes may be necessary.
• Advise the patient not to take any other drugs (prescription or OTC) without first consulting the doctor.
• Whenever possible, patient should take full dose at bedtime. Warn the patient about the possibility of morning orthostatic hypotension.
• Has been used successfully to treat intractable hiccups and chronic severe pain.

amoxapine
Asendin♦

Pregnancy Risk Category: C

MECHANISM OF ACTION
Increases the amount of norepinephrine or serotonin, or both, in the CNS by blocking their reuptake by the presynaptic neurons. This action allows these neurotransmitters to accumulate.

INDICATIONS & DOSAGE
Treatment of depression—
Adults: initial dose 50 mg P.O. t.i.d. May increase to 100 mg t.i.d. on third day of treatment. Increases above 300 mg daily should be made only if 300 mg daily has been ineffective during a trial period of at least 2 weeks. When effective dosage is established, entire dosage (not exceeding 300 mg) may be given at bedtime. Maximum dosage is 600 mg in hospitalized patients.

ADVERSE REACTIONS

CNS: *drowsiness, dizziness,* excitation, tremors, weakness, confusion, headache, nervousness, *tardive dyskinesia* (especially in elderly women).
CV: *orthostatic hypotension, tachycardia, ECG changes,* hypertension.
EENT: *blurred vision,* tinnitus, mydriasis.
GI: *dry mouth, constipation,* nausea, vomiting, anorexia, paralytic ileus.
GU: *urine retention, acute renal failure.*
Skin: rash, urticaria.
Other: *sweating,* weight gain and craving for sweets, allergy.
After abrupt withdrawal of long-term therapy: nausea, headache, malaise. (Does not indicate addiction.)

INTERACTIONS

Barbiturates: decrease tricyclic antidepressant (TCA) blood levels. Monitor for decreased antidepressant effect.
Cimetidine: may increase amoxapine serum levels. Monitor for increased adverse effects.
Epinephrine, norepinephrine: increase hypertensive effect. Use with caution.
MAO inhibitors: may cause severe excitation, hyperpyrexia, or seizures, usually with high dose. Use together cautiously.
Methylphenidate: increases TCA blood levels. Monitor for enhanced antidepressant effect.

NURSING CONSIDERATIONS

• Contraindicated in acute recovery phase of myocardial infarction, in patients with history of seizure disorders, and in prostatic hypertrophy. Use with caution in patients who are suicide risks; in urine retention, narrow-angle glaucoma, increased intraocular pressure, cardiovascular disease, impaired hepatic function, or hyperthyroidism; and in patients receiving thyroid medications, electroshock therapy, or elective surgery.
• Monitor for signs and symptoms of tardive dyskinesia, especially in elderly women.
• Reduce dosage in elderly or debilitated persons and adolescents.
• Do not withdraw drug abruptly.
• If psychotic signs increase, reduce dosage. Record mood changes. Watch for suicidal tendencies. Allow minimum supply of tablets to lessen suicide risk.
• Expect delay of 2 weeks or more before noticeable effect. Full effect may take 4 weeks or more.
• Check for urine retention and constipation. Increase fluids to lessen constipation. Suggest stool softener, if needed.
• Warn patient to avoid activities that require alertness and good psychomotor coordination until CNS effects of the drug are known. Drowsiness and dizziness usually subside after first few weeks.
• Dry mouth may be relieved with sugarless hard candy or gum. Saliva substitutes may be necessary.
• Whenever possible, patient should take full dose at bedtime.

---

desipramine hydrochloride
Norpramin♦**, Pertofrane♦
Pregnancy Risk Category: C

MECHANISM OF ACTION
Increases the amount of norepinephrine or serotonin, or both, in the CNS by blocking their reuptake by the presynaptic neurons. This action allows these neurotransmitters to accumulate.

INDICATIONS & DOSAGE
Treatment of depression—
Adults: 75 to 150 mg P.O. daily in divided doses, increasing to maximum of 300 mg daily. Alternatively, the entire dosage can be given at bedtime.

Elderly and adolescents: 25 to 50 mg P.O. daily, increasing gradually to maximum of 100 mg daily.

ADVERSE REACTIONS
CNS: *drowsiness, dizziness,* excitation, tremors, weakness, confusion, headache, nervousness.
CV: *orthostatic hypotension, tachycardia, ECG changes,* hypertension.
EENT: *blurred vision,* tinnitus, mydriasis.
GI: *dry mouth, constipation,* nausea, vomiting, anorexia, paralytic ileus.
GU: *urine retention.*
Skin: rash, urticaria.
Other: *sweating,* allergy.
After abrupt withdrawal of long-term therapy: nausea, headache, malaise. (Does not indicate addiction.)

INTERACTIONS
Barbiturates: decrease tricyclic antidepressant (TCA) blood levels. Monitor for decreased antidepressant effect.
Cimetidine: may increase desipramine serum levels. Monitor for increased adverse effects.
Epinephrine, norepinephrine: increase hypertensive effect. Use with caution.
MAO inhibitors: may cause severe excitation, hyperpyrexia, or seizures, usually with high dose. Use together cautiously.
Methylphenidate: increases TCA blood levels. Monitor for enhanced antidepressant effect.

NURSING CONSIDERATIONS
• Contraindicated during acute recovery phase of myocardial infarction, in patients with history of seizure disorders, and in prostatic hypertrophy. Use with caution in cardiovascular disease, urine retention, narrow-angle glaucoma, thyroid disease, blood dyscrasias, or impaired hepatic function; in patients who are suicide risks; and

in those receiving electroshock therapy, thyroid medication, or elective surgery.
• Reduce dosage in elderly or debilitated persons and adolescents.
• Do not withdraw drug abruptly.
• Orthostatic hypotension not as severe with this drug compared to other tricyclic antidepressants.
• If psychotic signs increase, dosage should be decreased. Record mood changes. Watch for suicidal tendencies. To lessen suicide risk, allow minimum supply of tablets.
• Check for urine retention and constipation. Increase fluids to lessen constipation. Suggest stool softener, if needed.
• Warn patient to avoid activities that require alertness and good psychomotor coordination until CNS effects of the drug are known. Drowsiness and dizziness usually subside after a few weeks.
• Dry mouth may be relieved with sugarless hard candy or gum. Saliva substitutes may be necessary.
• Drug has low potential for anticholinergic effects, is a metabolite of imipramine, and produces less sedation than amitriptyline or doxepin. Orthostatic hypotension is usually not a problem. Alcohol may antagonize effects of desipramine.
• Because it produces less tachycardia and other anticholinergic effects compared with other tricyclics, desipramine is often prescribed for cardiac patients.
• Expect delay of 2 weeks or more before noticeable effect. Full effect may take 4 weeks or more.
• Advise patient not to take any other drugs (prescription or OTC) without first consulting the doctor.
• Whenever possible, patient should take full dose at bedtime.

Italicized side effects are common or life-threatening.
*Liquid form contains alcohol.   **May contain tartrazine.

doxepin hydrochloride
Adapin**, Sinequan♦, Triadapin♦♦

Pregnancy Risk Category: C

MECHANISM OF ACTION
Increases the amount of norepinephrine or serotonin, or both, in the CNS by blocking their reuptake by the presynaptic neurons. This action allows these neurotransmitters to accumulate.

INDICATIONS & DOSAGE
Treatment of depression—
Adults: initially, 50 to 75 mg P.O. daily in divided doses, to maximum of 300 mg daily. Alternatively, entire dosage may be given at bedtime.

ADVERSE REACTIONS
CNS: *drowsiness, dizziness,* excitation, tremors, weakness, confusion, headache, nervousness.
CV: *orthostatic hypotension, tachycardia, ECG changes,* hypertension.
EENT: *blurred vision,* tinnitus, glossitis, mydriasis.
GI: *dry mouth, constipation,* nausea, vomiting, anorexia, paralytic ileus.
GU: *urine retention.*
Skin: rash, urticaria.
Other: *sweating,* allergy.
After abrupt withdrawal of long-term therapy: nausea, headache, malaise. (Does not indicate addiction.)

INTERACTIONS
Barbiturates: decrease tricyclic depressant (TCA) blood levels. Monitor for decreased antidepressant effect.
Cimetidine: may increase doxepin serum levels. Monitor for increased adverse effects.
MAO inhibitors: may cause severe excitation, hyperpyrexia, or seizures, usually with high dose. Use together cautiously.
Methylphenidate: increases TCA blood levels. Monitor for enhanced antidepressant effect.

NURSING CONSIDERATIONS
• Contraindicated in urine retention, narrow-angle glaucoma, or prostatic hypertrophy. Use with caution in suicide risks.
• Reduce dose in elderly or debilitated patients, adolescents, and those receiving other medications (especially anticholinergics).
• Dilute oral concentrate with 120 ml water, milk, or juice (orange, grapefruit, tomato, prune, or pineapple). Incompatible with carbonated beverages.
• If psychotic symptoms increase, dosage should be decreased. Record mood changes. Watch for suicidal tendencies.
• Check for urine retention and constipation. Increase fluids to lessen constipation. Suggest stool softener, if needed.
• Warn patient to avoid activities that require alertness and good psychomotor coordination until CNS effects of the drug are known. Drowsiness and dizziness usually subside after a few weeks.
• Expect delay of 2 weeks or more before noticeable effect. Full effect may take 4 weeks or more.
• Dry mouth may be relieved with sugarless hard candy or gum. Saliva substitutes may be necessary.
• Has strong anticholinergic effects; one of the most sedating tricyclic antidepressants. Avoid combining with alcohol or other depressants.
• Advise patient not to take any other drugs (OTC or prescription) without first consulting the doctor.
• Liquid formulation available.
• Whenever possible, patient should take full dose at bedtime. Warn patient about the possibility of morning orthostatic hypotension.
• Especially well tolerated by elderly patients.
• May be useful for chronic, severe

Unmarked trade names available in the United States only.
♦ Also available in Canada.   ♦♦ Available in Canada only.   ◊ Also available OTC.

neurogenic pain.

fluoxetine hydrochloride
Prozac

Pregnancy Risk Category: B

MECHANISM OF ACTION
CNS neuronal uptake of serotonin.

INDICATIONS & DOSAGE
Short-term management of depressive illness—
Adults: initially, 20 mg P.O. in the morning; dosage increased according to patient response. May be given b.i.d. in the morning and at noon. Maximum dosage is 80 mg/day.

ADVERSE REACTIONS
CNS: *nervousness, anxiety, insomnia, headache, drowsiness, tremor, dizziness,* abnormal dreams.
CV: palpitations, flushing, bradycardia, dysrhythmias.
EENT: flu-like syndrome, nasal congestion, upper respiratory infection, pharyngitis, cough sinusitis, visual disturbances, tinnitus, respiratory distress.
GI: *nausea, diarrhea, dry mouth, anorexia, dyspepsia,* constipation, abdominal pain, vomiting, taste change, flatulence, increased appetite.
GU: sexual dysfunction, urine retention.
Other: muscle pain, *weight loss, rash, pruritus, urticaria, asthenia,* edema, lymphadenopathy.

INTERACTIONS
Diazepam: half-life may be prolonged. Drugs highly bound to plasma proteins (warfarin, digitoxin) can cause displacement of drug and potential toxic effects.
Tryptophan: agitation, GI distress, and restlessness.

NURSING CONSIDERATIONS
• Because this drug commonly causes

nervousness and insomnia, patient should avoid taking this drug in the afternoon to prevent sleep disturbances.
• May cause dizziness or drowsiness in some patients. Warn patient to avoid driving or other hazardous activities that require alertness until CNS effects of the drug are known.
• Elderly or debilitated patients and patients with renal or hepatic dysfunction may require lower dosages or less frequent dosing.
• Fluoxetine and its active metabolite have a long elimination half-life. Clinical effects of dosage changes may not be evident for weeks; full antidepressant effects may not appear for 4 or more weeks of treatment.

imipramine hydrochloride
Apo-Imipramine♦♦, Impril♦♦, Janimine**, Novo-Pramine♦♦, Tripramine, Tofranil♦**

imipramine pamoate
Tofranil-PM**

Pregnancy Risk Category: D

MECHANISM OF ACTION
Increases the amount of norepinephrine or serotonin, or both, in the CNS by blocking their reuptake by the presynaptic neurons. This action allows these neurotransmitters to accumulate.

INDICATIONS & DOSAGE
Treatment of depression—
Adults: 75 to 100 mg P.O. or I.M. daily in divided doses, with 25- to 50-mg increments up to 200 mg. Maximum dosage is 300 mg daily. Alternatively, the entire dosage may be given at bedtime. (I.M. route rarely used.)
Childhood enuresis—
25 to 75 mg P.O. daily.

ADVERSE REACTIONS
CNS: *drowsiness, dizziness,* excita-

tion, tremors, weakness, confusion, headache, nervousness.

CV: *orthostatic hypotension, tachycardia, ECG changes,* hypertension.

EENT: *blurred vision,* tinnitus, mydriasis.

GI: *dry mouth, constipation,* nausea, vomiting, anorexia, paralytic ileus.

GU: *urine retention.*

Skin: rash, urticaria.

Other: *sweating,* allergy.

After abrupt withdrawal of long-term therapy: nausea, headache, malaise. (Does not indicate addiction.)

INTERACTIONS

Barbiturates: decrease tricyclic antidepressant (TCA) blood levels. Monitor for decreased antidepressant effect.

Cimetidine: may increase imipramine serum levels. Monitor for increased adverse effects.

Epinephrine, norepinephrine: increase hypertensive effect. Use with caution.

MAO inhibitors: may cause severe excitation, hyperpyrexia, or seizures, usually with high dose. Use together cautiously.

Methylphenidate: increases TCA blood levels. Monitor for enhanced antidepressant effect.

NURSING CONSIDERATIONS

• Contraindicated during acute recovery phase of myocardial infarction, in prostatic hypertrophy, and in patients with history of seizure disorders. Use with extreme caution in cardiovascular disease, urine retention, narrow-angle glaucoma or increased intraocular pressure, thyroid disease, blood dyscrasias, or impaired hepatic function; in patients who are suicide risks; and in those receiving electroshock therapy, thyroid medication, or elective surgery.

• Reduce dosage in elderly or debilitated persons, adolescents, and pa-

tients with aggravated psychotic symptoms.

• Do not withdraw drug abruptly.

• If psychotic signs increase, dosage should be reduced. Record mood changes. Watch for suicidal tendencies. To lessen suicide risk, allow minimum supply of tablets.

• Check for urine retention and constipation. Increase fluids to lessen constipation. Suggest stool softener, if needed.

• Warn patient to avoid activities that require alertness and good psychomotor coordination until CNS effects of the drug are known.. Drowsiness and dizziness usually subside after a few weeks.

• Expect delay of 2 weeks or more before noticeable effect. Full effect may take 4 weeks or more.

• Dry mouth may be relieved with sugarless hard candy or gum. Saliva substitutes may be necessary.

• Avoid combining with alcohol or other depressants.

• Advise patient not to take any other drugs (prescription or OTC) without first consulting the doctor.

• Imipramine has a high potential for inducing orthostatic hypotension. Whenever possible, patient should take full dose at bedtime. Warn patient about the possibility of morning orthostatic hypotension.

• May be useful for chronic, severe neurogenic pain.

---

isocarboxazid
Marplan♦

Pregnancy Risk Category: C

MECHANISM OF ACTION
Promotes accumulation of neurotransmitters by inhibiting MAO.

INDICATIONS & DOSAGE
Treatment of depression—

Adults: 30 mg P.O. daily in divided doses. Reduce to 10 to 20 mg daily when condition improves. Not recommended for children under 16 years.

ADVERSE REACTIONS
CNS: *dizziness,* vertigo, weakness, headache, overactivity, hyperreflexia, tremors, muscle twitching, mania, *insomnia,* confusion, memory impairment, fatigue.
CV: *orthostatic hypotension,* dysrhythmias, paradoxical hypertension.
EENT: blurred vision.
GI: dry mouth, *anorexia,* nausea, diarrhea, constipation.
Skin: rash.
Other: peripheral edema, sweating, weight changes, altered libido.

INTERACTIONS
Amphetamines, ephedrine, levodopa, meperidine, metaraminol, methotrimeprazine, methylphenidate, phenylephrine, phenylpropanolamine: pressor effects of these drugs are enhanced by isocarboxazid. Use together very cautiously.
Alcohol, barbiturates, and other sedatives; narcotics; dextromethorphan; tricyclic antidepressants: unpredictable interaction. Use with caution and in reduced dosage.
Insulin, oral hypoglycemic agents: isocarboxazid may alter requirements for antidiabetic medications.

NURSING CONSIDERATIONS
• Contraindicated in elderly or debilitated patients; and in severe hepatic or renal impairment, CHF, pheochromocytoma; hypertensive, cardiovascular, or cerebrovascular disease; severe or frequent headaches. Also contraindicated with foods containing tryptophan or tyramine. Also during therapy with other MAO inhibitors (including pargyline hydrochloride, phenelzine sulfate, tranylcypromine sulfate) or within 10 days of such therapy; within 10 days of elective surgery requiring general anesthetic, cocaine, or local anesthetic containing sympathomimetic vasoconstrictors. Use cautiously with other psychotropic drugs or with spinal anesthetic; in hyperactive, agitated, or schizophrenic patients; in suicide risks; and in patients with diabetes or epilepsy.
• Avoid combining with alcohol or other depressant.
• Use only when tricyclic antidepressant or electroshock therapy is ineffective or contraindicated.
• If patient develops symptoms of overdosage (palpitations, frequent headaches, or severe orthostatic hypotension), hold dose and notify doctor.
• Watch for suicidal tendencies.
• Dosage is usually reduced to maintenance level as soon as possible.
• Do not withdraw drug abruptly.
• Weigh patient biweekly; check for edema and urine retention.
• Warn patient to avoid foods high in tyramine or tryptophan (aged cheese, Chianti wine, beer, avocados, chicken livers, chocolate, bananas, soy sauce, meat tenderizers, salami, bologna); large amounts of caffeine; and self-medication with OTC cold, hay fever, or diet preparations.
• Incidence of orthostatic hypotension is high. Supervise walking. Tell patient to get out of bed slowly, sitting up first for 1 minute.
• Have phentolamine (Regitine) available to counteract severe hypertension.
• Continue precautions 10 days after stopping drug because it has long-lasting effects.
• Expect delay of 2 weeks or more before noticeable effect. Full effect may take 4 weeks or more.
• Obtain baseline blood pressure readings, CBC, and liver function tests before beginning therapy, and continue to monitor throughout treatment.

Italicized side effects are common or life-threatening.
*Liquid form contains alcohol.   **May contain tartrazine.

maprotiline hydrochloride
Ludiomil♦

Pregnancy Risk Category: B

MECHANISM OF ACTION
Increases the amount of norepinephrine or serotonin, or both, in the CNS by blocking their reuptake by the presynaptic neurons. This action allows these neurotransmitters to accumulate.

INDICATIONS & DOSAGE
Treatment of depression—
Adults: initial dose of 75 mg daily for patients with mild to moderate depression. The dosage may be increased as required to a dose of 150 mg daily. Maximum dosage is 225 mg in patients who are not hospitalized. More severely depressed, hospitalized patients may receive up to 300 mg daily.

ADVERSE REACTIONS
CNS: *drowsiness, dizziness,* excitation, *seizures,* tremors, weakness, confusion, headache, nervousness.
CV: orthostatic hypotension, tachycardia, *ECG changes,* hypertension.
EENT: *blurred vision,* tinnitus, mydriasis.
GI: *dry mouth, constipation,* nausea, vomiting, anorexia, paralytic ileus.
GU: *urine retention.*
Skin: rash, urticaria.
Other: *sweating,* allergy.
After abrupt withdrawal of long-term therapy: nausea, headache, malaise. (Does not indicate addiction.)

INTERACTIONS
Barbiturates: decrease maprotiline blood levels. Monitor for decreased antidepressant effect.
Cimetidine: may increase maprotiline serum levels. Monitor for increased adverse effects.
Epinephrine, norepinephrine: increase hypertensive effect. Use with caution.
MAO inhibitors: may cause severe excitation, hyperpyrexia, or seizures, usually with high dose. Use together cautiously.
Methylphenidate: increases maprotiline blood levels. Monitor for enhanced antidepressant effect.

NURSING CONSIDERATIONS
• Contraindicated during acute recovery phase of myocardial infarction, in prostatic hypertrophy, and in patients with history of seizure disorders. Use with caution in CV disease, urine retention, narrow-angle glaucoma, thyroid disease or medication, blood dyscrasias, and impaired hepatic functon; in patients with a history of seizures; in patients who are suicide risks; and in those receiving electroshock therapy or elective surgery.
• Reduce dosage in elderly or debilitated persons and adolescents.
• Do not withdraw drug abruptly.
• If psychotic signs increase, reduce dosage. Record mood changes. Watch for suicidal tendencies. To lessen suicide risk, allow minimum supply of tablets.
• Check for urine retention and constipation. Increase fluids to lessen constipation. Suggest stool softener, if needed.
• Warn patient to avoid activities that require alertness and good psychomotor coordination until CNS effects of the drug are known. Drowsiness and dizziness usually subside after a few weeks.
• Dry mouth may be relieved with sugarless hard candy or gum, but maprolitine usually has a low potential for inducing anticholinergic effects. Saliva substitutes may be necessary.
• Whenever possible, patient should take full dose at bedtime.
• The first "tetracyclic" antidepressant.

nortriptyline hydrochloride
Aventyl♦*, Pamelor

Pregnancy Risk Category: D

MECHANISM OF ACTION
Increases the amount of norepinephrine or serotonin, or both, in the CNS by blocking their reuptake by the presynaptic neurons. This action allows these neurotransmitters to accumulate.

INDICATIONS & DOSAGE
Treatment of depression—
Adults: 25 mg P.O. t.i.d. or q.i.d., gradually increasing to maximum of 150 mg daily. Alternatively, entire dose may be given at bedtime.

ADVERSE REACTIONS
CNS: *drowsiness, dizziness,* excitation, seizures, tremors, weakness, confusion, headache, nervousness.
CV: *tachycardia, ECG changes,* hypertension.
EENT: *blurred vision,* tinnitus, mydriasis.
GI: *dry mouth, constipation,* nausea, vomiting, anorexia, paralytic ileus.
GU: *urine retention.*
Skin: rash, urticaria.
Other: *sweating,* allergy.
After abrupt withdrawal of long-term therapy: nausea, headache, malaise. (Does not indicate addiction.)

INTERACTIONS
Barbiturates: decrease tricyclic depressant (TCA) blood levels. Monitor for decreased antidepressant effect.
Cimetidine: may increase nortriptyline serum levels. Monitor for increased adverse effects.
Epinephrine, norepinephrine: increase hypertensive effect. Use with caution.
MAO inhibitors: may cause severe excitation, hyperpyrexia, or seizures, usually with high dose. Use together cautiously.
Methylphenidate: increases TCA blood levels. Monitor for enhanced antidepressant effect.

NURSING CONSIDERATIONS
• Contraindicated during acute recovery phase of myocardial infarction, in prostatic hypertrophy, and in patients with history of seizure disorders. Use with caution in CV disease, urine retention, glaucoma, thyroid disease, impaired hepatic function, or blood dyscrasias; in patients who are suicide risks; or in those receiving electroshock therapy, thyroid medication, or elective surgery.
• Reduce dosage in elderly or debilitated persons and adolescents.
• Do not withdraw drug abruptly.
• If psychotic signs increase, dosage should be reduced. Record mood changes. Watch for suicidal tendencies. To lessen suicide risk, allow minimum tablet supply.
• Check for urine retention and constipation. Increase fluids to lessen constipation. Suggest stool softener, if needed.
• Warn patient to avoid activities that require alertness and good psychomotor coordination until CNS effects of the drug are known. Drowsiness and dizziness usually subside after a few weeks.
• Expect delay of 2 weeks or more before noticeable effect. Full effect may take 4 weeks or more.
• Dry mouth may be relieved with sugarless hard candy or gum. Saliva substitutes may be necessary.
• Drug is tricyclic antidepressant, similar in anticholinergic effects to other cyclics. Has low potential for orthostatic hypotension. Avoid combining with alcohol or other depressants.
• Advise patient not to use other drugs (prescription or OTC) without first consulting the doctor.
• Liquid formulation available.

Italicized side effects are common or life-threatening.
*Liquid form contains alcohol.   **May contain tartrazine.

• Whenever possible, patient should take full dose at bedtime.

phenelzine sulfate
Nardil♦

Pregnancy Risk Category: C

MECHANISM OF ACTION
Promotes accumulation of neurotransmitters by inhibiting MAO.

INDICATIONS & DOSAGE
Treatment of depression—
Adults: 45 mg P.O. daily in divided doses, increasing rapidly to 60 mg daily. Then dosage can usually be reduced to 15 mg daily. Maximum is 90 mg daily.

ADVERSE REACTIONS
CNS: *dizziness,* vertigo, headache, overactivity, hyperreflexia, tremors, muscle twitching, mania, jitters, *insomnia,* confusion, memory impairment, drowsiness, weakness, fatigue.
CV: paradoxical hypertension, *orthostatic hypotension,* dysrhythmias.
GI: dry mouth, *anorexia,* nausea, constipation.
Other: peripheral edema, sweating, weight changes.

INTERACTIONS
Alcohol, barbiturates, and other sedatives; narcotics; dextromethorphan; tricyclic antidepressants: unpredictable interaction. Use with caution and in reduced dosage.
Amphetamines, ephedrine, levodopa, meperidine, metaraminol, methotrimeprazine, methylphenidate, phenylephrine, phenylpropanolamine: enhance pressor effects. Use together cautiously.
Insulin, oral hypoglycemic agents: phenelzine may alter requirements for antidiabetic medications.

NURSING CONSIDERATIONS
• Contraindicated in elderly or debilitated patients, and in hepatic impairment, CHF, pheochromocytoma, hypertension, cardiovascular or cerebrovascular disease, or severe or frequent headaches. Also contraindicated with foods containing tryptophan (broad beans) or tyramine; during therapy with other MAO inhibitors (including pargyline HCl, isocarboxazid, tranylcypromine sulfate) or within 10 days of such therapy; within 10 days of elective surgery requiring general anesthetic, cocaine, or local anesthetic containing sympathomimetic vasoconstrictors; and in hyperactive, agitated, or schizophrenic patients. Use cautiously with antihypertensive drugs containing thiazide diuretics or with spinal anesthetic; and in patients with suicide risk or diabetes.
• Avoid combining with alcohol or other depressant.
• Use only when tricyclic antidepressant or electroshock therapy is ineffective or contraindicated.
• If patient develops symptoms of overdose (severe hypotension, palpitations, or frequent headaches), hold dose and notify doctor.
• Watch for suicidal tendencies.
• Dosage is usually reduced to maintenance level as soon as possible.
• Store drug in tight container, away from heat and light.
• Have phentolamine (Regitine) available to counteract severe hypertension.
• Warn patient to avoid foods high in tyramine or tryptophan (aged cheese, Chianti wine, beer, avocados, chicken livers, chocolate, bananas, soy sauce, meat tenderizers, salami, bologna) and self-medication with OTC cold, hay fever, or diet preparations.
• Incidence of orthostatic hypotension is high. Supervise walking. Tell patient to get out of bed slowly, sitting up first for 1 minute.
• Continue precautions 10 days after stopping drug because it has long-lasting effects.

- Expect delay of 2 weeks or more before noticeable effect. Full effect may take 4 weeks or more.
- Obtain baseline blood pressure readings, CBC, and liver function tests before therapy, and continue to monitor throughout treatment.

---

protriptyline hydrochloride
Triptil♦♦, Vivactil

Pregnancy Risk Category: C

MECHANISM OF ACTION
Increases the amount of norepinephrine or serotonin, or both, in the CNS by blocking their reuptake by the presynaptic neurons. This action allows these neurotransmitters to accumulate.

INDICATIONS & DOSAGE
Treatment of depression—
Adults: 15 to 40 mg P.O. daily in divided doses, increasing gradually to maximum of 60 mg daily.

ADVERSE REACTIONS
CNS: excitation, seizures, tremors, weakness, confusion, headache, nervousness.
CV: *orthostatic hypotension, tachycardia, ECG changes,* hypertension.
EENT: *blurred vision,* tinnitus, mydriasis.
GI: *dry mouth, constipation,* nausea, vomiting, anorexia, paralytic ileus.
GU: *urine retention.*
Skin: rash, urticaria.
Other: *sweating,* allergy.
After abrupt withdrawal of long-term therapy: nausea, headache, malaise. (Does not indicate addiction.)

INTERACTIONS
Barbiturates: decrease tricyclic antidepressant (TCA) blood levels. Monitor for decreased antidepressant effect.
Epinephrine, norepinephrine: in-

crease hypertensive effect. Use with caution.
Cimetidine: may increase protriptyline serum levels. Monitor for increased adverse effects.
MAO inhibitors: may cause severe excitation, hyperpyrexia, or seizures, and death, usually with high dose. Use together cautiously.
Methylphenidate: increases TCA blood levels. Monitor for enhanced antidepressant effect.

NURSING CONSIDERATIONS
- Contraindicated during acute recovery phase of myocardial infarction, in prostatic hypertrophy, and in patients with history of seizure disorders. Use with caution in elderly patients and in CV disease, urine retention, increased intraocular tension, thyroid disease, or blood dyscrasias; in suicide risks; and in those receiving electroshock therapy, thyroid medication, or elective surgery.
- Protriptyline has low potential for producing orthostatic hypotension, and is the least sedating of the tricyclic antidepressants. It may even have amphetamine-like effects. Avoid late-day dosing to prevent insomnia.
- Reduce dosage in elderly or debilitated patients and adolescents.
- Do not withdraw drug abruptly.
- Watch for increased psychotic signs, anxiety, agitation, or CV reactions; dosage should be reduced if they occur. Record mood changes. Watch for suicidal tendencies. To lessen suicide risk, allow minimum supply of tablets.
- Check for urine retention and constipation. Increase fluids to lessen constipation. Suggest stool softener, if needed.
- Protriptylene has high anticholinergic effects. Dry mouth may be relieved with sugarless hard candy or gum. Saliva substitutes may be necessary.
- Expect delay of 2 weeks or more

---

before noticeable effect. Full effect may take 4 weeks or more.
• Advise patient not to use other drugs (prescription or OTC) without first consulting the doctor. Avoid combining with alcohol or other depressants.
• Used investigationally to treat obstructive sleep apnea.

---

tranylcypromine sulfate
Parnate♦

Pregnancy Risk Category: C

MECHANISM OF ACTION
Promotes accumulation of neurotransmitters by inhibiting MAO.

INDICATIONS & DOSAGE
Treatment of depression—
Adults: 10 mg P.O. b.i.d. Increase to maximum of 30 mg daily, if necessary, after 2 weeks. Not recommended for children under 16 years.

ADVERSE REACTIONS
CNS: *dizziness,* vertigo, headache, overactivity, hyperreflexia, tremors, muscle twitching, mania, jitters, confusion, memory impairment, fatigue.
CV: *orthostatic hypotension,* dysrhythmias, paradoxical hypertension.
EENT: blurred vision.
GI: dry mouth, *anorexia,* nausea, diarrhea, constipation, abdominal pain.
GU: impotence.
Skin: rash.
Other: peripheral edema, sweating, weight changes, chills, altered libido.

INTERACTIONS
Alcohol, barbiturates, and other sedatives; narcotics; dextromethorphan; tricyclic antidepressants: use with caution and in reduced dosage.
Amphetamines, ephedrine, levodopa, meperidine, metaraminol, methotrimeprazine, methylphenidate, phenylephrine, phenylpropanolamine: pressor effects of these drugs are enhanced by tranylcypromine. Use together cautiously.
Insulin, oral hypoglycemic agents: tranylcypromine may alter requirements of antidiabetic medications.

NURSING CONSIDERATIONS
• Contraindicated in severe hepatic or renal impairment; CHF; pheochromocytoma, hypertension, or cardiovascular or cerebrovascular disease; severe or frequent headaches; in patients taking antihypertensive drugs or diuretics; in elderly or debilitated patients; in patients for whom close supervision is not possible; and in hyperactive, agitated, or schizophrenic patients. Also contraindicated with foods containing tryptophan or tyramine. Also contraindicated during therapy with other MAO inhibitors (including pargyline, phenelzine sulfate, isocarboxazid) or within 7 days of such therapy; within 7 days of elective surgery requiring general anesthetic, cocaine, or local anesthetic containing sympathomimetic vasoconstrictors. Use cautiously with antiparkinsonian drugs, spinal anesthetics; in renal disease, diabetes, epilepsy, hyperthyroidism; and in suicide risks.
• MAO inhibitor most often reported to cause hypertensive crisis with high-tyramine ingestion.
• Avoid combining with alcohol or other depressants.
• Use only when tricyclic antidepressant or electroshock therapy is ineffective or contraindicated.
• If patient develops symptoms of overdose (palpitations, severe hypotension, or frequent headaches), hold dose and notify doctor.
• Watch for suicidal tendencies.
• Dosage is usually reduced to maintenance level as soon as possible.
• Do not withdraw drug abruptly.
• Have phentolamine (Regitine) available to counteract severe hyper-

---

tension.
• Warn patient to avoid foods high in tyramine or tryptophan (aged cheese, Chianti wine, beer, avocados, chicken livers, chocolate, bananas, soy sauce, meat tenderizers, salami, bologna) and self-medication with OTC cold, hay fever, or reducing preparations.
• Tell patient to get out of bed slowly, sitting up for 1 minute.
• Continue precautions for 7 days after stopping drug; effects last that long.
• Expect delay of 2 weeks or more before noticeable effect. Full effect may take 4 weeks or more.
• More rapid onset of action than isocarboxazid or phenelzine sulfate.
• Obtain baseline blood pressure readings, CBC, and liver function tests before beginning therapy, and continue to monitor throughout treatment.

---

trazodone hydrochloride
Desyrel♦, Trazon, Trialodine
Pregnancy Risk Category: C

MECHANISM OF ACTION
Inhibits serotonin uptake in the brain.

INDICATIONS & DOSAGE
Treatment of depression—
Adults: Initial dosage is 150 mg daily in divided doses, which can be increased by 50 mg daily q 3 to 4 days. Average dosage ranges from 150 mg to 400 mg daily. Maximum dosage is 600 mg.

ADVERSE REACTIONS
CNS: *drowsiness, dizziness,* nervousness, fatigue, confusion, tremors, weakness.
CV: orthostatic hypotension, tachycardia.
EENT: blurred vision, tinnitus.
GI: dry mouth, constipation, nausea, vomiting, anorexia.
GU: urine retention, priapism possi-

bly leading to impotence.
Skin: rash, urticaria.
Other: sweating.

INTERACTIONS
Alcohol, CNS depressants: enhanced CNS depression.
Antihypertensives: added hypotensive effect of trazodone. Dose of antihypertensive drug may have to be decreased.
Digoxin, phenytoin: trazodone may increase serum levels of these drugs. Monitor for toxicity.
MAO inhibitors: No clinical experience. Use together very cautiously.

NURSING CONSIDERATIONS
• Should not be used during initial recovery phase of myocardial infarction. Avoid concurrent administration with electroshock therapy. Drug may be discontinued before surgery.
• Use cautiously with preexisting cardiac disease.
• Priapism is a potential problem in men taking trazodone. Be sure to note if patient complains of prolonged and painful erections. May need surgical intervention.
• Watch for suicidal tendencies and record mood changes. Allow minimum amount of tablets to lessen suicide risk.
• Warn patient to avoid activities that require alertness and good psychomotor coordination until CNS effects of the drug are known. Drowsiness and dizziness usually subside after the first few weeks.
• Administer after meals or a light snack for optimal absorption and to decrease incidence of dizziness.
• Not chemically related to tricyclic antidepressants or MAO inhibitors.
• Anticholinergic and adverse cardiac effects are minimal.
• Expect delay of 2 weeks or more before noticeable effect. Full effect may take 4 weeks or more.

trimipramine maleate
Apo-Trimip♦♦, Surmontil♦

Pregnancy Risk Category: C

MECHANISM OF ACTION
Increases the amount of norepinephrine or serotonin, or both, in the CNS by blocking their reuptake by the presynaptic neurons. This action allows these neurotransmitters to accumulate.

INDICATIONS & DOSAGE
Treatment of depression—
Adults: 75 mg daily in divided doses, increased to 200 mg daily. Dosages over 300 mg daily not recommended.
Enuresis—
Children over 6 years: initial dosage 25 mg P.O. 1 hour before bedtime; if no response, increase dosage to 50 mg in children under 12 years, and to 75 mg in children over 12 years.

ADVERSE REACTIONS
CNS: *drowsiness, dizziness,* excitation, seizures, tremors, weakness, confusion, headache, nervousness.
CV: *orthostatic hypotension, tachycardia, ECG changes,* hypertension.
EENT: *blurred vision,* tinnitus, mydriasis.
GI: *dry mouth, constipation,* nausea, vomiting, anorexia, paralytic ileus.
GU: *urine retention.*
Skin: rash, urticaria.
Other: *sweating,* allergy.
After abrupt withdrawal of long-term therapy: nausea, headache, malaise. (Does not indicate addiction.)

INTERACTIONS
Barbiturates: decrease tricyclic antidepressant (TCA) blood levels. Monitor for decreased antidepressant effect.
Cimetidine: may increase trimipramine serum levels. Monitor for increased adverse effects.
Epinephrine, norepinephrine: increase hypertensive effect. Use with caution.
MAO inhibitors: may cause severe excitation, hyperpyrexia, or seizures, usually with high dose. Use together cautiously.
Methylphenidate: increases TCA blood levels. Monitor for enhanced antidepressant effects.

NURSING CONSIDERATIONS
• Contraindicated during acute recovery phase of myocardial infarction, in prostatic hypertrophy, and in patients with history of seizure disorders. Use with extreme caution in CV disease, urine retention, narrow-angle glaucoma or increased intraocular pressure, thyroid disease, blood dyscrasias, or impaired hepatic function. Also contraindicated in patients who are suicide risks and in those receiving electroshock therapy, thyroid medicaton, or elective surgery.
• Reduce dosage in elderly or debilitated persons and adolescents.
• Do not withdraw drug abruptly.
• Watch for increased psychotic signs; dosage should be reduced if they occur. Record mood changes. Watch for suicidal tendencies. Allow only minimum supply of tablets to lessen suicide risk.
• Check for urine retention and constipation. Increase fluids to lessen constipation. Suggest stool softener, if necessary.
• Warn patient to avoid activities that require alertness and good psychomotor coordination until CNS effects of the drug are known. Drowsiness and dizziness usually subside after a few weeks.
• Don't combine with alcohol or other depressants.
• Expect delay of 2 weeks or more before noticeable effect. Full effect may take 4 weeks or more.
• Dry mouth may be relieved with sugarless hard candy or gum. Saliva

---

substitutes may be necessary.

• Effectiveness in enuresis may decrease over time. Similar in anticholinergic effects to other tricyclic antidepressants.

• Advise patient not to use other drugs (prescription or OTC) without first consulting the doctor.

• Trimipramine has high sedative effect. Whenever possible, patient should take full dose at bedtime. Warn patient about possible morning orthostatic hypotension.

32

Antianxiety agents

alprazolam
buspirone hydrochloride
chlordiazepoxide
chlordiazepoxide hydrochloride
clorazepate dipotassium
diazepam
halazepam
hydroxyzine hydrochloride
hydroxyzine pamoate
lorazepam
meprobamate
oxazepam
prazepam

COMBINATION PRODUCTS

DEPROL**: meprobamate 400 mg and
benactyzine HCl 1 mg.
EQUAGESIC: meprobamate 200 mg
and aspirin 325 mg.
LIBRAX CAPSULES: chlordiazepoxide
hydrochloride 5 mg and clidinium
bromide 2.5 mg.
LIMBITROL 5-12.5: chlordiazepoxide
5 mg and amitriptyline (as HCl) 12.5
mg.
LIMBITROL 10-25: chlordiazepoxide
10 mg and amitriptyline (as HCl) 25
mg.
MENRIUM 5-2: chlordiazepoxide 5 mg
and esterified estrogens 0.2 mg.
MENRIUM 5-4: chlordiazepoxide 5 mg
and esterified estrogens 0.4 mg.
MENRIUM 10-4: chlordiazepoxide
10 mg and esterified estrogens 0.4
mg.
MILPREM-200: meprobamate 200 mg
and conjugated estrogens 0.45 mg.
MILPREM-400: meprobamate 400 mg
and conjugated estrogens 0.45 mg.
PMB 200: meprobamate 200 mg and
conjugated estrogens 0.45 mg.

PMB 400: meprobamate 400 mg and
conjugated estrogens 0.45 mg.

alprazolam
Xanax♦
Controlled Substance Schedule IV
Pregnancy Risk Category: D

MECHANISM OF ACTION
Depresses the CNS at the limbic and
subcortical levels of the brain.

INDICATIONS & DOSAGE
Anxiety and tension—
Adults: Usual starting dose is 0.25 to
0.5 mg t.i.d. Maximum total daily
dosage is 4 mg in divided doses. In elderly or debilitated patients, usual
starting dose is 0.25 mg b.i.d. or
t.i.d.

ADVERSE REACTIONS
CNS: *drowsiness, light-headedness,*
headache, confusion, hostility.
CV: transient hypotension, tachycar-
dia.
EENT: dry mouth.
GI: nausea, vomiting, constipation,
discomfort.

INTERACTIONS
Alcohol, other CNS depressants: increased CNS depression. Avoid concomitant use.
Cimetidine: increased sedation. Monitor carefully.
Tricyclic antidepressants: increased
plasma levels of tricyclic antidepressants.

Unmarked trade names available in the United States only.
♦ Also available in Canada.　　　♦♦ Available in Canada only.　　　◊ Also available OTC.

NURSING CONSIDERATIONS
• Contraindicated in acute narrow-angle glaucoma, psychoses, or anxiety-free psychiatric disorders.
• Reduce dosage in elderly or debilitated patients.
• Do not withdraw drug abruptly. Abuse or addiction is possible. Withdrawal symptoms may occur.
• Warn patient not to combine drug with alcohol or other depressants, and also to avoid activities that require alertness and psychomotor coordination until CNS effects of the drug are known.
• Caution patient against giving medication to others.
• Drug should not be prescribed for everyday stress.
• Drug is not for long-term use (more than 4 months).
• Warn patient not to discontinue drug without doctor's approval.
• Alprazolam is the first of a new type of benzodiazepine, known as a triazolo-benzodiazepine. It's more rapidly metabolized and excreted than most of the other drugs in the benzodiazepine class and has a lower incidence of lethargy than other drugs of this class.
• May also be effective for treatment of depression.

buspirone hydrochloride
Buspar

Pregnancy Risk Category: B

MECHANISM OF ACTION
Unknown. However, the drug may inhibit neuronal firing and reduce 5-HT turnover in cortical, amygdaloid, and septohippocampal tissue.

INDICATIONS & DOSAGE
Management of anxiety disorders; short-term relief of anxiety—
Adults: initially, 5 mg P.O. t.i.d. Dosage may be increased at 3-day intervals. Usual maintenance dosage is 20 to 30 mg daily in divided doses.

ADVERSE REACTIONS
CNS: *dizziness, drowsiness,* nervousness, insomnia, headache.
GI: nausea, dry mouth, diarrhea.
Other: fatigue.

INTERACTIONS
Alcohol, other CNS depressants: increased CNS depression. Avoid concomitant use.
MAO inhibitors: may elevate blood pressure.

NURSING CONSIDERATIONS
• Although buspirone is less sedating than other anxiolytics and does not produce any serious functional impairment, CNS effects in an individual patient may be unpredictable. Therefore, warn patients to avoid hazardous activities that require alertness and neuromuscular coordination until CNS effects of the drug are known.
• Unlike the benzodiazepines, buspirone is not an effective anticonvulsant or skeletal muscle relaxant. Its use is limited to the treatment of anxiety.
• Advise patient to take the drug with food.
• Before initiating buspirone therapy in patients already being treated with benzodiazepines, warn them against stopping the benzodiazepine abruptly. Abrupt discontinuation may cause a benzodiazepine withdrawal reaction.
• Signs of improvement with buspirone are usually evident within 7 to 10 days; optimal results are achieved after 3 to 4 weeks of therapy.
• This drug has shown no potential for abuse and has not been classified as a controlled substance. However, it is not recommended for use to relieve everyday stress.

Italicized side effects are common or life-threatening.
*Liquid form contains alcohol.   **May contain tartrazine.

chlordiazepoxide
Libritabs

chlordiazepoxide hydrochloride
Apo-Chlordiazepoxide♦♦,
Librium♦, Lipoxide, Medilium♦♦,
Mitran, Novopoxide♦♦, Reposans,
Sereen, Solium♦♦
Controlled Substance Schedule IV

Pregnancy Risk Category: D

MECHANISM OF ACTION
Depresses the CNS at the limbic and
subcortical levels of the brain.

INDICATIONS & DOSAGE
Mild to moderate anxiety and tension—
Adults: 5 to 10 mg t.i.d. or q.i.d.
Children over 6 years: 5 mg P.O.
b.i.d. to q.i.d. Maximum dosage is
10 mg P.O. b.i.d. to t.i.d.
Severe anxiety and tension—
Adults: 20 to 25 mg t.i.d. or q.i.d.
Withdrawal symptoms of acute alcoholism—
Adults: 50 to 100 mg P.O., I.M., or
I.V. Maximum dosage is 300 mg
daily.
Preoperative apprehension and anxiety—
Adults: 5 to 10 mg P.O. t.i.d. or
q.i.d. on day preceding surgery; or 50
to 100 mg I.M. 1 hour before surgery.
   Note: Parenteral form not recommended in children under 12 years.

ADVERSE REACTIONS
CNS: *drowsiness, lethargy, hangover,*
fainting.
CV: *transient hypotension.*
GI: nausea, vomiting, abdominal discomfort.
Local: *pain at injection site.*

INTERACTIONS
Alcohol, other CNS depressants: increased CNS depression. Avoid concomitant use.

Cimetidine: increased sedation. Monitor carefully.

NURSING CONSIDERATIONS
• Use with caution in mental depression, psychiatric disturbances, blood
dyscrasias, porphyria, hepatic or
renal disease, or in those undergoing
anticoagulant therapy.
• Dosage should be reduced in elderly or debilitated patients.
• Possibility of abuse and addiction.
Do not withdraw drug abruptly; withdrawal symptoms may occur.
• Warn patient to avoid activities that
require alertness and good psychomotor coordination until CNS effects of
the drug are known.
• Warn patient not to combine drug
with alcohol or other depressants.
• Although package recommends
I.M. use only, this drug may be given
I.V.
• Injectable form (as hydrochloride)
comes as two ampules—diluent and
powdered drug. Read directions carefully. For I.M., add 2 ml of diluent to
powder and agitate gently until clear.
Use immediately. I.M. form may be
erratically absorbed.
• For I.V., use 5 ml of saline injection
or sterile water for injection as diluent; do not give packaged diluent I.V.
Give slowly over 1 minute.
• Keep powder away from light; mix
just before use; discard remainder.
• Do not mix injectable form with
any other parenteral drug.
• Caution patient against giving medication to others.
• Drug should not be prescribed regularly for everyday stress.

clorazepate dipotassium
Gen-Xene, Novoclopate♦♦,
Tranxene♦, Tranxene-SD,
Tranxene-T-Tab
Controlled Substance Schedule IV

Pregnancy Risk Category: C

MECHANISM OF ACTION
Depresses the CNS at the limbic and subcortical levels of the brain. As an anticonvulsant, suppresses the spread of seizure activity produced by epileptogenic foci in the cortex, thalamus, and limbic structures.

INDICATIONS & DOSAGE
Acute alcohol withdrawal—
Adults: Day 1—30 mg P.O. initially, followed by 30 to 60 mg P.O. in divided doses; Day 2—45 to 90 mg P.O. in divided doses; Day 3—22.5 to 45 mg P.O. in divided doses; Day 4—15 to 30 mg P.O. in divided doses; gradually reduce daily dosage to 7.5 to 15 mg.
Anxiety—
Adults: 15 to 60 mg P.O. daily.
As an adjunct in epilepsy—
Adults and children over 12 years: Maximum recommended initial dosage is 7.5 mg P.O. t.i.d. Dosage increases should be no greater than 7.5 mg/week. Maximum daily dosage should not exceed 90 mg daily.
Children between 9 and 12 years: Maximum recommended initial dosage is 7.5 mg P.O. b.i.d. Dosage increases should be no greater than 7.5 mg/week. Maximum daily dosage should not exceed 60 mg/day.

ADVERSE REACTIONS
CNS: *drowsiness, lethargy, hangover,* fainting.
CV: transient hypotension.
GI: nausea, vomiting, abdominal discomfort.

INTERACTIONS
Alcohol, other CNS depressants: increased CNS depression. Avoid concomitant use.
Cimetidine: increased sedation. Monitor carefully.

NURSING CONSIDERATIONS
• Contraindicated in acute narrow-angle glaucoma, depressive neuroses, psychotic reactions, and in children under 18 years. Use with caution when hepatic or renal damage is present.
• Dosage should be reduced in elderly or debilitated patients.
• Possibility of abuse and addiction exists. Do not withdraw drug abruptly; withdrawal symptoms may occur.
• Warn patient to avoid activities requiring alertness and good psychomotor coordination until CNS effects of the drug are known.
• Warn patient not to combine drug with alcohol or other depressants.
• Suggest sugarless chewing gum or hard candy to relieve dry mouth.
• Caution patient against giving medication to others.
• Drug should not be prescribed regularly for everyday stress.

diazepam
Apo-Diazepam♦♦, Diazemuls♦♦,
Diazepam Intensol, E-Pam♦,
Meval♦♦, Novodipam♦♦, Q-Pam,
Rival♦♦, Valium♦, Valrelease,
Vasepam, Vivol♦♦, Zetran
Controlled Substance Schedule IV

Pregnancy Risk Category: D

MECHANISM OF ACTION
Depresses the CNS at the limbic and subcortical levels of the brain. As an anticonvulsant, suppresses the spread of seizure activity produced by epileptogenic foci in the cortex, thalamus, and limbic structures.

Italicized side effects are common or life-threatening.
*Liquid form contains alcohol.   **May contain tartrazine.

INDICATIONS & DOSAGE

Tension, anxiety, adjunct in seizure disorders or skeletal muscle spasm—
Adults: 2 to 10 mg P.O. t.i.d. or q.i.d. Or, 15 to 30 mg of extended-release capsule once daily.
Children over 6 months: 1 to 2.5 mg P.O. t.i.d. or q.i.d.
Tension, anxiety, muscle spasm, endoscopic procedures, seizures—
Adults: 5 to 10 mg I.V. initially, up to 30 mg in 1 hour or possibly more for cardioversion or status epilepticus, depending on response.
Children 5 years and older: 1 mg I.V. or I.M. slowly q 2 to 5 minutes to maximum of 10 mg. Repeat q 2 to 4 hours.
Children 30 days to 5 years: 0.2 to 0.5 mg I.V. or I.M. slowly q 2 to 5 minutes to maximum of 5 mg. Repeat q 2 to 4 hours.
Tetanic muscle spasms—
Children over 5 years: 5 to 10 mg I.M. or I.V. q 3 to 4 hours, p.r.n.
Infants over 30 days: 1 to 2 mg I.M. or I.V. q 3 to 4 hours, p.r.n.
Status epilepticus—
Adults: 5 to 20 mg slow I.V. push 2 to 5 mg/minute; may repeat q 5 to 10 minutes up to maximum total dose of 60 mg. Use 2 to 5 mg in elderly or debilitated patients. May repeat therapy in 20 to 30 minutes with caution if seizures recur.
Children: 0.1 to 0.3 mg/kg slow I.V. push (1 mg/minute over 3 minutes). May repeat q 15 minutes for 2 doses. Maximum single dose in children under 5 years is 5 mg; in children over 5 years, 10 mg.

ADVERSE REACTIONS

CNS: *drowsiness, lethargy, hangover, ataxia,* fainting, slurred speech, tremor.
CV: transient hypotension, bradycardia, *cardiovascular collapse*.
EENT: diplopia, blurred vision, nystagmus.
GI: nausea, vomiting, abdominal discomfort.
Skin: rash, urticaria.
Local: desquamation, *pain, phlebitis at injection site*.
Other: respiratory depression.

INTERACTIONS

Alcohol, other CNS depressants: increased CNS depression. Avoid concomitant use.
Cimetidine: increased sedation. Monitor carefully.
Phenobarbital: increased effects of both drugs. Use together cautiously.

NURSING CONSIDERATIONS

• Contraindicated in shock, coma, acute alcohol intoxication, acute narrow-angle glaucoma, psychoses, myasthenia gravis; in oral form for children under 6 months. Use with caution in blood dyscrasias, hepatic or renal damage, depression, open-angle glaucoma; in elderly and debilitated patients; and in those with limited pulmonary reserve.
• Dosage should be reduced in elderly or debilitated patients.
• Possibility of abuse and addiction exists. Do not withdraw drug abruptly; withdrawal symptoms may occur.
• Monitor CBC and hepatic function during long-term use.
• Warn patient to avoid activities that require alertness and good psychomotor coordination until CNS effects of the drug are known.
• Warn patient not to combine drug with alcohol or other depressants.
• Do not mix injectable form with other drugs because diazepam is incompatible with most drugs.
• There is considerable controversy about the use of diluted diazepam solutions for continuous I.V. infusion because of its low aqueous solubility. Under certain conditions, it may be compatible with sodium chloride 0.9% or Ringer's lactate injection, but the solution may not be stable. Con-

sult hospital pharmacy for further information.

• Avoid extravasation. Do not inject into small veins.

• Watch daily for phlebitis at injection site.

• Give I.V. slowly, at rate not exceeding 5 mg per minute. When injecting I.V., best to administer directly into the vein. If this is not possible, inject slowly through the infusion tubing as close as possible to the vein insertion site.

• Monitor respirations every 5 to 15 minutes and before each repeated I.V. dose. Have emergency resuscitative equipment and oxygen at bedside. Note that naloxone does not reverse the respiratory depression produced by diazepam.

• I.V. route is more reliable; I.M. administration is not recommended because absorption is variable and injection is painful (because the solution is highly alkaline).

• Drug of choice (I.V. form) for status epilepticus.

• Seizures may recur within 20 to 30 minutes of initial control, because of redistribution of the drug.

• Continuous infusions of 1 to 10 mg hourly have been used to prevent seizure recurrence.

• Do not store diazepam in plastic syringes.

• Caution patient against giving medication to others.

• Drug should not be prescribed regularly for everyday stress.

---

halazepam
Paxipam
Controlled Substance Schedule IV
Pregnancy Risk Category: D

MECHANISM OF ACTION
Depresses the CNS at the limbic and subcortical levels of the brain.

INDICATIONS & DOSAGE
Relief of anxiety and tension—
Adults: Usual dose is 20 to 40 mg P.O. t.i.d. or q.i.d. Optimal daily dosage is generally 80 to 160 mg. Daily dosages up to 600 mg have been given. In elderly or debilitated patients, initial dosage is 20 mg once or twice daily.

ADVERSE REACTIONS
CNS: *drowsiness, lethargy, hangover,* fainting.
CV: transient hypotension.
EENT: dry mouth.
GI: nausea and vomiting, discomfort.

INTERACTIONS
Alcohol, other CNS depressants: increased CNS depression. Avoid concomitant use.
Cimetidine: possible increased sedation. Monitor carefully.

NURSING CONSIDERATIONS
• Contraindicated in acute narrow-angle glaucoma, psychoses, or anxiety-free psychiatric disorders. Use with caution in hepatorenal impairment.

• Reduce dosage in elderly or debilitated patients.

• Do not withdraw drug abruptly.

• Abuse and addiction are possible. Withdrawal symptoms may occur.

• Warn patient not to combine drug with alcohol or other depressants, and to avoid activities that require alertness and psychomotor coordination until CNS effects of the drug are known.

• Caution patient against giving medication to others.

• Drug should not be prescribed for everyday stress.

• Halazepam is not for long-term use (more than 4 months).

Italicized side effects are common or life-threatening.
*Liquid form contains alcohol.   **May contain tartrazine.

hydroxyzine hydrochloride
Anxanil, Apo-Hydroxyzine♦♦,
Atarax♦*, Atozine, Durrax, E-Vista,
Hydroxacen, Hyzine-50,
Multipax♦♦, Hyzine-50,
Novohydroxyzin♦♦, Quiess,
Vistacon, Vistaject, Vistaquel,
Vistaril, Vistazine

hydroxyzine pamoate
Hy-Pam, Vamate, Vistaril (oral)

Pregnancy Risk Category: C

MECHANISM OF ACTION
A piperazine antihistamine. Depresses the CNS at the limbic and subcortical levels of the brain.

INDICATIONS & DOSAGE
Anxiety and tension—
Adults: 25 to 100 mg P.O. t.i.d. or q.i.d.
Anxiety, tension, hyperkinesia—
Children over 6 years: 50 to 100 mg P.O. daily in divided doses.
Children under 6 years: 50 mg P.O. daily in divided doses.
Preoperative and postoperative adjunctive therapy—
Adults: 25 to 100 mg I.M. q 4 to 6 hours.
Children: 1.1 mg/kg I.M. q 4 to 6 hours.
Rashes, pruritus—
Adults: 25 mg P.O. t..i.d. or q.i.d.
Children age 6 and over: 50 to 100 mg P.O. daily in divided doses.
Children under age 6: 50 mg P.O. daily in divided doses.

ADVERSE REACTIONS
CNS: *drowsiness,* involuntary motor activity.
GI: *dry mouth.*
Local: marked discomfort at site of I.M. injection.

INTERACTIONS
Alcohol, other CNS depressants: increased CNS depression. Avoid concomitant use.

NURSING CONSIDERATIONS
• Contraindicated in shock or comatose states.
• Dosage should be reduced in elderly or debilitated patients.
• Warn patient to avoid activities that require alertness and good psychomotor coordination until CNS effects of the drug are known.
• Warn patient not to combine drug with alcohol or other depressants.
• Observe for excessive sedation due to potentiation with other CNS drugs.
• Used perioperatively as an antiemetic and anxiolytic. Its sedative and antihistamine properties make it especially useful to treat pruritus that prevents sleep.
• Used in psychogenically induced allergic conditions, such as chronic urticaria and pruritus.
• Parenteral form (hydroxyzine hydrocholoride) for I.M. use only, never I.V. Z-track injection is preferred.
• Aspirate injection carefully to prevent inadvertent intravascular injection. Inject deep into a large muscle.
• Suggest sugarless hard candy or gum to relieve dry mouth.

lorazepam
Alzapam, Apo-Lorazepam♦♦,
Ativan♦, Loraz, Novolorazem♦♦
Controlled Substance Schedule IV

Pregnancy Risk Category: D

MECHANISM OF ACTION
Depresses the CNS at the limbic and subcortical levels of the brain.

INDICATIONS & DOSAGE
Anxiety, tension, agitation, irritability, especially in anxiety neuroses or organic (especially GI or CV) disorders—
Adults: 2 to 6 mg P.O. daily in divided doses. Maximum dosage is 10 mg daily.

Insomnia—
Adults: 2 to 4 mg P.O. h.s.
Premedication before operative procedure—
Adults: 0.05 mg/kg I.M. or I.V., not to exceed 4 mg.

ADVERSE REACTIONS
CNS: *drowsiness, lethargy, hangover,* fainting.
CV: transient hypotension.
GI: dry mouth, abdominal discomfort.

INTERACTIONS
Alcohol, other CNS depressants: increased CNS depression. Avoid comcomitant use.

NURSING CONSIDERATIONS
• Contraindicated in acute narrow-angle glaucoma, psychoses, or mental depression. Use with caution in organic brain syndrome, myasthenia gravis, and renal or hepatic impairment.
• Dosage should be reduced in elderly or debilitated patients. Preoperative I.V. dose should not exceed 2 mg in patients over 50.
• Possibility of abuse and addiction exists with long-term use. Do not withdraw drug abruptly: withdrawal symptoms may occur.
• When administering I.M., inject deep into muscle mass. Don't dilute.
• When administering I.V., dilute with an equal volume of sterile water for injection, sodium chloride injection, or dextrose 5% injection.
• Used as a preoperative premedication before surgery, lorazepam provides substantial preoperative amnesia.
• Warn patient to avoid activities that require alertness or good psychomotor coordination until CNS effects of the drug are known.
• Warn patient not to combine drug with alcohol or other depressants.
• Caution patient against giving med-

ication to others.
• Drug should not be prescribed regularly for everyday stress.
• Fewer cumulative effects than other benzodiazepines, due to short half-life.
• Store parenteral form in refrigerator to prolong shelf life.

---

meprobamate

Apo-Meprobamate♦♦, Equanil♦**,
Meditran♦, Meprospan, Miltown♦,
Neuramate, Novo-Mepro♦♦,
Sedabamate, Tranmep
Controlled Substance Schedule IV
Pregnancy Risk Category: D

MECHANISM OF ACTION
Depresses the CNS at the limbic and subcortical levels of the brain.

INDICATIONS & DOSAGE
Anxiety and tension—
Adults: 1.2 to 1.6 g P.O. in three or four equally divided doses. Maximum dosage is 2.4 g daily.
Children 6 to 12 years: 100 to 200 mg P.O. b.i.d. or t.i.d. Not recommended for children under 6 years.

ADVERSE REACTIONS
Blood: *thrombocytopenia, leukopenia,* eosinophilia.
CNS: *drowsiness,* ataxia, dizziness, slurred speech, headache, vertigo.
CV: palpitation, tachycardia, hypotension.
GI: anorexia, nausea, vomiting, diarrhea, stomatitis.
Skin: pruritus, urticaria, erythematous maculopapular rash.

INTERACTIONS
Alcohol, other CNS depressants: increased CNS depression. Avoid concomitant use.

NURSING CONSIDERATIONS
• Contraindicated in patients with hypersensitivity to meprobamate, cari-

---

Italicized side effects are common or life-threatening.
*Liquid form contains alcohol. **May contain tartrazine.

soprodol, mebutamate, tybamate, car-bromal; and in renal insufficiency or porphyria. Use with caution in impaired hepatic or renal function and in patients with suicidal tendencies.
• Dosage should be reduced in elderly or debilitated patients.
• Possibility of abuse and addiction exists with long-term use. Meprobamate should not be used for everyday stress. Withdraw drug gradually (over 2 weeks) or withdrawal symptoms may occur, including severe generalized tonic-clonic seizures.
• Warn patient to avoid activities that require alertness or good psychomotor coordination until CNS effects of the drug are known.
• Warn patient not to combine drug with alcohol or other depressants.
• Give drug with meals to reduce GI distress.
• Therapeutic blood levels 0.5 to 2 mg/100 ml; levels above 20 mg/100 ml may cause coma and death.
• Periodic evaluation of CBC and liver function tests are indicated in patients receiving high doses.

oxazepam
Apo-Oxazepam♦♦, Novoxapam♦♦, Ox-Pam♦♦, Serax♦**, Zapex♦♦
Controlled Substance Schedule IV
Pregnancy Risk Category: C

MECHANISM OF ACTION
Depresses the CNS at the limbic and subcortical levels of the brain.

INDICATIONS & DOSAGE
Alcohol withdrawal—
Adults: 15 to 30 mg P.O. t.i.d. or q.i.d.
Severe anxiety—
Adults: 15 to 30 mg P.O. t.i.d. or q.i.d.
Tension, mild to moderate anxiety—
Adults: 10 to 15 mg P.O. t.i.d. or q.i.d.

ADVERSE REACTIONS
Blood: *leukopenia*(rare).
CNS: *drowsiness, lethargy, hangover,* fainting.
CV: transient hypotension.
GI: nausea, vomiting, abdominal discomfort.
Metabolic: hepatic dysfunction.

INTERACTIONS
Alcohol, other CNS depressants: increased CNS depression. Avoid concomitant use.

NURSING CONSIDERATIONS
• Contraindicated in psychoses. Use cautiously in patients with history of convulsive disorders, drug allergies, blood dyscrasias, renal disease, and depression.
• Dose should be reduced in elderly or debilitated patients.
• Possibility of abuse and addiction exists. Don't stop drug abruptly; withdrawal symptoms may occur.
• Warn patient to avoid activities that require alertness or good psychomotor coordination until CNS effects of the drug are known.
• Warn patient not to combine drug with alcohol or other depressants.
• Fewer cumulative effects than many other benzodiazepines due to short half-life.
• Caution patient against giving medication to others.
• Monitor CBC and hepatic function periodically in patients on long-term therapy.
• Meprobamate should not be prescribed for everyday stress.

prazepam
Centrax
Controlled Substance Schedule IV
Pregnancy Risk Category: C

MECHANISM OF ACTION
Depresses the CNS at the limbic and subcortical levels of the brain.

INDICATIONS & DOSAGE
Anxiety—
Adults: 30 mg P.O. in divided doses. Range 20 to 60 mg daily. May be administered as single daily dose at bedtime. Start with 20 mg.

ADVERSE REACTIONS
CNS: *drowsiness, lethargy, hangover,* dizziness, ataxia, fainting.
CV: transient hypotension.
GI: dry mouth, nausea, vomiting, abdominal discomfort.
Skin: rash.

INTERACTIONS
Alcohol, other CNS depressants: increased CNS depression. Avoid concomitant use.
Cimetidine: increased sedation. Monitor carefully.

NURSING CONSIDERATIONS
• Contraindicated in acute narrow-angle glaucoma, psychoses, or anxiety-free psychiatric disorders. Use with caution in renal or hepatic impairment.
• Dosage should be reduced in elderly or debilitated patients.
• Possibility of abuse and addiction exists. Don't stop drug abruptly: withdrawal symptoms may occur.
• Warn patient to avoid activities that require alertness and good psychomotor coordination until CNS effects of the drug are known.
• Warn patient not to combine drug with alcohol or other depressants.
• Caution patient against giving medication to others.
• Prazepam should not be prescribed for everyday stress.

Italicized side effects are common or life-threatening.
*Liquid form contains alcohol.   **May contain tartrazine.

33

Antipsychotics

acetophenazine maleate
chlorpromazine hydrochloride
chlorprothixene
fluphenazine decanoate
fluphenazine enanthate
fluphenazine hydrochloride
haloperidol
haloperidol decanoate
loxapine hydrochloride
loxapine succinate
mesoridazine besylate
molindone hydrochloride
perphenazine
pimozide
prochlorperazine
   (See Chapter 49, EMETICS AND
   AMTIEMETICS.)
promazine hydrochloride
thioridazine hydrochloride
thiothixene
thiothixene hydrochloride
trifluoperazine hydrochloride
triflupromazine hydrochloride

COMBINATION PRODUCTS
ETRAFON 2-10: perphenazine 2 mg
and amitriptyline HCl 10 mg.
ETRAFON-A: perphenazine 2 mg and
amitriptyline HCl 25 mg.
ETRAFON-FORTE: perphenazine 4 mg
and amitriptyline HCl 25 mg.
TRIAVIL 2-10, TRIAVIL 4-10, TRIAVIL
2-25 are identical to Etrafon products
above; TRIAVIL 4-50: perphenazine 4
mg and amitriptyline HCl 50 mg.

acetophenazine maleate
Tindal

Pregnancy Risk Category: C

MECHANISM OF ACTION
Blocks postsynaptic dopamine receptors in the brain. A piperazine phenothiazine.

INDICATIONS & DOSAGE
Psychotic disorders—
Adults: initially, 20 mg P.O. t.i.d. or
q.i.d. Daily dosage ranges from 40 to
80 mg in outpatients, or 80 to 120 mg
in hospitalized patients, but in severe
psychotic states up to 600 mg daily
has been safely administered. Smallest effective dosage should be used at
all times.

ADVERSE REACTIONS
Blood: transient leukopenia, *agranulocytosis.*
CNS: *extrapyramidal reactions (high
incidence), tardive dyskinesia,* sedation (low incidence), pseudoparkinsonism, EEG changes, dizziness.
CV: *orthostatic hypotension,* tachycardia, ECG changes.
EENT: ocular changes, *blurred vision.*
GI: *dry mouth, constipation.*
GU: *urine retention,* dark urine, menstrual irregularities, gynecomastia,
inhibited ejaculation.
Hepatic: cholestatic jaundice, abnormal liver function tests.
Metabolic: hyperprolactinemia.
Skin: *mild photosensitivity,* dermal
allergic reactions.

Other: weight gain; increased appetite; rarely, *neuroleptic malignant syndrome* (fever, tachycardia, tachypnea, profuse diaphoresis).

After abrupt withdrawal of long-term therapy: gastritis, nausea, vomiting, dizziness, tremors, feeling of warmth or cold, sweating, tachycardia, headache, insomnia.

INTERACTIONS

Alcohol, other CNS depressants: increased CNS depression. Avoid concomitant use.

Antacids: inhibit absorption of oral phenothiazines. Separate antacid and phenothiazine doses by at least 2 hours.

Barbiturates: may decrease phenothiazine effect. Observe patient.

NURSING CONSIDERATIONS

• Contraindicated in CNS depression, bone marrow suppression, subcortical damage, and coma; also with use of spinal or epidural anesthetic, or adrenergic blocking agents. Use cautiously with other CNS depressants, anticholinergics; in elderly or debilitated patients; and in hepatic disease, arteriosclerosis or cardiovascular disease (may cause sudden drop in blood pressure), exposure to extreme heat or cold (including antipyretic therapy), respiratory disorders, hypocalcemia, seizure disorders (may lower seizure threshold), severe reactions to insulin or electroshock therapy, suspected brain tumor or intestinal obstruction, glaucoma, or prostatic hypertrophy.

• Tardive dyskinesia may occur after prolonged use. It may not appear until months or years later and may disappear spontaneously or persist for life despite discontinuation of drug.

• Acute dystonic reactions may be treated with I.V. diphenhydramine.

• Neuroleptic malignant syndrome is rare, but frequently fatal. It is not necessarily related to length of drug use or type of neuroleptic, but over 60% of affected patients are men. Watch for symptoms.

• Hold dose and notify doctor if patient develops symptoms of blood dyscrasias (fever, sore throat, infection, cellulitis, weakness), persistent (longer than a few hours) extrapyramidal reactions, or any such reaction during pregnancy.

• Dose of 20 mg is therapeutic equivalent of 100 mg chlorpromazine.

• Monitor therapy by weekly bilirubin tests during first month; periodic blood tests (CBC and liver function); and ophthalmic tests (long-term use).

• Have patient report urine retention or constipation.

• Tell patient to use sunscreening agents and protective clothing to avoid photosensitivity reactions.

• Warn against activities requiring alertness or good psychomotor coordination until CNS effects of the drug are known.

• Obtain baseline measures of blood pressure before starting therapy and monitor routinely. Watch for orthostatic hypotension. Advise patient to get up slowly.

• Dry mouth may be relieved with sugarless gum, sour hard candy, or rinsing with mouthwash.

• Do not withdraw drug abruptly unless required by severe side effects.

• Patient on maintenance may take medication at bedtime to facilitate sleep and decrease sedation during daytime.

chlorpromazine hydrochloride

Chlorpromanyl♦♦, Largactil♦♦, Novo-Chlorpromazine♦♦, Thorazine, Thor-Pram

Pregnancy Risk Category: C

MECHANISM OF ACTION

Blocks postsynaptic dopamine receptors in the brain. As an antiemetic, inhibits the medullary chemoreceptor

---

Italicized side effects are common or life-threatening.
*Liquid form contains alcohol.   **May contain tartrazine.

trigger zone. Aliphatic phenothiazine.

INDICATIONS & DOSAGE
Intractable hiccups—
Adults: 25 to 50 mg P.O. or I.M.
t.i.d. or q.i.d.
*Mild alcohol withdrawal, acute inter-
mittent porphyria, and tetanus—*
Adults: 25 to 50 mg I.M. t.i.d. or
q.i.d.
Psychosis—
Adults: 500 mg P.O. daily in divided
doses, increasing gradually to 2 g; or
25 to 50 mg I.M. q 1 to 4 hours, p.r.n.
Children: 0.25 mg/kg P.O. q 4 to 6
hours; or 0.25 mg/kg I.M. q 6 to 8
hours; or 0.5 mg/kg rectally q 6 to 8
hours. Maximum dose is 40 mg in
children under 5 years, and 75 mg in
children 5 to 12 years.
Nausea and vomiting—
Adults: 10 to 225 mg P.O. or I.M. q 4
to 6 hours, p.r.n.; or 50 to 100 mg
rectally q 6 to 8 hours, p.r.n.
Children: 0.25 mg/kg P.O. q 4 to 6
hours; or 0.25 mg/kg I.M. q 6 to 8
hours; or 0.5 mg/kg rectally q 6 to 8
hours.

ADVERSE REACTIONS
Blood: transient leukopenia, *agranulocytosis.*
CNS: *extrapyramidal reactions (moderate incidence), sedation (high incidence), tardive dyskinesia,* pseudoparkinsonism, EEG changes, dizziness.
CV: *orthostatic hypotension,* tachycardia, ECG changes.
EENT: ocular changes, *blurred vision.*
GI: *dry mouth, constipation.*
GU: *urine retention,* dark urine, menstrual irregularities, gynecomastia,
inhibited ejaculation.
Hepatic: cholestatic jaundice, abnormal liver function tests.
Metabolic: hyperprolactinemia.
Skin: *mild photosensitivity,* dermal
allergic reactions.
Local: *pain on I.M. injection,* sterile

abscess.
Other: weight gain; increased appetite; rarely, *neuroleptic malignant syndrome* (fever, tachycardia, tachypnea,
profuse diaphoresis).
**After abrupt withdrawal of long-
term therapy:** gastritis, nausea, vomiting, dizziness, tremors, feeling of
warmth or cold, sweating, tachycardia, headache, insomnia.

INTERACTIONS
Alcohol, other CNS depressants: increased CNS depression. Avoid concomitant use.
Antacids: inhibit absorption of oral
phenothiazines. Separate antacid and
phenothiazine doses by at least 2
hours.
*Anticholinergics (including antide-
pressant and antiparkinsonian
agents):* increased anticholinergic activity, aggravated parkinsonian symptoms. Use with caution.
Barbiturates, lithium: may decrease
phenothiazine effect. Observe patient.
Lithium: possible decreased response
to chlorpromazine. Observe patient.
*Centrally acting antihypertensive
agents:* decreased antihypertensive effect.
Oral anticoagulants: decreased anticoagulant effect.
Propranolol: increased levels of both
propranolol and chlorpromazine.

NURSING CONSIDERATIONS
• Contraindicated in CNS depression,
bone marrow suppresion, subcortical
damage, Reye's syndrome, and coma;
also contraindicated with use of
spinal or epidural anesthetic, or adrenergic blocking agents. Use cautiously with other CNS depressants,
anticholinergics; in elderly or debilitated patients; in hepatic disease, arteriosclerosis or CV disease (may
cause sudden drop in blood pressure),
exposure to extreme heat or cold (including antipyretic therapy), respira-

tory disorders, hypocalcemia, seizure disorders (may lower seizure threshold), severe reactions to insulin or electroshock therapy, suspected brain tumor or intestinal obstruction, glaucoma, or prostatic hypertrophy; and in acutely ill or dehydrated children. Use parenteral form cautiously in asthmatics and in patients allergic to sulfites.

• Tardive dyskinesia may occur after prolonged use. It may not appear until months or years later and may disappear spontaneously or persist for life despite discontinuation of drug.

• Neuroleptic malignant syndrome is rare, but frequently fatal. It is not necessarily related to length of drug use or type of neuroleptic, but over 60% of affected patients are men. Watch for symptoms.

• Acute dystonic reactions may be treated with I.V. diphenhydramine.

• Hold dose and notify doctor if patient develops jaundice, symptoms of blood dyscrasias (fever, sore throat, infection, cellulitis, weakness), persistent (longer than a few hours) extrapyramidal reactions, or any such reaction in pregnancy or in children.

• Monitor therapy by weekly bilirubin tests during first month; periodic blood tests (CBC and liver function); and ophthalmic tests (long-term use).

• Have patient report urine retention or constipation.

• Tell patient to use sunscreening agents and protective clothing to avoid photosensitivity reactions. Chlorpromazine causes higher incidence of photosensitivity than any other drug in its class.

• Warn against activities that require alertness or good psychomotor coordination until CNS effects of the drug are known. Drowsiness and dizziness usually subside after first few weeks.

• Obtain baseline measures of blood pressure before starting therapy and monitor regularly. Watch for orthostatic hypotension, especially with parenteral administration. Monitor blood pressure before and after I.M. administration. Keep patient supine for 1 hour afterward. Advise patient to get up slowly.

• Give deep I.M. only in upper outer quadrant of buttocks. Massage slowly afterward to prevent sterile abscess. Injection stings.

• Liquid (oral) and parenteral forms of drug can cause contact dermatitis. If susceptible, wear gloves when preparing solutions of this drug, and prevent any contact with skin and clothing.

• Protect liquid concentrate from light. Dilute with fruit juice, milk, or semisolid food just before administration.

• Slight yellowing of injection or concentrate is common; does not affect potency. Discard markedly discolored solutions.

• Do not withdraw drug abruptly unless required by severe side effects.

• Dry mouth may be relieved by sugarless gum, sour hard candy, or rinsing with mouthwash.

• Also available as a rectal suppository.

---

chlorprothixene
Taractan**, Tarasan♦♦
Pregnancy Risk Category: C

MECHANISM OF ACTION
Blocks postsynaptic dopamine receptors in the brain. A thioxanthene.

INDICATIONS & DOSAGE
Psychotic disorders—
Adults: initially, 10 mg P.O. t.i.d. or q.i.d. Increase gradually to maximum of 600 mg daily.
Children over 6 years: 10 to 25 mg P.O. t.i.d. or q.i.d.
Agitation of severe neurosis, depression, schizophrenia—
Adults: 25 to 50 mg P.O. or I.M. t.i.d. or q.i.d. Increase as needed up

---

to maximum of 600 mg.

ADVERSE REACTIONS
Blood: transient leukopenia, *agranulocytosis.*
CNS: extrapyramidal reactions (low incidence), tardive dyskinesia, *sedation,* pseudoparkinsonism, EEG changes, dizziness.
CV: *orthostatic hypotension,* tachycardia, ECG changes.
EENT: ocular changes, *blurred vision.*
GI: *dry mouth, constipation.*
GU: *urine retention,* dark urine, menstrual irregularities, gynecomastia, inhibited ejaculation.
Hepatic: cholestatic jaundice, abnormal liver function tests.
Metabolic: hyperprolactinemia.
Skin: *mild photosensitivity,* dermal allergic reactions.
Local: pain on I.M. injection, sterile abscess.
Other: weight gain; increased appetite; rarely, *neuroleptic malignant syndrome* (fever, tachycardia, tachypnea, profuse diaphoresis).
After abrupt withdrawal of long-term therapy: gastritis, nausea, vomiting, dizziness, tremors, feeling of warmth or cold, sweating, tachycardia, headache, insomnia.

INTERACTIONS
Alcohol, other CNS depressants: increased CNS depression. Avoid concomitant use.
Anticholinergics: potentiated central anticholinergic effects.
Centrally acting antihypertensives: decreased antihypertensive effect.

NURSING CONSIDERATIONS
• Contraindicated in coma, CNS depression, bone marrow suppression, circulatory collapse, CHF, cardiac decompensation, coronary artery or cerebrovascular disorders, subcortical damage; with use of spinal or epidural anesthetic, or adrenergic blocking agents. Use cautiously with other CNS depressants, anticholinergics; in elderly or debilitated patients; in hepatic or renal disease, arteriosclerosis or CV disease (may cause sudden drop in blood pressure), exposure to extreme heat or cold (including antipyretic therapy), respiratory disorders, hypocalcemia, seizure disorders (may lower seizure threshold), severe reactions to insulin or electroshock therapy, suspected brain tumor or intestinal obstruction, glaucoma, or prostatic hypertrophy; and in acutely ill or dehydrated children.
• Tardive dyskinesia may occur after prolonged use. It may not appear until months or years later and may disappear spontaneously or persist for life despite discontinuation of drug.
• Neuroleptic malignant syndrome is rare, but frequently fatal. It is not necessarily related to length of drug use or type of neuroleptic, but over 60% of affected patients are men. Watch for symptoms.
• Acute dystonic reactions may be treated with I.V. diphenhydramine.
• Hold dose and notify doctor if patient develops symptoms of blood dyscrasias (fever, sore throat, infection, cellulitis, weakness), jaundice, persistent (longer than a few hours) extrapyramidal reactions, or any such reactions in children.
• Monitor therapy by weekly bilirubin tests during first month; periodic blood tests (CBC and liver function) before and during therapy; and ophthalmic tests (long-term therapy).
• Have patient report urine retention or constipation.
• Tell patient to use sunscreening agents and protective clothing to avoid photosensitivity reactions.
• Warn against activities that require alertness or good psychomotor coordination until CNS effects of the drug are known. Drowsiness and dizziness usually subside after first few weeks.
• Obtain baseline measures of blood

pressure before starting therapy and monitor regularly. Watch for orthostatic hypotension, especially with parenteral administration, since adrenergic blockage is high. Keep patient in a supine position for 1 hour afterward. Advise patient to change positions slowly.

• Give deep I.M. only in upper outer quadrant of buttocks or midlateral thigh. Massage slowly afterward to prevent sterile abscess. Injection stings.

• Dilute liquid concentrate with fruit juice, milk, or semisolid food just before administration.

• Protect medication from light. Slight yellowing of injection or concentrate is common; does not affect potency. Discard markedly discolored solutions.

• Do not withdraw drug abruptly unless required by severe side effects.

• Prevent contact dermatitis by keeping drug off patient's skin and clothes. Wear gloves when preparing liquid forms of the drug.

• Dry mouth may be relieved by sugarless gum, sour hard candy, or rinsing with mouthwash.

• Dose of 100 mg is the therapeutic equivalent of 100 mg chlorpromazine.

---

fluphenazine decanoate
Modecate Decanoate♦♦, Prolixin Decanoate

fluphenazine enanthate
Moditen Enanthate♦♦, Prolixin Enanthate

fluphenazine hydrochloride
Apo-Fluphenazine♦♦, Moditen HCl♦♦, Moditen HCl-HP♦♦, Permitil♦***, Prolixin ***

Pregnancy Risk Category: C

MECHANISM OF ACTION
Blocks postsynaptic dopamine receptors in the brain. A piperazine phenothiazine.

INDICATIONS & DOSAGE
Psychotic disorders—
Adults: initially, 0.5 to 10 mg fluphenazine hydrochloride P.O. daily in divided doses q 6 to 8 hours; may increase cautiously to 20 mg. Higher doses (50 to 100 mg) have been given. Maintenance dosage is 1 to 5 mg P.O. daily. I.M. doses are ⅓ to ½ oral doses. Lower dosages for geriatric patients (1 to 2.5 mg daily).
Children: 0.25 to 3.5 mg fluphenazine HCl P.O. daily in divided doses q 4 to 6 hours; or ⅓ to ½ of oral dose I.M.; maximum dosage is 10 mg daily.
Adults and children over 12 years: 12.5 to 25 mg of long-acting esters (fluphenazine decanoate and enanthate) I.M. or S.C. q 1 to 6 weeks. Maintenance dosage is 25 to 100 mg, p.r.n.

ADVERSE REACTIONS
Blood: transient leukopenia, *agranulocytosis.*
CNS: *extrapyramidal reactions (high incidence), tardive dyskinesia,* sedation (low incidence), pseudoparkinsonism, EEG changes, dizziness.
CV: *orthostatic hypotension,* tachycardia, ECG changes.
EENT: ocular changes, *blurred vision.*
GI: *dry mouth, constipation.*
GU: *urine retention,* dark urine, menstrual irregularities, gynecomastia, inhibited ejaculation.
Hepatic: cholestatic jaundice, abnormal liver function tests.
Metabolic: hyperprolactinemia.
Skin: *mild photosensitivity,* dermal allergic reactions.
Other: weight gain; increased appetite; rarely, *neuroleptic malignant syndrome* (fever, tachycardia, tachypnea, profuse diaphoresis).
After abrupt withdrawal of long-term therapy: gastritis, nausea, vom-

---

Italicized side effects are common or life-threatening.
*Liquid form contains alcohol.   **May contain tartrazine.

iting, dizziness, tremors, feeling of warmth or cold, sweating, tachycardia, headache, insomnia.

INTERACTIONS
Alcohol, other CNS depressants: increased CNS depression. Avoid concomitant use.
Antacids: inhibit absorption of oral phenothiazines. Separate antacid and phenothiazine doses by at least 2 hours.
Barbiturates, lithium: may decrease phenothiazine effect. Observe patient.
Centrally acting antihypertensives: decreased antihypertensive effect.

NURSING CONSIDERATIONS
• Contraindicated in coma, CNS depression, bone marrow suppression or other blood dyscrasia, subcortical damage, hepatic damage, renal insufficiency; and with use of spinal or epidural anesthetic, or adrenergic blocking agents. Use cautiously with other CNS depressants, anticholinergics; in elderly or debilitated patients; in acutely ill or dehydrated children; and in hepatic disease, pheochromocytoma, arteriosclerotic, cerebrovascular, or CV disease (may cause sudden drop in blood pressure), peptic ulcer, exposure to extreme heat or cold (including antipyretic therapy), respiratory disorders, hypocalcemia, seizure disorders (may lower seizure threshold), severe reactions to insulin or electroshock therapy, suspected brain tumor or intestinal obstruction, glaucoma, or prostatic hypertrophy. Use parenteral form cautiously in asthmatic patients and patients allergic to sulfites.
• For long-acting forms (decanoate and enanthate), which are oil preparations, use a dry needle of at least 21 gauge. Allow 24 to 96 hours for onset of action. Note and report adverse side effects in patients taking the long-acting drug forms.

• Tardive dyskinesia may occur after prolonged use. It may not appear until months or years later and may disappear spontaneously or persist for life despite discontinuation of drug.
• Neuroleptic malignant syndrome is rare, but frequently fatal. It is not necessarily related to length of drug use or type of neuroleptic, but over 60% of affected patients are men. Watch for symptoms.
• Acute dystonic reactions may be treated with I.V. diphenhydramine.
• Hold dose and notify doctor if patient develops symptoms of blood dyscrasias (fever, sore throat, infection, cellulitis, weakness), persistent (longer than a few hours) extrapyramidal reactions, or any such reactions in pregnancy or in children.
• Monitor therapy by weekly bilirubin tests during first month; periodic blood tests (CBC and liver function); periodic renal function and ophthalmic tests (long-term use).
• Have patient report urine retention or constipation.
• Tell patient to use sunscreening agents and protective clothing to avoid photosensitivity reactions.
• Warn against activities that require alertness and good psychomotor coordination until CNS effects of the drug are known. Drowsiness and dizziness usually subside after first few weeks.
• Decanoate and enanthate may be given subcutaneously.
• Liquid (oral) and parenteral forms can cause contact dermatitis. If susceptible, wear gloves when preparing solutions of this drug, and prevent any contact with skin and clothing.
• Dilute liquid concentrate with water, fruit juice, milk, or semisolid food just before administration.
• Protect medication from light. Slight yellowing of injection or concentrate is common; does not affect potency. Discard markedly discolored solutions.
• Dry mouth may be relieved by sug-

---

arless gum, sour hard candy, or rinsing with mouthwash.
• Do not withdraw drug abruptly unless required by severe side effects.
• Dose of 2 mg is therapeutic equivalent of 100 mg chlorpromazine.
• Note that Prolixin Concentrate and Permitil Concentrate are 10 times more concentrated than Prolixin Elixir (5 mg/ml vs. 0.5 mg/ml).

haloperidol
Apo-Haloperidol♦♦, Haldol♦**,
Halperon, Novoperidol♦♦,
Peridol♦♦

haloperidol decanoate
Haldol Decanoate, Haldol LA♦♦

Pregnancy Risk Category: C

MECHANISM OF ACTION
Blocks postsynaptic dopamine receptors in the brain. A butyrophenone.

INDICATIONS & DOSAGE
Psychotic disorders—
Adults: dosage varies for each patient. Initial range is 0.5 to 5 mg P.O. b.i.d. or t.i.d.; or 2 to 5 mg I.M. q 4 to 8 hours, increasing rapidly if necessary for prompt control. Maximum dosage is 100 mg P.O. daily. Doses over 100 mg have been used for patients with severely resistant conditions.
Chronic psychotic patients who require prolonged therapy—
Adults: 50 to 100 mg I.M. haloperidol decanoate q 4 weeks.
Control of tics, vocal utterances in Gilles de la Tourette's syndrome—
Adults: 0.5 to 5 mg P.O. b.i.d. or t.i.d., increasing p.r.n.

ADVERSE REACTIONS
Blood: transient leukopenia and leukocytosis.
CNS: *high incidence of severe extrapyramidal reactions, tardive dyskinesia,* low incidence of sedation.
CV: low incidence of cardiovascular effects with therapeutic dosages.
EENT: *blurred vision, dry mouth.*
GU: urine retention, menstrual irregularities, gynecomastia.
Skin: rash.
Other: rarely, *neuroleptic malignant syndrome* (fever, tachycardia, tachypnea, profuse diaphoresis).

INTERACTIONS
Alcohol, other CNS depressants: increased CNS depression. Avoid concomitant use.
Lithium: lethargy and confusion with high doses. Observe patient.
Methyldopa: possible symptoms of dementia. Observe patient.

NURSING CONSIDERATIONS
• Contraindicated in parkinsonism, coma, or CNS depression. Use with caution in elderly and debilitated patients; in severe CV disorders, allergies, glaucoma, urine retention; and in conjunction with anticonvulsant, anticoagulant, antiparkinsonian, or lithium medications.
• Tardive dyskinesia may occur after prolonged use. It may not appear until months or years later and may disappear spontaneously or persist for life despite discontinuation of drug.
• Neuroleptic malignant syndrome is rare, but frequently fatal. It is not necessarily related to length of drug use or type of neuroleptic, but over 60% of affected patients are men. Watch for symptoms.
• Acute dystonic reactions may be treated with I.V. diphenhydramine.
• Elderly patients usually require lower initial doses and a more gradual dosage titration.
• Haloperidol is the least sedating of the antipsychotic agents. However, warn patient against activities that require alertness and good psychomotor coordination until CNS effects of the drug are known. Drowsiness and dizziness usually subside after a few

---

Italicized side effects are common or life-threatening.
*Liquid form contains alcohol.   **May contain tartrazine.

weeks.
- Protect medication from light. Slight yellowing of injection or concentrate is common; does not affect potency. Discard markedly discolored solutions.
- Do not withdraw drug abruptly unless required by severe side effects.
- Dry mouth may be relieved by sugarless gum, sour hard candy, and rinsing with mouthwash.
- Dose of 2 mg is therapeutic equivalent of 100 mg chlorpromazine.
- Especially useful for agitation associated with senile dementia.
- When changing from tablets to decanoate injection, patient should receive 10 to 15 times the oral dose once a month (maximum 100 mg).
- Don't administer the decanoate form I.V.

---

loxapine hydrochloride
Loxapac♦♦, Loxitane C, Loxitane I.M.

loxapine succinate
Loxapac♦♦, Loxitane
Pregnancy Risk Category: C

MECHANISM OF ACTION
Blocks postsynaptic dopamine receptors in the brain. A dibenzoxazepine.

INDICATIONS & DOSAGE
Psychotic disorders—
Adults: 10 mg P.O. or I.M. b.i.d. to q.i.d., rapidly increasing to 60 to 100 mg P.O. daily for most patients; dosage varies from patient to patient.

ADVERSE REACTIONS
Blood: transient leukopenia.
CNS: *extrapyramidal reactions (moderate incidence), sedation (moderate incidence), tardive dyskinesia,* pseudoparkinsonism, EEG changes, dizziness.
CV: *orthostatic hypotension,* tachycardia, ECG changes.

EENT: *blurred vision.*
GI: *dry mouth, constipation.*
GU: *urine retention,* dark urine, menstrual irregularities, gynecomastia.
Skin: *mild photosensitivity,* dermal allergic reactions.
Other: weight gain; increased appetite; rarely, *neuroleptic malignant syndrome* (fever, tachycardia, tachypnea, profuse diaphoresis).

INTERACTIONS
Alcohol, other CNS depressants: increased CNS depression. Avoid concomitant use.

NURSING CONSIDERATIONS
- Contraindicated in coma, severe CNS depression, or drug-induced depressed states. Use with caution in epilepsy, CV disorders, glaucoma, urine retention, suspected intestinal obstruction or brain tumor, and renal damage.
- Tardive dyskinesia may occur after prolonged use. It may not appear until months or years later and may disappear spontaneously or persist for life despite discontinuation of drug.
- Neuroleptic malignant syndrome is rare, but frequently fatal. It is not necessarily related to length of drug use or type of neuroleptic, but over 60% of affected patients are men. Watch for symptoms.
- Acute dystonic reactions may be treated with I.V. diphenhydramine.
- Warn against activities that require alertness and good psychomotor coordination until CNS effects of the drug are known. Drowsiness and dizziness usually subside after first few weeks.
- Obtain baseline measures of blood pressure before starting therapy and monitor regularly. Advise patient to get up slowly to avoid orthostatic hypotension.
- Dilute liquid concentrate with orange or grapefruit juice just before giving.
- Dry mouth may be relieved by sug-

---

arless gum, sour hard candy, or rinsing with mouthwash.
• Periodic eye examinations are recommended.
• Tricyclic dibenzoxazepine; the only dibenzoxazepine derivative.
• Dose of 10 mg is therapeutic equivalent of 100 mg chlorpromazine.

---

mesoridazine besylate
Serentil♦* **

Pregnancy Risk Category: C

MECHANISM OF ACTION
Blocks postsynaptic dopamine receptors in the brain. It is a piperidine phenothiazine and the major sulfoxide metabolite of thioridazine.

INDICATIONS & DOSAGE
Alcoholism—
Adults and children over 12 years: 25 mg P.O. b.i.d. up to maximum of 200 mg daily.
Behavioral problems associated with chronic brain syndrome—
Adults and children over 12 years: 25 mg P.O. t.i.d. up to maximum of 300 mg daily.
Psychoneurotic manifestations (anxiety)—
Adults and children over 12 years: 10 mg P.O. t.i.d. up to maximum of 150 mg daily.
Schizophrenia—
Adults and children over 12 years: initially, 50 mg P.O. t.i.d. or 25 mg I.M. repeated in 30 to 60 minutes, p.r.n.

ADVERSE REACTIONS
Blood: transient leukopenia, *agranulocytosis.*
CNS: extrapyramidal reactions (low incidence), *tardive dyskinesia, sedation (high incidence),* EEG changes, dizziness.
CV: *orthostatic hypotension,* tachycardia, ECG changes.
EENT: *ocular changes, blurred vi-*

sion, pigmentary retinopathy.
GI: *dry mouth, constipation.*
GU: *urine retention,* dark urine, menstrual irregularities, gynecomastia, inhibited ejaculation.
Hepatic: cholestatic jaundice, abnormal liver function tests.
Metabolic: hyperprolactinemia.
Skin: *mild photosensitivity,* dermal allergic reactions.
Local: pain at I.M. injection site, sterile abscess.
Other: weight gain; increased appetite; rarely, *neuroleptic malignant syndrome* (fever, tachycardia, tachypnea, profuse diaphoresis).
After abrupt withdrawal of long-term therapy: gastritis, nausea, vomiting, dizziness, tremors, feeling of warmth or cold, sweating, tachycardia, headache, insomnia.

INTERACTIONS
Alcohol, other CNS depressants: increased CNS depression. Avoid concomitant use.
Antacids: inhibit absorption of oral phenothiazines. Separate antacid and phenothiazine doses by at least 2 hours.
Barbiturates: may decrease phenothiazine effect. Observe patient.

NURSING CONSIDERATIONS
• Contraindicated in coma, CNS depression, bone marrow suppression, subcortical damage, and with use of spinal or epidural anesthetic or adrenergic blocking agents. Use cautiously with other CNS depressants, anticholinergics; in elderly or debilitated patients; in acutely ill or dehydrated children; and in hepatic disease, arteriosclerosis or CV disease (may cause sudden drop in blood pressure), exposure to extreme heat or cold (including antipyretic therapy), respiratory disorders, hypocalcemia, seizure disorders, severe reactions to insulin or electroshock therapy, suspected brain tumor or intestinal obstruction, glau-

---

Italicized side effects are common or life-threatening.
*Liquid form contains alcohol.   **May contain tartrazine.

coma, and prostatic hypertrophy.
• Tardive dyskinesia may occur after prolonged use. It may not appear until months or years later and may disappear spontaneously or persist for life despite discontinuation of drug.
• Neuroleptic malignant syndrome is rare, but frequently fatal. It is not necessarily related to length of drug use or type of neuroleptic, but over 60% of affected patients are men. Watch for symptoms.
• Acute dystonic reactions may be treated with I.V. diphenhydramine.
• Hold dose and notify doctor if patient develops jaundice, symptoms of blood dyscrasias (fever, sore throat, infection, cellulitis, weakness), persistent (longer than a few hours) extrapyramidal reactions, or any such reactions in pregnancy or in children.
• Monitor therapy by weekly bilirubin tests during first month; periodic blood tests (CBC and liver function); and ophthalmic tests (long-term use).
• Have patient report urine retention or constipation.
• Tell patient to use sunscreening agents and protective clothing to avoid photosensitivity reactions.
• Warn against activities that require alertness and good psychomotor coordination until CNS effects of the drug are known. Drowsiness and dizziness usually subside after a few weeks.
• Obtain baseline measures of blood pressure before starting therapy and monitor regularly. Watch for orthostatic hypotension, especially with parenteral administration. Advise patient to change positions slowly.
• Give deep I.M. only in upper outer quadrant of buttocks. Massage slowly afterward to prevent sterile abscess. Injection may sting.
• Protect medication from light. Slight yellowing of injection or concentrate is common; does not affect potency. Discard markedly discolored solutions.
• Liquid (oral) and parenteral forms

may cause contact dermatitis. If susceptible, wear gloves when preparing solutions of this drug, and prevent contact with skin and clothing.
• Dry mouth may be relieved with sugarless gum, sour hard candy, or rinsing with mouthwash.
• Do not withdraw drug abruptly unless required by severe side effects.
• Dose of 50 mg is therapeutic equivalent of 100 mg chlorpromazine.

molindone hydrochloride
Moban

Pregnancy Risk Category: C

MECHANISM OF ACTION
Blocks postsynaptic dopamine receptors in the brain. A dihydroindolone.

INDICATIONS & DOSAGE
Psychotic disorders—
Adults: 50 to 75 mg P.O. daily, increasing to maximum of 225 mg daily. Doses up to 400 mg may be required.

ADVERSE REACTIONS
Blood: transient leukopenia.
CNS: *extrapyramidal reactions (moderate incidence), tardive dyskinesia, sedation (moderate incidence),* pseudoparkinsonism, EEG changes, dizziness.
CV: *orthostatic hypotension,* tachycardia, ECG changes.
EENT: *blurred vision.*
GI: *dry mouth, constipation.*
GU: *urine retention,* dark urine, menstrual irregularities, gynecomastia, inhibited ejaculation.
Hepatic: cholestatic jaundice, abnormal liver function tests.
Metabolic: hyperprolactinemia.
Skin: *mild photosensitivity,* dermal allergic reactions.
Other: rarely, *neuroleptic malignant syndrome* (fever, tachycardia, tachypnea, profuse diaphoresis).

INTERACTIONS
Alcohol, other CNS depressants: increased CNS depression. Avoid concomitant use.

NURSING CONSIDERATIONS
• Contraindicated in coma or severe CNS depression. Use with caution when increased physical activity would be harmful, as this agent increases activity; in seizures (may lower seizure threshold), suicide risk, suspected brain tumor, or intestinal obstruction.
• Tardive dyskinesia may occur after prolonged use. It may not appear until months or years later and may disappear spontaneously or persist for life despite discontinuation of drug.
• Neuroleptic malignant syndrome is rare, but frequently fatal. It is not necessarily related to length of drug use or type of neuroleptic, but over 60% of affected patients are men. Watch for symptoms.
• Acute dystonic reactions may be treated with I.V. diphenhydramine.
• Warn against activities that require alertness or good psychomotor coordination until CNS effects of the drug are known. Drowsiness and dizziness usually subside after first few weeks.
• Dry mouth may be relieved with sugarless gum, sour hard candy, or rinsing with mouthwash.
• Drug is the only dihydroindolone derivative.
• Dose of 20 mg is therapeutic equivalent of 100 mg chlorpromazine.
• No injection available.
• Liquid oral concentrate is available.
• May be administered in a single daily dose.

perphenazine
Apo-Perphenazine♦♦,
Phenazine♦♦, Trilafon♦

Pregnancy Risk Category: C

MECHANISM OF ACTION
Blocks postsynaptic dopamine receptors in the brain. As an antiemetic, inhibits the medullary chemoreceptor trigger zone.

INDICATIONS & DOSAGE
Hospitalized psychiatric patients—
Adults: initially, 8 to 16 mg P.O. b.i.d., t.i.d., or q.i.d., increasing to 64 mg daily.
Children over 12 years: 6 to 12 mg P.O. daily in divided doses.
Mental disturbances, acute alcoholism, nausea, vomiting, hiccups—
Adults and children over 12 years: 5 to 10 mg I.M., p.r.n. Maximum 15 mg daily in ambulatory patients, 30 mg daily in hospitalized patients.

ADVERSE REACTIONS
Blood: transient leukopenia, *agranulocytosis.*
CNS: *extrapyramidal reactions (high incidence), tardive dyskinesia,* sedation (low incidence), pseudoparkinsonism, EEG changes, dizziness.
CV: *orthostatic hypotension,* tachycardia, ECG changes.
EENT: ocular changes, *blurred vision.*
GI: *dry mouth, constipation.*
GU: *urine retention,* dark urine, menstrual irregularities, gynecomastia, inhibited ejaculation.
Hepatic: cholestatic jaundice, abnormal liver function tests.
Metabolic: hyperprolactinemia.
Skin: *mild photosensitivity,* dermal allergic reactions.
Local: pain at I.M. injection site, sterile abscess.
Other: weight gain; increased appetite; rarely, *neuroleptic malignant syndrome* (fever, tachycardia, tachypnea,

---

Italicized side effects are common or life-threatening.
*Liquid form contains alcohol.   **May contain tartrazine.

profuse diaphoresis).

After abrupt withdrawal of long-term therapy: gastritis, nausea, vomiting, dizziness, tremors, feeling of warmth or cold, sweating, tachycardia, headache, insomnia.

INTERACTIONS

Alcohol, other CNS depressants: increased CNS depression. Avoid concomitant use.

Antacids: inhibit absorption of oral phenothiazines. Separate antacid and phenothiazine doses by at least 2 hours.

Barbiturates: may decrease phenothiazine effect. Observe patient.

NURSING CONSIDERATIONS

• Contraindicated in coma, CNS depression, bone marrow suppression, subcortical damage, use of spinal or epidural anesthetic or adrenergic blocking agents. Use cautiously with other CNS depressants, anticholinergics; in elderly or debilitated patients; in acutely ill or dehydrated children; and in hepatic disease, arteriosclerosis or CV disease (may cause sudden drop in blood pressure), exposure to extreme heat or cold (including antipyretic therapy), respiratory disorders, hypocalcemia, seizure disorders (may lower seizure threshold), severe reactions to insulin or electroshock therapy, suspected brain tumor or intestinal obstruction, glaucoma, prostatic hypertrophy.

• Tardive dyskinesia may occur after prolonged use. It may not appear until months or years later and may disappear spontaneously or persist for life despite discontinuation of drug.

• Neuroleptic malignant syndrome is rare, but frequently fatal. It is not necessarily related to length of drug use or type of neuroleptic, but over 60% of affected patients are men. Watch for symptoms.

• Acute dystonic reactions may be treated with I.V. diphenhydramine.

• Hold dose and notify doctor if patient develops jaundice, symptoms of blood dyscrasias (fever, sore throat, infection, cellulitis, weakness), persistent (longer than a few hours) extrapyramidal reactions, or any such reactions in pregnancy or in children.

• Monitor therapy by weekly bilirubin tests during first month; periodic blood tests (CBC and liver function); and ophthalmic tests (long-term use).

• Have patient report urine retention or constipation.

• Tell patient to use sunscreening agents and protective clothing to avoid photosensitivity reactions.

• Warn against activities that require alertness or good psychomotor coordination until CNS effects of the drug are known. Drowsiness and dizziness usually subside after a few weeks.

• Obtain baseline measures of blood pressure before starting therapy and monitor regularly. Watch for orthostatic hypotension, especially with parenteral administration. Keep patient supine for 1 hour afterward. Advise patient to change positions slowly.

• Give deep I.M. only in upper outer quadrant of buttocks. Massage slowly afterward to prevent sterile abscess. Injection may sting.

• Do not withdraw drug abruptly unless required by severe side effects.

• Protect drug from light. Slight yellowing of injection or concentrate is common; does not affect potency. Discard markedly discolored solutions.

• Prevent contact dermatitis by keeping drug off patient's skin and clothes. Wear gloves when preparing liquid forms of the drug.

• Dilute liquid concentrate with fruit juice, milk, carbonated beverage, or semisolid food just before giving. Exceptions: Oral concentrate causes turbidity or precipitation in colas, black coffee, grape or apple juice, or tea. Do not mix with these liquids.

Unmarked trade names available in the United States only.
♦Also available in Canada.   ♦♦Available in Canada only.   ◊Also available OTC.

• Dry mouth may be relieved with sugarless gum, sour hard candy, or rinsing with mouthwash.
• Dose of 8 mg is therapeutic equivalent of 100 mg chlorpromazine.

pimozide
Orap♦

Pregnancy Risk Category: C

MECHANISM OF ACTION
Blocks dopaminergic receptors.

INDICATIONS & DOSAGE
Suppression of severe motor and phonic tics in patients with Tourette's disorder—
Adults and children over 12 years: initially, 1 to 2 mg daily in divided doses. Then, increase dosage every other day. Maintenance dosage ranges from 7 to 16 mg daily.

ADVERSE REACTIONS
CNS: *parkinsonian-like symptoms,* other extrapyramidal symptoms (dystonia, akathisia, hyperreflexia, opisthotonus, oculogyric crisis), *tardive dyskinesia, sedation.*
CV: *ECG changes (prolonged Q-T interval),* hypotension.
EENT: visual disturbances.
GI: *dry mouth, constipation.*
GU: impotence.
Other: rarely, *neuroleptic malignant syndrome* (fever, tachycardia, tacypnea, profuse diaphoresis), muscle tightness.

INTERACTIONS
Alcohol, other CNS depressants: increased CNS depression.
Phenothiazines, tricyclic antidepressants, antiarrhythmics: increased incidence of ECG abnormalities.

NURSING CONSIDERATIONS
• Contraindicated in congenital long Q-T syndrome or history of cardiac dysrhythmias, severe toxic CNS depression, or in coma. Use cautiously in hepatic or renal dysfunction, glaucoma, and prostatic hypertrophy.
• Tardive dyskinesia may occur after prolonged use. It may not appear until months or years later and may disappear spontaneously or persist for life despite discontinuation of drug.
• Neuroleptic malignant syndrome is rare, but frequently fatal. It is not necessarily related to length of drug use or type of neuroleptic, but over 60% of affected patients are men. Watch for symptoms.
• Acute dystonic reactions may be treated with I.V. diphenhydramine.
• Pimozide is not recommended for treatment of simple tics except those associated with Tourette's disorder. Don't use in drug-induced motor and phonic tics.
• Avoid concurrent administration of other drugs that prolong the Q-T interval, such as antiarrhythmic agents.
• Perform an ECG before treatment begins and periodically thereafter. Monitor for prolonged Q-T interval.
• Monitor patients who are also taking anticonvulsants for increased seizure activity. Pimozide may lower the seizure threshold.
• Because pimozide may cause serious adverse effects, the patient and his family should be thoroughly informed before deciding whether he should take the drug. Pimozide is indicated only in patients who have failed to respond satisfactorily to standard treatment.
• Warn patient not to stop taking drug abruptly and not to exceed prescribed dose.
• Tell patient to use sugarless hard candy, gum, and liquids, as needed, to relieve dry mouth.

Italicized side effects are common or life-threatening.
*Liquid form contains alcohol.   **May contain tartrazine.

promazine hydrochloride
Sparine♦**

Pregnancy Risk Category: C

MECHANISM OF ACTION
Blocks postsynaptic dopamine receptors in the brain. An aliphatic phenothiazine.

INDICATIONS & DOSAGE
Psychosis—
Adults: 25 to 200 mg P.O. or I.M. q 4 to 6 hours, up to 1 g daily. I.V. dose in concentrations no greater than 25 mg/ml for acutely agitated patients. Initial dose is 50 to 150 mg; repeat within 5 to 10 minutes if necessary.
Children over 12 years: 10 to 25 mg P.O. or I.M. q 4 to 6 hours.

ADVERSE REACTIONS
Blood: transient leukopenia, *agranulocytosis.*
CNS: *extrapyramidal reactions (moderate incidence), tardive dyskinesia, sedation (high incidence),* pseudoparkinsonism, EEG changes, dizziness.
CV: *orthostatic hypotension,* tachycardia, ECG changes.
EENT: ocular changes, *blurred vision.*
GI: *dry mouth, constipation.*
GU: *urine retention,* dark urine, menstrual irregularities, gynecomastia, inhibited ejaculation.
Hepatic: cholestatic jaundice, abnormal liver function tests.
Metabolic: hyperprolactinemia.
Skin: *mild photosensitivity,* dermal allergic reactions.
Local: pain at I.M. injection site, sterile abscess.
Other: weight gain; increased appetite; rarely, *neuroleptic malignant syndrome* (fever, tachycardia, tachypnea, profuse diaphoresis).
After abrupt withdrawal of long-term therapy: gastritis, nausea, vomiting, dizziness, tremors, feeling of warmth or cold, sweating, tachycardia, headache, insomnia.

INTERACTIONS
Alcohol, other CNS depressants: increased CNS depression. Avoid concomitant use.
Antacids: inhibit absorption of oral phenothiazines. Separate antacid and phenothiazine doses by at least 2 hours.
Anticholinergics (including antidepressant and antiparkinsonian agents): increased anticholinergic activity, aggravated parkinsonian symptoms. Use with caution.
Barbiturates, lithium: may decrease phenothiazine effect. Observe patient.
Centrally acting antihypertensives: decreased antihypertensive effect.
Oral anticoagulants: decreased effectiveness.
Propranolol: increased serum levels of propranolol and promazine.

NURSING CONSIDERATIONS
• Contraindicated in coma, CNS depression, bone marrow suppression, subcortical damage, and with use of spinal or epidural anesthetic or adrenergic blocking agents. Use cautiously with other CNS depressants, anticholinergics; in elderly or debilitated patients; in hepatic disease, arteriosclerosis or CV disease (may cause sudden drop in blood pressure), exposure to extreme heat or cold (including antipyretic therapy), respiratory disorders, hypocalcemia, seizure disorders (may lower seizure threshold), severe reactions to insulin or electroshock therapy, suspected brain tumor or intestinal obstruction, glaucoma, prostatic hypertrophy; and in acutely ill or dehydrated children.
• Tardive dyskinesia may occur after prolonged use. It may not appear until months or years later and may disappear spontaneously or persist for life despite discontinuation of drug.
• Neuroleptic malignant syndrome is

rare, but frequently fatal. It is not necessarily related to length of drug use or type of neuroleptic, but over 60% of affected patients are men. Watch for symptoms.
• Acute dystonic reactions may be treated with I.V. diphenhydramine.
• Hold dose and notify doctor if patient develops jaundice, symptoms of blood dyscrasias (fever, sore throat, infection, cellulitis, weakness), persistent (longer than a few hours) extrapyramidal reactions, or such reactions during pregnancy or in children.
• Monitor therapy by weekly bilirubin tests during first month; periodic blood tests (CBC and liver function); and ophthalmic tests (long-term use).
• Have patient report urine retention or constipation.
• Tell patient to use sunscreening agents and protective clothing to avoid photosensitivity reactions.
• Warn against activities that require alertness or good psychomotor coordination until CNS effects of the drug are known. Drowsiness and dizziness usually subside after a few weeks.
• Monitor blood pressure with patient lying and standing before starting therapy, and routinely throughout course of treatment.
• Watch for orthostatic hypotension, especially with parenteral administration. Keep patient supine for 1 hour afterward. Advise patient to change positions slowly.
• Give deep I.M. only in upper outer quadrant of buttocks. Massage slowly afterward to prevent sterile abscess. Injection may sting.
• Protect drug from light. Slight yellowing of injection or concentrate is common; does not affect potency. Discard markedly discolored solutions.
• Prevent contact dermatitis by keeping drug off patient's skin and clothes. Wear gloves when preparing liquid forms of the drug.
• Dilute liquid concentrate with fruit juice, milk, semisolid food, or chocolate-flavored drinks just before giving. For best taste, use at least 10 ml diluent per 25 mg drug.
• Do not withdraw drug abruptly unless required by severe side effects.
• Dry mouth may be relieved with sugarless gum, sour hard candy, or rinsing with mouthwash.

---

thioridazine hydrochloride
Apo-Thioridazine♦♦, Mellaril♦*, Mellaril-S, Novoridazine♦♦, PMS Thioridazine♦♦

Pregnancy Risk Category: C

MECHANISM OF ACTION
Blocks postsynaptic dopamine receptors in the brain. A piperidine phenothiazine.

INDICATIONS & DOSAGE
Psychosis—
Adults: initially, 50 to 100 mg P.O. t.i.d., with gradual increments up to 800 mg daily in divided doses, if needed. Dosage varies.
Adults over 65 years: initial dose, 25 mg t.i.d.
Depressive neurosis, alcohol withdrawal, dementia in geriatric patients, behavioral problems in children—
Adults: initially, 25 mg P.O. t.i.d. Maintenance dosage is 20 to 200 mg daily.
Children over 2 years: 0.5 to 3 mg/kg daily in divided doses.

ADVERSE REACTIONS
Blood: transient leukopenia, *agranulocytosis.*
CNS: extrapyramidal reactions (low incidence), *tardive dyskinesia, sedation (high incidence),* EEG changes, dizziness.
CV: *orthostatic hypotension,* tachycardia, ECG changes.
EENT: *ocular changes, blurred vision,* pigmentary retinopathy.

Italicized side effects are common or life-threatening.
*Liquid form contains alcohol.   **May contain tartrazine.

GI: *dry mouth, constipation*.
GU: *urine retention*, dark urine, menstrual irregularities, gynecomastia, inhibited ejaculation.
Hepatic: cholestatic jaundice.
Metabolic: hyperprolactinemia.
Skin: *mild photosensitivity*, dermal allergic reactions.
Other: weight gain; increased appetite; rarely, *neuroleptic malignant syndrome* (fever, tachycardia, tachypnea, profuse diaphoresis).
After abrupt withdrawal of long-term therapy: gastritis, nausea, vomiting, dizziness, tremors, feeling of warmth or cold, sweating, tachycardia, headache, insomnia.

INTERACTIONS

Alcohol, other CNS depressants: increased CNS depression. Avoid concomitant use.
Antacids: inhibit absorption of oral phenothiazines. Separate antacid and phenothiazine doses by at least 2 hours.
Barbiturates, lithium: may decrease phenothiazine effect. Observe patient.
Centrally acting antihypertensives: decreased antihypertensive effect.

NURSING CONSIDERATIONS

• Contraindicated in coma, CNS depression, bone marrow suppression, hypertensive or hypotensive cardiac disease, subcortical damage, and with use of spinal or epidural anesthetic or adrenergic blocking agents. Use cautiously with other CNS depressants, anticholinergics; in elderly or debilitated patients; in hepatic disease, arteriosclerosis or CV disease (may cause sudden drop in blood pressure), exposure to extreme heat or cold (including antipyretic therapy), respiratory disorders, hypocalcemia, seizure disorders, severe reactions to insulin or electroshock therapy, suspected brain tumor or intestinal obstruction, glaucoma, or prostatic hypertrophy;

and in acutely ill or dehydrated children.
• Tardive dyskinesia may occur after prolonged use. It may not appear until months or years later and may disappear spontaneously or persist for life despite discontinuation of drug.
• Neuroleptic malignant syndrome is rare, but frequently fatal. It is not necessarily related to length of drug use or type of neuroleptic, but over 60% of affected patients are men. Watch for symptoms.
• Acute dystonic reactions may be treated with I.V. diphenhydramine.
• Hold dose and notify doctor if patient develops jaundice, symptoms of blood dyscrasias (fever, sore throat, infection, cellulitis, weakness), persistent (longer than a few hours) extrapyramidal reactions, or such reactions during pregnancy or in children.
• Monitor therapy by weekly bilirubin tests during first month; periodic blood tests (CBC and liver function); and ophthalmic tests (long-term therapy).
• Have patient report urine retention or constipation.
• Watch for blurred vision, dry mouth; high incidence of anticholinergic effects.
• Tell patient to use sunscreening agents and protective clothing to avoid photosensitivity reactions.
• Monitor blood pressure.
• Warn against activities that require alertness or good psychomotor coordination until CNS effects of the drug are known. Drowsiness and dizziness usually subside after a few weeks.
• Watch for orthostatic hypotension, especially with parenteral administration. Advise patient to change positions slowly.
• Prevent contact dermatitis by keeping drug off patient's skin and clothes. Wear gloves when preparing liquid forms of the drug.
• Caution: There are four different liquid formulations available (two

concentrates and two suspensions).
• Not available in injectable form.
Mesoridazine is prescribed when parenteral use of a thioridazine-like drug is desirable.
• Dilute liquid concentrate with water or fruit juice just before giving.
• Do not withdraw abruptly unless required by severe side effects.
• Dry mouth may be relieved with sugarless gum, sour hard candy, or rinsing with mouthwash.
• Dose of 100 mg is the therapeutic equivalent of 100 mg chlorpromazine.
• Dosage above 800 mg may be associated with ocular toxicity (pigmentary retinopathy).

thiothixene
Navane♦

thiothixene hydrochloride
Navane♦*

Pregnancy Risk Category: C

MECHANISM OF ACTION
Blocks postsynaptic dopamine receptors in the brain. A thioxanthene.

INDICATIONS & DOSAGE
Acute agitation—
Adults: 4 mg I.M. b.i.d. to q.i.d. Maximum dosage is 30 mg daily I.M. Change to P.O. as soon as possible.
Mild to moderate psychosis—
Adults: initially, 2 mg P.O. t.i.d. May increase gradually to 15 mg daily.
Severe psychosis—
Adults: initially, 5 mg P.O. b.i.d. May increase gradually to 15 to 30 mg daily. Maximum recommended daily dose is 60 mg. Not recommended in children under 12 years.

ADVERSE REACTIONS
Blood: transient leukopenia, *agranulocytosis.*
CNS: *extrapyramidal reactions (high incidence), tardive dyskinesia,* sedation (low incidence), pseudoparkin-

sonism, EEG changes, dizziness.
CV: *orthostatic hypotension,* tachycardia, ECG changes.
EENT: ocular changes, *blurred vision.*
GI: *dry mouth, constipation.*
GU: *urine retention,* dark urine, menstrual irregularities, gynecomastia, inhibited ejaculation.
Hepatic: cholestatic jaundice.
Metabolic: hyperprolactinemia.
Skin: *mild photosensitivity,* dermal allergic reactions.
Local: pain at I.M. injection site, sterile abscess.
Other: weight gain; increased appetite; rarely, *neuroleptic malignant syndrome* (fever, tachycardia, tachypnea, profuse diaphoresis).
After abrupt withdrawal of long-term therapy: gastritis, nausea, vomiting, dizziness, tremors, feeling of warmth or cold, sweating, tachycardia, headache, insomnia.

INTERACTIONS
Alcohol, other CNS depressants: increased CNS depression. Avoid concomitant use.

NURSING CONSIDERATIONS
• Contraindicated in convulsive seizures, circulatory collapse, coma, CNS depression, blood dyscrasias, bone marrow suppression, alcohol withdrawal, akathisia or restlessness, subcortical damage, and with use of spinal or epidural anesthetic or adrenergic blocking agents. Use cautiously with other CNS depressants, anticholinergics; in elderly or debilitated patients; and in hepatic disease, arteriosclerosis or CV disease (may cause sudden drop in blood pressure), exposure to extreme heat or cold (including antipyretic therapy) or undue sunlight, respiratory disorders, hypocalcemia, severe reactions to insulin or electroshock therapy, suspected brain tumor or intestinal obstruction, glaucoma, and prostatic hypertrophy.

Italicized side effects are common or life-threatening.
*Liquid form contains alcohol.   **May contain tartrazine.

• Tardive dyskinesia may occur after prolonged use. It may not appear until months or years later and may disappear spontaneously or persist for life despite discontinuation of drug.
• Neuroleptic malignant syndrome is rare, but frequently fatal. It is not necessarily related to length of drug use or type of neuroleptic, but over 60% of affected patients are men. Watch for symptoms.
• Acute dystonic reactions may be treated with I.V. diphenhydramine.
• Hold dose and notify doctor if patient develops jaundice, symptoms of blood dyscrasias (fever, sore throat, infection, cellulitis, weakness), persistent (longer than a few hours) extrapyramidal reactions, or any such reactions during pregnancy.
• Monitor therapy by weekly bilirubin tests during first month; periodic blood tests (CBC and liver function); and ophthalmic tests (long-term use).
• Have patient report urine retention or constipation.
• Tell patient to use sunscreening agents and protective clothing to avoid photosensitivity reactions.
• Warn against activities that require alertness or good psychomotor coordination until CNS effects of the drug are known. Drowsiness and dizziness usually subside after a few weeks.
• Watch for orthostatic hypotension, especially with parenteral administration. Keep patient in a supine position for 1 hour afterward. Advise patient to change positions slowly.
• Give I.M. only in upper outer quadrant of buttocks or midlateral thigh. Massage slowly afterward to prevent sterile abscess. Injection may sting.
• I.M. form must be stored in refrigerator.
• Slight yellowing of injection or concentrate is common; does not affect potency. Discard markedly discolored solutions.
• Prevent contact dermatitis by keeping drug off patient's skin and clothes.

Wear gloves when preparing liquid forms of the drug.
• Dilute liquid concentrate with fruit juice, milk, or semisolid food just before giving.
• Do not withdraw abruptly unless required by severe side effects.
• Dry mouth may be relieved with sugarless gum, sour hard candy, or rinsing with mouthwash.
• Dose of 4 mg is therapeutic equivalent of 100 mg chlorpromazine.

trifluoperazine hydrochloride
Apo-Trifluoperazine♦♦, Novo-Flurazine♦♦, Solazine♦♦, Stelazine♦, Suprazine, Terfluzine♦♦

Pregnancy Risk Category: C

MECHANISM OF ACTION
Blocks postsynaptic dopamine receptors in the brain. A piperazine phenothiazine.

INDICATIONS & DOSAGE
Anxiety states—
Adults: 1 to 2 mg P.O. b.i.d.
Schizophrenia and other psychotic disorders—
Adults: *outpatients*—1 to 2 mg P.O. b.i.d., up to 4 mg daily; *hospitalized*—2 to 5 mg P.O. b.i.d.; may gradually increase to 40 mg daily. 1 to 2 mg I.M. q 4 to 6 hours, p.r.n.
Children 6 to 12 years (hospitalized or under close supervision): 1 mg P.O. daily or b.i.d.; may increase gradually to 15 mg daily.

ADVERSE REACTIONS
Blood: transient leukopenia, *agranulocytosis.*
CNS: *extrapyramidal reactions (high incidence), tardive dyskinesia,* sedation (low incidence), pseudoparkinsonism, EEG changes, dizziness.
CV: *orthostatic hypotension,* tachycardia, ECG changes.
EENT: ocular changes, *blurred vi-*

EENT: ocular changes, *blurred vision*.
GI: *dry mouth, constipation*.
GU: *urine retention*, dark urine, menstrual irregularities, gynecomastia, inhibited ejaculation.
Hepatic: cholestatic jaundice.
Metabolic: hyperprolactinemia.
Skin: *mild photosensitivity*, dermal allergic reactions.
Local: pain at I.M. injection site, sterile abscess.
Other: weight gain; increased appetite; rarely, *neuroleptic malignant syndrome* (fever, tachycardia, tachypnea, profuse diaphoresis).
After abrupt withdrawal of long-term therapy: gastritis, nausea, vomiting, dizziness, tremors, feeling of warmth or cold, sweating, tachycardia, headache, insomnia.

INTERACTIONS
Alcohol, other CNS depressants: increased CNS depression. Avoid concomitant use.
Antacids: inhibit absorption of oral phenothiazines. Separate antacid and phenothiazine doses by at least 2 hours.
Barbiturates, lithium: may decrease phenothiazine effect. Observe patient.
Centrally acting antihypertensives: decreased antihypertensive effect.

NURSING CONSIDERATIONS
• Contraindicated in coma, CNS depression, bone marrow suppression, subcortical damage, and with use of spinal or epidural anesthetic or adrenergic blocking agents. Use cautiously with other CNS depressants, anticholinergics; in elderly or debilitated patients; in hepatic disease, arteriosclerosis or CV disease (may cause drop in blood pressure), exposure to extreme heat or cold (including antipyretic therapy), respiratory disorders, hypocalcemia, seizure disorders, severe reactions to insulin or electro-

shock therapy, suspected brain tumor or intestinal obstruction, glaucoma, or prostatic hypertrophy; and in acutely ill or dehydrated children.
• Tardive dyskinesia may occur after prolonged use. It may not appear until months or years later and may disappear spontaneously or persist for life despite discontinuation of drug.
• Neuroleptic malignant syndrome is rare, but frequently fatal. It is not necessarily related to length of drug use or type of neuroleptic, but over 60% of affected patients are men. Watch for symptoms.
• Acute dystonic reactions may be treated with I.V. diphenhydramine.
• Hold dose and notify doctor if patient develops jaundice, symptoms of blood dyscrasias (fever, sore throat, infection, cellulitis, weakness), persistent (longer than a few hours) extrapyramidal reactions, or any such reactions during pregnancy or in children.
• Monitor therapy by weekly bilirubin tests during first month; periodic blood tests (CBC and liver function); and ophthalmic tests (long-term use).
• Have patient report urine retention or constipation.
• Tell patient to use sunscreening agents and protective clothing to avoid photosensitivity reactions.
• Warn against activities that require alertness or good psychomotor coordination until CNS effects of the drug are known. Drowsiness and dizziness usually subside after a few weeks.
• Watch for orthostatic hypotension, especially with parenteral administration. Keep patient supine for 1 hour afterward. Advise patient to change positions slowly.
• Give deep I.M. only in upper outer quadrant of buttocks. Massage slowly afterward to prevent sterile abscess. Injection may sting.
• Protect drug from light. Slight yellowing of injection or concentrate is common; does not affect potency.

Italicized side effects are common or life-threatening.
*Liquid form contains alcohol.   **May contain tartrazine.

Discard markedly discolored solutions.
• Prevent contact dermatitis by keeping drug off patient's skin and clothes. Wear gloves when preparing liquid forms of the drug.
• Dilute liquid concentrate with 60 ml tomato or fruit juice, carbonated beverages, coffee, tea, milk, water, or semisolid food just before giving.
• Do not withdraw abruptly unless required by severe side effects.
• Dry mouth may be relieved with sugarless gum, sour hard candy, or rinsing with mouthwash.
• Drug is a prototype piperazine phenothiazine.
• Dose of 5 mg is therapeutic equivalent of 100 mg chlorpromazine.

triflupromazine hydrochloride
Vesprin

Pregnancy Risk Category: C

MECHANISM OF ACTION
Blocks postsynaptic dopamine receptors in the brain. An aliphatic phenothiazine.

INDICATIONS & DOSAGE
Acute, severe agitation—
Adults: 60 to 150 mg I.M. in two or three divided doses.
Children over 2½ years: 0.2 to 0.25 mg/kg in divided doses. Maximum dosage is 10 mg daily.
Nausea and vomiting—
Adults: 1 to 3 mg I.V. daily; or 5 to 15 mg I.M. daily up to maximum of 60 mg daily.
Children: 0.2 mg/kg I.M. up to maximum of 10 mg daily.

ADVERSE REACTIONS
Blood: transient leukopenia, *agranulocytosis.*
CNS: *extrapyramidal reactions (moderate incidence), tardive dyskinesia, sedation (high incidence),* pseudopar-
kinsonism, EEG changes, dizziness.
CV: *orthostatic hypotension,* tachycardia, ECG changes.
EENT: ocular changes, *blurred vision.*
GI: *dry mouth, constipation.*
GU: *urine retention,* dark urine, menstrual irregularities, gynecomastia, inhibited ejaculation.
Hepatic: cholestatic jaundice.
Metabolic: hyperprolactinemia.
Skin: *mild photosensitivity,* dermal allergic reactions.
Local: pain at I.M. injection site, sterile abscess.
Other: weight gain; increased appetite; rarely, *neuroleptic malignant syndrome* (fever, tachycardia, tachypnea, profuse diaphoresis).
After abrupt withdrawal of long-term therapy: gastritis, nausea, vomiting, dizziness, tremors, feeling of warmth or cold, sweating, tachycardia, headache, insomnia.

INTERACTIONS
Alcohol, other CNS depressants: increased CNS depression. Avoid concomitant use.
Anticholinergics (including antidepressant and antiparkinsonian agents): increased anticholinergic activity, aggravated parkinsonian symptoms. Use with caution.
Barbiturates, lithium: may decrease phenothiazine effect. Observe patient.
Centrally acting antihypertensives: decreased antihypertensive effect.

NURSING CONSIDERATIONS
• Contraindicated in coma, CNS depression, blood dyscrasias, bone marrow suppression, subcortical brain damage, and with use of spinal or epidural anesthetic or adrenergic blocking agents. Use cautiously with other CNS depressants, anticholinergics; in elderly or debilitated patients; in hepatic disease, arteriosclerosis or CV disease (may cause sudden drop in

heat or cold (including antipyretic therapy), respiratory disorders, pheochromocytoma, hypocalcemia, seizure disorders, severe reactions to insulin or electroshock therapy, suspected brain tumor or intestinal obstruction, glaucoma, prostatic hypertrophy; and in acutely ill or dehydrated children.

• Tardive dyskinesia may occur after prolonged use. It may not appear until months or years later and may disappear spontaneously or persist for life despite discontinuation of drug.

• Neuroleptic malignant syndrome is rare, but frequently fatal. It is not necessarily related to length of drug use or type of neuroleptic, but over 60% of affected patients are men. Watch for symptoms.

• Acute dystonic reactions may be treated with I.V. diphenhydramine.

• Hold dose and notify doctor if patient develops jaundice, symptoms of blood dyscrasias (fever, sore throat, infection, cellulitis, weakness), persistent (longer than a few hours) extrapyramidal reactions, or any such reactions during pregnancy or in children.

• Monitor therapy by weekly bilirubin tests during first month; periodic blood tests (CBC and liver function); and ophthalmic tests in long-term use.

• Have patient report urine retention or constipation.

• Tell patient to use sunscreening agents and protective clothing to avoid photosensitivity reactions.

• Warn against activities that require alertness or good psychomotor coordination until CNS effects of the drug are known. Drowsiness and dizziness usually subside after a few weeks.

• Watch for orthostatic hypotension, especially with parenteral administration. Keep patient supine for 1 hour afterward. Advise patient to change positions slowly.

• Give I.M. only in upper outer quadrant of buttocks. Massage slowly afterward to prevent sterile abscess. Injection may sting.

• Protect drug from light. Slight yellowing of injection or concentrate is common; does not affect potency. Discard markedly discolored solutions.

• Prevent contact dermatitis by avoiding contact with skin.

• Do not withdraw abruptly unless required by severe side effects.

• Dry mouth may be relieved with sugarless gum, sour hard candy, or rinsing with mouthwash.

• Dose of 25 mg is therapeutic equivalent of 100 mg chlorpromazine.

34

Miscellaneous psychotherapeutics

lithium carbonate
lithium citrate

COMBINATION PRODUCTS
None.

lithium carbonate
Carbolith♦♦, Duralith♦♦, Eskalith, Eskalith CR, Lithane♦**, Lithizine♦♦, Lithobid, Lithonate, Lithotabs

lithium citrate
Cibalith-S

Pregnancy Risk Category: D

MECHANISM OF ACTION
Alters chemical transmitters in the CNS, possibly by interfering with ionic pump mechanisms in brain cells. Its exact mechanism of action in mania, however, is unknown.

INDICATIONS & DOSAGE
Prevention or control of mania—
Adults: 300 to 600 mg P.O. up to q.i.d., increasing on the basis of blood levels to achieve optimal dosage. Recommended therapeutic lithium blood levels: 1 to 1.5 mEq/liter for acute mania; 0.6 to 1.2 mEq/liter for maintenance therapy; and 2 mEq/liter as maximum.
    Note: 5 ml lithium citrate (liquid) contains 8 mEq lithium equal to 300 mg lithium carbonate.

ADVERSE REACTIONS
Blood: *leukocytosis of 14,000 to 18,000 (reversible).*

CNS: tremors, drowsiness, headache, confusion, restlessness, dizziness, psychomotor retardation, stupor, lethargy, coma, blackouts, epileptiform seizures, EEG changes, worsened organic brain syndrome, impaired speech, ataxia, muscle weakness, incoordination, hyperexcitability.
CV: *reversible ECG changes,* dysrhythmias, hypotension, peripheral circulatory collapse, allergic vasculitis, ankle and wrist edema.
EENT: tinnitus, impaired vision.
GI: nausea, vomiting, anorexia, diarrhea, dry mouth, *thirst,* metallic taste.
GU: *polyuria,* glycosuria, incontinence, renal toxicity with long-term use.
Metabolic: transient hyperglycemia, goiter, hypothyroidism (lowered T_3, T_4, and protein-bound iodine, but elevated ^{131}I uptake), hyponatremia.
Skin: pruritus, rash, diminished or lost sensation, drying and thinning of hair.

INTERACTIONS
Aminophylline, sodium bicarbonate, and sodium chloride: ingestion of these salts increases lithium excretion. Avoid salt loads and monitor lithium levels.
Carbamazepine, probenecid, indomethacin, methyldopa and piroxicam: increased effect of lithium. Monitor for lithium toxicity.
Diuretics: increased reabsorption of lithium by kidneys, with possible toxic effect. Use with extreme caution, and monitor lithium and electro-

lyte levels (especially sodium).
Haloperidol and thioridazine: encephalopathic syndrome (lethargy, tremors, extrapyramidal symptoms).
Watch for syndrome, and stop drug if it occurs.
Thyroid hormones: lithium may induce hypothyroidism.

NURSING CONSIDERATIONS
• Contraindicated if therapy cannot be closely monitored. Use with caution with haloperidol, other antipsychotics, neuromuscular blocking agents, and diuretics; in elderly or debilitated persons; and in thyroid disease, epilepsy, renal or cardiovascular disease, brain damage, severe debilitation or dehydration, and sodium depletion.
• Monitor baseline ECG, thyroid, and renal studies, and electrolyte levels. Monitor lithium blood levels 8 to 12 hours after first dose, usually before morning dose, two or three times weekly first month, then weekly to monthly on maintenance.
• Determination of lithium blood concentration is crucial to the safe use of the drug. Shouldn't be used in patients who can't have regular lithium blood level checks.
• Explain to patient that lithium has a narrow therapeutic margin of safety. A blood level that is even slightly too high can be dangerous.
• When blood levels of lithium are below 1.5 mEq/liter, adverse reactions usually remain mild.
• Check fluid intake/output, especially when surgery is scheduled.
• Warn patient and family to watch for signs of toxicity (diarrhea, vomiting, drowsiness, muscular weakness, ataxia) and to expect transient nausea, polyuria, thirst, and discomfort during first few days. Patient should withhold one dose and call doctor if toxic symptoms appear, but not stop drug abruptly.
• Expect lag of 1 to 3 weeks before drug's beneficial effects are noticed.
• Weigh patient daily; check for signs of edema or sudden weight gain.
• Adjust fluid and salt ingestion to compensate if excessive loss occurs through protracted sweating or diarrhea. Under normal conditions, patients should have fluid intake of 2,500 to 3,000 ml daily and a balanced diet with adequate salt intake.
• Have outpatient follow-up of thyroid and renal functions every 6 to 12 months. Palpate thyroid to check for enlargement.
• Patient should carry identification/instruction card (available from pharmacy) with toxicity and emergency information.
• Warn ambulatory patient to avoid activities that require alertness and good psychomotor coordination until CNS effects of the drug are known.
• Administer with plenty of water, and after meals to minimize GI upset.
• Check urine for specific gravity and report level below 1.005, which may indicate diabetes insipidus syndrome.
• May alter glucose tolerance in diabetics. Monitor blood glucose closely.
• Tell patient not to switch brands of lithium or to take other drugs (prescription or OTC) without doctor's guidance.
• Investigationally used to increase white cells in patients undergoing cancer chemotherapy.
• Also used investigationally for treatment of cluster headaches, aggression, organic brain syndrome, and tardive dyskinesia. Has been used to treat syndrome of inappropriate antidiuretic hormone.

Italicized side effects are common or life-threatening.
*Liquid form contains alcohol.   **May contain tartrazine.

35

Cerebral stimulants

amphetamine sulfate
benzphetamine hydrochloride
caffeine◇
dextroamphetamine sulfate
diethylpropion hydrochloride
fenfluramine hydrochloride
mazindol
methamphetamine hydrochloride
methylphenidate hydrochloride
pemoline
phendimetrazine tartrate
phenmetrazine hydrochloride
phentermine hydrochloride

COMBINATION PRODUCTS
BIPHETAMINE 12½: dextroamphetamine 6.25 mg and amphetamine
6.25 mg.
BIPHETAMINE 20: dextroamphetamine
10 mg and amphetamine 10 mg.

---

amphetamine sulfate
Controlled Substance Schedule II

Pregnancy Risk Category: C

MECHANISM OF ACTION
Main site of activity appears to be the
cerebral cortex and the reticular activating system. Promotes nerve impulse transmission by releasing stored
norepinephrine from nerve terminals
in the brain. In children with hyperkinesia, amphetamines have a paradoxical calming effect.

INDICATIONS & DOSAGE
*Attention deficit disorder with hyper-
activity (ADDH)—*
Children 6 years and older: 5 mg
P.O. daily, with 5-mg increments

weekly, p.r.n.
Children 3 to 5 years: 2.5 mg P.O.
daily, with 2.5-mg increments
weekly, p.r.n.
Narcolepsy—
Adults: 5 to 60 mg P.O. daily in divided doses.
Children over 12 years: 10 mg P.O.
daily, with 10-mg increments weekly,
p.r.n.
Children 6 to 12 years: 5 mg P.O.
daily, with 5-mg increments weekly,
p.r.n.
*Short-term adjunct in exogenous obe-
sity—*
Adults: single 10- or 15-mg long-acting capsule daily, or 2 if needed, up to
30 mg daily; or 5 to 30 mg daily in divided doses 30 to 60 minutes before
meals. Not recommended for children
under 12 years.

ADVERSE REACTIONS
CNS: *restlessness,* tremor, *hyperactivity, talkativeness, insomnia,* irritability, dizziness, headache, chills, overstimulation, dysphoria.
CV: *tachycardia, palpitations,* hypertension, hypotension.
GI: nausea, vomiting, cramps, dry
mouth, diarrhea, constipation, metallic taste, anorexia, weight loss.
Other: urticaria, impotence, altered
libido.

INTERACTIONS
MAO inhibitors: severe hypertension;
possible hypertensive crisis. Don't
use together.
*Antacids, sodium bicarbonate, acet-
azolamide:* increased renal reabsorp-

---

tion. Monitor for enhanced effect.
Ammonium chloride, ascorbic acid:
observe for decreased amphetamine
effect.
Phenothiazines, haloperidol: observe
for decreased amphetamine effect.

NURSING CONSIDERATIONS
• Contraindicated in symptomatic
CV diseases, hyperthyroidism, nephritis, angina pectoris, moderate to
severe hypertension, parkinsonism
due to arteriosclerosis, certain types
of glaucoma, advanced arteriosclerosis, in agitated states, or patients with
history of drug abuse. Use with caution in diabetes mellitus and in elderly, debilitated, or hyperexcitable
patients.
• Use cautiously in children with
Tourette's disorder.
• Psychic dependence or habituation
may occur, especially in patients with
history of drug addiction. Avoid prolonged administration. When used
long-term, lower dosage gradually to
prevent acute rebound depression.
• Not recommended for first-line
treatment of obesity. Use as an anorexigenic agent is prohibited in some
states.
• When used for obesity, make sure
patient is also on a weight-reduction
program. Give drug 30 to 60 minutes
before meals. Monitor dietary intake.
Do calorie counts, if necessary.
• Fatigue may result as drug effects
wear off. Patient will need more rest.
• Tell patient to avoid drinks containing caffeine, which increase the effects of amphetamines and related
amines.
• Have patient report signs of excessive stimulation.
• Urine acidification enhances renal
excretion; urine alkalinization enhances renal reabsorption and recycling.
• When tolerance to anorexigenic effect develops, dosage should not be
increased, but drug discontinued.

• Should not be used to combat fatigue.
• Warn patient to avoid activities that
require alertness or good psychomotor coordination until CNS effects of
the drug are known.
• May alter daily insulin needs in patients with diabetes. Monitor blood
and urine sugars.
• Use as analeptic is usually discouraged, since CNS stimulation superimposed on CNS depression can lead to
neuronal instability and seizures.
• May reverse beneficial effect of antihypertensives. Monitor blood pressure.
• Give at least 6 hours before bedtime
to avoid sleep interference.

benzphetamine hydrochloride
Didrex**
Controlled Substance Schedule III
Pregnancy Risk Category: X

MECHANISM OF ACTION
Main site of activity appears to be the
cerebral cortex and the reticular activating system. Promotes nerve impulse transmission by releasing stored
norepinephrine from nerve terminals
in the brain.

INDICATIONS & DOSAGE
*Short-term adjunct in exogenous obe-
sity—*
Adults: 25 to 50 mg P.O. daily,
b.i.d., or t.i.d.

ADVERSE REACTIONS
CNS: *restlessness,* tremor, *hyperactivity, talkativeness, insomnia,* irritability, dizziness, headache, chills, overstimulation, dysphoria.
CV: *tachycardia, palpitations,* hypertension, hypotension.
GI: nausea, vomiting, cramps, dry
mouth, diarrhea, constipation, metallic taste, anorexia, weight loss.
Skin: urticaria.

Italicized side effects are common or life-threatening.
*Liquid form contains alcohol.   **May contain tartrazine.

Other: impotence, altered libido.

INTERACTIONS
MAO inhibitors: severe hypertension; possible hypertensive crisis. Don't use together.
Antacids, sodium bicarbonate, acetazolamide: increased renal reabsorption. Monitor for enhanced effects.
Ammonium chloride, ascorbic acid: observe for decreased benzphetamine effects.
Phenothiazines, haloperidol: observe for decreased benzphetamine effects.

NURSING CONSIDERATIONS
• Contraindicated in symptomatic CV diseases, hyperthyroidism, nephritis, angina pectoris, moderate to severe hypertension, parkinsonism due to arteriosclerosis, certain types of glaucoma, advanced arteriosclerosis, agitated states, or patients with history of drug abuse. Use with caution in diabetes mellitus and in elderly, debilitated, or hyperexcitable patients.
• Psychic dependence or habituation may occur, especially in patients with history of drug addiction. Avoid prolonged administration. When used long-term, lower dosage gradually to prevent acute rebound depression.
• Use in conjunction with weight-reduction program. Monitor dietary intake. Do calorie counts, if necessary. Give 30 to 60 minutes before meals.
• Fatigue may result as drug effects wear off. Patient will need more rest.
• Tell patient to avoid drinks containing caffeine, which increase the effects of amphetamines and related amines.
• Have patient report signs of excessive stimulation.
• Urine acidification enhances renal excretion; urine alkalinization enhances renal reabsorption and recycling.
• When tolerance to anorexigenic effect develops, dosage should not be increased, but drug discontinued.
• Warn patient to avoid activities that require alertness or good psychomotor coordination until CNS effects of the drug are known.
• May alter daily insulin needs in patients with diabetes. Monitor blood and urine sugars.
• Give at least 6 hours before bedtime to avoid sleep interference.

---

caffeine◇
Caffedrine, Dexitac, No Doz, Quick Pep, Tirend, Vivarin♦

Pregnancy Risk Category: B

MECHANISM OF ACTION
Inhibits phosphodiesterase, the enzyme that degrades cyclic adenosine monophosphate.

INDICATIONS & DOSAGE
CNS stimulant—
Adults: 100 to 200 mg anhydrous caffeine P.O.
Neonatal apnea—
Neonates: 5 to 10 mg/kg P.O., I.M., or I.V. as a loading dose, then 2.5 to 5 mg. P.O., I.M., or I.V. daily, according to patient tolerance and serum caffeine levels (therapeutic range is 5 to 20 mcg/ml).

ADVERSE REACTIONS
CNS: *stimulation, insomnia,* restlessness, nervousness, mild delirium, headache, excitement, agitation, muscle tremors, twitches.
CV: *tachycardia.*
GI: nausea, vomiting.
GU: *diuresis.*
Skin: hyperesthesia.

INTERACTIONS
Theophylline, beta-adrenergic agonists: Excessive CNS stimulation.

NURSING CONSIDERATIONS
• Contraindicated in gastric or duo-

---

denal ulcer, dysrhythmias, or postmyocardial infarction.
• Caffeine-containing beverages should be restricted in patients who experience dysrhythmic symptoms.
• Tolerance or psychological dependence may develop.
• Be alert for signs of overdose: GI pain, mild delirium, insomnia, diuresis, dehydration, and fever. Treat with short-acting barbiturates, gastric emesis, or lavage.
• Single dose should not exceed 1 g.
• Caffeine content in cola beverages, 17 to 55 mg/180 ml; tea, 40 to 100 mg/180 ml; instant coffee, 60 to 180 mg/180 ml; brewed coffee, 100 to 150 mg/180 ml; decaffeinated coffee, 1 to 6 mg/180 ml.
• Caffeine does not reverse alcohol intoxication or depressant effects of alcohol. Overvigorous therapy with caffeine may aggravate depression in an already depressed patient.
• Sudden discontinuation of caffeine may cause headache and irritability.
• Caffeine is included in many OTC analgesic preparations. There's conflicting evidence regarding whether it increases pain relief.
• Treatment of neonatal apnea is an unlabeled indication. Solution may have to be made in pharmacy because most commercially available parenteral caffeine injections contain sodium benzoate, a preservative that may cause kernicterus in neonates.

---

dextroamphetamine sulfate
Dexedrine♦***, Ferndex, Oxydess II, Robese, Spancap #1
Controlled Substance Schedule II

Pregnancy Risk Category: C

MECHANISM OF ACTION
Main site of activity appears to be the cerebral cortex and the reticular activating system. Promotes nerve impulse transmission by releasing stored norepinephrine from nerve terminals in the brain. In children with hyperkinesia, amphetamines have a paradoxical calming effect.

INDICATIONS & DOSAGE
Narcolepsy—
Adults: 5 to 60 mg P.O. daily in divided doses.
Children over 12 years: 10 mg P.O. daily, with 10-mg increments weekly, p.r.n.
Children 6 to 12 years: 5 mg P.O. daily, with 5-mg increments weekly, p.r.n.
Short-term adjunct in exogenous obesity—
Adults: single 10- to 15-mg long-acting capsule, up to 30 mg daily; or in divided doses, 5 to 10 mg half hour before meals.
Attention deficit disorders with hyperactivity (ADDH)—
Children 6 years and older: 5 mg once daily or b.i.d., with 5-mg increments weekly, p.r.n.
Children 3 to 5 years: 2.5 mg P.O. daily, with 2.5-mg increments weekly, p.r.n.

ADVERSE REACTIONS
CNS: *restlessness,* tremor, *hyperactivity, talkativeness, insomnia,* irritability, dizziness, headache, chills, overstimulation, dysphoria.
CV: *tachycardia, palpitations,* hypertension, hypotension.
GI: nausea, vomiting, cramps, dry mouth, diarrhea, constipation, metallic taste, anorexia, weight loss.
Skin: urticaria.
Other: impotence, altered libido.

INTERACTIONS
Ammonium chloride, ascorbic acid: observe for decreased amphetamine effects.
Antacids, sodium bicarbonate, acetazolamide: increased renal reabsorption. Monitor for enhanced amphetamine effects.
MAO inhibitors: severe hypertension;

Italicized side effects are common or life-threatening.
*Liquid form contains alcohol.   **May contain tartrazine.

possible hypertensive crisis. Don't
use together.
Phenothiazines, haloperidol: observe
for decreased amphetamine effects.

NURSING CONSIDERATIONS
• Contraindicated in hyperthyroidism, nephritis, severe hypertension,
angina pectoris or other severe CV
disease, some types of glaucoma, or
history of drug abuse. Use with caution in diabetes mellitus and in elderly, debilitated, or hyperexcitable
patients.
• Use cautiously in children with
Tourette's disorder.
• Psychic dependence or habituation
may occur, especially in patients with
history of drug addiction. Avoid prolonged administration. When used
long-term, lower dosage gradually to
prevent acute rebound depression.
• Not recommended for first-line
treatment of obesity. Use as an anorexigenic agent is prohibited in some
states.
• When used for obesity, be sure patient is also on a weight-reduction
program. Give 30 to 60 minutes before meals. Avoid giving within 6
hours of bedtime.
• Fatigue may result as drug effects
wear off. Patient will need more rest.
• Tell patient to avoid drinks containing caffeine, which increase the effects of amphetamines and related
amines.
• Have patient report signs of excessive stimulation.
• Urine acidification enhances renal
excretion; urine alkalinization enhances renal reabsorption and recycling.
• When tolerance to anorexigenic effect develops, dosage should not be
increased, but drug discontinued.
• Should not be used to prevent fatigue.
• Warn patient to avoid activities that
require alertness or good psychomotor coordination until CNS effects of
the drug are known.
• May alter daily insulin needs in patients with diabetes. Monitor blood
and urine sugars.
• Use as analeptic is usually discouraged, since CNS stimulation superimposed on CNS depression can lead to
neuronal instability and seizures.
• Give at least 6 hours before bedtime
to avoid sleep interference.

diethylpropion hydrochloride
Nobesine♦♦, Propion♦♦, Tenuate♦,
Tenuate Dospan, Tepanil, Tepanil
Ten-Tab
Controlled Substance Schedule IV
Pregnancy Risk Category: B

MECHANISM OF ACTION
Main site of activity appears to be the
cerebral cortex and the reticular activating system. Promotes nerve impulse transmission by releasing stored
norepinephrine from nerve terminals
in the brain.

INDICATIONS & DOSAGE
Short-term adjunct in exogenous obesity—
Adults: 25 mg P.O. before meals,
t.i.d.; or 75 mg controlled-release
tablet P.O. in mid-morning.

ADVERSE REACTIONS
CNS: headache, *nervousness,* dizziness.
CV: *tachycardia, palpitations,* rise in
blood pressure.
EENT: blurred vision.
GI: nausea, abdominal cramps, dry
mouth, diarrhea, constipation.
Skin: urticaria.
Other: impotence, altered libido,
menstrual changes.

INTERACTIONS
MAO inhibitors: hypertension; possible hypertensive crisis. Don't use together.

NURSING CONSIDERATIONS
• Contraindicated in hyperthyroidism, hypertension, angina pectoris, severe CV disease, glaucoma, or history of drug abuse. Use with caution in epilepsy, diabetes mellitus, and hyperexcitability states. May alter insulin requirements. Monitor blood and urine sugars.
• When tolerance to anorexigenic effect develops, dosage should not be increased, but drug discontinued.
• Habituation or psychic dependence may occur.
• Be sure patient is also on a weight-reduction program.
• Can be used to stop nighttime eating. Rarely causes insomnia.
• Fatigue may result as drug effects wear off. Patient will need more rest.
• Tell patient to avoid drinks containing caffeine, which increase the effects of amphetamines and related amines.
• Have patient report signs of excessive stimulation.
• Urine acidification enhances renal excretion; urine alkalinization enhances renal reabsorption and recycling.
• Use as analeptic is usually discouraged, since CNS stimulation superimposed on CNS depression can lead to neuronal instability and seizures.
• Give at least 6 hours before bedtime to avoid sleep interference.

---

fenfluramine hydrochloride
Ponderal♦♦, Ponderal Pacaps♦♦, Pondimin♦, Pondimin Extentabs♦
Controlled Substance Schedule IV
Pregnancy Risk Category: C

MECHANISM OF ACTION
Stimulates ventromedial nucleus of the hypothalamus. May also affect serotonin metabolism.

INDICATIONS & DOSAGE
Short-term adjunct in exogenous obesity—
Adults: initially, 20 mg P.O. t.i.d. before meals. Maximum dosage is 40 mg t.i.d. Adjust dosage according to patient's response.

ADVERSE REACTIONS
CNS: *drowsiness,* dizziness, incoordination, headache, euphoria or depression, anxiety, *insomnia,* weakness, fatigue, agitation.
CV: *palpitations,* hypotension, hypertension, chest pain.
EENT: eye irritation, blurred vision.
GI: *diarrhea, dry mouth,* nausea, vomiting, abdominal pain, constipation.
GU: dysuria, increased urinary frequency, impotence.
Skin: rashes, urticaria, burning sensation.
Other: sweating, chills, fever, increased libido.

INTERACTIONS
Alcohol, CNS depressants: enhanced CNS depression.
Centrally acting antihypertensives: decreased antihypertensive effect.
MAO inhibitors: severe hypertension; possible hypertensive crisis. Don't use together.

NURSING CONSIDERATIONS
• Contraindicated in glaucoma, hypersensitivity to sympathomimetic amines, symptomatic cardiovascular disease, alcoholism, or history of drug abuse. Use with caution in hypertension, history of mental depression, and diabetes mellitus.
• Because of possible hypoglycemia, patients with diabetes may have altered insulin or sulfonylurea requirements. Monitor blood and urine sugars.
• Differs pharmacologically from amphetamines in that it produces CNS depression more often than stimulation.
• Have patient report signs of excessive sedation, depression, or excessive

---

Italicized side effects are common or life-threatening.
*Liquid form contains alcohol.   **May contain tartrazine.

stimulation. Closely monitor blood pressure.
• Be sure patient is on a weight-reduction program.
• Tolerance or dependence may occur. Avoid prolonged administration.
• Tell patient to avoid drinks containing caffeine, which increase the effects of amphetamines and related amines.
• Fenfluramine should not be discontinued abruptly; may precipitate an acute depressive reaction.
• Has been proven effective for treating autistic children.

mazindol
Mazanor, Sanorex♦
Controlled Substance Schedule IV

Pregnancy Risk Category: C

MECHANISM OF ACTION
Inhibits neuronal uptake of norepinephrine and dopamine.

INDICATIONS & DOSAGE
Short-term adjunct in exogenous obesity—
Adults: 1 mg P.O. t.i.d. 1 hour before meals, or 2 mg daily 1 hour before lunch. Use lowest effective dosage.

ADVERSE REACTIONS
CNS: *nervousness,* restlessness, dizziness, *insomnia,* dysphoria, headache, depression, drowsiness, weakness, tremor.
CV: *palpitations, tachycardia.*
GI: dry mouth, nausea, constipation, diarrhea, unpleasant taste.
GU: difficulty initiating micturition, impotence.
Skin: rash, clamminess, pallor.
Other: shivering, excessive sweating, altered libido.

INTERACTIONS
Centrally acting antihypertensives: decreased antihypertensive effect.
MAO inhibitors: severe hypertension;

possible hypertensive crisis. Don't use together.

NURSING CONSIDERATIONS
• Contraindicated in glaucoma, CV disease including dysrhythmias, agitated states, or history of drug abuse. Use with caution in diabetes mellitus, hypertension, and hyperexcitability states.
• Warn patient to avoid activities that require alertness or good psychomotor coordination until CNS effects of the drug are known.
• Fatigue may result as drug effects wear off. Patient will need more rest.
• Tell patient to avoid drinks containing caffeine, which increase the effects of amphetamines and related amines.
• Have patient report signs of excessive stimulation.
• Tolerance or dependence may develop. Avoid prolonged use.
• Be sure patient is also on a weight-reduction program.
• May alter insulin needs in patients with diabetes. Monitor blood and urine sugars.
• Give at least 6 hours before bedtime to avoid sleep interference.

methamphetamine hydrochloride
Desoxyn, Desoxyn Gradumet
Controlled Substance Schedule II

Pregnancy Risk Category: C

MECHANISM OF ACTION
Main site of activity appears to be the cerebral cortex and the reticular activating system. Promotes nerve impulse transmission by releasing stored norepinephrine from nerve terminals in the brain. In children with hyperkinesia, amphetamines have a paradoxical calming effect.

INDICATIONS & DOSAGE
Attention deficit disorder with hyper-

activity (ADDH)—
Children 6 years and older: 2.5 to 5 mg P.O. once daily or b.i.d., with 5-mg increments weekly, p.r.n. Usual effective dosage is 20 to 25 mg daily.
Short-term adjunct in exogenous obesity—
Adults: 2.5 to 5 mg P.O. once to t.i.d. 30 minutes before meals; or 1 long-acting 5- to 15-mg tablet daily before breakfast.

ADVERSE REACTIONS
CNS: *nervousness, insomnia,* irritability, *talkativeness,* dizziness, headache, hyperexcitability, tremor.
CV: hypertension, hypotension, *tachycardia, palpitations,* cardiac dysrhythmias.
EENT: blurred vision, mydriasis.
GI: nausea, vomiting, abdominal cramps, diarrhea, constipation, dry mouth, anorexia, metallic taste.
Skin: urticaria.
Other: impotence, altered libido.

INTERACTIONS
Ammonium chloride, ascorbic acid: observe for decreased amphetamine effects.
Antacids, sodium bicarbonate, acetazolamide: increased renal reabsorption. Monitor for enhanced effects.
MAO inhibitors: severe hypertension; possible hypertensive crisis. Don't use together.
Phenothiazines, haloperidol: observe for decreased amphetamine effects.

NURSING CONSIDERATIONS
• Contraindicated in hypertension, hyperthyroidism, nephritis, angina pectoris or other severe CV disease, glaucoma, parkinsonism due to arteriosclerosis, agitated states, or history of drug abuse. Use with caution in diabetes mellitus; and in patients who are elderly, debilitated, asthenic, psychopathic, or who have a history of suicidal or homicidal tendencies.
• Use cautiously in children with

Tourette's disorder.
• Warn that potential for abuse is high. Should not be used to prevent fatigue.
• May alter insulin needs in patients with diabetes. Monitor blood and urine sugars.
• Not recommended for first-line treatment of obesity. Use as an anorexigenic agent is prohibited in some states.
• When used for obesity, be sure patient is on a weight-reduction program.
• Tell patient to avoid drinks containing caffeine, which increase the effects of amphetamines and related amines.
• Have patient report signs of excessive stimulation.
• Urine acidification enhances renal excretion; urine alkalinization enhances renal reabsorption and recycling.
• When tolerance to anorexigenic effect develops, dosage should not be increased, but drug discontinued.
• Warn patient to avoid activities that require alertness or good psychomotor coordination until CNS effects of the drug are known.
• Give at least 6 hours before bedtime to avoid sleep interference.

methylphenidate hydrochloride
Ritalin♦, Ritalin SR
Controlled Substance Schedule II

Pregnancy Risk Category: C

MECHANISM OF ACTION
Main site of activity appears to be the cerebral cortex and the reticular activating system. Promotes nerve impulse transmission by releasing stored norepinephrine from nerve terminals in the brain. In children with hyperkinesia, amphetamines have a paradoxical calming effect.

Italicized side effects are common or life-threatening.
*Liquid form contains alcohol.   **May contain tartrazine.

INDICATIONS & DOSAGE

Attention deficit disorder with hyperactivity (ADDH)—

Children 6 years and older: initial dose 5 to 10 mg P.O. daily before breakfast and lunch, with 5- to 10-mg increments weekly as needed, up to 60 mg daily.

Narcolepsy—

Adults: 10 mg P.O. b.i.d. or t.i.d. half hour before meals. Dosage varies with patient needs. Dosage range is 5 to 50 mg daily.

ADVERSE REACTIONS

Blood: thrombocytopenia.
CNS: *nervousness, insomnia,* dizziness, headache, akathisia, dyskinesia, *Tourette's disorder.*
CV: *palpitations,* angina, *tachycardia,* changes in blood pressure and pulse rate.
EENT: difficulty with accommodation and blurring of vision.
GI: nausea, dry throat, abdominal pain, anorexia, weight loss.
Skin: rash, urticaria, *exfoliative dermatitis,* erythema multiforme, thrombocytopenic purpura.
Other: growth suppression.

INTERACTIONS

Anticonvulsants, tricyclic antidepressants, oral anticoagulants: methylphenidate may increase plasma levels of these drugs and enhance their pharmacologic effects.
Centrally acting antihypertensives: decreased antihypertensive effect.
MAO inhibitors: severe hypertension; possible hypertensive crisis. Don't use together.

NURSING CONSIDERATIONS

• Contraindicated in symptomatic cardiac disease; hyperthyroidism; moderate to severe hypertension; angina pectoris; advanced arteriosclerosis; severe depression of either endogenous or exogenous form; glaucoma; parkinsonism; history of drug abuse or dependency; or history of marked anxiety, tension, or agitation. Use with caution in elderly, debilitated, or hyperexcitable patients, and those with history of CV disease, diabetes, or seizures.

• May precipitate Tourette's disorder in children. Monitor especially at start of therapy.

• Closely monitor blood pressure. Observe for signs of excessive stimulation.

• Should not be used to prevent fatigue.

• Observe for interactions, as treatment of other disease states may be affected. May alter daily insulin needs in patients with diabetes. Monitor blood and urine sugars. May decrease seizure threshold in patients with seizure disorders.

• Drug of choice for ADDH. Usually stopped after puberty.

• Periodic CBC, differential, and platelet counts advised with long-term use.

• Tolerance, psychic dependence, or habituation may develop, especially in patients with history of drug addiction. High abuse potential. Avoid prolonged administration. When used long-term, lower dosage gradually to prevent acute rebound depression.

• Fatigue may result as drug effects wear off. Patient will need more rest.

• Tell patient to avoid drinks containing caffeine, which increase the effects of amphetamines and related amines.

• Warn patient to avoid activities that require alertness or good psychomotor coordination until CNS effects of the drug are known.

• Monitor height and weight in children on prolonged therapy because drug has been associated with growth suppression. Recent evidence suggests it may delay "growth spurt", but children will attain normal height when drug is discontinued.

• Now available in a sustained-release

form (duration, 6 to 8 hours). Warn patient against chewing these tablets.
• Give at least 6 hours before bedtime to prevent insomnia. Administer after meals to reduce appetite-suppressive effects.

pemoline
Cylert♦, Cylert Chewable
Controlled Substance Schedule IV

Pregnancy Risk Category: B

MECHANISM OF ACTION
Main site of activity appears to be the cerebral cortex and the reticular activating system. Promotes nerve impulse transmission by releasing stored norepinephrine from nerve terminals in the brain.

INDICATIONS & DOSAGE
Attention deficit disorder with hyperactivity (ADDH)—
Children 6 years and older: initially, 37.5 mg P.O. given in the morning. Daily dose can be raised by 18.75 mg weekly. Effective dosage range is 56.25 to 75 mg daily; maximum dosage is 112.5 mg daily.

ADVERSE REACTIONS
CNS: *insomnia,* malaise, irritability, fatigue, mild depression, dizziness, headache, drowsiness, hallucinations, nervousness (large doses), seizures, *Tourette's disorder,* psychosis.
CV: *tachycardia (large doses).*
GI: anorexia, abdominal pain, nausea, diarrhea.
Hepatic: elevated liver enzymes.
Skin: rash.

INTERACTIONS
Insulin, oral hypoglycemics: pemoline may alter requirements of antidiabetic agents.

NURSING CONSIDERATIONS
• Contraindicated in patients with hepatic dysfunction, and in children under 6 years. Use with caution in patients with impaired renal function or a history of Tourette's disorder. Drug may accumulate.
• May precipitate Tourette's disorder in children. Monitor especially at start of therapy.
• Closely monitor patients on long-term therapy for possible blood or hepatic function abnormalities and for growth suppression.
• Structurally dissimilar to amphetamines or methylphenidate. However, may produce similar adverse reactions, including lowered seizure threshold. Also, has a greater potential for drug abuse and dependence than previously thought.
• Therapeutic effects may not be evident for up to 3 to 4 weeks.
• Give at least 6 hours before bedtime to avoid sleep interference.

phendimetrazine tartrate
Adipost, Adphen, Anorex, Bacarate, Bontril PDM, Bontril Slow Release, Dyrexan OD, Melfiat, Metra, Obalan, Obeval, Phenazine-35, Phenzine, Plegine, Prelu-2, Slyn-LL, Sprx-105, Statobex**, Trimtabs, Trimstat, Wehless, Weightrol, X-Trozine, X-Trozine LA
Controlled Substance Schedule IV

Pregnancy Risk Category: C

MECHANISM OF ACTION
Main site of activity appears to be the cerebral cortex and the reticular activating system. Promotes nerve impulse transmission by releasing stored norepinephrine from nerve terminals in the brain.

INDICATIONS & DOSAGE
Short-term adjunct in exogenous obesity—
Adults: 35 mg P.O. b.i.d. to t.i.d. 1 hour before meals. Maximum dosage is 70 mg t.i.d. Use lowest effective dosage. Adjust dose to individual re-

---

Italicized side effects are common or life-threatening.
*Liquid form contains alcohol.   **May contain tartrazine.

sponse.

ADVERSE REACTIONS
CNS: *nervousness,* dizziness, *insomnia,* tremor, headache.
CV: *tachycardia, palpitations,* rise in blood pressure.
EENT: blurred vision
GI: dry mouth, nausea, abdominal cramps, diarrhea, constipation.
GU: dysuria.

INTERACTIONS
Ammonium chloride, ascorbic acid: observe for decreased phendimetrazine effects.
Antacids, sodium bicarbonate, acetazolamide: increased renal reabsorption. Monitor for enhanced effects.
MAO inhibitors: severe hypertension; possible hypertensive crisis. Don't use together.
Phenothiazines, haloperidol: observe for decreased effect.

NURSING CONSIDERATIONS
• Contraindicated in hyperthyroidism, hypertension, angina pectoris or other severe CV disease, or glaucoma. Use with caution in hyperexcitability states or with history of drug addiction.
• Warn patient to avoid activities that require alertness or good psychomotor coordination until CNS effects of the drug are known.
• Be sure patient is following weight-reduction program.
• Tolerance or dependence can develop. Not advised for prolonged use.
• Fatigue may result as drug effects wear off. Patient will need more rest.
• Tell patient to avoid drinks containing caffeine, which increase the effects of amphetamines and related amines.
• Have patient report signs of excessive stimulation.
• Urine acidification enhances renal excretion; urine alkalinization enhances renal reabsorption and recy-

cling.
• May alter daily insulin needs in patients with diabetes. Monitor blood urine sugars.
• Give at least 6 hours before bedtime to avoid sleep interference.

phenmetrazine hydrochloride
Preludin**
Controlled Substance Schedule II
Pregnancy Risk Category: C

MECHANISM OF ACTION
Main site of activity appears to be the cerebral cortex and the reticular activating system. Promotes nerve impulse transmission by releasing stored norepinephrine from nerve terminals in the brain.

INDICATIONS & DOSAGE
Short-term adjunct in exogenous obesity—
Adults: 25 mg P.O. b.i.d. or t.i.d. 1 hour before meals, up to 75 mg daily; or single 50- to 75-mg extended-release tablet daily in midmorning.

ADVERSE REACTIONS
CNS: *nervousness,* dizziness, *insomnia,* headache.
CV: *tachycardia, palpitations,* increased blood pressure.
EENT: blurred vision.
GI: dry mouth, nausea, abdominal cramps, constipation.
Skin: urticaria.
Other: altered libido, impotence.

INTERACTIONS
Ammonium chloride, ascorbic acid: observe for decreased phenmetrazine effects.
Antacids, sodium bicarbonate, acetazolamide: increased renal reabsorption. Monitor for enhanced effects.
MAO inhibitors: severe hypertension; possible hypertensive crisis. Don't use together.

Phenothiazines, haloperidol: observe for decreased effect.

NURSING CONSIDERATIONS
• Contraindicated in patients with hyperthyroidism, hypertension, angina pectoris or other CV disease, glaucoma, or history of drug addiction. Use with caution in hyperexcitability states.
• Tolerance or dependence may develop. High abuse potential. Not advised for prolonged use.
• Be sure patient is also following weight-reduction program.
• Fatigue may result as drug effects wear off. Patient will need more rest.
• Tell patient to avoid drinks containing caffeine, which increase the effects of amphetamines and related amines.
• Have patient report signs of excessive stimulation.
• Urine acidification enhances renal excretion; urine alkalinization enhances renal reabsorption and recycling.

---

phentermine hydrochloride
Adipex-P, Dapex, Fastin, Ionamin♦, Obe-Nix, Obephen, Obermine, Obestin, Oby-Trim, Parmine, Phentrol, Span R/D, Teramine, Unifast
Controlled Substance Schedule IV

Pregnancy Risk Category: C

MECHANISM OF ACTION
Main site of activity appears to be the cerebral cortex and the reticular activating system. Promotes nerve impulse transmission by releasing stored norepinephrine from nerve terminals in the brain.

INDICATIONS & DOSAGE
Short-term adjunct in exogenous obesity—
Adults: 8 mg P.O. t.i.d. half hour before meals; or 15 to 30 mg daily before breakfast (resin complex).

ADVERSE REACTIONS
CNS: *nervousness,* dizziness, *insomnia.*
CV: *palpitations, tachycardia,* increased blood pressure.
GI: dry mouth, unpleasant taste, nausea, constipation, diarrhea.
Skin: urticaria.
Other: altered libido, impotence.

INTERACTIONS
MAO inhibitors: severe hypertension; possible hypertensive crisis. Don't use together.
Antacids, sodium bicarbonate, acetazolamide: increased renal reabsorption. Monitor for enhanced effects.
Ammonium chloride, ascorbic acid: observe for decreased phentermine effects.
Phenothiazines, haloperidol: observe for decreased effects.

NURSING CONSIDERATIONS
• Contraindicated in hyperthyroidism, hypertension, angina pectoris or other severe CV disease, or glaucoma. Use with caution in hyperexcitability states or history of drug addiction.
• Tolerance or dependence may develop. Avoid prolonged administration.
• Use with weight-reduction program. Give 30 minutes before meals.
• Fatigue may result as drug effects wear off. Patient will need more rest.
• Tell patient to avoid drinks containing caffeine, which increase the effects of amphetamines and related amines.
• Have patient report signs of excessive stimulation.
• Urine acidification enhances renal excretion; urine alkalinization enhances renal reabsorption and recycling.
• Give at least 6 hours before bedtime to avoid sleep interference.

Italicized side effects are common or life-threatening.
*Liquid form contains alcohol.   **May contain tartrazine.

36

Respiratory stimulants

ammonia, aromatic spirits◊
doxapram hydrochloride

COMBINATION PRODUCTS
None.

---

ammonia, aromatic spirits◊

Pregnancy Risk Category: C

MECHANISM OF ACTION
Irritates the sensory receptors in the nasal membranes, producing reflex stimulation of the respiratory centers.

INDICATIONS & DOSAGE
Fainting—
Adults and children: inhale as needed.

ADVERSE REACTIONS
None reported.

INTERACTIONS
None significant.

NURSING CONSIDERATIONS
• Avoid inhaling vapors when administering drug.

---

doxapram hydrochloride
Dopram♦

Pregnancy Risk Category: C

MECHANISM OF ACTION
Acts either directly on the central respiratory centers in the medulla or indirectly on the chemoreceptors.

INDICATIONS & DOSAGE
Postanesthesia respiratory stimulation, drug-induced CNS depression, and chronic pulmonary disease associated with acute hypercapnia—
Adults: 0.5 to 1 mg/kg of body weight (up to 2 mg/kg in CNS depression), I.V. injection or infusion. Maximum dosage is 4 mg/kg, up to 3 g/day. Infusion rate is 1 to 3 mg/minute (initial: 5 mg/minute for postanesthesia).
Chronic obstructive pulmonary disease—
Adults: infusion, 1 to 2 mg/minute. Maximum is 3 mg/minute for a maximum duration of 2 hours.

ADVERSE REACTIONS
CNS: *seizures, headache,* dizziness, apprehension, disorientation, pupillary dilation, bilateral Babinski's signs, flushing, sweating, paresthesias.
CV: *chest pain and tightness, variations in heart rate, hypertension,* lowered T waves.
GI: nausea, vomiting, diarrhea.
GU: urine retention, or stimulation of the bladder with incontinence.
Other: sneezing, coughing, laryngospasm, bronchospasm, hiccups, rebound hypoventilation, pruritus.

INTERACTIONS
MAO inhibitors, sympathomimetics: potentiate adverse cardiovascular effects. Use together cautiously.

NURSING CONSIDERATIONS
• Contraindicated in seizure disor-

Unmarked trade names available in the United States only.
♦Also available in Canada.   ♦♦Available in Canada only.   ◊Also available OTC.

ders; head injury; cardiovascular disorders; frank uncompensated heart failure; severe hypertension; CVA; respiratory failure or incompetence secondary to neuromuscular disorders, muscle paresis, flail chest, obstructed airway, pulmonary embolism, pneumothorax, restrictive respiratory disease, acute bronchial asthma, extreme dyspnea; or hypoxia not associated with hypercapnia. Use with caution in bronchial asthma, severe tachycardia or cardiac dysrhythmias, cerebral edema or increased cerebrospinal fluid pressure, hyperthyroidism, pheochromocytoma, and metabolic disorders.

• Doxapram's use as an analeptic is strongly discouraged by most doctors.

• Establish adequate airway before administering drug. Prevent patient from aspirating vomitus by placing him on his side.

• Monitor blood pressure, heart rate, deep tendon reflexes, and arterial blood gases before giving drug and every 30 minutes afterward.

• Be alert for signs of overdosage: hypertension, tachycardia, dysrhythmias, skeletal muscle hyperactivity, dyspnea. Discontinue if patient shows signs of increased arterial carbon dioxide or oxygen tension, or if mechanical ventilation is started. May give I.V. injection of anticonvulsant.

• Use only in surgical or emergency room situations.

• Do not combine with alkaline solutions such as thiopental sodium; doxapram is acidic.

• Extravasation may lead to thrombophlebitis and local skin irritation.

• Rapid infusion may cause hemolysis.

Italicized side effects are common or life-threatening.
*Liquid form contains alcohol.   **May contain tartrazine.

37

Cholinergics (parasympathomimetics)

ambenonium chloride
bethanechol chloride
edrophonium chloride
neostigmine bromide
neostigmine methylsulfate
physostigmine salicylate
(eserine)
pyridostigmine bromide

COMBINATION PRODUCTS
None.

---

ambenonium chloride
Mytelase♦

Pregnancy Risk Category: C

MECHANISM OF ACTION
Inhibits the destruction of acetylcholine released from the parasympathetic and somatic efferent nerves. Acetylcholine accumulates, promoting increased stimulation of the receptor.

INDICATIONS & DOSAGE
Symptomatic treatment of myasthenia gravis in patients who cannot take neostigmine bromide and pyridostigmine bromide—
Adults: dosage must be individualized for each patient, but usually ranges from 5 to 25 mg P.O. t.i.d. to q.i.d. Starting dose usually is 5 mg P.O. t.i.d. to q.i.d. Increase gradually and adjust at 1- to 2-day intervals to avoid drug accumulation and overdosage. May range from 5 mg to as much as 75 mg per dose.

ADVERSE REACTIONS
CNS: headache, dizziness, muscle weakness, seizures, mental confusion, jitters, sweating.
CV: bradycardia, hypotension.
EENT: miosis, blurred vision.
GI: *nausea, vomiting, diarrhea, abdominal cramps,* increased salivation.
GU: urinary frequency, incontinence.
Other: bronchospasm, *muscle cramps,* bronchoconstriction, increased bronchial secretions, *respiratory paralysis.*

INTERACTIONS
Corticosteroids, magnesium, procainamide, quinidine: may impair drug effect. Observe for lack of drug effect.

NURSING CONSIDERATIONS
• Contraindicated in mechanical obstruction of intestine or urinary tract, bradycardia, or hypotension.
• Use with extreme caution in bronchial asthma.
• Use cautiously in epilepsy, recent coronary occlusion, vagotonia, hyperthyroidism, cardiac dysrhythmias, and peptic ulcer.
• Avoid large dose in patients with decreased GI motility or megacolon.
• Discontinue all other cholinergics before administering this drug.
• Watch patient very closely for side effects, particularly if total dosage is greater than 200 mg daily. Side effects may indicate drug toxicity. Notify doctor immediately if they develop.
• Monitor and document vital signs

---

frequently, being especially careful to check respirations. Always have atropine injection readily available and be prepared to give atropine 0.5 mg subcutaneously or slow I.V. push as ordered, and provide respiratory support as needed.

• Administer each dose exactly as ordered, on time. Amount and frequency of dosage should vary with patient's activity level. The doctor will probably order larger doses to be given when patient is fatigued, for example, in the afternoon and at mealtime.

• If muscle weakness is severe, doctor must determine if this is caused by drug toxicity or exacerbation of myasthenia gravis. A test dose of edrophonium I.V. will aggravate drug-induced weakness but will temporarily relieve weakness that results from the disease.

• Weakness occurring 30 to 60 minutes after taking dose is a warning sign of drug toxicity. Notify doctor immediately.

• Observe and record the patient's variations in muscle strength. Show him how to do it himself.

• When given for myasthenia gravis, explain to patient that this drug will relieve symptoms of ptosis, double vision, difficulty in chewing and swallowing, and trunk and limb weakness. Stress the importance of taking this drug exactly as ordered. Explain to patient and his family that he may have to take this drug for the rest of his life. Teach them about the disease and the drug's effect on symptoms.

• Patient may develop resistance to drug.

• Seek approval when indicated for hospitalized patient to have bedside supply of tablets to take himself. Patients with long-standing disease often insist on this.

• Give with milk or food to produce fewer muscarinic side effects.

• Advise patient to wear identification tag indicating he has myasthenia gravis.

bethanechol chloride
Duvoid♦, Urabeth, Urecholine♦

Pregnancy Risk Category: C

MECHANISM OF ACTION
Binds to cholinergic (muscarinic) receptors, mimicking the action of acetylcholine.

INDICATIONS & DOSAGE
Acute postoperative and postpartum nonobstructive (functional) urine retention, neurogenic atony of urinary bladder with retention, abdominal distention, megacolon—
Adults: 10 to 30 mg P.O. t.i.d. or q.i.d. Or, 2.5 to 10 mg S.C. Never give I.M. or I.V. When used for urine retention, some patients may require 50 to 100 mg P.O. per dose. Use such doses with extreme caution.

Test dose is 2.5 mg S.C. repeated at 15- to 30-minute intervals to total of 4 doses to determine the minimal effective dose; then use minimal effective dose q 6 to 8 hours. All doses must be adjusted individually.

ADVERSE REACTIONS
Dose-related:
CNS: headache, malaise.
CV: bradycardia, hypotension, *cardiac arrest,* reflex tachycardia.
EENT: lacrimation, miosis.
GI: *abdominal cramps, diarrhea,* salivation, nausea, vomiting, belching, borborygmus.
GU: urinary urgency.
Skin: flushing, sweating.
Other: bronchoconstriction, increased bronchial secretions.

INTERACTIONS
Atropine, anticholinergic agents, procainamide, quinidine: may reverse cholinergic effects. Observe for lack of drug effect.

NURSING CONSIDERATIONS
• Contraindicated in patients with uncertain strength or integrity of bladder wall; when increased muscular activity of GI or urinary tract is harmful; in mechanical obstructions of GI or urinary tract; in hyperthyroidism, peptic ulcer, latent or active bronchial asthma, cardiac or coronary artery disease, vagotonia, epilepsy, Parkinson's disease, bradycardia, chronic obstructive pulmonary disease, hypotension. Use cautiously in hypertension, vasomotor instability, peritonitis, and other acute inflammatory conditions of GI tract.
• *Never* give I.M. or I.V.; could cause circulatory collapse, hypotension, severe abdominal cramping, bloody diarrhea, shock, or cardiac arrest.
• Should stop all other cholinergics before giving this drug.
• Watch closely for side effects that may indicate drug toxicity, especially with S.C. administration.
• Monitor vital signs frequently, being especially careful to check respirations. Always have atropine injection readily available and be prepared to give atropine 0.5 mg subcutaneously or slow I.V. push as ordered, and provide respiratory support if needed.
• If used to treat urine retention, make sure bedpan is readily available. Monitor intake/output.
• When used to prevent abdominal distention and GI distress, the doctor may also order a rectal tube inserted to help passage of gas.
• Poor and variable oral absorption requires larger oral doses. Oral and S.C. doses are *not* interchangeable.
• Drug usually effective 5 to 15 minutes after injection and 30 to 90 minutes after oral use.
• Give on empty stomach; if taken after meals, may cause nausea and vomiting.

edrophonium chloride
Enlon, Reversol, Tensilon♦
Pregnancy Risk Category: C

MECHANISM OF ACTION
Inhibits the destruction of acetylcholine released from the parasympathetic and somatic efferent nerves. Acetylcholine accumulates, promoting increased stimulation of the receptor.

INDICATIONS & DOSAGE
As a curare antagonist (to reverse neuromuscular blocking action)—
Adults: 10 mg I.V. given over 30 to 45 seconds. Dose may be repeated as necessary to 40 mg maximum dosage. Larger dosages may potentiate rather than antagonize effect of curare.
Diagnostic aid in myasthenia gravis (Tensilon test)—
Adults: 1 to 2 mg I.V. within 15 to 30 seconds, then 8 mg if no response (increase in muscular strength).
Children over 34 kg: 2 mg I.V. If no response within 45 seconds, give 1 mg q 45 seconds to maximum of 10 mg.
Children up to 34 kg: 1 mg I.V. If no response within 45 seconds, give 1 mg q 45 seconds to maximum of 5 mg.
Infants: 0.5 mg I.V.
To differentiate myasthenic crisis from cholinergic crisis—
Adults: 1 mg I.V. If no response in 1 minute, repeat dose once. Increased muscular strength confirms myasthenic crisis; no increase or exaggerated weakness confirms cholinergic crisis.
Paroxysmal supraventricular tachycardia—
Adults: 5 to 10 mg I.V. given over 1 minute or less.
Children: 2 mg I.V. Administer slowly.

ADVERSE REACTIONS
CNS: seizures, weakness, dysphagia, respiratory paralysis, sweating.
CV: hypotension, bradycardia.
EENT: excessive lacrimation, diplopia, miosis.
GI: nausea, vomiting, *diarrhea, abdominal cramps,* excessive salivation.
GU: urinary frequency.
Other: increased bronchial secretions, bronchospasm, muscle cramps, muscle fasciculation.

INTERACTIONS
Procainamide, quinidine: may reverse cholinergic effects. Observe for lack of drug effect.

NURSING CONSIDERATIONS
• Contraindicated in mechanical obstruction of intestine or urinary tract, bradycardia, or hypotension. Use cautiously in hyperthyroidism, cardiac disease, peptic ulcer, and bronchial asthma.
• Should stop all other cholinergics before giving this drug.
• Watch closely for side effects; may indicate toxicity.
• Monitor vital signs frequently, being especially careful to check respirations. Always have atropine injection readily available and be prepared to give atropine 0.5 mg subcutaneously or slow I.V. push as ordered, and provide respiratory support as needed.
• When giving drug to differentiate myasthenic crisis from cholinergic crisis, observe patient's muscle strength closely.
• Edrophonium not effective against muscle relaxation induced by decamethonium bromide and succinylcholine chloride.
• This cholinergic has the most rapid onset but shortest duration; therefore, not used for treatment of myasthenia gravis.
• For easier parenteral administration, use a tuberculin syringe with an I.V. needle.
• I.M. route may be used in children because of difficulty with I.V. route: for children under 34 kg, inject 2 mg I.M.; children over 34 kg, 5 mg I.M. Expect same reactions as with I.V. test, but these appear after 2- to 10-minute delay.

---

neostigmine bromide
Prostigmin Bromide♦

neostigmine methylsulfate
Prostigmin♦

Pregnancy Risk Category: C

MECHANISM OF ACTION
Inhibits the destruction of acetylcholine released from the parasympathetic and somatic efferent nerves. Acetylcholine accumulates, promoting increased stimulation of the receptor.

INDICATIONS & DOSAGE
Antidote for tubocurarine—
Adults: 0.5 to 2 mg I.V. slowly. Repeat p.r.n. Give 0.6 to 1.2 mg atropine sulfate I.V. before antidote dose.
Postoperative abdominal distention and bladder atony—
Adults: 0.5 to 1 mg I.M. or S.C. q 4 to 6 hours.
Postoperative ileus—
Adults: 0.25 to 1 mg I.M. or S.C. q 4 to 6 hours.
Treatment of myasthenia gravis—
Adults: 15 to 30 mg P.O. t.i.d. (range is 15 to 375 mg daily); or 0.5 to 2 mg I.M. or I.V. q 1 to 3 hours. Dosage must be individualized, depending on response and tolerance of side effects. Therapy may be required day and night.
Children: 7.5 to 15 mg P.O. t.i.d. to q.i.d.
Note: 1:1,000 solution of injectable solution contains 1 mg/ml; 1:2,000 solution contains 0.5 mg/ml.

Italicized side effects are common or life-threatening.
*Liquid form contains alcohol.　　　**May contain tartrazine.

ADVERSE REACTIONS
CNS: dizziness, muscle weakness, mental confusion, jitters, sweating, respiratory depression.
CV: bradycardia, hypotension.
EENT: miosis.
GI: *nausea, vomiting, diarrhea, abdominal cramps,* excessive salivation.
GU: urinary frequency.
Skin: rash (bromide).
Other: bronchospasm, *muscle cramps,* muscle fasciculations, bronchoconstriction.

INTERACTIONS
Atropine, anticholinergic agents, procainamide, aminoglycosides, quinidine: may reverse cholinergic effect on muscle. Observe for lack of drug effect.

NURSING CONSIDERATIONS
• Contraindicated in hypersensitivity to cholinergics or to bromide, mechanical obstruction of the intestine or urinary tract, bradycardia, or hypotension. Use with extreme caution in bronchial asthma. Use cautiously in epilepsy, recent coronary occlusion, peritonitis, vagotonia, hyperthyroidism, cardiac dysrhythmias, and peptic ulcer.
• Should stop all other cholinergics before giving this drug.
• Monitor vital signs frequently, being especially careful to check respirations. Have atropine injection readily available and be prepared to give as ordered, and provide respiratory support as needed.
• Difficult to judge optimum dosage. Help doctor by documenting patient's response after each dose. Observe closely for improvement in strength, vision, and ptosis 45 to 60 minutes after each dose. Show patient how to observe and record variations in muscle strength.
• When using for myasthenia gravis, explain that this drug will relieve ptosis, double vision, difficulty in chewing and swallowing, trunk and limb weakness. Stress importance of taking drug exactly as ordered. Explain that drug may have to be taken for life.
• In myasthenia gravis, schedule the largest dose before periods of fatigue. For example, if patient has dysphagia, schedule dose 30 minutes before each meal.
• When used to prevent abdominal distention and GI distress, the doctor may order a rectal tube inserted to help passage of gas.
• Patients sometimes develop a resistance to neostigmine.
• If muscle weakness is severe, doctor determines if it is caused by drug-induced toxicity or exacerbation of myasthenia gravis. Test dose of edrophonium I.V. will aggravate drug-induced weakness but will temporarily relieve weakness caused by disease.
• Hospitalized patient with long-standing myasthenia may request bedside supply of tablets. This will enable patient to take each dose precisely as ordered. Seek approval for self-medication program according to hospital policy, but continue to oversee medication regimen.
• GI side effects may be reduced by taking drug with milk or food.
• Advise patient to wear an identification tag indicating that he has myasthenia gravis.
• I.M. neostigmine may be used instead of edrophonium to diagnose myasthenia gravis. May be preferable to edrophonium when limb weakness is the only symptom.

---

physostigmine salicylate (eserine)
Antilirium♦

Pregnancy Risk Category: C

MECHANISM OF ACTION
Inhibits the destruction of acetylcholine released from the parasympathetic and somatic efferent nerves.

Acetylcholine accumulates, promoting increased stimulation of the receptor.

INDICATIONS & DOSAGE

Tricyclic antidepressant and anticholinergic poisoning—
Adults: 0.5 to 2 mg I.M. or I.V. (1 mg/minute I.V.) repeated as necessary if life-threatening signs recur (coma, seizures, dysrhythmias).
Senile dementia (Alzheimer's)—
Adults: initially, 0.5 mg P.O. q 2 hours, increased to 2 to 2.5 mg P.O. q 2 hours 6 or 7 times daily (maximum is 16 mg/day).

ADVERSE REACTIONS

CNS: seizures, hallucinations, muscular twitching, muscle weakness, ataxia, *restlessness, excitability, sweating*.
CV: irregular pulse, palpitations.
EENT: miosis.
GI: nausea, vomiting, epigastric pain, *diarrhea, excessive salivation*.
Other: bronchospasm, bronchial constriction, dyspnea.

INTERACTIONS

Atropine, anticholinergic agents, procainamide, quinidine: may reverse cholinergic effects. Observe for lack of drug effect.

NURSING CONSIDERATIONS

• Use cautiously in preexisting conditions: mechanical obstruction of intestine or urogenital tract, bronchial asthma, gangrene, diabetes, cardiovascular disease, vagotonia, bradycardia, hypotension, epilepsy, Parkinson's disease, hyperthyroidism, and peptic ulcer.
• Watch closely for side effects, particularly CNS disturbances. Use side rails if patient becomes restless or hallucinates. Side effects may indicate drug toxicity.
• Monitor vital signs frequently, being especially careful to check respirations. Position patient to make breathing easier. Always have atropine injection readily available and be prepared to give atropine 0.5 mg subcutaneously or slow I.V. push as ordered, and provide respiratory support as needed. Best administered in presence of doctor.
• Use only clear solution. Darkening may indicate loss of potency.
• Give I.V. at controlled rate; use slow, direct injection at no more than 1 mg/minute.
• Only cholinergic that crosses blood-brain barrier; therefore the only one useful for treating CNS effects of anticholinergic or tricyclic antidepressant toxicity.
• Effectiveness often immediate and dramatic but may be transient and may require repeat dose.
• Is used investigationally to improve cognitive function in patients with Alzheimer's disease.

pyridostigmine bromide

Mestinon♦*, Mestinon Supraspan♦♦, Mestinon Timespan, Regonol♦

Pregnancy Risk Category: C

MECHANISM OF ACTION

Inhibits the destruction of acetylcholine released from the parasympathetic and somatic efferent nerves. Acetylcholine accumulates, promoting increased stimulation of the receptor.

INDICATIONS & DOSAGE

Curariform antagonist postoperatively—
Adults: 10 to 20 mg I.V. preceded by atropine sulfate 0.6 to 1.2 mg I.V.
Myasthenia gravis—
Adults: 60 to 120 mg P.O. q 3 or 4 hours. Usual dosage is 600 mg daily but higher dosage may be needed (up to 1,500 mg daily). Give ⅟₃₀ of oral dose I.M. or I.V. Dosage must be ad-

---

Italicized side effects are common or life-threatening.
*Liquid form contains alcohol.   **May contain tartrazine.

justed for each patient, depending on response and tolerance of adverse reactions. Alternatively, may give 180 to 540 mg timed-release tablets (1 to 3 tablets) b.i.d., with at least 6 hours between doses.

ADVERSE REACTIONS
CNS: headache (with high doses), weakness, sweating, seizures.
CV: bradycardia, hypotension.
EENT: miosis.
GI: abdominal cramps, nausea, vomiting, diarrhea, excessive salivation.
Skin: rash.
Local: thrombophlebitis.
Other: bronchospasm, bronchoconstriction, increased bronchial secretions, muscle cramps, muscle fasciculations.

INTERACTIONS
Atropine, anticholinergic agents, procainamide, quinidine: may reverse cholinergic effects. Observe for lack of drug effect.

NURSING CONSIDERATIONS
• Contraindicated in mechanical obstruction of intestine or urinary tract, bradycardia, or hypotension. Use with extreme caution in bronchial asthma. Use cautiously in epilepsy, recent coronary occlusion, vagotonia, hyperthyroidism, cardiac dysrhythmias, and peptic ulcer. Avoid large doses in decreased GI motility.
• Difficult to judge optimum dosage. Help doctor by recording patient's response after each dose.
• Should stop all other cholinergics before giving this drug.
• Monitor vital signs frequently, being especially careful to check respirations. Position patient to make breathing easier. Have atropine injection readily available and be prepared to give as ordered, and provide respiratory support as needed.
• If muscle weakness is severe, doctor determines if it is caused by drug-induced toxicity or exacerbation of myasthenia gravis. Test dose of edrophonium I.V. will aggravate drug-induced weakness but will temporarily relieve weakness caused by disease.
• When using for myasthenia gravis, stress importance of taking drug exactly as ordered, on time, in evenly spaced doses. If doctor has ordered extended-release tablets, explain how these work. Patient must take them at the same time each day, at least 6 hours apart. Explain that he may have to take this drug for life.
• Has longest duration of the cholinergics used for myasthenia gravis.
• Used by the oral route in the treatment of senility associated with Alzheimer's disease.
• Don't crush the timed-release (Timespan or Supraspan) tablets.
• Available as a syrup for patients who have difficulty swallowing. Syrup is very sweet; give over ice chips if patient can't tolerate flavor.
• Store tablets in a tightly capped bottle, away from moisture.

38

Cholinergic blockers (parasympatholytics)

atropine sulfate◇
   (See Chapter 20, ANTIARRHYTHMICS.)
benztropine mesylate
biperiden hydrochloride
biperiden lactate
glycopyrrolate
ipratropium bromide
procyclidine hydrochloride
scopolamine butylbromide
scopolamine hydrobromide◇
trihexyphenidyl hydrochloride

COMBINATION PRODUCTS
Cholinergic blocking agents are available in tablets and capsules, combined with varying amounts of sedatives.

---

benztropine mesylate
Apo-Benztropine♦♦, Bensylate♦♦,
Cogentin♦, PMS Benztropine♦♦

Pregnancy Risk Category: C

MECHANISM OF ACTION
Blocks central cholinergic receptors, helping to balance cholinergic activity in the basal ganglia.

INDICATIONS & DOSAGE
Acute dystonic reaction—
Adults: 2 mg I.V. or I.M. followed by 1 to 2 mg P.O. b.i.d. to prevent recurrence.
Parkinsonism—
Adults: 0.5 to 6 mg P.O. daily. Initial dose is 0.5 mg to 1 mg. Increase 0.5 mg q 5 to 6 days. Adjust dosage to meet individual requirements.

ADVERSE REACTIONS
CNS: disorientation, restlessness, ir-ritability, incoherence, hallucinations, headache, sedation, depression, muscular weakness.
CV: palpitations, tachycardia, paradoxical bradycardia.
EENT: dilated pupils, blurred vision, photophobia, difficulty swallowing.
GI: *constipation, dry mouth,* nausea, vomiting, epigastric distress.
GU: urinary hesitancy, urine retention.
   Some side effects may be due to pending atropine-like toxicity and are dose related.

INTERACTIONS
Amantadine, phenothiazines, tricyclic antidepressants: additive anticholinergic side effects, such as confusion and hallucinations. Reduce dosage before administering amantadine.

NURSING CONSIDERATIONS
• Contraindicated in narrow-angle glaucoma. Use cautiously in prostatic hypertrophy, tendency to tachycardia, and in elderly or debilitated patients; produces atropine-like side effects and may aggravate tardive dyskinesia.
• Monitor vital signs carefully. Watch closely for side effects, especially in elderly or debilitated patients. Call doctor promptly.
• Never discontinue this drug abruptly. Dosage must be reduced gradually.
• Warn patient to avoid activities that require alertness until CNS effects of the drug are known. If patient is to receive single daily dose, give at bedtime.

Italicized side effects are common or life-threatening.
*Liquid form contains alcohol.   **May contain tartrazine.

• Explain that drug may take 2 to 3 days to exert full effect.
• Advise patient to report signs of urinary hesitancy or urine retention.
• Watch for intermittent constipation, distention, abdominal pain; may be onset of paralytic ileus.
• Relieve dry mouth with cool drinks, ice chips, sugarless gum or hard candy.
• To help prevent GI distress, administer after meals.
• Advise patient to limit activities during hot weather because drug-induced anhydrosis may result in hyperthermia.

biperiden hydrochloride
Akineton♦

biperiden lactate
Akineton Lactate
Pregnancy Risk Category: C

MECHANISM OF ACTION
Blocks central cholinergic receptors, helping to balance cholinergic activity in the basal ganglia.

INDICATIONS & DOSAGE
Extrapyramidal disorders—
Adults: 2 to 6 mg P.O. daily, b.i.d., or t.i.d., depending on severity. Usual dose is 2 mg daily, or 2 mg I.M. or I.V. q half hour, not to exceed 4 doses or 8 mg total daily.
Parkinsonism—
Adults: 2 mg P.O. t.i.d. to q.i.d.

ADVERSE REACTIONS
CNS: disorientation, euphoria, restlessness, irritability, incoherence, dizziness, increased tremor.
CV: transient postural hypotension.
EENT: blurred vision.
GI: *constipation, dry mouth,* nausea, vomiting, epigastric distress.
GU: urinary hesitancy, urine retention.
Side effects are dose-related and

may resemble atropine toxicity.

INTERACTIONS
Phenothiazines, tricyclic antidepressants: excessive CNS anticholinergic effects.

NURSING CONSIDERATIONS
• Use with caution in prostatism, cardiac dysrhythmias, narrow-angle glaucoma, and epilepsy.
• Monitor vital signs carefully. Watch closely for adverse reactions, especially in elderly or debilitated patients. Call doctor promptly.
• Give oral doses with or after meals to decrease GI adverse reactions.
• When giving parenterally, keep patient in a supine position. Parenteral administration may cause transient postural hypotension and coordination disturbances.
• I.V. injections should be made very slowly.
• Because of possible dizziness, help patient when he gets out of bed.
• Tolerance may develop, requiring increased dosage.
• In severe parkinsonism, tremors may increase as spasticity is relieved.
• Warn patient to avoid activities that require alertness until CNS effects of the drug are known.
• Advise patient to report signs of urinary hesitancy or urine retention.
• Relieve dry mouth with cool drinks, ice chips, sugarless gum, or hard candy.

glycopyrrolate
Robinul♦, Robinul Forte♦
Pregnancy Risk Category: B

MECHANISM OF ACTION
Inhibits cholinergic (muscarinic) actions of acetylcholine on autonomic effectors innervated by postganglionic cholinergic nerves.

INDICATIONS & DOSAGE

To reverse neuromuscular blockade—
Adults: 0.2 mg I.V. for each 1 mg neostigmine or equivalent dose of pyridostigmine. May be given I.V. without dilution or may be added to dextrose injection and given by infusion.
Preoperatively to diminish secretions and block cardiac vagal reflexes—
Adults: 0.002 mg/lb of body weight I.M. 30 to 60 minutes before anesthesia.
Adjunctive therapy in peptic ulcers and other GI disorders—
Adults: 1 to 2 mg P.O. t.i.d. or 0.1 mg I.M. t.i.d. or q.i.d. Dosage should be individualized.

ADVERSE REACTIONS

CNS: disorientation, irritability, incoherence, weakness, nervousness, drowsiness, dizziness, headache.
CV: palpitations, tachycardia, paradoxical bradycardia.
EENT: *dilated pupils, blurred vision,* photophobia, increased intraocular pressure, difficulty swallowing.
GI: *constipation, dry mouth,* nausea, vomiting, epigastric distress.
GU: *urinary hesitancy, urine retention,* impotence.
Skin: urticaria, decreased sweating or anhidrosis, other dermal manifestations.
Local: burning at injection site.
Other: bronchial plugging, fever.

INTERACTIONS

None significant.

NURSING CONSIDERATIONS

• Contraindicated in narrow-angle glaucoma, obstructive uropathy, obstructive disease of the GI tract, myasthenia gravis, paralytic ileus, intestinal atony, unstable cardiovascular status in acute hemorrhage, or toxic megacolon. Use with caution in patients with autonomic neuropathy, hyperthyroidism, coronary artery disease, cardiac dysrhythmias, CHF, hypertension, hiatal hernia associated with reflux esophagitis, hepatic or renal disease, and ulcerative colitis; and in patients over 40 years because of increased incidence of glaucoma. Use with caution in hot or humid environments. Drug-induced heatstroke possible.
• Check all dosages carefully. Even slight overdose could lead to toxicity.
• Don't mix with I.V. solution containing sodium chloride or bicarbonate.
• Monitor vital signs carefully. Watch closely for side effects, especially in elderly or debilitated patients. Call doctor promptly.
• Advise patient to report signs of urinary hesitancy or urine retention.
• Warn patient to avoid activities that require alertness until CNS effects of the drug are known.
• Administer 30 minutes to 1 hour before meals.
• Administer smaller doses to elderly patients.

ipratropium bromide
Atrovent♦

Pregnancy Risk Category: B

MECHANISM OF ACTION

Inhibits vagally mediated reflexes by antagonizing acetylcholine. An anticholinergic.

INDICATIONS & DOSAGE

Maintenance treatment of bronchospasm associated with chronic obstructive pulmonary disease—
Adults: 2 inhalations (26 mcg) q.i.d. Additional inhalations may be needed. However, total inhalations should not exceed 12 in 24 hours.

ADVERSE REACTIONS

CNS: nervousness, dizziness, headache.
CV: palpitations.
EENT: cough, blurred vision.

GI: nausea, GI distress, dry mouth.
Skin: rash.

INTERACTIONS
None significant.

NURSING CONSIDERATIONS
• Use cautiously in patients with narrow-angle glaucoma, prostatic hypertrophy, and bladder-neck obstruction.
• Warn patient that this drug is not effective in the treatment of acute episodes of bronchospasm where rapid response is required.
• Teach patient to use the inhaler correctly, as follows: Enclose mouthpiece with lips and hold the base of the canister vertically. Exhale deeply, then inhale slowly through the mouth and, at the same time, firmly press once on the up-ended canister base. Hold your breath for a few seconds, then remove mouthpiece from the mouth and exhale slowly. Wait 15 seconds, then repeat inhalation.
• Tell patient to avoid accidentally spraying into eyes. Temporary blurring of vision may result.
• Ipratropium is the first anticholinergic bronchodilator available as an aerosol. Works by a different mechanism from either the adrenergics or theophylline compounds.

---

procyclidine hydrochloride
Kemadrin♦, PMS Procyclidine♦♦, Procyclid♦♦

Pregnancy Risk Category: C

MECHANISM OF ACTION
Blocks central cholinergic receptors, helping to balance cholinergic activity in the basal ganglia.

INDICATIONS & DOSAGE
Parkinsonism, muscle rigidity—
Adults: initially, 2 to 2.5 mg P.O. t.i.d., after meals. Increase as needed to maximum of 60 mg daily.

Also used to relieve extrapyramidal dysfunction that accompanies treatment with phenothiazines and rauwolfia derivatives. Also controls excessive salivation from neuroleptic medications.

ADVERSE REACTIONS
CNS: light-headedness, giddiness.
EENT: blurred vision, mydriasis.
GI: *constipation, dry mouth,* nausea, vomiting, epigastric distress.
Skin: rash.
Other: muscle weakness.

INTERACTIONS
None significant.

NURSING CONSIDERATIONS
• Contraindicated in narrow-angle glaucoma. Use cautiously in tachycardia, hypotension, urine retention, and prostatic hypertrophy.
• Watch closely for mental confusion, disorientation, agitation, hallucinations, and psychotic symptoms, especially in the elderly. Call doctor promptly if these occur.
• In severe parkinsonism, tremors may increase as spasticity is relieved.
• Give after meals to minimize GI distress.
• Warn patient to avoid activities that require alertness until CNS effects of the drug are known.
• Relieve dry mouth with cool drinks, ice chips, sugarless gum, or hard candy.

---

scopolamine butylbromide
Buscospan♦♦

scopolamine hydrobromide◊

Pregnancy Risk Category: C

MECHANISM OF ACTION
Inhibits muscarinic actions of acetylcholine on autonomic effectors innervated by postganglionic cholinergic

neurons.

INDICATIONS & DOSAGE
Postencephalitic parkinsonism and other spastic states—
Adults: 0.5 to 1 mg P.O. t.i.d. to q.i.d.; 0.3 to 0.6 mg S.C., I.M., or I.V. (with suitable dilution) t.i.d. to q.i.d.
Children: 0.006 mg/kg P.O. or S.C. t.i.d. to q.i.d.; or 0.2 mg/m².
Preoperatively to reduce secretions—
Adults: 0.4 to 0.6 mg S.C.

ADVERSE REACTIONS
CNS: disorientation, restlessness, irritability, dizziness, drowsiness, headache.
CV: palpitations, tachycardia, paradoxical bradycardia.
EENT: dilated pupils, blurred vision, photophobia, increased intraocular pressure, difficulty swallowing.
GI: constipation, *dry mouth, nausea, vomiting, epigastric distress.*
GU: urinary hesitancy, urine retention.
Skin: rash, flushing, dryness.
Other: bronchial plugging, fever, depressed respirations.
    Adverse reactions may be caused by pending atropine-like toxicity and are dose related. Individual tolerance varies greatly.

INTERACTIONS
Alcohol, CNS depressants: increased CNS depression.
Centrally acting anticholinergics (tricyclic antidepressants, phenothiazines): increased CNS adverse effects.
Digoxin: increased digoxin levels.

NURSING CONSIDERATIONS
• Contraindicated in narrow-angle glaucoma, obstructive uropathy, obstructive disease of the GI tract, asthma, chronic pulmonary disease, myasthenia gravis, paralytic ileus, intestinal atony, unstable cardiovascular status in acute hemorrhage, or toxic megacolon. Use with caution in patients with autonomic neuropathy, hyperthyroidism, coronary artery disease, cardiac dysrhythmias, CHF, hypertension, hiatal hernia associated with reflux esophagitis, hepatic or renal disease, ulcerative colitis; in patients over 40 years because of the increased incidence of glaucoma; and in children under 6 years. Use with caution in hot or humid environments. Drug-induced heatstroke possible.
• Some patients become temporarily excited or disoriented. Symptoms disappear when sedative effect is complete. Raise side rails as a precaution.
• In therapeutic doses, scopolamine may produce amnesia, drowsiness, and euphoria. These effects are desirable when used as an adjunct to anesthesia. May need to reorient patient.
• Warn patient to avoid activities requiring alertness until CNS effects of the drug are known.
• Advise patient to report signs of urinary hesitancy or urine retention.
• Tolerance may develop when given over a long period of time.
• Many of the side effects (such as dry mouth, constipation) are an expected extension of the drug's pharmacologic activity.
• To determine m² for dosage calculation in children, use a nomogram.

trihexyphenidyl hydrochloride
Aparkane♦♦, Apo-Trihex♦♦, Artane♦*, Artane Sequels, Novohexidyl♦♦, Trihexane, Trihexy-2, Trihexy-5

Pregnancy Risk Category: C

MECHANISM OF ACTION
Blocks central cholinergic receptors, helping to balance cholinergic activity in the basal ganglia.

INDICATIONS & DOSAGE
Drug-induced parkinsonism—
Adults: 1 mg P.O. 1st day, 2 mg 2nd day, then increases by 2 mg q 3 to 5 days until total of 6 to 10 mg is given daily. Usually given t.i.d. with meals and, if needed, q.i.d. (last dose should be before bedtime) or may switch to extended-release form b.i.d. Postencephalitic parkinsonism may require 12 to 15 mg total daily dosage.

ADVERSE REACTIONS
CNS: nervousness, dizziness, headache, restlessness, agitation, hallucinations, euphoria, delusion, amnesia.
CV: tachycardia.
EENT: blurred vision, mydriasis, increased intraocular pressure.
GI: constipation, *dry mouth, nausea*.
GU: urinary hesitancy, urine retention.
Adverse reactions are dose-related.

INTERACTIONS
Amantadine: additive anticholinergic adverse reactions, such as confusion and hallucinations. Reduce dosage before administering amantadine.

NURSING CONSIDERATIONS
• Use cautiously in patients with narrow-angle glaucoma; cardiac, hepatic, or renal disorders; hypertension; obstructive disease of the GI and GU tracts; possible prostatic hypertrophy; patients over 60 years; and those with arteriosclerosis or history of drug hypersensitivities. Side effects are usually mild and transient.
• Warn patient to avoid activities that require alertness until CNS effects of the drug are known.
• Causes nausea if given before meals.
• Relieve dry mouth with cool drinks, ice chips, sugarless gum, or hard candy.
• Patient may develop a tolerance to this drug, so dosage may need to be gradually increased.
• Advise patient to report signs of urinary hesitancy or urine retention.
• Gonioscopic evaluation and close monitoring of intraocular pressure is advised, especially in patients over 40 years.

39

Adrenergics (sympathomimetics)

albuterol (salbutamol)
bitolterol mesylate
dobutamine hydrochloride
dopamine hydrochloride
ephedrine sulfate◊
epinephrine◊
epinephrine bitartrate◊
epinephrine hydrochloride
ethylnorepinephrine
   hydrochloride
isoetharine hydrochloride◊
isoetharine mesylate
isoproterenol
isoproterenol hydrochloride
isoproterenol sulfate
mephentermine sulfate
metaproterenol sulfate◊
metaraminol bitartrate
norepinephrine injection
   (levarterenol bitartrate)
phenylephrine hydrochloride◊
pirbuterol
pseudoephedrine
   hydrochloride◊
pseudoephedrine sulfate
terbutaline sulfate

COMBINATION PRODUCTS
Only a few of the many combinations are included here as examples of this group.

Inhalants
DUO-MEDIHALER: isoproterenol hydrochloride 0.16 mg and phenylephrine bitartrate 0.24 mg per dose.

Oral bronchodilators
BRONCHOBID DURACAPS: theophylline 260 mg and ephedrine HCl 35 mg.
MARAX♦*: theophylline 130 mg, ephedrine sulfate 25 mg, and hydroxyzine HCl 10 mg.
QUADRINAL♦: theophylline calcium salicylate 65 mg, ephedrine hydrochloride 24 mg, potassium iodide 320 mg, and phenobarbital 24 mg.
QUIBRON PLUS*: theophylline 150 mg, ephedrine hydrochloride 25 mg, guaifenesin 100 mg, and butabarbital 20 mg.
TEDRAL SA♦: theophylline 180 mg, ephedrine hydrochloride 48 mg, and phenobarbital 25 mg.
TEDRAL◊: theophylline 130 mg, ephedrine hydrochloride 24 mg, and phenobarbital 8 mg.
THALFED◊: theophylline 120 mg, ephedrine hydrochloride 25 mg, and phenobarbital 8 mg.

Decongestants
ACTIFED◊: pseudoephedrine hydrochloride 60 mg and triprolidine hydrochloride 2.5 mg.
CONGESPRIN◊: phenylephrine hydrochloride 1.25 mg and aspirin 81 mg.
DRISTAN◊: phenylephrine hydrochloride 5 mg, chlorpheniramine maleate 2 mg, aspirin 325 mg, and caffeine 16.2 mg.
HISTASPAN-PLUS: phenylephrine hydrochloride 20 mg and chlorpheniramine maleate 8 mg.
NALDECON: phenylpropanolamine hydrochloride 40 mg, phenylephrine hydrochloride 10 mg, chlorpheniramine maleate 5 mg, and phenyltoloxamine citrate 15 mg.
ORNEX◊: phenylpropanolamine hydrochloride 18 mg and acetaminophen 325 mg.
PHENERGAN-D: pseudoephedrine hydrochloride 60 mg and promethazine

---

Italicized side effects are common or life-threatening.
*Liquid form contains alcohol.   **May contain tartrazine.

hydrochloride 6.25 mg.
TRIAMINIC◇: phenylpropanolamine hydrochloride 50 mg, pyrilamine maleate 25 mg, and pheniramine maleate 25 mg.

---

albuterol (salbutamol)
Proventil, Proventil Syrup, Ventolin♦

Pregnancy Risk Category: C

MECHANISM OF ACTION
Relaxes bronchial smooth muscle by acting on beta$_2$-adrenergic receptors.

INDICATIONS & DOSAGE
Prevention and treatment of bronchospasm in patients with reversible obstructive airway disease—
Adults and children over 13 years: 1 to 2 inhalations q 4 to 6 hours. More frequent administration or a greater number of inhalations is not recommended.
*Oral tablets—*2 to 4 mg t.i.d. or q.i.d. Maximum dosage is 8 mg q.i.d.
*Sustained-release tablets—*4 to 8 mg q 12 hours. Maximum dosage is 16 mg b.i.d.
Children 6 to 13 years: 2 mg (1 teaspoonful) t.i.d. or q.i.d.
Children 2 to 5 years: 0.1 mg/kg t.i.d., not to exceed 2 mg (1 teaspoonful) t.i.d.
Adults over 65 years: 2 mg t.i.d. or q.i.d.
To prevent exercise-induced asthma—
Adults: 2 inhalations 15 minutes before exercise.

ADVERSE REACTIONS
CNS: *tremor, nervousness,* dizziness, insomnia, headache.
CV: tachycardia, palpitations, hypertension.
EENT: drying and irritation of nose and throat (with inhaled form).
GI: heartburn, nausea, vomiting.
Other: muscle cramps.

INTERACTIONS
Propranolol and other beta blockers: mutual antagonism. Monitor patient carefully.
MAO inhibitors, tricyclic antidepressants: increased adverse cardiovascular effects.

NURSING CONSIDERATIONS
• Use cautiously in cardiovascular disorders, including coronary insufficiency and hypertension; in hyperthyroidism or diabetes mellitus; and in patients who are unusually responsive to adrenergics.
• Warn patient about the possibility of paradoxical bronchospasm. If this occurs, the drug should be discontinued immediately.
• Patients may use tablets and aerosol concomitantly. Monitor closely for toxicity.
• Albuterol reportedly produces less cardiac stimulation than other sympathomimetics, especially isoproterenol.
• Elderly patients usually require a lower dosage.
• May be prescribed for use 15 minutes before exercise to prevent exercise-induced bronchospasm.
• Teach patient how to administer metered dose correctly. Have him shake container; exhale through nose; administer aerosol while inhaling deeply on mouthpiece of inhaler; and hold breath for a few seconds, then exhale slowly. Tell him to allow 2 minutes between inhalations and not to use more than the prescribed amount.
• Pleasant-tasting syrup may be taken by children as young as age 2. Contains no alcohol or sugar.
• Store drug in light-resistant container.

---

bitolterol mesylate
Tornalate

Pregnancy Risk Category: C

MECHANISM OF ACTION
Relaxes bronchial smooth muscle by acting on beta$_2$-adrenergic receptors.

INDICATIONS & DOSAGE
To prevent and treat bronchial asthma and bronchospasm—
Adults and children over 12 years: to treat bronchospasm, two inhalations at an interval of at least 1 to 3 minutes followed by a third inhalation, if needed. To prevent bronchospasm, the usual dose is two inhalations q 8 hours. In either case, dose should never exceed three inhalations q 6 hours or two inhalations q 4 hours.

ADVERSE REACTIONS
CNS: *tremors,* nervousness, headache, dizziness, light-headedness.
CV: palpitations, chest discomfort, tachycardia.
EENT: throat irritation, cough.
GI: nausea.
Other: dyspnea, *hypersensitivity.*

INTERACTIONS
None significant.

NURSING CONSIDERATIONS
• Use cautiously in ischemic heart disease or hypertension, hyperthyroidism, diabetes mellitus, cardiac dysrhythmias, and seizure disorders.
• Monitor blood pressure regularly.
• Advise patients not to exceed recommended dosages. Too frequent use may cause tachycardia.
• Remind patients that beneficial effects last for up to 8 hours, longer than most other similar bronchodilators.
• Has rapid onset of action (about 3 to 4 minutes). Peak effect occurs in 30 to 60 minutes.
• Show patient how to use inhaler correctly.

dobutamine hydrochloride
Dobutrex♦

Pregnancy Risk Category: C

MECHANISM OF ACTION
Directly stimulates beta$_1$ receptors of the heart to increase myocardial contractility and stroke volume, resulting in increased cardiac output.

INDICATIONS & DOSAGE
Refractory heart failure and as adjunct in cardiac surgery—
Adults: 2.5 to 10 mcg/kg/minute as an I.V. infusion. Rarely, infusion rates up to 40 mcg/kg/minute may be needed.

ADVERSE REACTIONS
CNS: headache.
CV: *increased heart rate, hypertension, premature ventricular contractions,* angina, nonspecific chest pain.
GI: nausea, vomiting.
Other: shortness of breath.

INTERACTIONS
Beta blockers: may antagonize dobutamine effects. Do not use together.
General anesthetics: greater incidence of ventricular dysrhythmias.

NURSING CONSIDERATIONS
• Contraindicated in idiopathic hypertrophic subaortic stenosis.
• A unique agent. Increases contractility of failing heart without inducing marked tachycardia, except at high doses.
• Hypovolemia should be corrected with plasma volume expanders before initiating therapy with dobutamine.
• Dobutamine is chemical modification of isoproterenol.
• Often used with nitroprusside for additive effects.
• ECG, blood pressure, pulmonary wedge pressure, and cardiac output

should be monitored continuously. Also monitor urine output.
• Incompatible with alkaline solutions. Do not mix with sodium bicarbonate injection.
• Infusions of up to 72 hours produce no more adverse effects than shorter infusions.
• Oxidation of drug may slightly discolor admixtures containing dobutamine. This does not indicate a significant loss of potency.
• I.V. solutions remain stable for 24 hours.

dopamine hydrochloride
Intropin♦, Revimine♦♦

Pregnancy Risk Category: C

MECHANISM OF ACTION
Stimulates dopaminergic, beta-adrenergic, and alpha-adrenergic receptors of the sympathetic nervous system.

INDICATIONS & DOSAGE
To treat shock and correct hemodynamic imbalances; to improve perfusion to vital organs; to increase cardiac output; to correct hypotension—
Adults: 2 to 5 mcg/kg/minute I.V. infusion, up to 50 mcg/kg/minute. Titrate the dosage to the desired hemodynamic and/or renal response.

ADVERSE REACTIONS
CNS: headache.
CV: ectopic beats, tachycardia, anginal pain, palpitations, *hypotension*. Less frequently, bradycardia, widening of QRS complex, conduction disturbances, vasoconstriction.
GI: nausea, vomiting.
Local: necrosis and tissue sloughing with extravasation.
Other: piloerection, dyspnea.

INTERACTIONS
Beta blockers: may antagonize dopamine's effects.
Ergot alkaloids: extreme elevations in blood pressure. Don't use together.
MAO inhibitors: may cause hypertensive crisis. Avoid if possible.
Phenytoin: may lower blood pressure of dopamine-stabilized patients. Monitor carefully.

NURSING CONSIDERATIONS
• Contraindicated in uncorrected tachydysrhythmias, pheochromocytoma, or ventricular fibrillation. Use cautiously in patients with occlusive vascular disease, cold injuries, diabetic endarteritis, and arterial embolism; also, in pregnant patients and those taking MAO inhibitors.
• Not a substitute for blood or fluid volume deficit. Volume deficit should be replaced before vasopressors are administered.
• Use large vein, as in the antecubital fossa, to minimize risk of extravasation. Watch site carefully for signs of extravasation. If it occurs, stop infusion immediately and call doctor. He may want to counteract effect by infiltrating the area with 5 to 10 mg phentolamine and 10 to 15 ml normal saline solution.
• Monitor blood pressure, cardiac output, pulse rate, urine output, and extremity color and temperature often during infusion. Titrate infusion rate according to findings, using doctor's guidelines. Use a continuous infusion pump to regulate flow rate.
• Observe patient closely for adverse effects. If adverse effects develop, dosage may need to be adjusted or discontinued.
• If a disproportionate rise in the diastolic pressure (a marked decrease in pulse pressure) is observed in patients receiving dopamine, decrease infusion rate and observe carefully for further evidence of predominant vasoconstrictor activity, unless such an effect is desired.
• Most patients satisfactorily maintained on less than 20 mcg/kg/minute.
• If doses exceed 50 mcg/kg/minute,

check urine output often. If urine flow decreases without hypotension, consider reducing dose.
• If drug is stopped, watch closely for sudden drop in blood pressure.
• Don't mix with alkaline solutions. Use dextrose 5% in water, normal saline solution, or combination of dextrose 5% in water and saline solution. Mix just before use.
• Dopamine solutions deteriorate after 24 hours. Discard at that time or earlier if solution is discolored.
• Do not mix other drugs in I.V. container with dopamine.
• Do not give alkaline drugs (e.g., sodium bicarbonate, phenytoin sodium) through I.V. line containing dopamine.
• Acidosis decreases effectiveness of dopamine.

---

ephedrine sulfate◇
Ephed II

Pregnancy Risk Category: C

MECHANISM OF ACTION
Both a direct- and indirect-acting sympathomimetic that stimulates alpha- and beta-adrenergic receptors.

INDICATIONS & DOSAGE
To correct hypotensive states; to support ventricular rate in Adams-Stokes syndrome—
Adults: 25 to 50 mg I.M. or S.C., or 10 to 25 mg I.V. p.r.n. to maximum of 150 mg/24 hours.
Children: 3 mg/kg S.C. or I.V. daily, in four to six divided doses.
Bronchodilator or nasal decongestant—
Adults: 12.5 to 50 mg P.O. b.i.d., t.i.d., or q.i.d. Maximum dosage is 400 mg daily in six to eight divided doses.
Children: 2 to 3 mg/kg P.O. daily in four to six divided doses.

ADVERSE REACTIONS
CNS: *insomnia, nervousness,* dizziness, headache, muscle weakness, sweating, euphoria, confusion, delirium.
CV: *palpitations,* tachycardia, hypertension.
EENT: dryness of nose and throat.
GI: nausea, vomiting, anorexia.
GU: urine retention, painful urination due to visceral sphincter spasm.

INTERACTIONS
Alpha-adrenergic blocking agents: unopposed beta-adrenergic effects, resulting in hypotension.
Antihypertensives: decreased effects.
Beta-adrenergic blocking agents: unopposed alpha-adrenergic effects, resulting in hypertension.
Digitalis glycosides, general anesthetics (halogenated hydrocarbons): increased risk of ventricular dysrhythmias.
Ergot alkaloids: enhanced vasoconstrictor activity.
Guanadrel, guanethidine: enhanced pressor effects of ephedrine.
Levodopa: enhanced risk of ventricular dysrhythmias.
MAO inhibitors and tricyclic antidepressants: when given with sympathomimetics, may cause severe hypertension (hypertensive crisis).
Methyldopa: may inhibit effects of ephedrine. Use together cautiously.

NURSING CONSIDERATIONS
• Contraindicated in porphyria, severe coronary artery disease, cardiac dysrhythmias, narrow-angle glaucoma, or psychoneurosis; and in patients on MAO-inhibitor therapy. Use with caution in elderly patients and those with hypertension, hyperthyroidism, nervous or excitable states, cardiovascular disease, and prostatic hypertrophy.
• Not a substitute for blood or fluid volume deficit. Volume deficit should be replaced before vasopressors are

---

Italicized side effects are common or life-threatening.
*Liquid form contains alcohol.   **May contain tartrazine.

administered.
- Give I.V. injection slowly.
- Hypoxia, hypercapnia, and acidosis, which may reduce effectiveness or increase the incidence of adverse effects, must be identified and corrected before or during ephedrine administration.
- Effectiveness decreases after 2 to 3 weeks. Then increased dosage may be needed. Tolerance develops, but drug is not known to cause addiction.
- To prevent insomnia, avoid giving within 2 hours before bedtime.
- Warn patient not to take OTC drugs that contain ephedrine without informing doctor.

epinephrine◇
Inhalants:
Adrenalin, Bronkaid Mist, Bronkaid Mistometer♦♦, Dysne-Inhal♦♦, Primatene Mist Solution

epinephrine bitartrate◇
Inhalants: AsthmaHaler, Broniten Mist, Bronkaid Mist Suspension, Medihaler-Epi♦, Primatene Mist Suspension

epinephrine hydrochloride
Injections: Adrenalin♦, Epi-Pen, Epi-Pen Jr., Sus-Phrine♦

Pregnancy Risk Category: C

MECHANISM OF ACTION
Stimulates alpha- and beta-adrenergic receptors within the sympathetic nervous system.

INDICATIONS & DOSAGE
Bronchospasm, hypersensitivity reactions, anaphylaxis—
Adults: 0.1 to 0.5 ml of 1:1,000 S.C. or I.M. Repeat q 10 to 15 minutes, p.r.n. Or 0.1 to 0.25 ml 1:1,000 I.V.
Children: 0.01 ml (10 mcg) of 1:1,000/kg S.C. Repeat q 20 minutes to 4 hours, p.r.n.; 0.005 ml/kg of 1:200 (Sus-Phrine). Repeat q 8 to 12

hours, p.r.n.
Hemostasis—
Adults: 1:50,000 to 1:1,000, applied topically.
Acute asthmatic attacks (inhalation)—
Adults and children: 1 or 2 inhalations of 1:100 or 2.25% racemic, every 1 to 5 minutes until relief is obtained; 0.2 mg/dose usual content.
To prolong local anesthetic effect—
Adults and children: 0.2 to 0.4 ml of 1:1,000 intraspinal; 1:500,000 to 1:50,000 local mixed with local anesthetic.
To restore cardiac rhythm in cardiac arrest—
Adults: 0.5 to 1 mg I.V. or into endotracheal tube. May be given intracardiac if no I.V. route or intratracheal route available. Following initial I.V. administration, may be infused I.V. at a rate of 1 to 4 mcg/minute.
Children: 10 mcg/kg I.V. or 5 to 10 mcg (0.05 to 0.1 ml of 1:10,000)/kg intracardiac.
   Note: 1 mg = 1 ml of 1:1,000 or 10 ml of 1:10,000.

ADVERSE REACTIONS
CNS: *nervousness,* tremor, euphoria, anxiety, coldness of extremities, vertigo, *headache,* sweating, disorientation, agitation. In patients with Parkinson's disease, the drug increases rigidity and tremor.
CV: *palpitations;* widened pulse pressure; hypertension; *tachycardia; ventricular fibrillation; CVA;* anginal pain; ECG changes, including a decrease in the T wave amplitude.
Metabolic: *hyperglycemia,* glycosuria.
Other: pulmonary edema, dyspnea, *pallor.*

INTERACTIONS
Alpha-adrenergic blocking agents: hypotension due to unopposed beta-adrenergic effects.
Beta blockers, such as propranolol: vasoconstriction and reflex bradycar-

dia. Monitor patient carefully.

Digitalis glycosides, general anesthetics (halogenated hydrocarbons): increased risk of ventricular dysrhythmias.

Doxapram, mazindol, methylphenidate: enhanced CNS stimulation or pressor effects.

Ergot alkaloids: enhanced vasoconstrictor activity.

Guanadrel, guanethidine: enhanced pressor effects of epinephrine.

Levodopa: enhanced risk of cardiac dysrhythmias.

MAO inhibitors: increased risk of hypertensive crisis.

Tricyclic antidepressants, antihistamines, thyroid hormones: when given with sympathomimetics, may cause severe adverse cardiac effects. Avoid giving together.

NURSING CONSIDERATIONS
• Contraindicated in narrow-angle glaucoma, shock (other than anaphylactic shock), organic brain damage, cardiac dilatation, or coronary insufficiency. Also contraindicated during general anesthesia with halogenated hydrocarbons or cyclopropane and in labor (may delay second stage). Use with extreme caution in long-standing bronchial asthma and emphysema who have developed degenerative heart disease. Use with caution in elderly patients, and those with hyperthyroidism, angina, hypertension, psychoneurosis, and diabetes.
• Don't mix with alkaline solutions. Use dextrose 5% in water, normal saline solution, or a combination of dextrose 5% in water and saline solution. Mix just before use.
• When administered I.V., monitor blood pressure, heart rate, and ECG when therapy is initiated and frequently thereafter.
• Epinephrine is rapidly destroyed by oxidizing agents, such as iodine, chromates, nitrates, nitrites, oxygen, and salts of easily reducible metals (such as iron).
• Epinephrine solutions deteriorate after 24 hours. Discard after that time or before if solution is discolored or contains precipitate. Keep solution in light-resistant container, and don't remove before use.
• Massage site after injection to counteract possible vasoconstriction. Repeated local injection can cause necrosis at site from vasoconstriction.
• Avoid I.M. administration of oil injection into buttocks. Gas gangrene may occur because epinephrine reduces oxygen tension of the tissues, encouraging the growth of contaminating organisms.
• This drug may widen patient's pulse pressure.
• In the event of a sharp blood pressure rise, rapid-acting vasodilators, such as nitrites or alpha-adrenergic blocking agents, can be given to counteract the marked pressor effect of large doses of epinephrine.
• Observe patient closely for adverse effects. If adverse effects develop, dosage may need to be adjusted or discontinued.
• If patient has acute hypersensitivity reactions, it may be necessary to instruct him to self-inject epinephrine at home.
• Drug of choice in emergency treatment of acute anaphylactic reactions, including anaphylactic shock.

ethylnorepinephrine hydrochloride
Bronkephrine

Pregnancy Risk Category: C

MECHANISM OF ACTION
Relaxes bronchial smooth muscle by acting on beta-adrenergic receptors.

INDICATIONS & DOSAGE
To relieve bronchospasm caused by asthma—
Adults: 0.6 to 2 mg S.C. or I.M.

Children: 0.2 to 1 mg S.C. or I.M.

ADVERSE REACTIONS
CNS: *headache,* dizziness.
CV: changes in blood pressure, *elevation in pulse rate,* palpitations.
GI: nausea.

INTERACTIONS
Beta blockers: mutual inhibition of clinical effects.
CNS stimulants, xanthine derivatives: enhanced CNS stimulation.
Digitalis glycosides, levodopa, inhalation anesthetics: increased risk of cardiac dysrhythmias.
Nitrates, antihypertensives: decreased effects of these agents.
Rauwolfia alkaloids, sympathomimetics: enhanced effects.
Thyroid hormones: increased risk of coronary insufficiency.

NURSING CONSIDERATIONS
• Use with caution in cardiovascular disease or history of stroke.
• Safer than epinephrine for use in hypertensive or severely ill patients in whom significant pressor effects are undesirable.
• Valuable when used in children because of low incidence of adverse effects; may be useful in diabetic asthmatics due to low glycogenolytic activity.
• Choose anatomic injection site carefully to avoid inadvertent intraneural or intravascular injection.

isoetharine hydrochloride◊
Arm-a-Med Isoetharine, Beta-2, Bisorine, Bronkosol, Dey-Dose Isoetharine, Dey-Dose Isoetharine S/F, Dey-Lute Isoetharine, Dispos-a-Med Isoetharine

isoetharine mesylate
Bronkometer
Pregnancy Risk Category: C

MECHANISM OF ACTION
Relaxes bronchial smooth muscle by acting on beta$_2$-adrenergic receptors.

INDICATIONS & DOSAGE
Bronchial asthma and reversible bronchospasm that may occur with bronchitis and emphysema—
Adults (hydrochloride): administered by hand nebulizer, oxygen aerosolization, or IPPB.

Method	Dose	Dilution
Hand	3 to 7 inhalations	undiluted
Oxygen aerosolization	0.5 ml	1:3 with saline
IPPB	0.5 ml	1:3 with saline

Adults (mesylate): 1 to 2 inhalations. Occasionally, more may be required.

ADVERSE REACTIONS
CNS: *tremor, headache,* dizziness, excitement.
CV: *palpitations,* increased heart rate.
GI: nausea, vomiting.

INTERACTIONS
Propranolol and other beta blockers: blocked bronchodilating effect of isoetharine. Monitor patient carefully if used together.

NURSING CONSIDERATIONS
• Use cautiously in hyperthyroidism, hypertension, or coronary disease, and in patients with sensitivity to sympathomimetics.

Unmarked trade names available in the United States only.
♦ Also available in Canada. ♦ ♦ Available in Canada only. ◊ Also available OTC.

- Excessive use can lead to decreased effectiveness.
- Monitor for severe paradoxical bronchoconstriction after excessive use. Discontinue immediately if bronchoconstriction occurs.
- Although isoetharine has minimal effects on the heart, use cautiously in patients receiving general anesthetics that sensitize the myocardium to sympathomimetic drugs.
- Instruct patient in the use of aerosol and mouthpiece.
- Due to oxidation of drug when diluted with water, pink sputum mimicking hemoptysis may occur after inhaling isoetharine solution. Tell patient not to be concerned.

isoproterenol
Aerolone, Dey-Dose Isoproterenol, Dispos-a-Med Isoproterenol, Isuprel♦, Vapo-Iso

isoproterenol hydrochloride
Isuprel♦, Isuprel Mistometer♦, Norisodrine Aerotrol

isoproterenol sulfate
Medihaler-Iso♦

Pregnancy Risk Category: C

MECHANISM OF ACTION
Relaxes bronchial smooth muscle by acting on beta$_2$-adrenergic receptors. As a cardiac stimulant, acts on beta$_1$-adrenergic receptors in the heart.

INDICATIONS & DOSAGE
Bronchial asthma and reversible bronchospasm (hydrochloride)—
Adults: 10 to 20 mg S.L. q 6 to 8 hours.
Children: 5 to 10 mg S.L. q 6 to 8 hours. Not recommended for children under 6 years.
Bronchospasm (sulfate)—
Adults and children: acute dyspneic episodes: 1 inhalation initially. May repeat if needed after 2 to 5 minutes.

Maintenance dosage is 1 to 2 inhalations q.i.d. to 6 times daily. May repeat once more 10 minutes after second dose. Not more than 3 doses should be administered for each attack.
Heart block and ventricular dysrhythmias (hydrochloride)—
Adults: initially, 0.02 to 0.06 mg I.V. Subsequent doses 0.01 to 0.2 mg I.V. or 5 mcg/minute I.V.; or 0.2 mg I.M. initially, then 0.02 to 1 mg, p.r.n.
Children: may give half of initial adult dose.
Shock (hydrochloride)—
Adults and children: 0.5 to 5 mcg/minute by continuous I.V. infusion. Usual concentration is 1 mg (5 ml) in 500 ml dextrose 5% in water. Adjust rate according to heart rate, central venous pressure, blood pressure, and urine flow.

ADVERSE REACTIONS
CNS: *headache,* mild tremor, weakness, dizziness, nervousness, insomnia.
CV: *palpitations, tachycardia, anginal pain; blood pressure may rise and then fall.*
GI: nausea, vomiting.
Metabolic: hyperglycemia.
Other: sweating, flushing of face, bronchial edema and inflammation.

INTERACTIONS
Epinephrine: increased risk of dysrhythmias.
Propranolol and other beta blockers: blocked bronchodilating effect of isoproterenol. Monitor patient carefully if used together.

NURSING CONSIDERATIONS
- Contraindicated in tachycardia caused by digitalis intoxication and in preexisting dysrhythmias, especially tachycardia, because chronotropic effect on the heart may aggravate such disorders. Contraindicated in recent myocardial infarction. Use cautiously

---

Italicized side effects are common or life-threatening.
*Liquid form contains alcohol.   **May contain tartrazine.

ADRENERGICS (SYMPATHOMIMETICS)** **387**

in coronary insufficiency, diabetes, or hyperthyroidism.

• Not a substitute for blood or fluid volume deficit. Volume deficit should be replaced before vasopressors are administered.

• If heart rate exceeds 110 beats/minute, it may be advisable to decrease infusion rate or temporarily stop infusion. Doses sufficient to increase the heart rate to more than 130 beats/minute may induce ventricular dysrhythmias.

• If precordial distress or anginal pain occurs, stop drug immediately.

• When administering I.V. isoproterenol for shock, closely monitor blood pressure, central venous pressure, ECG, arterial blood gas measurements, and urine output. Carefully adjust infusion rate according to these measurements.

• Oral and sublingual tablets are poorly and erratically absorbed.

• Teach patient how to take sublingual tablet properly. Tell him to hold tablet under tongue until it dissolves and is absorbed and not to swallow saliva until that time. Prolonged use of sublingual tablets can cause tooth decay. Instruct patient to rinse mouth with water between doses. Will also help prevent dryness of oropharynx.

• If possible, don't give at bedtime because it interrupts sleep patterns.

• This drug may cause a slight rise in systolic blood pressure and a slight to marked drop in diastolic blood pressure.

• Use a continuous infusion pump to regulate infusion flow rate.

• Observe patient closely for side effects. Dosage may need to be adjusted or discontinued.

• Tell patient to discontinue the drug if it causes an increase in airway resistance.

• Teach patient to perform oral inhalation correctly. Give the following instructions for using a metered-dose nebulizer:

—Clear nasal passages and throat.
—Breathe out, expelling as much air from lungs as possible.
—Place mouthpiece well into mouth as dose from nebulizer is released, and inhale deeply.
—Hold breath for several seconds, remove mouthpiece, and exhale slowly.

• Instructions for metered powder nebulizer are the same, except that deep inhalation is not necessary.

• Patient may develop a tolerance to this drug. Warn against overuse.

• Warn patient using oral inhalant that drug may turn sputum and saliva pink.

• May aggravate ventilation perfusion abnormalities; even while ease of breathing is improved, arterial oxygen tension may fall paradoxically.

• If ordered via inhalation with oxygen, be sure oxygen concentration will not suppress respiratory drive.

• Discard inhalation solution if it is discolored or contains precipitate.

mephentermine sulfate
Wyamine♦

Pregnancy Risk Category: C

MECHANISM OF ACTION
Indirectly stimulates beta- and alpha-adrenergic receptors by releasing norepinephrine.

INDICATIONS & DOSAGE
Hypotension following spinal anesthesia—
Adults: 30 to 45 mg I.V. in a single injection, then 30 mg I.V. repeated p.r.n. Maintenance of blood pressure: continuous I.V. infusion of 0.1% solution of mephentermine in dextrose 5% in water.
Children: 0.4 mg/kg I.M. or I.V.
Hypotension following spinal anesthesia during obstetric procedures—
Adults: initially 15 mg I.V. p.r.n.
Prevention of hypotension during

Unmarked trade names available in the United States only.
♦Also available in Canada.   ♦♦Available in Canada only.   ◊Also available OTC.

spinal anesthesia—
Adults: 30 to 45 mg I.M. 10 to 20 minutes before anesthesia.

ADVERSE REACTIONS
CNS: euphoria, nervousness, anxiety, tremor, incoherence, drowsiness, seizures.
CV: *dysrhythmias, marked elevation of blood pressure (with large doses).*

INTERACTIONS
Antihypertensives, nitrates: decreased effects of these adrenergic blocking agents.
Beta-adrenergic blocking agents, rauwolfia alkaloids: mutual inhibition of therapeutic effects.
CNS stimulants, mazindol, methylphenidate, sympathomimetics: increased CNS stimulation.
Digitalis glycosides, levodopa, inhalation anesthetics: increased risk of cardiac dysrhythmias.
Ergot alkaloids, oxytocin: enhanced vasoconstriction.
MAO inhibitors: may cause severe hypertension (hypertensive crisis) or dysrhythmias. Don't use together.
Thyroid hormones: enhanced risk of coronary insufficiency.
Tricyclic antidepressants, maprotiline: decreased pressure of mephentermine.

NURSING CONSIDERATIONS
• Contraindicated in concealed hemorrhage or hypotension from hemorrhage, except in emergencies; also in patients receiving phenothiazines, or who have received MAO inhibitors within 2 weeks. Use cautiously in arteriosclerosis, cardiovascular disease, hyperthyroidism, hypertension, chronic illness.
• Not a substitute for blood or fluid volume deficit. If deficit exists, it should be replaced before vasopressors are administered.
• During infusion, check blood pressure every 2 minutes until stabilized;

then every 10 to 15 minutes.
• Observe patient closely for adverse effects. If adverse effects develop, dosage may need to be adjusted or discontinued.
• Monitor blood pressure even after stopping drug.
• I.M. route may be used since drug is not irritating to tissue.
• I.V. drug is not irritating to tissue, and extravasation is not dangerous. To prepare 0.1% I.V. solution; add 16.6 ml mephentermine (30 mg/ml) to 500 ml dextrose 5% in water.
• Can be given I.V. undiluted.
• Don't mix with I.V. hydralazine or epinephrine because they are physically incompatable with mephentermine.
• May increase uterine contractions during third trimester of pregnancy.
• Hypercapnia, hypoxia, acidosis may reduce effectiveness or increase adverse effects. Identify and correct before and during administration.

---

metaproterenol sulfate◊
Alupent♦, Arm-A-Med
Metaproterenol, Dey-Dose
Metaproterenol, Dey-Med
Metaproterenol, Metaprel

Pregnancy Risk Category: C

MECHANISM OF ACTION
Relaxes bronchial smooth muscle by acting on $beta_2$-adrenergic receptors.

INDICATIONS & DOSAGE
Acute episodes of bronchial asthma—
Adults and children: 2 to 3 inhalations. Should not repeat inhalations more often than q 3 to 4 hours. Should not exceed 12 inhalations daily.
Bronchial asthma and reversible bronchospasm—
Adults: 20 mg P.O. q 6 to 8 hours.
Children over 9 years or over 27 kg: 20 mg P.O. q 6 to 8 hours (0.4 mg to 0.9 mg/kg/dose t.i.d.).
Children 6 to 9 years or less than 27

kg: 10 mg P.O. q 6 to 8 hours (0.4 mg to 0.9 mg/kg/dose t.i.d.).

Not recommended for children under 6 years.

ADVERSE REACTIONS
CNS: nervousness, weakness, drowsiness, tremor.
CV: tachycardia, hypertension, palpitations; *with excessive use, cardiac arrest*.
GI: vomiting, nausea, bad taste in mouth.
Other: paradoxical bronchiolar constriction with excessive use.

INTERACTIONS
Propranolol and other beta blockers: blocked bronchodilating effect of metaproterenol. Monitor patient carefully if used together.

NURSING CONSIDERATIONS
• Contraindicated in tachycardia and dysrhythmias associated with tachycardia. Use with caution in hypertension, coronary artery disease, hyperthyroidism, and diabetes.
• Safe use of inhalant in children under 12 years not established.
• Teach patient how to administer metered dose correctly. Instructions: shake container; exhale through nose; administer aerosol while inhaling deeply on mouthpiece of inhaler; and hold breath for a few seconds, then exhale slowly. Allow 2 minutes between inhalations. Store drug in light-resistant container.
• Metaproterenol inhalations should precede steroid inhalations (when prescribed) by 10 to 15 minutes to maximize therapy.
• Warn patient about the possibility of paradoxical bronchospasm. If this occurs, the drug should be discontinued immediately.
• Patients may use tablets and aerosol concomitantly. Monitor closely for toxicity.
• Metaproterenol reportedly pro-

duces less cardiac stimulation than other sympathomimetics, especially isoproterenol.
• Inhalant solution can be administered by IPPB diluted in saline solution or via a hand nebulizer at full strength.
• Tell patient to notify doctor if no response is derived from dosage. Warn against changing dose without calling doctor.

---

metaraminol bitartrate
Aramine
Pregnancy Risk Category: D

MECHANISM OF ACTION
Predominantly stimulates alpha-adrenergic receptors within the sympathetic nervous system.

INDICATIONS & DOSAGE
Prevention of hypotension—
Adults: 2 to 10 mg I.M. or S.C.
Severe shock—
Adults: 0.5 to 5 mg direct I.V. followed by I.V. infusion.
Treatment of hypotension caused by shock—
Adults: 15 to 100 mg in 500 ml normal saline solution or dextrose 5% in water I.V. infusion. Adjust rate to maintain blood pressure.
All indications—
Children: 0.01 mg/kg as single I.V. injection; 1 mg/25 ml dextrose 5% in water as I.V. infusion. Adjust rate to maintain blood pressure in normal range. 0.1 mg/kg I.M. as single dose, p.r.n. Allow at least 10 minutes to elapse before increasing dose because maximum effect is not immediately apparent.

ADVERSE REACTIONS
CNS: apprehension, restlessness, dizziness, headache, tremor, weakness; with excessive use, seizures.
CV: hypertension; hypotension; precordial pain; palpitations; dysrhyth-

mias, including sinus or ventricular tachycardia; bradycardia; premature supraventricular contractions; atrioventricular dissociation.
GI: nausea, vomiting.
GU: decreased urine output.
Metabolic: hyperglycemia.
Skin: flushing, pallor, sweating.
Local: abscess, necrosis, and sloughing upon extravasation.
Other: *metabolic acidosis in hypovolemia, increased body temperature, respiratory distress.*

INTERACTIONS

General anesthetics: increased risk of adverse cardiac effects. Monitor closely.
MAO inhibitors: may cause severe hypertension (hypertensive crisis). Don't use together.

NURSING CONSIDERATIONS

• Contraindicated in peripheral or mesenteric thrombosis, pulmonary edema, hypercarbia, or acidosis; also during anesthesia with cyclopropane and halogenated hydrocarbon anesthetics. Use cautiously in hypertension, thyroid disease, diabetes, cirrhosis, malaria, or sulfite sensitivity, and those receiving digitalis.
• Not a substitute for blood or fluid volume deficit. Volume deficit should be replaced before vasopressors are administered.
• Keep solution in light-resistant container, away from heat.
• Use large veins, as in the antecubital fossa, to minimize risk of extravasation. Watch infusion site carefully for signs of extravasation. If it occurs, stop infusion immediately and call doctor.
• During infusion, check blood pressure every 5 minutes until stabilized; then every 15 minutes. Check pulse rates, urine output, and color and temperature of extremities. Titrate infusion rate according to findings, using doctor's guidelines.

• Use a continuous infusion pump to regulate infusion flow rate.
• Observe patient closely for adverse effects. If adverse effects develop, dosage may need to be adjusted or discontinued.
• For I.V. therapy, use two-bottle setup so I.V. can continue if this drug is stopped.
• Blood pressure should be raised to slightly less than the patient's normal level. Be careful to avoid excessive blood pressure response. Rapidly induced hypertensive response can cause acute pulmonary edema, dysrhythmias, and cardiac arrest.
• Because of prolonged action, a cumulative effect is possible. With an excessive vasopressor response, elevated blood pressure may persist after the drug is stopped.
• Urine output may decrease initially, then increase as blood pressure reaches normal level. Report persistent decreased urine output.
• When discontinuing therapy with this drug, slow infusion rate gradually. Continue monitoring vital signs, watching for possible severe drop in blood pressure. Keep equipment nearby to start drug again, if necessary. Pressor therapy should not be reinstated until the systolic blood pressure falls below 70 to 80 mm Hg.
• Keep emergency drugs on hand to reverse effects of metaraminol: atropine for reflex bradycardia; phentolamine to decrease vasopressor effects; and propranolol for dysrhythmias.
• Closely monitor patients with diabetes. Adjustment in insulin dose may be needed.
• Metaraminol should not be mixed with other drugs.

Italicized side effects are common or life-threatening.
*Liquid form contains alcohol.   **May contain tartrazine.

norepinephrine injection (levarterenol bitartrate)
Levophed♦

Pregnancy Risk Category: D

MECHANISM OF ACTION
Stimulates alpha- and beta-adrenergic receptors within the sympathetic nervous system.

INDICATIONS & DOSAGE
To restore blood pressure in acute hypotensive states—
Adults: initially, 8 to 12 mcg/minute I.V. infusion, then adjust to maintain normal blood pressure. Average maintenance dosage is 2 to 4 mcg/minute.

ADVERSE REACTIONS
CNS: *headache,* anxiety, weakness, dizziness, tremor, restlessness, insomnia.
CV: bradycardia, severe hypertension, marked increase in peripheral resistance, decreased cardiac output, dysrhythmias, *ventricular tachycardia, fibrillation,* bigeminal rhythm, atrioventricular dissociation, precordial pain.
GU: *decreased urine output.*
Metabolic: *metabolic acidosis,* hyperglycemia, increased glycogenolysis.
Local: irritation with extravasation.
Other: fever, respiratory difficulty.

INTERACTIONS
Alpha-adrenergic blocking agents: may antagonize drug effects.
MAO inhibitors: increased risk of hypertensive crisis.
Tricyclic antidepressants: when given with sympathomimetics, may cause severe hypertension (hypertensive crisis). Don't give together.

NURSING CONSIDERATIONS
• Contraindicated in mesenteric or peripheral vascular thrombosis, pregnancy, profound hypoxia, hypercarbia, hypotension from blood volume deficits; and during cyclopropane and halothane anesthesia. Use cautiously in hypertension, hyperthyroidism, severe cardiac disease, and sulfite sensitivity. Use with extreme caution in patients receiving MAO inhibitors or tricyclic antidepressants.
• Not a substitute for blood or fluid volume deficit. Volume deficit should be replaced before vasopressors are administered.
• Norepinephrine solutions deteriorate after 24 hours.
• Use large vein, as in the antecubital fossa, to minimize risk of extravasation. Check site frequently for signs of extravasation. If it occurs, stop infusion immediately and call doctor. He may counteract effect by infiltrating area with 5 to 10 mg phentolamine and 10 to 15 ml normal saline solution. Also check for blanching along course of infused vein; may progress to superficial sloughing.
• During infusion, check blood pressure every 2 minutes until stabilized; then every 5 minutes. Also check pulse rates, urine output, and color and temperature of extremities. Titrate infusion rate according to findings, using doctor's guidelines. In previously hypertensive patients, blood pressure should be raised no more than 40 mm Hg below preexisting systolic pressure.
• Never leave patient unattended during infusion.
• Use a continuous infusion pump to regulate infusion flow rate.
• For I.V. therapy, use two-bottle setup with Y port so I.V. can continue if norepinephrine is stopped.
• Report decreased urine output to doctor immediately.
• If prolonged I.V. therapy is necessary, change injection site frequently.
• When stopping drug, slow infusion rate gradually. Monitor vital signs, even after drug is stopped. Watch for severe drop in blood pressure.

• Keep emergency drugs on hand to reverse effects of norepinephrine: atropine for reflex bradycardia; phentolamine for increased vasopressor effects; and propranolol for dysrhythmias.

• Administer in dextrose 5% in water and saline solution; saline solution alone is not recommended.

phenylephrine hydrochloride◇
Neo-Synephrine◆

Pregnancy Risk Category: C

MECHANISM OF ACTION
Predominantly stimulates alpha-adrenergic receptors in the sympathetic nervous system.

INDICATIONS & DOSAGE
Hypotensive emergencies during spinal anesthesia—
Adults: initially, 0.2 mg I.V., then subsequent doses of 0.1 to 0.2 mg.
Maintenance of blood pressure during spinal or inhalation anesthesia—
Adults: 2 to 3 mg S.C. or I.M. 3 or 4 minutes before anesthesia.
Children: 0.04 mg to 0.088 mg/kg S.C. or I.M.
Mild to moderate hypotension—
Adults: 2 to 5 mg S.C. or I.M.; 0.1 to 0.5 mg I.V. Not to be repeated more often than 10 to 15 minutes.
Paroxysmal supraventricular tachycardia—
Adults: initially, 0.5 mg rapid I.V.; subsequent doses should not exceed the preceding dose by more than 0.1 to 0.2 mg and should not exceed 1 mg.
Prolongation of spinal anesthesia—
Adults: 2 to 5 mg added to anesthetic solution.
Severe hypotension and shock (including drug-induced)—
Adults: 10 mg in 500 ml dextrose 5% in water. Start 100 to 180 drops per minute I.V. infusion, then 40 to 60

drops per minute. Adjust to patient response.
Vasoconstrictor for regional anesthesia—
Adults: 1 mg phenylephrine added to 20 ml local anesthetic.

ADVERSE REACTIONS
CNS: *headache, restlessness, lightheadedness, weakness.*
CV: palpitations, bradycardia, dysrhythmias, hypertension, anginal pain.
EENT: blurred vision.
Skin: goose bumps, feeling of coolness.
Local: tissue sloughing with extravasation.
Other: tachyphylaxis may occur with continued use.

INTERACTIONS
MAO inhibitors: may cause severe hypertension (hypertensive crisis). Don't use together.
Oxytocics, tricyclic antidepressants: increased pressor response. Observe patient.

NURSING CONSIDERATIONS
• Contraindicated in narrow-angle glaucoma, hypotension, ventricular tachycardia, severe coronary disease, or cardiovascular disease (including myocardial infarction), and in patients who are taking MAO inhibitors or tricyclic antidepressants. Use with extreme caution in patients with heart disease, hyperthyroidism, diabetes, severe atherosclerosis, bradycardia, partial heart block, myocardial disease, sulfite sensitivity, and in elderly patients.
• Longer acting than ephedrine and epinephrine.
• Causes little or no CNS stimulation.
• Monitor blood pressure frequently. Avoid excessive rise in blood pressure. Maintain blood pressure at slightly below the patient's normal level. In previously normotensive pa-

tients, maintain systolic blood pressure at 80 to 100 mm Hg; in previously hypertensive patients, maintain systolic blood pressure at 30 to 40 mm Hg below their usual level.
• May reverse severe increase in blood pressure with phentolamine.
• With I.V. infusions, avoid abrupt withdrawal. Monitor blood pressure throughout. Reverse therapy if blood pressure falls too rapidly.

pirbuterol
Maxair

Pregnancy Risk Category: C

MECHANISM OF ACTION
Relaxes bronchial smooth muscle by acting on beta$_2$-adrenergic receptors.

INDICATIONS AND DOSAGE
Prevention and reversal of bronchospasm, asthma—
Adults: 1 or 2 inhalations (0.2 to 0.4 mg) repeated every 4 to 6 hours. Not to exceed 12 inhalations daily.

ADVERSE REACTIONS
CNS: tremors, nervousness, dizziness, insomnia, headache.
CV: tachycardia, palpitations, increased blood pressure.
EENT: drying or irritation of throat.

INTERACTIONS
Propranolol and other beta-adrenergic blocking agents: decreased bronchodilating effects.

NURSING CONSIDERATIONS
• Contraindicated in hypersensitivity to pirbuterol or other adrenergics, and in patients with digitalis toxicity or cardiac dysrhythmias associated with tachycardia.
• Tell patient to call the doctor if he experiences increased bronchospasm after using the drug.
• Teach patient how to administer metered dose correctly. Have him shake container; exhale through nose; administer aerosol while inhaling deeply on mouthpiece of inhaler; and hold breath for a few seconds, then exhale slowly. Tell him to allow 2 minutes between inhalations and to wait at least 5 minutes before using his steroid inhalant (if he's taking concomitant corticosteroid inhalants).
• Advise patient to seek medical attention if a previously effective dosage does not control symptoms because this may signify a worsening of the disease.

pseudoephedrine hydrochloride◊
Cenafed, Children's Sudafed Liquid, Decofed, Dorcol Children's Decongestant, Eltor♦♦, Genaphed, Halofed, NeoFed, Robidrine, Ornex Cold♦♦, Pediacare Infant's Oral Decongestant Drops, Pseudofrin♦♦, Pseudogest, Sinufed, Sudafed, Sudafed 12-Hour, Sudrin, Sufedrin

pseudoephedrine sulfate
Afrinol Repetabs

Pregnancy Risk Category: C

MECHANISM OF ACTION
Stimulates alpha-adrenergic receptors in the respiratory tract, producing vasoconstriction.

INDICATIONS & DOSAGE
Nasal and eustachian tube decongestant—
Adults: 60 mg P.O. q 4 hours. Maximum dosage is 240 mg daily.
Children 6 to 12 years: 30 mg P.O. q 4 hours. Maximum dosage is 120 mg daily.
Children 2 to 6 years: 15 mg P.O. q 4 hours. Maximum dosage is 60 mg/day.
Extended-relief tablets and capsules:
Adults and children over 12 years:

60 to 120 mg P.O. q 12 hours. This form is contraindicated for children under 12 years.
Relief of nasal congestion—
Adults: 120 mg q 12 hours.

ADVERSE REACTIONS
CNS: *anxiety,* transient stimulation, tremors, dizziness, headache, insomnia, *nervousness.*
CV: dysrhythmias, *palpitations,* tachycardia.
EENT: dry mouth.
GI: anorexia, nausea, vomiting.
GU: difficulty in urinating.
Skin: pallor.

INTERACTIONS
MAO inhibitors: may cause severe hypertension (hypertensive crisis). Don't use together.
Antihypertensives: hypotensive effect may be attenuated.

NURSING CONSIDERATIONS
• Contraindicated in severe hypertension or severe coronary artery disease; in patients receiving MAO inhibitors; and in breast-feeding women. Use cautiously in hypertension, cardiac disease, diabetes, glaucoma, hyperthyroidism, and prostatic hypertrophy.
• Elderly patients are more sensitive to the drug's effects.
• Tell patient to stop drug if he becomes unusually restless and to notify doctor promptly.
• Warn against using OTC products containing other sympathomimetic amines.
• Tell patient not to take drug within 2 hours of bedtime because it can cause insomnia.
• Tell patient to relieve dry mouth with sugarless gum or sour hard candy.

terbutaline sulfate
Brethaire, Brethine, Bricanyl♦
Pregnancy Risk Category: B

MECHANISM OF ACTION
Relaxes bronchial smooth muscle by acting on beta$_2$-adrenergic receptors. Also relaxes uterine muscle.

INDICATIONS & DOSAGE
Relief of bronchospasm in patients with reversible obstructive airway disease—
Adults and children over 11 years: 2 inhalations separated by a 60-second interval, repeated q 4 to 6 hours. May also administer 2.5 to 5 mg P.O. q 8 hours or 0.25 mg S.C.
Treatment of premature labor—
0.01 mg/minute by I.V. infusion. Increase by 0.005 mg q 10 minutes up to 0.025 mg/minute or until contractions cease. Or, give 0.25 mg S. C. hourly until contractions cease. Maintenance dosage is 5 mg P.O. q 4 hours for 48 hours, then 5 mg q 6 hours.

ADVERSE REACTIONS
CNS: *nervousness, tremors, headache,* drowsiness, sweating.
CV: palpitations, increased heart rate.
EENT: drying and irritation of nose and throat (with inhaled form).
GI: vomiting, nausea.

INTERACTIONS
MAO inhibitors: when given with sympathomimetics, may cause severe hypertension (hypertensive crisis). Don't use together.
Propranolol and other beta blockers: blocked bronchodilating effects of terbutaline.

NURSING CONSIDERATIONS
• Use cautiously in patients with diabetes, hypertension, hyperthyroidism, severe cardiac disease, and car-

diac dysrhythmias.
• Protect injection from light. Do not
use if discolored.
• Make sure patient and his family
understand why drug is necessary.
• Give S.C. injections in lateral deltoid area.
• Tolerance may develop with prolonged use.
• Warn patient about the possibility
of paradoxical bronchospasm. If this
occurs, the drug should be discontinued immediately.
• Patient may use tablets and aerosol
concomitantly. Monitor closely for
toxicity.
• Teach patient how to administer
metered dose correctly. Have him
shake container; exhale through nose;
administer aerosol while inhaling
deeply on mouthpiece of inhaler; and
hold breath for a few seconds, then
exhale slowly.
• Although not approved by the FDA
for treatment of preterm labor, it is
considered very effective and is used
in many hospitals. Monitor neonates
for hypoglycemia.

40

Adrenergic blockers (sympatholytics)

dihydroergotamine mesylate
ergotamine tartrate
methysergide maleate
phenoxybenzamine
hydrochloride
(See Chapter 22, ANTIHYPERTENSIVES.)
propranolol hydrochloride
(See Chapter 21, ANTIANGINALS.)

COMBINATION PRODUCTS
CAFERGOT: ergotamine tartrate 1 mg and caffeine 100 mg.
CAFERGOT SUPPOSITORIES: ergotamine tartrate 2 mg and caffeine 100 mg.
ERGOCAFF: ergotamine tartrate 1 mg and caffeine 100 mg.
MIGRAL: ergotamine tartrate 1 mg, caffeine 50 mg, and cyclizine HCl 25 mg.
WIGRAINE♦: ergotamine tartrate 1 mg, caffeine 100 mg, levorotatory belladonna alkaloids 0.1 mg, and phenacetin 130 mg.
WIGRAINE SUPPOSITORIES: ergotamine tartrate 2 mg, caffeine 100 mg, and tartaric acid 21.5 mg.

---

dihydroergotamine mesylate
D.H.E. 45

Pregnancy Risk Category: X

MECHANISM OF ACTION
Inhibits the effects of epinephrine, norepinephrine, and other sympathomimetic amines. Also has antiserotonin effects.

INDICATIONS & DOSAGE
Vascular or migraine headache—
Adults: 1 mg I.M. or I.V. May repeat q 1 to 2 hours, p.r.n., up to total of 3 mg. Maximum weekly dosage is 6 mg.

ADVERSE REACTIONS
CV: numbness and tingling in fingers and toes, transient tachycardia or bradycardia, precordial distress and pain, increased arterial pressure.
GI: *nausea, vomiting.*
Skin: itching.
Other: weakness in legs, muscle pains in extremities, localized edema.

INTERACTIONS
Propranolol and other beta blockers: blocked natural pathway for vasodilation in patients receiving ergot alkaloids and thus could result in excessive vasoconstriction. Watch closely if drugs are used together.

NURSING CONSIDERATIONS
• Contraindicated in pregnancy and in peripheral and occlusive vascular disease, coronary artery disease, hypertension, hepatic or renal dysfunction, sepsis.
• Avoid prolonged administration; don't exceed recommended dosage.
• Tell patient to report any feeling of coldness in extremities or tingling of fingers and toes from vasoconstriction. Severe vasoconstriction may result in tissue damage.
• Most effective when used at first sign of migraine or soon after onset. Provide a quiet, low-light environ-

---

ment to help patient relax.
• Help patient evaluate underlying causes of stress.
• Protect ampules from heat and light. Discard if solution is discolored.
• Best results are obtained by adjusting the dose in order to determine the most effective, minimal dose.
• Ergotamine rebound, or an increase in frequency and duration of headache, may occur when the drug is stopped.
• For short-term use only.

---

ergotamine tartrate
Ergomar♦, Ergostat, Gynergen♦♦, Medihaler-Ergotamine♦

Pregnancy Risk Category: X

MECHANISM OF ACTION
Inhibits the effects of epinephrine, norepinephrine, and other sympathomimetic amines. Also has antiserotonin effects.

INDICATIONS & DOSAGE
Vascular or migraine headache—
Adults: initially, 2 mg P.O. S.L., then 1 to 2 mg P.O. q hour or S.L. q ½ hour, to maximum of 6 mg daily and 10 mg weekly. Maximum dosage is 0.5 mg/24 hours and 1 mg/week; or 1 inhalation initially; if not relieved in 5 minutes, use another inhalation. May repeat inhalations at least 5 minutes apart up to maximum of 6 per 24 hours. As a suppository, 2 mg initially; if not relieved, give another 2 mg in 1 hour. Maximum dosage is 4 mg per attack or 10 mg/week.

ADVERSE REACTIONS
CV: numbness and tingling in fingers and toes, transient tachycardia or bradycardia, precordial distress and pain, increased arterial pressure, angina pectoris.
GI: nausea, vomiting, diarrhea, abdominal cramps.

Skin: itching.
Other: weakness in legs, muscle pains in extremities, localized edema.

INTERACTIONS
Propranolol and other beta blockers: blocked natural pathway for vasodilation in patients receiving ergot alkaloids and thus could result in excessive vasoconstriction. Watch closely if drugs are used together.

NURSING CONSIDERATIONS
• Contraindicated in pregnancy and in peripheral and occlusive vascular diseases, coronary artery disease, hypertension, hepatic or renal dysfunction, sepsis.
• Avoid prolonged administration; don't exceed recommended dosage.
• Most effective when used during prodromal stage of headache or as soon as possible after onset.
• Provide a quiet, low-light environment to help patient relax.
• Help patient evaluate underlying causes of physical or emotional stress, which may precipitate attacks.
• Prolonged exposure to cold weather should be avoided whenever possible. Cold may increase many of the side effects.
• Instruct patient on long-term therapy to check for and report feeling of coldness in extremities or tingling of fingers and toes due to vasoconstriction. Severe vasoconstriction may result in tissue damage.
• Store drug in light-resistant container.
• Sublingual tablet is preferred during early stage of attack because of its rapid absorption.
• Warn patient not to increase dosage without first consulting the doctor.
• Obtain an accurate dietary history from patient to determine if a relationship exists between certain foods and onset of headache.
• Ergotamine rebound, or an increase in frequency and duration of head-

---

ache, may occur if the drug is stopped.
• Instruct patient how to use the inhaler correctly.

---

methysergide maleate
Sansert♦**

Pregnancy Risk Category: C

MECHANISM OF ACTION
Specifically blocks serotonin (a neurotransmitter).

INDICATIONS & DOSAGE
Prevention of frequent, severe, uncontrollable, or disabling migraine or vascular headache—
Adults: 4 to 8 mg P.O. daily with meals.

ADVERSE REACTIONS
Blood: neutropenia, eosinophilia.
CNS: insomnia, drowsiness, *euphoria, vertigo,* ataxia, *light-headedness,* hyperesthesia, weakness, *hallucinations or feelings of dissociation.*
CV: *fibrotic thickening of cardiac valves and aorta, inferior vena cava, and common iliac branches (retroperitoneal fibrosis);* vasoconstriction, causing chest pain, abdominal pain, vascular insufficiency of lower limbs; cold, numb, painful extremities with or without paresthesias and diminished or absent pulses; postural hypotension; tachycardia; peripheral edema; murmurs; bruits.
EENT: nasal stuffiness.
GI: nausea, vomiting, diarrhea, constipation, epigastric pain.
Skin: hair loss, dermatitis, sweating, flushing, rash.
Other: *retroperitoneal fibrosis,* causing general malaise, fatigue, weight gain, backache, low-grade fever, urinary obstruction; *pulmonary fibrosis,* causing dyspnea, tightness and pain in chest, pleural friction rubs and effusion, arthralgia, myalgia.

INTERACTIONS
None significant.

NURSING CONSIDERATIONS
• Contraindicated in severe hypertension, arteriosclerosis, peripheral vascular insufficiency, renal or hepatic disease, severe coronary artery diseases, thromboembolic disorders, phlebitis or cellulitis of lower limbs, fibrotic processes, valvular heart disease; and in debilitated patients. Use cautiously in peptic ulcers or suspected coronary artery disease. ECG and cardiac status evaluation advisable before giving to patients over 40 years.
• GI effects may be prevented by gradual introduction of medication and by administering with meals.
• Obtain laboratory studies of cardiac and renal function, blood count, and sedimentation rate before and during therapy.
• Drug may be gradually withdrawn every 6 months; then restart after at least 3 or 4 weeks.
• Tell patient not to stop drug abruptly; may cause rebound headaches. Stop gradually over 2 to 3 weeks.
• Patient should keep daily weight record and report unusually rapid weight gain. Teach him to check for peripheral edema. Explain and suggest low-salt diet if necessary.
• Give drug for 3 weeks before evaluating effectiveness.
• Tell patient to report to doctor promptly if he experiences cold, numb, or painful hands and feet; leg cramps when walking; pelvic, chest, or flank pain.
• Not for treatment of migraine or vascular headache in progress or for treatment of tension (muscle contraction) headaches.
• Indicated only for patients who are unresponsive to other drugs and who can be kept under close medical supervision.

Italicized side effects are common or life-threatening.
*Liquid form contains alcohol.   **May contain tartrazine.

41

Skeletal muscle relaxants

baclofen
carisoprodol
chlorphenesin carbamate
chlorzoxazone
cyclobenzaprine
dantrolene sodium
methocarbamol
orphenadrine citrate

COMBINATION PRODUCTS
BLANEX: chlorzoxazone 250 mg and acetaminophen 300 mg.
CHLOROFON-F: chlorzoxazone 250 mg and acetaminophen 300 mg.
CHLORZONE FORTE: chlorzoxazone 250 mg and acetaminophen 300 mg.
LOBAC: chlorzoxazone 250 mg and acetaminophen 300 mg.
MUS-LAX: chlorzoxazone 250 mg and acetaminophen 300 mg.
NORGESIC: orphenadrine citrate 25 mg, aspirin 385 mg, and caffeine 30 mg.
NORGESIC FORTE: orphenadrine citrate 50 mg, aspirin 770 mg, and caffeine 60 mg.
PARACET FORTE: chlorzoxazone 250 mg and acetaminophen 300 mg.
POLYFLEX: chlorzoxazone 250 mg and acetaminophen 300 mg.
ROBAXISAL♦: methocarbamol 400 mg and aspirin 325 mg.
SKELEX: chlorazoxazone 250 mg and acetaminophen 300 mg.
SOMA COMPOUND♦: carisoprodol 200 mg and aspirin 325 mg.
SOMA COMPOUND WITH CODEINE: carisoprodol 200 mg, aspirin 325 mg, caffeine 32 mg, and codeine phosphate 16 mg.
ZOXAPHEN: chlorzoxazone 250 mg and acetaminophen 300 mg.

baclofen
Lioresal♦, Lioresal DS
Pregnancy Risk Category: C

MECHANISM OF ACTION
Reduces transmission of impulses from the spinal cord to skeletal muscle.

INDICATIONS & DOSAGE
Spasticity in multiple sclerosis, spinal cord injury—
Adults: initially, 5 mg t.i.d. for 3 days, 10 mg t.i.d. for 3 days, 15 mg t.i.d. for 3 days, 20 mg t.i.d. for 3 days. Increase according to response up to maximum of 80 mg daily.

ADVERSE REACTIONS
CNS: *drowsiness, dizziness,* headache, *weakness, fatigue,* confusion, insomnia.
CV: hypotension.
EENT: nasal congestion.
GI: *nausea,* constipation.
GU: urinary frequency.
Hepatic: increased AST (SGOT) and alkaline phosphatase.
Metabolic: hyperglycemia.
Skin: rash, pruritus.
Other: ankle edema, excessive perspiration, weight gain.

INTERACTIONS
Alcohol, CNS depressants: increased CNS depression.

NURSING CONSIDERATIONS
• Use cautiously in impaired renal

Unmarked trade names available in the United States only.
♦Also available in Canada.　　　　♦♦Available in Canada only.　　　　◊Also available OTC.

function, stroke (minimal benefit, poor tolerance), epilepsy, and when spasticity is used to maintain motor function.
• Give with meals or milk to prevent GI distress.
• Amount of relief determines if dosage (and drowsiness) can be reduced.
• Tell patient to avoid activities that require alertness until CNS effects of the drug are known. Drowsiness is usually transient.
• Watch for increased incidence of seizures in epileptics.
• Watch for sensitivity reactions, such as fever, skin eruptions, and respiratory distress.
• Advise patient to follow doctor's orders regarding rest and physical therapy.
• Do not withdraw abruptly unless required by severe adverse effects; may precipitate hallucinations or rebound spasticity.
• Overdosage treatment is supportive only; do not induce emesis or use a respiratory stimulant in obtunded patients.
• Used investigationally for treatment of unstable bladder.

---

carisoprodol
Rela, Sodol, Soma•, Soprodol, Soridol

Pregnancy Risk Category: C

MECHANISM OF ACTION
Reduces transmission of impulses from the spinal cord to skeletal muscle.

INDICATIONS & DOSAGE
As an adjunct in acute, painful musculoskeletal conditions—
Adults and children over 12 years: 350 mg P.O. t.i.d. and h.s.
    Not recommended for children under 12 years.

ADVERSE REACTIONS
CNS: *drowsiness, dizziness,* vertigo, ataxia, tremor, agitation, irritability, headache, depressive reactions, insomnia.
CV: orthostatic hypotension, tachycardia, facial flushing.
GI: nausea, vomiting, hiccups, increased bowel activity, epigastric distress.
Skin: rash, *erythema multiforme,* pruritus.
Other: asthmatic episodes, fever, angioneurotic edema, *anaphylaxis.*

INTERACTIONS
Alcohol, CNS depressants: increased CNS depression.

NURSING CONSIDERATIONS
• Contraindicated in hypersensitivity to related compounds (e.g., meprobamate, tybamate) or intermittent porphyria. Use with caution in impaired hepatic or renal function.
• Watch for idiosyncratic reactions after first to fourth dose (weakness, ataxia, visual and speech difficulties, fever, skin eruptions, and mental changes) or severe reactions, including bronchospasm, hypotension, and anaphylactic shock. Withhold dose and notify doctor immediately of any unusual reactions.
• Record amount of relief to determine whether dosage can be reduced.
• Warn patient to avoid activities that require alertness until CNS effects of the drug are known. Drowsiness is transient.
• Avoid combining with alcohol or other depressants.
• Advise patient to follow doctor's orders regarding rest and physical therapy.
• Do not stop drug abruptly, mild withdrawal effects, such as insomnia, headache, nausea, and abdominal cramps, may result.

Italicized side effects are common or life-threatening.
*Liquid form contains alcohol.   **May contain tartrazine.

chlorphenesin carbamate
Maolate**

Pregnancy Risk Category: C

MECHANISM OF ACTION
Reduces transmission of impulses from the spinal cord to skeletal muscle.

INDICATIONS & DOSAGE
As an adjunct in short-term, acute, painful musculoskeletal conditions—
Adults: initial dose is 800 mg P.O. t.i.d. Maintenance dose is 400 mg P.O. q.i.d. for maximum of 8 weeks.

ADVERSE REACTIONS
Blood: thrombocytopenia, leukopenia, *agranulocytosis.*
CNS: *drowsiness, dizziness,* confusion, headache, weakness. Dose-related side effects include paradoxical stimulation, agitation, insomnia, nervousness, headache.
GI: *nausea, GI distress.*
Other: *anaphylaxis.*

INTERACTIONS
Alcohol and CNS depressants: increased CNS depression.

NURSING CONSIDERATIONS
• Use cautiously in hepatic disease or impaired renal function, and in patients hypersensitive to aspirin.
• Safe use for periods over 8 weeks not established.
• Take with meals or milk to prevent GI distress.
• Amount of relief determines if dosage (and drowsiness) can be reduced.
• Watch for sensitivity reactions, such as fever, skin eruptions, and respiratory distress. Withhold dose and notify doctor of unusual reactions.
• Monitor CBC and platelet studies in patients on long-term therapy. Watch for unusual bleeding and infections that may indicate blood dyscrasia.
• Tell patient to avoid activities that require mental alertness (such as driving or operating heavy machinery) until adverse CNS effects of the drug are known.

chlorzoxazone
Paraflex, Parafon Forte DSC, Strifon Forte DSC

Pregnancy Risk Category: C

MECHANISM OF ACTION
Reduces transmission of impulses from the spinal cord to skeletal muscle.

INDICATIONS & DOSAGE
As an adjunct in acute, painful musculoskeletal conditions—
Adults: 250 to 750 mg t.i.d. or q.i.d.
Children: 20 mg/kg daily in divided doses t.i.d. or q.i.d.

ADVERSE REACTIONS
Blood: anemia, granulocytopenia.
CNS: *drowsiness, dizziness, lightheadedness,* malaise, headache, overstimulation.
GI: anorexia, nausea, vomiting, heartburn, abdominal distress, constipation, diarrhea.
GU: urine discoloration (orange or purple-red).
Hepatic: hepatic dysfunction.
Skin: urticaria, redness, itching, petechiae, bruising.

INTERACTIONS
Alcohol and CNS depressants: increased CNS depression.

NURSING CONSIDERATIONS
• Contraindicated in impaired hepatic function. Use cautiously in history of drug allergies.
• Amount of relief determines if dosage (and drowsiness) can be reduced.
• Watch for signs of hepatic dysfunction. Withhold dose and notify doctor.
• Warn patient to avoid activities that require alertness until CNS effects of the drug are known. Drowsiness is usually mild and transient.

- Avoid combining with alcohol or other depressants.
- Tell patient that the drug may discolor urine orange or purple-red.
- Advise patient to follow doctor's orders regarding rest and physical therapy.
- Give with meals or milk to prevent GI distress.

---

cyclobenzaprine
Flexeril♦

Pregnancy Risk Category: B

MECHANISM OF ACTION
Reduces transmission of impulses from the spinal cord to skeletal muscle.

INDICATIONS & DOSAGE
Short-term treatment of muscle spasm—
Adults: 10 mg P.O. t.i.d. for 7 days. Maximum dosage is 60 mg daily for 2 to 3 weeks.

ADVERSE REACTIONS
CNS: *drowsiness,* euphoria, weakness, headache, insomnia, nightmares, paresthesias, dizziness, depression, visual disturbances, precipitation of seizures.
CV: tachycardia.
EENT: blurred vision, dry mouth.
GI: abdominal pain, dyspepsia, peculiar taste, constipation.
GU: urine retention.
Skin: rash, urticaria, pruritus.
Other: in high doses, watch for adverse reactions like those of other tricyclic drugs (e.g., amitriptyline, imipramine).

INTERACTIONS
None significant.

NURSING CONSIDERATIONS
- Contraindicated in patients who have received MAO inhibitors within 14 days; during acute recovery phase of myocardial infarction; in heart block, dysrhythmias, conduction disturbances, or CHF. Use cautiously in urine retention, narrow-angle glaucoma, increased intraocular pressure, cardiovascular disease, impaired hepatic function, and seizures; and in elderly or debilitated patients.
- Withdrawal symptoms (nausea, headache, and malaise) may occur if drug is stopped abruptly after long-term use.
- Watch for symptoms of overdose, including possible cardiotoxicity. Notify doctor immediately and have physostigmine available.
- Advise patient to report urinary hesitancy or urine retention. If constipation is a problem, increase fluid intake and get an order for a stool softener.
- Warn patient to avoid activities that require alertness until CNS effects of the drug are known. Drowsiness and dizziness usually subside after 2 weeks.
- Avoid combining alcohol or other depressants with cyclobenzaprine.
- Tell patient that dry mouth may be relieved with sugarless candy or gum.

---

dantrolene sodium
Dantrium♦, Dantrium I.V.♦

Pregnancy Risk Category: C

MECHANISM OF ACTION
Acts directly on skeletal muscle to interfere with intracellular calcium movement.

INDICATIONS & DOSAGE
Spasticity and sequelae secondary to severe chronic disorders (multiple sclerosis, cerebral palsy, spinal cord injury, stroke)—
Adults: 25 mg P.O. daily. Increase gradually in increments of 25 mg at 4- to 7-day intervals, up to 100 mg b.i.d. to q.i.d., to maximum of 400 mg daily.
Children: 1 mg/kg daily P.O. b.i.d.

Italicized side effects are common or life-threatening.
*Liquid form contains alcohol.   **May contain tartrazine.

to q.i.d. Increase gradually as needed by 1 mg/kg daily to maximum of 100 mg q.i.d.

Management of malignant hyperthermia—

Adults and children: 1 mg/kg I.V. initially; may repeat dose up to cumulative dose of 10 mg/kg.

Prevention or attenuation of malignant hyperthermia in susceptible patients who require surgery—

Adults: 4 to 8 mg/kg P.O. daily given in three to four divided doses for 1 to 2 days before procedure. Administer final dose 3 to 4 hours before procedure.

Prevention of recurrence of malignant hyperthermia—

Adults: 4 to 8 mg/kg/day given in four divided doses for up to 3 days following hyperthermic crisis.

ADVERSE REACTIONS

CNS: *muscle weakness, drowsiness,* dizziness, light-headedness, malaise, headache, confusion, nervousness, insomnia.
CV: tachycardia, blood pressure changes.
EENT: excessive tearing, visual disturbances.
GI: anorexia, constipation, cramping, dysphagia, *severe diarrhea.*
GU: urinary frequency, incontinence, nocturia, dysuria, crystalluria, difficulty achieving erection.
Hepatic: *hepatitis.*
Skin: eczematous eruption, pruritus, urticaria, photosensitivity.
Other: abnormal hair growth, drooling, sweating, pleural effusion, myalgia, chills, fever.

INTERACTIONS

Alcohol, CNS depressants: increased CNS depression. Monitor for decreased alertness.
Verapamil (I.V.): may result in cardiovascular collapse. Stop drug before administering I.V. dantrolene.

NURSING CONSIDERATIONS

The following are considerations for the P.O. form only:
• Contraindicated when spasticity is used to maintain motor function; in spasms in rheumatic disorders; and in lactation. Use with caution in severely impaired cardiac or pulmonary function or preexisting hepatic disease; in women; and in patients over 35 years.
• Safety and efficacy in long-term use not established; value may be determined by therapeutic trial. Do not give more than 45 days if no benefits are obtained.
• Give with meals or milk to prevent GI distress.
• Prepare oral suspension for single dose by dissolving capsule contents in juice or other suitable liquid. For multiple doses, use acid vehicle, such as citric acid in USP syrup; refrigerate. Use within several days.
• Amount of relief determines if dosage (and drowsiness) can be reduced.
• Liver function tests should be performed at the beginning of therapy.
• Watch for hepatitis (fever and jaundice), severe diarrhea, severe weakness, or sensitivity reactions (fever and skin eruptions). Withhold dose and notify doctor.
• Warn patient to avoid driving and other hazardous activities until CNS effects of the drug are known. Side effects should subside after 4 days.
• Tell patient to avoid combining with alcohol or other depressants; to avoid photosensitivity reactions by using sunscreening agents and protective clothing; to report abdominal discomfort or GI problems immediately; and to follow doctor's orders regarding rest and physical therapy.
The following are considerations for the I.V. form only:
• Administer as soon as malignant hyperthermia reaction is recognized.
• Reconstitute each vial by adding 60 ml of sterile water for injection and shaking vial until clear. Don't use a

diluent that contains a bacteriostatic agent.
• Protect contents from light and use within 6 hours.
• Be careful to avoid extravasation.

---

methocarbamol
Carbacot, Delaxin, Marbaxin, Robamol, Robaxin♦, Robomol-500, Robomol-750

Pregnancy Risk Category: C

MECHANISM OF ACTION
Reduces transmission of impulses from the spinal cord to skeletal muscle.

INDICATIONS & DOSAGE
As an adjunct in acute, painful musculoskeletal conditions—
Adults: 1.5 g P.O. for 2 to 3 days, then 1 g P.O. q.i.d., or not more than 500 mg (5 ml) I.M. into each gluteal region. May repeat q 8 hours. Or 1 to 3 g daily (10 to 30 ml) I.V. directly into vein at 3 ml/minute, or 10 ml may be added to no more than 250 ml of dextrose 5% in water or normal saline solution. Maximum dosage is 3 g daily.
Supportive therapy in tetanus management—
Adults: 1 to 2 g into tubing of running I.V. or 1 to 3 g in infusion bottle q 6 hours.
Children: 15 mg/kg I.V. q 6 hours.

ADVERSE REACTIONS
Blood: hemolysis, increased hemoglobin (I.V. only).
CNS: drowsiness, dizziness, lightheadedness, headache, syncope, mild muscular incoordination (I.M. or I.V. only), *seizures* (I.V. only).
CV: hypotension, bradycardia (I.M. or I.V. only).
GI: nausea, anorexia, GI upset.
GU: hematuria (I.V. only), discoloration of urine.
Skin: urticaria, pruritus, rash.
Local: thrombophlebitis, extravasa-

tion (I.V. only).
Other: fever, metallic taste, flushing, *anaphylactic reactions* (I.M. or I.V. only).

INTERACTIONS
Alcohol and CNS depressants: increased CNS depression.

NURSING CONSIDERATIONS
• Contraindicated in impaired renal function (injectable form), myasthenia gravis, epilepsy (injectable form); in children under 12 years (except in tetanus); and in patients receiving anticholinesterase agents.
• I.V. irritates veins, may cause phlebitis, aggravate seizures, and may cause fainting if injected rapidly.
• Give I.V. slowly. Maximum rate 300 mg (3 ml)/minute. Give I.M. deeply, only in upper outer quadrant of buttocks, with maximum of 5 ml in each buttock, and inject slowly. Do not give subcutaneously.
• In tetanus management, use methocarbamol with tetanus antitoxin, penicillin, tracheotomy, and aggressive supportive care. Long course of I.V. methocarbamol required.
• Watch for sensitivity reactions, such as fever and skin eruptions.
• Warn patient to avoid activities that require alertness until CNS effects of the drug are known. Drowsiness subsides.
• Avoid combining with alcohol or other depressants.
• Advise patient to follow doctor's orders regarding rest and physical therapy.
• Tell patient urine may turn green, black, or brown.
• Give with meals or milk to prevent GI distress.
• Watch for orthostatic hypotension, especially with parenteral administration. Keep patient supine for 15 minutes afterward, and supervise ambulation. Advise patient to get up slowly.
• Have epinephrine, antihistamines,

Italicized side effects are common or life-threatening.
*Liquid form contains alcohol.   **May contain tartrazine.

and corticosteroids available.
• Prepare liquid by crushing tablets into water or saline solution. Give through nasogastric tube.
• Obtain CBC periodically during prolonged therapy.
• May interfere with urine tests for 5-hydroxyindoleacetic acid (5-HIAA) and vanillylmandelic acid (VMA).

orphenadrine citrate

Banflex, Blanex, Flexagin, Flexain, Flexoject, Flexon, K-Flex, Marflex, Myolin, Myotrol, Neocyten, Noradex, Norflex♦, O-Flex, Orflagen, Orphenate, Tega-Flex

Pregnancy Risk Category: C

MECHANISM OF ACTION
Reduces transmission of impulses from the spinal cord to skeletal muscle.

INDICATIONS & DOSAGE
Adjunctive treatment in painful, acute musculoskeletal conditions—
Adults: 100 mg P.O. b.i.d., or 60 mg I.V. or I.M. q 12 hours, p.r.n. For maintenance, switch to oral therapy beginning 12 hours after last parenteral dose.

ADVERSE REACTIONS
Blood: *aplastic anemia.*
CNS: disorientation, restlessness, irritability, weakness, *drowsiness,* headache, dizziness.
CV: palpitations, tachycardia.
EENT: dilated pupils, blurred vision, difficulty swallowing.
GI: constipation, *dry mouth,* nausea, vomiting, paralytic ileus, epigastric distress.
GU: urinary hesitancy or urine retention.

INTERACTIONS
Alcohol, other CNS depressants: increased CNS depression.

NURSING CONSIDERATIONS
• Contraindicated in narrow-angle glaucoma; prostatic hypertrophy; pyloric, duodenal, or bladder-neck obstruction; myasthenia gravis; tachycardia; severe hepatic or renal disease; or ulcerative colitis. Use cautiously in elderly or debilitated patients with cardiac disease, dysrhythmias, sulfite sensitivity, and those exposed to high temperatures.
• Check all dosages carefully. Even a slight overdose can lead to toxicity. Early signs are excessive dry mouth, dilated pupils, blurred vision, skin flushing, and fever.
• Monitor vital signs carefully.
• With I.V. administration, inject the drug over a period of approximately 5 minutes while patient is supine. Wait 5 to 10 minutes and then help patient to sit up.
• When given I.V., may cause paradoxical initial bradycardia. Usually disappears in 2 minutes.
• Have patient report urinary hesitancy and urine retention. Orphenadrine is an anticholinergic. Have patient void before taking the drug.
• Relieve dry mouth with cool drinks, sugarless gum, or hard candy.
• Monitor CBC and urinalysis in patients receiving drug over extended periods.
• Advise patients to avoid hazardous tasks (such as driving or operating heavy machinery) until CNS effects of the drug are known.

42

Neuromuscular blockers

atracurium besylate
gallamine triethiodide
hexafluorenium bromide
metocurine iodide
pancuronium bromide
succinylcholine chloride
  (suxamethonium chloride)
tubocurarine chloride
vecuronium bromide

COMBINATION PRODUCTS
None.

---

atracurium besylate
Tracrium♦

Pregnancy Risk Category: C

MECHANISM OF ACTION
Prevents acetylcholine from binding
to the receptors on the muscle end
plate, thus blocking depolarization.
Nondepolarizing agent.

INDICATIONS & DOSAGE
*Adjunct to general anesthesia, to fa-
cilitate endotracheal intubation and to
provide skeletal muscle relaxation
during surgery or mechanical ventilation—*
Dose depends on anesthetic used, individual needs, and response. Doses
are representative and must be adjusted.
Adults and children over 2 years:
0.4 to 0.5 mg/kg by I.V. bolus. Maintenance dose of 0.08 to 0.10 mg/kg
within 20 to 45 minutes of initial dose
should be administered during prolonged surgical procedures. Maintenance doses may be administered q 12

to 25 minutes in patients receiving
balanced anesthesia.
Children 1 month to 2 years: initial
dose, 0.3 to 0.4 mg/kg. Frequent
maintenance doses may be needed.

ADVERSE REACTIONS
CV: bradycardia.
Skin: skin flush, erythema, pruritus,
urticaria.
Other: *prolonged dose-related apnea,
wheezing, increased bronchial secretions.*

INTERACTIONS
*Aminoglycoside antibiotics (including
amikacin, gentamicin, kanamycin,
neomycin, streptomycin); polymyxin
antibiotics (polymyxin B sulfate, colistin); clindamycin; quinidine; general
anesthetics such as halothane, enflurane, and isoflurane:* potentiated neuromuscular blockade, leading to increased skeletal muscle relaxation and
possible respiratory paralysis. Use
cautiously during surgical and postoperative periods.
Lithium, narcotic analgesics: potentiated neuromuscular blockade, leading to increased skeletal muscle relaxation and possible respiratory paralysis. Use with extreme caution and reduce dose of atracurium.

NURSING CONSIDERATIONS
• Use cautiously in cardiovascular
disease, severe electrolyte disorders,
bronchogenic carcinoma, and neuromuscular diseases.
• Atracurium should only be used by
personnel experienced in airway man-

Italicized side effects are common or life-threatening.
*Liquid form contains alcohol.   **May contain tartrazine.

agement.
• Keep airway clear. Have emergency respiratory support equipment (endotracheal equipment, ventilator, oxygen, atropine, edrophonium, neostigmine, and epinephrine) on hand.
• Prior administration of succinylcholine does not prolong duration of action, but it quickens onset and may deepen neuromuscular blockade.
• Atracurium facilitates intubation within 2 to 2½ minutes. The duration of effect is 20 to 35 minutes.
• Once spontaneous recovery starts, atracurium-induced neuromuscular blockade may be reversed with an anticholinesterase agent (such as neostigmine or edrophonium). Usually administered together with an anticholinergic drug (such as atropine or glycopyrollate).
• Don't administer by I.M. injection.
• Don't mix with alkaline solutions such as barbiturates (precipitate may form).
• Monitor respirations closely until patient is fully recovered from neuromuscular blockade, as evidenced by tests of muscle strength (hand grip, head lift, and ability to cough).
• Atracurium has a longer duration of action than succinylcholine and a shorter duration of action than *d*-tubocurarine or pancuronium.

---

gallamine triethiodide
Flaxedil♦

Pregnancy Risk Category: C

MECHANISM OF ACTION
Prevents acetylcholine from binding to the receptors on the muscle end plate, thus blocking depolarization. Nondepolarizing agent.

INDICATIONS & DOSAGE
Adjunct to anesthesia to induce skeletal muscle relaxation; facilitate intubation, reduction of fractures and dislocations; lessen muscle contractions

in pharmacologically or electrically induced seizures; assist with mechanical ventilation—
Dosage depends on anesthetic used, individual needs, and response. Dosages are representative and must be adjusted.
Adults and children over 1 month: initially, 1 mg/kg I.V. to maximum of 100 mg, regardless of patient's weight; then 0.5 mg to 1 mg/kg q 30 to 40 minutes.
Children under 1 month but over 5 kg (11 lb): initially, 0.25 to 0.75 mg/kg I.V., then may give additional doses of 0.1 to 0.5 mg/kg q 30 to 40 minutes.

ADVERSE REACTIONS
CV: tachycardia.
Other: *respiratory paralysis, dose-related prolonged apnea,* residual muscle weakness, increased oropharyngeal secretions, allergic or idiosyncratic hypersensitivity reactions.

INTERACTIONS
Aminoglycoside antibiotics (amikacin, gentamicin, kanamycin, neomycin, streptomycin); polymyxin antibiotics (polymyxin B sulfate, colistin); clindamycin; quinidine; general anesthetics (such as halothane, enflurane, isoflurane: potentiated neuromuscular blockade, leading to increased skeletal muscle relaxation and possible respiratory paralysis. Use cautiously during surgical and postoperative periods.
Narcotic analgesics, I.V. diazepam: potentiated neuromuscular blockade, leading to increased skeletal muscle relaxation and possible respiratory paralysis. Use with extreme caution, and reduce dose of gallamine.

NURSING CONSIDERATIONS
• Contraindicated in patients with hypersensitivity to iodides, impaired renal function, myasthenia gravis; patients in shock; and patients in whom

tachycardia may be hazardous. Use cautiously in elderly or debilitated patients; in hepatic or pulmonary impairment, respiratory depression, myasthenic syndrome of lung cancer or bronchogenic carcinoma, dehydration, thyroid disorders, collagen diseases, porphyria, and electrolyte disturbances; in patients sensitive to sulfites; and in patients undergoing cesarean section.
• Gallamine should only be used by personnel experienced in airway management.
• Keep airway clear. Have emergency respiratory support equipment (endotracheal equipment, ventilator, oxygen, atropine, edrophonium, neostigmine, and epinephrine) on hand.
• Monitor baseline electrolyte determinations (electrolyte imbalance can potentiate neuromuscular effects).
• Take vital signs every 15 minutes, especially for developing tachycardia. Notify doctor immediately of significant changes.
• Measure intake and output (renal dysfunction prolongs duration of action, since drug is unchanged before excretion).
• Monitor respirations closely until patient is fully recovered from neuromuscular blockade, as evidenced by tests of muscle strength (hand grip, head lift, and ability to cough).
• Determine whether patient has iodide allergy.
• Protect drug from light or excessive heat; use only fresh solutions.
• Do not mix solution with meperidine HCl or barbiturate solutions.
• Give I.V. slowly (over 30 to 90 seconds).
• May be preferred in patients who have bradycardia.
• Once spontaneous recovery starts, gallamine-induced neuromuscular blockade may be reversed with an anticholinesterase agent (such as neostigmine or edrophonium). Usually administered together with an anti-cholinergic drug (such as atropine or glycopyrrollate).

hexafluorenium bromide
Mylaxen
Pregnancy Risk Category: C

MECHANISM OF ACTION
Inhibits the enzymatic breakdown of succinylcholine, prolonging its duration.

INDICATIONS & DOSAGE
Adjunct for use with succinylcholine to prolong neuromuscular blockade and reduce muscular fasciculations—
Adults and children: use in ratio of 2 mg:1 mg succinylcholine and administer by I.V. push. Maximum dosage is hexafluorenium bromide 10 to 36 mg; should not be administered more frequently than q 15 to 30 minutes.

ADVERSE REACTIONS
CV: hypotension, hypertension, tachycardia, bradycardia, dysrhythmias, *cardiac arrest.*
EENT: increased intraocular pressure, salivation.
Other: increased bronchial tone, *bronchospasm, apnea, prolonged neuromuscular blockade,* hyperthermia.

INTERACTIONS
None reported for this drug alone; always used with succinylcholine. See succinylcholine.

NURSING CONSIDERATIONS
• Contraindicated in hypersensitivity to bromides, in bronchial asthma. Use cautiously in elderly or debilitated patient; in renal, hepatic, or pulmonary impairment, respiratory depression, myasthenia gravis, myasthenic syndrome of lung cancer or bronchogenic carcinoma, dehydration, thyroid disorders, collagen diseases, porphyria, electrolyte disturbances, and glaucoma; and during ocular surgery and

Italicized side effects are common or life-threatening.
*Liquid form contains alcohol.   **May contain tartrazine.

(in large doses) cesarean section.
- Monitor baseline electrolyte determinations (electrolyte imbalance potentiates neuromuscular effects) and vital signs (watch respirations closely).
- Keep airway clear. Have emergency respiratory support equipment (endotracheal equipment, ventilator, oxygen, atropine, edrophonium, neostigmine, and epinephrine) on hand.
- Reassure patient that postoperative stiffness is normal and will soon subside.
- Use only fresh solutions; do not give without direct supervision of doctor.

metocurine iodide
Metubine♦

Pregnancy Risk Category: C

MECHANISM OF ACTION
Prevents acetylcholine from binding to the receptors on the muscle end plate, thus blocking depolarization. Nondepolarizing agent.

INDICATIONS & DOSAGE
Adjunct to anesthesia to induce skeletal muscle relaxation; facilitate intubation, reduction of fractures and dislocations—
Dosage depends on anesthetic used, individual needs, and response. Dosages are representative and must be adjusted. Administer as sustained injection over 30 to 60 seconds.
Adults: given cyclopropane: 2 to 4 mg I.V. (2.68 mg average).
Given ether: 1.5 to 3 mg I.V. (2.1 mg average).
Given nitrous oxide: 4 to 7 mg I.V. (4.79 mg average). Supplemental injections of 0.5 to 1 mg in 25 to 90 minutes, repeated p.r.n.
Lessen muscle contractions in pharmacologically or electrically induced seizures—
Adults: 1.75 to 5.5 mg I.V.

ADVERSE REACTIONS
CV: hypotension secondary to histamine release, ganglionic blockade in rapid dose or overdose.
Other: *dose-related prolonged apnea,* residual muscle weakness, increased oropharyngeal secretions, allergic or idiosyncratic hypersensitivity reactions, *bronchospasm.*

INTERACTIONS
Aminoglycoside antibiotics (including amikacin, gentamicin, kanamycin, neomycin, streptomycin); polymyxin antibiotics (polymyxin B sulfate, colistin); clindamycin; quinidine; general anesthetics (such as halothane, enflurane, isoflurane), furosemide, thiazide diuretics, and beta-adrenergic blocking agents: potentiated neuromuscular blockade, leading to increased skeletal muscle relaxation and possible respiratory paralysis. Use cautiously during surgical and postoperative periods.
Narcotic analgesics: potentiated neuromuscular blockade, leading to increased skeletal muscle relaxation and possible respiratory paralysis. Use with extreme caution, and reduce dose of metocurine iodide.

NURSING CONSIDERATIONS
- Contraindicated in patients with hypersensitivity to iodides; and in whom histamine release is a hazard (asthmatic or atopic patients). Use cautiously in elderly or debilitated patients; and in renal, hepatic, or pulmonary impairment, respiratory depression, myasthenia gravis, myasthenic syndrome of lung cancer or bronchogenic carcinoma, dehydration, thyroid disorders, collagen diseases, porphyria, electrolyte disturbances, hyperthermia, and (in large doses) cesarean section.
- Metocurine should only be used by personnel experienced in airway management.
- Keep airway clear. Have emergency

respiratory support equipment (endo-tracheal equipment, ventilator, oxygen, atropine, edrophonium, epinephrine, and neostigmine) on hand.
• Once spontaneous recovery starts, metocurine-induced neuromuscular blockade may be reversed with an anticholinesterase agent (such as neostigmine or edrophonium). Usually administered together with an anticholinergic drug (such as atropine or glycopyrrollate).
• Dose of 1 mg is the therapeutic equivalent of 3 mg *d*-tubocurarine chloride.
• Monitor baseline electrolyte determinations (electrolyte imbalance, especially potassium, calcium, and magnesium, can potentiate neuromuscular effects) and vital signs, especially respiration.
• Measure intake and output (renal dysfunction prolongs duration of action, since drug is mainly unchanged before excretion).
• Monitor respirations closely until patient is fully recovered from neuromuscular blockade, as evidenced by tests of muscle strength (hand grip, head lift, and ability to cough).
• Determine whether patient has iodide allergy.
• Store solution away from heat, sunlight; do not mix with barbiturates (precipitate will form). Use fresh solutions only.

pancuronium bromide
Pavulon♦

Pregnancy Risk Category: C

MECHANISM OF ACTION
Prevents acetylcholine from binding to the receptors on the muscle end plate, thus blocking depolarization. Nondepolarizing agent.

INDICATIONS & DOSAGE
Adjunct to anesthesia to induce skeletal muscle relaxation; facilitate intu-bation; lessen muscle contractions in pharmacologically or electrically induced seizures; assist with mechanical ventilation—
Dosage depends on anesthetic used, individual needs, and response. Dosages are representative and must be adjusted.
Adults: initially, 0.04 to 0.1 mg/kg I.V.; then 0.01 mg/kg q 30 to 60 minutes.
Children over 10 years: initially, 0.04 to 0.1 mg/kg I.V., then ⅕ initial dose q 30 to 60 minutes.

ADVERSE REACTIONS
CV: tachycardia, increased blood pressure.
Local: burning sensation.
Skin: transient rashes.
Other: excessive sweating and salivation, *prolonged dose-related apnea,* wheezing, residual muscle weakness, allergic or idiosyncratic hypersensitivity reactions.

INTERACTIONS
Aminoglycoside antibiotics (including amikacin, gentamicin, kanamycin, neomycin, streptomycin); polymyxin antibiotics (polymyxin B sulfate, colistin); clindamycin; quinidine; general anesthetics (such as halothane, enflurane, isoflurane): potentiated neuromuscular blockade, leading to increased skeletal muscle relaxation and possible respiratory paralysis. Use cautiously during surgical and postoperative periods.
Lithium, narcotic analgesics: potentiated neuromuscular blockade, leading to increased skeletal muscle relaxation and possible respiratory paralysis. Use with extreme caution, and reduce dose of pancuronium.

NURSING CONSIDERATIONS
• Contraindicated in hypersensitivity to bromides; preexisting tachycardia; and in patients for whom even a minor increase in heart rate is undesirable.

Use cautiously in elderly or debilitated patients; renal, hepatic, or pulmonary impairment; respiratory depression; myasthenia gravis; myasthenic syndrome of lung cancer or bronchogenic carcinoma; dehydration; thyroid disorders; collagen diseases; porphyria; electrolyte disturbances; hyperthermia; toxemic states; and (in large doses) cesarean section.

• Pancuronium should only be used by personnel experienced in airway management.

• Have emergency respiratory support equipment (endotracheal equipment, ventilator, oxygen, atropine, edrophonium, epinephrine, and neostigmine) on hand.

• Causes no histamine release or hypotension.

• Dose of 1 mg is the approximate therapeutic equivalent of 5 mg *d*-tubocurarine chloride.

• Monitor baseline electrolyte determinations (electrolyte imbalance can potentiate neuromuscular effects) and vital signs (watch respiration and heart rate closely).

• Measure intake and output (renal dysfunction may prolong duration of action, since 25% of the drug is unchanged before excretion).

• Monitor respirations closely until patient is fully recovered from neuromuscular blockade, as evidenced by tests of muscle strength (hand grip, head lift, and ability to cough).

• Allow succinylcholine effects to subside before giving pancuronium.

• Store in refrigerator. Do not store in plastic containers or syringes, although plastic syringes may be used for administration.

• Do not mix with barbiturate solutions (precipitate will form); use only fresh solutions.

• Once spontaneous recovery starts, pancuronium-induced neuromuscular blockade may be reversed with an anticholinesterase agent (such as neostigmine or edrophonium). Usually administered together with an anticholinergic drug (such as atropine or glycopyrollate).

---

succinylcholine chloride (suxamethonium chloride)
Anectine♦, Anectine Flo-Pack, Quelicin, Sucostrin

Pregnancy Risk Category: C

MECHANISM OF ACTION
Prolongs depolarization of the muscle end plate. Depolarizing agent.

INDICATIONS & DOSAGE
Adjunct to anesthesia to induce skeletal muscle relaxation; facilitate intubation and assist with mechanical ventilation or orthopedic manipulations (drug of choice); lessen muscle contractions in pharmacologically or electrically induced seizures—
Dosage depends on anesthetic used, individual needs, and response. Dosages are representative and must be adjusted.
Adults: 25 to 75 mg I.V., then 2.5 mg/minute, p.r.n., or 2.5 mg/kg I.M. up to maximum of 150 mg I.M. in deltoid muscle.
Children: 1 to 2 mg/kg I.M. or I.V. Maximum I.M. dosage is 150 mg. (Children may be less sensitive to succinylcholine than adults.)

ADVERSE REACTIONS
CV: bradycardia, tachycardia, hypertension, hypotension, dysrhythmias.
EENT: increased intraocular pressure.
Other: *prolonged respiratory depression, apnea, malignant hyperthermia,* muscle fasciculation, *postoperative muscle pain,* myoglobinemia, excessive salivation, allergic or idiosyncratic hypersensitivity reactions.

INTERACTIONS
Aminoglycoside antibiotics (including amikacin, gentamicin, kanamycin,

neomycin, streptomycin); polymyxin antibiotics (polymyxin B sulfate, colistin); cholinesterase inhibitors such as neostigmine, pyridostigmine, edrophonium, physostigmine, or echothiophate; general anesthetics (such as halothane, enflurane, isoflurane): potentiated neuromuscular blockade, leading to increased skeletal muscle relaxation and possible respiratory paralysis. Use cautiously during surgical and postoperative periods.

Narcotic analgesics, methotrimeprazine: potentiated neuromuscular blockade, leading to increased skeletal muscle relaxation and possible respiratory paralysis. Use with extreme caution.

MAO inhibitors, lithium, cyclophosphamide: prolonged apnea. Use with caution.

Magnesium sulfate (parenterally): potentiated neuromuscular blockade, increased skeletal muscle relaxation, and possible respiratory paralysis. Use with caution, preferably with reduced doses.

Cardiac glycosides: possible cardiac dysrhythmias. Use together cautiously.

NURSING CONSIDERATIONS

• Contraindicated in abnormally low plasma pseudocholinesterase. Use with caution in patients with personal or family history of malignant hypertension or hyperthermia; elderly or debilitated patients; hepatic, renal, or pulmonary impairment; and in respiratory depression, severe burns or trauma, electrolyte imbalances, quinidine or digitalis therapy, hyperkalemia, paraplegia, spinal neuraxis injury, degenerative or dystrophic neuromuscular disease, myasthenia gravis, myasthenic syndrome of lung cancer or bronchogenic carcinoma, dehydration, thyroid disorders, collagen diseases, porphyria, fractures, muscle spasms, glaucoma, eye surgery or penetrating eye wounds, pheo-

chromocytoma, and (in large doses) cesarean section.

• Succinylcholine should only be used by personnel experienced in airway management.

• Keep airway clear. Have emergency respiratory support equipment (endotracheal equipment, ventilator, oxygen, atropine, and epinephrine) on hand.

• Unlike nondepolarizing agents, neostigmine or edrophonium may worsen neuromuscular blockade. Don't use reversing agents.

• Drug of choice for short procedures (less than 3 minutes) and for orthopedic manipulations; use caution in fractures or dislocations.

• Duration of action prolonged to 20 minutes by continuous I.V. infusion or single-dose administration, along with hexafluorenium bromide.

• Repeated or continuous infusions of succinylcholine alone not advised; may cause reduced response or prolonged muscle relaxation and apnea.

• Monitor baseline electrolyte determinations and vital signs (check respiration every 5 to 10 minutes during infusion).

• Reassure patient that postoperative stiffness is normal and will soon subside.

• Store injectable form in refrigerator. Store powder form at room temperature, tightly closed. Use immediately after reconstitution. Do not mix with alkaline solutions (thiopental, sodium bicarbonate, barbiturates).

• Give test dose (10 mg I.M. or I.V.) after patient has been anesthetized. Normal response (no respiratory depression or transient depression for up to 5 minutes) indicates drug may be given. Do not give if patient develops respiratory paralysis sufficient to permit endotracheal intubation. (Recovery within 30 to 60 minutes.)

• Monitor respirations closely until patient is fully recovered from neuromuscular blockade, as evidenced by

---

tests of muscle strength (hand grip, head lift, and ability to cough).
• If given I.M., give deep I.M., preferably high into the deltoid muscle.

tubocurarine chloride
Tubarine◆◆

Pregnancy Risk Category: C

MECHANISM OF ACTION
Prevents acetylcholine from binding to the receptors on the muscle end plate, thus blocking depolarization. Nondepolarizing agent.

INDICATIONS & DOSAGE
Adjunct to anesthesia to induce skeletal muscle relaxation; facilitate intubation, orthopedic manipulations—
Dosage depends on anesthetic used, individual needs, and response. Dosages listed are representative and must be adjusted.
Adults: 1 unit/kg or 0.15 mg/kg I.V. slowly over 60 to 90 seconds. Average, initially, 40 to 60 units I.V. May give 20 to 30 units in 3 to 5 minutes. For longer procedures, give 20 units, p.r.n.
Children: 1 unit/kg or 0.15 mg/kg.
Assist with mechanical ventilation—
Adults and children: initially, 0.0165 mg/kg I.V. (average 1 mg or 7 units), then adjust subsequent doses to patient's response.
Lessen muscle contractions in pharmacologically or electrically induced seizures—
Adults and children: 1 unit/kg or 0.15 mg/kg slowly over 60 to 90 seconds. Initial dose is 20 units (3 mg) less than calculated dose.

ADVERSE REACTIONS
CV: hypotension, circulatory depression.
Other: profound and prolonged muscle relaxation, *respiratory depression to the point of apnea,* hypersensitivity, idiosyncrasy, residual muscle weakness, increased salivation, *bronchospasm.*

INTERACTIONS
Aminoglycoside antibiotics (including amikacin, gentamicin, kanamycin, neomycin, streptomycin); polymyxin antibiotics (polymyxin B sulfate, colistin); general anesthetics (such as halothane, enflurane, isoflurane): potentiated neuromuscular blockade, leading to increased skeletal muscle relaxation and possible respiratory paralysis. Use cautiously during surgical and postoperative periods.
Quinidine: prolonged neuromuscular blockade. Use together with caution. Monitor closely.
Thiazide diuretics, furosemide, ethacrynic acid, amphotericin B, propranolol, methotrimeprazine, narcotic analgesics: potentiated neuromuscular blockade, leading to increased respiratory paralysis. Use with extreme caution during surgical and postoperative periods.

NURSING CONSIDERATIONS
• Contraindicated in patients for whom histamine release is a hazard (asthmatics). Use cautiously in elderly or debilitated patients; in hepatic or pulmonary impairment, respiratory depression, myasthenia gravis, myasthenic syndrome of lung cancer or bronchogenic carcinoma, dehydration, thyroid disorders, collagen diseases, porphyria, electrolyte disturbances, fractures, muscle spasms, and (in large doses) cesarean section.
• Tubocurarine should only be used by personnel experienced in airway management.
• Keep airway clear. Have emergency respiratory support equipment (endotracheal equipment, ventilator, oxygen, atropine, edrophonium, epinephrine, and neostigmine) on hand.
• Allow succinylcholine effects to subside before giving tubocurarine.

• Monitor baseline electrolyte determinations (electrolyte imbalance can potentiate neuromuscular effects).
• Monitor respirations closely until patient is fully recovered from neuromuscular blockade, as evidenced by tests of muscle strength (hand grip, head lift, and ability to cough).
• Check vital signs every 15 minutes. Notify doctor at once of changes.
• Measure intake and output (renal dysfunction prolongs duration of action, since much of drug is unchanged before excretion).
• Do not mix with barbiturates (precipitate will form). Use only fresh solutions and discard if discolored.
• Give I.V. slowly (60 to 90 seconds); give deep I.M. in deltoid muscle.
• Once spontaneous recovery starts, tubocurarine-induced neuromuscular blockade may be reversed with an anticholinesterase agent (such as neostigmine or edrophonium). Usually administered together with an anticholinergic drug (such as atropine or glycopyrrollate).

vecuronium bromide
Norcuron♦

Pregnancy Risk Category: C

MECHANISM OF ACTION
Prevents acetylcholine from binding to the receptors on the muscle end plate, thus blocking depolarization. Nondepolarizing agent.

INDICATIONS & DOSAGE
Adjunct to general anesthesia, to facilitate endotracheal intubation and to provide skeletal muscle relaxation during surgery or mechanical ventilation—
Dosage depends on anesthetic used, individual needs, and response. Dosages are representative and must be adjusted.
Adults and children over 9 years: Initially, 0.08 to 0.10 mg/kg I.V.

bolus. Maintenance doses of 0.010 to 0.015 mg/kg within 25 to 40 minutes of initial dose should be administered during prolonged surgical procedures. Maintenance doses may be given q 12 to 15 minutes in patients receiving balanced anesthesia.
Children under 10 years may require a slightly higher initial dose and may also require supplementation slightly more often than adults.

ADVERSE REACTIONS
CV: transient increases in heart rate.
Local: redness, itching, induration.
Other: *prolonged dose-related apnea.*

INTERACTIONS
Aminoglycoside antibiotics (including amikacin, gentamicin, kanamycin, neomycin, streptomycin); polymyxin antibiotics (polymyxin B sulfate, colistin); clindamycin; quinidine; general anesthetics (such as halothane, enflurane, isoflurane): potentiated neuromuscular blockade, leading to increased skeletal muscle relaxation and possible respiratory paralysis. Use cautiously during surgical and postoperative periods.
Narcotic analgesics: potentiated neuromuscular blockade, leading to increased skeletal muscle relaxation and possible respiratory paralysis. Use with extreme caution, and reduce dose of vecuronium.

NURSING CONSIDERATIONS
• Contraindicated in hypersensitivity to bromides. Use cautiously in altered circulation time from cardiovascular disease, old age, and edematous states; in hepatic disease; in severe obesity; in bronchogenic carcinoma; and in neuromuscular disease.
• Vecuronium should only be used by personnel experienced in airway management.
• Keep airway clear. Have emergency respiratory support equipment (endotracheal equipment, ventilator, oxy-

gen, atropine, edrophonium, epinephrine, and neostigmine) on hand.

• Unlike other nondepolarizing neuromuscular blockers, vecuronium has no effect on cardiovascular system. Also, the drug causes no histamine release and therefore no histamine-related hypersensitivity reactions, such as bronchospasm, hypotension, or tachycardia.

• The drug is well tolerated in renal failure.

• Prior administration of succinylcholine may enhance the neuromuscular blocking effect and duration of action.

• Vecuronium provides conditions for intubation within 2½ to 3 minutes. The duration of effect is 25 to 40 minutes.

• Once spontaneous recovery starts, vecuronium-induced neuromuscular blockade may be reversed with an anticholinesterase agent (such as neostigmine or edrophonium). Usually administered together with an anticholinergic drug (such as atropine or glycopyrollate).

• Monitor respirations closely until patient is fully recovered from neuromuscular blockade, as evidenced by tests of muscle strength (hand grip, head lift, and ability to cough).

• Store reconstituted solution in refrigerator. Discard after 24 hours.

43

Antihistamines

astemizole
azatadine maleate
brompheniramine maleate◊
carbinoxamine maleate
chlorpheniramine maleate◊
clemastine fumarate
cyproheptadine hydrochloride
dexchlorpheniramine maleate
diphenhydramine
    hydrochloride◊
methdilazine hydrochloride
promethazine hydrochloride◊
terfenadine
trimeprazine tartrate
tripelennamine citrate
tripelennamine hydrochloride
triprolidine hydrochloride◊

COMBINATION PRODUCTS

ALLEREST TABLETS◊: phenylpropanolamine hydrochloride 18.7 mg and
chlorpheniramine maleate 2 mg.
ALLERGESIC: phenylpropanolamine
18.7 mg and chlorpheniramine maleate 2 mg.
BROMFED-AT: brompheniramine maleate 2 mg, dextromethorphan hydrobromide 10 mg, and pseudoephedrine
hydrochloride 30 mg/5 ml.
CHLOR-TRIMETON DECONGESTANT◊:
chlorpheniramine maleate 4 mg and
pseudoephedrine sulfate 60 mg.
CHLOR-TRIMETON DECONGESTANT
REPETABS◊: chlorpheniramine maleate 8 mg and pseudoephedrine sulfate 120 mg.
CODIMAL DH*: hydrocodone bitartrate 1.66 mg, phenylephrine hydrochloride 5 mg, pyrilamine maleate
8.33 mg, potassium guaiacolsulfonate
83.3 mg, sodium citrate 216 mg, and

citric acid 50 mg.
CONDRIN-LA: phenylpropanolamine
HCl 75 mg and chlorpheniramine maleate 12 mg.
CONTAC CAPSULES◊: phenylpropanolamine 75 mg and chlorpheniramine
maleate 8 mg.
CONTAC 12-HOUR CAPLETS◊: phenylpropanolamine 75 mg and chlorpheniramine maleate 12 mg.
CORICIDIN TABLETS◊: chlorpheniramine maleate 2 mg and aspirin 325
mg.
DECONADE: phenylpropanolamine
HCl 75 mg and chlorpheniramine maleate 12 mg.
DECONAMINE: pseudoephedrine HCl
60 mg and chlorpheniramine maleate
4 mg.
DIMETAPP EXTENTABS: brompheniramine maleate 12 mg, and phenylpropanolamine hydrochloride 75 mg.
DISOPHROL CHRONOTABS◊: dexbrompheniramine maleate 6 mg and pseudoephedrine sulfate 120 mg.
DRIXORAL◊•: dexbrompheniramine
maleate 6 mg and pseudoephedrine
sulfate 120 mg.
DRIZE: phenylpropanolamine HCl 75
mg and chlorpheniramine maleate 12
mg.
FEDAHIST: pseudoephedrine HCl 60
mg and chlorpheniramine maleate 4
mg.
HISTABID DURACAPS: phenylpropanolamine 75 mg and chlorpheniramine
maleate 8 mg.
HISTASPAN-D: chlorpheniramine maleate 8 mg, phenylephrine hydrochloride 20 mg, and methscopolamine nitrate 2.5 mg.

NALDECON: phenylephrine hydrochloride 10 mg, phenylpropanolamine hydrochloride 40 mg, phenyltoloxamine citrate 15 mg, and chlorpheniramine maleate 5 mg.

NEOTEP-GRANUCAPS: chlorpheniramine maleate 9 mg and phenylephrine hydrochloride 21 mg.

NOLAMINE: chlorpheniramine maleate 4 mg, phenindamine tartrate 24 mg, and phenylpropanolamine hydrochloride 50 mg.

NOVAFED A: pseudoephedrine hydrochloride 120 mg and chlorpheniramine maleate 8 mg.

NOVAHISTINE ELIXIR◇*: phenylephrine 5 mg, chlorpheniramine maleate 2 mg, and alcohol 5%/5 ml.

ORAHIST: phenylpropanolamine HCl 75 mg and chlorpheniramine 12 mg.

ORNADE SPANSULES: phenylpropanolamine hydrochloride 75 mg and chlorpheniramine maleate 12 mg.

RHINEX D-LAY: acetaminophen 300 mg, salicylamide 300 mg, phenylpropanolamine hydrochloride 60 mg, and chlorpheniramine maleate 4 mg.

RONDEC: carbinoxamine maleate 4 mg and pseudoephedrine hydrochloride 60 mg.

SUDAFED PLUS◇: pseudoephedrine HCl 60 mg and chlorpheniramine maleate 4 mg.

TRIAMINIC-12: phenylpropanolamine HCl 75 mg and chlorpheniramine maleate 12 mg.

TRIAMINIC TABLETS: phenylpropanolamine hydrochloride 50 mg, pheniramine maleate 25 mg, and pyrilamine maleate 25 mg.

TRINALIN REPETABS: azatadine maleate 1 mg and pseudoephedrine sulfate 120 mg.

---

astemizole
Hismanal

Pregnancy Risk Category: C

MECHANISM OF ACTION
Blocks the effects of histamine at H_1 receptors. Astemizole is a nonsedating antihistamine because its chemical structure prevents entry into the CNS.

INDICATIONS AND DOSAGE
Relief of symptoms associated with chronic idiopathic urticaria and seasonal allergic rhinitis—
Adults and children over 12 years: 10 mg P.O. daily. A loading dose may be given in order to achieve steady-state plasma levels quickly. Begin therapy at 30 mg on the first day, followed by 20 mg on the second day, and 10 mg daily thereafter.

ADVERSE REACTIONS
CNS: headache, nervousness, dizziness.
EENT: dry mouth, pharyngitis, conjunctivitis.
GI: nausea, diarrhea, abdominal pain, increased appetite.
Other: arthralgia, weight gain.

INTERACTIONS
None significant.

NURSING CONSIDERATIONS
• Contraindicated in patients with hypersensitivity to astemizole.
• Instruct patient to take this drug on an empty stomach at least 2 hours after a meal and to avoid eating for at least 1 hour after dosing.
• Because of its potential for anticholinergic effects, use cautiously in patients with lower respiratory diseases (including asthma) because drying effects can increase the risk of bronchial mucous plug formation.
• Use with caution in patients with hepatic or renal disease. Astemizole is not believed to be dialysable.

---

azatadine maleate
Optimine♦

Pregnancy Risk Category: B

MECHANISM OF ACTION
Competes with histamine for H_1-receptor sites on effector cells. Prevents but does not reverse histamine-mediated responses.

INDICATIONS & DOSAGE
Rhinitis, allergy symptoms, chronic urticaria—
Adults: 1 to 2 mg P.O. b.i.d. Maximum dosage is 4 mg daily.
   Not intended for children under 12 years.

ADVERSE REACTIONS
Blood: thrombocytopenia.
CNS: (especially in elderly patients) *drowsiness, dizziness,* vertigo, disturbed coordination.
CV: hypotension, palpitations.
GI: anorexia, nausea, vomiting, *dry mouth and throat,* epigastric distress.
GU: urine retention.
Skin: urticaria, rash.
Other: thick bronchial secretions.

INTERACTIONS
CNS depressants: increased sedation. Use together cautiously.

NURSING CONSIDERATIONS
• Contraindicated in acute asthmatic attacks. Use cautiously in elderly patients and in increased intraocular pressure, hyperthyroidism, cardiovascular or renal disease, hypertension, bronchial asthma, urine retention, prostatic hypertrophy, bladder-neck obstruction, and stenosing peptic ulcers.
• Warn patient against drinking alcoholic beverages during therapy and against activities that require alertness until CNS response to drug is determined.
• Reduce GI distress by giving with food or milk.
• Coffee or tea may reduce drowsiness. Sugarless gum or sour hard candy, or ice chips may relieve dry mouth.
• If tolerance develops, another antihistamine may be substituted.
• Warn patient to stop taking drug 4 days before allergy skin tests to preserve accuracy of tests.
• Monitor blood counts during long-term therapy; watch for signs of blood dyscrasias.

brompheniramine maleate◇
Brombay, Bromphen*, Chlorphed, Codimal-A, Conjec-B, Cophene-B, Dehist, Diamine TD, Dimetane*♦, Dimetane Extertabs, Dimetane-Ten, Histaject Modified, Nasahist B, ND-Stat Revised, Oraminic II, Sinusol-B, Veltane

Pregnancy Risk Category: C

MECHANISM OF ACTION
Competes with histamine for H_1-receptor sites on effector cells. Prevents but does not reverse histamine-mediated responses.

INDICATIONS & DOSAGE
Rhinitis, allergy symptoms—
Adults: 4 to 8 mg P.O. t.i.d. or q.i.d.; or (timed-release) 8 to 12 mg P.O. b.i.d. or t.i.d.; or 5 to 20 mg q 6 to 12 hours I.M., I.V., or S.C. Maximum dosage is 40 mg daily.
Children over 6 years: 2 to 4 mg P.O. t.i.d. or q.i.d.; or (timed-release) 8 to 12 mg q 12 hours; or 0.5 mg/kg I.M., I.V., or S.C. daily divided t.i.d. or q.i.d.
Children under 6 years: 0.5 mg/kg P.O., I.M., I.V., or S.C. daily divided t.i.d. or q.i.d.
   Note: Children under 12 years should use only as directed by a doctor.

Italicized side effects are common or life-threatening.
*Liquid form contains alcohol.   **May contain tartrazine.

ADVERSE REACTIONS
Blood: thrombocytopenia, *agranulocytosis.*
CNS: (especially in elderly patients) dizziness, tremors, irritability, insomnia, *drowsiness, stimulation.*
CV: hypotension, palpitations.
GI: anorexia, nausea, vomiting, *dry mouth and throat.*
GU: urine retention.
Skin: urticaria, rash.
After parenteral administration: local reaction, sweating, syncope.

INTERACTIONS
CNS depressants: increased sedation. Use together cautiously.

NURSING CONSIDERATIONS
• Contraindicated in acute asthmatic attacks. Use cautiously in elderly patients, breast-feeding women, and in increased intraocular pressure, hyperthyroidism, cardiovascular or renal disease, hypertension, bronchial asthma, urine retention, prostatic hypertrophy, bladder-neck obstruction, and stenosing peptic ulcers.
• Warn patient against drinking alcoholic beverages during therapy and against activities that require alertness.
• Reduce GI distress by giving with food or milk.
• Causes less drowsiness than some other antihistamines.
• Coffee or tea may reduce drowsiness. Sugarless gum or sour hard candy, or ice chips may relieve dry mouth.
• If tolerance develops, another antihistamine may be substituted.
• Warn patient to stop taking drug 4 days before allergy skin tests to preserve accuracy of tests.
• Injectable form containing 10 mg/ml can be given diluted or undiluted very slowly I.V. The 100 mg/ml injection should not be given I.V.
• Monitor blood count during long-term therapy; observe for signs of blood dyscrasias.

---

carbinoxamine maleate
Clistin*

Pregnancy Risk Category: C

MECHANISM OF ACTION
Competes with histamine for H_1-receptor sites on effector cells. Prevents but does not reverse histamine-mediated responses.

INDICATIONS & DOSAGE
Rhinitis, allergy symptoms—
Adults: 4 to 8 mg P.O. t.i.d. or q.i.d.
Children over 6 years: 4 to 6 mg P.O. t.i.d. or q.i.d.
Children 3 to 6 years: 2 to 4 mg P.O. t.i.d. or q.i.d.
Children 1 to 3 years: 2 mg P.O. t.i.d. or q.i.d.
   Note: Children under 12 years should use only as directed by a doctor.

ADVERSE REACTIONS
CNS: (especially in elderly patients) *drowsiness, dizziness, stimulation.*
GI: anorexia, nausea, vomiting, *dry mouth.*
GU: urine retention.

INTERACTIONS
CNS depressants: increased sedation. Use together cautiously.

NURSING CONSIDERATIONS
• Contraindicated in acute asthmatic attacks. Use cautiously in elderly patients, and in increased intraocular pressure, hyperthyroidism, cardiovascular or renal disease, hypertension, bronchial asthma, urine retention, prostatic hypertrophy, bladder-neck obstruction, and stenosing peptic ulcers.
• Warn patient against drinking alcoholic beverages during therapy and against driving or other activities that require alertness until CNS response

to drug is determined.
• Reduce GI distress by giving with food or milk.
• Coffee or tea may reduce drowsiness. Sugarless gum or sour hard candy, or ice chips may relieve dry mouth.
• If tolerance develops, another antihistamine may be substituted.
• Warn patient to stop taking drug 4 days before allergy skin tests to preserve accuracy of tests.

---

chlorpheniramine maleate◦
Aller-Chlor*, Chlo-Amine, Chlorate, Chlor-100, Chlor-Niramine, Chlor-Pro, Chlor-Pro 10, Chlorspan-12, Chlortab-4, Chlortab-8, Chlor-Trimeton*, Chlor-Trimeton Repetabs, Chlor-Tripolon♦♦, Genallerate, Novopheniram♦♦, Pfeiffer's Allergy, Phenetron*, Phenetron Lanacaps, Pyranistan, Telachlor, Teldrin, Trymegen

Pregnancy Risk Category: B

MECHANISM OF ACTION
Competes with histamine for H_1-receptor sites on effector cells. Prevents but does not reverse histamine-mediated responses.

INDICATIONS & DOSAGE
Rhinitis, allergy symptoms—
Adults: 4 mg P.O. q 4 to 6 hours, not to exceed 24 mg/day; or (timed-release) 8 mg P.O. every 12 hours; or 5 to 40 mg I.M., I.V., or S.C. daily. Give I.V. injection over 1 minute.
Children 6 to 12 years: 2 mg P.O. q 4 to 6 hours, not to exceed 12 mg/day. Alternatively, may give 8 mg (timed-release) at bedtime.
Children 2 to 6 years: 1 mg P.O. q 4 to 6 hours.
Note: Children under 12 years should use only as directed by a doctor.

ADVERSE REACTIONS
CNS: *stimulation,* sedation, *drowsiness* (especially in elderly patients), excitability (in children).
CV: hypotension, palpitations.
GI: epigastric distress, *dry mouth.*
GU: urine retention.
Skin: rash, urticaria.
Other: thick bronchial secretions.
After parenteral administration: local stinging, burning sensation, pallor, weak pulse, transient hypotension.

INTERACTIONS
CNS depressants: increased sedation. Use together cautiously.

NURSING CONSIDERATIONS
• Contraindicated in acute asthmatic attacks. Use cautiously in elderly patients, and in increased intraocular pressure, hyperthyroidism, cardiovascular or renal disease, hypertension, bronchial asthma, urine retention, prostatic hypertrophy, bladder-neck obstruction and stenosing peptic ulcers.
• Warn patient against drinking alcoholic beverages and using other CNS depressants during therapy and against driving or other activities that require alertness until CNS response to drug is determined.
• Available as non-prescription item for self-medication by adults. However, use on children under 12 years is not recommended without doctor's supervision.
• Coffee or tea may reduce drowsiness. Sugarless gum or sour hard candy, or ice chips may relieve dry mouth.
• If tolerance develops, another antihistamine may be substituted.
• Warn patient to stop taking drug 4 days before allergy skin tests to preserve accuracy of tests.
• Only injectable forms *without* preservatives can be given I.V. Give *slowly.*
• If symptoms occur during or after

Italicized side effects are common or life-threatening.
*Liquid form contains alcohol.   **May contain tartrazine.

parenteral dose, discontinue drug. Notify doctor.

clemastine fumarate
Tavist*♦, Tavist-1

Pregnancy Risk Category: C

MECHANISM OF ACTION
Competes with histamine for H_1-receptor sites on effector cells. Prevents but does not reverse histamine-mediated responses.

INDICATIONS & DOSAGE
Rhinitis, allergy symptoms—
Adults: 1.34 to 2.68 mg P.O. b.i.d. or t.i.d. Maximum recommended daily dosage is 8.04 mg.
Children 6 to 12 years: 0.67 mg P.O. b.i.d. Maximum dosage is 4.02 mg/day.
Allergic skin manifestation of urticaria and angioedema—
Adults: 2.68 mg P.O. up to t.i.d. maximum.
Children 6 to 12 years: 1.34 mg P.O. b.i.d. Maximum dosage is 4.02 mg/day.
Note: Children under 12 years should use only as directed by a doctor.

ADVERSE REACTIONS
Blood: hemolytic anemia, thrombocytopenia, *agranulocytosis.*
CNS: (especially in elderly patients) *sedation, drowsiness.*
CV: hypotension, palpitations, tachycardia.
GI: epigastric distress, anorexia, nausea, vomiting, constipation, *dry mouth.*
GU: urine retention.
Skin: rash, urticaria.
Other: thick bronchial secretions.

INTERACTIONS
CNS depressants: increased sedation. Use together cautiously.

NURSING CONSIDERATIONS
• Contraindicated in acute asthmatic attacks. Use cautiously in elderly patients, and in increased intraocular pressure, hyperthyroidism, cardiovascular or renal disease, hypertension, bronchial asthma, urine retention, prostatic hypertrophy, bladder-neck obstruction, and stenosing peptic ulcers.
• Warn patient against drinking alcoholic beverages during therapy and against driving or other activities that require alertness until CNS response to drug is determined.
• Coffee or tea may reduce drowsiness. Sugarless gum or sour hard candy, or ice chips may relieve dry mouth.
• If tolerance develops, another antihistamine may be substituted.
• Warn patient to stop taking drug 4 days before allergy skin tests to preserve accuracy of tests.
• Monitor blood counts during long-term therapy; observe for signs of blood dyscrasias.

cyproheptadine hydrochloride
Periactin*♦

Pregnancy Risk Category: B

MECHANISM OF ACTION
Competes with histamine for H_1-receptor sites on effector cells. Prevents but does not reverse histamine-mediated responses.

INDICATIONS & DOSAGE
Allergy symptoms, pruritus—
Adults: 4 mg P.O. t.i.d. or q.i.d. Maximum dosage is 0.5 mg/kg daily.
Children 7 to 14 years: 4 mg P.O. b.i.d. or t.i.d. Maximum dosage is 16 mg daily.
Children 2 to 6 years: 2 mg P.O. b.i.d. or t.i.d. Maximum dosage is 12 mg daily.
Note: Children under 14 years

should use only as directed by a doctor.

ADVERSE REACTIONS
CNS: (especially in elderly patients) *drowsiness,* dizziness, headache, fatigue.
GI: nausea, vomiting, epigastric distress, *dry mouth.*
GU: urine retention.
Skin: rash.
Other: weight gain.

INTERACTIONS
CNS depressants: increased sedation. Use together cautiously.

NURSING CONSIDERATIONS
• Contraindicated in acute asthmatic attacks. Use cautiously in elderly patients, and in increased intraocular pressure, hyperthyroidism, cardiovascular or renal disease, hypertension, bronchial asthma, urine retention, prostatic hypertrophy, bladder-neck obstruction, and stenosing peptic ulcers.
• Warn patient against drinking alcoholic beverages during therapy and against driving or other activities that require alertness until CNS response to drug is determined.
• Reduce GI distress by giving with food or milk.
• Coffee or tea may reduce drowsiness. Sugarless gum or sour hard candy, or ice chips may relieve dry mouth.
• If tolerance develops, another antihistamine may be substituted.
• Warn patient to stop taking drug 4 days before allergy skin tests to preserve accuracy of tests.
• Used experimentally to stimulate appetite and increase weight gain in children.

dexchlorpheniramine maleate
Dexchlor, Poladex TD, Polaramine*•, Polaramine Repetabs, Polargen
Pregnancy Risk Category: B

MECHANISM OF ACTION
Competes with histamine for H_1-receptor sites on effector cells. Prevents but does not reverse histamine-mediated responses.

INDICATIONS & DOSAGE
Rhinitis, allergy symptoms, contact dermatitis, pruritus—
Adults: 2 mg P.O. q 4 to 6 hours, not to exceed 12 mg/day; or (timed-release) 4 to 6 mg b.i.d. or t.i.d.
Children 6 to 12 years: 1 mg P.O. q 4 to 6 hours, not to exceed 6 mg/day; or 4 mg (timed-release tablet) at bedtime.
Children 2 to 6 years: 0.5 mg P.O. q 4 to 6 hours, not to exceed 3 mg/day.
  Note: Children under 6 years should use only as directed by a doctor. Do not use timed-release tablets for children younger than 6 years.

ADVERSE REACTIONS
CNS: (especially in elderly patients) *drowsiness,* dizziness, *stimulation.*
GI: nausea, *dry mouth.*
GU: polyuria, dysuria, urine retention.

INTERACTIONS
CNS depressants: increased sedation. Use together cautiously.

NURSING CONSIDERATIONS
• Contraindicated in acute asthmatic attacks. Use cautiously in elderly patients, and with increased intraocular pressure, hyperthyroidism, cardiovascular or renal disease, hypertension, bronchial asthma, urine retention, prostatic hypertrophy, bladder-neck obstruction, and stenosing peptic ul-

Italicized side effects are common or life-threatening.
*Liquid form contains alcohol.   **May contain tartrazine.

cers.
• Warn patient against drinking alcoholic beverages during therapy and against driving or other activities that require alertness until CNS response to drug is determined.
• Available as non-prescription item for self-medication by adults. However, use in children under 6 years is not recommended without doctor's supervision.
• Causes less drowsiness than some other antihistamines.
• Coffee or tea may reduce drowsiness. Sugarless gum or sour hard candy, or ice chips may relieve dry mouth.
• If tolerance develops, another antihistamine may be substituted.
• Warn patient to stop taking drug 4 days before allergy skin tests to preserve accuracy of tests.

diphenhydramine hydrochloride◇
Allerdryl♦♦, AllerMax, Beldin*, Belix, Bena-D, Bena-D 50, Benadryl*♦, Benadryl Complete Allergy, Benahist 10, Benahist 50, Ben-Allergen-50, Benaphen, Benoject-10, Benoject-50, Benylin Cough*, Benylin Dietetic♦♦, Benylin Expectorant♦♦, Benylin Pediatric♦♦, Bydramine Cough, Compoz Diahist, Dihydrex, Diphenacen-50, Diphenadryl, Diphen Cough*, Diphenhist, Dormarex 2, Fenylhist, Fynex, Hydramine*, Hydril, Insomnal♦♦, Nervine Nighttime Sleep-Aid, Noradryl, Nordryl, Nytol with DPH, Sleep-Eze 3, Sominex, Sominex Liquid, Tusstat*, Twilite, Valdrene*, Wehdryl

Pregnancy Risk Category: C

MECHANISM OF ACTION
Competes with histamine for H_1-receptor sites on effector cells. Prevents but does not reverse histamine-mediated responses, particularly histamine's effects on the smooth muscle of the bronchial tubes, GI tract, uterus, and blood vessels. Structurally related to local anesthetics, diphenhydramine provides local anesthesia by preventing initiation and transmission of nerve impulses. Also suppresses the cough reflex by a direct effect in the medulla of the brain.

INDICATIONS & DOSAGE
Rhinitis, allergy symptoms, nighttime sedation, motion sickness, antiparkinsonism—
Adults: 25 to 50 mg P.O. t.i.d. or q.i.d.; or 10 to 50 mg deep I.M. or I.V. Maximum dosage is 400 mg daily.
Children under 12 years: 5 mg/kg daily P.O., deep I.M., or I.V. divided q.i.d. Maximum dosage is 300 mg daily.
Sedation—
Adults: 25 to 50 mg P.O., or deep I.M., p.r.n.
As a nighttime sleep aid—
Adults: 50 mg P.O. at bedtime.
Nonproductive cough—
Adults: 25 mg P.O. q 4 hours (not to exceed 100 mg daily).
Children 6 to 12 years: 12.5 mg P.O. q 4 hours (not to exceed 50 mg daily).
Children 2 to 6 years: 6.25 mg P.O. q 4 hours (not to exceed 25 mg daily).
Note: Children under 12 years should use only as directed by a doctor.

ADVERSE REACTIONS
CNS: (especially in elderly patients) *drowsiness,* confusion, insomnia, headache, vertigo.
CV: palpitations.
EENT: photosensitivity, diplopia, nasal stuffiness.
GI: *nausea,* vomiting, diarrhea, *dry mouth,* constipation.
GU: dysuria, urine retention.
Skin: urticaria.

INTERACTIONS
CNS depressants: increased sedation. Use together cautiously.

NURSING CONSIDERATIONS
• Contraindicated in acute asthmatic attacks. Use cautiously in narrow-angle glaucoma, prostatic hypertrophy, pyloroduodenal and bladder-neck obstruction, and stenosing peptic ulcers; in newborns; and in asthmatic, hypertensive, or cardiac patients.
• Alternate injection sites to prevent irritation. Administer deep I.M. into large muscle.
• Warn patient against drinking alcoholic beverages during therapy and against driving or other hazardous activities until CNS response to drug is determined.
• Reduce GI distress by giving with food or milk.
• Coffee or tea may reduce drowsiness. Sugarless gum or sour hard candy, or ice chips may relieve dry mouth.
• If tolerance develops, another antihistamine may be substituted.
• For use to prevent motion sickness, instruct patient to take 30 minutes before travel.
• Warn patient to stop taking drug 4 days before allergy skin tests to preserve accuracy of tests.
• Used with epinephrine in anaphylaxis.
• One of most sedating antihistamines; often used as a hypnotic.
• Warn patient of possible photosensitivity. Advise use of a sunscreen.

methdilazine hydrochloride
Dilosyn♦♦, Tacaryl*

Pregnancy Risk Category: C

MECHANISM OF ACTION
Competes with histamine for H_1-receptor sites on effector cells. Prevents but does not reverse histamine-mediated responses.

INDICATIONS & DOSAGE
Pruritus—
Adults: 8 mg P.O. b.i.d. to q.i.d. or (chewable tablets) 7.2 mg P.O. b.i.d. to q.i.d.
Children over 3 years: 4 mg P.O. b.i.d. to q.i.d. or (chewable tablets) 3.6 mg P.O. b.i.d. to q.i.d.

ADVERSE REACTIONS
CNS: (especially in elderly patients) *drowsiness,* dizziness, headache.
GI: nausea, *dry mouth and throat.*
GU: urine retention.
Hepatic: cholestatic jaundice.
Skin: rash.

INTERACTIONS
Phenothiazines: increased effects. Don't use together.
CNS depressants: increased sedation. Use together cautiously.

NURSING CONSIDERATIONS
• Contraindicated in acute asthmatic attacks. Use cautiously in elderly or debilitated patients; acutely ill or dehydrated children; and in pulmonary, hepatic, or cardiovascular disease, asthma, hypertension, prostatic hypertrophy, bladder-neck obstruction, CNS depression, and stenosing peptic ulcers.
• Warn patient against drinking alcoholic beverages during therapy and against driving or other activities that require alertness until CNS response to drug is determined.
• Reduce GI distress by giving with food or milk.
• Coffee or tea may reduce drowsiness. Sugarless gum or sour hard candy, or ice chips may relieve dry mouth.
• If tolerance develops, another antihistamine may be substituted.
• Available as chewable tablet for children. Instruct child to chew completely and swallow promptly; may cause local anesthetic effect in mouth, which increases the risk of

Italicized side effects are common or life-threatening.
*Liquid form contains alcohol.   **May contain tartrazine.

choking.
• Warn patient to stop taking drug 4 days before allergy skin tests to preserve accuracy of tests.

---

promethazine hydrochloride◊
Anergan 25, Anergan 50, Histanil♦♦, K-Phen, Mallergan, Pentazine, Phenameth, Phenazine 25, Phenazine 50, Phencen-50, Phenergan*♦, Phenergan-Fortis*, Phenergan-Plain*, Phenoject-50, PMS-Promethazine♦♦, Pro-50, Prometh-25, Prometh-50, Promethegan, Prothazine-25, Prothazine-50, Prothazine Plain, Remsed, V-Gan-25, V-Gan-50

Pregnancy Risk Category: C

MECHANISM OF ACTION
Competes with histamine for H_1-receptor sites on effector cells. Prevents but does not reverse histamine-mediated responses.

INDICATIONS & DOSAGE
Motion sickness—
Adults: 25 mg P.O. b.i.d.
Children: 12.5 to 25 mg P.O., I.M., or rectally b.i.d.
Nausea—
Adults: 12.5 to 25 mg P.O., I.M., or rectally q 4 to 6 hours, p.r.n.
Children: 0.25 to 0.5 mg/kg I.M. or rectally q 4 to 6 hours, p.r.n.
Rhinitis, allergy symptoms—
Adults: 12.5 mg P.O. q.i.d.; or 25 mg P.O. at bedtime.
Children: 6.25 to 12.5 mg P.O. t.i.d. or 25 mg P.O. or rectally at bedtime.
Sedation—
Adults: 25 to 50 mg P.O. or I.M. at bedtime or p.r.n.
Children: 12.5 to 25 mg P.O., I.M., or rectally at bedtime.
Routine preoperative or postoperative sedation or as an adjunct to analgesics—
Adults: 25 to 50 mg I.M., I.V., or

P.O.
Children: 12.5 to 25 mg I.M., I.V., or P.O.

ADVERSE REACTIONS
Blood: leukopenia, *agranulocytosis*.
CNS: (especially in elderly patients) *sedation,* confusion, restlessness, tremors, *drowsiness*.
CV: hypotension.
EENT: transient myopia, nasal congestion.
GI: anorexia, nausea, vomiting, constipation, *dry mouth*.
GU: urine retention.
Other: photosensitivity.

INTERACTIONS
Phenothiazines: increased effects. Don't give together.
CNS depressants: increased sedation. Use together cautiously.

NURSING CONSIDERATIONS
• Contraindicated in increased intraocular pressure, intestinal obstruction, prostatic hypertrophy, bladder-neck obstruction, epilepsy, bone-marrow depression, coma, CNS depression, stenosing peptic ulcers, and in newborns and acutely ill or dehydrated children. Use cautiously in pulmonary, hepatic, or cardiovascular disease; asthma; hypertension; bone-marrow depression; and in elderly or debilitated patients.
• Warn patient against drinking alcoholic beverages during therapy and against driving or other activities that require alertness until CNS response to drug is determined.
• Reduce GI distress by giving with food or milk.
• Coffee or tea may reduce drowsiness. Sugarless gum or sour hard candy, or ice chips may relieve dry mouth.
• Warn patient to stop taking drug 4 days before allergy skin tests to preserve accuracy of tests.
• Pronounced sedative effect limits

---

use in many ambulatory patients.
• May cause false-positive immunologic urine pregnancy test (Gravindex). Also may interfere with blood grouping in ABO system.
• When treating motion sickness, tell patient to take first dose 30 to 60 minutes before travel. On succeeding days of travel, he should take dose upon arising and with evening meal.
• Inject deep I.M. into large muscle mass. Don't administer S.C. Rotate injection sites.
• May be administered I.V., but don't give in a concentration greater than 25 mg/ml, nor at a rate exceeding 25 mg/minute. Shield I.V. infusion from direct light.
• May be safely mixed with meperidine (Demerol) in the same syringe.
• Warn patient about possible photosensitivity and precautions to avoid it.

INTERACTIONS
None significant.

NURSING CONSIDERATIONS
• May cause a mild anticholinergic drying effect in patients with lower airway disease, such as asthma. Keep patients well hydrated.
• Instruct patients not to exceed prescribed dose.
• Relief of symptoms begins within 1 hour.
• Terfenadine is a butyrophenone-derivative antihistamine. Significant lack of adverse reactions also makes it unique.
• Does not cause the degree of drowsiness and sedation associated with other antihistamines because drug does not cross blood-brain barrier; its anticholinergic and antiserotonin effects are mild.

terfenadine
Seldane♦

Pregnancy Risk Category: C

MECHANISM OF ACTION
Competes with histamine for H_1-receptor sites on effector cells. Prevents but does not reverse histamine-mediated responses.

INDICATIONS & DOSAGE
Rhinitis, allergy symptoms—
Adults and children over 12 years: 60 mg P.O. b.i.d.
Children 6 to 12 years: 30 to 60 mg P.O. b.i.d.
Children 3 to 5 years: 15 mg P.O. b.i.d.

ADVERSE REACTIONS
CNS: fatigue, dizziness, *headache,* sedation.
GI: abdominal distress, nausea.
EENT: dry throat and mouth, nasal stuffiness.

trimeprazine tartrate
Panectyl♦♦, Temaril*

Pregnancy Risk Category: C

MECHANISM OF ACTION
Competes with histamine for H_1-receptor sites on effector cells. Prevents but does not reverse histamine-mediated responses.

INDICATIONS & DOSAGE
Pruritus—
Adults: 2.5 mg P.O. q.i.d.; or (timed-release) 5 mg P.O. b.i.d.
Children 3 to 12 years: 2.5 mg P.O. at bedtime or t.i.d., p.r.n.
Children 6 months to 3 years: 1.25 mg P.O. at bedtime or t.i.d., p.r.n.
Note: Children under 12 years should use only as directed by a doctor.

ADVERSE REACTIONS
Blood: *agranulocytosis,* leukopenia.
CNS: (especially in elderly patients) drowsiness, dizziness, confusion, headache, restlessness, tremors, irri-

---

Italicized side effects are common or life-threatening.
*Liquid form contains alcohol.   **May contain tartrazine.

tability, insomnia; (in children) paradoxical excitation.
CV: hypotension, palpitations, tachycardia.
GI: anorexia, nausea, vomiting, *dry mouth and throat*.
GU: urinary frequency, urine retention.
Skin: urticaria, rash, *photosensitivity*.

INTERACTIONS
Phenothiazines: increased effects. Don't use together.
CNS depressants: increased sedation. Use together cautiously.

NURSING CONSIDERATIONS
• Contraindicated in acute asthmatic attacks. Use cautiously in pulmonary, hepatic, or cardiovascular disease; asthma; hypertension; narrow-angle glaucoma; intestinal obstruction; prostatic hypertrophy; bladder-neck obstruction; epilepsy; bone-marrow depression; coma; CNS depression; stenosing peptic ulcers; in elderly or debilitated patients; and in acutely ill or dehydrated children.
• Warn patient against drinking alcoholic beverages during therapy and against driving or other activities that require alertness until CNS response to drug is determined.
• Reduce GI distress by giving with food or milk.
• Coffee or tea may reduce drowsiness. Sugarless gum or sour hard candy, or ice chips may relieve dry mouth.
• Warn patient to stop taking drug 4 days before allergy skin tests to preserve accuracy of tests.
• Monitor blood counts during longterm therapy.
• Warn patient about risk of photosensitivity. Recommend use of a sunscreen. If photosensitivity occurs, tell patient to stop taking the drug and call the doctor.

tripelennamine citrate
PBZ*

tripelennamine hydrochloride
PBZ*, PBZ-SR, Pelamine, Pyribenzamine
Pregnancy Risk Category: B

MECHANISM OF ACTION
Competes with histamine for H_1-receptor sites on effector cells. Prevents but does not reverse histamine-mediated responses.

INDICATIONS & DOSAGE
Rhinitis, allergy symptoms—
Adults: 25 to 50 mg P.O. q 4 to 6 hours; or (timed-release) 100 mg b.i.d. or t.i.d. Maximum dosage is 600 mg daily.
Children over 5 years: 50 mg P.O. q 8 to 12 hours (timed-release).
Children under 5 years: 5 mg/kg P.O. daily in four to six divided doses. Maximum dosage is 300 mg daily.
  Note: Children under 12 years should use only as directed by a doctor.

ADVERSE REACTIONS
CNS: (especially in elderly patients) *drowsiness*, dizziness, confusion, restlessness, tremors, irritability, insomnia.
CV: palpitations.
GI: anorexia, diarrhea or constipation, *nausea, vomiting, dry mouth*.
GU: urinary frequency, urine retention.
Skin: urticaria, rash.
Other: thick bronchial secretions.

INTERACTIONS
CNS depressants: increased sedation. Use together cautiously.

NURSING CONSIDERATIONS
• Contraindicated in acute asthmatic attacks. Use cautiously in elderly pa-

tients, and in increased intraocular pressure, hyperthyroidism, cardiovascular or renal disease, hypertension, bronchial asthma, urine retention, prostatic hypertrophy, bladder-neck obstruction, and stenosing peptic ulcers.

• Warn patient against drinking alcoholic beverages during therapy and against driving or other activities that require alertness until CNS response to drug is determined.

• Reduce GI distress by giving with food or milk.

• Coffee or tea may reduce drowsiness. Sugarless gum or sour hard candy, or ice chips may relieve dry mouth.

• If tolerance develops, another antihistamine may be substituted.

• Warn patient to stop taking drug 4 days before allergy skin tests to preserve accuracy of tests.

triprolidine hydrochloride◇
Actidil*, Alleract, Myidyl

Pregnancy Risk Category: C

MECHANISM OF ACTION
Competes with histamine for H_1-receptor sites on effector cells. Prevents but does not reverse histamine-mediated responses.

INDICATIONS & DOSAGE
Colds and allergy symptoms—
Adults: 2.5 mg P.O. t.i.d. or q.i.d. Maximum dosage is 10 mg/day.
Children over 6 years: 1.25 mg P.O. t.i.d. or q.i.d. Maximum dosage is 5 mg/day.
Children 4 to 6 years: 0.9 mg P.O. t.i.d. or q.i.d. Maximum dosage is 3.75 mg/day.
Children 2 to 4 years: 0.6 mg P.O. t.i.d. or q.i.d. Maximum dosage is 2.5 mg/day.
Children 4 months to 2 years: 0.3 mg P.O. t.i.d. or q.i.d. Maximum dosage is 1.25 mg/day.

Note: Children under 12 years should use only as directed by a doctor.

ADVERSE REACTIONS
CNS: (especially in elderly patients) *drowsiness,* dizziness, confusion, restlessness, insomnia, *stimulation.*
GI: anorexia, diarrhea or constipation, nausea, vomiting, *dry mouth.*
GU: urinary frequency, urine retention.
Skin: urticaria, rash.

INTERACTIONS
CNS depressants: increased sedation.

NURSING CONSIDERATIONS
• Contraindicated in acute asthma attacks. Use cautiously in elderly patients, and in increased intraocular pressure, hyperthyroidism, cardiovascular or renal disease, hypertension, diabetes mellitus, bronchial asthma, urine retention, prostatic hypertrophy, bladder-neck obstruction, and stenosing peptic ulcers.

• Warn patient against drinking alcoholic beverages during therapy and against driving or other activities that require alertness until CNS response to drug is determined.

• Reduce GI distress by giving with food or milk.

• Coffee or tea may reduce drowsiness. Sugarless gum or sour hard candy, or ice chips may relieve dry mouth.

• Warn patient to stop taking drug 4 days before allergy skin tests to preserve accuracy of tests.

Expectorants and antitussives

Expectorants
acetylcysteine
ammonium chloride◇
(See Chapter 104, ACIDIFIERS AND
ALKALINIZERS.)
**guaifenesin (glyceryl
guaiacolate)**◇
iodinated glycerol
potassium iodide (SSKI)
terpin hydrate◇

Antitussives
benzonatate
codeine phosphate
(See Chapter 27, NARCOTIC AND OPIOID
ANALGESICS.)
codeine sulfate*
(See Chapter 27, NARCOTIC AND OPIOID
ANALGESICS.)
**dextromethorphan
hydrobromide**◇
**diphenhydramine
hydrochloride**◇
(See Chapter 43, ANTIHISTAMINES.)
hydromorphone hydrochloride
(See Chapter 27, NARCOTIC AND OPIOID
ANALGESICS.)

COMBINATION PRODUCTS
Preparations are available in the following combinations:
• expectorants with decongestants or antihistamines, or both
• antitussives with decongestants or antihistamines, or both
• expectorants and antitussives
• expectorants and antitussives with decongestants or antihistamines, or both.

acetylcysteine
Airbron♦♦, Mucomyst♦, Mucosol,
Parvolex♦♦

Pregnancy Risk Category: B

MECHANISM OF ACTION
Increases production of respiratory
tract fluids to help liquefy and reduce
the viscosity of thick, tenacious secretions. Also restores liver stores of
glutathione in the treatment of acetaminophen toxicity.

INDICATIONS & DOSAGE
*Pneumonia, bronchitis, tuberculosis,
cystic fibrosis, emphysema, atelectasis
(adjunct), complications of thoracic
surgery and CV surgery—*
Adults and children: 1 to 2 ml 10%
to 20% solution by direct instillation
into trachea as often as every hour; or
3 to 5 ml 20% solution, or 6 to 10 ml
10% solution, by mouthpiece t.i.d. or
q.i.d.
Acetaminophen toxicity—
140 mg/kg initially P.O., followed by
70 mg/kg q 4 hours for 17 doses (a total of 1,330 mg/kg).

ADVERSE REACTIONS
EENT: *rhinorrhea, hemoptysis.*
GI: *stomatitis, nausea.*
Other: *bronchospasm (especially in
asthmatics).*

INTERACTIONS
Activated charcoal: don't use together
in treating acetaminophen toxicity.
Limits acetylcysteine's effectiveness.

NURSING CONSIDERATIONS

• Use cautiously in asthma or severe respiratory insufficiency and in elderly or debilitated patients.
• Classified as a mucolytic.
• Use plastic, glass, stainless steel, or another nonreactive metal when administering by nebulization. Hand bulb nebulizers not recommended because output is too small and particle size too large.
• After opening, store in refrigerator; use within 96 hours.
• Incompatible with oxytetracycline, tetracycline, erythromycin lactobionate, amphotericin B, ampicillin, iodized oil, chymotrypsin, trypsin, and hydrogen peroxide. Administer separately.
• Monitor cough type and frequency. For maximum effect, instruct patient to clear his airway by coughing before aerosol administration.
• Dilute oral doses with cola, fruit juice, or water before administering.

benzonatate
Tessalon♦

Pregnancy Risk Category: C

MECHANISM OF ACTION
Suppresses the cough reflex by direct action on the cough center in the medulla (brain). Also has local anesthetic action.

INDICATIONS & DOSAGE
Nonproductive cough—
Adults and children over 10 years: 100 mg P.O. t.i.d.; up to 600 mg daily.
Children under 10 years: 8 mg/kg P.O. in 3 to 6 divided doses.

ADVERSE REACTIONS
CNS: dizziness, drowsiness, headache.
EENT: nasal congestion, sensation of burning in eyes.
GI: nausea, constipation.

Skin: rash.
Other: chills.

INTERACTIONS
None significant.

NURSING CONSIDERATIONS
• Patient should not chew capsules or leave in mouth to dissolve; local anesthesia will result. If capsules dissolve in mouth, CNS stimulation may cause restlessness, tremors, and possibly seizures.
• A nonnarcotic cough suppressant; don't use when cough is valuable as diagnostic sign or is beneficial (as after thoracic surgery).
• Monitor cough type and frequency.
• Use with percussion and chest vibration.
• Maintain fluid intake to help liquefy sputum.

dextromethorphan hydrobromide◊
Balminil D.M., Benylin DM , Broncho-Grippol-DM♦♦, Congespirin for Children, Cremacoat 1, DM Cough*, Hold, Koffex♦♦, Mediquell, Neo-DM♦♦, Pediacare 1, Pertussin 8 Hour Cough Formula, Robidex♦♦, Sedatuss♦♦, St. Joseph for Children, Sucrets Cough Control Formula. More commonly available in combination products such as Contac Cough Formula, Contac Cough and Sore Throat Formula, Contac Jr. Children's Cold Medicine, Contac Nighttime Cold Medicine, Contac Severe Cold Formula Caplets, Novahistine DMX Liquid, Phenergan with Dextromethorphan*, Robitussin-DM*, Rondec-DM*, Triaminicol Multi-Symptom Cold, Trind-DM Liquid*, Tussi-Organidin-DM Liquid*

Pregnancy Risk Category: C

Italicized side effects are common or life-threatening.
*Liquid form contains alcohol.   **May contain tartrazine.

MECHANISM OF ACTION
Suppresses the cough reflex by direct action on the cough center in the medulla (brain).

INDICATIONS & DOSAGE
Nonproductive cough—
Adults: 10 to 20 mg P.O. q 4 hours, or 30 mg q 6 to 8 hours. Or the controlled-release liquid twice daily (60 mg b.i.d.). Maximum 120 mg daily.
Children 6 to 12 years: 5 to 10 mg P.O. q 4 hours, or 15 mg q 6 to 8 hours. Or the controlled-release liquid twice daily (30 mg b.i.d.). Maximum 60 mg daily.
Children 2 to 6 years: 2.5 to 5 mg P.O. q 4 hours, or 7.5 mg q 6 to 8 hours. Maximum 30 mg daily.

ADVERSE REACTIONS
CNS: drowsiness, dizziness.
GI: nausea.

INTERACTIONS
MAO inhibitors: hypotension, coma, hyperpyrexia, and death have occurred. Do not use together.

NURSING CONSIDERATIONS
• Contraindicated in patients currently taking or within 2 weeks of discontinuing MAO inhibitors.
• Produces no analgesia or addiction and little or no CNS depression.
• An antitussive; don't use when cough is valuable diagnostic sign or beneficial (as after thoracic surgery).
• Use with percussion and chest vibration.
• Monitor cough type and frequency.
• Available in most OTC cough medicines.
• Dose of 15 to 30 mg dextromethorphan is equivalent to 8 to 15 mg codeine as an antitussive.

guaifenesin
(glyceryl guaiacolate)◇
Anti-Tuss*, Balminil Expectorant ♦♦, Baytussin, Breonesin, Colrex Expectorant*, Cremacoat 2, Gee-Gee, GG-CEN*, Glyate*, Glycotuss, Glytuss, Guiatuss*, Halotussin, Humibid L.A., Hytuss, Hytuss-2X, Malotuss, Naldecon Senior EX, Neo-Spec♦♦, Nortussin, Resyl♦♦, Robafen, Robitussin*, S-T Expectorant

Pregnancy Risk Category: C

MECHANISM OF ACTION
Increases production of respiratory tract fluids to help liquefy and reduce the viscosity of thick, tenacious secretions.

INDICATIONS & DOSAGE
As expectorant—
Adults: 200 to 400 mg P.O. q 4 hours. Maximum 2,400 mg daily.
Children: 12 mg/kg P.O. daily in 6 divided doses.

ADVERSE REACTIONS
CNS: drowsiness.
GI: vomiting and nausea occur with large doses.

INTERACTIONS
None significant.

NURSING CONSIDERATIONS
• May interfere with certain laboratory tests for 5-hydroxyindoleacetic acid and vanillylmandelic acid.
• Watch for bleeding gums, hematuria, and bruising if given to patients on heparin. Should such symptoms appear, guaifenesin should be discontinued.
• Liquefies thick, tenacious sputum; maintain fluid intake. Advise patient to take with a glass of water whenever possible.
• Monitor cough type and frequency.

• Encourage deep-breathing exercises.
• Although a popular expectorant, its efficacy has not been established.

iodinated glycerol
Iophen Elixir*, Myodine*,
Organidin*♦, R-Ger Elixir*

Pregnancy Risk Category: X

MECHANISM OF ACTION
Increases production of respiratory tract fluids to help liquefy and reduce the viscosity of thick, tenacious secretions.

INDICATIONS & DOSAGE
Bronchial asthma, bronchitis, emphysema (adjunct)—
Adults: 60 mg P.O. q.i.d. (tablets), or 20 drops (solution) P.O. q.i.d. with fluids, or 5 ml (elixir) P.O. q.i.d.
Children: up to half adult dose based on child's weight.

ADVERSE REACTIONS
After long-term use:
GI: *nausea,* gastrointestinal distress.
Skin: *eruptions.*
Other: acute parotitis, thyroid enlargement, hypothyroidism.

INTERACTIONS
None significant.

NURSING CONSIDERATIONS
• Contraindicated in hypothyroidism, iodine sensitivity, and during pregnancy and lactation.
• Skin rash or other hypersensitivity reaction may require stopping drug.
• May liquefy thick, tenacious sputum; maintain fluid intake.
• Monitor cough type and frequency.
• Encourage deep-breathing exercises.

potassium iodide (SSKI)
Pregnancy Risk Category: D

MECHANISM OF ACTION
Increases production of respiratory tract fluids to help liquefy and reduce the viscosity of thick secretions.

INDICATIONS & DOSAGE
As expectorant, chronic bronchitis, chronic pulmonary emphysema, bronchial asthma—
Adults: 0.3 to 0.6 ml P.O. q 4 to 6 hours.
Children: 0.25 to 0.5 ml P.O. of saturated solution (1 g/ml) b.i.d. to q.i.d.
Nuclear radiation protection—
Adults and children: 0.13 ml P.O. of SSKI immediately before or after initial exposure will block 90% of radioactive iodine. Same dose given 3 to 4 hours after exposure will provide 50% block. Should be administered for up to 10 days under medical supervision.
Infants under 1 year: ½ adult dose.

ADVERSE REACTIONS
GI: *nausea,* vomiting, *epigastric pain,* metallic taste.
Metabolic: goiter, hyperthyroid adenoma, hypothyroidism (with excessive use), collagen disease-like syndrome.
Skin: rash.
Other: drug fever.
Prolonged use: chronic iodine poisoning, soreness of mouth, coryza, sneezing, swelling of eyelids.

INTERACTIONS
Lithium carbonate: may cause hypothyroidism. Don't use together.

NURSING CONSIDERATIONS
• Contraindicated in iodine hypersensitivity, tuberculosis, hyperkalemia, acute bronchitis, hyperthyroidism.
• Maintain adequate fluid intake.
• Has strong, salty, metallic taste. Di-

Italicized side effects are common or life-threatening.
*Liquid form contains alcohol.   **May contain tartrazine.

lute with milk, fruit juice, or broth to
reduce GI distress and disguise taste.
• Sudden withdrawal may precipitate
thyroid storm.
• If skin rash appears, discontinue
use. Contact doctor.

terpin hydrate*◇
Pregnancy Risk Category: C

MECHANISM OF ACTION
Increases production of respiratory
tract fluids to help liquefy and reduce
the viscosity of thick secretions.

INDICATIONS & DOSAGE
Excessive bronchial secretions—
Adults: 5 to 10 ml P.O. of elixir q 4 to
6 hours.

ADVERSE REACTIONS
GI: nausea, vomiting.

INTERACTIONS
None significant.

NURSING CONSIDERATIONS
• Contraindicated in peptic ulcer or
severe diabetes mellitus.
• Don't give in large doses; *high alcoholic content of elixir* (86 proof).
• Monitor cough type and frequency.

45

Antacids, adsorbents, and antiflatulents

activated charcoal◇
aluminum carbonate◇
aluminum hydroxide◇
aluminum phosphate◇
calcium carbonate◇
dihydroxyaluminum sodium carbonate◇
magaldrate (aluminum-magnesium complex)◇
magnesium oxide◇
magnesium salts◇
   (See Chapter 48, LAXATIVES.)
magnesium trisilicate◇
simethicone◇
sodium bicarbonate◇
   (See Chapter 104, ACIDIFIERS AND ALKALINIZERS.)

COMBINATION PRODUCTS

ALKA-SELTZER, MEDI-SELTZER: sodium bicarbonate 1,916 mg, aspirin 325 mg, and citric acid 1,000 mg.
ALKA-SELTZER WITHOUT ASPIRIN: sodium bicarbonate 958 mg, citric acid 832 mg, and potassium bicarbonate 312 mg.
ALUDROX SUSPENSION: aluminum hydroxide 307 mg, magnesium hydroxide 103 mg.
CAMALOX TABLETS◆: aluminum hydroxide 225 mg, magnesium hydroxide 200 mg, and calcium carbonate 250 mg.
DELCID SUSPENSION: aluminum hydroxide 600 mg, magnesium hydroxide 665 mg.
DI-GEL LIQUID: aluminum hydroxide 200 mg, magnesium hydroxide 200 mg, simethicone 20 mg.
GAVISCON◆: aluminum hydroxide

31.7 mg, magnesium carbonate 137 mg.
GELUSIL◆: aluminum hydroxide 200 mg, magnesium hydroxide 200 mg, simethicone 25 mg.
GELUSIL-II: aluminum hydroxide 400 mg, magnesium hydroxide 400 mg, simethicone 30 mg.
GELUSIL-M: aluminum hydroxide 300 mg, magnesium hydroxide 200 mg, simethicone 25 mg.
MAALOX NO. 1: aluminum hydroxide 200 mg and magnesium hydroxide 200 mg.
EXTRA STRENGTH MAALOX TABLETS: aluminum hydroxide 400 mg and magnesium hydroxide 400 mg.
MAALOX PLUS TABLETS◆: aluminum hydroxide 200 mg, magnesium hydroxide 200 mg, simethicone 25 mg.
MAALOX TC TABLETS: aluminum hydroxide 600 mg, magnesium hydroxide 300 mg.
MAGNATRIL: aluminum hydroxide 260 mg, magnesium hydroxide 130 mg, and magnesium trisilicate 455 mg.
MYLANTA TABLETS◆: aluminum hydroxide 200 mg, magnesium hydroxide 200 mg, simethicone 20 mg.
MYLANTA-II TABLETS◆: aluminum hydroxide 400 mg, magnesium hydroxide 400 mg, simethicone 40 mg.
RIOPAN PLUS CHEW TABLETS: magaldrate 540 mg, simethicone 20 mg.
RIOPAN PLUS SUSPENSION: magaldrate 540 mg and simethicone 20 mg/5 ml.
SILAIN-GEL: aluminum hydroxide 282 mg, magnesium hydroxide 285 mg, simethicone 25 mg per 5 ml.
TITRALAC LIQUID: calcium carbonate

Italicized side effects are common or life-threatening.
*Liquid form contains alcohol.   **May contain tartrazine.

1,000 mg in glycine.
TITRALAC TABLETS: calcium carbonate 420 mg, glycine 150 mg.
UNIVOL♦♦: aluminum hydroxide and magnesium carbonate co-dried gel 300 mg and magnesium hydroxide 100 mg.
WINGEL: aluminum hydroxide 180 mg, magnesium hydroxide 160 mg.

activated charcoal◊
Actidose-Aqua, Charcoaide, Charcocaps, Liqui-Char, Superchar

Pregnancy Risk Category: C

MECHANISM OF ACTION
Adheres to many drugs and chemicals, inhibiting their absorption from the GI tract. An adsorbent.

INDICATIONS & DOSAGE
Flatulence or dyspepsia—
Adults: 600 mg to 5 g P.O. t.i.d. or q.i.d.
Poisoning—
Adults: initially, 1g/kg (30 to 100 g) P.O. or 5 to 10 times the amount of poison ingested as a suspension in 180 to 240 ml of water.
Children: 5 to 10 times estimated weight of drug or chemical ingested. Minimum dose is 30 g P.O. in 250 ml water to make a slurry. Give orally, preferably within 30 minutes of poisoning. Larger dose is necessary if food is in the stomach. For treating poisoning or overdosage with acetaminophen, amphetamines, aspirin, antimony, atropine, arsenic, barbiturates, camphor, cocaine, cardiac glycosides, glutethimide, ipecac, malathion, morphine, poisonous mushrooms, opium, oxalic acid, parathion, phenol, phenothiazines, potassium permanganate, propoxyphene, quinine, strychnine, sulfonamides, or tricyclic antidepressants.

ADVERSE REACTIONS
GI: black stools, nausea.

INTERACTIONS
ipecac: Ipecac rendered ineffective. Don't administer together.

NURSING CONSIDERATIONS
• Don't use in semiconscious or unconscious persons.
• Because activated charcoal absorbs and inactivates syrup of ipecac, give after emesis is complete.
• Don't give in ice cream, milk, or sherbert. Reduces absorptive capacity.
• Powder form is most effective. Mix with tap water to form consistency of thick syrup. May add small amount of fruit juice or flavoring to make more palatable.
• May need to repeat dose if patient vomits shortly after administration.
• Space doses at least 1 hour apart from other drugs if activated charcoal is being used for any indication other than poisoning.
• Warn patient that feces will be black.

aluminum carbonate◊
Basaljel

Pregnancy Risk Category: C

MECHANISM OF ACTION
Reduces total acid load in the GI tract and elevates gastric pH to reduce pepsin activity. Also strengthens the gastric mucosal barrier and increases esophageal sphincter tone. An antacid.

INDICATIONS & DOSAGE
As antacid—
Adults: suspension: 5 to 10 ml P.O., p.r.n. Extra-strength suspension: 2.5 to 5 ml, p.r.n. Tablets: 1 to 2, p.r.n. Capsules: 1 to 2, p.r.n.
To prevent formation of urinary phosphate stones (with low-phosphate

diet)—
Adults: suspension: 15 to 30 ml suspension in water or juice P.O. 1 hour after meals and h.s.; 5 to 15 ml extra-strength suspension in water or juice 1 hour after meals and h.s.; 2 to 6 tablets or capsules 1 hour after meals and h.s.

ADVERSE REACTIONS
GI: anorexia, *constipation*, intestinal obstruction.
Metabolic: hypophosphatemia.

INTERACTIONS
Tetracyclines: Decreased antibiotic effect. Separate administration times.

NURSING CONSIDERATIONS
• Use cautiously in elderly patients, especially those with decreased GI motility (those receiving antidiarrheals, antispasmodics, or anticholinergics), dehydration, fluid restriction, chronic renal disease, and suspected intestinal obstruction.
• Record amount and consistency of stools. Manage constipation with laxatives or stool softeners; alternate with magnesium-containing antacids (if patient does not have renal disease).
• Shake suspension well; give with small amount of water or fruit juice to ensure passage to stomach. When administering through nasogastric tube, be sure tube is placed correctly and is patent; follow antacid with water to clear tube.
• Watch long-term high-dose use in patient on restricted sodium intake.
• Warn patient not to take aluminum carbonate indiscriminately and not to switch antacids without doctor's advice.
• Because it contains aluminum, it is used in renal failure to help control hyperphosphatemia. Binds phosphate in GI tract.
• Monitor serum phosphate.
• Watch for symptoms of hypophos-

phatemia with prolonged use (anorexia, malaise, muscle weakness); can also lead to resorption of calcium and bone demineralization.
• May cause enteric-coated drugs to be released prematurely in stomach. Separate doses by 1 hour.
• Basaljel liquid contains no sugar.

---

aluminum hydroxide◊
ALternaGEL, Alu-Cap, Alu-Tab, Amphojel♦, Dialume, Nephrox
Pregnancy Risk Category: C

MECHANISM OF ACTION
Reduces total acid load in the GI tract and elevates gastric pH to reduce pepsin activity. Also strengthens the gastric mucosal barrier and increases esophageal sphincter tone. An antacid.

INDICATIONS & DOSAGE
Antacid—
Adults: 600 mg P.O. (5 to 10 ml of most products) 1 hour after meals and h.s.; 300- or 600-mg tablet, chewed before swallowing, taken with milk or water 5 to 6 times daily after meals and h.s.
Hyperphosphatemia in renal failure—
Adults: 500 mg to 2 g P.O. b.i.d. to q.i.d.

ADVERSE REACTIONS
GI: anorexia, *constipation*, intestinal obstruction.
Metabolic: hypophosphatemia.

INTERACTIONS
Tetracyclines: decreased antibiotic effect. Separate administration times.

NURSING CONSIDERATIONS
• Use cautiously in elderly patients, especially those with decreased GI motility (those receiving antidiarrheals, antispasmodics, or anticholinergics), dehydration, fluid restriction, chronic renal disease, and sus-

---

Italicized side effects are common or life-threatening.
*Liquid form contains alcohol.   **May contain tartrazine.

pected intestinal obstruction.
• Record amount and consistency of stools. Manage constipation with laxatives or stool softeners; alternate with magnesium-containing antacids (if patient does not have renal disease).
• Shake suspension well; give with small amount of milk or water to assure passage to stomach. When administering through nasogastric tube, make sure tube is placed correctly and is patent. After instilling antacid, flush tube with water.
• Watch long-term high-dose use in patient on restricted sodium intake.
• Warn patient not to take aluminum hydroxide indiscriminately or switch antacids without doctor's advice.
• Because it contains aluminum, it is used in renal failure to help control hyperphosphatemia. Binds phosphate in the GI tract.
• Monitor serum phosphate.
• Watch for symptoms of hypophosphatemia with prolonged use (anorexia, malaise, and muscle weakness); can also lead to resorption of calcium and bone demineralization.
• May cause enteric-coated drugs to be released prematurely in stomach. Separate doses by 1 hour.

---

aluminum phosphate◊
Phosphaljel♦

Pregnancy Risk Category: C

MECHANISM OF ACTION
Reduces total acid load in the GI tract and elevates gastric pH to reduce pepsin activity. Also strengthens the gastric mucosal barrier and increases esophageal sphincter tone. An antacid.

INDICATIONS & DOSAGE
Antacid—
Adults: 15 to 30 ml undiluted P.O. q 2 hours between meals and h.s.

ADVERSE REACTIONS
GI: *constipation*, intestinal obstruction.

INTERACTIONS
Tetracyclines: decreased antibiotic effect. Separate administration times.

NURSING CONSIDERATIONS
• Use cautiously in elderly patients, especially those with decreased GI motility (those receiving antidiarrheals, antispasmodics, or anticholinergics), dehydration, fluid restriction, chronic renal disease, and suspected intestinal obstruction.
• Record amount and consistency of stools. Manage constipation with laxatives or stool softeners; alternate with magnesium-containing antacids (if patient does not have renal disease).
• Shake well; give alone or with small amount of milk or water. When administering through nasogastric tube, make sure tube is placed correctly and is patent; after instilling, flush tube with water to facilitate passage to stomach and maintain tube patency.
• Watch long-term high-dose use in patient on restricted sodium intake.
• Warn patient not to take aluminum phosphate indiscriminately and not to switch antacids without doctor's advice.
• This drug is a very weak antacid.
• Can reverse hypophosphatemia induced by aluminum hydroxide.
• May cause enteric-coated drugs to be released prematurely in stomach. Separate doses by 1 hour.
• Phosphaljel contains no sugar.

---

calcium carbonate◇

Alka-Mints, Amitone, Calcilac, Calglycine, Chooz, Dicarbosil, Equilet, Genalac, Glycate, Gustalac, Mallamint, Pama No. 1, Titracid, Titralac, Tums, Tums E-X, Tums Liquid Extra Strength

Pregnancy Risk Category: C

MECHANISM OF ACTION

Reduces total acid load in the GI tract and elevates gastric pH to reduce pepsin activity. Also strengthens the gastric mucosal barrier and increases esophageal sphincter tone. An antacid.

INDICATIONS & DOSAGE

Antacid—
Adults: 1-g tablet, P.O. 4 to 6 times daily, chewed well and taken with water; or 1 g of suspension (5 ml of most products), 1 hour after meals and h.s.

ADVERSE REACTIONS

GI: *constipation,* gastric distention, flatulence, rebound hyperacidity, *nausea.*
Metabolic: *hypercalcemia, hypophosphatemia;* if taken with milk—milk-alkali syndrome.

INTERACTIONS

Tetracyclines: decreased antibiotic effect. Separate administration times.

NURSING CONSIDERATIONS

• Contraindicated in severe renal disease. Use cautiously in elderly patients, especially those with decreased GI motility (those receiving antidiarrheals, antispasmodics, or anticholinergics), dehydration, fluid restriction, chronic renal disease, and suspected intestinal obstruction.
• Do not administer with milk or other foods high in vitamin D. Can cause milk-alkali syndrome (headache, confusion, distaste for food,

nausea, vomiting, hypercalcemia, hypercalciuria, calcinosis, and hypophosphatemia).
• Record amount and consistency of stools. Manage constipation with laxatives or stool softeners.
• Watch for symptoms of hypercalcemia (nausea, vomiting, headache, mental confusion, and anorexia).
• Monitor serum calcium, especially in mild renal impairment.
• Warn patient not to take calcium carbonate indiscriminately and not to switch antacids without doctor's advice.
• May cause enteric-coated tablets to be released prematurely in stomach. Separate doses by 1 hour.

dihydroxyaluminum sodium carbonate◇

Rolaids♦

Pregnancy Risk Category: C

MECHANISM OF ACTION

Reduces total acid load in the GI tract and elevates gastric pH to reduce pepsin activity. Also strengthens the gastric mucosal barrier and increases esophageal sphincter tone. An antacid.

INDICATIONS & DOSAGE

Antacid—
Adults: chew 1 to 2 tablets (334 to 668 mg), p.r.n.

ADVERSE REACTIONS

GI: anorexia, *constipation,* intestinal obstruction.

INTERACTIONS

Tetracyclines: decreased antibiotic effect. Separate administration times.

NURSING CONSIDERATIONS

• Use cautiously in elderly patients, especially those with decreased GI motility (those receiving antidiarrheals, antispasmodics, or anticho-

---

Italicized side effects are common or life-threatening.
*Liquid form contains alcohol.   **May contain tartrazine.

linergics), dehydration, fluid restriction, chronic renal disease, and suspected intestinal obstruction.
• Has high sodium content and may increase sodium and water retention.
• Record amount and consistency of stools. Manage constipation with laxatives or stool softeners; alternate with magnesium-containing antacids (if patient does not have renal disease).
• Watch long-term high-dose use in patient on restricted sodium intake.
• Warn patient not to take dihydroxyaluminum sodium carbonate indiscriminately.
• May cause enteric-coated drugs to be released prematurely in stomach. Separate doses by 1 hour.

magaldrate (aluminum-magnesium complex)◊
Antiflux♦♦, Lowsium, Riopan♦
Pregnancy Risk Category: C

MECHANISM OF ACTION
Reduces total acid load in the GI tract and elevates gastric pH to reduce pepsin activity. Also strengthens the gastric mucosal barrier and increases esophageal sphincter tone. An antacid.

INDICATIONS & DOSAGE
Antacid—
Adults: suspension: 400 to 800 mg (5 to 10 ml) P.O. between meals and h.s. with water. Tablet: 400 to 800 mg (1 to 2 tablets) P.O. with water between meals and h.s. Chewable tablet: 400 to 800 mg (1 to 2 tablets) P.O. chewed before swallowing, between meals and h.s.

ADVERSE REACTIONS
GI: mild constipation or diarrhea.

INTERACTIONS
Tetracyclines: decreased antibiotic effect. Separate administration times.

NURSING CONSIDERATIONS
• Contraindicated in severe renal disease. Use cautiously in elderly patients, especially those with decreased GI motility (those receiving antidiarrheals, antispasmodics, or anticholinergics), dehydration, fluid restriction, and mild renal impairment.
• Record amount and consistency of stools.
• Shake suspension well; give with a little water to ensure passage to stomach. When giving through nasogastric tube, be sure tube is placed properly and is patent. After instilling, flush tube with water to ensure passage to stomach and maintain tube patency.
• Monitor serum magnesium in patients with mild renal impairment. Symptomatic hypermagnesemia usually occurs only in severe renal failure.
• Not usually used in renal failure (although it contains aluminum) to help control hypophosphatemia, because it contains magnesium, which may accumulate in renal failure.
• Good for patient on restricted sodium intake; very low sodium content.
• Warn patient not to take magaldrate indiscriminately and not to switch antacids without doctor's advice.
• May cause enteric-coated drugs to be released prematurely in stomach. Separate doses by 1 hour.
• Riopan, Riopan Plus liquid, and Riopan Swallow Tablet contain no sugar. Chewable tablets contain sugar.

magnesium oxide◊
Mag-Ox 400, Maox, Par-Mag, Uro-Mag
Pregnancy Risk Category: C

MECHANISM OF ACTION
Reduces total acid load in the GI tract and elevates gastric pH to reduce pepsin activity. Also strengthens the gastric mucosal barrier and increases

---

esophageal spincter tone. An antacid.

INDICATIONS & DOSAGE
Antacid—
Adults: 250 mg to 1 g P.O. with water or milk after meals and h.s.
Laxative—
Adults: 4 g P.O. with water or milk, usually h.s.
Oral replacement therapy in mild hypomagnesemia—
Adults: 650-mg to 1.3-g tablet or capsule P.O. daily. Monitor serum magnesium response.

ADVERSE REACTIONS
GI: *diarrhea,* nausea, abdominal pain.
Metabolic: hypermagnesemia.

INTERACTIONS
Tetracyclines: decreased antibiotic effect. Separate administration times.

NURSING CONSIDERATIONS
• Contraindicated in severe renal disease. Use cautiously in elderly patients, and in mild renal impairment.
• With prolonged use and some degree of renal impairment, watch for symptoms of hypermagnesemia (hypotension, nausea, vomiting, depressed reflexes, respiratory depression, and coma). Monitor serum magnesium.
• When used as laxative, do not give other oral drugs 1 to 2 hours before or after.
• If diarrhea occurs on antacid doses, suggest alternate preparation.
• Warn patient not to take magnesium oxide indiscriminately and not to switch antacid without doctor's advice.
• May cause enteric-coated drugs to be released prematurely in stomach. Separate doses by 1 hour.

magnesium trisilicate◊
Pregnancy Risk Category: C

MECHANISM OF ACTION
Reduces total acid load in the GI tract and elevates gastric pH to reduce pepsin activity. Also strengthens the gastric mucosal barrier and increases esophageal sphincter tone. An antacid.

INDICATIONS & DOSAGE
Antacid—
Adults: 1- to 4-g tablet P.O. t.i.d. chewed well and taken with half a glass of water.

ADVERSE REACTIONS
GI: *diarrhea,* gastric distention, flatulence, nausea, abdominal pain.
GU: possible formation of silica renal calculi with prolonged use.
Metabolic: hypermagnesemia.

INTERACTIONS
Tetracyclines: Decreased antibiotic effect. Separate administration times.

NURSING CONSIDERATIONS
• Contraindicated in severe renal disease. Use cautiously in elderly patients, and in mild renal impairment.
• With prolonged use and some degree of renal impairment, watch for symptoms of hypermagnesemia (hypotension, nausea, vomiting, depressed reflexes, respiratory depression, and coma). Monitor serum magnesium.
• If diarrhea occurs on antacid doses, suggest alternate preparation.
• Warn patient not to take magnesium trisilicate indiscriminately.
• Tell patient to chew tablet before swallowing.
• May cause enteric-coated drugs to be released prematurely in stomach. Separate doses by 1 hour.

simethicone◊
Extra Strength Gas-X, Gas-X,
Mylicon-80, Mylicon-125, Ovol-
40♦♦, Ovol-80♦♦, Phazyme,
Phazyme 55, Phazyme 95,
Phazyme 125, Silain

Pregnancy Risk Category: C

MECHANISM OF ACTION
By its defoaming action, disperses or
prevents formation of mucus-sur-
rounded gas pockets in the GI tract.

INDICATIONS & DOSAGE
*Flatulence, functional gastric bloat-
ing—*
Adults and children over 12 years:
40 to 125 mg after each meal and h.s.

ADVERSE REACTIONS
GI: expulsion of excessive liberated
gas as belching, rectal flatus.

INTERACTIONS
None significant.

NURSING CONSIDERATIONS
• Warn patient not to take simethicone indiscriminately.
• Tell patient to chew tablet before
swallowing.

Digestants

bentiromide
bile salts
chenodiol (chenodeoxycholic
acid)
dehydrocholic acid
glutamic acid hydrochloride
monooctanoin
pancreatin
pancrelipase
ursodiol

COMBINATION PRODUCTS
BILRON♦: bile salts and iron.
DONNAZYME TABLETS♦: pancreatin
300 mg, pepsin 150 mg, bile salts
150 mg, hyoscyamine sulfate 0.0518
mg, atropine sulfate 0.0097 mg,
hyoscine hydrobromide 0.0033 mg,
and phenobarbital 8.1 mg.
ENTOZYME TABLETS♦: pancreatin
300 mg, pepsin 250 mg, and bile salts
150 mg.
PANCREASE CAPSULES♦: lipase 4,000
units, protease 25,000 units, amylase
20,000 units, in enteric-coated micro-
spheres.

---

bentiromide
Chymex♦

Pregnancy Risk Category: B

MECHANISM OF ACTION
Biochemically broken down by pancreatic enzymes.

INDICATIONS & DOSAGE
*As a screening test for pancreatic exo-
crine insufficiency—*
Adults and children over 12 years:
Following overnight fast and morning
void, administer a single 500-mg dose
P.O. and follow with 250 ml of water.
Children under 12 years: Dose is 14
mg/kg followed with 250 ml of water.
   Give patient another glass of water
2 hours after dose. An additional 2
glasses of water are recommended
during post-dosing hours 2 to 6.

ADVERSE REACTIONS
CNS: headache.
GI: *diarrhea,* flatulence, nausea,
vomiting.
Other: weakness.

INTERACTIONS
None significant.

NURSING CONSIDERATIONS
• Effective use requires close attention to technical details of drug administration and urine collection,
handling of specimens, and assay of
arylamine.
• Encourage your patient to drink
water during post-dosing period to
promote diuresis.
• Collect urine during 0 to 6 hours
post-dosing. Measure volume of the
collection and retain a 10-ml sample
for analysis.
• If subsequent retesting is necessary,
wait at least 7 days.
• When testing diabetic patients, insulin dose may have to be adjusted
during the fasting procedure.

Italicized side effects are common or life-threatening.
*Liquid form contains alcohol.   **May contain tartrazine.

bile salts
Ox-Bile Extract Enseals
Pregnancy Risk Category: C

MECHANISM OF ACTION
Stimulate bile flow from the liver, promoting normal digestion and absorption of fats, fat-soluble vitamins, and cholesterol.

INDICATIONS & DOSAGE
Uncomplicated constipation—
Adults and children: 324 to 648 mg (enteric-coated tablets) P.O. b.i.d. or t.i.d. after meals; or 150- to 600-mg capsules with or after meals.

ADVERSE REACTIONS
GI: loose stools and mild cramping (with large doses).

INTERACTIONS
None significant.

NURSING CONSIDERATIONS
• Contraindicated in marked hepatic dysfunction and complete biliary obstruction, except in malnutrition with steatorrhea and vitamin K deficiency with hypoprothrombinemia.
• Use Ox-Bile Extract cautiously in obstructive jaundice.
• Don't use Ox-Bile Extract if other preparations are available, since it doesn't provide an adequate amount of conjugated bile salts.
• Has not been shown to effectively treat bile salt deficiency.

chenodiol (chenodeoxycholic acid)
Chenix
Pregnancy Risk Category: X

MECHANISM OF ACTION
Suppresses hepatic synthesis of both cholesterol and cholic acid. These actions contribute to biliary cholesterol desaturation and gradual dissolution of gallstones.

INDICATIONS & DOSAGE
Dissolution of radiolucent cholesterol stones (gallstones) when systemic disease or age precludes surgery—
Adults: 250 mg P.O. b.i.d. for the first 2 weeks, followed, as tolerated, by weekly increases of 250 mg/day, up to 13 to 16 mg/kg/day for up to 24 months.

ADVERSE REACTIONS
GI: *diarrhea,* cramps, heartburn, constipation, nausea, vomiting, anorexia, epigastric distress.
Hepatic: reversible elevated hepatic enzymes, possible liver toxicity.

INTERACTIONS
Cholestyramine, colestinol, estrogens, oral contraceptives, clofibrate: decreased chenodiol effect. Monitor patient carefully.

NURSING CONSIDERATIONS
• Contraindicated in known hepatocyte dysfunction; a gallbladder confirmed as nonvisualizing after two consecutive single doses of dye; radiopaque or radiolucent bile pigment stones; or gallstone complications or compelling reasons for gallbladder surgery, including unremitting acute cholecystitis, cholangitis, biliary obstruction, gallstone pancreatitis, or biliary GI fistula.
• Chenodiol treatment should be reserved for carefully selected patients.
• The drug is particularly effective in the dissolution of small, floatable gallstones.
• Monitor serum transaminase monthly for the first 3 months and thereafter every 3 months for duration of therapy.
• The final dosage shouldn't be less than 10 mg/kg/day; lower dosages are usually ineffective.
• Diarrhea occurs in 30% to 40% of all patients. Doctor may reduce dos-

age until diarrhea subsides. Antidiarrheals may also be prescribed. In
some patients, however, persistent
diarrhea will require discontinuation
of chenodiol therapy.
• Monitor oral cholecystogram or ul-
trasonogram every 6 to 9 months to
observe for gallstone dissolution.

dehydrocholic acid
Cholan-HMB, Decholin,
Hepahydrin

Pregnancy Risk Category: C

MECHANISM OF ACTION
Stimulates bile flow from the liver,
promoting normal digestion and absorption of fats, fat-soluble vitamins,
and cholesterol.

INDICATIONS & DOSAGE
*Constipation, biliary tract condi-
tions—*
Adults: 250 to 500 mg P.O. b.i.d. or
t.i.d. after meals for 4 to 6 weeks.

ADVERSE REACTIONS
GI: diarrhea with weakness (in large
doses).

INTERACTIONS
None significant.

NURSING CONSIDERATIONS
• Contraindicated in complete mechanical biliary obstruction.
• Do not use when patient is nau-
seated or vomiting, or has abdominal
pain.
• Simultaneous administration of bile
salts may be needed in biliary fistula.
• Used to prevent bacterial accumulation after biliary tract surgery.
• Probably much less effective than
natural bile salts in lowering surface
tension and promoting absorption.
• Don't use dehydrocholic acid to accelerate healing in jaundiced patients.
• Frequent use may result in dependence on laxatives.

glutamic acid hydrochloride
Acidulin♦

Pregnancy Risk Category: C

MECHANISM OF ACTION
Replaces gastric acid.

INDICATIONS & DOSAGE
Hypoacidity—
Adults: 1 to 3 capsules P.O. t.i.d. be-
fore meals.

ADVERSE REACTIONS
Metabolic: systemic acidosis in massive overdose.

INTERACTIONS
None significant.

NURSING CONSIDERATIONS
• Contraindicated in gastric hyperacidity or peptic ulcer.
• Use instead of hydrochloric acid so
tooth enamel won't be damaged; however, glutamic acid hydrochloride is
not as effective in decreasing gastric
pH.

monooctanoin
Moctanin

Pregnancy Risk Category: C

MECHANISM OF ACTION
Dissolves gallstones by rendering
them more soluble.

INDICATIONS & DOSAGE
*To solubilize cholesterol gallstones that
are retained in the biliary tract after
cholecystectomy—*
Adults: Administered as a continuous
infusion through a catheter inserted
directly into the common bile duct via
a T tube. Rate should not exceed 3 to
5 ml/hour at a pressure of 10 cm H_2O.
Duration of infusion is 7 to 21 days.

ADVERSE REACTIONS
GI: *GI pain and discomfort, nausea,*

vomiting, diarrhea, anorexia, indigestion.
Other: metabolic acidosis.

INTERACTIONS
None reported.

NURSING CONSIDERATIONS
• Contraindicated in clinical jaundice, significant biliary tract infection, or a history of recent duodenal ulcer or jejunitis.
• Because impaired liver function may lead to metabolic acidosis during administration of this drug, routine liver function tests should be done before perfusion therapy begins.
• Monooctanoin should only be started by individuals experienced in infusion therapy.
• Not to be administered parenterally. For biliary tract infusion only.
• Pressure *must* be kept below 15 cm H_2O. Keeping the pressure at 10 cm H_2O will help minimize GI and biliary tract irritation.
• Use a peristaltic infusion pump to regulate the infusion. Outpatients may use a battery-operated portable pump.
• Warm the solution to 60° to 80° F. (16° to 27° C.) before perfusion. Temperature of the solution should not fall below 65° F. (18° C.) during administration.
• GI symptoms may be reduced by slowing the infusion rate or discontinuing the infusion during meals.

pancreatin
Dizymes tablets, Hi-Vegi-Lip tablets, Pancreatin Enseals, Pancreatin tablets

Pregnancy Risk Category: C

MECHANISM OF ACTION
Replaces endogenous exocrine pancreatic enzymes and aids digestion of starches, fats, and proteins.

INDICATIONS & DOSAGE
Exocrine pancreatic secretion insufficiency, digestive aid in cystic fibrosis—
Adults and children: 1 to 3 tablets P.O. with meals.

ADVERSE REACTIONS
GI: nausea, diarrhea with high doses.
Other: hyperuricosuria (with high doses).

INTERACTIONS
Antacids: may negate pancreatin's beneficial effect. Don't use together.

NURSING CONSIDERATIONS
• Use cautiously in patients who are hypersensitive to pork. Bovine preparations are available for these patients, but are less effective.
• Minimal USP standards dictate that each milligram of bovine or porcine pancreatin contains lipase 2 units, protease 25 units, and amylase 25 units.
• Balance fat, protein, and starch intake properly to avoid indigestion. Dosage varies according to degree of maldigestion and malabsorption, amount of fat in diet, and enzyme activity of individual preparations.
• Adequate replacement decreases number of bowel movements and improves stool consistency.
• Use only after confirmed diagnosis of exocrine pancreatic insufficiency. Not effective in GI disorders unrelated to pancreatic enzyme deficiency.
• For infants, mix powder with applesauce and give with meals. Avoid inhalation of powder. Older children may swallow capsules with food.
• Enteric coating on some products may reduce availability of enzyme in upper portion of jejunum.
• Store in airtight containers at room temperature.

pancrelipase
Cotazym capsules♦, Cotazyme-S capsules, Creon capsules, Ilozyme tablets, Ku-Zyme HP capsules, Pancrease capsules♦, Viokase tablets, Viokase powder

Pregnancy Risk Category: C

MECHANISM OF ACTION
A combination of digestive enzymes that replaces endogenous exocrine pancreatic enzymes and aids digestion of starches, fats, and proteins.

INDICATIONS & DOSAGE
Dose must be titrated to patient's response. Exocrine pancreatic secretion insufficiency, cystic fibrosis in adults and children, steatorrhea and other disorders of fat metabolism secondary to insufficient pancreatic enzymes—
Adults and children: dosage ranges from 1 to 3 capsules or tablets P.O. before or with meals and 1 capsule or tablet with snack; or 1 to 2 powder packets before meals or snacks.

ADVERSE REACTIONS
GI: *nausea,* diarrhea with high doses.

INTERACTIONS
Antacids: may negate pancrelipase's beneficial effect. Don't use together.

NURSING CONSIDERATIONS
• Contraindicated in patients with severe pork hypersensitivity.
• Minimal USP standards dictate that each mg of pancrelipase contains 24 units lipase, 100 units protease, and 100 units amylase.
• Use only after confirmed diagnosis of exocrine pancreatic insufficiency. Not effective in GI disorders unrelated to enzyme deficiency.
• Lipase activity greater than with other pancreatic enzymes.
• For infants, mix powder with applesauce and give with meals. Avoid inhalation of powder. Older children may swallow capsules with food.
• Dosage varies with degree of maldigestion and malabsorption, amount of fat in diet, and enzyme activity of individual preparations.
• Adequate replacement decreases number of bowel movements and improves stool consistency.
• Enteric coating on some products may reduce availability of enzyme in upper portion of jejunum.
• Crushing or chewing of capsule interferes with the enteric coating.

ursodiol
Actigall

Pregnancy Risk Category: B

MECHANISM OF ACTION
Ursodiol is a naturally occurring bile acid that suppresses hepatic synthesis and secretion of cholesterol as well as intestinal cholesterol absorption. After long-term administration, it can solubilize cholesterol from gallstones.

INDICATIONS AND DOSAGE
Dissolution of gallstones less than 20 mm. in diameter in patients who are poor surgical candidates or refuse surgery—
Adults: 8 to 10 mg/kg P.O. daily in two or three divided doses. Most patients receive 300 mg P.O. b.i.d. Therapy is usually long-term, with ultrasound images of the gall bladder at 6 month intervals. If partial stone dissolution is not seen within 12 months, eventual success is unlikely. Safety of use for longer than 24 months has not been established.

ADVERSE REACTIONS
CNS: headache, fatigue, anxiety, depression, sleep disorders.
EENT: cough, rhinitis.
GI: nausea, vomiting, dyspepsia, metallic taste, abdominal pain, biliary pain, cholecystitis, diarrhea, constipation, stomatitis, flatulence.

Italicized side effects are common or life-threatening.
*Liquid form contains alcohol.   **May contain tartrazine.

Skin: pruritus, rash, dry skin, urticaria, itching, hair thinning.
Other: arthralgia, myalgia, back pain.

INTERACTIONS
Aluminum-containing antacids, cholestyramine, colestipol: bind ursodiol and prevent its absorption.
Estrogens, oral contraceptives, clofibrate: Increase hepatic cholesterol secretion and may counteract the effects of ursodiol.

NURSING CONSIDERATIONS
• Contraindicated in patients with hypersensitivity to ursodiol or other bile acids. Also contraindicated in chronic liver disease, acute cholecystitis, cholangitis, biliary obstruction, gallstone pancreatitis, or biliary-GI fistulae.
• Ursodiol will not dissolve calcified cholesterol stones, radiolucent bile pigment stones, or radio-opaque stones.
• Ursodiol therapy is long-term, requiring several months to produce an effect. The relapse rate after bile acid therapy may be as high as 50% after 5 years. Patients should be aware of alternative therapies, including 'watchful waiting' (no intervention) and cholecystectomy.
• Monitor liver function tests, including AST (SGOT) and ALT (SGPT) at the beginning of therapy, and after 1 month, 3 months and every 6 months while taking ursodiol. Abnormal tests may indicate a worsening of the disease. There is a theoretical risk of a hepatotoxic metabolite of ursodiol being formed in some patients.
• Ultrasound images of the gallbladder should be reviewed at least once every 6 months for the first year of therapy. Most patients who respond to ursodiol show significant improvement after 6 months of therapy.

47

Antidiarrheals

bismuth subgallate◇
bismuth subsalicylate◇
calcium polycarbophil
  (See Chapter 48, LAXATIVES.)
difenoxin hydrochloride
diphenoxylate hydrochloride
kaolin and pectin mixtures◇
lactobacillus◇
loperamide◇
opium tincture
opium tincture, camphorated
  (Paregoric)

COMBINATION PRODUCTS
DONNAGEL-PG*: powdered opium
24 mg, kaolin 6 g, pectin 142.8 mg,
hyoscyamine sulfate 0.1037 mg, atropine sulfate 0.0194 mg, hyoscine hydrobromide 0.0065 mg, and alcohol
5% in 30-ml suspension.
DONNAGEL SUSPENSION◆*: kaolin 6
g, pectin 142.8 mg, hyoscyamine sulfate 0.1037 mg, atropine sulfate
0.0194 mg, hyoscine hydrobromide
0.0065 mg, and alcohol 3.8% in 30-
ml suspension.
PAREPECTOLIN*: opium 15 mg
(equivalent to paregoric 3.7 ml), kaolin 5.85 g, pectin 162 mg, and alcohol 0.69% in 30-ml suspension.

bismuth subgallate◇
Devrom◆

bismuth subsalicylate◇
Pepto-Bismol
*Pregnancy Risk Category: C (D in
third trimester)*

MECHANISM OF ACTION
Has a mild water-binding capacity;
also may adsorb toxins and provide
protective coating for mucosa.

INDICATIONS & DOSAGE
Mild, nonspecific diarrhea—
Adults: 1 to 2 tablets P.O. chewed or
swallowed whole t.i.d. (subgallate).
Adults: 30 ml or 2 tablets P.O. q ½ to 1
hour up to a maximum of 8 doses and
for no longer than 2 days (subsalicylate).
Children 9 to 12 years: 20 ml or 1
tablet P.O.
Children 6 to 9 years: 10 ml or ⅔
tablet P.O.
Children 3 to 6 years: 5 ml or ⅓ tablet
P.O.
*Prevention and treatment of traveler's
diarrhea (turista)—*
Adults: Prophylactically, 60 ml
(Pepto-Bismol) P.O. q.i.d. during the
first 2 weeks of travel. During acute
illness, 30 to 60 ml P.O. q 30 minutes
for a total of 8 doses. Alternatively, 2
tablets P.O. q.i.d. for up to 3 weeks.

ADVERSE REACTIONS
GI: temporary darkening of tongue
and stools.
Other: salicylism (high doses).

Italicized side effects are common or life-threatening.
*Liquid form contains alcohol.   **May contain tartrazine.

INTERACTIONS
None significant.

NURSING CONSIDERATIONS
• Warn patient that bismuth subsalicylate contains a large amount of salicylate. Should be used cautiously in patients already taking aspirin.
• Instruct patient to chew tablets well.
• Both the liquid and tablet forms of Pepto-Bismol are effective against traveler's diarrhea. Tablets may be more convenient to carry.

---

difenoxin hydrochloride
Motofen

Pregnancy Risk Category: C

MECHANISM OF ACTION
Exerts a direct effect on the intestinal wall to slow motility.

INDICATIONS AND DOSAGE
Adjunct in acute nonspecific diarrhea, and acute exacerbations of chronic functional diarrhea—
Adults: Initially 2 mg P.O., then 1 mg P.O. after each loose bowel movement. Total dosage should not exceed 8 mg daily. Not recommended for use longer than 2 days.

ADVERSE REACTIONS
CNS: dizziness and light-headedness, drowsiness, headache, fatigue, nervousness, insomnia, confusion.
EENT: burning eyes, blurred vision.
GI: nausea, vomiting, dry mouth, epigastric distress, constipation.

INTERACTIONS
Alcohol, CNS depressants, tranquilizers, narcotics, barbiturates: enhanced CNS depression. Closely monitor patients.
MAO inhibitors: potential hypertensive crisis. Avoid concomitant use.

NURSING CONSIDERATIONS
• Contraindicated in patients with hypersensitivity to difenoxin or atropine, in children under 2 years, and in patients with diarrhea from pseudomembraneous colitis associated with antibiotics. Also contraindicated in patients with jaundice, or diarrhea from organisms that may penetrate the intestinal mucosa (including toxigenic *Escherichia coli, Salmonella,* or *Shigella*).
• Difenoxin is the principal metabolite of diphenoxylate (Lomotil) and is chemically related to meperidine. Use cautiously in patients with a history of drug abuse, or in those currently receiving drugs with a high abuse potential.
• Atropine has been added to difenoxin to prevent abuse. The small dosage of atropine is unlikely to cause any significant clinical problems, but patients may experience dry mouth, tachycardia, urine retention, and flushing. Monitor for these effects.
• Advise patients to avoid hazardous activities that may require mental alertness, such as driving or operating heavy machinery, until the CNS effects of the drug are known.
• Monitor patients closely for fluid and electrolyte imbalance. Difenoxin-induced decreases in peristalsis may result in fluid retention in the colon, with subsequent dehydration and possibly delayed difenoxin intoxication.
• Advise patient to adhere to dosing schedule. Overdose with difenoxin may result in respiratory depression and coma. Encourage proper storage to keep drug out of children's reach.
• Patients who overdose with difenoxin should be observed for at least 48 hours. Respiratory depression may occur up to 30 hours after ingestion. Gastric lavage, establishment of a patent airway, and mechanically assisted ventilation are advised. Naloxone will reverse the respiratory depression. Because difenoxin has a longer duration of action than naloxone, repeated injections of naloxone will be neces-

---

sary.

diphenoxylate hydrochloride
Diphenatol, Lofene, Logen, Lomanate, Lomotil*♦, Lonox, Lo-Trol, Low-Quel, Nor-Mil
Controlled Substance Schedule V

Pregnancy Risk Category: C

MECHANISM OF ACTION
Increases smooth muscle tone in the GI tract, inhibits motility and propulsion, and diminishes secretions.

INDICATIONS & DOSAGE
Acute, nonspecific diarrhea—
Adults: initially, 5 mg P.O. q.i.d., then adjust dosage.
Children 2 to 12 years: 0.3 to 0.4 mg/kg P.O. daily in 4 divided doses, using liquid form only. For maintenance, initial dose may be reduced by as much as 75%.
　Don't use in children under 2 years.

ADVERSE REACTIONS
CNS: *sedation, dizziness,* headache, drowsiness, lethargy, restlessness, depression, euphoria.
CV: tachycardia.
EENT: mydriasis.
GI: *dry mouth,* nausea, vomiting, abdominal discomfort or distention, *paralytic ileus,* anorexia, fluid retention in bowel (may mask depletion of extracellular fluid and electrolytes, especially in young children treated for acute gastroenteritis).
GU: urine retention.
Skin: pruritus, giant urticaria, rash.
Other: possibly physical dependence in long-term use, angioedema, respiratory depression.

INTERACTIONS
None significant.

NURSING CONSIDERATIONS
• Contraindicated in acute diarrhea

resulting from poison until toxic material is eliminated from GI tract; acute diarrhea caused by organisms that penetrate intestinal mucosa; diarrhea resulting from antibiotic-induced pseudomembranous enterocolitis; and in jaundiced patients. Use cautiously in children, in hepatic disease and narcotic dependence, and in pregnant women. Use cautiously in acute ulcerative colitis. Stop therapy immediately if abdominal distention or other signs of toxic megacolon develop.
• Risk of physical dependence increases with high dosage and long-term use. Atropine sulfate is included to discourage abuse.
• Not likely to be effective if there is no response within 48 hours.
• Patient should not use to treat acute diarrhea for longer than 2 days and should seek medical attention if diarrhea continues.
• Warn patient not to exceed recommended dosage.
• Dehydration, especially in young children, may increase risk of delayed toxicity. Correct fluid and electrolyte disturbances before starting drug.
• Dose of 2.5 mg is as effective as 5 ml camphorated tincture of opium.
• Not indicated in treatment of antibiotic-induced diarrhea.

kaolin and pectin mixtures◇
Donnagel-MB♦♦, Kao-Con♦♦, Kaopectate♦, Kaopectate Concentrate, Kao-tin, Kapectolin, K-C, K-P, K-Pek

Pregnancy Risk Category: C

MECHANISM OF ACTION
Decrease the stool's fluid content, although *total* water loss seems to remain the same.

INDICATIONS & DOSAGE
Mild, nonspecific diarrhea—
Adults: 60 to 120 ml P.O. after each bowel movement.

Italicized side effects are common or life-threatening.
*Liquid form contains alcohol.　　　**May contain tartrazine.

Children over 12 years: 60 ml P.O. after each bowel movement.
Children 6 to 12 years: 30 to 60 ml P.O. after each bowel movement.
Children 3 to 6 years: 15 to 30 ml P.O. after each bowel movement.

ADVERSE REACTIONS
GI: drug absorbs nutrients, drugs, and enzymes; fecal impaction or ulceration in infants and elderly or debilitated patients after chronic use; constipation.

INTERACTIONS
None significant.

NURSING CONSIDERATIONS
• Contraindicated in suspected obstructive bowel lesions.
• Don't use for more than 2 days.
• Don't use in place of specific therapy for underlying cause.
• May reduce absorption of other P.O. drugs, requiring dosage adjustments.
• It is a GI absorbent.

lactobacillus◊
Bacid♦, Lactinex♦
Pregnancy Risk Category: C

MECHANISM OF ACTION
Helps reestablish normal intestinal flora and suppresses the growth of pathogenic microorganisms.

INDICATIONS & DOSAGE
Diarrhea, especially that caused by antibiotics—
Adults: 2 capsules (Bacid) P.O. b.i.d., t.i.d., or q.i.d., preferably with milk; or 4 tablets or 1 packet (Lactinex) P.O. t.i.d. or q.i.d., preferably with food, milk, or juice.

ADVERSE REACTIONS
GI: (with Bacid) increased intestinal flatus at beginning of therapy; subsides with continued therapy.

INTERACTIONS
None significant.

NURSING CONSIDERATIONS
• Contraindicated in fever.
• Don't use for more than 2 days.
• Store in refrigerator.
• Diet containing large amounts of carbohydrate (up to 400 g), such as lactose, lactulose, and dextrin, may be more effective than lactobacillus in reestablishing normal flora after antibiotic therapy.
• Controversial form of diarrhea treatment.
• May be used prophylactically in patients with history of antibiotic-induced diarrhea.

loperamide◊
Imodium♦, Imodium A-D
Pregnancy Risk Category: B

MECHANISM OF ACTION
Inhibits peristaltic activity, prolonging transit of intestinal contents.

INDICATIONS & DOSAGE
Acute, nonspecific diarrhea—
Adults: initially, 4 mg P.O., then 2 mg after each unformed stool. Maximum 16 mg daily.
Children 8 to 12 years: 10 ml t.i.d. P.O. on first day. (Subsequent doses of 5 ml per 10 kg of body weight may be administered after each unformed stool.)
Children 5 to 8 years: 10 ml P.O. b.i.d. on first day.
Children 2 to 5 years: 5 ml P.O. t.i.d. on first day.
Chronic diarrhea—
Adults: initially, 4 mg P.O., then 2 mg after each unformed stool until diarrhea subsides. Adjust dosage to individual response.

ADVERSE REACTIONS
CNS: drowsiness, fatigue, dizziness.
GI: dry mouth; abdominal pain, dis-

tention, or discomfort; *constipation;* nausea; vomiting.
Skin: rash.

INTERACTIONS
None significant.

NURSING CONSIDERATIONS
• Contraindicated in acute diarrhea resulting from poison until toxic material is removed from GI tract, in acute diarrhea caused by organisms that penetrate intestinal mucosa, and when constipation must be avoided. Use cautiously in severe prostatic hypertrophy, hepatic disease, and history of narcotic dependence.
• Stop drug immediately if abdominal distention or other symptoms develop in acute colitis.
• In acute diarrhea, discontinue drug and seek medical attention if no improvement occurs within 48 hours; in chronic diarrhea, discontinue drug if no improvement occurs after giving 16 mg daily for at least 10 days.
• Warn patient not to exceed recommended dosage.
• Produces antidiarrheal action similar to diphenoxylate hydrochloride but without as many adverse CNS effects.

---

opium tincture*
Controlled Substance Schedule II

opium tincture, camphorated* (Paregoric)
Controlled Substance Schedule III

Pregnancy Risk Category: B (D for prolonged use or high doses at term)

MECHANISM OF ACTION
Increases smooth muscle tone in the GI tract, inhibits motility and propulsion, and diminishes secretions.

INDICATIONS & DOSAGE
Acute, nonspecific diarrhea—
Adults: 0.6 ml opium tincture (range 0.3 to 1 ml) P.O. q.i.d. Maximum dosage 6 ml daily; or 5 to 10 ml camphorated opium tincture daily b.i.d., t.i.d., or q.i.d. until diarrhea subsides.
Children: 0.25 to 0.5 ml/kg camphorated opium tincture daily, b.i.d., t.i.d., or q.i.d. until diarrhea subsides.

ADVERSE REACTIONS
GI: nausea, vomiting.
Other: physical dependence after long-term use.

INTERACTIONS
None significant.

NURSING CONSIDERATIONS
• Contraindicated in acute diarrhea resulting from poison until toxic material is removed from GI tract, and diarrhea caused by organisms that penetrate intestinal mucosa. Use cautiously in asthma, prostatic hypertrophy, hepatic disease, and narcotic dependence.
• Risk of physical dependence increases with long-term use.
• Don't use for more than 2 days.
• An effective and prompt-acting antidiarrheal; but unique because dosage can be adjusted precisely to patient's needs.
• Opium content of opium tincture 25 times greater than camphorated tincture of opium. Camphorated opium tincture is more dilute, and teaspoonful doses are easier to measure than dropper quantities of opium tincture.
• Milky fluid forms when camphorated opium tincture is added to water.
• Camphorated opium tincture 0.06 to 0.5 ml daily has been used to treat infants with mild narcotic physical dependence.
• Store in tightly capped, light-resistant container.

Italicized side effects are common or life-threatening.
*Liquid form contains alcohol.   **May contain tartrazine.

• Mix with sufficient water to ensure passage to stomach.
• Narcotic antagonist naloxone can reverse the respiratory depression resulting from overdose.

48

Laxatives

bisacodyl◊
calcium polycarbophil◊
cascara sagrada◊
cascara sagrada aromatic
   fluid extract◊
cascara sagrada fluid extract◊
castor oil◊
docusate calcium◊
docusate potassium◊
docusate sodium (dioctyl sodium
   sulfosuccinate)◊
glycerin◊
lactulose
magnesium salts◊
methylcellulose◊
mineral oil (liquid petrolatum)◊
phenolphthalein◊
polyethylene glycol-electrolyte
   solution
psyllium◊
senna◊
sodium biphosphate
sodium phosphate

COMBINATION PRODUCTS

AGORAL◊: mineral oil 28% and white
phenolphthalein 1.3% in emulsion,
with tragacanth, agar, egg albumin,
acacia, and glycerin.
DIALOSE-PLUS◊: docusate potassium
100 mg and casanthranol 30 mg.
DIOLAX◊: docusate sodium 100 mg
and casanthranol 50 mg.
DOXIDAN◊: docusate calcium 60 mg
and phenolphthalein 65 mg.
D-S-S PLUS◊: docusate sodium 100
mg and casanthranol 30 mg.
HALEY'S M-O◊: mineral oil (25%)
and magnesium hydroxide.
KONDREMUL WITH CASCARA◊♦:
heavy mineral oil 55%, cascara sa-

grada extract 660 mg/15 ml, and Irish
moss as emulsifier.
KONDREMUL WITH PHENOLPHTHA-
LEIN◊♦: heavy mineral oil 55%, white
phenolphthalein 150 mg/15 ml, and
Irish moss as emulsifier.
MODANE PLUS◊: docusate sodium 100
mg and phenolphthalein 60 mg.
PERI-COLACE◊♦ (capsules): docusate
sodium 100 mg and casanthranol 30
mg.
PERI-COLACE◊ (syrup): docusate sodium 60 mg and casanthranol 30 mg/
15 ml.
SENOKOT-S◊♦: docusate sodium 50
mg and standardized senna concentrate 187 mg.

---

bisacodyl◊
Bisacolax♦♦, Bisco-Lax**♦,
Dacodyl, Deficol, Dulcolax♦, Fleet
Bisacodyl, Fleet Bisacodyl Prep,
Laxit♦♦, Theralax

Pregnancy Risk Category: C

MECHANISM OF ACTION
Increases peristalsis by direct effect
on the smooth muscle of the intestine.
Thought either to irritate the musculature or to stimulate the colonic intramural plexus. Also promotes fluid
accumulation in the colon and small
intestine. A stimulant laxative.

INDICATIONS & DOSAGE
*Chronic constipation; preparation for
delivery, surgery, or rectal or bowel
examination—*
Adults: 10 to 15 mg P.O. in evening
or before breakfast. Up to 30 mg may

Italicized side effects are common or life-threatening.
*Liquid form contains alcohol.   **May contain tartrazine.

be used for thorough evacuation needed for examinations or surgery.
Children 6 years and older: 5 to 10 mg P.O.
Rectal:
Adults and children over 2 years: 10 mg.
Children under 2 years: 5 mg.

ADVERSE REACTIONS
CNS: muscle weakness in excessive use.
GI: *nausea, vomiting, abdominal cramps,* diarrhea with high doses, *burning sensation in rectum with suppositories.*
Metabolic: alkalosis, hypokalemia, tetany, protein-losing enteropathy in excessive use, fluid and electrolyte imbalance.
Other: laxative dependence in long-term or excessive use.

INTERACTIONS
None significant.

NURSING CONSIDERATIONS
• Contraindicated in patients with abdominal pain, nausea, vomiting, or other symptoms of appendicitis or acute surgical abdomen, or in rectal fissures or ulcerated hemorrhoids.
• Tell patient to swallow enteric-coated tablet whole to avoid GI irritation. Don't give within one hour of milk or antacid intake. Begins to act 6 to 12 hours after oral administration.
• Soft, formed stool usually produced 15 to 60 minutes after rectal administration. Time administration of drug so as not to interfere with scheduled activities or sleep.
• Tablets and suppositories may be used together to cleanse colon before and after surgery and before barium enema.
• Use for short-term treatment. A stimulant laxative, this type of laxative is most abused. Discourage excessive use.
• Before giving for constipation, de-

termine if patient has adequate fluid intake, exercise, and diet. Tell him that dietary sources of bulk include bran and other cereals, fresh fruit, and vegetables.
• Store tablets and suppositories at temperature below 86° F. (30° C.).
• Tell patient to report adverse effects to the doctor.

---

calcium polycarbophil ◇
Equalactin, Fibercon, Mitrolan ♦
Pregnancy Risk Category: C

MECHANISM OF ACTION
Absorbs water and expands to increase bulk and moisture content of the stool. The increased bulk encourages peristalsis and bowel movement. A bulk-forming laxative. As an antidiarrheal, absorbs free fecal water, thereby producing formed stools.

INDICATIONS & DOSAGE
Constipation (Mitrolan must be chewed before swallowing)—
Adults: 1 g P.O. q.i.d. as required. Maximum 6 g in 24-hour period.
Children 6 to 12 years: 500 mg P.O. t.i.d. as required. Maximum 3 g in 24-hour period.
Children 2 to 6 years: 500 mg P.O. b.i.d. as required. Maximum 1.5 g in 24-hour period.
Diarrhea associated with irritable bowel syndrome, as well as acute nonspecific diarrhea (Mitrolan must be chewed before swallowing)—
Adults: 1 g P.O. q.i.d. as required. Maximum 6 g in 24-hour period.
Children 6 to 12 years 500 mg P.O. t.i.d. as required. Maximum 3 g in 24-hour period.
Children 2 to 6 years: 500 mg P.O. b.i.d. as required. Maximum 1.5 g in 24-hour period.

ADVERSE REACTIONS
GI: abdominal fullness and increased flatus, intestinal obstruction.

Other: laxative dependence in long-term or excessive use.

INTERACTIONS
None significant.

NURSING CONSIDERATIONS
• Contraindicated in signs of GI obstruction.
• Rectal bleeding or failure to respond to therapy may indicate need for surgery.
• Before giving for constipation, determine if patient has adequate fluid intake, exercise, and diet. Tell him that dietary sources of bulk include bran and other cereals, fresh fruit, and vegetables.
• Advise patient to chew the Mitrolan tablets thoroughly and drink a full glass of water with each dose. However, when used as an antidiarrheal, tell patient *not* to drink a glass of water.
• For episodes of severe diarrhea, the dose may be repeated every half hour, but maximum daily dosage should not be exceeded.

---

cascara sagrada◇

cascara sagrada aromatic fluid extract*◇

cascara sagrada fluid extract*◇

Pregnancy Risk Category: C

MECHANISM OF ACTION
Increases peristalsis by direct effect on the smooth muscle of the intestine. Thought either to irritate the musculature or to stimulate the colonic intramural plexus. Also promotes fluid accumulation in the colon and small intestine. A stimulant laxative.

INDICATIONS & DOSAGE
Acute constipation; preparation for bowel or rectal examination—

Adults: 325 mg cascara sagrada tablets P.O. h.s.; or 1 ml fluid extract daily; or 5 ml aromatic fluid extract daily.
Children 2 to 12 years: ½ adult dose.
Children under 2 years: ¼ adult dose.

ADVERSE REACTIONS
GI: *nausea;* vomiting; diarrhea; loss of normal bowel function with excessive use; *abdominal cramps,* especially in severe constipation; malabsorption of nutrients; "cathartic colon" (syndrome resembling ulcerative colitis radiologically and pathologically) after chronic misuse; discoloration of rectal mucosa after long-term use.
Metabolic: hypokalemia, protein enteropathy, electrolyte imbalance in excessive use.
Other: laxative dependence in long-term or excessive use.

INTERACTIONS
None significant.

NURSING CONSIDERATIONS
• Contraindicated in abdominal pain, nausea, vomiting, or other symptoms of appendicitis or acute surgical abdomen; acute surgical delirium, fecal impaction, intestinal obstruction or perforation. Use cautiously when rectal bleeding is present.
• Aromatic cascara fluidextract is less active and less bitter than nonaromatic fluid extract.
• Liquid preparations more reliable than solid dosage forms.
• Before giving for constipation, determine if patient has adequate fluid intake, exercise, and diet. Tell him that dietary sources of bulk include bran and other cereals, fresh fruit, and vegetables.
• May turn alkaline urine red-pink and acidic urine yellow-brown.
• Monitor serum electrolytes during

Italicized side effects are common or life-threatening.
*Liquid form contains alcohol.   **May contain tartrazine.

prolonged use.
• Onset of action is 6 to 12 hours.

castor oil◊
Alphamul, Emulsoil, Fleet Flavored
Castor Oil, Kellogg's Castor Oil,
Neoloid♦, Purge

Pregnancy Risk Category: X

MECHANISM OF ACTION
Increases peristalsis by direct effect
on the smooth muscle of the intestine.
Thought either to irritate the musculature or to stimulate the colonic intramural plexus. Also promotes fluid
accumulation in the colon and small
intestine. A stimulant laxative.

INDICATIONS & DOSAGE
Preparation for rectal or bowel exami-
nation, or surgery; acute constipation
(rarely)—
Adults: 15 to 60 ml P.O.
Children over 2 years: 5 to 15 ml
P.O.
Children under 2 years: 1.25 to 7.5
ml P.O.
Infants: up to 4 ml P.O. Increased
dose produces no greater effect.

ADVERSE REACTIONS
GI: *nausea;* vomiting; diarrhea; loss
of normal bowel function with excessive use; *abdominal cramps,* especially in severe constipation; malabsorption of nutrients; "cathartic colon" (syndrome resembling ulcerative
colitis radiologically and pathologically) in chronic misuse. May cause
constipation after catharsis.
GU: pelvic congestion in menstruating women.
Metabolic: hypokalemia, protein-losing enteropathy, other electrolyte imbalance in excessive use.
Other: laxative dependence in long-
term or excessive use.

INTERACTIONS
None significant.

NURSING CONSIDERATIONS
• Contraindicated in ulcerative bowel
lesions; during menstruation; in abdominal pain, nausea, vomiting, or
other symptoms of appendicitis or
acute surgical abdomen; in anal or
rectal fissures, fecal impaction, intestinal obstruction or perforation; and in
pregnancy. Use cautiously in rectal
bleeding.
• Failure to respond may indicate
acute condition requiring surgery.
• Give with juice or carbonated beverage to mask oily taste. Patient
should stir mixture and drink it
promptly. Ice held in mouth before
taking drug will help prevent tasting
it.
• Shake emulsion well. Store below
40° F. (4.4° C.). Don't freeze.
• Give on empty stomach for best results.
• Produces complete evacuation after
3 hours. Tell patient that after castor
oil has emptied bowel he will not have
bowel movement for 1 to 2 days.
• Time drug administration so that it
doesn't interfere with scheduled activities or sleep.
• Monitor serum electrolytes during
prolonged use.
• Generally used before diagnostic
testing or therapy requiring thorough
evacuation of GI tract.
• Use for short-term treatment. Not
recommended for routine use; useful
for acute constipation not responsive
to milder laxatives.
• Before giving for constipation, determine if patient has adequate fluid
intake, exercise, and diet. Tell him
that dietary sources of bulk include
bran and other cereals, fresh fruit,
and vegetables.
• Increased intestinal motility lessens
absorption of concomitantly administered P.O. drugs. Reschedule dose.
• Castor oil affects the small intestine. Regular use may cause excessive
loss of water and salt.
• Castor oil emulsion is better toler-

Unmarked trade names available in the United States only.
♦ Also available in Canada.   ♦♦ Available in Canada only.   ◊ Also available OTC.

ated but is more expensive.

docusate calcium◇
Pro-Cal-Sof, Surfak

docusate potassium◇
Dialose, Diocto-K, Kasof

docusate sodium (dioctyl sodium sulfosuccinate)◇
Afko-Lube, Colace, Diocto, Dioeze, Diosuccin, Dio-Sul, Disonate, Di-Sosul, Doss, Doxinate, D-S-S, Duosol, Genasoft, Laxinate 100, Modane Soft, Pro-sof, Sof, Pro-Sof Liquid Concentrate, Regulax SS, Regutol, Stulex

Pregnancy Risk Category: C

MECHANISM OF ACTION
Reduces surface tension of interfacing liquid contents of the bowel. This detergent activity promotes incorporation of additional liquid into the stool, forming a softer mass. A stool softener.

INDICATIONS & DOSAGE
Stool softener—
Adults and older children: 50 to 300 mg (docusate sodium) P.O. daily or 50 to 300 mg (docusate calcium and docusate potassium) P.O. daily until bowel movements are normal.
Children 6 to 12 years: 40 to 120 mg (docusate sodium) P.O. daily.
Children 3 to 6 years: 20 to 60 mg (docusate sodium) P.O. daily.
Children under 3 years: 10 to 40 mg (docusate sodium) P.O. daily.
    Higher dosages are for initial therapy. Adjust dosage to individual response. Usual dosage in children and adults with minimal needs: 50 to 150 mg (docusate calcium) P.O. daily.

ADVERSE REACTIONS
EENT: throat irritation.
GI: bitter taste, mild abdominal cramping, diarrhea.
Other: laxative dependence in long-term or excessive use.

INTERACTIONS
Mineral oil: may increase mineral oil absorption and cause lipoid pneumonia. Don't administer together.

NURSING CONSIDERATIONS
• Should only be used occasionally. Don't use for more than 1 week without doctor's knowledge.
• Give liquid in milk, fruit juice, or infant formula to mask bitter taste.
• Not for use in treating existing constipation, but prevents constipation from developing.
• Laxative of choice in patients who should not strain during defecation, such as those recovering from myocardial infarction or rectal surgery; in disease of rectum and anus that makes passage of firm stool difficult; or in postpartum constipation.
• Acts within 24 to 48 hours to produce firm, semisolid stool.
• Instruct patient that dietary sources of bulk include bran and other cereals, fresh fruit, and vegetables.
• Doesn't stimulate intestinal peristaltic movements.
• Discontinue if severe cramping occurs.
• Store at 59° to 86° F. (15° to 30° C.). Protect liquid from light.
• Many doctors feel that the minimum effective dosage is 300 mg daily. A lower dosage may not produce satisfactory results.

glycerin◇
Fleet Babylax, Sani-Supp
Pregnancy Risk Category: C

MECHANISM OF ACTION
Draws water from the tissues into the feces and thus stimulates evacuation. A hyperosmolar laxative.

Italicized side effects are common or life-threatening.
*Liquid form contains alcohol.   **May contain tartrazine.

INDICATIONS & DOSAGE
Constipation—
Adults and children over 6 years:
3 g as a rectal suppository; or 5 to 15
ml as an enema.
Children under 6 years: 1 to 1.5 g as
a rectal suppository; or 2 to 5 ml as an
enema.

ADVERSE REACTIONS
GI: *cramping pain,* rectal discomfort,
hyperemia of rectal mucosa.

INTERACTIONS
None significant.

NURSING CONSIDERATIONS
• A hyperosmolar laxative used
mainly to reestablish proper toilet
habits in laxative-dependent patients.
• Must be retained for at least 15
minutes; usually acts within 1 hour.
Entire suppository need not melt to be
effective.

---

lactulose
Cephulac♦, Cholac, Chronulac♦,
Constilac, Lactulax♦♦
Pregnancy Risk Category: C

MECHANISM OF ACTION
Produces an osmotic effect in the colon. Resultant distention promotes
peristalsis. Also decreases blood ammonia, probably as a result of bacterial degradation, which decreases the
pH of colon contents.

INDICATIONS & DOSAGE
Treatment of constipation—
Adults: 15 to 30 ml P.O. daily.
*To prevent and treat portal-systemic
encephalopathy, including hepatic
precoma and coma in patients with severe hepatic disease—*
Adults: initially, 20 to 30 g P.O. (30
to 45 ml) t.i.d. or q.i.d., until two or
three soft stools are produced daily.
Usual dosage is 60 to 100 g daily in
divided doses. Can also be given by

retention
fluid.

ADV
GI: a
diarrhe
lence.
Metabolic: hy

INTERACTIONS
None significant.

NURSING CONSIDER
• Contraindicated in low-ga
diet. Use cautiously in diabete
tus.
• Reduce dosage if diarrhea occurs.
Replace fluid loss.
• Monitor serum sodium for possible
hypernatremia, especially when giving in higher doses to treat hepatic encephalopathy.
• Minimize drug's sweet taste by diluting with water or fruit juice or giving with food.
• Store at room temperature, preferably below 86° F. (30° C.). Don't
freeze.

---

magnesium salts◊
Concentrated Milk of Magnesia,
Magnesium Citrate, Magnesium
Sulfate, Milk of Magnesia
Pregnancy Risk Category: B

MECHANISM OF ACTION
Produces an osmotic effect in the
small intestine by drawing water into
the intestinal lumen. A saline laxative.

INDICATIONS & DOSAGE
*Constipation, to evacuate bowel be-
fore surgery—*
Adults and children over 6 years: 15
g magnesium sulfate P.O. in glass of
water; or 10 to 20 ml concentrated
Milk of Magnesia P.O.; or 15 to 60 ml
Milk of Magnesia P.O.; or 5 to 10 oz
magnesium citrate h.s.

Unmarked trade names available in the United States only.
♦Also available in Canada. ♦♦Available in Canada only. ◊Also available OTC.

ml Milk of Magnesia
...s.
...o 12 years: 15 to 30 ml
...agnesia P.O.
...2 to 6 years: 5 to 15 ml
...Magnesia P.O.

...RSE REACTIONS
...bdominal cramping, nausea.
...tabolic: fluid and electrolyte dis-
...bances if used daily.
...ther: laxative dependence in long-
term or excessive use.

INTERACTIONS
None significant.

NURSING CONSIDERATIONS
• Contraindicated in abdominal pain,
nausea, vomiting, or other symptoms
of appendicitis or acute surgical abdomen; and in myocardial damage,
heart block, imminent delivery, fecal
impaction, rectal fissures, intestinal
obstruction or perforation, or renal
disease. Use cautiously in rectal
bleeding.
• Shake suspension well; give with
large amount of water when used as
laxative. When administering through
nasogastric tube, make sure tube is
placed properly and is patent. After
instilling, flush tube with water to ensure passage to stomach and maintain
tube patency.
• For short-term therapy; don't use
longer than 1 week.
• When used as laxative, don't give
oral drugs 1 to 2 hours before or after
administration.
• As a saline laxative, drug produces
watery stool in 3 to 6 hours. Time
drug administration so that it doesn't
interfere with scheduled activities or
sleep.
• Magnesium sulfate is more potent
than other saline laxatives.
• Before giving for constipation, determine if patient has adequate fluid
intake, exercise, and diet. Tell him

that dietary sources of bulk include
bran and other cereals, fresh fruit,
and vegetables.
• Magnesium may accumulate in
renal insufficiency.
• Chilling before use may make magnesium citrate more palatable.
• Monitor serum electrolytes during
prolonged use.
• Frequent or prolonged use as a laxative may cause dependence.

methylcellulose◇
Citrucel, Cologel

Pregnancy Risk Category: C

MECHANISM OF ACTION
Absorbs water and expands to increase bulk and moisture content of
the stool. The increased bulk encourages peristalsis and bowel movement.
A bulk-forming laxative.

INDICATIONS & DOSAGE
Chronic constipation—
Adults: 5 to 20 ml liquid P.O. t.i.d.
with a glass of water; or 15 ml syrup
P.O. morning and evening.
Children: 5 to 10 ml P.O. daily or
b.i.d.

ADVERSE REACTIONS
GI: *nausea,* vomiting, diarrhea (all
after excessive use); esophageal, gastric, small intestinal, or colonic strictures when drug is chewed or taken in
dry form; *abdominal cramps,* especially in severe constipation.
Other: laxative dependence in long-
term or excessive use.

INTERACTIONS
None significant.

NURSING CONSIDERATIONS
• Contraindicated in abdominal pain,
nausea, vomiting, or other symptoms
of appendicitis or acute surgical abdomen; and in intestinal obstruction or
ulceration, disabling adhesion, or dif-

ficulty swallowing.
• Laxative effect usually takes 12 to 24 hours, but may be delayed 3 days.
• Tell patient to take drug with at least 8 oz (240 ml) of pleasant-tasting liquid to mask grittiness.
• Especially useful in postpartum constipation, debilitated patients, chronic laxative abuse, irritable bowel syndrome, diverticular disease, colostomies, and to empty colon before barium enema examinations.
• Before giving for constipation, determine if patient has adequate fluid intake, exercise, and diet. Tell him that dietary sources of bulk include bran and other cereals, fresh fruit, and vegetables.
• Not absorbed systemically; nontoxic.

mineral oil
(liquid petrolatum)◇
Agoral Plain♦, Fleet Mineral Oil, Kondremul Plain♦, Lansoyl, Milkinol, Neo-Cultol, Nujol, Petrogalar Plain, Zymenol

Pregnancy Risk Category: C

MECHANISM OF ACTION
Increases water retention in the stool by creating a barrier between colon wall and feces that prevents colonic reabsorption of fecal water. A lubricant laxative.

INDICATIONS & DOSAGE
Constipation; preparation for bowel studies or surgery—
Adults: 15 to 30 ml P.O. h.s.; or 120 ml enema.
Children: 5 to 15 ml P.O. h.s.; or 30 to 60 ml enema.

ADVERSE REACTIONS
GI: *nausea;* vomiting; diarrhea in excessive use; *abdominal cramps,* especially in severe constipation; decreased absorption of nutrients and fat-soluble vitamins, resulting in defi-

ciency; and slowed healing after hemorrhoidectomy.
Other: laxative dependence in long-term or excessive use, pruritus.

INTERACTIONS
Docusate salts: may increase mineral oil absorption and cause lipid pneumonia. Don't administer together.
Fat soluble vitamins (A,D,E,K): absorption may be decreased after prolonged administration.

NURSING CONSIDERATIONS
• Contraindicated in abdominal pain, nausea, vomiting, or other symptoms of appendicitis or acute surgical abdomen; and in fecal impaction, or intestinal obstruction or perforation. Use cautiously in young children; in elderly or debilitated patients because of susceptibility to lipid pneumonitis through aspiration, absorption, and transport from intestinal mucosa; and in rectal bleeding. Enema contraindicated in children under 2 years.
• Don't give drug with meals or immediately after, as it delays passage of food from stomach. More active on an empty stomach.
• To be taken only at bedtime. Warn patient not to take for more than 1 week.
• Give with fruit juices or carbonated drinks to disguise taste.
• Use when patient needs to ease the strain of evacuation.
• Warn patient of possible rectal leakage from excessive dosages so he can avoid soiling clothing.
• Before giving for constipation, determine if patient has adequate fluid intake, exercise, and diet. Tell him that dietary sources of bulk include bran and other cereals, fresh fruit, and vegetables.
• Onset of action is 6 to 8 hours.

phenolphthalein◊

Alophen**, Correctol, Espotabs, Evac-U-Gen, Evac-U-Lax, Ex-Lax, Ex-Lax Pills, Feen-A-Mint Gum, Modane, Modane Mild, Phenolax Wafers, Prulet

Pregnancy Risk Category: C

MECHANISM OF ACTION

Increases peristalsis by direct effect on the smooth muscle of the intestine. Thought either to irritate the musculature or to stimulate the colonic intramural plexus. Also promotes fluid accumulation in the colon and small intestine. A stimulant laxative.

INDICATIONS & DOSAGE

Constipation—
Adults and children over 12 years:
30 to 270 mg P.O., preferably h.s.
Children 6 to 11 years: 30 to 60 mg P.O. h.s.
Children 2 to 5 years: 15 to 30 mg P.O. h.s.

ADVERSE REACTIONS

GI: diarrhea; *colic in large doses;* factitious nausea; vomiting; loss of normal bowel function in excessive use; *abdominal cramps,* especially in severe constipation; malabsorption of nutrients; "cathartic colon" (syndrome resembling ulcerative colitis radiologically and pathologically) in chronic misuse; reddish discoloration in alkaline feces or urine.
Skin: dermatitis, pruritus, rash, pigmentation.
Other: laxative dependence in long-term or excessive use, *hypersensitivity*.

INTERACTIONS

None significant.

NURSING CONSIDERATIONS

• Contraindicated in abdominal pain, nausea, vomiting, or other symptoms of appendicitis or acute surgical abdo-

men; in fecal impaction, or intestinal obstruction or perforation. Use cautiously in rectal bleeding.
• Laxative effect may last up to 3 to 4 days.
• Produces semisolid stool within 6 to 8 hours. Time drug administration so that it doesn't interfere with scheduled activities or sleep.
• Warn patient with rash to avoid sun and discontinue use. Don't use any other product containing phenolphthalein.
• Before giving for constipation, determine if patient has adequate fluid intake, exercise, and diet. Tell him that dietary sources of bulk include bran and other cereals, fresh fruit, and vegetables.
• May discolor alkaline urine red-pink and acidic urine yellow-brown.
• Drug is available in many dosage forms. Most popular OTC laxative.
• Children may mistake for candy. Keep out of reach.
• Yellow phenolphthalein is two to three times as potent as white phenolphthalein.

---

polyethylene glycol-electrolyte solution

CoLyte, Glycoprep, GoLYTELY

Pregnancy Risk Category: C

MECHANISM OF ACTION

Polyethylene glycol 3350 (PEG 3350), a nonabsorbable solution, acts as an osmotic agent. Using sodium sulfate as the major sodium source, sodium absorption is greatly reduced. The electrolyte concentration results in virtually no net absorption or secretion of ions.

INDICATIONS & DOSAGE

Bowel preparation before GI examination—
Adults: 240 ml P.O. q 10 minutes until 4 liters are consumed. Usually administered 4 hours before examina-

---

tion, allowing 3 hours for drinking and 1 hour for bowel evacuation.

ADVERSE REACTIONS
GI: *nausea, bloating, cramps, vomiting.*

INTERACTIONS
None significant.

NURSING CONSIDERATIONS
• Contraindicated in GI obstruction or perforation, gastric retention, toxic colitis, or megacolon.
• If administered to semiconscious patients or to patients with impaired gag reflex, take care to prevent aspiration.
• No major shifts in fluid and electrolytes have been reported.
• Orally administered solution induces a diarrhea (onset 30 to 60 minutes) which rapidly cleanses the bowel, usually within 4 hours. The solution may be administered in the early morning, if the patient is scheduled for a mid-morning exam.
• May be less useful as a preparation for barium enema, because it may interfere with the barium coating of the colonic mucosa. To avoid such interference, administer solution the evening before the examination.
• Patient should fast for 3 to 4 hours before taking the solution, and thereafter ingest only clear fluids until the examination is complete.
• Tap water may be used to reconstitute powder. Shake vigorously to ensure that all powder is dissolved. Reconstituted solution may be refrigerated but should be used within 48 hours.
• Do not add flavoring or additional ingredients to the solution, and do not administer chilled solution. Hypothermia has been reported after ingestion of large amounts of chilled solution.

psyllium◊
Cillium, Konsyl, Metamucil♦,
Metamucil Instant Mix♦, Metamucil
Sugar Free, Naturacil, Perdiem
Plain, Siblin♦, Syllact

Pregnancy Risk Category: C

MECHANISM OF ACTION
Absorbs water and expands to increase bulk and moisture content of the stool. The increased bulk encourages peristalsis and bowel movement. A bulk-forming laxative.

INDICATIONS & DOSAGE
Constipation; bowel management—
Adults: 1 to 2 rounded teaspoonfuls P.O. in full glass of liquid daily, b.i.d. or t.i.d., followed by second glass of liquid; or 1 packet P.O. dissolved in water daily, b.i.d. or t.i.d.
Children over 6 years: 1 level teaspoonful P.O. in half a glass of liquid h.s.

ADVERSE REACTIONS
GI: nausea, vomiting, diarrhea, all after excessive use; esophageal, gastric, small intestinal, or colonic strictures when drug taken in dry form; abdominal cramps, especially in severe constipation.

INTERACTIONS
None significant.

NURSING CONSIDERATIONS
• Contraindicated in abdominal pain, nausea, vomiting, or other symptoms of appendicitis; and in intestinal obstruction or ulceration, disabling adhesion, or difficulty swallowing.
• In diabetic patients, use brand of psyllium that does not contain sugar. Check label.
• Mix with at least 8 oz (240 ml) of cold, pleasant-tasting liquid such as orange juice to mask grittiness, and stir only a few seconds. Patient should drink it immediately or mixture will

congeal. Follow with additional glass of liquid.

• Before giving for constipation, determine if patient has adequate fluid intake, exercise, and diet. Tell him that dietary sources of bulk include bran and other cereals, fresh fruit, and vegetables.

• May reduce appetite if taken before meals.

• Laxative effect usually seen in 12 to 24 hours, but may be delayed 3 days.

• Not absorbed systemically; nontoxic. Especially useful in postpartum constipation, debilitated patients, chronic laxative abuse, irritable bowel syndrome, diverticular disease, and in combination with other laxatives to empty colon before barium enema examinations.

---

senna◇
Black-Draught, Senokot♦, X-Prep Liquid*

Pregnancy Risk Category: C

MECHANISM OF ACTION
Increases peristalsis by direct effect on the smooth muscle of the intestine. Thought either to irritate the musculature or to stimulate the colonic intramural plexus. Also promotes fluid accumulation in the colon and small intestine. A stimulant laxative.

INDICATIONS & DOSAGE
Acute constipation, preparation for bowel or rectal examination—
Adults: Dosage range for Senokot: 1 to 8 tablets P.O.; ½ to 4 teaspoonfuls of granules added to liquid; 1 to 2 suppositories h.s.; 1 to 4 teaspoonfuls syrup h.s. Black-Draught: 2 tablets or ¼ to ½ level teaspoonfuls of granules mixed with water.
Children over 27 kg: half adult dose of tablets, granules, or syrup (except Black-Draught tablets and granules not recommended for children).
Children 1 month to 1 year: 1.25 to

2.5 ml Senokot syrup P.O. h.s.

X-Prep used solely as single dose for preradiographic bowel evacuation. Give 20 g powder dissolved in juice or 75 ml liquid between 2 p.m. and 4 p.m. on day before X-ray procedure. May be given in divided doses for elderly or debilitated patients.

ADVERSE REACTIONS
GI: *nausea;* vomiting; diarrhea; loss of normal bowel function in excessive use; *abdominal cramps,* especially in severe constipation; malabsorption of nutrients; "cathartic colon" (syndrome resembling ulcerative colitis radiologically) in chronic misuse; may cause constipation after catharsis; yellow, yellow-green cast to feces; diarrhea in nursing infants of mothers receiving senna; darkened pigmentation of rectal mucosa in long-term use, which is usually reversible within 4 to 12 months after stopping drug.
GU: red-pink discoloration in alkaline urine; yellow-brown color to acidic urine.
Metabolic: hypokalemia, protein-losing enteropathy, electrolyte imbalance with excessive use.
Other: laxative dependence in long-term or excessive use.

INTERACTIONS
None significant.

NURSING CONSIDERATIONS
• Contraindicated in ulcerative bowel lesions; in nausea, vomiting, abdominal pain, or other symptoms of appendicitis or acute surgical abdomen; fecal impaction; or intestinal obstruction or perforation.
• Use for short-term treatment.
• More potent than cascara sagrada. Acts in 6 to 10 hours. X-Prep Liquid gives thorough, strong bowel action beginning in 6 hours.
• Avoid exposing to excessive heat or light.
• Before giving for constipation, de-

---

termine if patient has adequate fluid intake, exercise, and diet. Tell him that dietary sources of bulk include bran and other cereals, fresh fruit, and vegetables.
• After X-Prep Liquid is taken, diet should be confined to clear liquids.
• Senna is one of the most effective laxatives for counteracting constipation caused by narcotic analgesics.

sodium biphosphate
Fleet Enema♦, Phospho-Soda**

sodium phosphate
Pregnancy Risk Category: C

MECHANISM OF ACTION
Produces an osmotic effect in the small intestine by drawing water into the intestinal lumen. A saline laxative.

INDICATIONS & DOSAGE
Constipation—
Adults: 5 to 20 ml liquid P.O. with water; or 4 g powder P.O. dissolved in warm water; or 20 to 46 ml solution mixed with 120 ml cold water; or 60 to 135 ml enema.

ADVERSE REACTIONS
GI: *abdominal cramping.*
Metabolic: fluid and electrolyte disturbances (hypernatremia, hyperphosphatemia) if used daily.
Other: laxative dependence in long-term or excessive use.

INTERACTIONS
None significant.

NURSING CONSIDERATIONS
• Contraindicated in abdominal pain, nausea, vomiting, or other symptoms of appendicitis or acute surgical abdomen; intestinal obstruction or perforation; edema; congestive heart failure; megacolon; impaired renal function; and in patients on salt-restricted diets.

• Use with caution in patients with large hemorrhoids or anal excoriations.
• Available in oral and rectal forms.
• Before giving for constipation, determine if patient has adequate fluid intake, exercise, and diet. Tell him that dietary sources of bulk include bran and other cereals, fresh fruit, and vegetables.
• Saline laxative; up to 10% of sodium content may be absorbed.
• Enema form elicits response in 5 to 10 minutes.
• Used in preparation for barium enema, sigmoidoscopy, and for treatment of fecal impaction.
• Also prescribed to treat hypercalcemia or as a phosphate replacement.

49

Emetics and antiemetics

apomorphine hydrochloride
benzquinamide hydrochloride
buclizine hydrochloride
chlorpromazine hydrochloride
(See Chapter 33, ANTIPSYCHOTICS.)
cyclizine hydrochloride◊
cyclizine lactate
dimenhydrinate◊
diphenidol
dronabinol
   (tetrahydrocannabinol)
ipecac syrup◊
meclizine hydrochloride◊
metoclopramide hydrochloride
nabilone
prochlorperazine
prochlorperazine edisylate◊
prochlorperazine maleate
scopolamine◊
trimethobenzamide
   hydrochloride

COMBINATION PRODUCTS
None.

---

apomorphine hydrochloride
Controlled Substance Schedule II

Pregnancy Risk Category: C

MECHANISM OF ACTION
Acts directly on the chemoreceptor
trigger zone in the medulla oblongata
to induce vomiting.

INDICATIONS & DOSAGE
To induce vomiting in poisoning—
Adults: 5 to 6 mg S.C. preceded by
200 to 300 ml water or, preferably,
evaporated milk. Don't repeat.
Children: 0.07 to 0.1 mg/kg S.C.

preceded by up to 2 glasses of water
or, preferably, evaporated milk.

ADVERSE REACTIONS
CNS: *depression, euphoria,* restlessness, tremor.
CV: *acute circulatory failure in elderly or debilitated patients,* tachycardia.
Other: *depressed respiratory center in
large or repeated doses.*

INTERACTIONS
*Antiemetics (such as antihistamines,
phenothiazines):* decreased emetic response, possibly with increased CNS
depression.

NURSING CONSIDERATIONS
• Contraindicated in patients with hypersensitivity to narcotics; impending
shock; corrosive poisoning; narcosis
resulting from opiates, barbiturates,
alcohol, or other CNS depressants;
and in patients too inebriated to stand
unaided. Use cautiously in children
and in patients who are debilitated,
have cardiac decompensation, or are
predisposed to nausea and vomiting.
• Don't give after ingestion of petroleum distillates (for example, kerosene, gasoline) or volatile oils; retching and vomiting may cause aspiration
and lead to bronchospasm, pulmonary
edema, or aspiration pneumonitis.
Vegetable oil will delay absorption of
these substances.
• Emetic action is increased if dosage
is followed immediately by water or
evaporated milk. Evaporated milk is
preferred because studies show that

Italicized side effects are common or life-threatening.
*Liquid form contains alcohol.   **May contain tartrazine.

water may increase absorption of toxic substances.

• Don't give after ingestion of caustic substances, such as lye; additional injury to the esophagus and mediastinum can occur.

• Keep narcotic antagonists, such as naloxone, available to help stop vomiting and to alleviate drowsiness.

• If delay in giving emetic is expected, give activated charcoal P.O. immediately. When absorbable poison is ingested, give activated charcoal P.O. immediately after apomorphine hydrochloride.

• Vomiting occurs in 5 to 10 minutes in adults. If vomiting doesn't occur within 15 minutes, gastric lavage should begin. Apomorphine is emetic of choice when rapid removal of poisons is necessary, and when identification of enteric-coated tablets or other ingested toxic material in vomitus is important. Stomach contents are usually expelled completely; vomitus may also contain material from upper portion of intestinal tract.

• Don't administer if solution for injection is discolored green or precipitate is present.

benzquinamide hydrochloride
Emete-Con

Pregnancy Risk Category: C

MECHANISM OF ACTION
Acts on the chemoreceptor trigger zone to inhibit nausea and vomiting.

INDICATIONS & DOSAGE
Nausea and vomiting associated with anesthesia and surgery—
Adults: 50 mg I.M. (0.5 mg/kg to 1 mg/kg). May repeat in 1 hour, and thereafter q 3 to 4 hours, p.r.n.; or 25 mg (0.2 mg/kg to 0.4 mg/kg) I.V. as single dose, administered slowly.

ADVERSE REACTIONS
CNS: *drowsiness,* fatigue, insomnia, restlessness, headache, excitation, tremors, twitching, dizziness.
CV: sudden rise in blood pressure and transient dysrhythmias (premature atrial and ventricular contractions, atrial fibrillation) after I.V. administration; hypertension; hypotension.
EENT: dry mouth, salivation, blurred vision.
GI: anorexia, nausea.
Skin: urticaria, rash.
Other: muscle weakness, flushing, hiccups, sweating, chills, fever. May mask symptoms of ototoxicity, brain tumor, or intestinal obstruction.

INTERACTIONS
None significant.

NURSING CONSIDERATIONS
• I.V. use contraindicated in cardiovascular disease. Don't give I.V. within 15 minutes of preanesthetic or cardiovascular drugs.

• Give I.M. injections in large muscle mass. Use deltoid area only if well developed. Be sure to aspirate syringe for I.M. injection to avoid inadvertent I.V. injection.

• Reconstituted solution is stable for 14 days at room temperature. Store dry powder and reconstituted solution in a light-resistant container.

• Precipitation occurs if reconstituted with 0.9% sodium chloride injection.

• Monitor blood pressure frequently.

• Excellent alternative if prochlorperazine (Compazine) is contraindicated.

buclizine hydrochloride
Bucladin-S**

Pregnancy Risk Category: C

MECHANISM OF ACTION
May affect neural pathways originating in the labyrinth to inhibit nausea and vomiting, but the exact mechanism of action is unknown.

INDICATIONS & DOSAGE

Motion sickness (prevention)—
Adults: 50 mg P.O. at least one half hour before beginning travel. If needed, may repeat another 50 mg P.O. after 4 to 6 hours.
Vertigo—
Adults: 50 mg P.O., up to 150 mg P.O. daily in severe cases. Maintenance dose is 50 mg b.i.d.

ADVERSE REACTIONS

CNS: *drowsiness,* headache, dizziness, jitters.
EENT: blurred vision, dry mouth.
GU: urine retention.
Other: may mask symptoms of ototoxicity, intestinal obstruction, or brain tumor.

INTERACTIONS

None significant.

NURSING CONSIDERATIONS

• Use cautiously in patients with glaucoma, GU or GI obstruction, and in elderly males with possible prostatic hypertrophy.
• Warn patient against driving and other activities that require alertness until CNS effects of the drug are known.
• Tablets may be placed in mouth and allowed to dissolve without water. May also be chewed or swallowed whole.
• Classified as an antihistamine.

---

cyclizine hydrochloride◇
Marezine

cyclizine lactate
Marezine, Marzine◆◆

Pregnancy Risk Category: B

MECHANISM OF ACTION

May affect neural pathways originating in the labyrinth to inhibit nausea and vomiting, but the exact mechanism of action is unknown.

INDICATIONS & DOSAGE

Motion sickness (prevention and treatment)—
Adults: 50 mg P.O. (hydrochloride) one half hour before travel, then q 4 to 6 hours, p.r.n., to maximum of 200 mg daily; or 50 mg I.M. (lactate) q 4 to 6 hours, p.r.n.
Postoperative vomiting (prevention)—
Adults: 50 mg I.M. (lactate) preoperatively or 20 to 30 minutes before expected termination of surgery; then postoperatively 50 mg I.M. (lactate) q 4 to 6 hours, p.r.n.
Motion sickness and postoperative vomiting—
Children 6 to 12 years: 3 mg/kg (lactate) I.M. divided t.i.d., or 25 mg (hydrochloride) P.O. q 4 to 6 hours p.r.n. to a maximum of 75 mg daily.

ADVERSE REACTIONS

CNS: *drowsiness,* dizziness, auditory and visual hallucinations.
CV: hypotension.
EENT: blurred vision, dry mouth.
GI: constipation.
GU: urine retention.
Other: may mask symptoms of ototoxicity, brain tumor, or intestinal obstruction.

INTERACTIONS

None significant.

NURSING CONSIDERATIONS

• Use cautiously in glaucoma, GU or GI obstruction, and in elderly males with possible prostatic hypertrophy.
• Warn patient against driving and other activities that require alertness until CNS effects of the drug are known.
• Classified as an antihistamine.
• Store in cool place. When stored at room temperature, injection may turn slightly yellow, but this color change does not indicate loss of potency.

Italicized side effects are common or life-threatening.
*Liquid form contains alcohol.   **May contain tartrazine.

dimenhydrinate◊

Apo-Dimenhydrinate♦♦, Calm X,
Dimentabs, Dinate, Dommanate,
Dramamine*♦, Dramamine
Chewable, Dramamine Liquid,
Dramanate, Dramilin, Dramocen,
Dramoject, Dymenate, Gravol♦♦,
Hydrate, Marmine, Motion-Aid,
Nauseatol♦♦, Novodimenate♦♦,
PMS-Dimenhydrinate♦♦,
Reidamine, Travamine♦♦, Triptone,
Wehamine

Pregnancy Risk Category: B

MECHANISM OF ACTION
May affect neural pathways originating in the labyrinth to inhibit nausea and vomiting, but the exact mechanism of action is unknown.

INDICATIONS & DOSAGE
Nausea, vomiting, dizziness of motion sickness (treatment and prevention)—
Adults: 50 mg P.O. q 4 hours, or 100 mg q 4 hours if drowsiness is not objectionable; or 50 mg I.M., p.r.n.; or 50 mg I.V. diluted in 10 ml sodium chloride solution, injected over 2 minutes.
Children: 5 mg/kg P.O. or I.M., divided q.i.d. Maximum dosage is 300 mg daily. Don't use in children under 2 years.

ADVERSE REACTIONS
CNS: *drowsiness,* headache, incoordination, dizziness.
CV: palpitations, hypotension.
EENT: blurred vision, tinnitus, dry mouth and respiratory passages.
Other: may mask symptoms of ototoxicity, brain tumor, or intestinal obstruction.

INTERACTIONS
None significant.

NURSING CONSIDERATIONS
• Use cautiously in seizures, narrow-angle glaucoma, and enlargement of prostate gland.
• Undiluted solution is irritating to veins; may cause sclerosis.
• Classified as an antihistamine.
• Warn patient against driving and other activities that require alertness until CNS effects of the drug are known.
• May mask ototoxicity of aminoglycoside antibiotics.
• Avoid mixing parenteral preparation with other drugs; incompatible with many solutions.

diphenidol

Vontrol**♦

Pregnancy Risk Category: C

MECHANISM OF ACTION
Influences the chemoreceptor trigger zone to inhibit nausea and vomiting.

INDICATIONS & DOSAGE
Peripheral (labyrinthine) dizziness—
Adults: 25 to 50 mg P.O. q 4 hours, p.r.n.
Nausea and vomiting—
Adults: 25 to 50 mg P.O. q 4 hours, p.r.n.
Children over 23 kg: 0.88 mg/kg q 4 hours, not to exceed 5.5 mg/kg/24 hours. Usual dosage is 25 mg.

ADVERSE REACTIONS
CNS: *drowsiness,* dizziness, sleep disturbances, *confusion;* auditory and visual hallucinations, disorientation occur within 3 days of starting drug; subside within 3 days after stopping drug.
CV: transient hypotension.
GI: dry mouth, nausea, indigestion, heartburn.
Skin: urticaria.
Other: antiemetic effect may mask symptoms of ototoxicity, brain tumor, intestinal obstruction, or other conditions.

INTERACTIONS
None significant.

NURSING CONSIDERATIONS
• Contraindicated in anuria. Use cautiously in glaucoma, pyloric stenosis, pylorospasm, obstructive lesions of GI or GU tract, prostatic hypertrophy, or organic cardiospasm.
• Used in Ménière's disease, following middle and inner ear surgery, labyrinthine disturbances, and to control nausea and vomiting associated with infectious diseases, cancers, radiation sickness, general anesthetics, and antineoplastic agents.
• Drug should be stopped if auditory or visual hallucinations or disorientation or confusion occurs.
• Closely supervise patient. Patients are usually hospitalized when receiving this drug. Monitor intake/output; report any changes.
• Treatment of toxicity is symptomatic and supportive.

dronabinol
(tetrahydrocannabinol)
Marinol
Controlled Substance Schedule II
Pregnancy Risk Category: B

MECHANISM OF ACTION
Unknown.

INDICATIONS & DOSAGE
Treatment of nausea and vomiting associated with cancer chemotherapy—
Adults: 5 mg/m² P.O. 1 to 3 hours before administration of chemotherapy. Then give same dose q 2 to 4 hours after chemotherapy is administered for a total of 4 to 6 doses per day. Dosage may be increased in increments of 2.5 mg/m² to a maximum of 15 mg/m² per dose.

ADVERSE REACTIONS
CNS: *drowsiness, euphoria, dizziness, anxiety, muddled thinking, perceptual difficulties, impaired coordination,* irritability, depression, weakness, headache, hallucinations, ataxia, paresthesias, visual disturbances, confusion.
CV: tachycardia, orthostatic hypotension.
GI: dry mouth, diarrhea.
Other: muscular pains.

INTERACTIONS
CNS depressants: may increase CNS adverse reactions. Avoid concomitant use.

NURSING CONSIDERATIONS
• Contraindicated for nausea and vomiting from any cause other than cancer chemotherapy; contraindicated in patients hypersensitive to sesame oil.
• Use cautiously in elderly patients and those with hypertension, heart disease, and psychiatric illness.
• Warn patients against hazardous activities that require alertness until CNS effects of the drug are known.
• This drug is to be prescribed only for patients who have not responded satisfactorily to other antiemetics.
• Effects of this drug may persist for days after treatment ends. Duration of persistent effect varies greatly among patients. Therefore, patient should be supervised for untoward responses until it's certain that he's no longer experiencing the drug's effects.
• Dronabinol is the principal active substance present in *Cannabis sativa* (marijuana). Therefore, this can produce both physical and psychic dependence and has high potential for abuse.
• CNS effects are intensified at higher drug dosages.
• To prevent panic and anxiety, tell patients this drug may induce unusual changes in mood or other adverse behavioral effects.
• Impress upon family members that patient should be under supervision

by a responsible person during and immediately after the treatment.

ipecac syrup◇

Pregnancy Risk Category:C

MECHANISM OF ACTION
Induces vomiting by acting locally on the gastric mucosa and centrally on the chemoreceptor trigger zone.

INDICATIONS & DOSAGE
To induce vomiting in poisoning—
Adults: 15 ml P.O., followed by 200 to 300 ml of water.
Children 1 year or older: 15 ml P.O., followed by about 200 ml of water or milk.
Children under 1 year: 5 to 10 ml P.O., followed by 100 to 200 ml of water or milk. May repeat dose once after 20 minutes, if necessary.

ADVERSE REACTIONS
CNS: depression.
CV: *cardiac dysrhythmias, bradycardia, hypotension, atrial fibrillation, or fatal myocarditis after ingestion of excessive dose.*
GI: diarrhea.

INTERACTIONS
Activated charcoal: neutralized emetic effect. Don't give together but may give activated charcoal after vomiting has occurred.

NURSING CONSIDERATIONS
• Contraindicated in semicomatose or unconscious patients, or those with severe inebriation, seizures, shock, or loss of gag reflex.
• Don't give after ingestion of petroleum distillates (for example, kerosene, gasoline) or volatile oils; retching and vomiting may cause aspiration and lead to bronchospasm, pulmonary edema, or aspiration pneumonitis. Vegetable oil will delay absorption of these substances.

• Don't give after ingestion of caustic substances, such as lye; additional injury to the esophagus and mediastinum can occur.
• Clearly indicate ipecac *syrup,* not single word "ipecac," to avoid confusion with fluid extract. Fluid extract is 14 times more concentrated and, if inadvertently used instead of syrup, may cause death.
• Induces vomiting within 30 minutes in more than 90% of patients; average time usually less than 20 minutes.
• Stomach is usually emptied completely; vomitus may contain some intestinal material as well.
• In antiemetic toxicity, ipecac syrup is usually effective if less than 1 hour has passed since ingestion of antiemetic.
• Recommend that 1 oz (30 ml) of syrup be readily available in the home when child becomes 1 year old for immediate use in case of emergency.
• No systemic toxicity with doses of 30 ml or less.
• If two doses do not induce vomiting, gastric lavage is necessary.
• Now commonly abused by bulimics who practice "binge-purge."

meclizine hydrochloride◇

Antivert♦, Antivert/25, Antivert/50, Bonamine♦♦, Bonine, Ru-Vert M

Pregnancy Risk Category: B

MECHANISM OF ACTION
May affect neural pathways originating in the labyrinth to inhibit nausea and vomiting, but the exact mechanism of action is unknown.

INDICATIONS & DOSAGE
Dizziness—
Adults: 25 to 100 mg P.O. daily in divided doses. Dosage varies with patient response.
Motion sickness—
Adults: 25 to 50 mg P.O. 1 hour before travel, repeated daily for duration

---

of journey.

ADVERSE REACTIONS
CNS: *drowsiness,* fatigue.
EENT: dry mouth, blurred vision.
Other: may mask symptoms of oto-
toxicity, brain tumor, or intestinal ob-
struction.

INTERACTIONS
CNS depressants: increased drowsiness.

NURSING CONSIDERATIONS
• Use cautiously in glaucoma, GU or
GI obstruction, and in elderly males
with possible prostatic hypertrophy.
• Warn patient against driving and
other activities that require alertness
until CNS effects of the drug are
known.
• This antihistamine has a slower onset and longer duration of action than
other antihistamine antiemetics.

---

metoclopramide hydrochloride
Maxeran♦♦, Reglan♦

Pregnancy Risk Category: B

MECHANISM OF ACTION
Stimulates motility of the upper GI
tract by increasing lower esophageal
sphincter tone. Also blocks dopamine
receptors at the chemoreceptor trigger
zone.

INDICATIONS & DOSAGE
*Preventing or reducing nausea and
vomiting induced by cisplatin and
other chemotherapy—*
Adults: 2 mg/kg I.V. q 2 hours for 5
doses, beginning 30 minutes prior to
cisplatin administration.
*To facilitate small-bowel intubation
and to aid in radiologic examinations—*
Adults: 10 mg (2 ml) I.V. as a single
dose over 1 to 2 minutes.
Children 6 to 14 years: 2.5 to 5 mg

(0.5 to 1 ml).
Children under 6 years: 0.1 mg/kg.
*Delayed gastric emptying secondary
to diabetic gastroparesis—*
Adults: 10 mg P.O. 30 minutes before
meals and h.s. for 2 to 8 weeks, depending on response.
*Treatment of gastroesophageal re-
flux—*
Adults: 10 to 15 mg P.O. q.i.d.,
p.r.n. Take 30 minutes before meals.

ADVERSE REACTIONS
CNS: *restlessness, anxiety, drowsiness,* fatigue, *lassitude,* insomnia,
headache, dizziness, *extrapyramidal
symptoms, tardive dyskinesia, dystonic reactions,* sedation.
CV: transient hypertension.
GI: nausea, bowel disturbances.
Skin: rash.
Other: fever, prolactin secretion, loss
of libido.

INTERACTIONS
Anticholinergics, narcotic analgesics:
antagonize effects of metoclopramide.
Use together cautiously.

NURSING CONSIDERATIONS
• Contraindicated whenever stimulation of GI motility might be dangerous (hemorrhage, obstruction, or perforation), and in pheochromocytoma
or epilepsy.
• Diphenhydramine 25 mg I.V. may
be prescribed to counteract the extrapyramidal side effects associated with
high metoclopramide doses.
• Elderly patients are more likely to
experience extrapyramidal symptoms
and tardive dyskinesia.
• Safety and effectiveness have not
been established for therapy that continues longer than 12 weeks.
• Monitor blood pressure frequently
in patients receiving I.V. dosage.
• I.V. infusions should be given
slowly over at least 15 minutes. Protection from light is unnecessary if
the infusion mixture is administered

Italicized side effects are common or life-threatening.
*Liquid form contains alcohol.   **May contain tartrazine.

within 24 hours.
• Warn patient to avoid activities requiring alertness for 2 hours after taking each dose.
• Now available in syrup form. Contains 5 mg/5 ml.
• Oral form is being used investigationally to treat nausea and vomiting.

nabilone
Cesamet♦
Controlled Substance Schedule II
Pregnancy Risk Category: B

MECHANISM OF ACTION
Unknown.

INDICATIONS & DOSAGE
Treatment of nausea and vomiting associated with cancer chemotherapy—
Adults: 1 to 2 mg P.O. b.i.d. On the day of chemotherapy, the first dose should be given 1 to 3 hours before chemotherapy is administered. Maximum daily dosage is 6 mg divided t.i.d.

ADVERSE REACTIONS
CNS: *drowsiness, vertigo, euphoria, anxiety, decreased ability to concentrate, disorientation, depression,* ataxia, headache, visual disturbances, paresthesias, hallucinations.
CV: orthostatic hypotension, tachycardia.
GI: *dry mouth,* increased appetite.

INTERACTIONS
CNS depressants: may increase CNS adverse reactions. Avoid concomitant use.

NURSING CONSIDERATIONS
• Contraindicated for nausea and vomiting from any cause other than cancer chemotherapy.
• Use cautiously in elderly patients and those with hypertension, heart disease, or psychiatric illness.
• Warn patients to avoid driving and

other hazardous activities that require mental alertness until CNS effects of the drug are known.
• This drug is to be prescribed only for patients who have not responded satisfactorily to other antiemetics.
• Effects of nabilone may persist for a variable and unpredictable period of time after its administration. Adverse psychological reactions can persist for 48 to 72 hours after treatment ends.
• Nabilone is a synthetic cannabinoid. It is chemically similar to dronabinol (tetrahydrocannabinol), the active substance in marijuana.
• CNS effects are intensified at higher dosages.
• To prevent panic and anxiety, tell patients this drug may induce unusual changes in mood or other adverse behavioral effects.
• Impress upon family members that patient should be under supervision by a responsible person during and immediately after the treatment.

prochlorperazine
Compazine, Stemetil♦♦

prochlorperazine edisylate◊
Compazine

prochlorperazine maleate
Chlorpazine, Compazine, Stemetil♦♦
Pregnancy Risk Category: C

MECHANISM OF ACTION
Acts on the chemoreceptor trigger zone to inhibit nausea and vomiting, and in larger doses, partially depresses the vomiting center as well.

INDICATIONS & DOSAGE
Preoperative nausea control—
Adults: 5 to 10 mg I.M. 1 to 2 hours before induction of anesthetic, repeat once in 30 minutes, if necessary; or 5 to 10 mg I.V. 15 to 30 minutes before induction of anesthetic (repeat once if

necessary); or 20 mg/liter dextrose 5% in water and 0.9% sodium chloride solution by I.V. infusion, added to infusion 15 to 30 minutes before induction. Maximum parenteral dosage is 40 mg daily.

Severe nausea, vomiting—
Adults: 5 to 10 mg P.O. t.i.d. or q.i.d.; or 15 mg sustained-release form P.O. on arising; or 10 mg sustained-release form P.O. q 12 hours; or 25 mg rectally b.i.d.; or 5 to 10 mg I.M. injected deeply into upper outer quadrant of gluteal region. Repeat q 3 to 4 hours, p.r.n. Maximum I.M. dosage is 40 mg daily.

Children 18 to 39 kg: 2.5 mg P.O. or rectally t.i.d.; or 5 mg P.O. or rectally b.i.d. Maximum dosage is 15 mg daily; or 0.132 mg/kg deep I.M. injection. (Control usually obtained with 1 dose.)

Children 14 to 17 kg: 2.5 mg P.O. or rectally b.i.d. or t.i.d. Maximum dosage is 10 mg daily; or 0.132 mg/kg deep I.M. injection. (Control usually obtained with 1 dose.)

Children 9 to 13 kg: 2.5 mg P.O. or rectally daily or b.i.d. Maximum dosage is 7.5 mg daily; or 0.132 mg/kg deep I.M. injection. (Control usually obtained with 1 dose.)

Symptomatic management of psychotic disorders—
Adults: 5 to 10 mg, P.O. t.i.d. or q.i.d.

Children 2 to 12 years: 2.5 mg P.O. or P.R. b.i.d. or t.i.d. Do not exceed 10 mg on day 1. Increase dosage gradually to recommended maximum (if necessary).

Children 6 to 10 years: maximum 25 mg daily.

Children 2 to 5 years: maximum 20 mg daily.

Symptomatic management of severe psychoses—
Adults: 10 to 20 mg I.M. May be repeated in 1 to 4 hours. Rarely, patients may receive 10 to 20 mg q 4 to 6 hours. Oral therapy should be insti-

tuted after symptoms are controlled.
Children: 0.13 mg/kg I.M.
Management of excessive anxiety—
Adults: 5 to 10 mg by deep I.M. injection every 3 to 4 hours, not to exceed 40 mg daily; or 5 to 10 mg P.O. t.i.d. or q.i.d.; alternatively, give 15 mg (as the extended-release capsule) once daily, or 10 mg (extended-release capsule) q 12 hours.

ADVERSE REACTIONS
Blood: *transient leukopenia, agranulocytosis.*
CNS: *extrapyramidal reactions,* sedation, pseudoparkinsonism, EEG changes, dizziness.
CV: *orthostatic hypotension,* tachycardia, ECG changes.
EENT: *ocular changes, blurred vision.*
GI: *dry mouth, constipation.*
GU: *urine retention,* dark urine, menstrual irregularities, gynecomastia, inhibited ejaculation.
Hepatic: *cholestatic jaundice.*
Metabolic: hyperprolactinemia.
Skin: *mild photosensitivity,* dermal allergic reactions, *exfoliative dermatitis.*
Other: weight gain, increased appetite.

INTERACTIONS
Anticholinergics, including antidepressants and antiparkinsonian agents: increased anticholinergic activity and aggravated parkinsonian symptoms. Use together cautiously.
Antacids: inhibited absorption of oral phenothiazines. Separate antacid and phenothiazine doses by at least 2 hours.
Barbiturates: may decrease phenothiazine effect. Monitor patient for decreased antiemetic effect.

NURSING CONSIDERATIONS
• Contraindicated in phenothiazine hypersensitivity, CNS depression, bone marrow suppression, or subcort-

ical damage; during pediatric surgery, use of spinal or epidural anesthetic or adrenergic blocking agents, alcohol usage, and those in a coma or depression. Use with caution in combination with other CNS depressants; in hepatic disease, arteriosclerosis or cardiovascular disease (may cause sudden drop in blood pressure), exposure to extreme heat or cold (including antipyretic therapy), respiratory disorders, hypocalcemia, convulsive disorders or severe reactions to insulin or electroshock therapy, suspected brain tumor or intestinal obstruction, glaucoma, or prostatic hypertrophy; in acutely ill, dehydrated, or vomiting children; and in elderly or debilitated patients.
• Elderly patients should usually receive dosages in the lower range.
• Store in light-resistant container. Slight yellowing does not affect potency; discard very discolored solutions.
• Use only when vomiting can't be controlled by other measures, or when only a few doses are required. If more than 4 doses needed in 24-hour period, notify doctor.
• Not effective in motion sickness.
• To prevent contact dermatitis, avoid getting concentrate or injection solution on hands or clothing.
• Dilute oral solution with tomato or fruit juice, milk, coffee, carbonated beverage, tea, water, soup, or pudding.
• Monitor CBC and liver function studies during prolonged therapy. Warn patients to wear protective clothing when exposed to sunlight.
• Watch for orthostatic hypotension, especially when giving I.V.
• Do not give subcutaneously or mix in syringe with another drug. Give deep I.M.

scopolamine◊
Transderm-Scōp, Transderm-V♦♦
Pregnancy Risk Category: C

MECHANISM OF ACTION
May affect neural pathways originating in the labyrinth to inhibit nausea and vomiting, but the exact mechanism of action is unknown.

INDICATIONS & DOSAGE
Prevention of nausea and vomiting associated with motion sickness—
Adults: One Transderm-Scōp system (a circular flat unit) programmed to deliver 0.5 mg scopolamine over 3 days (72 hours), applied to the skin behind the ear several hours before the antiemetic is required.
    Not recommended for children.

ADVERSE REACTIONS
CNS: *drowsiness,* restlessness, disorientation, confusion.
EENT: *dry mouth,* transient impairment of eye accommodation.

INTERACTIONS
None significant.

NURSING CONSIDERATIONS
• Use cautiously in patients with glaucoma, pyloric obstruction, or urinary bladder-neck obstruction.
• Wash and dry hands thoroughly before applying the system on dry skin behind the ear. After removing the system, discard it, then wash both the hands and application site thoroughly.
• If the system becomes displaced, remove and replace it with another system on a fresh skin site in the postauricular area.
• Caution patient to wash hands after applying transdermal patch, particularly before touching eye. May cause pupil to dilate.
• A patient brochure is available with this product; tell patient to request it from the pharmacist.

• Warn patient against driving and other activities that require alertness until CNS effects of the drug are known.

• Sugarless hard candy may be helpful in minimizing dry mouth.

• Transderm-Scōp is effective if applied 2 to 3 hours before experiencing motion, but more effective if used 12 hours before. Therefore, advise patient to apply system the night before a planned trip.

• Transdermal method of administration releases a controlled therapeutic amount of scopolamine.

---

trimethobenzamide hydrochloride
Tebamide, Tegamide, Ticon, Tigan♦, Tiject-20

Pregnancy Risk Category: C

MECHANISM OF ACTION
Acts on the chemoreceptor trigger zone to inhibit nausea and vomiting.

INDICATIONS & DOSAGE
Nausea and vomiting (treatment)—
Adults: 250 mg P.O. t.i.d. or q.i.d.; or 200 mg I.M. or rectally t.i.d. or q.i.d.
Postoperative nausea and vomiting (prevention)—
Adults: 200 mg I.M. or rectally (single dose) before or during surgery; may repeat 3 hours after termination of anesthesia, p.r.n.
Children 13 to 40 kg: 100 to 200 mg P.O. or rectally t.i.d. or q.i.d.
Children under 13 kg: 100 mg rectally t.i.d. or q.i.d. Limited to prolonged vomiting of known etiology.

ADVERSE REACTIONS
CNS: *drowsiness,* dizziness (in large doses).
CV: hypotension.
GI: diarrhea, exaggeration of preexisting nausea (in large doses).
Hepatic: *liver toxicity.*

Local: pain, stinging, burning, redness, swelling at I.M. injection site.
Skin: skin hypersensitivity reactions.
Other: antiemetic effect may mask signs of overdosage of toxic agents, or intestinal obstruction, brain tumor, or other conditions.

INTERACTIONS
None significant.

NURSING CONSIDERATIONS
• Contraindicated in children with viral illness (a possible cause of vomiting in children); may contribute to the development of Reye's syndrome, a potentially fatal acute childhood encephalopathy, characterized by fatty degeneration of the liver.

• Suppositories contraindicated in hypersensitivity to benzocaine hydrochloride or similar local anesthetic.

• Stop drug if allergic skin reaction occurs.

• Give I.M. dose by deep injection into upper outer quadrant of gluteal region to reduce pain and local irritation.

• Warn patient of the possibility of drowsiness and dizziness, and caution him against driving or other activities requiring alertness until CNS effects of the drug are known.

• Store suppositories in refrigerator.

• Has little or no value in preventing motion sickness; limited value as antiemetic.

Italicized side effects are common or life-threatening.
*Liquid form contains alcohol.   **May contain tartrazine.

50

Gastrointestinal anticholinergics

Belladonna alkaloids
atropine sulfate
(See Chapter 20, ANTIARRHYTHMICS.)
belladonna leaf
hyoscyamine
hyoscyamine sulfate
hyoscyamine and scopolamine
Quaternary anticholinergics
anisotropine methylbromide
clidinium bromide
glycopyrrolate
(See Chapter 38, CHOLINERGIC BLOCKERS.)
hexocyclium methylsulfate
isopropamide iodide
mepenzolate bromide
methantheline bromide
methscopolamine bromide
oxyphenonium bromide
propantheline bromide

Tertiary synthetics
(antispasmodics)
dicyclomine hydrochloride
oxyphencyclimine hydrochloride

COMBINATION PRODUCTS

BARBIDONNA ELIXIR*: atropine sulfate 0.034 mg/5 ml, phenobarbital 21.6 mg/5 ml, hyoscyamine hydrobromide or sulfate 0.174 mg/5 ml, hyoscine hydrobromide 0.01 mg/5 ml, and alcohol 15%.
BARBIDONNA TABLETS: atropine sulfate 0.025 mg, hyoscine hydrobromide 0.0074 mg, hyoscyamine hydrobromide or sulfate 0.1286 mg, and phenobarbital 16 mg.
BARBIDONNA NO. 2 TABLETS: atropine sulfate 0.025 mg, hyoscine hydrobromide 0.0074 mg, hyoscyamine hydrobromide or sulfate 0.1286 mg,

and phenobarbital 32 mg.
BELLADENAL TABLETS♦: L-alkaloids of belladonna 0.25 mg and phenobarbital 50 mg.
CHARDONNA-2: belladonna extract 15 mg and phenobarbital 15 mg.
DONNATAL ELIXIR•♦: atropine sulfate 0.0194 mg/5 ml, hyoscine hydrobromide 0.0065 mg/5 ml, alcohol 23%, hyoscyamine hydrobromide or sulfate 0.1037 mg/5 ml and phenobarbital 16 mg/5 ml.
DONNATAL EXTENTABS♦: atropine sulfate 0.0582 mg, hyoscine hydrobromide 0.0195 mg, hyoscyamine sulfate 0.3111 mg, and phenobarbital 48.6 mg.
DONNATAL TABLETS AND CAPSULES♦: atropine sulfate 0.0194 mg, hyoscine hydrobromide 0.0065 mg, hyoscyamine hydrobromide or sulfate 0.1037 mg, and phenobarbital 16 mg.
DONNATAL NO. 2 TABLETS: atropine sulfate 0.0194 mg, hyoscine hydrobromide 0.0065 mg, hyoscyamine hydrobromide or sulfate 0.1037 mg, and phenobarbital 32.4 mg.
KINESED TABLETS: atropine sulfate 0.02 mg, hyoscine hydrobromide 0.007 mg, hyoscyamine hydrobromide or sulfate 0.1 mg, and phenobarbital 16 mg.
LIBRAX CAPSULES: clidinium bromide 2.5 mg and chlordiazepoxide hydrochloride 5 mg.
ROBINUL FORTE TABLETS♦: glycopyrrolate 2 mg and phenobarbital 16.2 mg.
ROBINUL TABLETS♦: glycopyrrolate 1 mg and phenobarbital 16.2 mg.
VISTRAX 10 TABLETS: oxyphencycli-

---

mine hydrochloride 10 mg and hydroxyzine hydrochloride 25 mg.

anisotropine methylbromide
Valpin 50♦

Pregnancy Risk Category: C

MECHANISM OF ACTION
Competitively blocks acetylcholine, which decreases GI motility and inhibits gastric acid secretion.

INDICATIONS & DOSAGE
Adjunctive treatment of peptic ulcer—
Adults: 50 mg P.O. t.i.d. To be effective, should be titrated to individual patient's needs.

ADVERSE REACTIONS
CNS: headache, insomnia, drowsiness, dizziness, *confusion or excitement in elderly patients,* nervousness, weakness.
CV: *palpitations,* tachycardia.
EENT: *blurred vision,* mydriasis, increased ocular tension, cycloplegia, photophobia.
GI: *dry mouth,* dysphagia, heartburn, loss of taste, nausea, vomiting, *paralytic ileus, constipation.*
GU: *urinary hesitancy, urine retention,* impotence.
Skin: urticaria, decreased sweating and possible anhidrosis, other dermal manifestations.
Other: fever, allergic reactions.
Overdosage may cause curare-like symptoms.

INTERACTIONS
None significant.

NURSING CONSIDERATIONS
• Contraindicated in narrow-angle glaucoma, obstructive uropathy, obstructive disease of the GI tract, severe ulcerative colitis, myasthenia gravis, hypersensitivity to anticholinergics, paralytic ileus, intestinal atony, unstable cardiovascular status in acute hemorrhage, or toxic megacolon. Use cautiously in autonomic neuropathy, hyperthyroidism, coronary artery disease, cardiac dysrhythmias, CHF, hypertension, hiatal hernia associated with reflux esophagitis, hepatic or renal disease, and ulcerative colitis, or in patients over 40 years because of increased incidence of glaucoma.
• Use with caution in hot or humid environments. Drug-induced heatstroke can develop.
• Give 30 minutes to 1 hour before meals.
• Administer smaller doses to elderly patients.
• Monitor patient's vital signs and urine output carefully.
• Instruct patient to avoid driving and other hazardous activities if he is drowsy, dizzy, or has blurred vision; to drink plenty of fluids to help prevent constipation; to report any skin rash or local eruption.
• Gum or sugarless hard candy may relieve dry mouth.

belladonna leaf
(used to prepare extract and tincture)
Belladonna Tincture USP*

Pregnancy Risk Category: C

MECHANISM OF ACTION
Competitively blocks acetylcholine, which decreases GI motility and inhibits gastric acid secretion.

INDICATIONS & DOSAGE
Adjunctive therapy for peptic ulcer, irritable bowel syndrome, functional gastrointestinal disorders, and neurogenic bowel disturbances—
Adults: 15 mg P.O. t.i.d. or q.i.d. of the extract; 0.3 to 1 ml t.i.d. or q.i.d. of tincture.

ADVERSE REACTIONS
CNS: headache, insomnia, drowsiness, dizziness, *confusion or excitement in elderly patients,* nervousness, weakness.
CV: *palpitations,* tachycardia.
EENT: *blurred vision,* mydriasis, increased ocular tension, cycloplegia, photophobia.
GI: *dry mouth,* dysphagia, heartburn, loss of taste, *constipation,* nausea, vomiting.
GU: *urinary hesitancy, urine retention,* impotence.
Skin: urticaria, decreased sweating or possible anhidrosis, other dermal manifestations.
Other: fever, allergic reactions.
Overdosage may cause curare-like symptoms.

INTERACTIONS
None significant.

NURSING CONSIDERATIONS
• Contraindicated in narrow-angle glaucoma, obstructive uropathy, obstructive disease of GI tract, severe ulcerative colitis, myasthenia gravis, hypersensitivity to anticholinergics, paralytic ileus, intestinal atony, unstable cardiovascular status in acute hemorrhage, or toxic megacolon. Use cautiously in autonomic neuropathy, hyperthyroidism, coronary artery disease, cardiac dysrhythmias, CHF, hypertension, hiatal hernia associated with reflux esophagitis, hepatic or renal disease, and ulcerative colitis, or in patients over 40 years because of increased incidence of glaucoma.
• Give 30 minutes to 1 hour before meals and at bedtime. Bedtime dose can be larger and should be given at least 2 hours after last meal of day.
• Administer smaller doses to elderly patients.
• Use with caution in hot or humid environments. Drug-induced heatstroke can develop.
• Monitor patient's vital signs and urine output carefully.
• Instruct patient to avoid driving and other hazardous activities if he is drowsy, dizzy, or has blurred vision; to drink plenty of fluids to help prevent constipation; to report any skin rash or local eruption.
• Gum or sugarless hard candy may relieve dry mouth.

clidinium bromide
Quarzan
Pregnancy Risk Category: C

MECHANISM OF ACTION
Competitively blocks acetylcholine, which decreases GI motility and inhibits gastric acid secretion.

INDICATIONS & DOSAGE
Adjunctive therapy for peptic ulcers— Dosage should be individualized according to severity of symptoms and occurrence of adverse reactions.
Elderly or debilitated patients: 2.5 to 5 mg P.O. t.i.d. or q.i.d. before meals and h.s.

ADVERSE REACTIONS
CNS: headache, insomnia, drowsiness, dizziness, *confusion or excitement in elderly patients,* nervousness, weakness.
CV: *palpitations,* tachycardia.
EENT: *blurred vision,* mydriasis, increased ocular tension, cycloplegia, photophobia.
GI: *dry mouth,* dysphagia, heartburn, loss of taste, nausea, vomiting, *paralytic ileus, constipation.*
GU: *urinary hesitancy, urine retention,* impotence.
Skin: urticaria, decreased sweating or possible anhidrosis, other dermal manifestations.
Other: fever, allergic reactions.
Overdosage may cause curare-like symptoms.

INTERACTIONS
None significant.

NURSING CONSIDERATIONS
• Contraindicated in narrow-angle glaucoma, obstructive uropathy, obstructive disease of GI tract, severe ulcerative colitis, myasthenia gravis, hypersensitivity to anticholinergics, paralytic ileus, intestinal atony, unstable cardiovascular status in acute hemorrhage, or toxic megacolon. Use cautiously in autonomic neuropathy, hyperthyroidism, coronary artery disease, cardiac dysrhythmias, CHF, hypertension, hiatal hernia associated with reflux esophagitis, hepatic or renal disease, and ulcerative colitis, or in patients over 40 years, because of increased incidence of glaucoma.
• Give 30 minutes to 1 hour before meals and at bedtime. Bedtime dose can be larger and should be given at least 2 hours after last meal of day.
• Use with caution in hot or humid environments. Drug-induced heatstroke may develop.
• Monitor patient's vital signs and urine output carefully.
• Instruct patient to avoid driving and other hazardous activities if he is drowsy, dizzy, or has blurred vision; to drink plenty of fluids to help prevent constipation; and to report any rash or skin eruption.
• Gum or sugarless hard candy may relieve dry mouth.
• Dysphagia may cause aspiration.
• There is no conclusive evidence that clidinium aids in healing, decreases recurrence of, or prevents complications of peptic ulcers.

dicyclomine hydrochloride
Antispas, A-Spas, Bentyl, Bentylol♦♦, Byclomine, Dibent, Dicen, Di-Cyclonex, Di-Spaz, Formulex♦♦, Lomine♦♦, Neoquess, Or-Tyl, Spasmoban♦♦, Spasmoject, Viscerol♦♦

Pregnancy Risk Category: B

MECHANISM OF ACTION
Exerts a nonspecific, direct spasmolytic action on smooth muscle. Also possesses local anesthetic properties that may be partly responsible for spasmolysis.

INDICATIONS & DOSAGE
Adjunctive therapy for peptic ulcers and other functional GI disorders—
Adults: 10 to 20 mg P.O. t.i.d. or q.i.d.; 20 mg I.M. q 4 to 6 hours.
 Always adjust dosage according to patient's needs and response.

ADVERSE REACTIONS
CNS: *headache,* insomnia, drowsiness, *dizziness.*
CV: *palpitations,* tachycardia.
GI: nausea, *constipation,* vomiting, *paralytic ileus.*
GU: *urinary hesitancy, urine retention, impotence.*
Skin: urticaria, decreased sweating or possible anhidrosis, other dermal manifestations.
Other: fever, allergic reactions.
 Overdosage may cause curare-like symptoms.

INTERACTIONS
None significant.

NURSING CONSIDERATIONS
• Contraindicated in obstructive uropathy, obstructive disease of GI tract, severe ulcerative colitis, myasthenia gravis, hypersensitivity to anticholinergics, paralytic ileus, intestinal atony, unstable cardiovascular status in acute hemorrhage, or toxic mega-

colon. Use cautiously in autonomic neuropathy, narrow-angle glaucoma, hyperthyroidism, coronary artery disease, cardiac dysrhythmias, CHF, hypertension, hiatal hernia associated with reflux esophagitis, hepatic or renal disease, and ulcerative colitis.

• Use with caution in hot or humid environments. Drug-induced heat-stroke can develop.

• Give 30 minutes to 1 hour before meals and at bedtime. Bedtime dose can be larger and should be given at least 2 hours after last meal of day.

• Monitor patient's vital signs and urine output carefully.

• Instruct patient to avoid driving and other hazardous activities if he is drowsy, dizzy, or has blurred vision; to drink plenty of fluids to help prevent constipation; and to report any rash or skin eruption.

• Gum or sugarless hard candy may relieve dry mouth.

• A synthetic tertiary derivative that may have fewer atropine-like adverse reactions.

• Not for I.V. use.

hexocyclium methylsulfate
Tral Filmtabs**

Pregnancy Risk Category: C

MECHANISM OF ACTION
Competitively blocks acetylcholine, which decreases GI motility and inhibits gastric acid secretion.

INDICATIONS & DOSAGE
Adjunctive therapy in peptic ulcer and other GI disorders—
Adults: 25 mg q.i.d. before meals and h.s.

ADVERSE REACTIONS
CNS: headache, insomnia, drowsiness, dizziness, *confusion or excitement in elderly patients,* nervousness, weakness.
CV: *palpitations,* tachycardia.

EENT: *blurred vision,* mydriasis, increased ocular tension, cycloplegia, photophobia.
GI: *dry mouth,* dysphagia, heartburn, loss of taste, nausea, *constipation,* vomiting, *paralytic ileus.*
GU: *urinary hesitancy, urine retention,* impotence.
Skin: urticaria, decreased sweating or possible anhidrosis, other dermal manifestations.
Other: fever, allergic reactions.
Overdosage may cause curare-like symptoms.

INTERACTIONS
None significant.

NURSING CONSIDERATIONS
• Contraindicated in narrow-angle glaucoma, obstructive uropathy, obstructive disease of GI tract, severe ulcerative colitis, myasthenia gravis, hypersensitivity to anticholinergics, paralytic ileus, intestinal atony, unstable cardiovascular status in acute hemorrhage, or toxic megacolon. Use cautiously in autonomic neuropathy, hyperthyroidism, coronary artery disease, cardiac dysrhythmias, CHF, hypertension, hiatal hernia associated with reflux esophagitis, hepatic or renal disease, and ulcerative colitis, or in patients over 40 years because of increased incidence of glaucoma.

• Use with caution in hot or humid environments. Drug-induced heat-stroke can develop.

• Give 30 minutes to 1 hour before meals and at bedtime. Bedtime dose can be larger and should be given at least 2 hours after last meal of day.

• Monitor patient's vital signs and urine output carefully.

• Instruct patient to avoid driving and other hazardous activities if he is drowsy, dizzy, or has blurred vision; to drink plenty of fluids to help prevent constipation; and to report any rash or skin eruption.

• Gum or sugarless hard candy may

relieve dry mouth.

hyoscyamine
Cystospaz

hyoscyamine sulfate
Anaspaz, Bellaspaz, Cystospaz-M, Levsin, Levsinex Timecaps, Neoquess

Pregnancy Risk Category: C

MECHANISM OF ACTION
Competitively blocks acetylcholine, which decreases GI motility and inhibits gastric acid secretion.

INDICATIONS & DOSAGE
Treatment of GI tract disorders caused by spasm; adjunctive therapy for peptic ulcers—
Adults: 0.125 to 0.25 mg P.O. or sublingually t.i.d. or q.i.d. before meals and h.s.; sustained-release form 0.375 mg P.O. q 12 hours; or 0.25 to 0.5 mg (1 or 2 ml) I.M., I.V., or S.C. q 6 hours. (Substitute oral medication when symptoms are controlled.)
Children 2 to 10 years: half of adult dose P.O.

ADVERSE REACTIONS
CNS: headache, insomnia, drowsiness, dizziness, *confusion or excitement in elderly patients,* nervousness, weakness.
CV: *palpitations,* tachycardia.
EENT: *blurred vision,* mydriasis, increased ocular tension, cycloplegia, photophobia.
GI: *dry mouth,* dysphagia, *constipation,* heartburn, loss of taste, nausea, vomiting, *paralytic ileus.*
GU: *urinary hesitancy, urine retention,* impotence.
Skin: urticaria, decreased sweating or possible anhidrosis, other dermal manifestations.
Other: fever, allergic reactions.
Overdosage may cause curare-like symptoms.

INTERACTIONS
None significant.

NURSING CONSIDERATIONS
• Contraindicated in narrow-angle glaucoma, obstructive uropathy, obstructive disease of GI tract, severe ulcerative colitis, myasthenia gravis, hypersensitivity to anticholinergics, paralytic ileus, intestinal atony, unstable cardiovascular status in acute hemorrhage, or toxic megacolon. Use cautiously in autonomic neuropathy, hyperthyroidism, coronary artery disease, cardiac dysrhythmias, CHF, hypertension, hiatal hernia associated with reflux esophagitis, hepatic or renal disease, and ulcerative colitis, or in patients over 40 years, because of the increased incidence of glaucoma.
• Use with caution in hot or humid environments. Drug-induced heatstroke can develop.
• Give 30 minutes to 1 hour before meals and at bedtime. Bedtime dose can be larger and should be given at least 2 hours after the last meal of the day.
• Monitor patient's vital signs and urine output carefully.
• Instruct patient to avoid driving and other hazardous activities if he is drowsy, dizzy, or has blurred vision; to drink plenty of fluids to help prevent constipation; and to report any rash or skin eruption.
• Gum or sugarless hard candy may relieve dry mouth.

hyoscyamine and scopolamine
Bellafoline

Pregnancy Risk Category: C

MECHANISM OF ACTION
Competitively blocks acetylcholine, which decreases GI motility and inhibits gastric acid secretion.

Italicized side effects are common or life-threatening.
*Liquid form contains alcohol.   **May contain tartrazine.

INDICATIONS & DOSAGE
Adjunctive therapy for peptic ulcer, irritable bowel syndrome, and functional GI disorders—
Adults: 0.25 to 0.5 mg P.O. t.i.d.
Children over 6 years: 0.125 to 0.25 mg P.O. t.i.d.

ADVERSE REACTIONS
CNS: headache, insomnia, drowsiness, dizziness, *confusion or excitement in elderly patients,* nervousness, weakness.
CV: *palpitations,* tachycardia.
EENT: *blurred vision,* mydriasis, increased ocular tension, cycloplegia, photophobia.
GI: *dry mouth,* dysphagia, heartburn, loss of taste, *constipation, paralytic ileus.*
GU: *urinary hesitancy, urine retention,* impotence.
Skin: urticaria, decreased sweating or possible anhidrosis, other dermal manifestations.
Other: fever, allergic reactions.
Overdosage may cause curare-like symptoms.

INTERACTIONS
None significant.

NURSING CONSIDERATIONS
• Contraindicated in narrow-angle glaucoma, obstructive uropathy, obstructive disease of GI tract, severe ulcerative colitis, myasthenia gravis, hypersensitivity to anticholinergics, paralytic ileus, intestinal atony, unstable cardiovascular status in acute hemorrhage, or toxic megacolon. Use cautiously in autonomic neuropathy, hyperthyroidism, coronary artery disease, cardiac dysrhythmias, CHF, hypertension, hiatal hernia associated with reflux esophagitis, hepatic or renal disease, and ulcerative colitis, or in patients over 40 years because of increased incidence of glaucoma.
• Use with caution in hot or humid environments. Drug-induced heat-

stroke can develop.
• Administer 30 minutes to 1 hour before meals.
• Monitor patient's vital signs and urine output carefully.
• Instruct patient to avoid driving and other hazardous activities if he is drowsy, dizzy, or has blurred vision; to drink plenty of fluids to help prevent constipation; to report any rash or skin eruption.
• Gum or sugarless hard candy may relieve dry mouth.

isopropamide iodide
Darbid♦

Pregnancy Risk Category: C

MECHANISM OF ACTION
Competitively blocks acetylcholine, which decreases GI motility and inhibits gastric acid secretion.

INDICATIONS & DOSAGE
Adjunctive therapy for peptic ulcer, irritable bowel syndrome—
Adults and children over 12 years: 5 mg P.O. q 12 hours. Some patients may require 10 mg or more b.i.d.
Dosage should be individualized to patient's need.

ADVERSE REACTIONS
CNS: headache, insomnia, drowsiness, dizziness, *confusion or excitement in elderly patients,* nervousness, weakness.
CV: *palpitations,* tachycardia.
EENT: *blurred vision,* mydriasis, increased ocular tension, cycloplegia, photophobia.
GI: *dry mouth,* dysphagia, heartburn, loss of taste, nausea, vomiting, *constipation, paralytic ileus.*
GU: *urinary hesitancy, urine retention,* impotence.
Skin: urticaria, decreased sweating or possible anhidrosis, other dermal manifestations, iodine skin rash.
Other: fever, allergic reactions.

Overdosage may cause curare-like symptoms.

INTERACTIONS
None significant.

NURSING CONSIDERATIONS
• Contraindicated in hypersensitivity to iodine, narrow-angle glaucoma, obstructive uropathy, obstructive disease of GI tract, severe ulcerative colitis, myasthenia gravis, hypersensitivity to anticholinergics, paralytic ileus, intestinal atony, unstable cardiovascular status in acute hemorrhage, or toxic megacolon. Use cautiously in autonomic neuropathy, hyperthyroidism, coronary artery disease, cardiac dysrhythmias, CHF, hypertension, hiatal hernia associated with reflux esophagitis, hepatic or renal disease, and ulcerative colitis, or in patients over 40 years because of increased incidence of glaucoma.
• Use with caution in hot or humid environments. Drug-induced heatstroke can develop.
• Give 30 minutes to 1 hour before meals and at bedtime. Bedtime dose can be larger and should be given at least 2 hours after the last meal of the day.
• Monitor patient's vital signs and urine output carefully.
• Instruct patient to avoid driving and other hazardous activities if he is drowsy, dizzy, or has blurred vision; to drink plenty of fluids to help prevent constipation; and to report any rash or skin eruption.
• Gum or sugarless hard candy may relieve dry mouth.
• Single dose produces 10- to 12-hour antisecretory effect and GI antispasmodic effect.
• Discontinue 1 week before thyroid function tests.

mepenzolate bromide
Cantil**
Pregnancy Risk Category: C

MECHANISM OF ACTION
Competitively blocks acetylcholine, which decreases GI motility and inhibits gastric acid secretion.

INDICATIONS & DOSAGE
Adjunctive therapy in treating peptic ulcer, irritable bowel syndrome, and neurologic bowel disturbances—
Adults: 25 to 50 mg P.O. q.i.d. with meals and at bedtime. Adjust dosage to individual patient's needs.

ADVERSE REACTIONS
CNS: headache, insomnia, drowsiness, dizziness, *confusion or excitement in elderly patients,* nervousness, weakness.
CV: *palpitations,* tachycardia.
EENT: *blurred vision,* mydriasis, increased ocular tension, cycloplegia, photophobia.
GI: *dry mouth,* dysphagia, heartburn, loss of taste, nausea, *constipation,* vomiting, *paralytic ileus.*
GU: *urinary hesitancy, urine retention,* impotence.
Skin: urticaria, decreased sweating or possible anhidrosis, other dermal manifestations.
Other: fever, allergic reactions.
Overdosage may cause curare-like symptoms.

INTERACTIONS
None significant.

NURSING CONSIDERATIONS
• Contraindicated in narrow-angle glaucoma, obstructive uropathy, obstructive disease of GI tract, severe ulcerative colitis, myasthenia gravis, hypersensitivity to anticholinergics, paralytic ileus, intestinal atony, unstable cardiovascular status in acute hemorrhage, or toxic megacolon. Use

---

Italicized side effects are common or life-threatening.
*Liquid form contains alcohol.   **May contain tartrazine.

cautiously in autonomic neuropathy, hyperthyroidism, coronary artery disease, cardiac dysrhythmias, CHF, hypertension, hiatal hernia associated with reflux esophagitis, hepatic or renal disease, and ulcerative colitis, or in patients over 40 years, because of increased incidence of glaucoma.
• Use with caution in hot or humid environments. Drug-induced heatstroke can develop.
• Give with meals and at bedtime.
• Monitor patient's vital signs and urine output carefully.
• Instruct patient to avoid driving and other hazardous activities if he is drowsy, dizzy, or has blurred vision; to drink plenty of fluids to help prevent constipation; and to report any rash or skin eruption.
• Gum or sugarless hard candy may relieve dry mouth.

methantheline bromide
Banthine

Pregnancy Risk Category: C

MECHANISM OF ACTION
Competitively blocks acetylcholine, which decreases GI motility and inhibits gastric acid secretion.

INDICATIONS & DOSAGE
Adjunctive therapy in peptic ulcer, pylorospasm, spastic colon, biliary dyskinesia, pancreatitis, and certain forms of gastritis—
Adults: 50 to 100 mg P.O. q 6 hours.
Children over 1 year: 12.5 to 50 mg q.i.d.
Children under 1 year: 12.5 to 25 mg q.i.d.
Neonates: 12.5 mg b.i.d., then t.i.d.

ADVERSE REACTIONS
CNS: headache, insomnia, drowsiness, dizziness, *confusion or excitement in elderly patients,* nervousness, weakness.
CV: *palpitations,* tachycardia.

EENT: *blurred vision,* mydriasis, increased ocular tension, cycloplegia, photophobia.
GI: *dry mouth,* dysphagia, *constipation,* heartburn, loss of taste, nausea, vomiting, *paralytic ileus.*
GU: *urinary hesitancy, urine retention,* impotence.
Skin: urticaria, decreased sweating or possible anhidrosis, other dermal manifestations.
Other: fever, allergic reactions.
Overdosage may cause curare-like symptoms.

INTERACTIONS
None significant.

NURSING CONSIDERATIONS
• Contraindicated in narrow-angle glaucoma, obstructive uropathy, obstructive disease of GI tract, severe ulcerative colitis, myasthenia gravis, hypersensitivity to anticholinergics, paralytic ileus, intestinal atony, unstable cardiovascular status in acute hemorrhage, or toxic megacolon. Use cautiously in autonomic neuropathy, hyperthyroidism, coronary artery disease, cardiac dysrhythmias, CHF, hypertension, hiatal hernia associated with reflux esophagitis, hepatic or renal disease, and ulcerative colitis, or in patients over 40 years because of the increased incidence of glaucoma.
• Use with caution in hot or humid environments. Drug-induced heatstroke can develop.
• Give 30 minutes to 1 hour before meals and at bedtime. Bedtime dose can be larger and should be given at least 2 hours after the last meal of the day.
• If patient is also taking antihistamines, he may experience increased dryness of mouth.
• Monitor patient's vital signs and urine output carefully.
• Instruct patient to avoid driving and other hazardous activities if he is drowsy, dizzy, or has blurred vision;

to drink plenty of fluids to help prevent constipation; and to report any rash or skin eruption.
• Gum or sugarless hard candy may relieve dry mouth.
• Therapeutic effects appear in 30 to 45 minutes; persist for 4 to 6 hours after oral administration.

methscopolamine bromide
Pamine

Pregnancy Risk Category: C

MECHANISM OF ACTION
Competitively blocks acetylcholine, which decreases GI motility and inhibits gastric acid secretion.

INDICATIONS & DOSAGE
Adjunctive therapy in peptic ulcer—
Adults: 2.5 to 5 mg P.O. half hour before meals and h.s.

ADVERSE REACTIONS
CNS: headache, insomnia, dizziness, *confusion or excitement in elderly patients,* nervousness, weakness.
CV: *palpitations,* tachycardia.
EENT: *blurred vision,* mydriasis, increased ocular tension, cycloplegia, photophobia.
GI: *dry mouth,* dysphagia, *constipation,* heartburn, loss of taste, nausea, vomiting, *paralytic ileus.*
GU: *urinary hesitancy, urine retention,* impotence.
Skin: urticaria, decreased sweating or possible anhidrosis, other dermal manifestations.
Other: fever, allergic reactions.
Overdosage may cause curare-like symptoms.

INTERACTIONS
None significant.

NURSING CONSIDERATIONS
• Contraindicated in narrow-angle glaucoma, obstructive uropathy, obstructive disease of GI tract, severe ulcerative colitis, myasthenia gravis, hypersensitivity to anticholinergics, paralytic ileus, intestinal atony, unstable cardiovascular status in acute hemorrhage, or toxic megacolon. Use cautiously in autonomic neuropathy, hyperthyroidism, coronary artery disease, cardiac dysrhythmias, CHF, hypertension, hiatal hernia associated with reflux esophagitis, hepatic or renal disease, and ulcerative colitis, or in patients over 40 years because of increased incidence of glaucoma.
• Use with caution in hot or humid environments. Drug-induced heatstroke can develop.
• Give 30 minutes to 1 hour before meals and at bedtime. Bedtime dose can be larger and should be given at least 2 hours after the last meal of the day.
• Monitor patient's vital signs and urine output carefully.
• Instruct patient to avoid driving and other hazardous activities if he is drowsy, dizzy, or has blurred vision; to drink plenty of fluids to help prevent constipation; and to report any rash or skin eruption.
• Gum or sugarless hard candy may relieve dry mouth.

oxyphencyclimine hydrochloride
Daricon

Pregnancy Risk Category: C

MECHANISM OF ACTION
Exerts a nonspecific, direct spasmolytic action on smooth muscle. Also possesses local anesthetic properties that may be partly responsible for spasmolysis.

INDICATIONS & DOSAGE
Adjunctive treatment of peptic ulcer—
Adults: 10 mg P.O. b.i.d. in the morning and at bedtime, or 5 mg b.i.d. or t.i.d.

Italicized side effects are common or life-threatening.
*Liquid form contains alcohol.   **May contain tartrazine.

ADVERSE REACTIONS
CNS: *headache*, insomnia, drowsiness, *dizziness*.
CV: *palpitations*, tachycardia.
EENT: *blurred vision*, mydriasis, increased ocular tension, cycloplegia, photophobia.
GI: *constipation*, nausea, vomiting, *paralytic ileus*.
GU: *urinary hesitancy, urine retention, impotence*.
Skin: urticaria, decreased sweating or possible anhidrosis, other dermal manifestations.
Other: fever, allergic reactions.
   Overdosage may cause curare-like symptoms.

INTERACTIONS
None significant.

NURSING CONSIDERATIONS
• Contraindicated in narrow-angle glaucoma, obstructive uropathy, obstructive disease of GI tract, severe ulcerative colitis, myasthenia gravis, hypersensitivity to anticholinergics, paralytic ileus, intestinal atony, unstable cardiovascular status in acute hemorrhage, or toxic megacolon.
• Use cautiously in autonomic neuropathy, hyperthyroidism, coronary artery disease, cardiac dysrhythmias, CHF, hypertension, hiatal hernia associated with reflux esophagitis, hepatic or renal disease, and ulcerative colitis, or in patients over 40 years because of increased incidence of glaucoma.
• Use with caution in hot or humid environments. Drug-induced heatstroke can develop.
• Give 30 minutes to 1 hour before breakfast and at bedtime.
• Monitor patient's vital signs and urine output carefully.
• Instruct patient to avoid driving and other hazardous activities if he is drowsy, dizzy, or has blurred vision; to drink plenty of fluids to help prevent constipation; and to report any rash or skin eruption.
• Gum or sugarless hard candy may relieve dry mouth.
• A synthetic tertiary derivative that may have fewer atropine-like adverse reactions.

---

oxyphenonium bromide
Antrenyl

Pregnancy Risk Category: C

MECHANISM OF ACTION
Competitively blocks acetylcholine, which decreases GI motility and inhibits gastric acid secretion.

INDICATIONS & DOSAGE
Adjunctive treatment of peptic ulcer—
Adults: 10 mg P.O. q.i.d. for several days, then reduced according to patient response.

ADVERSE REACTIONS
CNS: headache, insomnia, drowsiness, dizziness, *confusion or excitement in elderly patients,* nervousness, weakness.
CV: *palpitations,* tachycardia.
EENT: *blurred vision,* mydriasis, increased ocular tension, cycloplegia, photophobia.
GI: *dry mouth,* dysphagia, *constipation,* heartburn, loss of taste, nausea, vomiting, *paralytic ileus*.
GU: *urinary hesitancy, urine retention,* impotence.
Skin: urticaria, decreased sweating or possible anhidrosis, other dermal manifestations.
Other: fever, allergic reactions.
   Overdosage may cause curare-like symptoms.

INTERACTIONS
None significant.

NURSING CONSIDERATIONS
• Contraindicated in narrow-angle glaucoma, obstructive uropathy, obstructive disease of GI tract, severe

ulcerative colitis, myasthenia gravis, hypersensitivity to anticholinergics, paralytic ileus, intestinal atony, unstable cardiovascular status in acute hemorrhage, or toxic megacolon.

• Use cautiously in autonomic neuropathy, hyperthyroidism, coronary artery disease, cardiac dysrhythmias, CHF, hypertension, hiatal hernia associated with reflux esophagitis, hepatic or renal disease, and ulcerative colitis, or in patients over 40 years because of increased incidence of glaucoma.

• Use with caution in hot or humid environments. Drug-induced heatstroke can develop.

• Give 30 minutes to 1 hour before meals and at bedtime. Bedtime dose can be larger and should be given at least 2 hours after the last meal of the day.

• Monitor patient's vital signs and urine output carefully.

• Instruct patient to avoid driving and other hazardous activities if he is drowsy, dizzy, or has blurred vision; to drink plenty of fluids to help prevent constipation; and to report any skin rash or local eruption.

• Gum or sugarless hard candy may relieve dry mouth.

---

propantheline bromide
Norpanth, Pro-Banthine♦, Propanthel♦♦

Pregnancy Risk Category: C

MECHANISM OF ACTION
Competitively blocks acetylcholine, which decreases GI motility and inhibits gastric acid secretion.

INDICATIONS & DOSAGE
Adjunctive treatment of peptic ulcer, irritable bowel syndrome, and other gastrointestinal disorders; to reduce duodenal motility during diagnostic radiologic procedures—
Adults: 15 mg P.O. t.i.d. before

meals, and 30 mg h.s. up to 60 mg q.i.d. For elderly patients, 7.5 mg P.O. t.i.d. before meals.

ADVERSE REACTIONS
CNS: headache, insomnia, drowsiness, dizziness, *confusion or excitement in elderly patients,* nervousness, weakness.
CV: *palpitations,* tachycardia.
EENT: *blurred vision,* mydriasis, increased ocular tension, cycloplegia, photophobia.
GI: *dry mouth,* dysphagia, constipation, heartburn, loss of taste, nausea, vomiting, paralytic ileus.
GU: *urinary hesitancy, urine retention,* impotence.
Skin: urticaria, decreased sweating or possible anhidrosis, other dermal manifestations.
Other: fever, allergic reactions.
  Overdosage may cause curare-like symptoms.

INTERACTIONS
None significant.

NURSING CONSIDERATIONS
• Contraindicated in narrow-angle glaucoma, obstructive uropathy, obstructive disease of GI tract, severe ulcerative colitis, myasthenia gravis, hypersensitivity to anticholinergics, paralytic ileus, intestinal atony, unstable cardiovascular status in acute hemorrhage, or toxic megacolon. Use cautiously in autonomic neuropathy, hyperthyroidism, coronary artery disease, cardiac dysrhythmias, congestive heart failure, hypertension, hiatal hernia associated with reflux esophagitis, hepatic or renal disease, and ulcerative colitis, or in patients over 40 years because of the increased incidence of glaucoma.

• Use with caution in hot or humid environments. Drug-induced heatstroke can develop.

• Give 30 minutes to 1 hour before meals and at bedtime. Bedtime dose

---

Italicized side effects are common or life-threatening.
*Liquid form contains alcohol.   **May contain tartrazine.

can be larger and should be given at least 2 hours after the last meal of the day.
• Monitor patient's vital signs and urine output carefully.
• Instruct patient to avoid driving and other hazardous activities if he is drowsy, dizzy, or has blurred vision; to drink plenty of fluids to help prevent constipation; and to report any rash or skin eruption.
• Gum or sugarless hard candy may relieve dry mouth.

51

Antiulcer agents

cimetidine
famotidine
misoprostol
nizatidine
ranitidine
sucralfate

COMBINATION PRODUCTS
None.

cimetidine
Tagamet♦

Pregnancy Risk Category: B

MECHANISM OF ACTION
Competitively inhibits the action of histamine (H_2) at receptor sites of the parietal cells, decreasing gastric acid secretion.

INDICATIONS & DOSAGE
Duodenal ulcer (short-term treatment)—
Adults and children over 16 years: 300 mg P.O. q.i.d. with meals and h.s. Alternatively, may give 400 mg P.O. b.i.d. or 800 mg once daily h.s. Continue treatment for 4 to 6 weeks unless endoscopy shows healing. Maintenance therapy: 400 mg h.s. Parenteral: 300 mg diluted to 20 ml with 0.9% normal saline solution or other compatible I.V. solution by I.V. push over 1 to 2 minutes q 6 hours. Or 300 mg diluted in 50 ml dextrose 5% solution or other compatible I.V. solution by I.V. infusion over 15 to 20 minutes q 6 hours. Or 300 mg I.M. q 6 hours (no dilution necessary). To increase dose, give 300 mg doses more

frequently to maximum daily dosage of 2,400 mg.
Duodenal ulcer prophylaxis—
Adults and children over 16 years: 400 mg P.O. h.s.
Active benign gastric ulcer—
Adults: 300 mg q.i.d. with meals and h.s. for up to 8 weeks.
Pathologic hypersecretory conditions (such as Zollinger-Ellison syndrome, systemic mastocytosis, and multiple endocrine adenomas)—
Adults and children over 16 years: 300 mg P.O. q.i.d. with meals and h.s.; adjust to individual needs. Maximum daily dosage is 2,400 mg. Parenteral: 300 mg diluted to 20 ml with 0.9% normal saline solution or other compatible I.V. solutions by I.V. push over 1 to 2 minutes q 6 hours. Or 300 mg diluted in 50 ml dextrose 5% solution or other compatible I.V. solution by I.V. infusion over 15 to 20 minutes q 6 hours. To increase dosage, give 300-mg doses more frequently to maximum daily dosage of 2,400 mg.

ADVERSE REACTIONS
Blood: *agranulocytosis, neutropenia, thrombocytopenia, aplastic anemia (rare).*
CNS: mental confusion, dizziness, headaches, peripheral neuropathy.
CV: bradycardia.
GI: *mild and transient diarrhea.*
GU: transient elevations in serum creatinine.
Hepatic: jaundice (rare).

Italicized side effects are common or life-threatening.
*Liquid form contains alcohol.   **May contain tartrazine.

Skin: acne-like rash, urticaria.
Other: hypersensitivity, muscle pain, mild gynecomastia after use longer than 1 month.

INTERACTIONS

Antacids: interfere with absorption of cimetidine. Separate cimetidine and antacids by at least 1 hour if possible.

Cimetidine may inhibit hepatic microsomal enzyme metabolism of some drugs, like warfarin, phenytoin, some benzodiazepines, lidocaine, theophylline, and propranolol. Monitor serum levels of these drugs closely during cimetidine therapy.

NURSING CONSIDERATIONS

• I.M. route of administration may be painful.
• I.V. solutions compatible for dilution with cimetidine: 0.9% sodium chloride solution, dextrose 5% and 10% (and combinations of these) in water solutions, lactated Ringer's solution, and 5% sodium bicarbonate injection. Do not dilute with sterile water for injection.
• Hemodialysis reduces blood levels of cimetidine. Schedule cimetidine dose at end of hemodialysis treatment.
• Up to 10 g overdosage has been reported without adverse effects.
• Effectiveness in treatment of gastric ulcers not as great as in duodenal ulcer. Cimetidine may prove useful but is still unapproved in pancreatic insufficiency, short-bowel syndrome, psoriasis, prevention and treatment of GI bleeding, relief of symptoms and acid sensitivity in reflux esophagitis, and prevention of gastric inactivation of oral enzyme preparations by gastric acid and pepsin.
• Taking tablets with meals will ensure a more consistent therapeutic effect.
• Remind patient that if he's taking cimetidine once daily, he should take it at bedtime for best results.

• Available in liquid form (300 mg/5 ml).
• Tablets available in four strengths: 200 mg, 300 mg, 400 mg, and 800 mg. All tablets are pale blue-green. Identify tablet strength when obtaining a drug history.
• Blue dye in Tagamet tablets may produce a false-positive Hemoccult test for blood in gastric juice. This can be avoided by administering the tablet at least 15 minutes before obtaining gastric juice by aspiration or by administering the liquid form.
• Elderly or debilitated patients may be more susceptible to cimetidine-induced mental confusion.
• I.V. cimetidine often used in critically ill patients prophylactically to prevent GI bleeding.
• Don't infuse I.V. too rapidly. May cause bradycardia.
• Urge patient to avoid cigarette smoking, as this may increase gastric acid secretion and worsen disease.
• When administering cimetidine I.V. in 100 ml of diluent solution, do not infuse so rapidly that circulatory overload is produced. Some authorities recommend that the drug be infused over at least 30 minutes, to minimize the risk of adverse cardiac effects.
• Has many investigational uses. Used before anesthesia for prophylaxis of aspiration pneumonitis; also used to treat hyperparathyroidism, herpes zoster, chronic hives, and as an adjunct in the treatment of acetaminophen overdose.

famotidine
Pepcid

Pregnancy Risk Category: B

MECHANISM OF ACTION
Competitively inhibits the action of histamine (H_2) at receptor sites of the parietal cells, decreasing gastric acid secretion.

INDICATIONS & DOSAGE
Duodenal ulcer—
Adults: For acute therapy, 40 mg P.O. once daily h.s. For maintenance therapy, 20 mg P.O. once daily h.s.
Pathologic hypersecretory conditions (such as Zollinger-Ellison syndrome)—
Adults: 20 mg P.O. q 6 hours. As much as 160 mg q 6 hours may be administered.
Hospitalized patients with intractable ulcers or hypersecretory conditions, or patients who cannot take oral medication—
Adults: 20 mg I.V. q 12 hours.

ADVERSE REACTIONS
Blood: thrombocytopenia (rare).
CNS: *headache,* dizziness, hallucinations.
GI: diarrhea, constipation, nausea, flatulence.
GU: increased BUN and creatinine.
Skin: acne, pruritus, rash.
Local: transient irritation at I.V. site.

INTERACTIONS
None significant.

NURSING CONSIDERATIONS
• Gastric cancer must be ruled out before famotidine therapy.
• Advise patient not to take the drug for longer than 8 weeks unless doctor specifically orders it.
• Especially at the beginning of therapy when pain is severe and with doctor's knowledge, patient may take antacids concomitantly.
• Urge patient to avoid cigarette smoking as this may increase gastric acid secretion and worsen disease.
• Patient may take famotidine with a snack if he desires. Remind patient that this drug is most effective if taken at bedtime.
• Some patients may have this drug prescribed to be taken 20 mg twice daily instead of 40 mg at bedtime. This alternate dosing schedule is also effective. However, at least one dose

should be taken at bedtime.
• Unlike cimetidine, which has a weak androgenic effect, famotidine has not been reported to cause gynecomastia in males. Unlike cimetidine and ranitidine, famotidine is not known to cause significant drug interactions.

misoprostol
Cytotec

Pregnancy Risk Category: X

MECHANISM OF ACTION
A synthetic prostaglandin E_1 analog, misoprostol replaces gastric prostaglandins that are depleted by NSAID therapy. It also decreases basal and stimulated gastric acid secretion, and may increase gastric mucus and bicarbonate production.

INDICATIONS AND DOSAGE
Prevention of NSAID-induced gastric ulcers in elderly or debilitated patients at high risk of complications from gastric ulcer, and patients with a history of NSAID-induced ulcers—
Adults: 200 mcg P.O. q.i.d. with food. If this dosage isn't tolerated, it may be decreased to 100 mcg P.O. q.i.d.

ADVERSE REACTIONS
CNS: headache.
GI: diarrhea, abdominal pain, nausea, flatulence, dyspepsia, vomiting, constipation.
GU: hypermenorrhea, dysmenorrhea, spotting, cramps, menstrual disorders.

INTERACTIONS
Antacids: reduced plasma levels when administered concomitantly. Not considered significant.

NURSING CONSIDERATIONS
• Misoprostol is an abortifacient and is contraindicated for use in pregnant

---

women. Misoprostol is also contraindicated in patients who have a history of an allergic response to prostaglandins.

• Misoprostol should not be routinely administered to women of childbearing age unless they are at high risk of developing ulcers or complications from NSAID-induced ulcers.

• Special precautions must be taken to prevent the use of this drug during pregnancy. The patient must be fully aware of the dangers of misoprostol to a fetus, and must receive both oral and written warnings regarding these dangers. She must be capable of complying with effective contraceptive means, and must have a negative serum pregnancy test within 2 weeks of initiating therapy.

• Misoprostol therapy must not begin until the second or third day of the next normal menstrual period.

• Instruct *ALL* patients not to share misoprostol with anyone else. They should be aware that when taken by a pregnant patient this drug may cause miscarriage, often with potentially life threatening bleeding. Concomitant ingestion of food or antacids seems to reduce maximal plasma concentrations of misoprostol, but this doesn't appear to impair the drug's effectiveness.

• Misoprostol appears to reduce the bioavailability of concomitantly administered aspirin, but this effect is not considered clinically significant.

nizatidine
Axid

Pregnancy Risk Category: C

MECHANISM OF ACTION
Competitively inhibits the action of histamine at H_2 receptor sites of the parietal cells, decreasing gastric acid secretion.

INDICATIONS & DOSAGE
Active duodenal ulcer treatment—
Adults: 300 mg once daily at bedtime. Alternatively, patient may receive 150 mg b.i.d.
Maintenance therapy of duodenal ulcer—
Adults: 150 mg once daily h.s.

ADVERSE REACTIONS
Blood: *thrombocytopenia.*
CNS: *somnolence.*
CV: dysrhythmias.
Skin: *sweating,* rash, urticaria, *exfoliative dermatitis.*
Other: hepatic damage, hyperuricemia, gynecomastia.

INTERACTIONS
Aspirin: nizatidine may elevate serum salicylate levels in patients taking high doses of aspirin.

NURSING CONSIDERATIONS
• Contraindicated in patients with hypersensitivity to H_2-receptor antagonists.

• Dosage should be reduced in patients with impaired renal function. Patients with a creatinine clearance of 20 to 50 ml/minute should receive 150 mg daily for treatment of active duodenal ulcer, or 150 mg every other day for maintenance therapy. Patients with a creatinine clearance below 20 ml/minute should receive 150 mg every other day for treatment or 150 mg every third day for maintenance.

• False-positive test results for urobilinogen may occur.

• Nizatidine has not been associated with antiandrogenic activity and does not appear to affect hepatic drug-metabolizing enzyme systems.

• Urge patient to avoid cigarette smoking, which will increase gastric acid secretion and worsen disease.

ranitidine
Zantac♦

Pregnancy Risk Category: B

MECHANISM OF ACTION
Competitively inhibits the action of histamine (H_2) at receptor sites of the parietal cells, decreasing gastric acid secretion.

INDICATIONS & DOSAGE
Duodenal and gastric ulcer (short-term treatment); pathological hypersecretory conditions, such as Zollinger-Ellison syndrome—
Adults: 150 mg P.O. b.i.d. or 300 mg once daily h.s. Dosages up to 6 g/day may be prescribed in patients with Zollinger-Ellison syndrome. May also be administered parenterally: 50 mg I.V. or I.M. q 6 to 8 hours. When administering I.V. push, dilute to a total volume of 20 ml and inject over a period of 5 minutes. No dilution necessary when administering I.M. May also be administered by intermittent I.V. infusion. Dilute 50 mg ranitidine in 100 ml of dextrose 5% in water and infuse over 15 to 20 minutes.
Maintenance therapy of duodenal ulcer—
Adults: 150 mg P.O. h.s.
Gastroesophageal reflux disease (GERD)—
Adults: 150 mg P.O. b.i.d.

ADVERSE REACTIONS
Blood: neutropenia, thrombocytopenia.
CNS: headache, malaise, dizziness, confusion.
CV: bradycardia.
GI: nausea, constipation.
Hepatic: elevated liver enzymes, jaundice.
Skin: rash.
Local: burning and itching at injection site.

INTERACTIONS
Antacids: interfere with absorption of ranitidine. Separate ranitidine and antacids dosage by at least 1 hour, if possible.

NURSING CONSIDERATIONS
• Use cautiously in hepatic dysfunction. Dosage should be adjusted in patients with impaired renal function.
• Does not interact with other drugs to the extent that cimetidine does.
• Due to decreased renal clearance, elderly patients are more likely to experience adverse reactions.
• Can be taken without regard to meals. Absorption not affected by food.
• Remind patient that if he's taking ranitidine once daily, he should take it at bedtime for best results.
• Urge patient to avoid smoking, as this may increase gastric acid secretion and worsen disease.
• Most patients show healing of ulcer within 4 weeks. Additional treatment after this interval has not been demonstrated.

sucralfate
Carafate, Sulcrate♦♦

Pregnancy Risk Category: B

MECHANISM OF ACTION
Adheres to and protects the ulcer surface by forming a barrier.

INDICATIONS & DOSAGE
Short-term (up to 8 weeks) treatment of duodenal ulcer—
Adults: 1 g P.O. q.i.d. 1 hour before meals and h.s.

ADVERSE REACTIONS
CNS: dizziness, sleepiness.
GI: *constipation,* nausea, gastric discomfort, diarrhea, bezoar formation.

INTERACTIONS
Antacids: may decrease binding of

ANTIULCER AGENTS 495

drug to gastroduodenal mucosa, impairing effectiveness. Don't give within 30 minutes of each other.

NURSING CONSIDERATIONS
• No known contraindications.
• Drug is minimally absorbed. Incidence of adverse reactions is low.
• Tell patient for best results to take sucralfate on an empty stomach (1 hour before each meal and at bedtime).
• Pain and ulcer symptoms may subside within first few weeks of therapy. However, for complete healing, be sure patient continues on prescribed regimen.
• Monitor for severe, persistent constipation.
• Studies suggest that drug is as effective as cimetidine in healing duodenal ulcers.
• Drug has been used to treat gastric ulcers, but effectiveness of this use is still under investigation.
• Drug contains aluminum but isn't classified as an antacid.
• Urge patient to avoid smoking, as this may increase gastric acid secretion and worsen disease.

52

Corticosteroids

Glucocorticoids
beclomethasone dipropionate
betamethasone
betamethasone acetate and betamethasone sodium phosphate
betamethasone disodium phosphate
betamethasone sodium phosphate
cortisone acetate
dexamethasone
dexamethasone acetate
dexamethasone sodium phosphate
flunisolide
hydrocortisone
hydrocortisone acetate
hydrocortisone cypionate
hydrocortisone sodium phosphate
hydrocortisone sodium succinate
methylprednisolone
methylprednisolone acetate
methylprednisolone sodium succinate
paramethasone acetate
prednisolone
prednisolone acetate
prednisolone sodium phosphate
prednisolone tebutate
prednisone
triamcinolone
triamcinolone acetonide
triamcinolone diacetate
triamcinolone hexacetonide

Mineralocorticoids
fludrocortisone acetate

COMBINATION PRODUCTS
DECADRON WITH XYLOCAINE: dexamethasone phosphate 4 mg and lidocaine hydrochloride 10 mg/ml.

---

beclomethasone dipropionate
Beclovent♦, Beclovent Rotacaps ♦♦, Vanceril♦

Pregnancy Risk Category: C

MECHANISM OF ACTION
Decreases inflammation, mainly by stabilizing leukocyte lysosomal membranes. Also suppresses the immune response, stimulates bone marrow, and influences protein, fat, and carbohydrate metabolism.

INDICATIONS & DOSAGE
Steroid-dependent asthma—
Adults: 2 to 4 inhalations t.i.d. or q.i.d. Maximum dosage is 20 inhalations daily.
Children 6 to 12 years: 1 to 2 inhalations t.i.d. or q.i.d. Maximum dosage is 10 inhalations daily.

ADVERSE REACTIONS
EENT: hoarseness, fungal infections of mouth and throat.
GI: dry mouth.

INTERACTIONS
None significant.

NURSING CONSIDERATIONS
• Contraindicated in status asthmaticus. Not for use in asthma controlled by bronchodilators or other noncor-

---

Italicized side effects are common or life-threatening.
*Liquid form contains alcohol.   **May contain tartrazine.

ticosteroids alone, or for nonasthmatic bronchial diseases.

• Oral glucocorticoid therapy should be tapered slowly. Acute adrenal insufficiency and death have occurred in asthmatics who changed abruptly from oral corticosteroids to beclomethasone.

• During times of stress (trauma, surgery, or infection) systemic corticosteroids may be needed to prevent adrenal insufficiency in previously steroid-dependent patients.

• Instruct patient to carry a card indicating his need for supplemental systemic glucocorticoids during stress.

• Patient requiring bronchodilator should use it several minutes before beclomethasone.

• Tell patient to allow 1 minute to elapse before taking subsequent puffs of medication, and to hold breath for a few seconds to enhance action of drug.

• Inform patient that beclomethasone doesn't provide relief for emergency asthma attacks.

• Instruct patient to contact doctor if he notices a decreased response. Dose may have to be adjusted. Patient shouldn't exceed recommended dose on his own.

• Check mucous membranes frequently for signs of fungal infection.

• Oral fungal infections can be prevented by following inhalations with glass of water.

• Tell patient to keep inhaler clean and unobstructed. Wash with warm water and dry thoroughly.

betamethasone
Betnelan♦♦, Celestone♦*

betamethasone acetate and betamethasone sodium phosphate
Celestone Soluspan♦

betamethasone sodium phosphate
Betameth, Betnesol♦♦, B.S.P., Celestone Phosphate♦, Cel-U-Jec, Prelestone, Selestoject

Pregnancy Risk Category: C

MECHANISM OF ACTION
Decreases inflammation, mainly by stabilizing leukocyte lysosomal membranes. Also suppresses the immune response, stimulates bone marrow, and influences protein, fat, and carbohydrate metabolism.

INDICATIONS & DOSAGE
Severe inflammation or immunosuppression—
Adults: 0.6 to 7.2 mg P.O. daily; or 0.5 to 9 mg (sodium phosphate) I.M., I.V., or into joint or soft tissue daily; or 1.5 to 12 mg (sodium phosphate-acetate suspension) into joint or soft tissue q 1 to 2 weeks, p.r.n.
Prevention of neonatal respiratory distress syndrome—
Adults (pregnant women): 12 mg I.M. Celestone Soluspan 36 to 48 hours before premature delivery. Repeat in 24 hours.

ADVERSE REACTIONS
Most adverse reactions of corticosteroids are dose- or duration-dependent.
CNS: *euphoria, insomnia,* psychotic behavior, pseudotumor cerebri.
CV: *CHF,* hypertension, edema.
EENT: cataracts, glaucoma.
GI: *peptic ulcer,* GI irritation, increased appetite.
Metabolic: *possible hypokalemia, hy-*

perglycemia and carbohydrate intolerance, growth suppression in children.
Skin: delayed wound healing, acne, various skin eruptions.
Other: muscle weakness, pancreatitis, hirsutism, susceptibility to infections. Acute adrenal insufficiency may follow increased stress (infection, surgery, or trauma) or abrupt withdrawal after long-term therapy. *Withdrawal symptoms:* rebound inflammation, fatigue, weakness, arthralgia, fever, dizziness, lethargy, depression, fainting, orthostatic hypotension, dyspnea, anorexia, hypoglycemia. *Sudden withdrawal may be fatal.*

INTERACTIONS
Barbiturates, phenytoin, rifampin: decreased corticosteroid effect. Corticosteroid dose may need to be increased.
Indomethacin, aspirin: increased risk of GI distress and bleeding. Give together cautiously.

NURSING CONSIDERATIONS
• Contraindicated in systemic fungal infections. Use cautiously in patients with GI ulceration or renal disease, hypertension, osteoporosis, varicella, vaccinia, exanthema, diabetes mellitus, Cushing's syndrome, thromboembolic disorders, seizures, myasthenia gravis, CHF, tuberculosis, ocular herpes simplex, hypoalbuminemia, emotional instability, and psychotic tendencies.
• Don't use for alternate-day therapy.
• Adrenal suppression may last up to 1 year after drug is stopped. Gradually reduce drug dosage after long-term therapy. Tell patient not to stop drug abruptly or without doctor's consent.
• Always titrate to lowest effective dose.
• To prevent muscle atrophy, give I.M. injection deeply.
• Monitor blood sugar and serum po-

tassium regularly. Diabetic patients may require adjustments in insulin dosage.
• Teach patients about the effects of the drug. Warn those on long-term therapy about cushingoid symptoms.
• Observe for signs of infection, especially after steroid withdrawal. Tell patients to report slow healing.
• Instruct patient to carry a card indicating his need for supplemental glucocorticoids during stress.
• Give a daily dosage in the morning for better results and less toxicity.
• Give with milk or food to reduce GI irritation.
• A glucocorticoid with little mineralocorticoid effect.
• Watch for additional potassium depletion from diuretics and amphotericin B.
• Immunizations may show decreased antibody response.
• Obtain baseline weight before starting therapy, and weigh patient daily; report any sudden weight gain to doctor.
• Betamethasone sometimes prescribed to treat respiratory distress syndrome in premature infants.

cortisone acetate
Cortone Acetate♦
Pregnancy Risk Category: D

MECHANISM OF ACTION
Decreases inflammation, mainly by stabilizing leukocyte lysosomal membranes. Also suppresses the immune response, stimulates bone marrow, and influences protein, fat, and carbohydrate metabolism.

INDICATIONS & DOSAGE
Adrenal insufficiency, allergy, inflammation—
Adults: 25 to 300 mg P.O. or I.M. daily or on alternate days. Dosages highly individualized, depending on severity of disease.

ADVERSE REACTIONS

Most adverse reactions of corticosteroids are dose- or duration-dependent.

CNS: *euphoria, insomnia,* psychotic behavior, pseudotumor cerebri.
CV: *CHF,* hypertension, edema.
EENT: cataracts, glaucoma.
GI: *peptic ulcer,* GI irritation, increased appetite.
Metabolic: *possible hypokalemia, hyperglycemia and carbohydrate intolerance,* growth suppression in children.
Skin: delayed wound healing, acne, various skin eruptions.
Local: atrophy at I.M. injection sites.
Other: muscle weakness, pancreatitis, hirsutism, susceptibility to infections. Acute adrenal insufficiency may follow increased stress (infection, surgery, or trauma) or abrupt withdrawal after long-term therapy. *Withdrawal symptoms:* rebound inflammation, fatigue, weakness, arthralgia, fever, dizziness, lethargy, depression, fainting, orthostatic hypotension, dyspnea, anorexia, hypoglycemia. *Sudden withdrawal may be fatal.*

INTERACTIONS

Barbiturates, phenytoin, rifampin: decreased corticosteroid effect. Corticosteroid dose may need to be increased.
Indomethacin, aspirin: increased risk of GI distress and bleeding. Give together cautiously.

NURSING CONSIDERATIONS

• Contraindicated in systemic fungal infections. Use cautiously in patients with GI ulceration or renal disease, hypertension, osteoporosis, varicella, vaccinia, exanthema, diabetes mellitus, Cushing's syndrome, thromboembolic disorders, seizures, myasthenia gravis, congestive heart failure, tuberculosis, ocular herpes simplex, hypoalbuminemia, emotional instability, and psychotic tendencies.

• Gradually reduce drug dosage after long-term therapy. Tell patient not to discontinue drug abruptly or without doctor's consent.
• Always titrate to lowest effective dose.
• Patient may need low-sodium diet and potassium supplement.
• I.M. route causes slow onset of action. Don't use in acute conditions where rapid effect required. May use on a twice-daily schedule matching diurnal variation.
• A glucocorticoid with potent mineralocorticoid effect; report sudden weight gain or edema to doctor.
• Observe for signs of infection, especially after steroid withdrawal. Tell patient to report slow healing.
• Drug of choice for replacement therapy in adrenal insufficiency.
• Monitor serum electrolytes and blood sugar.
• Warn patients on long-term therapy about cushingoid symptoms.
• Give with milk or food to reduce GI irritation.
• Instruct patient to carry a card indicating his need for supplemental glucocorticoids during stress.
• Give a daily dosage in the morning for better results and less toxicity.
• Not for I.V. use.
• Watch for additional potassium depletion from diuretics and amphotericin B.
• Immunizations may show decreased antibody response.

dexamethasone
Decadron♦, Deronil, Dexasone♦♦, Dexone, Hexadrol♦, Mymethasone

dexamethasone acetate
Dalalone D.P., Dalalone L.A., Decadron L.A., Decaject-L.A., Decameth L.A., Dexacen LA, Dexasone-LA, Dexone LA, Dexon LA, Solurex-LA

dexamethasone sodium phosphate
Ak-Dex, Dalalone, Decadrol, Decadron Phosphate♦, Decaject, Decameth, Dex, Dexacen, Dexasone, Dexon, Dexone, Hexadrol Phosphate♦, Solurex

Pregnancy Risk Category: C

MECHANISM OF ACTION
Decreases inflammation, mainly by stabilizing leukocyte lysosomal membranes. Also suppresses the immune response, stimulates bone marrow, and influences protein, fat, and carbohydrate metabolism.

INDICATIONS & DOSAGE
Cerebral edema—
Adults: initially, 10 mg (phosphate) I.V., then 4 to 6 mg I.M. q 6 hours for 2 to 4 days, then tapered over 5 to 7 days.
Children: 0.2 mg/kg P.O. daily in divided doses.
Inflammatory conditions, allergic reactions, neoplasias—
Adults: 0.25 to 4 mg P.O. b.i.d., t.i.d., or q.i.d.; or 4 to 16 mg (acetate) I.M. into joint or soft tissue q 1 to 3 weeks; or 0.8 to 1.6 mg (acetate) into lesions q 1 to 3 weeks.
Shock—
Adults: 1 to 6 mg/kg (phosphate) I.V. single dosage; or 40 mg I.V. q 2 to 6 hours, p.r.n.
Dexamethasone suppression test—
Adults: 0.5 mg P.O. q 6 hours for 48 hours.

ADVERSE REACTIONS
Most adverse reactions of corticosteroids are dose- or duration-dependent.
CNS: *euphoria, insomnia,* psychotic behavior, pseudotumor cerebri.
CV: *CHF,* hypertension, edema.
EENT: cataracts, glaucoma.
GI: *peptic ulcer,* GI irritation, increased appetite.
Metabolic: *possible hypokalemia, hyperglycemia and carbohydrate intolerance,* growth suppression in children.
Skin: delayed wound healing, acne, various skin eruptions.
Local: atrophy at I.M. injection sites.
Other: muscle weakness, pancreatitis, hirsutism, susceptibility to infections. Acute adrenal insufficiency may follow increased stress (infection, surgery, or trauma) or abrupt withdrawal after long-term therapy. *Withdrawal symptoms:* rebound inflammation, fatigue, weakness, arthralgia, fever, dizziness, lethargy, depression, fainting, orthostatic hypotension, dyspnea, anorexia, hypoglycemia. *Sudden withdrawal may be fatal.*

INTERACTIONS
Barbiturates, phenytoin, rifampin: decreased corticosteroid effect. Corticosteroid dose may need to be increased.
Indomethacin, aspirin: increased risk of GI distress and bleeding. Give together cautiously.

NURSING CONSIDERATIONS
• Contraindicated in systemic fungal infections and for alternate-day therapy. Use cautiously in GI ulceration or renal disease, hypertension, osteoporosis, varicella, vaccinia, exanthema, diabetes mellitus, Cushing's syndrome, thromboembolic disorders, seizures, myasthenia gravis, metastatic cancer, congestive heart failure, tuberculosis, ocular herpes simplex, hypoalbuminemia, emotional insta-

---

Italicized side effects are common or life-threatening.
*Liquid form contains alcohol.   **May contain tartrazine.

bility, and psychotic tendencies, and in children.

• Gradually reduce drug dosage after long-term therapy. Tell patient not to discontinue drug abruptly or without doctor's consent.

• Always titrate to lowest effective dose.

• Monitor patient's weight, blood pressure, serum electrolytes.

• Instruct patient to carry a card indicating his need for supplemental systemic glucocorticoids during stress, especially as dosage is decreased.

• Give a daily dosage in the morning for better results and less toxicity.

• Teach patient signs of early adrenal insufficiency: fatigue, muscular weakness, joint pain, fever, anorexia, nausea, dyspnea, dizziness, and fainting.

• May mask or exacerbate infections.

• Watch for depression or psychotic episodes, especially in high-dose therapy.

• Inspect patient's skin for petechiae. Warn patient about easy bruising.

• Patients with diabetes may need increased insulin; monitor blood glucose.

• Monitor growth in infants and children on long-term therapy.

• Give I.M. injection deep into gluteal muscle. Avoid S.C. injection, as atrophy and sterile abscesses may occur.

• Give P.O. dose with food when possible.

• Warn patients on long-term therapy about cushingoid symptoms.

• Watch for additional potassium depletion from diuretics and amphotericin B.

• Immunizations may show decreased antibody response.

• Not used for alternate-day therapy.

• Dexamethasone most recently used in the diagnosis of depression. It is also an effective antiemetic.

fludrocortisone acetate
Florinef ♦

Pregnancy Risk Category: C

MECHANISM OF ACTION
Increases sodium reabsorption, and potassium and hydrogen secretion at the nephron's distal convoluted tubule.

INDICATIONS & DOSAGE
Adrenal insufficiency (partial replacement), adrenogenital syndrome—
Adults: 0.1 to 0.2 mg P.O. daily.

ADVERSE REACTIONS
CV: *sodium and water retention,* hypertension, cardiac hypertrophy, edema.
Metabolic: hypokalemia.

INTERACTIONS
None significant.

NURSING CONSIDERATIONS
• Contraindicated in hypertension, CHF, or cardiac disease. Use cautiously in Addison's disease.

• Monitor patient's blood pressure and serum electrolytes. Weigh patient daily; report sudden weight gain to doctor.

• Warn patient that mild peripheral edema is common.

• Unless contraindicated, give low-sodium diet high in potassium and protein. Potassium supplement may be needed.

• Has potent mineralocorticoid effects. Little glucocorticoid effect with usual doses.

• Used with cortisone or hydrocortisone in adrenal insufficiency.

• Watch for additional potassium depletion from diuretics and amphotericin B.

• Fludrocortisone is also prescribed to treat severe orthostatic hypotension.

---

flunisolide
AeroBid Inhaler

Pregnancy Risk Category: C

MECHANISM OF ACTION
Decreases inflammation, mainly by stabilizing leukocyte lysosomal membranes. Also suppresses the immune response, stimulates bone marrow, and influences protein, fat, and carbohydrate metabolism.

INDICATIONS & DOSAGE
Steroid-dependent asthma—
Adults and children over 6 years: AeroBid Inhaler 2 inhalations (500 mcg) b.i.d. Don't exceed 4 inhalations b.i.d.

ADVERSE REACTIONS
EENT: hoarseness, fungal infections of mouth and throat.
GI: dry mouth.

INTERACTIONS
None significant.

NURSING CONSIDERATIONS
• Contraindicated in status asthmaticus. Not recommended for use in asthma controlled by bronchodilators or other noncorticosteroids alone, or for nonasthmatic bronchial diseases.
• Oral glucocorticoid therapy should be tapered slowly.
• During times of stress (trauma, surgery, or infection), systemic corticosteroids may be needed to prevent adrenal insufficiency in previously steroid-dependent patients.
• Instruct patient to carry a card indicating his need for supplemental systemic glucocorticoids during stress.
• Check mucous membranes frequently for signs of fungal infection. Tell patient to follow inhalations with glass of water to help prevent fungal infections.
• Tell patient to keep inhaler clean and unobstructed. Wash with warm water and dry thoroughly after use.
• Patient requiring bronchodilator should use it several minutes before flunisolide.
• Tell patient to allow 1 minute to elapse before repeating inhalations, and to hold breath for a few seconds to enhance action of drug.
• Inform patient that flunisolide doesn't relieve emergency asthma attacks.

hydrocortisone
Cortef♦, Cortenema, Hycort♦♦, Hydrocortone♦

hydrocortisone acetate
Biosone, Cortifoam♦, Hydrocortone Acetate♦

hydrocortisone cypionate
Cortef

hydrocortisone sodium phosphate
Hydrocortone Phosphate

hydrocortisone sodium succinate
A-HydroCort, Solu-Cortef♦

Pregnancy Risk Category: C

MECHANISM OF ACTION
Decreases inflammation, mainly by stabilizing leukocyte lysosomal membranes. Also suppresses the immune response, stimulates bone marrow, and influences protein, fat, and carbohydrate metabolism.

INDICATIONS & DOSAGE
Severe inflammation, adrenal insufficiency—
Adults: 5 to 30 mg P.O. b.i.d., t.i.d., or q.i.d. (as much as 80 mg P.O. q.i.d. may be given in acute situations); or initially, 100 to 250 mg (succinate) I.M. or I.V., then 50 to 100 mg I.M., as indicated; or 15 to 240 mg (phosphate) I.M. or I.V. q 12

hours; or 5 to 75 mg (acetate) into joints and soft tissue. Dosage varies with size of joint. Often local anesthetics are injected with dose.
Shock—
Adults: 500 mg to 2 g (succinate) q 2 to 6 hours.
Children: 0.16 to 1 mg/kg (phosphate or succinate) I.M. or I.V., b.i.d. or t.i.d.
Adjunctive treatment of ulcerative colitis and proctitis—
Adults: 1 enema (100 mg) nightly for 21 days.

ADVERSE REACTIONS
Most adverse reactions of corticosteroids are dose- or duration-dependent.
CNS: *euphoria, insomnia,* psychotic behavior, pseudotumor cerebri.
CV: *CHF,* hypertension, edema.
EENT: cataracts, glaucoma.
GI: *peptic ulcer,* GI irritation, increased appetite.
Metabolic: *possible hypokalemia, hyperglycemia and carbohydrate intolerance,* growth suppression in children.
Skin: delayed wound healing, acne, various skin eruptions.
Other: muscle weakness, pancreatitis, hirsutism, susceptibility to infections. Acute adrenal insufficiency may occur with increased stress (infection, surgery, or trauma) or abrupt withdrawal after long-term therapy.
Withdrawal symptoms: rebound inflammation, fatigue, weakness, arthralgia, fever, dizziness, lethargy, depression, fainting, orthostatic hypotension, dyspnea, anorexia, hypoglycemia. *Sudden withdrawal may be fatal.*

INTERACTIONS
Barbiturates, phenytoin, rifampin: decreased corticosteroid effect. Corticosteroid dose may need to be increased.
Indomethacin, aspirin: increased risk of GI distress and bleeding. Give to-

gether cautiously.

NURSING CONSIDERATIONS
• Contraindicated in systemic fungal infections. Use cautiously in patients with GI ulceration or renal disease, hypertension, osteoporosis, varicella, vaccinia, exanthema, diabetes mellitus, Cushing's syndrome, thromboembolic disorders, seizures, myasthenia gravis, metastatic cancer, congestive heart failure, tuberculosis, ocular herpes simplex, hypoalbuminemia, emotional instability, and psychotic tendencies, and in children.
• Gradually reduce drug dosage after long-term therapy. Tell patient not to discontinue drug abruptly or without doctor's consent.
• Always titrate to lowest effective dose.
• Has a glucocorticoid and mineralocorticoid effect.
• Monitor patient's weight, blood pressure, and serum electrolytes.
• May mask or exacerbate infections.
• Stress (fever, trauma, surgery, and emotional problems) may increase adrenal insufficiency. Dose may have to be increased.
• Instruct patient to carry a card identifying his need for supplemental systemic glucocorticoids during stress.
• Give a daily dosage in the morning for better results and less toxicity.
• Teach patient signs of early adrenal insufficiency: fatigue, muscular weakness, joint pain, fever, anorexia, nausea, dyspnea, dizziness, and fainting.
• Watch for depression or psychotic episodes, especially in high-dose therapy.
• Inspect patient's skin for petechiae. Warn patient about easy bruising.
• Patients with diabetes may need increased insulin; monitor blood glucose.
• Monitor growth in infants and children on long-term therapy.
• Give I.M. injection deep into glu-

teal muscle. Avoid S.C. injection as atrophy and sterile abscesses may occur.
- Unless contraindicated, give low-sodium diet high in potassium and protein. Potassium supplement may be needed. Watch for additional potassium depletion from diuretics and amphotericin B.
- Give P.O. dose with food when possible.
- Warn patients on long-term therapy about cushingoid symptoms.
- Acetate form not for I.V. use.
- Enema may produce same systemic effects as other forms of hydrocortisone. If enema therapy must exceed 21 days, discontinue gradually by reducing administration to every other night for 2 or 3 weeks.
- Immunizations may show decreased antibody response.
- Do not confuse Solu-Cortef with Solu-Medrol.
- Injectable forms not used for alternate-day therapy.

---

methylprednisolone
Medrol**♦, Meprolone

methylprednisolone acetate
depMedalone, Depoject, Depo-Medrol♦, Depopred, Depo-Predate, D-Med, Duralone, Durameth, Medralone, Medrol Enpak, Medrone, Methylone, M-Prednisol, Rep-Pred

methylprednisolone sodium succinate
A-Metha-pred, Solu-Medrol♦

Pregnancy Risk Category: C

MECHANISM OF ACTION
Decreases inflammation, mainly by stabilizing leukocyte lysosomal membranes. Also suppresses the immune response, stimulates bone marrow, and influences protein, fat, and carbohydrate metabolism.

INDICATIONS & DOSAGE
Severe inflammation or immunosuppression—
Adults: 2 to 60 mg P.O. in four divided doses; or 40 to 80 mg (acetate) daily, I.M. or 10 to 250 mg (succinate) I.M. or I.V. q 4 hours; or 4 to 30 mg (acetate) into joints and soft tissue, p.r.n.
Children: 117 mcg to 1.66 mg/kg (succinate) I.V. in three or four divided doses.
Shock—
Adults: 100 to 250 mg (succinate) I.V. at 2- to 6-hour intervals.

ADVERSE REACTIONS
Most adverse reactions of corticosteroids are dose- or duration-dependent.
CNS: *euphoria, insomnia,* psychotic behavior, pseudotumor cerebri.
CV: *CHF,* hypertension, edema.
EENT: cataracts, glaucoma.
GI: *peptic ulcer,* GI irritation, increased appetite.
Metabolic: *possible hypokalemia, hyperglycemia and carbohydrate intolerance,* growth suppression in children.
Skin: delayed wound healing, acne, various skin eruptions.
Other: muscle weakness, pancreatitis, hirsutism, susceptibility to infections. Acute adrenal insufficiency may occur with increased stress (infection, surgery, or trauma) or abrupt withdrawal after long-term therapy. *Withdrawal symptoms:* rebound inflammation, fatigue, weakness, arthralgia, fever, dizziness, lethargy, depression, fainting, orthostatic hypotension, dyspnea, anorexia, hypoglycemia. *Sudden withdrawal may be fatal.*

INTERACTIONS
Barbiturates, phenytoin, rifampin: decreased corticosteroid effect. Corticosteroid dose may need to be increased.
Indomethacin, aspirin: increased risk

Italicized side effects are common or life-threatening.
*Liquid form contains alcohol.   **May contain tartrazine.

of GI distress and bleeding. Give together cautiously.

NURSING CONSIDERATIONS
• Contraindicated in systemic fungal infections. Use cautiously in patients with GI ulceration or renal disease, hypertension, osteoporosis, varicella, vaccinia, exanthema, diabetes mellitus, Cushing's syndrome, thromboembolic disorders, seizures, myasthenia gravis, metastatic cancer, CHF, tuberculosis, ocular herpes simplex, hypoalbuminemia, emotional instability, and psychotic tendencies.
• Gradually reduce drug dosage after long-term therapy. Tell patient not to discontinue drug abruptly or without doctor's consent.
• Always titrate to lowest effective dose.
• A glucocorticoid with little mineralocorticoid effect.
• Discard reconstituted solutions after 48 hours.
• Don't use acetate salt when immediate onset of action is needed.
• Dermal atrophy may occur with large doses of acetate salt. Use multiple small injections rather than a single large dose.
• Monitor weight, blood pressure, serum electrolytes, and sleep patterns. Euphoria may initially interfere with sleep, but patient generally adjusts to the medication after 1 to 3 weeks.
• May mask or exacerbate infections.
• Instruct patient to carry a card identifying his need for supplemental systemic glucocorticoids during stress.
• Give a daily dosage in the morning for better results and less toxicity.
• Teach patient signs of early adrenal insufficiency: fatigue, muscular weakness, joint pain, fever, anorexia, nausea, dyspnea, dizziness, and fainting.
• Watch for depression or psychotic episodes, especially in high-dose therapy.
• Patients with diabetes may need increased insulin; monitor blood glucose.
• Give I.M. injection deep into gluteal muscle. Avoid S.C. injection, as atrophy and sterile abscesses may occur.
• Unless contraindicated, give low-sodium diet high in potassium and protein. Potassium supplement may be needed. Watch for additional potassium depletion from diuretics and amphotericin B.
• Give P.O. dose with food when possible. Critically ill patients may require concomitant antacid therapy.
• Give I.V. dose slowly over 1 minute; in shock, give massive I.V. doses over at least 10 minutes to prevent cardiac dysrhythmias and circulatory collapse.
• Warn patients on long-term therapy about cushingoid symptoms.
• Acetate form not for I.V. use.
• Do not confuse Solu-Medrol with Solu-Cortef.
• Immunizations may show decreased antibody response.
• May be used for alternate-day therapy.

paramethasone acetate
Haldrone

Pregnancy Risk Category: C

MECHANISM OF ACTION
Decreases inflammation, mainly by stabilizing leukocyte lysosomal membranes. Also suppresses the immune response, stimulates bone marrow, and influences protein, fat, and carbohydrate metabolism.

INDICATIONS & DOSAGE
Inflammatory conditions—
Adults: 0.5 to 6 mg P.O. t.i.d. or q.i.d.
Children: 58 to 800 mcg/kg P.O. daily divided t.i.d. or q.i.d.

ADVERSE REACTIONS
Most adverse reactions of corticosteroids are dose- or duration-dependent.
CNS: *euphoria, insomnia,* psychotic behavior, pseudotumor cerebri.
CV: *CHF,* hypertension, edema.
EENT: cataracts, glaucoma.
GI: *peptic ulcer,* GI irritation, increased appetite.
Metabolic: *possible hypokalemia, hyperglycemia and carbohydrate intolerance,* growth suppression in children.
Skin: delayed wound healing, acne, various skin eruptions.
Other: muscle weakness, pancreatitis, hirsutism, susceptibility to infections. Acute adrenal insufficiency may occur with increased stress (infection, surgery, or trauma) or abrupt withdrawal after long-term therapy. *Withdrawal symptoms:* rebound inflammation, fatigue, weakness, arthralgia, fever, dizziness, lethargy, depression, fainting, orthostatic hypotension, dyspnea, anorexia, hypoglycemia. *Sudden withdrawal may be fatal.*

INTERACTIONS
Barbiturates, phenytoin, rifampin: decreased corticosteroid effect. Corticosteroid dose may need to be increased.
Indomethacin, aspirin: increased risk of GI distress and bleeding. Give together cautiously.

NURSING CONSIDERATIONS
• Contraindicated in systemic fungal infections and alternate-day therapy. Use cautiously in GI ulceration or renal disease, hypertension, osteoporosis, varicella, vaccinia, exanthema, diabetes mellitus, Cushing's syndrome, thromboembolic disorders, seizures, myasthenia gravis, metastatic cancer, CHF, tuberculosis, ocular herpes simplex, hypoalbuminemia, emotional instability, and psychotic tendencies.

• Gradually reduce drug dosage after long-term therapy. Tell patient not to discontinue drug abruptly or without doctor's consent.
• Titrate to lowest effective dose.
• Has little mineralocorticoid effect.
• Monitor patient's weight, blood pressure, and serum electrolytes.
• May mask or exacerbate infections.
• Instruct patient to carry a card identifying his need for supplemental systemic glucocorticoids during stress.
• Give a daily dosage in the morning for better results and less toxicity.
• Teach patient signs of early adrenal insufficiency: fatigue, muscular weakness, joint pain, fever, anorexia, nausea, dyspnea, dizziness, and fainting.
• Watch for depression or psychotic episodes with high-dose therapy.
• Patients with diabetes may need increased insulin; monitor blood glucose.
• Monitor growth in infants and children on long-term therapy.
• Unless contraindicated, give low-sodium diet high in potassium and protein. Potassium supplement may be needed.
• Watch for additional hypokalemia from diuretics and amphotericin B.
• Give P.O. dose with food when possible, especially if GI irritation occurs.
• Warn patients on long-term therapy about cushingoid symptoms.
• Immunizations may show decreased antibody response.

prednisolone
Cortalone, Delta-Cortef, Novo-
prednisolone♦♦, Prelone

prednisolone acetate
Articulose, Key-Pred, Niscort,
Predaject, Predalone, Predate,
Predcor, Predicort

prednisolone sodium phosphate
Codesol, Hydeltrasol, Key-Pred-SP,
Pediapred, Predate-S, Predicort RP

prednisolone tebutate
Hydeltra-TBA, Metalone-TBA, Nor-
Pred TBA, Predalone TBA, Predate
TBA, Predcor TBA, Prednisol TBA

Pregnancy Risk Category: B

MECHANISM OF ACTION
Decreases inflammation, mainly by
stabilizing leukocyte lysosomal membranes. Also suppresses the immune
response, stimulates bone marrow,
and influences protein, fat, and carbohydrate metabolism.

INDICATIONS & DOSAGE
*Severe inflammation or immunosup-
pression—*
Adults: 2.5 to 15 mg P.O. b.i.d.,
t.i.d., or q.i.d.; 2 to 30 mg I.M. (acetate, phosphate), or I.V. (phosphate) q
12 hours; or 2 to 30 mg (phosphate)
into joints, lesions, and soft tissue; or
4 to 40 mg (tebutate) into joints and
lesions; or 0.25 to 1 ml (acetate-phos-
phate suspension) into joints weekly,
p.r.n.

ADVERSE REACTIONS
Most adverse reactions of corticoste-
roids are dose- or duration-depen-
dent.
CNS: *euphoria, insomnia,* psychotic
behavior, pseudotumor cerebri.
CV: *CHF,* hypertension, edema.
EENT: cataracts, glaucoma.
GI: *peptic ulcer,* GI irritation, in-

creased appetite.
Metabolic: *possible hypokalemia, hyperglycemia and carbohydrate intolerance,* growth suppression in children.
Skin: delayed wound healing, acne,
various skin eruptions.
Other: muscle weakness, pancreatitis, hirsutism, susceptibility to infections. Acute adrenal insufficiency
may occur with increased stress (infection, surgery, or trauma) or abrupt
withdrawal after long-term therapy.
Withdrawal symptoms: rebound inflammation, fatigue, weakness, arthralgia, fever, dizziness, lethargy,
depression, fainting, orthostatic hypotension, dyspnea, anorexia, hypoglycemia. *Sudden withdrawal may be
fatal.*

INTERACTIONS
Barbiturates, phenytoin, rifampin: decreased corticosteroid effect. Corticosteroid dose may need to be increased.
Indomethacin, aspirin: increased risk
of GI distress and bleeding. Give together cautiously.

NURSING CONSIDERATIONS
• Contraindicated in systemic fungal
infections. Use cautiously in GI ulceration or renal disease, hypertension,
osteoporosis, varicella, vaccinia, exanthema, diabetes mellitus, Cushing's
syndrome, thromboembolic disorders,
seizures, myasthenia gravis, metastatic cancer, CHF, tuberculosis, ocular herpes simplex, hypoalbuminemia, emotional instability, and psychotic tendencies.
• Gradually reduce drug dosage after
long-term therapy. Tell patient not to
discontinue drug abruptly or without
doctor's consent.
• Always titrate to lowest effective
dose.
• A glucocorticoid with slight mineralocorticoid action.
• Prednisolone salts (acetate, sodium
phosphate, and tebutate) are used par-

enterally less often than other corticosteroids that have more potent anti-inflammatory action.

• May be used for alternate-day therapy.

• Monitor patient's weight, blood pressure, and serum electrolytes.

• May mask or exacerbate infections. Tell patient to report slow healing.

• Instruct patient to carry a card identifying his need for supplemental systemic glucocorticoids during stress.

• Teach patient signs of early adrenal insufficiency: fatigue, muscular weakness, joint pain, fever, anorexia, nausea, dyspnea, dizziness, and fainting.

• Watch for depression or psychotic episodes, especially in high-dose therapy.

• Patients with diabetes may need increased insulin; monitor blood glucose.

• Give I.M. injection deep into gluteal muscle. Avoid S.C. injection, as atrophy and sterile abscesses may occur.

• Unless contraindicated, give low-sodium diet high in potassium and protein. Potassium supplement may be needed.

• Give P.O. dose with food when possible to reduce GI irritation.

• Warn patients on long-term therapy about cushingoid symptoms.

• Acetate form not for I.V. use.

• Watch for additional potassium depletion from diuretics and amphotericin B.

• Immunizations may show decreased antibody response.

prednisone

Apo-Prednisone♦♦, Deltasone♦, Liquid Pred, Meticorten, Novo-prednisone♦♦, Orasone, Panasol, Prednicen-M, Sterapred, Winpred♦♦

Pregnancy Risk Category: B

MECHANISM OF ACTION

Decreases inflammation, mainly by stabilizing leukocyte lysosomal membranes. Also suppresses the immune response, stimulates bone marrow, and influences protein, fat, and carbohydrate metabolism.

INDICATIONS & DOSAGE

Severe inflammation or immunosuppression—
Adults: 2.5 to 15 mg P.O. b.i.d., t.i.d., or q.i.d. Maintenance dosage given once daily or every other day. Dosage must be individualized.
Children: 0.14 to 2 mg/kg P.O. daily divided q.i.d.
Acute exacerbations of multiple sclerosis—
Adults: 200 mg P.O. daily for 1 week, then 80 mg every other day for 1 month.

ADVERSE REACTIONS

Most adverse reactions of corticosteroids are dose- or duration-dependent.
CNS: *euphoria, insomnia,* psychotic behavior, pseudotumor cerebri.
CV: *CHF,* hypertension, edema.
EENT: cataracts, glaucoma.
GI: *peptic ulcer,* GI irritation, increased appetite.
Metabolic: *possible hypokalemia, hyperglycemia and carbohydrate intolerance,* growth suppression in children.
Skin: delayed wound healing, acne, various skin eruptions.
Other: muscle weakness, pancreatitis, hirsutism, susceptibility to infections. Acute adrenal insufficiency may occur with increased stress (in-

---

Italicized side effects are common or life-threatening.
*Liquid form contains alcohol.   **May contain tartrazine.

fection, surgery, or trauma) or abrupt withdrawal after long-term therapy. *Withdrawal symptoms:* rebound inflammation, fatigue, weakness, arthralgia, fever, dizziness, lethargy, depression, fainting, orthostatic hypotension, dyspnea, anorexia, hypoglycemia. *Sudden withdrawal may be fatal.*

INTERACTIONS
Barbiturates, phenytoin, rifampin: decreased corticosteroid effect. Corticosteroid dose may need to be increased.
Indomethacin, aspirin: increased risk of GI distress and bleeding. Give together cautiously.

NURSING CONSIDERATIONS
• Contraindicated in systemic fungal infections. Use cautiously in GI ulceration or renal disease, hypertension, osteoporosis, varicella, vaccinia, exanthema, diabetes mellitus, Cushing's syndrome, thromboembolic disorders, seizures, myasthenia gravis, metastatic cancer, CHF, tuberculosis, ocular herpes simplex, hypoalbuminemia, emotional instability, and psychotic tendencies.
• Gradually reduce drug dosage after long-term therapy. Tell patient not to discontinue drug abruptly or without doctor's consent.
• Always titrate to lowest effective dose.
• Monitor patient's blood pressure, sleep patterns, and serum potassium.
• Weigh patient daily; report sudden weight gain to doctor.
• May mask or exacerbate infections. Tell patient to report slow healing.
• Instruct patient to carry a card identifying his need for supplemental systemic glucocorticoids during stress.
• Give a daily dosage in the morning for better results and less toxicity.
• Teach patient signs of early adrenal insufficiency: fatigue, muscular weakness, joint pain, fever, anorexia,

nausea, dyspnea, dizziness, and fainting.
• Watch for depression or psychotic episodes, especially in high-dose therapy.
• Patients with diabetes may need increased insulin; monitor blood glucose.
• Monitor growth in infants and children on long-term therapy.
• Unless contraindicated, give low-sodium diet high in potassium and protein. Potassium supplement may be needed.
• Unless contraindicated, give P.O. dose with food when possible to reduce GI irritation.
• May be used for alternate-day therapy.
• Watch for additional potassium depletion from diuretics and amphotericin B.
• Warn patients on long-term therapy about cushingoid symptoms.
• Immunizations may show decreased antibody response.
• Now available in oral solution form.

triamcinolone
Aristocort♦, Atolone, Kenacort**♦, Tricilone

triamcinolone acetonide
Cenocort A, Cinonide, Kenaject, Kenalog♦, Kenalone, Tramacort, Triam-A, Triamonide, Tri-Kort, Trilog

triamcinolone diacetate
Amcort, Aristocort Forte, Aristocort Intralesional♦ ,Articulose-L.A., Cenocort Forte, Cinalone, Kenacort, Triam-Forte, Trilone, Tristoject

triamcinolone hexacetonide
Aristospan Intra-articular♦, Aristospan Intralesional♦

Pregnancy Risk Category: C

MECHANISM OF ACTION
Decreases inflammation, mainly by stabilizing leukocyte lysosomal membranes. Also suppresses the immune response, stimulates bone marrow, and influences protein, fat, and carbohydrate metabolism.

INDICATIONS & DOSAGE
Severe inflammation or immunosuppression—
Adults: 4 to 48 mg P.O. daily divided b.i.d., t.i.d., or q.i.d., or 40 mg I.M. (diacetate or acetonide) weekly; or 5 to 48 mg (diacetate or acetonide) into lesions; or 2 to 40 mg (diacetate or acetonide) into joints and soft tissue; or up to 0.5 mg (hexacetonide) per square inch of affected skin intralesional; or 2 to 20 mg (hexacetonide) intra-articular or intrasynovial into soft tissue or into joint or lesion. Often, a local anesthetic is injected into the joint with triamcinolone.
Steroid-dependent asthma—
Adults: 2 inhalations t.i.d. to q.i.d. Maximum 16 inhalations daily.
Children 6 to 12 years: 1 to 2 inhalations t.i.d. to q.i.d. Maximum 12 inhalations daily.

ADVERSE REACTIONS
Most adverse reactions of corticosteroids are dose- or duration-dependent.
CNS: *euphoria, insomnia,* psychotic behavior, pseudotumor cerebri.
CV: *CHF,* hypertension, edema.
EENT: cataracts, glaucoma.
GI: *peptic ulcer,* GI irritation, increased appetite.
Metabolic: *possible hypokalemia, hyperglycemia and carbohydrate intolerance,* growth suppression in children.
Skin: delayed wound healing, acne, various skin eruptions.
Other: muscle weakness, pancreatitis, hirsutism, susceptibility to infections. Acute adrenal insufficiency may occur with increased stress (infection, surgery, or trauma) or abrupt withdrawal after long-term therapy.
Withdrawal symptoms: rebound inflammation, fatigue, weakness, arthralgia, fever, dizziness, lethargy, depression, fainting, orthostatic hypotension, dyspnea, anorexia, hypoglycemia. *Sudden withdrawal may be fatal.*
Inhalation:
EENT: hoarseness, fungal infections of mouth and throat.
GI: dry mouth.

INTERACTIONS
Systemic:
Barbiturates, phenytoin, rifampin: decreased corticosteroid effect. Corticosteroid dose may need to be increased.
Indomethacin, aspirin: increased risk of GI distress and bleeding. Give together cautiously.

NURSING CONSIDERATIONS
Systemic:
• Contraindicated in systemic fungal infections. Use cautiously in GI ulceration or renal disease, hypertension, osteoporosis, varicella, vaccinia, ex-

anthema, diabetes mellitus, Cushing's syndrome, thromboembolic disorders, seizures, myasthenia gravis, metastatic cancer, CHF, tuberculosis, ocular herpes simplex, hypoalbuminemia, emotional instability, and psychotic tendencies.
• Gradually reduce drug dosage after long-term therapy. Tell patient not to discontinue drug abruptly or without doctor's consent.
• Always titrate to lowest effective dose.
• Monitor patient's weight, blood pressure, and serum electrolytes.
• May mask or exacerbate infections. Tell patient to report slow healing.
• Instruct patient to carry a card identifying his need for supplemental systemic glucocorticoids during stress.
• Give a daily dosage in the morning for better results and less toxicity.
• Teach patient signs of early adrenal insufficiency: fatigue, muscular weakness, joint pain, fever, anorexia, nausea, dyspnea, dizziness, and fainting.
• Watch for depression or psychotic episodes, especially in high-dose therapy.
• Patients with diabetes may need increased insulin; monitor blood glucose.
• Give I.M. injection deep into gluteal muscle.
• Unless contraindicated, give low-sodium diet high in potassium and protein. Potassium supplement may be needed. Watch for additional potassium depletion from diuretics and amphotericin B.
• Give P.O. dose with food when possible to reduce GI irritation.
• Don't use diluents that contain preservatives. Flocculation may occur.
• Warn patients on long-term therapy about cushingoid symptoms.
• Immunizations may show decreased antibody response.
• Not used for alternate-day therapy.

Inhalation:
• Contraindicated in status asthmaticus. Not for use in asthma controlled by bronchodilators or other noncorticosteroids alone, or for nonasthmatic bronchial diseases.
• Oral therapy should be tapered slowly.
• Instruct patient to carry a card indicating his need for supplemental systemic glucocorticoids during stress.
• Patient requiring bronchodilator should use it several minutes before triamcinolone.
• Tell patient to allow 1 minute to elapse before repeat inhalations, and hold breath for a few seconds to enhance action of drug.
• Inform patient that triamcinolone doesn't provide relief for emergency asthma attacks.
• Instruct patient to contact doctor if he notices a decreased response. Dose may have to be adjusted. Patient shouldn't exceed recommended dose on his own.
• Check mucous membranes frequently for signs of fungal infection. Tell patient to follow inhalations with glass of water to help prevent fungal infections.
• Tell patient to keep inhaler clean and unobstructed. Wash with warm water and dry thoroughly after use.

53

Androgens and anabolic steroids

danazol
ethylestrenol
fluoxymesterone
methyltestosterone
nandrolone decanoate
nandrolone phenpropionate
oxandrolone
oxymetholone
stanozolol
testosterone
testosterone cypionate
testosterone enanthate
testosterone propionate

COMBINATION PRODUCTS

DELADUMONE ♦: testosterone enanthate 90 mg/ml, estradiol valerate 4 mg/ml, and chlorobutanol 0.5% in sesame oil.
DEPO-TESTADIOL (oil): testosterone cypionate 50 mg, estradiol cypionate 2 mg, and chlorobutanol 0.5%.
DITATE-DS: estradiol valerate 8 mg, and testosterone enanthate 180 mg.
ESTRATEST: esterified estrogens 1.25 mg, and methyltestosterone 2.5 mg.
ESTRATEST H.S.: esterified estrogens 0.625 mg, and methyltestosterone 1.25 mg.
PREMARIN WITH METHYLTESTOSTERONE♦: conjugated estrogens 0.625 mg and methyltestosterone 5 mg.

---

danazol
Cyclomen♦♦, Danocrine
Pregnancy Risk Category: C

MECHANISM OF ACTION
Gonadotropin inhibitor that suppresses the pituitary-ovarian axis. Also acts on estrogen receptors to inhibit estrogenic effects.

INDICATIONS & DOSAGE
Mild endometriosis—
Women: Initially, 100 to 200 mg P.O. b.i.d. Subsequent dosage based upon patient response.
Moderate to severe endometriosis—
Women: 400 mg P.O. b.i.d. uninterrupted for 3 to 6 months; may continue for 9 months.
Fibrocystic breast disease—
Women: 100 to 400 mg P.O. daily in 2 divided doses uninterrupted for 2 to 6 months.
Prevention of hereditary angio-edema—
Adults: 200 mg P.O. 2 to 3 times a day, continued until favorable response is achieved. Then dosage should be decreased by half at 1- to 3-month intervals.

ADVERSE REACTIONS
Androgenic: acne, edema, *weight gain, hirsutism,* hoarseness, clitoral enlargement, *decrease in breast size,* changes in libido, male pattern baldness, *oiliness of skin or hair.*
Blood: thrombocytopenia.
CNS: dizziness, headache, sleep disorders, fatigue, tremor, irritability, excitation, lethargy, mental depression, chills, paresthesias.
CV: elevated blood pressure.
EENT: visual disturbances.
GI: gastric irritation, nausea, vomiting, diarrhea, constipation, change in appetite.
GU: hematuria.

Italicized side effects are common or life-threatening.
*Liquid form contains alcohol.   **May contain tartrazine.

Hepatic: reversible jaundice.
Hypoestrogenic: flushing; sweating; vaginitis, including itching, dryness, burning, and vaginal bleeding; nervousness, emotional lability, menstrual irregularities.
Other: muscle cramps or spasms.

INTERACTIONS
None significant.

NURSING CONSIDERATIONS
• Contraindicated in undiagnosed abnormal genital bleeding; impaired renal, cardiac, or hepatic function. Use cautiously in epilepsy or migraine headache.
• Use with diet high in calories and protein unless contraindicated.
• Monitor closely for signs of virilization. Some androgenic effects, such as deepening of voice, may not be reversible upon discontinuation of drug.
• Advise patient who is taking danazol for fibrocystic disease to examine breasts regularly. If breast nodule enlarges during treatment, tell patient to call doctor immediately.
• Instruct patient to wear cotton underwear only.
• Washing after intercourse is recommended to decrease the risk of vaginitis.
• Has been used investigationally with impressive results in treating hemophilia and Christmas disease; has also been used to decrease symptoms of systemic lupus erythematosus in women and to treat gynecomastia in men.

---

ethylestrenol
Maxibolin*♦

Pregnancy Risk Category: X

MECHANISM OF ACTION
Anabolic steroid that promotes tissue-building processes and reverses catabolism. Also stimulates erythropoiesis.

INDICATIONS & DOSAGE
Promote weight gain and combat tissue depletion, refractory anemias, catabolic effects of corticosteroid therapy, osteoporosis, prolonged immobilization, and debilitated states—
Adults: 4 to 8 mg P.O. daily, reduced to minimum levels at first evidence of clinical response.
Children: 1 to 3 mg P.O. daily; dosage is highly individualized.
A single course of therapy in both adults and children should not exceed 6 weeks; may be reinstituted after 4-week interval.

ADVERSE REACTIONS
Androgenic: in women—*acne, edema, oily skin, weight gain, hirsutism, hoarseness,* clitoral enlargement, changes in libido. In men—prepubertal: premature epiphyseal closure, acne, priapism, growth of body and facial hair, phallic enlargement; postpubertal: testicular atrophy, oligospermia, decreased ejaculatory volume, impotence, gynecomastia, epididymitis.
CV: edema.
GI: gastroenteritis, nausea, vomiting, diarrhea, constipation, change in appetite.
GU: bladder irritability.
Hepatic: reversible jaundice, hepatotoxicity.
Hypoestrogenic: in women—flushing; sweating; vaginitis with itching, drying, burning, or bleeding; menstrual irregularities.
Other: hypercalcemia.

INTERACTIONS
None significant.

NURSING CONSIDERATIONS
• Contraindicated in prostatic hypertrophy with obstruction; carcinoma of male breast; hypercalcemia; prostatic cancer; cardiac, hepatic, or renal decompensation; nephrosis; and in premature infants. Use cautiously in pre-

pubertal males; patients with diabetes or coronary disease; patients taking ACTH, corticosteroids, or anticoagulants.

• Hypercalcemia symptoms may be difficult to distinguish from symptoms of condition being treated unless anticipated and thought of as a symptom cluster. Hypercalcemia is particularly likely to occur in patients with metastatic breast cancer and may indicate bone metastases.

• Tell women to report menstrual irregularities; therapy should be discontinued pending etiologic determination.

• Watch for signs of virilization; may be irreversible despite prompt discontinuation of therapy. Doctor must decide if benefits outweigh effects.

• Closely monitor boys under 7 years for precocious development of male sexual characteristics.

• In children: therapy should be preceded by X-ray of wrist bones to establish level of bone maturation. During treatment, bone maturation may proceed more rapidly than linear growth; dosage should be intermittent and X-rays taken periodically.

• Edema is generally controllable with salt restriction or diuretics. Monitor weight routinely.

• Watch for symptoms of jaundice. Dosage adjustment may reverse condition. If liver function tests are abnormal, discontinue therapy.

• Observe patient on concomitant anticoagulant therapy for ecchymotic areas, petechiae, or abnormal bleeding. Monitor prothrombin time.

• Watch for symptoms of hypoglycemia in patients with diabetes. Dosage of antidiabetic drug may need adjustment.

• Use with diet high in calories and protein unless contraindicated. Give small, frequent feedings.

• Take with food or meals if GI upset occurs.

• Anabolic steroids may alter many laboratory studies during therapy and for 2 to 3 weeks after therapy is stopped.

• Involve the patient, family members, and a dietitian in developing a dietary regimen suitable to the anorexic or debilitated patient.

fluoxymesterone
Android F, Halotestin**♦, Ora-Testryl

Pregnancy Risk Category: X

MECHANISM OF ACTION
Stimulates target tissues to develop normally in androgen-deficient men.

INDICATIONS & DOSAGE
Hypogonadism and impotence caused by testicular deficiency—
Adults: 2 to 10 mg P.O. daily.
Palliation of breast cancer in women—
15 to 30 mg P.O. daily in divided doses. All dosages should be individualized and reduced to minimum when effect is noted.
Postpartum breast engorgement—
2.5 mg P.O. followed by 5 to 10 mg daily for 5 days.

ADVERSE REACTIONS
Androgenic: in women—*acne, edema, oily skin, weight gain, hirsutism, hoarseness,* clitoral enlargement, change in libido. In men—prepubertal: premature epiphyseal closure, acne, priapism, growth of body and facial hair, phallic enlargement; postpubertal: testicular atrophy, oligospermia, decreased ejaculatory volume, impotence, gynecomastia, epididymitis.
CV: edema.
GI: gastroenteritis, nausea, vomiting, constipation, change in appetite, diarrhea.
GU: bladder irritability.
Hepatic: reversible jaundice.
Hypoestrogenic: in women—flushing; sweating; vaginitis with itching,

---

Italicized side effects are common or life-threatening.
*Liquid form contains alcohol.   **May contain tartrazine.

drying, burning, or bleeding; menstrual irregularities; emotional lability.
Other: hypercalcemia.

INTERACTIONS
None significant.

NURSING CONSIDERATIONS
• Contraindicated in prostatic hypertrophy with obstruction; carcinoma of male breast; prostatic cancer; cardiac, hepatic, or renal decompensation; nephrosis; hypercalcemia; and in premature infants. Use cautiously in prepubertal males; patients with diabetes or coronary disease; and patients taking ACTH, corticosteroids, or anticoagulants.
• Hypercalcemia symptoms may be difficult to distinguish from symptoms associated with condition being treated unless anticipated and thought of as a symptom cluster. Hypercalcemia is particularly likely to occur in patients with metastatic breast cancer and may indicate bone metastases.
• Explain to patient on drug for palliation of breast cancer that virilization usually occurs at dosage used. Give emotional support. Tell patient to report androgenic effects immediately. Stopping drug will prevent further androgenic changes but will probably not reverse those already existing.
• When used in breast cancer, subjective effects may not be seen for about 1 month; objective symptoms not for 3 months.
• Tell women to report menstrual irregularities; therapy should be discontinued pending etiologic determination.
• Edema is generally controllable with salt restriction or diuretics. Monitor weight routinely.
• Watch for symptoms of jaundice. Dosage adjustment may reverse condition. If liver function tests are abnormal, therapy should be stopped.

• Observe patient on concomitant anticoagulant therapy for ecchymotic areas, petechiae, or abnormal bleeding. Monitor prothrombin time.
• Watch for symptoms of hypoglycemia in patients with diabetes. Dosage of antidiabetic drug may need adjustment.
• Use with diet high in calories and protein unless contraindicated. Give small, frequent feedings.
• Take with food or meals if GI upset occurs.

methyltestosterone
Android, Metandren**◆, Metandren Linguets◆, Oreton Methyl, Testred, Virilon

Pregnancy Risk Category: X

MECHANISM OF ACTION
Stimulates target tissues to develop normally in androgen-deficient males.

INDICATIONS & DOSAGE
Adults:
Breast engorgement of nonnursing mothers—80 mg P.O. daily, or 40 mg buccal daily for 3 to 5 days.
Breast cancer in women 1 to 5 years postmenopausal—200 mg P.O. daily; or 100 mg buccal daily.
Eunuchoidism and eunuchism, male climacteric symptoms—10 to 40 mg P.O. daily; or 5 to 20 mg buccal daily.
Postpubertal cryptorchidism—30 mg P.O. daily; or 15 mg buccal daily.

ADVERSE REACTIONS
Androgenic: in women—*acne, edema, oily skin, weight gain, hirsutism, hoarseness,* clitoral enlargement, changes in libido. In men—prepubertal: premature epiphyseal closure, acne, priapism, growth of body and facial hair, phallic enlargement; postpubertal: testicular atrophy, oligospermia, decreased ejaculatory volume, impotence, gynecomastia, epididymitis.

CV: edema.
GI: gastroenteritis, constipation, nausea, vomiting, diarrhea, change in appetite.
GU: bladder irritability.
Hepatic: reversible jaundice.
Hypoestrogenic: in women—flushing; sweating; vaginitis with itching, drying, burning, or bleeding; menstrual irregularities.
Local: irritation of oral mucosa with buccal administration.
Other: hypercalcemia.

INTERACTIONS
None significant.

NURSING CONSIDERATIONS
• Contraindicated in women of childbearing potential (possible masculinization of female infant); in elderly, asthenic men who may react adversely to androgen overstimulation; in hypercalcemia; cardiac, hepatic, or renal decompensation; prostatic or breast cancer in men; benign prostatic hypertrophy with obstruction; conditions aggravated by fluid retention; hypertension; and in premature infants. Use cautiously in myocardial infarction or coronary artery disease.
• Treatment of breast cancer usually restricted to patients 1 to 5 years postmenopausal.
• Edema is generally controllable with salt restriction or diuretics.
• Periodic serum cholesterol and calcium determinations, and cardiac and liver function tests recommended. Usually only used for intermittent therapy. Because of the potential for hepatotoxicity, watch closely for jaundice.
• In metastatic breast cancer, hypercalcemia may indicate progression of bone metastases. Report signs of hypercalcemia.
• Therapeutic response in breast cancer is usually apparent within 3 months. Therapy should be stopped if signs of disease progression appear.

• Enhances hypoglycemia; teach patient signs of hypoglycemia, and instruct him to report immediately if they occur.
• Watch for ecchymoses, petechiae, and abnormal bleeding in patients receiving concomitant anticoagulants.
• Promptly report signs of virilization in women.
• Use with diet high in calories and protein unless contraindicated. Give small, frequent feedings.
• Buccal tablets twice as potent as oral tablets. Tell patient to avoid eating, drinking, chewing, or smoking while buccal tablet is in place, and that tablet is not to be swallowed. Place in upper or lower buccal pouch between cheek and gum. Tablet requires 30 to 60 minutes to dissolve. Instruct patient to change tablet absorption site with each dose to minimize risk of buccal irritation.
• Erroneously thought to enhance athletic ability.

nandrolone decanoate
Anabolin LA, Androlone-D, Deca-Durabolin♦, Decolone, Hybolin Decanoate, Kabolin, Nandrobolic L.A., Neo-Durabolic

nandrolone phenpropionate
Anabolin IM, Androlone, Durabolin♦, Hybolin Improved, Nandrobolic
Pregnancy Risk Category: X

MECHANISM OF ACTION
Anabolic steroid that promotes tissue-building processes and reverses catabolism. Also stimulates erythropoiesis.

INDICATIONS & DOSAGE
Severe debility or disease states, refractory anemias (decanoate)—
Adults: 100 to 200 mg I.M. weekly. Therapy should be intermittent.
Tissue-building (decanoate)—
Adults: 50 to 100 mg I.M. q 3 to 4

weeks.
Children 2 to 13 years: 25 to 50 mg
I.M. q 3 to 4 weeks.
*Control of metastatic breast cancer
(phenpropionate)—*
Adults: 25 to 50 mg I.M. weekly.
Children 2 to 13 years: 12.5 to 25
mg I.M. every 2 to 4 weeks.

ADVERSE REACTIONS
Androgenic: in women—*acne,
edema, oily skin, weight gain, hirsutism, hoarseness,* clitoral enlargement,
decreased or increased libido. In
men—prepubertal: premature epiphyseal closure, acne, priapism, growth
of body and facial hair, phallic enlargement; postpubertal: testicular
atrophy, oligospermia, decreased
ejaculatory volume, impotence, gynecomastia, epididymitis.
CV: edema.
GI: gastroenteritis, nausea, vomiting,
diarrhea, change in appetite.
GU: bladder irritability.
Hepatic: reversible jaundice, hepatotoxicity.
Hypoestrogenic: in women—flushing; sweating; vaginitis with itching,
drying, burning, or bleeding; menstrual irregularities with large doses.
Local: pain at injection site, induration.
Other: hypercalcemia, hypercalciuria.

INTERACTIONS
None significant.

NURSING CONSIDERATIONS
• Contraindicated in prostatic hypertrophy with obstruction; male breast
and prostatic cancer; cardiac, hepatic,
or renal decompensation; nephrosis;
and in premature infants. Use cautiously in prepubertal males; patients
with diabetes or coronary disease; patients taking ACTH, corticosteroids,
or anticoagulants.
• Inject drug deep I.M., preferably
into upper outer quadrant of gluteal

muscle in adults.
• Hypercalcemia is most likely to occur in patients with mammary carcinoma; these patients should have
quantitative urine and serum calcium
level determinations.
• Tell women to report menstrual irregularities; therapy should be discontinued pending etiologic determination.
• Watch for signs of virilization; they
may be irreversible despite prompt
discontinuation of therapy.
• Closely observe boys under 7 years
for precocious development of male
sexual characteristics.
• In children, therapy should be
preceded by X-ray of wrist bones to
establish level of bone maturation.
During treatment, bone maturation
may proceed more rapidly than linear
growth; dosage should be intermittent
and X-rays taken periodically.
• Edema is generally controllable
with salt restrictions or diuretics.
• Watch for symptoms of jaundice.
Dosage adjustment may reverse condition. If liver function tests are abnormal, therapy should be stopped.
• Observe patients receiving concomitant anticoagulant therapy for ecchymotic areas, petechiae, or abnormal
bleeding. Monitor prothrombin time.
• Watch for symptoms of hypoglycemia in patients with diabetes. Dosage
of antidiabetic drug may need adjustment.
• Use with diet high in calories and
protein unless contraindicated. Give
small, frequent feedings.
• Erroneously thought to enhance
athletic ability.
• Considered an adjunctive therapy.
• Anabolic steroids may alter many
laboratory studies during therapy and
for 2 to 3 weeks after therapy is
stopped.

---

oxandrolone
Anavar

Pregnancy Risk Category: X

MECHANISM OF ACTION
Anabolic steroid that promotes tissue-building processes and reverses catabolism. Also stimulates erythropoiesis.

INDICATIONS & DOSAGE
To combat catabolic effects of corticosteroid therapy, osteoporosis, prolonged immobilization and debilitated states—
Adults: 2.5 mg P.O. b.i.d., t.i.d., or q.i.d.; up to 20 mg daily for 2 to 4 weeks.
Children: 0.25 mg/kg daily P.O. for 2 to 4 weeks.
   Continuous therapy should not exceed 3 months.

ADVERSE REACTIONS
Androgenic: in women—*acne, edema, oily skin, weight gain, hirsutism, hoarseness,* clitoral enlargement, decreased or increased libido. In men—prepubertal: premature epiphyseal closure, acne, priapism, growth of body and facial hair, phallic enlargement; postpubertal: testicular atrophy, oligospermia, decreased ejaculatory volume, impotence, gynecomastia, epididymitis.
CV: edema.
GI: gastroenteritis, nausea, vomiting, constipation or diarrhea, change in appetite.
GU: bladder irritability.
Hepatic: reversible jaundice, hepatotoxicity.
Hypoestrogenic: in women—flushing; sweating; vaginitis with itching, drying, burning, or bleeding; menstrual irregularities.
Other: hypercalcemia.

INTERACTIONS
None significant.

NURSING CONSIDERATIONS
• Contraindicated in prostatic hypertrophy with obstruction; prostatic and male breast cancer; cardiac, hepatic, or renal decompensation; nephrosis; and in premature infants. Use cautiously in prepubertal males; patients with diabetes or coronary disease; patients taking ACTH, corticosteroids, or anticoagulants.
• Hypercalcemia symptoms may be difficult to distinguish from symptoms of condition being treated unless anticipated and thought of as a cluster. Hypercalcemia most likely to occur with metastatic breast cancer and may indicate bone metastases.
• Tell women to report menstrual irregularities; therapy should be discontinued pending etiologic determination.
• Watch for signs of virilization; may be irreversible despite prompt discontinuation of therapy. Doctor must decide if benefits outweigh effects.
• Boys under 7 years should be closely observed for precocious development of male sexual characteristics.
• In children, therapy should be preceded by X-ray of wrist bones to establish level of bone maturation. During treatment, bone maturation may proceed more rapidly than linear growth; dosage should be intermittent and X-rays taken periodically.
• Edema is generally controllable with salt restriction or diuretics. Monitor weight routinely.
• Watch for symptoms of jaundice. Dosage adjustment may reverse condition. Periodic liver function tests are recommended.
• Observe patient on concomitant anticoagulant therapy for ecchymotic areas, petechiae, or abnormal bleeding. Monitor prothrombin time.
• Watch for symptoms of hypoglycemia in patients with diabetes. Dosage of antidiabetic drug may need adjustment.

Italicized side effects are common or life-threatening.
*Liquid form contains alcohol.   **May contain tartrazine.

- Use with diet high in calories and protein unless contraindicated. Give small, frequent feedings.
- Take with food or meals if GI upset occurs.
- Erroneously thought to enhance athletic ability.
- Anabolic steroids may alter many laboratory studies during therapy and for 2 to 3 weeks after therapy is stopped.

---

oxymetholone
Anadrol, Anapolon♦♦

Pregnancy Risk Category: X

MECHANISM OF ACTION
Anabolic steroid that promotes tissue-building processes and reverses catabolism. Also stimulates erythropoiesis.

INDICATIONS & DOSAGE
Aplastic anemia—
Adults and children: 1 to 5 mg/kg P.O. daily. Dosage highly individualized; response not immediate. Trial of 3 to 6 months required.
Osteoporosis, catabolic conditions—
Adults: 5 to 15 mg P.O. daily, or up to 30 mg P.O. daily.
Children over 6 years: up to 10 mg P.O. daily.
Children under 6 years: 1.25 mg P.O. daily or up to q.i.d. Continuous therapy should not exceed 30 days in children; 90 days in any patient.

ADVERSE REACTIONS
Androgenic: in women—*acne, edema, oily skin, weight gain, hirsutism, hoarseness,* clitoral enlargement, decreased or increased libido, male pattern baldness. In men—prepubertal: premature epiphyseal closure, acne, priapism, growth of body and facial hair; phallic enlargement; postpubertal: testicular atrophy, oligospermia, decreased ejaculatory volume, impotence, gynecomastia, epididymitis.

CV: edema.
GI: gastroenteritis, nausea, vomiting, constipation, diarrhea, change in appetite.
GU: bladder irritability.
Hepatic: reversible jaundice, hepatotoxicity.
Hypoestrogenic: in women—flushing; sweating; vaginitis with itching, drying, burning, or bleeding; menstrual irregularities.
Other: hypercalcemia.

INTERACTIONS
None significant.

NURSING CONSIDERATIONS
- Contraindicated in prostatic hypertrophy with obstruction; prostatic and male breast cancer; cardiac, hepatic, or renal decompensation; nephrosis; and in premature infants. Use cautiously in prepubertal males; patients with diabetes or coronary diseases; patients taking ACTH, corticosteroids, or anticoagulants.
- Hypercalcemia symptoms may be difficult to distinguish from symptoms of condition being treated unless anticipated and thought of as a cluster. Hypercalcemia most likely to occur in metastatic breast cancer and may indicate bone metastases.
- Supportive treatment of anemias (transfusions, correction of iron, folic acid, vitamin B_{12}, or pyridoxine deficiency). Give 3 to 6 months for response.
- Effects in osteoporosis usually seen in 4 to 6 weeks.
- Tell women to report menstrual irregularities; therapy should be discontinued pending etiologic determination.
- Watch for signs of virilization; may be irreversible despite prompt discontinuation of therapy. Doctor must decide if benefits outweigh effects.
- Boys under 7 years should be closely observed for precocious development of male sexual characteris-

tics.
- In children, therapy should be preceded by X-ray of wrist bones to establish level of bone maturation. During treatment, bone maturation may proceed more rapidly than linear growth; dosage should be intermittent and X-rays taken periodically. Epiphyseal development may continue 6 months after stopping therapy.
- Edema is generally controllable with salt restriction or diuretics. Monitor weight routinely.
- Watch for symptoms of jaundice. Dosage adjustment may reverse condition; if liver function tests are abnormal, therapy should be stopped.
- Observe patient on concomitant anticoagulant therapy for ecchymotic areas, petechiae, or abnormal bleeding. Monitor prothrombin time.
- Watch for symptoms of hypoglycemia in patients with diabetes. Dosage of antidiabetic drug may need adjustment.
- Use with diet high in calories and protein unless contraindicated. Give small, frequent feedings.
- Take with food or meals if GI upset occurs.
- Erroneously thought to enhance athletic ability.
- Anabolic steroids may alter many laboratory studies during therapy and for 2 to 3 weeks after therapy is stopped.
- Has also been used to prevent hereditary angioedema.

---

stanozolol
Winstrol♦

Pregnancy Risk Category: X

MECHANISM OF ACTION
Anabolic steroid that promotes tissue-building processes and reverses catabolism. Also stimulates erythropoiesis.

INDICATIONS & DOSAGE
Prevention of hereditary angio-
edema—
Adults: 2 mg P.O. t.i.d. to 4 mg P.O. q.i.d for 5 days initially. Dosage is gradually reduced at intervals of 1 to 3 months to a dosage of 2 mg daily.
Children age 6 to 12: Administer up to 2 mg P.O. daily.
Children under age 6: 1 mg. P.O. daily
Note: Stanozolol should be used in children only during an acute attack.

ADVERSE REACTIONS
Androgenic: in women—*acne, edema, oily skin, weight gain, hirsutism, hoarseness,* clitoral enlargement, decreased or increased libido. In men— prepubertal: premature epiphyseal closure, acne, priapism, growth of body and facial hair, phallic enlargement; postpubertal: testicular atrophy, oligospermia, decreased ejaculatory volume, impotence, gynecomastia, epididymitis.
CV: edema.
GI: gastroenteritis, nausea, vomiting, constipation, diarrhea, change in appetite.
GU: bladder irritability.
Hepatic: reversible jaundice, hepatotoxicity.
Hypoestrogenic: in women—flushing; sweating; vaginitis with itching, drying, burning or bleeding; menstrual irregularities.
Other: hypercalcemia.

INTERACTIONS
None significant.

NURSING CONSIDERATIONS
- Contraindicated in prostatic hypertrophy with obstruction; prostatic and male breast cancer; cardiac, hepatic, or renal decompensation; nephrosis; and in premature infants. Use cautiously in prepubertal males; patients with diabetes or coronary disease; patients taking ACTH, corticosteroids, or anticoagulants.
- A lower dosage in young women (2

Italicized side effects are common or life-threatening.
*Liquid form contains alcohol.   **May contain tartrazine.

mg b.i.d.) is recommended to avoid virilization. Watch for these adverse reactions; may be irreversible despite prompt discontinuation of therapy. Doctor must decide if benefits outweigh adverse effects.

• Tell women to report menstrual irregularities; therapy should be discontinued pending etiologic determination.

• Boys under 7 years should be closely observed for precocious development of male sexual characteristics.

• In children, therapy should be preceded by X-ray of wrist bones to establish level of bone maturation. During treatment, bone maturation may proceed more rapidly than linear growth; dosage should be intermittent and X-rays taken periodically.

• Edema is generally controllable with salt restriction or diuretics. Monitor weight routinely.

• Watch for symptoms of jaundice. Dosage adjustment may reverse condition; check liver function tests regularly. If abnormal, therapy should be discontinued.

• Observe patient on concomitant anticoagulant therapy for ecchymotic areas, petechiae, or abnormal bleeding. Monitor prothrombin time.

• Watch for symptoms of hypoglycemia in patients with diabetes. Dosage of antidiabetic drug may need adjustment.

• Use with diet high in calories and protein unless contraindicated. Give small, frequent feedings.

• Administer before or with meals to minimize GI distress.

• Monitor serum cholesterol in cardiac patients.

• Erroneously thought to enhance athletic ability.

• Anabolic steroids may alter many laboratory studies during therapy and for 2 to 3 weeks after therapy is stopped.

testosterone
Andro, Andronaq, Histerone, Malogen♦, Testaqua, Testoject
Pregnancy Risk Category: X

MECHANISM OF ACTION
Stimulates target tissues to develop normally in androgen-deficient men.

INDICATIONS & DOSAGE
Eunuchoidism, eunuchism, male climacteric symptoms—
Adults: 10 to 25 mg I.M. 2 to 5 times weekly.
Breast engorgement of nonnursing mothers—
25 to 50 mg I.M. daily for 3 to 4 days, starting at delivery.
Breast cancer in women 1 to 5 years postmenopausal—
100 mg I.M. 3 times weekly as long as improvement maintained.

ADVERSE REACTIONS
Androgenic: in women—*acne, edema, oily skin, weight gain, hirsutism, hoarseness,* clitoral enlargement, decreased or increased libido. In men—prepubertal: premature epiphyseal closure, acne, priapism, growth of body and facial hair, phallic enlargement; postpubertal: testicular atrophy, oligospermia, decreased ejaculatory volume, impotence, gynecomastia, epididymitis.
CV: edema.
GI: gastroenteritis, nausea, vomiting, constipation, diarrhea, change in appetite.
GU: bladder irritability.
Hepatic: reversible jaundice.
Hypoestrogenic: in women—flushing; sweating; vaginitis with itching, drying, burning, or bleeding; menstrual irregularities.
Local: pain at injection site, induration, irritation and sloughing with pellet implantation, edema.
Other: hypercalcemia.

Unmarked trade names available in the United States only.
♦Also available in Canada.   ♦♦Available in Canada only.   ◊Also available OTC.

INTERACTIONS
None significant.

NURSING CONSIDERATIONS
• Contraindicated in women of child-bearing potential (possible masculinization of female infant); in elderly, asthenic men who may react adversely to androgen overstimulation; in hypercalcemia; cardiac, hepatic, or renal decompensation; prostatic or breast cancer in males; benign prostatic hypertrophy with obstruction; conditions aggravated by fluid retention; hypertension; and in premature infants. Use cautiously in myocardial infarction or coronary artery disease, and in prepubertal males.
• Periodic liver function tests should be performed.
• In metastatic breast cancer, hypercalcemia usually indicates progression of bone metastases. Report signs of hypercalcemia.
• Therapeutic response in breast cancer is usually apparent within 3 months. Stop therapy if signs of disease progression appear.
• Enhances hypoglycemia; tell patient to report signs of hyperinsulinism.
• Instruct men to report priapism, reduced ejaculatory volume, and gynecomastia. Withdraw drug if these occur.
• Report signs of virilization in females; reevaluate treatment.
• Monitor prepubertal men by X-ray for rate of bone maturation.
• Edema is generally controllable with salt restriction or diuretics. Monitor weight routinely.
• Use with diet high in calories and protein unless contraindicated. Give small, frequent feedings.
• Store I.M. preparations at room temperature. If crystals appear, warming and shaking the bottle will usually disperse them.
• Inject deep into upper outer quadrant of gluteal muscle.
• Watch for ecchymotic areas, petechiae, or abnormal bleeding in patients on concomitant anticoagulant therapy. Monitor prothrombin time.
• Many laboratory studies may be altered during therapy and for 2 to 3 weeks after therapy is stopped.

testosterone cypionate
Andro-Cyp, Andronaq-LA, Andronate, dep Andro, Depotest, Depo-Testosterone♦, Duratest, T-Cypionate, Tesionate, Testa-C, Testoject-LA, Testred Cypionate, Virilon IM

testosterone enanthate
Android-T, Andro-LA, Andryl, Delatestryl♦, Durathate, Everone, Malogex♦♦, Testone LA, Testrin PA,

testosterone propionate
Malogen♦♦, Testex

Pregnancy Risk Category: X

MECHANISM OF ACTION
Stimulates target tissues to develop normally in androgen-deficient men.

INDICATIONS & DOSAGE
Eunuchism, eunuchoidism, deficiency after castration and male climacteric—
Adults: 200 to 400 mg (cypionate or enanthate) I.M. q 4 weeks.
Oligospermia—
Adults: 100 to 200 mg (cypionate or enanthate) I.M. q 4 to 6 weeks for development and maintenance of testicular function.
Eunuchism and eunuchoidism, male climacteric, impotence—
Adults: 10 to 25 mg (propionate) I.M. 2 to 4 times weekly.
Metastatic breast cancer in women—
50 to 100 mg (propionate) I.M. 3 times weekly. 200 to 400 mg (cypionate or enanthate) I.M. q 2 to 4 weeks.
Postmenopausal or primary osteoporosis—

Adults: 200 to 400 mg (enanthate) I.M. q 4 weeks.

ADVERSE REACTIONS
Androgenic: in women—*acne, edema, oily skin, weight gain, hirsutism, hoarseness,* clitoral enlargement, changes in libido. In men—prepubertal: premature epiphyseal closure, acne, priapism, growth of body and facial hair, phallic enlargement; postpubertal: testicular atrophy, oligospermia, decreased ejaculatory volume, impotence, gynecomastia, epididymitis.
CV: edema.
GI: gastroenteritis, nausea, vomiting, constipation, diarrhea, change in appetite.
GU: bladder irritability.
Hepatic: reversible jaundice.
Local: pain at injection site, induration, postinjection furunculosis.
Other: hypercalcemia.

INTERACTIONS
None significant.

NURSING CONSIDERATIONS
• Contraindicated in women of childbearing potential (possible masculinization of female infant); in patients with hypercalcemia; cardiac, hepatic, or renal decompensation; prostatic or breast cancer in men; benign prostatic hypertrophy with obstruction; conditions aggravated by fluid retention; hypertension; elderly, asthenic men who may react adversely to androgen overstimulation; and in premature infants. Use cautiously in myocardial infarction or coronary artery disease, and in prepubertal males.
• Periodic liver function tests should be performed.
• In metastatic breast cancer, hypercalcemia usually indicates progression of bone metastases. Report signs of hypercalcemia.
• Response in breast cancer is usually apparent within 3 months. Stop therapy if signs of disease progression appear.
• Enhances hypoglycemia; teach signs of hypoglycemia, and instruct the patient to report immediately if they occur.
• Instruct men to report priapism, reduced ejaculatory volume, and gynecomastia. Withdraw drug.
• Watch for signs of ecchymoses, petechiae with concomitant anticoagulant therapy. Monitor prothrombin time.
• Inject deep into upper outer quadrant of gluteal muscle. Report soreness at site; possibility of postinjection furunculosis.
• Report signs of virilization in women; reevaluate treatment.
• Monitor prepubertal males by X-ray for rate of bone maturation.
• Edema is generally controllable with salt restriction or diuretics. Monitor weight routinely.
• Use with diet high in calories and protein unless contraindicated. Give small, frequent feedings.
• Daily requirements best administered in divided doses.
• May alter many laboratory studies during therapy and for 2 to 3 weeks after therapy is stopped.

54

Oral contraceptives

estrogen with progestogen

COMBINATION PRODUCTS
None.

---

estrogen with progestogen
Brevicon, Demulen♦, Enovid,
Loestrin 1/20, Loestrin 1.5/30♦, Lo/
Ovral, Min-Ovral♦♦, Modicon,
Nordette, Norinyl 1 + 35, Norinyl 1
+ 50♦, Norinyl 1 + 80♦, Norinyl 2
mg♦, Norlestrin♦, Norlestrin 1/50,
Norlestrin 2.5/50, Ortho-Novum 1/
50♦, Ortho-Novum 7/7/7, Ortho-
Novum 10/11, Ovcon 35**, Ovcon
50**, Ovral, Ovulen♦, Trilevlen, Tri-
Norinyl, Triphasil

Pregnancy Risk Category: X

MECHANISM OF ACTION
Oral contraceptives inhibit ovulation
through a negative feedback mechanism directed at the hypothalamus.
They may also prevent transport of
the ovum through the fallopian tubes.

Estrogen suppresses secretion of
follicle-stimulating hormone, blocking follicular development and ovulation.

Progestogen suppresses luteinizing
hormone secretion so ovulation can't
occur even if the follicle develops.
Progestogen thickens cervical mucus,
which interferes with sperm migra-
tion, and also causes endometrial
changes that prevent implantation of
the fertilized ovum.

INDICATIONS & DOSAGE
Contraception—

Women: 1 tablet P.O. daily, beginning on day 5 of menstrual cycle (first
day of menstrual flow is day 1). With
20- and 21-tablet packages, new dosing cycle begins 7 days after last tablet
taken. With 28-tablet packages, dosage is 1 tablet daily without interruption; extra tablets are placebos or contain iron. If only 1 or 2 doses are
missed, dosage may continue on
schedule. If 3 or more doses are
missed, remaining tablets in monthly
package must be discarded and another contraceptive method substituted. If next menstrual period
doesn't begin on schedule, rule out
pregnancy before starting new dosing
cycle. If menstrual period begins,
start new dosing cycle 7 days after
last tablet was taken. If all doses have
been taken on schedule and 1 menstrual period is missed, continue dosing cycle. If 2 consecutive menstrual
periods are missed, pregnancy test is
required before new dosing cycle is
started.
*Biphasic oral contraceptives (Ortho-
Novum 10/11)—*
1 color tablet P.O. daily for 10 days,
then next color tablet for 11 days.
*Triphasic oral contraceptives (Ortho-
Novum 7/7/7, Tri-Norinyl, Triphasil)—*
1 tablet P.O. daily in the sequence
specified by the brand.
Endometriosis—
Women: Enovid 5 mg or 10 mg—1
tablet P.O. daily for 2 weeks starting on
day 5 of menstrual cycle. Continue
without interruption for 6 to 9 months,
increasing dose by 5 to 10 mg q 2

Italicized side effects are common or life-threatening.
*Liquid form contains alcohol.   **May contain tartrazine.

weeks, up to 20 mg daily. Up to 40 mg daily may be needed if breakthrough bleeding occurs.

ADVERSE REACTIONS
CNS: *headache, dizziness,* depression, libido changes, lethargy, migraine.
CV: *thromboembolism,* hypertension, edema.
EENT: worsening of myopia or astigmatism, intolerance to contact lenses.
GI: *nausea,* vomiting, abdominal cramps, bloating, diarrhea, constipation, anorexia, changes in appetite, weight gain, *bowel ischemia,* pancreatitis.
GU: *breakthrough bleeding, granulomatous colitis,* dysmenorrhea, amenorrhea, cervical erosion or abnormal secretions, enlargement of uterine fibromas, vaginal candidiasis.
Hepatic: gallbladder disease, cholestatic jaundice, liver tumors.
Metabolic: hyperglycemia, hypercalcemia, folic acid deficiency.
Skin: rash, acne, seborrhea, oily skin, erythema multiforme, hyperpigmentation.
Other: *breast tenderness,* enlargement, secretion.
  Adverse effects may be more serious, frequent, and rapid in onset with high-dose than with low-dose combinations.

INTERACTIONS
Barbiturates, anticonvulsants, rifampin: may diminish contraceptive effectiveness. Use supplemental form of contraception.

NURSING CONSIDERATIONS
• Contraindicated in thromboembolic disorders, cerebrovascular or coronary artery disease, myocardial infarction, known or suspected cancer of breasts or reproductive organs, benign or malignant liver tumors, undiagnosed abnormal vaginal bleeding, known or suspected pregnancy, lacta-tion; and in adolescents with incomplete epiphyseal closure. Also contraindicated in women 35 years or older who smoke more than 15 cigarettes a day, and in all women over 40 years. Use cautiously in patients with systemic lupus erythematosus, hypertension, mental depression, migraine, epilepsy, asthma, diabetes mellitus, amenorrhea, scanty or irregular periods, fibrocystic breast disease, family history (mother, grandmother, sister) of breast or genital tract cancer, renal or gallbladder disease. Report development or worsening of these conditions to doctor. Prolonged therapy inadvisable in women who plan to become pregnant.
• Discontinue if patient develops granulomatous colitis while on oral contraceptives.
• Discontinue at least 1 week before surgery to decrease risk of thromboembolism. Use an alternate method of birth control.
• If one menstrual period is missed and tablets have been taken on schedule, tell patient to continue taking them. If two consecutive menstrual periods are missed, tell patient to stop drug and to have pregnancy test. Progestogens may cause birth defects if taken early in pregnancy.
• Missed doses in midcycle greatly increase likelihood of pregnancy.
• If one tablet is missed, tell patient to take it as soon as remembered, or take two tablets the next day and continue regular schedule. If patient misses 2 consecutive days, she should take two tablets daily for 2 days, and resume normal schedule. Patient should use an additional method of birth control for 7 days after two missed doses.
• Warn patient that headache, nausea, dizziness, breast tenderness, spotting, and breakthrough bleeding are common at first. These should diminish after 3 to 6 dosing cycles (months). However, breakthrough

bleeding in patients taking high-dose estrogen-progestogen combinations for menstrual disorders may necessitate dosage adjustment.

• Warn patient to immediately report abdominal pain; numbness, stiffness, or pain in legs or buttocks; pressure or pain in chest; shortness of breath; severe headache; visual disturbances, such as blind spots, blurriness, or flashing lights; undiagnosed vaginal bleeding or discharge; two consecutive missed menstrual periods; lumps in the breast; swelling of hands or feet; severe pain in the abdomen (tumor rupture in the liver).

• Advise patient to use an additional method of birth control for the first week of administration in the initial cycle. Some doctors instruct patients to also use condoms or a diaphragm with spermicide.

• Tell patient to take tablets at same time each day; nighttime dosing may reduce nausea and headaches.

• Advise patient not to take same drug for longer than 18 months without consulting doctor. Stress importance of Pap smears and annual gynecologic examinations.

• Warn the patient of possible delay in achieving pregnancy when drug is discontinued.

• Many doctors recommend that women not become pregnant within 2 months after stopping drug. Advise patient to check with her doctor about how soon pregnancy may be attempted after hormonal therapy is stopped.

• Teach the patient how to perform a breast self-examination.

• Advise the patient of increased risks associated with simultaneous use of cigarettes and oral contraceptives.

• Many laboratory tests are affected by oral contraceptives; some include: increase in serum bilirubin, alkaline phosphatase, AST (SGOT), ALT (SGPT), and protein-bound iodine; decrease in glucose tolerance and urinary excretion of 17-hydroxycorticosteroids (17-OHCS).

• Estrogens and progestogens may alter glucose tolerance, thus changing requirements for antidiabetic drugs. Monitor blood glucose levels.

• Instruct patient to weigh herself at least twice a week and to report any sudden weight gain or edema to doctor.

• Warn patient to avoid exposure to ultraviolet light or prolonged exposure to sunlight.

• Many doctors advise women on prolonged therapy with oral contraceptives (5 years or longer) to stop drug and use other birth control methods in order to periodically reassess patient while off hormone therapy.

• The Centers for Disease Control (CDC) report that the use of oral contraceptives *may decrease* the incidence of ovarian and endometrial cancer. Also, oral contraceptives do not appear to increase a woman's risk of breast cancer. However, FDA reports that they may be linked to an increased risk of cervical cancer.

• Ovral has been prescribed as a postcoital contraceptive ("morning-after" pill). Patients are given 2 tablets at the initial visit and 2 tablets 12 hours later.

• Triphasic oral contraceptives may cause fewer side effects such as breakthrough bleeding and spotting.

Italicized side effects are common or life-threatening.
*Liquid form contains alcohol.   **May contain tartrazine.

55

Estrogens

chlorotrianisene
dienestrol
diethylstilbestrol (stilboestrol)
diethylstilbestrol diphosphate
esterified estrogens
estradiol
estradiol cypionate
estradiol valerate
estrogens, conjugated
estrone
ethinyl estradiol
quinestrol

COMBINATION PRODUCTS

MENRIUM 5-2♦: chlordiazepoxide 5 mg and esterified estrogens 0.2 mg.
MENRIUM 5-4♦: chlordiazepoxide 5 mg and esterified estrogens 0.4 mg.
MENRIUM 10-4♦: chlordiazepoxide 10 mg and esterified estrogens 0.4 mg.
MILPREM-200: conjugated estrogens 0.45 mg and meprobamate 200 mg.
MILPREM-400: conjugated estrogens 0.45 mg and meprobamate 400 mg.
PMB 200: conjugated estrogens 0.45 mg and meprobamate 200 mg.
PMB 400: conjugated estrogens 0.45 mg and meprobamate 400 mg.
(See Chapter 54, ORAL CONTRACEPTIVES.)

---

chlorotrianisene
TACE♦

Pregnancy Risk Category: X

MECHANISM OF ACTION
Increases the synthesis of DNA, RNA, and protein in responsive tissues. Also reduces FSH and LH release from the pituitary.

INDICATIONS & DOSAGE
Men:
Prostatic cancer—
12 to 25 mg P.O. daily.
Nonnursing mothers:
Postpartum breast engorgement—
72 mg P.O. b.i.d. for 2 days; or 50 mg q 6 hours for 6 doses; or 12 mg q.i.d. for 7 days. Start dosing within 8 hours after delivery.
Women:
Menopausal symptoms—
12 to 25 mg P.O. daily for 30 days or cyclic (3 weeks on, 1 week off).
Female hypogonadism—
12 to 25 mg P.O. for 21 days, followed by 1 dose of progesterone 100 mg I.M. or 5 days of oral progestogen given concurrently with last 5 days of chlorotrianisene (for example, medroxyprogesterone 5 to 10 mg).
Atrophic vaginitis—
12 to 25 mg P.O. daily for 30 to 60 days.

ADVERSE REACTIONS
CNS: headache, dizziness, chorea, migraine, depression, libido changes.
CV: thrombophlebitis; *thromboembolism;* hypertension; edema; *increased risk of stroke, pulmonary embolism, and myocardial infarction.*
EENT: worsening of myopia or astigmatism, intolerance to contact lenses.
GI: *nausea,* vomiting, abdominal cramps, bloating, diarrhea, constipation, anorexia, increased appetite, excessive thirst, weight changes, pan-

---

creatitis.

GU: in women—breakthrough bleeding, altered menstrual flow, dysmenorrhea, amenorrhea, cervical erosion or abnormal secretions, enlargement of uterine fibromas, vaginal candidiasis. In men—*gynecomastia, testicular atrophy, impotence.*

Hepatic: cholestatic jaundice.

Metabolic: hyperglycemia, hypercalcemia, folic acid deficiency.

Skin: melasma, urticaria, acne, seborrhea, oily skin, hirsutism or loss of hair.

Other: leg cramps, purpura, breast changes (tenderness, enlargement, secretion).

INTERACTIONS
None significant.

NURSING CONSIDERATIONS
• Contraindicated in thrombophlebitis or thromboembolic disorders; cancer of breast, reproductive organs, or genitals; undiagnosed abnormal genital bleeding; and pregnancy. Use cautiously in hypertension, asthma, mental depression, bone diseases, blood dyscrasias, gallbladder disease, migraine, seizures, diabetes mellitus, amenorrhea, heart failure, hepatic or renal dysfunction, and family history (mother, grandmother, sister) of breast or genital tract cancer. Development or worsening of these conditions may require discontinuation of the drug.
• Patient package insert that describes estrogen's adverse effects is available. However, provide verbal explanation also.
• Warn patient to report immediately: abdominal pain; pain, numbness, or stiffness in legs or buttocks; pressure or pain in chest; shortness of breath; severe headaches; visual disturbances, such as blind spots, flashing lights, blurriness; vaginal bleeding or discharge; breast lumps; swelling of hands or feet; yellow skin and sclera;

dark urine; and light-colored stools.
• Not used for menstrual disorders because duration of action is very long.
• Pathologist should be advised of estrogen therapy when specimen is sent.
• Patients with diabetes should report elevated blood glucose test results so antidiabetic medication dose can be adjusted.
• Teach women how to perform routine breast self-examination.
• Explain to patient on cyclic therapy for postmenopausal symptoms that, although withdrawal bleeding may occur during week off drug, fertility has not been restored. Pregnancy is not possible since she has not ovulated.

---

dienestrol
DV♦ , Estraguard, Ortho Dienestrol♦
Pregnancy Risk Category: X

MECHANISM OF ACTION
Increases the synthesis of DNA, RNA, and protein in responsive tissues. Also reduces FSH and LH release from the pituitary.

INDICATIONS & DOSAGE
Postmenopausal women:
Atrophic vaginitis and kraurosis vulvae—
1 to 2 intravaginal applications of cream daily for 1 to 2 weeks (as directed), then half that dose for the same period. A maintenance dosage of 1 applicatorful one to three times a week may be ordered.

ADVERSE REACTIONS
GU: vaginal discharge; with excessive use, uterine bleeding.
Local: increased discomfort, burning sensation. Systemic effects possible.
Other: breast tenderness.

INTERACTIONS
None significant.

NURSING CONSIDERATIONS

• Contraindicated in thrombophlebitis or thromboembolic disorders; cancer of breast, reproductive organs, or genitals; undiagnosed abnormal genital bleeding; and pregnancy. Use cautiously in menstrual irregularities or endometriosis.
• Instruct patient to apply drug at bedtime to increase effectiveness.
• Prolonged therapy with estrogen-containing products is contraindicated.
• Patient package insert that describes estrogen's adverse effects is available. However, provide verbal explanation also.
• Systemic reactions possible with normal intravaginal use. Monitor closely.
• Warn patient not to exceed the prescribed dose.
• Withdrawal bleeding may occur if estrogen is suddenly stopped.
• Patient shouldn't wear tampon while receiving vaginal therapy. She may need to wear sanitary pad to protect clothing.
• Teach patient how to insert suppositories or cream. Wash vaginal area with soap and water before application.
• Instruct patient to remain recumbent for 30 minutes after administration to prevent loss of drug.
• Teach patient how to perform breast self-examination.

---

diethylstilbestrol (stilboestrol)
DES

diethylstilbestrol diphosphate
Honvol♦♦, Stilphostrol

Pregnancy Risk Category: X

MECHANISM OF ACTION
Increases the synthesis of DNA, RNA, and protein in responsive tissues. Also reduces FSH and LH release from the pituitary.

INDICATIONS & DOSAGE
Women:
Hypogonadism, castration, primary ovarian failure—
0.2 to 0.5 mg P.O. daily.
Menopausal symptoms—
0.1 to 2 mg P.O. daily in cycles of 3 weeks on and 1 week off.
Postcoital contraception ("morning-after pill")—
25 mg P.O. b.i.d. for 5 days, starting within 72 hours after coitus.
Postpartum breast engorgement—
5 mg P.O. daily or t.i.d. up to total dose of 30 mg.
Men:
Prostatic cancer—
initially, 1 to 3 mg P.O. daily; may be reduced to 1 mg P.O. daily, or 5 mg I.M. twice weekly initially, followed by up to 4 mg I.M. twice weekly. Or 50 to 200 mg (diphosphate) P.O. t.i.d.; or 0.25 to 1 g I.V. daily for 5 days, then once or twice weekly.
Men and postmenopausal women:
Breast cancer—
15 mg P.O. daily.

ADVERSE REACTIONS
CNS: headache, dizziness, chorea, depression, lethargy.
CV: *thrombophlebitis; thromboembolism;* hypertension; edema; *increased risk of stroke, pulmonary embolism, and myocardial infarction.*
EENT: worsening of myopia or astigmatism, intolerance to contact lenses.
GI: *nausea,* vomiting, abdominal cramps, bloating, diarrhea, constipation, anorexia, increased appetite, excessive thirst, weight changes, pancreatitis.
GU: in women—breakthrough bleeding, altered menstrual flow, dysmenorrhea, amenorrhea, cervical erosion, altered cervical secretions, enlargement of uterine fibromas, vaginal candidiasis, loss of libido. In men—gy-

---

necomastia, testicular atrophy, impotence.
Hepatic: cholestatic jaundice.
Metabolic: hyperglycemia, hypercalcemia, folic acid deficiency.
Skin: melasma, urticaria, acne, seborrhea, oily skin, hirsutism or loss of hair.
Other: leg cramps, breast tenderness or enlargement.

INTERACTIONS
None significant.

NURSING CONSIDERATIONS
• Contraindicated in thrombophlebitis or thromboembolic disorders; undiagnosed abnormal genital bleeding; and pregnancy. Use cautiously in hypertension, asthma, mental depression, bone disease, migraine, seizures, blood dyscrasias, diabetes mellitus, gallbladder disease, amenorrhea, heart failure, hepatic or renal dysfunction, and family history (mother, grandmother, sister) of breast or genital tract cancer. Development or worsening of these conditions may require discontinuation of the drug.
• Patient package insert that describes estrogen's adverse effects is available. However, provide verbal explanation also.
• Only the 25-mg tablet is approved by FDA as the "morning-after pill." To be effective, it must be taken within 72 hours after coitus. Nausea and vomiting are common with this large dose.
• Warn patient to stop taking drug immediately if she becomes pregnant, since it can affect the fetus adversely.
• Warn patient to report immediately: abdominal pain; pain, numbness, or stiffness in legs or buttocks; pressure or pain in chest; shortness of breath; severe headache; visual disturbances, such as blind spots, flashing lights, or blurriness; vaginal bleeding or discharge; breast lumps; sudden weight gain; swelling of hands or feet; yellow sclera or skin; dark urine or light-colored stools.
• Pathologist should be advised of estrogen therapy when specimen is sent.
• Patients with diabetes should report elevated blood glucose test results so antidiabetic medication dose can be adjusted.
• High incidence of gross nonmalignant genital changes in offspring of women taking drug during pregnancy. Female offspring have higher than normal risk of developing cervical and vaginal adenocarcinoma. Male offspring may have higher than normal risk of developing testicular tumors, epididymal cysts, and impaired fertility.
• Increased number of cardiovascular deaths reported in men taking diethylstilbestrol tablet (5 mg daily) for prostatic cancer over long period of time. This effect not associated with 1-mg daily dose.
• Teach women how to perform routine breast self-examination.
• Explain to patient on cyclic therapy for postmenopausal symptoms that, although withdrawal bleeding may occur during week off drug, fertility has not been restored. Pregnancy is not possible since she has not ovulated.
• Use of estrogens associated with increased risk of endometrial cancer. Possible increased risk of breast cancer.

esterified estrogens
Estratab, Estromed♦♦, Menest, Neo-Estrone♦♦
Pregnancy Risk Category: X

MECHANISM OF ACTION
Increases the synthesis of DNA, RNA, and protein in responsive tissues. Also reduces FSH and LH release from the pituitary.

INDICATIONS & DOSAGE
Men:
Inoperable prostatic cancer—
1.25 to 2.5 mg P.O. t.i.d.
Men and postmenopausal women:
Breast cancer—
10 mg P.O. t.i.d. for 3 or more
months.
Women:
*Hypogonadism, castration, primary
ovarian failure—*
2.5 mg P.O. daily to t.i.d. in cycles of
3 weeks on, 1 week off.
Menopausal symptoms—
average 0.3 to 3.75 mg P.O. daily in
cycles of 3 weeks on, 1 week off.

ADVERSE REACTIONS
CNS: headache, dizziness, chorea,
depression, libido changes, lethargy.
CV: thrombophlebitis; *thromboembolism;* hypertension; edema; *increased
risk of stroke, pulmonary embolism,
and myocardial infarction.*
EENT: worsening of myopia or astigmatism, intolerance to contact lenses.
GI: *nausea,* vomiting, abdominal
cramps, bloating, diarrhea, constipation, anorexia, increased appetite,
weight changes, pancreatitis.
GU: in women—breakthrough bleeding, altered menstrual flow, dysmenorrhea, amenorrhea, cervical erosion,
altered cervical secretions, enlargement of uterine fibromas, vaginal candidiasis. In men—gynecomastia, testicular atrophy, impotence.
Hepatic: cholestatic jaundice.
Metabolic: hyperglycemia, hypercalcemia, folic acid deficiency.
Skin: melasma, rash, acne, hirsutism
or hair loss, seborrhea, oily skin.
Other: breast changes (tenderness,
enlargement, secretion).

INTERACTIONS
None significant.

NURSING CONSIDERATIONS
• Contraindicated in thrombophlebitis or thromboembolic disorders; undiagnosed abnormal genital bleeding;
and pregnancy. Use cautiously in patients with history of hypertension,
mental depression, gallbladder disease, migraine, seizures, diabetes
mellitus, amenorrhea, or family history (mother, grandmother, sister) of
breast or genital tract cancer. Development or worsening of these conditions may require discontinuation of
the drug.
• Patient package insert that describes estrogen's adverse effects is
available. However, provide verbal
explanation also.
• Warn patient to report immediately:
abdominal pain; pain, numbness, or
stiffness in legs or buttocks; pressure
or pain in chest; shortness of breath;
severe headaches; visual disturbances, such as blind spots, flashing
lights, or blurriness; vaginal bleeding
or discharge; breast lumps; swelling
of hands or feet; yellow skin or sclera;
dark urine or light-colored stools.
• Pathologist should be advised of estrogen therapy when specimen is sent.
• Patients with diabetes should report
elevated blood glucose test results so
antidiabetic medication dosage can be
adjusted.
• Explain to patient on cyclic therapy
for postmenopausal symptoms that,
although she may experience withdrawal bleeding during week off drug,
fertility has not been restored. Pregnancy cannot occur since she has not
ovulated.
• Teach women how to perform routine breast self-examination.

estradiol
Estrace**♦, Estrace Vaginal Cream,
Estraderm

estradiol cypionate
Depanate, Depestro, depGynogen,
Depo-Estradiol, Depogen, Dura-
Estrin, E-Cypionate, E-Ionate P.A.,
Estra-D, Estro-Cyp, Estrofem,
Estroject-L.A., Estronol-LA,
Hormogen Depot

estradiol valerate
Delestrogen♦, Dioval, Duragen,
Estradiol L.A., Estra-L, Estraval,
Estraval P.A., Feminate, Femogex,
Gynogen L.A., L.A.E., Menaval,
Valergen

Pregnancy Risk Category: X

MECHANISM OF ACTION
Increases the synthesis of DNA,
RNA, and protein in responsive tissues. Also reduces FSH and LH release from the pituitary.

INDICATIONS & DOSAGE
Women:
*Menopausal symptoms, hypogonad-
ism, castration, primary ovarian failure—*
1 to 2 mg P.O. daily, in cycles of 21
days on and 7 days off, or cycles of 5
days on and 2 days off; or 0.2 to 1 mg
I.M. weekly.
Kraurosis vulvae—
1 to 1.5 mg I.M. once or more per
week.
Atrophic vaginitis—
2 to 4 g intravaginal applications of
cream daily for 1 to 2 weeks. When
vaginal mucosa is restored, begin
maintenance dosage of 1 g one to
three times weekly.
Menopausal symptoms—
1 to 5 mg (cypionate) I.M. q 3 to 4
weeks. Or 5 to 20 mg (valerate) I.M.,
repeated once after 2 to 3 weeks.
Postpartum breast engorgement—
10 to 25 mg (valerate) I.M. at end of
first stage of labor.
*Inoperable breast cancer (oral estra-
diol)—*
10 mg P.O. t.i.d. for 3 months.
*Treatment of moderate to severe symp-
toms of menopause, female hypogonadism, female castration, primary
ovarian failure, and atrophic conditions caused by deficient endogenous
estrogen production—*
Place one Estraderm transdermal
patch on trunk of the body twice
weekly. Administer on an intermittent
cyclic schedule (3 weeks of therapy
followed by discontinuation for 1
week).
Men:
Inoperable prostatic cancer—
30 mg (valerate) I.M. q 1 to 2 weeks.
Or, 1 to 2 mg (oral estradiol) t.i.d.

ADVERSE REACTIONS
CNS: headache, dizziness, chorea,
depression, libido changes, lethargy.
CV: thrombophlebitis, *thromboembolism,* hypertension, edema.
EENT: worsening of myopia or astigmatism, intolerance to contact lenses.
GI: *nausea,* vomiting, abdominal
cramps, bloating, diarrhea, constipation, anorexia, increased appetite,
weight changes, pancreatitis.
GU: in women—breakthrough bleeding, altered menstrual flow, dysmenorrhea, amenorrhea, cervical erosion,
altered cervical secretions, enlargement of uterine fibromas, vaginal candidiasis. In men—gynecomastia, testicular atrophy, impotence.
Hepatic: cholestatic jaundice.
Metabolic: hyperglycemia, hypercalcemia, folic acid deficiency.
Skin: melasma, urticaria, acne, seborrhea, oily skin, hirsutism or hair
loss.
Other: breast changes (tenderness,
enlargement, secretion), leg cramps.

INTERACTIONS
None significant.

Italicized side effects are common or life-threatening.
*Liquid form contains alcohol.   **May contain tartrazine.

NURSING CONSIDERATIONS
• Contraindicated in thrombophlebitis or thromboembolic disorders; cancer of breast, reproductive organs; undiagnosed abnormal genital bleeding; and pregnancy. Use cautiously in hypertension, mental depression, bone diseases, blood dyscrasias, migraine, seizures, diabetes mellitus, amenorrhea, heart failure, hepatic or renal dysfunction, or family history (mother, grandmother, sister) of breast or genital tract cancer. Development or worsening of these conditions may require discontinuation of the drug.
• Patient package insert that describes estrogen's adverse effects is available. However, provide verbal explanation also.
• Warn patient to report immediately: abdominal pain; pain, numbness, or stiffness in legs or buttocks; pressure or pain in chest; shortness of breath; severe headaches; visual disturbances, such as blind spots, flashing lights, or blurriness; vaginal bleeding or discharge; breast lumps; swelling of hands or feet; yellow skin or sclera; dark urine or light-colored stools.
• Risk of endometrial cancer is increased in postmenopausal women who take estrogens for more than 1 year.
• Patients with diabetes should report elevated blood glucose test results so antidiabetic medication dosage can be adjusted.
• Pathologist should be advised of estrogen therapy when specimen is sent.
• Estradiol available as aqueous suspension or solution in peanut oil.
• Estradiol cypionate available as solution in cottonseed oil or vegetable oil.
• Estradiol valerate available as solution in castor oil, sesame oil, and vegetable oil. Check for allergy.
• Before injection, make sure drug is well dispersed in solution by rolling vial between palms. Inject deep I.M.

into large muscle.
• In women who are currently taking oral estrogen, treatment with the Estraderm transdermal patch can begin 1 week after withdrawal of oral therapy or sooner if symptoms appear before the end of the week.
• Teach women how to perform routine breast self-examination.
• Explain to patient on cyclic therapy for postmenopausal symptoms that, although withdrawal bleeding may occur during week off drug, fertility has not been restored. Pregnancy cannot occur since she has not ovulated.

---

estrogens, conjugated
C.E.S.♦♦, Conjugated Estrogens
C.S.D.♦♦, Premarin♦, Premarin
Intravenous♦, Progens

Pregnancy Risk Category: X

MECHANISM OF ACTION
Increases the synthesis of DNA, RNA, and protein in responsive tissues. Also reduces FSH and LH release from the pituitary.

INDICATIONS & DOSAGE
Women:
Abnormal uterine bleeding (hormonal imbalance)—
25 mg I.V. or I.M. Repeat in 6 to 12 hours.
Breast cancer (at least 5 years after menopause)—
10 mg P.O. t.i.d. for 3 months or more.
Castration, primary ovarian failure, and osteoporosis—
1.25 mg P.O. daily in cycles of 3 weeks on, 1 week off.
Hypogonadism—
2.5 mg P.O. b.i.d. or t.i.d. for 20 consecutive days each month.
Menopausal symptoms—
0.3 to 1.25 mg P.O. daily in cycles of 3 weeks on, 1 week off.
Postpartum breast engorgement—
3.75 mg P.O. q 4 hours for 5 doses or

1.25 mg q 4 hours for 5 days.
Men:
Inoperable prostatic cancer—
1.25 to 2.5 mg P.O. t.i.d.

ADVERSE REACTIONS
CNS: headache, dizziness, chorea, depression, libido changes, lethargy.
CV: thrombophlebitis; *thromboembolism;* hypertension; edema; *increased risk of stroke, pulmonary embolism, and myocardial infarction.*
EENT: worsening of myopia or astigmatism, intolerance to contact lenses.
GI: *nausea,* vomiting, abdominal cramps, bloating, diarrhea, constipation, anorexia, increased appetite, weight changes, pancreatitis.
GU: in women—breakthrough bleeding, altered menstrual flow, dysmenorrhea, amenorrhea, cervical erosion, altered cervical secretions, enlargement of uterine fibromas, vaginal candidiasis. In men—gynecomastia, testicular atrophy, impotence.
Hepatic: cholestatic jaundice.
Metabolic: hyperglycemia, hypercalcemia, folic acid deficiency.
Skin: melasma, urticaria, acne, seborrhea, oily skin, flushing (when given rapidly I.V.), hirsutism or loss of hair.
Other: breast changes (tenderness, enlargement, secretion), leg cramps.

INTERACTIONS
None significant.

NURSING CONSIDERATIONS
• Contraindicated in thrombophlebitis or thromboembolic disorders; undiagnosed abnormal genital bleeding; and pregnancy. Use cautiously in hypertension, gallbladder disease, bone diseases, blood dyscrasias, migraine, seizures, diabetes mellitus, amenorrhea, heart failure, hepatic or renal dysfunction, or family history (mother, grandmother, sister) of breast or genital tract cancer. Development or worsening of these condi-

tions may require discontinuation of the drug.
• Patient package insert that describes estrogen's adverse effects is available. However, provide verbal explanation also.
• Warn patient to report immediately: abdominal pain; pain, numbness, or stiffness in legs or buttocks; pressure or pain in chest; shortness of breath; severe headaches; visual disturbances, such as blind spots, flashing lights, or blurriness; vaginal bleeding or discharge; breast lumps; swelling of hands or feet; yellow skin or sclera; dark urine or light-colored stools.
• I.M. or I.V. use preferred for rapid treatment of dysfunctional uterine bleeding or reduction of surgical bleeding.
• Refrigerate before reconstituting. Agitate gently after adding diluent.
• Pathologist should be advised of estrogen therapy when specimen is sent.
• Patients with diabetes should report elevated blood glucose test results so antidiabetic medication dosage can be adjusted.
• Use associated with increased risk of endometrial cancer. Possible increased risk of breast cancer.
• Teach women how to perform routine breast self-examination.
• Explain to patient on cyclic therapy for postmenopausal symptoms that, although withdrawal bleeding may occur during week off drug, fertility has not been restored. Pregnancy cannot occur since she has not ovulated.

Italicized side effects are common or life-threatening.
*Liquid form contains alcohol.   **May contain tartrazine.

estrone

Bestrone, Estaqua, Estrofol,
Estroject, Estrone-A, Estronol,
Femogen♦♦, Foygen Aqueous,
Gynogen, Hormogen-A, Kestrin
Aqueous, Kestrone, Theelin
Aqueous, Theogen, Unigen,
Wehgen

Pregnancy Risk Category: X

MECHANISM OF ACTION
Increases the synthesis of DNA,
RNA, and protein in responsive tissues. Also reduces FSH and LH release from the pituitary.

INDICATIONS & DOSAGE
Women:
*Atrophic vaginitis and menopausal
symptoms—*
0.1 to 0.5 mg I.M. two or three times
weekly.
*Female hypogonadism and primary
ovarian failure—*
0.1 to 1 mg I.M. weekly in single or
divided doses.
Men:
Inoperable prostatic cancer—
2 to 4 mg I.M. 2 to 3 times weekly.

ADVERSE REACTIONS
CNS: headache, dizziness, chorea,
depression, libido changes, lethargy.
CV: thrombophlebitis, *thromboembolism,* hypertension, edema.
EENT: worsening of myopia or astigmatism, intolerance to contact lenses.
GI: *nausea,* vomiting, abdominal
cramps, bloating, diarrhea, constipation, anorexia, increased appetite,
weight changes, pancreatitis.
GU: in women—breakthrough bleeding, altered menstrual flow, dysmenorrhea, amenorrhea, cervical erosion,
altered cervical secretions, enlargement of uterine fibromas, vaginal candidiasis. In men—gynecomastia, testicular atrophy, impotence.
Hepatic: cholestatic jaundice.
Metabolic: hyperglycemia, hypercalcemia, folic acid deficiency.
Skin: melasma, urticaria, acne, seborrhea, oily skin, hirsutism or hair
loss.
Other: breast changes (tenderness,
enlargement, secretion), leg cramps.

INTERACTIONS
None significant.

NURSING CONSIDERATIONS
• Contraindicated in thrombophlebitis or thromboembolic disorders; cancer of breast or reproductive organs;
undiagnosed abnormal genital bleeding; and pregnancy. Use cautiously in
hypertension, mental depression, migraine, seizures, diabetes mellitus,
amenorrhea, hepatic or renal dysfunction, or family history (mother,
grandmother, sister) of breast or genital tract cancer. Development or worsening of these conditions may require
discontinuation of the drug.
• Estrone must be administered I.M.
• Patient package insert that describes estrogen's adverse effects is
available. However, provide verbal
explanation also.
• Warn patient to report immediately:
abdominal pain; pain, numbness, or
stiffness in legs or buttocks; pressure
or pain in chest; shortness of breath;
severe headaches; visual disturbances, such as blind spots, flashing
lights, or blurriness; vaginal bleeding
or discharge; breast lumps; swelling
of hands or feet.
• Pathologist should be advised of estrogen therapy when specimen is sent.
• Patients with diabetes should report
elevated blood glucose test results so
antidiabetic medication dosage can be
adjusted.
• Teach women how to perform routine breast self-examination.
• Use of estrogens associated with increased risk of endometrial cancer.
Possible increased risk of breast cancer.
• Explain to patient on cyclic therapy

for postmenopausal symptoms that, although withdrawal bleeding may occur during week off drug, fertility has not been restored. Pregnancy cannot occur since she has not ovulated.

ethinyl estradiol

Estinyl**♦, Feminone

Pregnancy Risk Category: X

MECHANISM OF ACTION
Increases the synthesis of DNA, RNA, and protein in responsive tissues. Also reduces FSH and LH release from the pituitary.

INDICATIONS & DOSAGE
Women:

Breast cancer (at least 5 years after menopause)—
1 mg P.O. t.i.d.

Hypogonadism—
0.05 mg P.O. daily to t.i.d. for 2 weeks a month, followed by 2 weeks progesterone therapy; continue for 3 to 6 monthly dosing cycles, followed by 2 months off.

Menopausal symptoms—
0.02 to 0.05 mg P.O. daily for cycles of 3 weeks on, 1 week off.

Postpartum breast engorgement—
0.5 to 1 mg P.O. daily for 3 days, then taper over 7 days to 0.1 mg and discontinue.

Men:

Inoperable prostatic cancer—
0.15 to 2 mg P.O. daily.

ADVERSE REACTIONS
CNS: headache, dizziness, chorea, depression, libido changes, lethargy.
CV: thrombophlebitis, *thromboembolism,* hypertension, edema.
EENT: worsening of myopia or astigmatism, intolerance to contact lenses.
GI: *nausea,* vomiting, abdominal cramps, bloating, diarrhea, constipation, anorexia, increased appetite, weight changes.
GU: in women—breakthrough bleeding, altered menstrual flow, dysmenorrhea, amenorrhea, cervical erosion, altered cervical secretions, enlargement of uterine fibromas, vaginal candidiasis. In men—gynecomastia, testicular atrophy, impotence.
Hepatic: cholestatic jaundice.
Metabolic: hyperglycemia, hypercalcemia, folic acid deficiency.
Skin: melasma, urticaria, acne, seborrhea, oily skin, hirsutism or hair loss.
Other: breast changes (tenderness, enlargement, secretion), leg cramps.

INTERACTIONS
None significant.

NURSING CONSIDERATIONS
• Contraindicated in thrombophlebitis or thromboembolic disorders; undiagnosed abnormal genital bleeding; and pregnancy. Use cautiously in hypertension, mental depression, bone diseases, migraine, seizures, blood dyscrasias, diabetes mellitus, amenorrhea, heart failure, hepatic or renal dysfunction, or family history (mother, grandmother, sister) of breast or genital tract cancer. Development or worsening of these conditions may require discontinuation of the drug.
• Patient package insert that describes estrogen's adverse effects is available. However, provide verbal explanation also.
• Warn patient to report immediately: abdominal pain; pain, numbness, or stiffness in legs or buttocks; pressure or pain in chest; shortness of breath; severe headaches; visual disturbances, such as blind spots, flashing lights, or blurriness; vaginal bleeding or discharge; breast lumps; swelling of hands or feet; yellow skin or sclera; dark urine or light-colored stools.
• Pathologist should be advised of estrogen therapy when specimen is sent.
• Patients with diabetes should report elevated blood glucose test results so

---

Italicized side effects are common or life-threatening.
*Liquid form contains alcohol.   **May contain tartrazine.

antidiabetic medication dosage can be adjusted.

• Teach women how to perform routine breast self-examination.

• Use of estrogens associated with increased risk of endometrial cancer. Possible increased risk of breast cancer.

• Explain to patient on cyclic therapy for postmenopausal symptoms that, although withdrawal bleeding may occur during week off drug, fertility has not been restored. Pregnancy cannot occur because she has not ovulated.

---

quinestrol
Estrovis

Pregnancy Risk Category: X

MECHANISM OF ACTION
Increases the synthesis of DNA, RNA, and protein in responsive tissues. Also reduces FSH and LH release from the pituitary.

INDICATIONS & DOSAGE
Women:
Moderate to severe vasomotor symptoms associated with menopause, and for atrophic vaginitis, kraurosis vulvae, female hypogonadism, female castration, and primary ovarian failure—
100 mcg P.O. once daily for 7 days, followed by 100 mcg weekly as maintenance dosage beginning 2 weeks after start of treatment. Dosage may be increased to 200 mcg weekly.

ADVERSE REACTIONS
CNS: headache, dizziness, chorea, migraine, depression, libido changes.
CV: thrombophlebitis; *thromboembolism;* hypertension; edema; *increased risk of stroke, pulmonary embolism, and myocardial infarction.*
EENT: worsening of myopia or astigmatism, intolerance to contact lenses.
GI: *nausea,* vomiting, abdominal cramps, bloating, diarrhea, constipa-

tion, anorexia, increased appetite, excessive thirst, weight changes.
GU: breakthrough bleeding, altered menstrual flow, dysmenorrhea, amenorrhea, cervical erosion or abnormal secretions, enlargement of uterine fibromas, vaginal candidiasis.
Hepatic: cholestatic jaundice.
Metabolic: hyperglycemia, hypercalcemia, folic acid deficiency.
Skin: melasma, urticaria, acne, seborrhea, oily skin, hirsutism or loss of hair.
Other: leg cramps, purpura, breast changes (tenderness, enlargement, secretion).

INTERACTIONS
None significant.

NURSING CONSIDERATIONS
• Contraindicated in thrombophlebitis or thromboembolic disorders; cancer of breast or reproductive organs; undiagnosed abnormal genital bleeding; and pregnancy. Use cautiously in hypertension, mental depression, migraine, seizures, diabetes mellitus, amenorrhea, hepatic or renal dysfunction, or family history (mother, grandmother, sister) of breast or genital tract cancer. Development or worsening of these may require discontinuation of the drug.

• Patient package insert that describes estrogen's adverse effects is available. However, provide verbal explanation also.

• Warn patient to report immediately: abdominal pain; pain, numbness, or stiffness in legs or buttocks; pressure or pain in chest; shortness of breath; severe headaches; visual disturbances, such as blind spots, flashing lights, or blurriness; vaginal bleeding or discharge; breast lumps; swelling of hands or feet; yellow skin or sclera; dark urine or light-colored stools.

• Pathologist should be advised of estrogen therapy when specimen is sent.

• Patients with diabetes should report

elevated blood glucose test results so antidiabetic medication dosage can be adjusted.

• Attempts to discontinue medication should be made at 3- to 6-month intervals.

• Similar in effectiveness to conjugated estrogens in treating postmenopausal symptoms. Biggest advantage is that quinestrol can be taken once a week.

• Use of estrogens associated with increased risk of endometrial cancer.

• Explain to patients on replacement therapy for postmenopausal symptoms that, although menstrual-like bleeding or spotting may occur, fertility has not been restored.

• Teach women how to perform breast self-examination.

56

Progestogens

hydroxyprogesterone caproate
medroxyprogesterone acetate
norethindrone
norethindrone acetate
norgestrel
progesterone

COMBINATION PRODUCTS
See Chapter 54, ORAL CONTRACEP-TIVES.

---

hydroxyprogesterone caproate
Delalutin♦♦, Duralutin, Gesterol L.A., Hy-Gesterone, Hylutin, Hyprogest, Hyproval P.A., Hyroxon, Pro-Depo, Prodrox

Pregnancy Risk Category: X

MECHANISM OF ACTION
Suppresses ovulation, possibly by inhibiting pituitary gonadotropin secretion. Also forms a thick cervical mucus.

INDICATIONS & DOSAGE
Women:
Menstrual disorders—
125 to 375 mg I.M. q 4 weeks. Stop after 4 cycles.
Uterine cancer—
1 to 5 g I.M. weekly.

ADVERSE REACTIONS
CNS: dizziness, migraine headache, lethargy, depression.
CV: hypertension, thrombophlebitis, *pulmonary embolism, edema.*
GI: nausea, vomiting, abdominal cramps.
GU: breakthrough bleeding, dysmenorrhea, amenorrhea, cervical erosion, or abnormal secretions, uterine fibromas, vaginal candidiasis.
Hepatic: cholestatic jaundice.
Local: irritation and pain at injection site.
Metabolic: hyperglycemia.
Skin: melasma, rash.
Other: breast tenderness, enlargement, or secretion; decreased libido.

INTERACTIONS
Rifampin: decreased progestogen effects. Monitor for diminished therapeutic response.

NURSING CONSIDERATIONS
• Contraindicated in thromboembolic disorders, breast cancer, undiagnosed abnormal vaginal bleeding, severe hepatic disease, missed abortion, or in pregnant women. Use cautiously in diabetes mellitus, seizure disorder, migraine, cardiac or renal disease, asthma, and mental illness.
• FDA regulations require that, before receiving first dose, patients read package insert explaining possible progestogen adverse effects. Provide verbal explanation also. Patient should report any unusual symptoms immediately and should stop drug and call doctor if visual disturbances or migraine occurs.
• Hydroxyprogesterone should not be used to induce withdrawal bleeding or as a test for pregnancy; drug may cause birth defects and masculinization of female fetus.
• Warn patient that edema and weight

Unmarked trade names available in the United States only.
♦ Also available in Canada.   ♦ ♦ Available in Canada only.   ◊ Also available OTC.

gain are likely.

• Give oil solutions (sesame oil and castor oil) deep I.M. in gluteal muscle.

• Effect lasts 7 to 14 days.

• Teach patient how to perform a monthly breast self-examination.

• Instruct patient that normal menstrual cycles may not resume for 2 to 3 months after drug is stopped.

medroxyprogesterone acetate
Amen, Curretab, Cycrin, Depo-Provera♦, Provera♦

Pregnancy Risk Category: X

MECHANISM OF ACTION
Suppresses ovulation, possibly by inhibiting pituitary gonadotropin secretion. Also forms a thick cervical mucus.

INDICATIONS & DOSAGE
Women:
Abnormal uterine bleeding due to hormonal imbalance—
5 to 10 mg P.O. daily for 5 to 10 days beginning on the 16th day of menstrual cycle. If patient has received estrogen—10 mg P.O. daily for 10 days beginning on 16th day of cycle.
Secondary amenorrhea—
5 to 10 mg P.O. daily for 5 to 10 days.
Endometrial or renal carcinoma—
Adults: 400 to 1,000 mg/week I.M.

ADVERSE REACTIONS
CNS: dizziness, migraine headache, lethargy, depression.
CV: hypertension, thrombophlebitis, *pulmonary embolism, edema.*
GI: nausea, vomiting, abdominal cramps.
GU: breakthrough bleeding, dysmenorrhea, amenorrhea, cervical erosion, or abnormal secretions, uterine fibromas, vaginal candidiasis.
Hepatic: cholestatic jaundice.
Metabolic: hyperglycemia.

Skin: melasma, rash.
Local: pain, induration, sterile abscesses.
Other: breast tenderness, enlargement, or secretion; decreased libido.

INTERACTIONS
Rifampin: decreased progestogen effects. Monitor for diminished therapeutic response.

NURSING CONSIDERATIONS
• Contraindicated in thromboembolic disorders, breast cancer, undiagnosed abnormal vaginal bleeding, missed abortion, hepatic dysfunction, or in pregnant women. Use cautiously in diabetes mellitus, seizure disorder, migraine, cardiac or renal disease, asthma, and mental illness.

• I.M. injection may be painful. Monitor sites for evidence of sterile abscess.

• FDA regulations require that, before receiving first dose, patients read package insert explaining possible progestogen adverse effects. Provide verbal explanation also. Patient should report any unusual symptoms immediately and should stop drug and call doctor if visual disturbances or migraine occurs.

• Don't use as test for pregnancy; drug may cause birth defects and masculinization of female fetus.

• Teach patient how to perform a monthly breast self-examination.

• Has been used effectively to treat obstructive sleep apnea.

norethindrone
Micronor♦, Norlutin, Nor-Q.D.

Pregnancy Risk Category: X

MECHANISM OF ACTION
Suppresses ovulation, possibly by inhibiting pituitary gonadotropin secretion. Also forms a thick cervical mucus.

Italicized side effects are common or life-threatening.
*Liquid form contains alcohol.   **May contain tartrazine.

INDICATIONS & DOSAGE
Women:
Amenorrhea, abnormal uterine bleeding—
5 to 20 mg P.O. daily on days 5 to 25 of menstrual cycle.
Endometriosis—
10 mg P.O. daily for 14 days, then increase by 5 mg P.O. daily q 2 weeks up to 30 mg daily.

ADVERSE REACTIONS
CNS: dizziness, migraine headache, lethargy, depression.
CV: hypertension, thrombophlebitis, *pulmonary embolism, edema.*
GI: nausea, vomiting, abdominal cramps.
GU: breakthrough bleeding, dysmenorrhea, amenorrhea, cervical erosion, or abnormal secretions, uterine fibromas, vaginal candidiasis.
Hepatic: cholestatic jaundice.
Metabolic: hyperglycemia.
Skin: melasma, rash.
Other: breast tenderness, enlargement, or secretion; decreased libido.

INTERACTIONS
Rifampin: decreased progestogen effects. Monitor for diminished therapeutic response.

NURSING CONSIDERATIONS
• Contraindicated in thromboembolic disorders, breast cancer, undiagnosed abnormal vaginal bleeding, severe hepatic disease, missed abortion, or in pregnant women. Use cautiously in diabetes mellitus, seizure disorder, migraine, cardiac or renal disease, asthma, and mental illness.
• Don't use as test for pregnancy; drug may cause birth defects and masculinization of female fetus.
• FDA regulations require that, before receiving first dose, patients read package insert explaining possible progestogen adverse effects. Provide verbal explanation also. Patient should report any unusual symptoms

immediately and should stop drug and call doctor if visual disturbances or migraine occurs.
• Watch patient carefully for signs of edema.
• Preliminary estrogen treatment is usually needed in menstrual disorders.
• Teach the patient how to perform a monthly breast self-examination.

norethindrone acetate
Aygestin, Norlutate♦
Pregnancy Risk Category: X

MECHANISM OF ACTION
Suppresses ovulation, possibly by inhibiting pituitary gonadotropin secretion. Also forms a thick cervical mucus.

INDICATIONS & DOSAGE
Women:
Amenorrhea, abnormal uterine bleeding—
2.5 to 10 mg P.O. daily on days 5 to 25 of menstrual cycle.
Endometriosis—
5 mg P.O. daily for 14 days, then increase by 2.5 mg daily q 2 weeks up to 15 mg daily.

ADVERSE REACTIONS
CNS: dizziness, migraine headache, lethargy, depression.
CV: hypertension, thrombophlebitis, *pulmonary embolism, edema.*
GI: nausea, vomiting, abdominal cramps.
GU: breakthrough bleeding, dysmenorrhea, amenorrhea, cervical erosion, or abnormal secretions, uterine fibromas, vaginal candidiasis.
Hepatic: cholestatic jaundice.
Metabolic: hyperglycemia.
Skin: melasma, rash.
Other: breast tenderness, enlargement, or secretion; decreased libido.

INTERACTIONS

Rifampin: decreased progestogen effects. Monitor for diminished therapeutic response.

NURSING CONSIDERATIONS

• Contraindicated in thromboembolic disorders, breast cancer, undiagnosed abnormal vaginal bleeding, severe hepatic disease, missed abortion, or in pregnant women. Use cautiously in diabetes mellitus, seizure disorder, migraine, cardiac or renal disease, asthma, and mental illness.

• FDA regulations require that, before receiving first dose, patients read package insert explaining possible progestogen adverse effects. Provide verbal explanation also. Patient should report any unusual symptoms immediately and should stop drug and call doctor if visual disturbances or migraine occurs.

• Don't use as test for pregnancy; drug may cause birth defects and masculinization of female fetus.

• Preliminary estrogen treatment is usually needed in menstrual disorders.

• Twice as potent as norethindrone.

• Teach patient how to perform a monthly breast self-examination.

norgestrel
Ovrette**

Pregnancy Risk Category: X

MECHANISM OF ACTION

Suppresses ovulation, possibly by inhibiting pituitary gonadotropin secretion. Also forms a thick cervical mucus.

INDICATIONS & DOSAGE
Women:

Contraception—
1 tablet P.O. daily.

ADVERSE REACTIONS

CNS: cerebral thrombosis or hemorrhage, migraine headache, lethargy, depression.

CV: hypertension, thrombophlebitis, *pulmonary embolism, edema.*

GI: nausea, vomiting, abdominal cramps, gallbladder disease.

GU: *breakthrough bleeding, change in menstrual flow,* dysmenorrhea, spotting, amenorrhea, cervical erosion, vaginal candidiasis.

Hepatic: cholestatic jaundice.

Skin: melasma, rash.

Other: breast tenderness, enlargement, or secretion.

INTERACTIONS

Rifampin: decreased progestogen effects. Monitor for diminished therapeutic response.

NURSING CONSIDERATIONS

• Contraindicated in thromboembolic disorders, breast cancer, undiagnosed abnormal vaginal bleeding, severe hepatic disease, missed abortion, or in pregnant women. Use cautiously in diabetes mellitus, seizure disorder, migraine, cardiac or renal disease, asthma, and mental illness.

• FDA regulations require that, before receiving first dose, patients read package insert explaining possible progestogen adverse effects. Provide verbal explanation also. Patient should report any unusual symptoms immediately and should stop drug and call doctor if visual disturbances, migraine, or numbness or tingling in limbs occurs.

• Tell patient to take pill every day, even if menstruating. Pill should be taken at the same time every day.

• A progestogen-only oral contraceptive known as "minipill."

• Teach the patient how to perform a monthly breast self-examination.

• Women using oral contraceptives should be advised of the increased risk of serious cardiovascular side effects associated with heavy cigarette smoking (15 or more cigarettes per

---

Italicized side effects are common or life-threatening.
*Liquid form contains alcohol.   **May contain tartrazine.

day). These risks are quite marked in women over 35 years.

• Risk of pregnancy increases with each tablet missed. A patient who misses one tablet should take it as soon as she remembers; she should then take the next tablet at the regular time. A patient who misses two tablets should take one as soon as she remembers and then take the next regular dose at the usual time; she should use a nonhormonal method of contraception in addition to norgestrel until 14 tablets have been taken. A patient who misses three or more tablets should discontinue the drug and use a nonhormonal method of contraception until after her menses. If her menstrual period does not occur within 45 days, pregnancy testing is necessary.

• Instruct the patient to immediately report excessive bleeding or bleeding between menstrual cycles.

---

progesterone
Femotrone, Gesterol, Progestaject, Progestilin♦♦

Pregnancy Risk Category: X

MECHANISM OF ACTION
Suppresses ovulation, possibly by inhibiting pituitary gonadotropin secretion. Also forms a thick cervical mucus.

INDICATIONS & DOSAGE
Women:
Amenorrhea—
5 to 10 mg I.M. daily for 6 to 8 days.
Dysfunctional uterine bleeding—
5 to 10 mg I.M. daily for 6 doses.
Contraception (as an intrauterine device)—
Progestasert system inserted into uterine cavity. Replace after 1 year.
Management of premenstrual syndrome (PMS)—
200 to 400 mg as a suppository administered either rectally or vaginally.

ADVERSE REACTIONS
CNS: dizziness, migraine headache, lethargy, depression.
CV: hypertension, thrombophlebitis, *pulmonary embolism, edema.*
GI: nausea, vomiting, abdominal cramps.
GU: breakthrough bleeding, dysmenorrhea, amenorrhea, cervical erosion, or abnormal secretions, uterine fibromas, vaginal candidiasis.
Hepatic: cholestatic jaundice.
Local: pain at injection site.
Metabolic: hyperglycemia.
Skin: melasma, rash.
Other: breast tenderness, enlargement, or secretion; decreased libido.

INTERACTIONS
Rifampin: decreased progestogen effects. Monitor for diminished therapeutic response.

NURSING CONSIDERATIONS
• Contraindicated in thromboembolic disorders, breast cancer, undiagnosed abnormal vaginal bleeding, severe hepatic disease, or missed abortion. Use cautiously in diabetes mellitus, seizure disorder, migraine, cardiac or renal disease, asthma, and mental illness.
• FDA regulations require that, before receiving first dose, patients read package insert explaining possible progestogen adverse effects. Provide verbal explanation also. Patient should report any unusual symptoms immediately and should stop drug and call doctor if visual disturbances or migraine occurs.
• Give oil solutions (peanut oil or sesame oil) deep I.M. Check sites frequently for irritation. Rotate injection sites.
• A progesterone-containing IUD (Progestasert) available that releases 65 mcg progesterone daily for 1 year.
• Instruct patient with Progestasert IUD how to check for proper IUD placement. Also, advise patient that

---

Unmarked trade names available in the United States only.
♦Also available in Canada. ♦♦Available in Canada only. ◊Also available OTC.

she may experience cramps for several days after insertion and menstrual periods may be heavier. Patient should report excessively heavy menses and bleeding between menses to the doctor.

• Tell patient with Progestasert IUD that the progesterone supply is depleted in 1 year and the device must be changed. Pregnancy risk increases after 1 year if patient relies on progesterone-depleted device for contraception.

• Patients considering IUD contraception should be advised of adverse effects, including uterine perforation, increased risk of infection, pelvic inflammatory disease, ectopic pregnancy, abdominal cramping, increased menstrual flow, and expulsion of the device.

• Preliminary estrogen treatment is usually needed in menstrual disorders.

• Teach the patient how to perform a monthly breast self-examination.

Gonadotropins

gonadorelin hydrochloride
(luteinizing hormone-releasing
hormone, LHRH)
gonadotropin, chorionic (HCG)
menotropins

COMBINATION PRODUCTS
None.

---

gonadorelin hydrochloride (luteinizing hormone-releasing hormone, LHRH)
Factrel♦

Pregnancy Risk Category: B

MECHANISM OF ACTION
A synthetic luteinizing hormone that
releases LHRH.

INDICATIONS & DOSAGE
*Evaluation of the functional capacity
and response of gonadotropic hormones—*
Adults: 100 mcg S.C. or I.V. In
women for whom the phase of the
menstrual cycle can be established,
perform the test between day 1 and
day 7.

ADVERSE REACTIONS
Local: swelling, occasionally with
pain and pruritus when administered
S.C.; skin rash after chronic S.C. administration.
Systemic: headache, nausea, light-
headedness, abdominal discomfort.

INTERACTIONS
Levodopa, spironolactone: may elevate gonadotropin levels. Monitor results carefully.
Digoxin, oral contraceptives: may de-
press gonadotropin levels. Monitor results carefully.

NURSING CONSIDERATIONS
• Although no hypersensitivity reactions have been reported to date, use
cautiously in patients who are allergic
to other drugs. Keep epinephrine
readily available.
• The gonadorelin test can be performed concomitantly with other
post-treatment evaluations.
• For specific test methodology and
interpretation of test results, refer to
the manufacturer's full product information. Ask pharmacist for a copy.
• Reconstitute vial with 1 ml of accompanying sterile diluent. Prepare
solution immediately before use. After reconstitution, store at room temperature and use within 1 day. Discard unused reconstituted solution
and diluent.
• As a single injection, gonadorelin
can evaluate the functional capacity
and response of the gonadotropins of
the anterior pituitary. Prolonged or repeated administration may be necessary to measure pituitary gonadotropic reserve.

---

gonadotropin, chorionic (HCG)

Antuitrin, A.P.L.♦, Chorex, Follutein, Pregnyl, Profasi HP♦

Pregnancy Risk Category: C

MECHANISM OF ACTION
Serves as a substitute for luteinizing hormone to stimulate ovulation of an human menopausal gonadotropin–prepared follicle. Also promotes secretion of gonadal steroid hormones by stimulating production of androgen by the interstitial cells of the testes (Leydig's cells).

INDICATIONS & DOSAGE
Anovulation and infertility—
Women: 10,000 units I.M. 1 day after last dose of menotropins.
Hypogonadism—
Men: 500 to 1,000 units I.M. 3 times weekly for 3 weeks, then twice weekly for 3 weeks; or 4,000 units I.M. 3 times weekly for 6 to 9 months, then 2,000 units 3 times weekly for 3 more months.
Nonobstructive cryptorchidism—
Boys 4 to 9 years: 5,000 units I.M. every other day for 4 doses.

ADVERSE REACTIONS
CNS: headache, fatigue, irritability, restlessness, depression.
GU: early puberty (growth of testes, penis, pubic and axillary hair; voice change; down on upper lip; growth of body hair).
Local: *pain at injection site*.
Other: gynecomastia, edema.

INTERACTIONS
None significant.

NURSING CONSIDERATIONS
• Contraindicated in pituitary hypertrophy or tumor, prostatic cancer, and early puberty (usual onset between 10 and 13 years of age). Use cautiously in epilepsy, migraine, asthma, and cardiac or renal disease.
• When used with menotropins to induce ovulation, multiple births are possible.
• Usually used only after failure of clomiphene in anovulatory patients.
• In infertility, encourage daily intercourse from day before chorionic gonadotropin is given until ovulation occurs.
• Inspect genitalia of boys for signs of early puberty.
• Be alert to symptoms of ectopic pregnancy. Usually evident between week 8 to 12 of gestation.

menotropins

Pergonal♦

Pregnancy Risk Category: C

MECHANISM OF ACTION
Menotropins, when administered to women who have not had primary ovarian failure, mimics follicle-stimulating hormone (FSH) in inducing follicular growth and luteinizing hormone (LH) in aiding follicular maturation.

INDICATIONS & DOSAGE
Anovulation—
Women: 75 international units (IU) each FSH and LH I.M. daily for 9 to 12 days, followed by 10,000 units chorionic gonadotropin I.M. 1 day after last dose of menotropins. Repeat for 1 to 3 menstrual cycles until ovulation occurs.
Infertility with ovulation—
Women: 75 IU each of FSH and LH I.M. daily for 9 to 12 days, followed by 10,000 units chorionic gonadotropin I.M. 1 day after last dose of menotropins. Repeat for 2 menstrual cycles and then increase to 150 IU each FSH and LH I.M. daily for 9 to 12 days, followed by 10,000 units chorionic gonadotropin I.M. 1 day after last dose of menotropins. Repeat for 2 menstrual cycles.

Italicized side effects are common or life-threatening.
*Liquid form contains alcohol.   **May contain tartrazine.

Infertility—
Men: 1 ampul I.M. 3 times weekly (given concomitantly with HCG 2,000 units twice weekly) for at least 4 months.

Menotropins are available in ampuls containing 75 IU each FSH and LH.

ADVERSE REACTIONS
Blood: hemoconcentration with fluid loss into abdomen.
GI: nausea, vomiting, diarrhea.
GU: women; *ovarian enlargement with pain and abdominal distention,* multiple births, ovarian hyperstimulation syndrome (sudden ovarian enlargement, ascites with or without pain, or pleural effusion).
GU: *gynecomastia in men.*
Other: fever.

INTERACTIONS
None significant.

NURSING CONSIDERATIONS
• Contraindicated in ovarian failure, high urinary gonadotropin levels, thyroid or adrenal dysfunction, pituitary tumor, abnormal uterine bleeding, ovarian cysts or enlargement, and pregnancy.
• Close monitoring of patient response is critical to ensure adequate ovarian stimulation without hyperstimulation.
• Tell patient that there is a possibility of multiple births.
• In infertility, encourage daily intercourse from day before chorionic gonadotropin is given until ovulation occurs.
• Pregnancy usually occurs 4 to 6 weeks after therapy.
• Reconstitute with 1 to 2 ml sterile saline injection. Use immediately.

58

Antidiabetic agents and glucagon

acetohexamide
chlorpropamide
glipizide
glucagon
glyburide
insulins◇
tolazamide
tolbutamide

COMBINATION PRODUCTS
MIXTARD INJECTION◇: 100 mg/ml isophane purified pork insulin suspension and purified pork insulin injection.

---

acetohexamide
Dimelor♦♦, Dymelor
Pregnancy Risk Category: D

MECHANISM OF ACTION
Stimulates insulin release from the pancreatic beta cells and reduces glucose output by the liver. An extrapancreatic effect increases peripheral sensitivity to insulin. A sulfonylurea.

INDICATIONS & DOSAGE
Adjunct to diet to lower the blood glucose in patients with non-insulin-dependent diabetes mellitus (type II)—
Adults: initially, 250 mg P.O. daily before breakfast; may increase dosage q 5 to 7 days (by 250 to 500 mg) as needed to maximum of 1.5 g daily, divided b.i.d. to t.i.d. before meals.
To replace insulin therapy—
If insulin dosage is less than 20 units daily, insulin may be stopped and oral therapy started with 250 mg P.O. daily, before breakfast, increased as

above if needed. If insulin dosage is 20 to 40 units daily, start oral therapy with 250 mg P.O. daily, before breakfast, while reducing insulin dosage 25% to 30% daily or every other day, depending on response to oral therapy.

ADVERSE REACTIONS
GI: nausea, heartburn, vomiting.
Metabolic: sodium loss, *hypoglycemia.*
Skin: rash, pruritus, facial flushing.
Other: hypersensitivity reactions.

INTERACTIONS
Anabolic steroids, chloramphenicol, clofibrate, guanethidine, MAO inhibitors, oral anticoagulants, phenylbutazone, salicylates, sulfonamides: increased hypoglycemic activity. Monitor blood glucose level.
Beta blockers, clonidine: prolonged hypoglycemic effect and masked symptoms of hypoglycemia. Use together cautiously.
Corticosteroids, glucagon, rifampin, thiazide diuretics: decreased hypoglycemic response. Monitor blood glucose level.

NURSING CONSIDERATIONS
• Contraindicated in treating type I (insulin-dependent) diabetes mellitus (IDDM); in diabetes adequately controlled by diet; and in type II diabetes complicated by ketosis, acidosis, diabetic coma, Raynaud's disease, gangrene, renal or hepatic impairment, or thyroid or other endocrine dysfunction. Use cautiously in patients with

---

Italicized side effects are common or life-threatening.
*Liquid form contains alcohol.   **May contain tartrazine.

sulfonamide hypersensitivity.
• Instruct patient about nature of disease; importance of following therapeutic regimen, adhering to specific diet, weight reduction, exercise, and personal hygiene programs, and avoiding infection; how and when to perform self-monitoring of blood glucose level; and recognition of hypoglycemia and hyperglycemia.
• Make sure patient understands that therapy relieves symptoms but doesn't cure the disease.
• Patient transferring from another oral sulfonylurea antidiabetic drug usually needs no transition period.
• Patient transferring from insulin therapy to an oral antidiabetic requires blood glucose monitoring at least t.i.d. before meals. Patient may require hospitalization during transition.
• During periods of increased stress, such as infection, fever, surgery, or trauma, patient may require insulin therapy. Monitor patient closely for hyperglycemia in these situations.
• Advise patient to avoid moderate to large intake of alcohol; disulfiram-like reaction possible.
• The possibility of increased cardiovascular mortality is associated with the use of sulfonylureas.

---

chlorpropamide

Apo-Chlorpropamide♦♦,
Diabinese♦, Glucamide, Novo-propamide♦♦

Pregnancy Risk Category: D

MECHANISM OF ACTION

Stimulates insulin release from the pancreatic beta cells and reduces glucose output by the liver. An extrapancreatic effect increases peripheral sensitivity to insulin. Also exerts an antidiuretic effect in patients with pituitary-deficient diabetes insipidus. A sulfonylurea.

INDICATIONS & DOSAGE

Adjunct to diet to lower blood glucose in patients with non-insulin-dependent diabetes mellitus (type II)—
Adults: 250 mg P.O. daily with breakfast or in divided doses if GI disturbances occur. First dosage increase may be made after 5 to 7 days because of extended duration of action, then dosage may be increased q 3 to 5 days by 50 to 125 mg, if needed, to maximum of 750 mg daily.
Adults over 65 years: initial dose should be in the range of 100 to 125 mg daily.
To change from insulin to oral therapy—
If insulin dosage is less than 40 units daily, insulin may be stopped and oral therapy started as above. If insulin dosage is 40 units or more daily, start oral therapy as above with insulin reduced 50%. Further insulin reductions should be made according to patient response.

ADVERSE REACTIONS

GI: nausea, heartburn, vomiting.
GU: tea-colored urine.
Metabolic: prolonged hypoglycemia, *dilutional hyponatremia*.
Skin: rash, pruritus, facial flushing.
Other: *hypersensitivity reactions*.

INTERACTIONS

Anabolic steroids, chloramphenicol, clofibrate, guanethidine, MAO inhibitors, oral anticoagulants, phenylbutazone, salicylates, sulfonamides: increased hypoglycemic activity. Monitor blood glucose level.
Beta blockers, clonidine: prolonged hypoglycemic effect and masked symptoms of hypoglycemia. Use together cautiously.
Corticosteroids, glucagon, rifampin, thiazide diuretics: decreased hypoglycemic response. Monitor blood glucose level.

NURSING CONSIDERATIONS
• Contraindicated in treating type I (insulin-dependent) diabetes mellitus (IDDM); in diabetes adequately controlled by diet; and in type II diabetes complicated by fever, ketosis, acidosis, diabetic coma, major surgery, severe trauma, Raynaud's disease, gangrene, renal or hepatic impairment, or thyroid or other endocrine dysfunction. Use cautiously in patients with sulfonamide hypersensitivity.
• Elderly patients may be more sensitive to this drug's adverse reactions.
• Instruct patient about nature of the disease; importance of following therapeutic regimen, adhering to specific diet, weight reduction, exercise, and personal hygiene programs, and avoiding infection; how and when to perform self-monitoring of blood glucose level; and recognition of and intervention for hypoglycemia and hyperglycemia.
• Make sure patient understands that therapy relieves symptoms but doesn't cure the disease.
• Adverse effects, especially hypoglycemia, may be more frequent or severe than with some other sulfonylurea drugs (acetohexamide, tolazamide, and tolbutamide) because of its long duration of effect (36 hours).
• If hypoglycemia occurs, patient should be monitored closely for a minimum of 3 to 5 days.
• Patient transferring from another oral sulfonylurea antidiabetic drug usually needs no transition period.
• Patient may require hospitalization during transition from insulin therapy to an oral antidiabetic. Monitor patient for blood glucose levels at least t.i.d., before meals; emphasize the need for a double-voided specimen.
• Drug may accumulate in patients with renal insufficiency.
• Advise patient to avoid intake of alcohol. Chlorpropamide-alcohol flush (CPAF) is characterized by facial flushing, light-headedness, headache, and occasional breathlessness. Even very small amounts of alcohol can produce this reaction.
• Watch for signs of impending renal insufficiency, such as dysuria, anuria, and hematuria, and report them to the doctor immediately.
• May potentiate antidiuretic hormone. Sometimes used to treat diabetes insipidus.
• The possibility of increased cardiovascular mortality is associated with the use of sulfonylureas.

---

glipizide
Glucotrol

Pregnancy Risk Category: C

MECHANISM OF ACTION
Stimulates insulin release from the pancreatic beta cells and reduces glucose output by the liver. An extrapancreatic effect increases peripheral sensitivity to insulin. A sulfonylurea.

INDICATIONS & DOSAGE
Adjunct to diet to lower the blood glucose in patients with non-insulin-dependent diabetes mellitus (type II)—
Adults: initially, 5 mg P.O. daily given before breakfast. Elderly patients or those with liver disease may be started on 2.5 mg. Usual maintenance dosage is 10 to 15 mg. Maximum recommended daily dosage is 40 mg.
To replace insulin therapy—
If insulin dosage is more than 20 units daily, patient may be started at usual dosage in addition to 50% of the insulin. If insulin dosage is less than 20 units, insulin may be discontinued.

ADVERSE REACTIONS
CNS: dizziness.
GI: nausea, vomiting, constipation.
Hepatic: *cholestatic jaundice.*
Metabolic: *hypoglycemia.*
Skin: rash, pruritus, facial flushing.

Italicized side effects are common or life-threatening.
*Liquid form contains alcohol.   **May contain tartrazine.

INTERACTIONS

Anabolic steroids, chloramphenicol, clofibrate, guanethidine, MAO inhibitors, oral anticoagulants, phenylbutazone, salicylates, sulfonamides: increased hypoglycemic activity. Monitor blood glucose level.

Beta blockers, clonidine: prolonged hypoglycemic effect and masked symptoms of hypoglycemia. Use together cautiously.

Corticosteroids, glucagon, rifampin, thiazide diuretics: decreased hypoglycemic response. Monitor blood glucose level.

NURSING CONSIDERATIONS

• Contraindicated in diabetic ketoacidosis, with or without coma. Use cautiously in renal and hepatic disease and sulfonamide hypersensitivity.

• Elderly patients may be more sensitive to this drug's adverse effects.

• Patient transferring from insulin therapy to an oral antidiabetic requires blood glucose monitoring at least t.i.d. before meals. Patient may require hospitalization during transition.

• During periods of increased stress, such as infection, fever, surgery, or trauma, patient may require insulin therapy. Monitor patient closely for hyperglycemia in these situations.

• Instruct patient about nature of disease; importance of following therapeutic regimen, adhering to specific diet, weight reduction, exercise, and personal hygiene programs, and avoiding infection; how and when to perform self-monitoring of blood glucose level; recognition of hypoglycemia and hyperglycemia.

• Some patients taking glipizide may be effectively controlled on a once-daily regimen, while others show better response with divided dosing.

• Give approximately 30 minutes before meals.

• Glipizide is a second-generation sulfonylurea oral hypoglycemic. The frequency of adverse effects appears to be lower than with first-generation drugs such as chlorpropamide and tolbutamide.

• Glipizide has a mild diuretic effect. May be useful in patients who have CHF or cirrhosis.

• The possibility of increased cardiovascular mortality is associated with the use of sulfonylureas.

glucagon

Pregnancy Risk Category: B

MECHANISM OF ACTION

Raises blood glucose level by promoting catalytic depolymerization of hepatic glycogen to glucose.

INDICATIONS & DOSAGE

Coma of insulin-shock therapy—
Adults: 0.5 to 1 mg S.C., I.M., or I.V. 1 hour after coma develops; may repeat within 25 minutes, if necessary. In very deep coma, also give glucose 10% to 50% I.V. for faster response. When patient responds, give additional carbohydrate immediately.

Severe insulin-induced hypoglycemia during diabetic therapy—
Adults and children: 0.5 to 1 mg S.C., I.M., or I.V.; may repeat q 20 minutes for 2 doses, if necessary. If coma persists, give glucose 10% to 50% I.V.

Diagnostic aid for radiologic examination—
Adults: 0.25 to 2 mg I.V. or I.M. before initiation of radiologic procedure.

ADVERSE REACTIONS

GI: nausea, vomiting.
Other: hypersensitivity.

INTERACTIONS

Phenytoin: inhibited glucagon-induced insulin release. Use cautiously.

NURSING CONSIDERATIONS

• Unstable hypoglycemic diabetics may not respond to glucagon. Give dextrose I.V. instead.

• It is vital to arouse the patient from coma as quickly as possible and to give additional carbohydrates orally to prevent secondary hypoglycemic reactions.

• For I.V. drip infusion, glucagon is compatible with dextrose solution, but forms a precipitate in chloride solutions.

• Instruct the patient and family in proper glucagon administration, recognition of hypoglycemia, and urgency of calling a doctor immediately in emergencies.

• May be used as diagnostic aid in radiologic examination of the stomach, duodenum, small bowel, and colon when a hypotonic state is advantageous.

• Has a positive inotropic and chronotropic action on the heart. May be used to treat overdosage of beta-adrenergic blockers.

---

glyburide

DiaBeta**, Euglucon♦♦, Micronase

Pregnancy Risk Category: B

MECHANISM OF ACTION

Stimulates insulin release from the pancreatic beta cells and reduces glucose output by the liver. An extrapancreatic effect increases peripheral sensitivity to insulin. A sulfonylurea.

INDICATIONS & DOSAGE

Adjunct to diet to lower the blood glucose in patients with non-insulin-dependent diabetes mellitus (type II)—
Adults: initially, 2.5 to 5 mg P.O. daily administered with breakfast. Patients who are more sensitive to hypoglycemic drugs should be started at 1.25 mg daily. Usual maintenance dosage is 1.25 to 20 mg daily, given either as a single dose or in divided

doses.
To replace insulin therapy—
If insulin dosage is more than 40 units daily, patient may be started on 5 mg glyburide daily in addition to 50% of the insulin dosage.

ADVERSE REACTIONS

GI: nausea, epigastric fullness, heartburn.
Hepatic: *cholestatic jaundice.*
Metabolic: *hypoglycemia.*
Skin: rash, pruritus, facial flushing.

INTERACTIONS

Anabolic steroids, chloramphenicol, clofibrate, guanethidine, MAO inhibitors, oral anticoagulants, phenylbutazone, salicylates, sulfonamides: increased hypoglycemic activity. Monitor blood glucose level.
Beta blockers, clonidine: prolonged hypoglycemic effect and masked symptoms of hypoglycemia. Use together cautiously.
Corticosteroids, glucagon, rifampin, thiazide diuretics: decreased hypoglycemic response. Monitor blood glucose level.

NURSING CONSIDERATIONS

• Contraindicated in diabetic ketoacidosis, with or without coma. Use cautiously in sulfonamide hypersensitivity and severe renal impairment.

• Elderly patients may be more sensitive to this drug's adverse effects.

• Patient transferring from insulin therapy to an oral antidiabetic requires blood glucose monitoring at least t.i.d. before meals. Patient may require hospitalization during transition.

• During periods of increased stress, such as infection, fever, surgery, or trauma, patient may require insulin therapy. Monitor patient closely for hyperglycemia in these situations.

• Instruct patient about nature of disease; importance of following therapeutic regimen, adhering to specific

---

Italicized side effects are common or life-threatening.
*Liquid form contains alcohol.　　**May contain tartrazine.

diet, weight reduction, exercise, and personal hygiene programs, and avoiding infection; how and when to perform self-monitoring of blood glucose level; recognition of hypoglycemia and hyperglycemia.

• A maintenance dosage of 5 mg glyburide provides approximately the same degree of blood glucose control as 250 to 375 mg chlorpropamide, 250 to 375 mg tolazamide, 500 to 750 mg acetohexamide, or 1,000 to 1,500 mg tolbutamide.

• Although most patients may take glyburide once daily, patients taking more than 10 mg daily may achieve better results with twice-daily dosage.

• Glyburide is a second-generation sulfonylurea oral hypoglycemic. The frequency of adverse effects appears to be lower than with first-generation drugs such as chlorpropamide and tolbutamide.

• Glyburide exerts a mild diuretic effect. May be useful in patients who have CHF or cirrhosis.

• The possibility of increased cardiovascular mortality is associated with the use of sulfonylureas.

insulins◇

regular insulin
Beef Regular Iletin II, Pork Regular Iletin II, Regular, Regular (concentrated) Iletin II, Regular Iletin I♦, Regular Iletin II♦ U-500, Velosulin♦

human insulin
Humulin R♦, Novolin R, Velosulin Human

human insulin, buffered
Humulin BR♦

prompt insulin zinc suspension
Iletin Semilente♦♦, Semilente Iletin I, Semilente Insulin, Semilente Purified Pork

isophane insulin suspension (NPH)
Beef NPH Iletin II, Insulatard NPH♦, NPH Iletin I, NPH Iletin II, Pork NPH Iletin II

isophane insulin, human, suspension
Humulin N, Insulatard NPH Human, Novolin N

isophane insulin suspension and regular insulin
Mixtard♦, Novolin 70/30

isophane insulin, human, suspension and regular human insulin injection
Mixtard Human♦, Novolin 70/30

insulin zinc suspension
Lente, Lente Iletin I, Lente Iletin II

insulin zinc, human, suspension
Humulin L, Novolin L

protamine zinc insulin (PZI) suspension
Protamine Zinc & Iletin I, Protamine Zinc & Iletin II

extended insulin zinc suspension
Ultralente, Ultralente Iletin I

Pregnancy Risk Category: B

MECHANISM OF ACTION
Increases glucose transport across muscle and fat cell membranes to reduce blood glucose level. Promotes conversion of glucose to its storage form, glycogen; triggers amino acid

uptake and conversion to protein in muscle cells and inhibits protein degradation; stimulates triglyceride formation and inhibits release of free fatty acids from adipose tissue; and stimulates lipoprotein lipase activity, which converts circulating lipoproteins to fatty acids.

INDICATIONS & DOSAGE

Diabetic ketoacidosis (use regular insulin only)—
Adults: 25 to 150 units I.V. immediately, then additional doses may be given q 1 hour based on blood sugar level until patient is out of acidosis; then give S.C. q 6 hours thereafter. Alternative dosage schedule: 50 to 100 units I.V. and 50 to 100 units S.C. stat; additional doses may be given q 2 to 6 hours based on blood sugar levels; or 0.33 units/kg I.V. bolus, followed by 7 to 10 units/hour I.V. by continuous infusion. Continue infusion until blood sugar drops to 250 mg/dl, then start S.C. insulin q 6 hours.
Children: 0.5 to 1 unit/kg in two divided doses, 1 given I.V. and the other S.C., followed by 0.5 to 1 unit/kg I.V. q 1 to 2 hours; or 0.1 unit/kg I.V. bolus, then 0.1 unit/kg hourly continuous I.V. infusion until blood sugar drops to 250 mg/dl, then start S.C. insulin. Preparation of infusion: add 100 units regular insulin and 1 g albumin to 100 ml 0.9% saline solution. Insulin concentration will be 1 unit/ml. (The albumin will adsorb to plastic, preventing loss of the insulin to plastic.)
Type I (insulin-dependent) diabetes mellitus, ketosis-prone diabetics, diabetes mellitus inadequately controlled by diet and oral hypoglycemics—
Adults and children: therapeutic regimen prescribed by doctor and adjusted according to patient's blood and urine glucose concentrations.

ADVERSE REACTIONS

Metabolic: *hypoglycemia, hyperglycemia (rebound, or Somogyi, effect).*
Skin: *urticaria.*
Local: *lipoatrophy, lipohypertrophy,* itching, swelling, redness, stinging, warmth at site of injection.
Other: *anaphylaxis.*

INTERACTIONS

Alcohol, beta blockers, clofibrate, fenfluramine, MAO inhibitors, salicylates, tetracycline: prolonged hypoglycemic effect. Monitor blood glucose level carefully.
Corticosteroids, thiazide diuretics: diminished insulin response. Monitor for hyperglycemia.

NURSING CONSIDERATIONS

• Use only regular insulin in patients with circulatory collapse, diabetic ketoacidosis, or hyperkalemia. Do not use regular insulin concentrated I.V. Do not use intermediate or long-acting insulins for coma or other emergency requiring rapid drug action.
• Accuracy of measurement is very important, especially with regular insulin concentrated. Aids, such as magnifying sleeve, dose magnifier, or cornwall syringe, may help improve accuracy.
• Dosage is always expressed in USP units.
• Don't interchange single-source beef or pork insulins; a dosage adjustment may be required.
• Lente, semilente, and ultralente insulins may be mixed in any proportion.
• Regular insulin may be mixed with NPH or lente insulins in any proportion.
• Regular insulin *should not* be mixed with globin insulin.
• Advise patient not to alter the order of mixing insulins or change the model or brand of syringe or needle.
• Note that switching from separate

injections to a prepared mixture may alter patient's response. Whenever NPH or lente is mixed with regular insulin in the same syringe, be sure to administer immediately to avoid binding.
• Store insulin in cool area. Refrigeration desirable but not essential, except with regular insulin concentrated.
• Don't use insulin that has changed color or becomes clumped or granular in appearance.
• Check expiration date on vial before using contents.
• Administration route is S.C. because absorption rate and pain are less than with I.M. injections.
• Ketosis-prone type I diabetics, severely ill, and newly diagnosed diabetics with very high blood sugar level may require hospitalization and I.V. treatment with regular fast-acting insulin.
• Ketosis-resistant diabetics may be treated as outpatients with intermediate-acting insulin and instructions on how to alter dosage according to self-performed blood glucose determinations.
• Instruct patients on proper use of equipment for performing self-monitoring of blood glucose.
• Press but do not rub site after injection. Rotate injection sites and chart to avoid overuse of one area. However, unstable diabetics may achieve better control if injection site is rotated within same anatomic region.
• To mix insulin suspension, swirl vial gently or rotate between palms or between palm and thigh. Don't shake vigorously: this causes bubbling and air in syringe.
• Insulin requirements increase, sometimes drastically, in pregnant diabetics, then decline immediately postpartum.
• Be sure the patient knows that therapy relieves symptoms but doesn't cure the disease.

• Instruct patient about nature of disease; the importance of following the therapeutic regimen, adhering to specific diet, weight reduction, exercise, and personal hygiene programs, and avoiding infection; and timing of injection and eating. Emphasize that meals must not be omitted. Teach that self-monitoring of blood glucose tests and urine ketone tests are essential guides to dosage and success of therapy; important to recognize hypoglycemic symptoms because insulin-induced hypoglycemia is hazardous and may cause brain damage if prolonged; most adverse effects are self-limiting and temporary.
• Advise patient to wear medical identification alert at all times; to carry ample insulin supply and syringes on trips; to have carbohydrates (lump of sugar or candy) on hand for emergency; to take note of time zone changes for dose schedule when traveling.
• Marijuana use may increase insulin requirements.
• Cigarette smoking decreases the amount of absorption of insulin administered subcutaneously. Advise patient not to smoke within 30 minutes after insulin injection.
• Some patients may develop insulin resistance and require large insulin doses to control symptoms of diabetes. U-500 insulin is available for such patients as Purified Pork Iletin Regular Insulin, U500. Although every pharmacy may not normally stock it, it is readily available. Patient should notify pharmacist several days before refill of prescription is needed. Nurse should give hospital pharmacy sufficient notice before needing to refill in-house prescription. Never store U-500 insulin in same area with other insulin preparations because of danger of severe overdose if given accidentally to other patients. U-500 insulin must be administered with a U-100 syringe since no syringes are

made for this drug.
• Humulin is synthesized by a strain of *Escherichia coli* that has been genetically altered. Novolin is derived from enzymatic alteration of pork insulin.

tolazamide
Tolamide, Tolinase

Pregnancy Risk Category: C

MECHANISM OF ACTION
Stimulates insulin release from the pancreatic beta cells and reduces glucose output by the liver. An extrapancreatic effect increases peripheral sensitivity to insulin. A sulfonylurea.

INDICATIONS & DOSAGE
Adjunct to diet to lower the blood glucose in patients with non-insulin-dependent diabetes mellitus (type II)—
Adults: initially, 100 mg P.O. daily with breakfast if fasting blood sugar (FBS) under 200 mg/dl; or 250 mg if FBS is over 200 mg/dl. May adjust dosage at weekly intervals by 100 to 250 mg. Maximum dosage is 500 mg b.i.d. before meals.
Adults over 65: 100 mg once daily.
To change from insulin to oral therapy—
If insulin dosage is under 20 units daily, insulin may be stopped and oral therapy started at 100 mg P.O. daily with breakfast. If insulin dosage is 20 to 40 units daily, insulin may be stopped and oral therapy started at 250 mg P.O. daily with breakfast. If insulin dosage is over 40 units daily, decrease insulin 50% and start oral therapy at 250 mg P.O. daily with breakfast. Increase dosages as above.

ADVERSE REACTIONS
GI: nausea, vomiting.
Metabolic: hypoglycemia.
Skin: rash, urticaria, facial flushing.
Other: hypersensitivity reactions.

INTERACTIONS
Anabolic steroids, chloramphenicol, clofibrate, guanethidine, MAO inhibitors, oral anticoagulants, phenylbutazone, salicylates, sulfonamides: increased hypoglycemic activity. Monitor blood glucose level.
Beta blockers, clonidine: prolonged hypoglycemic effect and masked symptoms of hypoglycemia. Use together cautiously.
Corticosteroids, glucagon, rifampin, thiazide diuretics: decreased hypoglycemic response. Monitor blood glucose level.

NURSING CONSIDERATIONS
• Contraindicated in treating type I (insulin-dependent) diabetes mellitus (IDDM); in diabetes adequately controlled by diet; and in type II diabetes complicated by fever, ketosis, acidosis, or coma, major surgery, severe trauma, Raynaud's disease, renal or hepatic impairment, or thyroid or other endocrine dysfunction. Use cautiously in sulfonamide hypersensitivity and in elderly, debilitated, or malnourished patients.
• Elderly patients may be more sensitive to this drug's adverse effects.
• Instruct patient about nature of disease; importance of following therapeutic regimen, adhering to specific diet, weight reduction, exercise, and personal hygiene programs, and avoiding infection; how and when to perform self-monitoring of blood glucose level; and recognition of hypoglycemia and hyperglycemia.
• Be sure patient knows that therapy relieves symptoms but doesn't cure disease.
• Patient transferring from another oral sulfonylurea antidiabetic drug usually needs no transition period.
• Patient transferring from insulin therapy to an oral hypoglycemic should test for blood glucose at least t.i.d. before meals. Hospitalization may be required during the transition.

Italicized side effects are common or life-threatening.
*Liquid form contains alcohol.   **May contain tartrazine.

- Advise patient to avoid moderate to large intake of alcohol; disulfiram-like reaction possible.
- The possibility of increased cardiovascular mortality is associated with the use of sulfonylureas.

---

tolbutamide
Apo-Tolbutamide, Mobenol♦♦, Novobutamide♦♦, Oramide, Orinase♦

Pregnancy Risk Category: C

MECHANISM OF ACTION
Stimulates insulin release from the pancreatic beta cells and reduces glucose output by the liver. An extrapancreatic effect increases peripheral sensitivity to insulin. A sulfonylurea.

INDICATIONS & DOSAGE
Stable, maturity-onset (Type II) nonketotic diabetes mellitus uncontrolled by diet alone and previously untreated—
Adults: initially, 1 to 2 g P.O. daily as single dose or divided b.i.d. to t.i.d. May adjust dosage to maximum of 3 g daily.
To change from insulin to oral therapy—
If insulin dosage is under 20 units daily, insulin may be stopped and oral therapy started at 1 to 2 g daily. If insulin dosage is 20 to 40 units daily, insulin is reduced 30% to 50% and oral therapy started as above. If insulin dosage is over 40 units daily, insulin is decreased 20% and oral therapy started as above. Further reductions in insulin are based on patient's response to oral therapy.

ADVERSE REACTIONS
GI: nausea, heartburn.
Metabolic: hypoglycemia, dilutional hyponatremia.
Skin: rash, pruritus, facial flushing.
Other: hypersensitivity reactions.

INTERACTIONS
Anabolic steroids, chloramphenicol, clofibrate, guanethidine, MAO inhibitors, oral anticoagulants, phenylbutazone, salicylates, sulfonamides: increased hypoglycemic activity. Monitor blood glucose level.
Beta blockers, clonidine: prolonged hypoglycemic effect and masked symptoms of hypoglycemia. Use together cautiously.
Corticosteroids, glucagon, rifampin, thiazide diuretics: decreased hypoglycemic response. Monitor blood glucose level.

NURSING CONSIDERATIONS
- Contraindicated in treating type I (insulin-dependent) diabetes mellitus (IDDM); in diabetes mellitus adequately controlled by diet; and in type II diabetes complicated by fever, ketosis, acidosis, or coma, major surgery, severe trauma, Raynaud's disease, renal or hepatic impairment, thyroid or other endocrine dysfunction, or pregnancy. Use cautiously in patients with sulfonamide hypersensitivity.
- Elderly patients may be more sensitive to this drug's adverse effects.
- Instruct patient about nature of disease; importance of following therapeutic regimen, adhering to specific diet, weight reduction, exercise, and personal hygiene program, and avoiding infection; how and when to perform self-monitoring of blood glucose level; and recognition of hypoglycemia and hyperglycemia.
- Be sure patient knows that therapy relieves symptoms but doesn't cure disease.
- Patient transferring from another oral sulfonylurea antidiabetic drug usually needs no transition period.
- Patient transferring from insulin therapy to an oral hypoglycemic should test for blood glucose at least t.i.d. before meals. Hospitalization may be required during the transition.
- Advise patient to avoid moderate to

---

large intake of alcohol: disulfiram-like reaction possible.

• The possibility of increased cardiovascular mortality is associated with the use of sulfonylureas.

59

Thyroid hormones

levothyroxine sodium (T₄ or
  L-thyroxine sodium)
liothyronine sodium (T₃)
liotrix
thyroglobulin
thyroid USP (desiccated)
thyrotropin (thyroid-stimulating
  hormone, or TSH)

COMBINATION PRODUCTS
EUTHROID-½: levothyroxine sodium
30 mcg and liothyronine sodium 7.5
mcg.
EUTHROID-1: levothyroxine sodium
60 mcg and liothyronine sodium 15
mcg.
EUTHROID-2: levothyroxine sodium
120 mcg and liothyronine sodium 30
mcg.
EUTHROID-3: levothyroxine sodium
180 mcg and liothyronine sodium
45 mcg.
THYROLAR-¼: levothyroxine sodium
12.5 mcg and liothyronine sodium
3.1 mcg.
THYROLAR-½♦: levothyroxine sodium 25 mcg and liothyronine sodium
6.25 mcg.
THYROLAR-1♦: levothyroxine sodium
50 mcg and liothyronine sodium 12.5
mcg.
THYROLAR-2♦: levothyroxine sodium
100 mcg and liothyronine sodium
25 mcg.
THYROLAR-3♦: levothyroxine sodium
150 mcg and liothyronine sodium
37.5 mcg.

levothyroxine sodium
(T₄ or L-thyroxine sodium)
Eltroxin♦♦, Levoid, Levothroid,
Levoxine, Synthroid**♦

Pregnancy Risk Category: A

MECHANISM OF ACTION
Stimulates the metabolism of all body
tissues by accelerating the rate of cellular oxidation.

INDICATIONS & DOSAGE
Cretinism in children under 1 year—
initially, 0.025 to 0.05 mg P.O. daily,
increased by 0.05 mg P.O. q 2 to 3
weeks to total daily dosage of 0.1 to
0.4 mg P.O.
Myxedema coma—
Adults: 0.2 to 0.5 mg I.V. If no response in 24 hours, additional 0.1 to
0.3 mg I.V. After condition stabilized, oral maintenance.
Thyroid hormone replacement—
Adults: initially, 0.025 to 0.1 mg
P.O. daily, increased by 0.05 to 0.1
mg P.O. q 1 to 4 weeks until desired
response. Maintenance dosage is 0.1
to 0.4 mg daily. May be administered
I.V. or I.M. when P.O. ingestion is
precluded for long periods.
Adults over 65 years: 0.025 mg P.O.
daily. May be increased by 0.025 mg
at 3- to 4-week intervals depending on
response.
Children: initially, maximum 0.05
mg P.O. daily, gradually increased by
0.025 to 0.05 mg P.O. q 1 to 4 weeks
until desired response.

Unmarked trade names available in the United States only.
♦ Also available in Canada.　　　♦♦ Available in Canada only.　　　◊ Also available OTC.

ADVERSE REACTIONS

Adverse reactions of thyroid hormones are extensions of their pharmacologic properties and reflect patient sensitivity to them.

Signs of overdosage:

CNS: *nervousness, insomnia, tremor.*
CV: *tachycardia, palpitations, dysrhythmias, angina pectoris,* hypertension.
GI: change in appetite, nausea, diarrhea.
Other: headache, leg cramps, weight loss, sweating, heat intolerance, fever, menstrual irregularities.

INTERACTIONS

Cholestyramine and colestipol: levothyroxine absorption impaired. Separate doses by 4 to 5 hours.
I.V. phenytoin: free thyroid released. Monitor for tachycardia.

NURSING CONSIDERATIONS

• Contraindicated in myocardial infarction, thyrotoxicosis (except with antithyroid drugs), or uncorrected adrenal insufficiency (thyroid hormones increase tissue demand for adrenocortical hormone and may cause acute adrenal crisis). Use with extreme caution in angina pectoris, hypertension, or other cardiovascular disorders; renal insufficiency; and ischemic states.
• Thyroid hormone replacement requirements are about 25% lower in patients over 60 years than in young adults.
• Use carefully in myxedema; patients are unusually sensitive to thyroid hormone. Dose varies widely among patients; start at lowest and titrate in higher doses according to patient's symptoms and laboratory data until euthyroid state is reached.
• Rapid replacement in patients with arteriosclerosis may precipitate angina, coronary occlusion, or stroke. Use cautiously in these patients.
• In patients with coronary artery disease who must receive thyroid, observe carefully for possible coronary insufficiency if catecholamines must be given.
• Potentially dangerous; not indicated to relieve such vague symptoms as physical and mental sluggishness, irritability, depression, nervousness, and ill-defined pains; to treat obesity in euthyroid persons; to treat metabolic insufficiency not associated with thyroid insufficiency; or to treat menstrual disorders or male infertility, unless associated with hypothyroidism.
• When changing from levothyroxine to liothyronine, stop levothyroxine and begin liothyronine. Increase in small increments after residual effects of levothyroxine have disappeared. When changing from liothyronine to levothyroxine, start levothyroxine several days before withdrawing liothyronine to avoid relapse.
• Different brands of levothyroxine may not be bioequivalent. Once the patient has been stabilized on one brand, warn him not to switch to another. Also advise him to avoid "generic" levothyroxine.
• Warn patient (especially elderly patients) to tell doctor at once if chest pain, palpitations, sweating, nervousness, or other signs of overdosage occur. Also notify doctor immediately if any signs of aggravated cardiovascular disease develop (chest pain, dyspnea, and tachycardia).
• Tell patient to take thyroid hormones at the same time each day to maintain constant hormone levels.
• Suggest morning dosage to prevent insomnia.
• Monitor pulse rate and blood pressure.
• Prepare I.V. dosage immediately before injection.
• Thyroid hormones alter thyroid function test results. Monitor prothrombin time; patients taking these hormones usually require less antico-

---

Italicized side effects are common or life-threatening.
*Liquid form contains alcohol.   **May contain tartrazine.

agulant. Alert patients to report unusual bleeding and bruising.
• Patients taking levothyroxine who need to have radioactive iodine uptake studies must discontinue drug 4 weeks before test.

liothyronine sodium (T₃)
Cytomel♦
Pregnancy Risk Category: A

MECHANISM OF ACTION
Stimulates the metabolism of all body tissues by accelerating the rate of cellular oxidation.

INDICATIONS & DOSAGE
Cretinism—
Children 3 years and older: 50 to 100 mcg P.O. daily.
Children under 3 years: 5 mcg P.O. daily, increased by 5 mcg q 3 to 4 days until desired response occurs.
Myxedema—
Adults: initially, 5 mcg daily, increased by 5 to 10 mcg q 1 or 2 weeks. Maintenance dosage is 50 to 100 mcg daily.
Nontoxic goiter—
Adults: initially, 5 mcg P.O. daily; may be increased by 12.5 to 25 mcg daily q 1 to 2 weeks. Usual maintenance dosage is 75 mcg daily.
Adults over 65 years: initially, 5 mcg P.O. daily, increased by 5-mcg increments at weekly intervals until desired response.
Children: initially, 5 mcg P.O. daily, increased by 5-mcg increments at weekly intervals until desired response.
Thyroid hormone replacement—
Adults: initially, 25 mcg P.O. daily, increased by 12.5 to 25 mcg q 1 to 2 weeks until satisfactory response. Usual maintenance dosage is 25 to 75 mcg daily.
T₃ suppression test to differentiate hyperthyroidism from euthyroidism—

Adults: 75 to 100 mcg daily for 7 days.

ADVERSE REACTIONS
Adverse reactions of thyroid hormones are extensions of their pharmacologic properties and reflect patient sensitivity to them.
CNS: hyperirritability, *nervousness, insomnia,* twitching, *tremors,* headache.
CV: increased cardiac output, *tachycardia,* cardiac dysrhythmias, *angina pectoris,* increased blood pressure, *cardiac decompensation and collapse.*
GI: diarrhea, abdominal cramps, vomiting.
Other: weight loss, heat intolerance, hyperhidrosis, menstrual irregularities; in infants and children—accelerated rate of bone maturation.

INTERACTIONS
Cholestyramine and colestipol: liothyronine absorption impaired. Separate doses by 4 to 5 hours.
I.V. phenytoin: free thyroid released. Monitor for tachycardia.

NURSING CONSIDERATIONS
• Contraindicated in myocardial infarction, thyrotoxicosis (except with antithyroid drugs), or uncorrected adrenal insufficiency (thyroid hormones increase tissue demand for adrenocortical hormone and may cause acute adrenal crisis). Use with extreme caution in angina pectoris, hypertension, or other cardiovascular disorders; renal insufficiency; and ischemic states.
• Thyroid hormone replacement requirements are about 25% lower in patients over 60 years than in young adults.
• Rapid replacement in patients with arteriosclerosis may precipitate angina, coronary occlusion, or stroke. Use cautiously in these patients.
• In patients with coronary artery disease who must receive thyroid hor-

mones, observe carefully for possible coronary insufficiency if catecholamines must be given.
- Use carefully in myxedema; these patients are unusually sensitive to thyroid hormone.
- Potentially dangerous; not indicated to relieve vague symptoms, such as physical and mental sluggishness, irritability, depression, nervousness, and ill-defined aches and pains; to treat obesity in euthyroid persons; to treat metabolic insufficiency; or to treat menstrual disorders or male infertility, unless asssociated with hypothyroidism.
- When changing from levothyroxine to liothyronine, stop levothyroxine and begin liothyronine. Increase in small increments after residual effects of levothyroxine have disappeared. When changing from liothyronine to levothyroxine, start levothyroxine several days before withdrawing liothyronine to avoid relapse.
- Warn patient (especially elderly patients) to tell doctor at once if chest pain, palpitations, sweating, nervousness, or other signs of overdosage occur. Also notify doctor immediately if any signs of aggravated cardiovascular disease develop (chest pain, dyspnea, and tachycardia).
- Tell patient to take thyroid hormones at the same time each day, to maintain constant hormone levels.
- Suggest morning dosage to prevent insomnia.
- Monitor pulse rate and blood pressure.
- Thyroid hormones alter thyroid function tests. Monitor prothrombin time; patients taking these hormones usually require less anticoagulant. Alert patients to report unusual bleeding and bruising.
- Patients taking liothyronine who need to have radioactive iodine uptake studies must discontinue drug 7 to 10 days before test.

liotrix
Euthroid**◆, Thyrolar◆
Pregnancy Risk Category: A

MECHANISM OF ACTION
Stimulates the metabolism of all body tissues by accelerating the rate of cellular oxidation.

INDICATIONS & DOSAGE
Hypothyroidism—dosages are expressed in thyroid equivalents and must be individualized to approximate the deficit in the patient's thyroid secretion.
Adults and children: initially, 15 to 30 mg P.O. daily, increasing by 15 to 30 mg q 1 to 2 weeks to desired response; increments in children's dosage q 2 weeks.
Adults over 65 years: initially, 15 to 30 mg. Usual adult dosage doubled q 6 to 8 weeks to desired response.

ADVERSE REACTIONS
Adverse reactions of thyroid hormones are extensions of their pharmacologic properties and reflect patient sensitivity to them.
CNS: hyperirritability, *nervousness, insomnia,* twitching, *tremors.*
CV: increased cardiac output, *tachycardia,* cardiac dysrhythmias, *angina pectoris,* increased blood pressure, *cardiac decompensation and collapse.*
GI: diarrhea, abdominal cramps, vomiting.
Other: weight loss, menstrual irregularities, heat intolerance, hyperhidrosis; infants and children—accelerated rate of bone maturation.

INTERACTIONS
Cholestyramine and colestipol: liotrix absorption impaired. Separate doses by 4 to 5 hours.
I.V. phenytoin: free thyroid released. Monitor for tachycardia.

Italicized side effects are common or life-threatening.
*Liquid form contains alcohol.   **May contain tartrazine.

NURSING CONSIDERATIONS

• Contraindicated in myocardial infarction, thyrotoxicosis (except with antithyroid drugs), or uncorrected adrenal insufficiency (thyroid hormones increase tissue demand for adrenocortical hormone and may cause acute adrenal crisis). Use with extreme caution in angina pectoris, hypertension, or other cardiovascular disorders; renal insufficiency; and ischemic states.

• Thyroid hormone replacement requirements are about 25% lower in patients over 60 years than in young adults.

• Rapid replacement in arteriosclerosis may precipitate angina, coronary occlusion, or stroke. Use cautiously in these patients.

• Use carefully in myxedema; these patients are unusually sensitive to thyroid hormone.

• In patients with coronary artery disease who must receive thyroid hormones, observe carefully for possible coronary insufficiency if catecholamines must be given. Also observe carefully during surgery, since cardiac dysrhythmias can be precipitated.

• Potentially dangerous; not indicated to relieve vague symptoms, such as physical and mental sluggishness, irritability, depression, nervousness, and ill-defined pains; to treat obesity in euthyroid persons; to treat metabolic insufficiency not associated with thyroid insufficiency; or to treat menstrual disorders for male infertility, unless associated with hypothyroidism.

• Tell patient to take thyroid hormones at the same time each day, preferably before breakfast, to maintain constant hormone levels.

• Warn patient (especially elderly patients) to tell doctor at once if chest pain, palpitations, sweating, nervousness, or other signs of overdosage occur. Also notify doctor immediately if any signs of aggravated cardiovascular disease develop (chest pain, dyspnea, and tachycardia).

• The two commercially prepared liotrix drugs contain different amounts of each ingredient; do not change from one brand to the other without considering the differences in potency: Thyrolar-½ contains 25 mcg T_4 and 6.25 mcg T_3; Euthroid-½ contains 30 mcg T_4 and 7.5 mcg T_3.

• Monitor pulse rate and blood pressure.

• Thyroid hormones alter thyroid function test results. Monitor prothrombin time; patients taking these hormones usually require less anticoagulant. Alert patients to report unusual bleeding and bruising.

thyroglobulin
Proloid♦

Pregnancy Risk Category: A

MECHANISM OF ACTION
Stimulates the metabolism of all body tissues by accelerating the rate of cellular oxidation.

INDICATIONS & DOSAGE
Cretinism and juvenile hypothyroidism—
Children 1 year and older: dosage may approach adult dosage (60 to 180 mg P.O. daily), depending on response.
Children 4 to 12 months: 60 to 80 mg P.O. daily.
Children 1 to 4 months: initially, 15 to 30 mg P.O. daily, increased at 2-week intervals. Usual maintenance dosage is 30 to 45 mg P.O. daily.
Hypothyroidism or myxedema—
Adults: initially, 15 to 30 mg P.O. daily, increased by 15 to 30 mg at 2-week intervals until desired response. Usual maintenance dosage is 60 to 180 mg P.O. daily, as a single dose.
Adults over 65 years: initially, 7.5 to 15 mg P.O. daily; dosage is doubled at

6- to 8-week intervals until desired response is obtained.

ADVERSE REACTIONS
Adverse reactions of thyroid hormones are extensions of their pharmacologic properties and reflect patient sensitivity to them.
CNS: hyperirritability, *nervousness, insomnia,* twitching, *tremors,* headache.
CV: increased cardiac output, *tachycardia,* cardiac dysrhythmias, *angina pectoris,* increased blood pressure, *cardiac decompensation and collapse.*
GI: diarrhea, abdominal cramps, vomiting.
Other: weight loss, heat intolerance, hyperhidrosis, menstrual irregularities; in infants and children—accelerated rate of bone maturation.

INTERACTIONS
Cholestyramine and colestipol: thyroglobulin absorption impaired. Separate doses by 4 to 5 hours.
I.V. phenytoin: free thyroid released. Monitor for tachycardia.

NURSING CONSIDERATIONS
• Contraindicated in myocardial infarction, thyrotoxicosis (except with antithyroid drugs), or uncorrected adrenal insufficiency (thyroid hormones increase tissue demand for adrenocortical hormone and may cause acute adrenal crisis). Use with extreme caution in angina pectoris, hypertension, or other cardiovascular disorders; renal insufficiency; and ischemic states.
• Thyroid hormone replacement requirements are about 25% lower in patients over 60 years than in young adults.
• In patients with coronary artery disease who must receive thyroid hormones, observe carefully for possible coronary insufficiency if catecholamines must be given.
• Use carefully in myxedema; these

patients are unusually sensitive to thyroid hormone.
• Potentially dangerous; not indicated to relieve vague symptoms, such as physical and mental sluggishness, irritability, depression, nervousness, and ill-defined pains; to treat obesity in euthyroid persons; to treat metabolic insufficiency not associated with thyroid insufficiency; or to treat menstrual disorders or male infertility, unless associated with hypothyroidism.
• Tell patient to take thyroid hormones at the same time each day, to maintain constant hormone levels.
• Warn patient (especially elderly patients) to tell doctor at once if chest pain, palpitations, sweating, nervousness, or other signs of overdosage occur. Also notify doctor immediately if any signs of aggravated cardiovascular disease develop (chest pain, dyspnea, and tachycardia).
• Suggest morning dosage to prevent insomnia.
• Monitor pulse rate and blood pressure.
• Thyroid hormones alter thyroid function test results. Monitor prothrombin time; patients taking these hormones usually require less anticoagulant. Alert patients to report unusual bleeding and bruising.

---

thyroid USP (desiccated)
Pregnancy Risk Category: A

MECHANISM OF ACTION
Stimulates the metabolism of all body tissues by accelerating the rate of cellular oxidation.

INDICATIONS & DOSAGE
Adult hypothyroidism—
Adults: initially, 60 mg P.O. daily, increased by 60 mg q 30 days until desired response. Usual maintenance dosage is 60 to 180 mg P.O. daily, as a

---

Italicized side effects are common or life-threatening.
*Liquid form contains alcohol.   **May contain tartrazine.

single dose.
Adults over 65 years: 7.5 to 15 mg
P.O. daily; dosage is doubled at 6- to
8-week intervals.
Adult myxedema—
Adults: 16 mg P.O. daily. May double
dosage q 2 weeks to maximum 120
mg.
*Cretinism and juvenile hypothyroid-
ism—*
Children 1 year and older: dosage
may approach adult dosage (60 to 180
mg) daily, depending on response.
Children 4 to 12 months: 30 to 60
mg P.O. daily.
Children 1 to 4 months: initially, 15
to 30 mg P.O. daily, increased at 2-
week intervals. Usual maintenance
dosage is 30 to 45 mg P.O. daily.

ADVERSE REACTIONS
Adverse reactions of thyroid hormones are extensions of their pharmacologic properties and reflect patient
sensitivity to them.
CNS: *hyperirritability, nervousness,
insomnia,* twitching, tremors, headache.
CV: increased cardiac output, *tachycardia,* cardiac dysrhythmias, *angina
pectoris,* increased blood pressure,
cardiac decompensation and collapse.
GI: diarrhea, abdominal cramps,
vomiting.
Other: weight loss, heat intolerance,
hyperhidrosis, menstrual irregularities; in infants and children—accelerated rate of bone maturation.

INTERACTIONS
Cholestyramine: thyroid absorption
impaired. Separate doses by 4 to 5
hours.
I.V. phenytoin: free thyroid released.
Monitor for tachycardia.

NURSING CONSIDERATIONS
• Contraindicated in myocardial infarction, thyrotoxicosis (except with
antithyroid drugs), or uncorrected adrenal insufficiency (thyroid hormones

increase tissue demand for adrenocortical hormone and may cause acute
adrenal crisis). Use with extreme caution in angina pectoris, hypertension,
or other cardiovascular disorders;
renal insufficiency; and ischemic
states.
• Thyroid hormone replacement requirements are about 25% lower in
patients over 60 years than in young
adults.
• Use carefully in myxedema; these
patients are unusually sensitive to thyroid hormone.
• In patients with coronary artery
disease who must receive thyroid hormones, observe carefully for possible
coronary insufficiency if catecholamines must be given.
• Potentially dangerous; not indicated
to relieve vague symptoms, such as
physical and mental sluggishness, irritability, depression, nervousness,
and ill-defined pains; to treat obesity
in euthyroid persons; to treat metabolic insufficiency not associated with
thyroid insufficiency; or to treat menstrual disorders or male infertility,
unless associated with hypothyroidism.
• Tell patient to take thyroid hormones at the same time each day to
maintain constant hormone levels.
• Warn patient (especially elderly patients) to tell doctor at once if chest
pain, palpitations, sweating, nervousness, or other signs of overdosage occur. Also notify doctor immediately if
any signs of aggravated cardiovascular disease develop (chest pain, dyspnea, and tachycardia).
• Suggest morning dosage to prevent
insomnia.
• Monitor pulse rate and blood pressure.
• In children, sleeping pulse rate and
basal morning temperature are guides
to treatment.
• Thyroid hormones alter thyroid
function test results. Monitor prothrombin time; patients taking these

hormones usually require less anticoagulant. Alert patients to report unusual bleeding and bruising.

thyrotropin
(thyroid-stimulating hormone, or TSH)
Thytropar♦

Pregnancy Risk Category: C

MECHANISM OF ACTION
Stimulates the uptake of radioactive iodine in patients with thyroid carcinoma. Also promotes thyroid hormone production by the anterior pituitary.

INDICATIONS & DOSAGE
Diagnosis of thyroid cancer remnant with ¹³¹I after surgery—
10 international units I.M. or S.C. for 3 to 7 days.
Differential diagnosis of primary and secondary hypothyroidism—
10 units I.M. or S.C. for 1 to 3 days.
In PBI or ¹³¹I uptake determinations for differential diagnosis of subclinical hypothyroidism or low thyroid reserve—
10 units I.M. or S.C.
Therapy for thyroid carcinoma (local or metastatic) with ¹³¹I—
10 units I.M. or S.C. for 3 to 8 days.
To determine thyroid status of patient receiving thyroid—
10 units I.M. or S.C. for 1 to 3 days.

ADVERSE REACTIONS
CNS: headache.
CV: *tachycardia,* atrial fibrillation, *angina pectoris, CHF,* hypotension.
GI: nausea, vomiting.
Other: thyroid hyperplasia (large doses), fever, menstrual irregularities, allergic reactions (postinjection flare, urticaria, *anaphylaxis*).

INTERACTIONS
None significant.

NURSING CONSIDERATIONS
• Contraindicated in coronary thrombosis and untreated Addison's disease. Use cautiously in angina pectoris, CHF, hypopituitarism, and adrenocortical suppression.
• May cause thyroid hyperplasia.
• Diagnostic use: to identify subclinical hypothyroidism or low thyroid reserve, to evaluate need for thyroid therapy, to distinguish between primary and secondary hypothyroidism, and to detect thyroid remnants and metastases of thyroid carcinoma.
• Therapeutic use: management of certain types of thyroid carcinoma and resulting metastases, and in conjunction with radioactive ¹³¹I to enhance uptake of ¹³¹I by the thyroid.
• Three-day dosage schedule may be used in long-standing pituitary myxedema or with prolonged use of thyroid medication.

Italicized side effects are common or life-threatening.
*Liquid form contains alcohol.   **May contain tartrazine.

Thyroid hormone antagonists

methimazole
potassium iodide
propylthiouracil (PTU)
radioactive iodine (sodium
    iodide) ¹³¹I

COMBINATION PRODUCTS
None.

---

methimazole
Tapazole♦

Pregnancy Risk Category: D

MECHANISM OF ACTION
Inhibits oxidation of iodine in the thyroid gland, blocking iodine's ability to combine with tyrosine to form thyroxine. May also prevent the coupling of monoiodotyrosine and diiodotyrosine to form thyroxine and triiodothyronine.

INDICATIONS & DOSAGE
Hyperthyroidism—
Adults: 5 mg P.O. t.i.d. if mild; 10 to 15 mg P.O. t.i.d. if moderately severe; and 20 mg P.O. t.i.d. if severe. Continue until patient is euthyroid, then start maintenance dosage of 5 mg daily to t.i.d. Maximum dosage 150 mg daily.
Children: 0.4 mg/kg daily divided q 8 hours. Continue until patient is euthyroid, then start maintenance dosage of 0.2 mg/kg daily divided q 8 hours.
Preparation for thyroidectomy—
Adults and children: same doses as for hyperthyroidism until patient is euthyroid; then iodine may be added for 10 days before surgery.
Thyrotoxic crisis—
Adults and children: same doses as for hyperthyroidism, with concomitant iodine therapy and propranolol.

ADVERSE REACTIONS
Blood: *agranulocytosis,* leukopenia, granulopenia, thrombocytopenia (appear to be dose-related).
CNS: headache, drowsiness, vertigo.
GI: diarrhea, nausea, vomiting (may be dose-related).
Hepatic: jaundice.
Skin: rash, urticaria, skin discoloration.
Other: arthralgia, myalgia, salivary gland enlargement, loss of taste, drug fever, lymphadenopathy.

INTERACTIONS
None significant.

NURSING CONSIDERATIONS
• Use cautiously in pregnancy. Pregnant women may require less drug as pregnancy progresses. Monitor thyroid function studies closely. Thyroid may be added to regimen. Drugs may be stopped during last few weeks of pregnancy.
• Watch for signs of hypothyroidism (mental depression; cold intolerance; hard, nonpitting edema). Dosage may need to be adjusted.
• Monitor CBC periodically to detect impending leukopenia, thrombocytopenia, and agranulocytosis.
• Doses of over 30 mg/day increase the risk of agranulocytosis.
• Warn patient to report immediately:

fever, sore throat, or mouth sores (possible signs of developing agranulocytosis). Agranulocytosis can develop too rapidly to be detected by periodic blood cell counts. Tell patient also to immediately report skin eruptions (sign of hypersensitivity).
• Drug should be stopped if severe rash or enlarged cervical lymph nodes develop.
• Tell patient to ask doctor about using iodized salt and eating shellfish during treatment.
• Warn patient against over-the-counter cough medicines; many contain iodine.
• Give with meals to reduce GI side effects.
• Store in light-resistant container.

---

potassium iodide
Iostat, Thyro-Block♦
Potassium Iodide Solution, USP
Strong Iodine Solution, USP
(Lugol's Solution)

Pregnancy Risk Category: D

MECHANISM OF ACTION
Inhibits thyroid hormone formation by blocking iodotyrosine and iodothyronine synthesis. It also limits iodide transport into the thyroid gland and blocks thyroid hormone release.

INDICATIONS & DOSAGE
Preparation for thyroidectomy—
Adults and children: Strong Iodine Solution, USP, 0.1 to 0.3 ml t.i.d., or Potassium Iodide Solution, USP, 5 drops in water t.i.d. after meals for 2 to 3 weeks before surgery.
Thyrotoxic crisis—
Adults and children: Strong Iodine Solution, USP, 1 ml in water P.O. t.i.d. after meals.

ADVERSE REACTIONS
EENT: acute rhinitis, inflammation of salivary glands, periorbital edema, conjunctivitis, hyperemia.

GI: burning, irritation, *nausea,* vomiting, *metallic taste.*
Skin: acneiform rash, mucous membrane ulceration.
Other: fever, frontal headache, tooth discoloration, *hypersensitivity, including symptoms resembling serum sickness.*

INTERACTIONS
Lithium carbonate: hypothyroidism may occur. Use with caution.

NURSING CONSIDERATIONS
• Contraindicated in tuberculosis, iodide hypersensitivity, hyperkalemia; after meals that contain excessive starch; in laryngeal edema, swelling of salivary glands.
• Earliest signs of delayed hypersensitivity caused by iodides are irritation and swelling of the eyelids.
• Dilute oral doses in water, milk, or fruit juice, and give after meals to prevent gastric irritation, to hydrate the patient, and to mask the very salty taste.
• Tell patient to ask the doctor about using iodized salt and eating shellfish during treatment. Iodine-rich foods may not be permitted.
• Warn the patient that sudden withdrawal may precipitate thyroid storm.
• Store in light-resistant container.
• Give iodides through straw to avoid tooth discoloration.
• Usually given with other antithyroid drugs.

---

propylthiouracil (PTU)
Propyl-Thyracil♦♦

Pregnancy Risk Category: D

MECHANISM OF ACTION
Inhibits oxidation of iodine in the thyroid gland, blocking iodine's ability to combine with tyrosine to form thyroxine. May also prevent the coupling of monoiodotyrosine and diiodotyrosine to form thyroxine and triiodothyro-

---

Italicized side effects are common or life-threatening.
*Liquid form contains alcohol.   **May contain tartrazine.

nine.

INDICATIONS & DOSAGE
Hyperthyroidism—
Adults: 100 mg P.O. t.i.d.; up to 300 mg q 8 hours have been used in severe cases. Continue until patient is euthyroid, then start maintenance dosage of 100 mg daily to t.i.d.
Children over 10 years: 100 mg P.O. t.i.d. Continue until patient is euthyroid, then start maintenance dosage of 25 mg t.i.d. to 100 mg b.i.d.
Children 6 to 10 years: 50 to 150 mg P.O. divided doses q 8 hours.
Preparation for thyroidectomy—
Adults and children: same doses as for hyperthyroidism, then iodine may be added 10 days before surgery.
Thyrotoxic crisis—
Adults and children: same doses as for hyperthyroidism, with concomitant iodine therapy and propranolol.

ADVERSE REACTIONS
Blood: *agranulocytosis,* leukopenia, thrombocytopenia (appear to be dose-related).
CNS: headache, drowsiness, vertigo.
EENT: visual disturbances.
GI: diarrhea, *nausea, vomiting* (may be dose-related).
Hepatic: jaundice, *hepatotoxicity.*
Skin: rash, urticaria, skin discoloration, pruritus.
Other: arthralgia, myalgia, salivary gland enlargement, loss of taste, drug fever, lymphadenopathy, vasculitis.

INTERACTIONS
None significant.

NURSING CONSIDERATIONS
• Use cautiously in pregnancy. Pregnant women may require less drug as pregnancy progresses. Monitor thyroid function studies closely. Thyroid may be added to regimen. Drugs may be stopped during last few weeks of pregnancy.
• Watch for signs of hypothyroidism (mental depression; cold intolerance; hard, nonpitting edema). Dosage may need to be adjusted.
• Monitor CBC periodically to detect impending leukopenia, thrombocytopenia, and agranulocytosis.
• Warn patient to report immediately: fever, sore throat, or mouth sores (possible signs of developing agranulocytosis). Agranulocytosis can develop too rapidly to be detected by periodic blood cell counts. Tell patient to also report skin eruptions (sign of hypersensitivity) immediately.
• Drug should be stopped if severe rash or enlarged cervical lymph nodes develop.
• Tell patient to ask doctor about using iodized salt and eating shellfish during treatment.
• Warn patient against over-the-counter cough medicines; many contain iodine.
• Give with meals to reduce GI side effects.
• Store in light-resistant container.

radioactive iodine (sodium iodide) ¹³¹I
Iodotope Therapeutic
Pregnancy Risk Category: X

MECHANISM OF ACTION
Limits thyroid hormone secretion by destroying thyroid tissue. The affinity of thyroid tissue for radioactive iodine facilitates uptake of the drug by cancerous thyroid tissue that has metastasized to other sites in the body.

INDICATIONS & DOSAGE
Hyperthyroidism—
Adults: usual dosage is 4 to 10 millicuries P.O. Dosage based on estimated weight of thyroid gland and thyroid uptake. Treatment may be repeated after 6 weeks, according to serum thyroxine.
Thyroid cancer—
Adults: 50 to 150 millicuries P.O.

Dosage based on estimated malignant thyroid tissue and metastatic tissue as determined by total body scan. Treatment may be repeated according to clinical status.

ADVERSE REACTIONS
EENT: *feeling of fullness in neck,* metallic taste, "radiation mumps."
Endocrine: hypothyroidism, radiation thyroiditis.
GU: possible increased risk of birth defects in offspring after sufficient ^{131}I dose for thyroid ablation following cancer surgery.
Other: possible increased risk of developing leukemia later in life after sufficient ^{131}I dose for thyroid ablation following cancer surgery.

INTERACTIONS
Lithium carbonate: hypothyroidism may occur. Use with caution.

NURSING CONSIDERATIONS
• Contraindicated in pregnancy and lactation unless used to treat thyroid cancer.
• Stop all antithyroid medications, thyroid preparations, and iodine-containing preparations 1 week before ^{131}I dose. If medications are not stopped, patient may receive thyroid-stimulating hormone for 3 days before ^{131}I dose. When treating women of childbearing age, give dose during menstruation or within 7 days after menstruation.
• Food may delay absorption. Patient should fast overnight before administration.
• After therapy for hyperthyroidism, patient should not resume antithyroid drugs, but should continue propranolol or other drugs used to treat symptoms of hyperthyroidism until onset of full ^{131}I effect (usually 6 weeks).
• Monitor thyroid function with serum thyroxine.
• After dose for hyperthyroidism, patient's urine and saliva are slightly radioactive for 24 hours; vomitus is highly radioactive for 6 to 8 hours. Institute full radiation precautions during this time. Instruct patient to use appropriate disposal methods when coughing and expectorating.
• After dose for thyroid cancer, patient's urine, saliva, and perspiration remain radioactive for 3 days. Isolate patient and observe the following precautions: pregnant personnel should not take care of patient; disposable eating utensils and linens should be used; instruct patient to save all urine in lead containers for 24 to 48 hours so amount of radioactive material excreted can be determined. Patient should drink as much fluid as possible for 48 hours after drug administration to facilitate excretion. Limit contact with patient to 30 minutes per shift per person the first day. May increase time to 1 hour second day and longer on third day.
• If patient is discharged less than 7 days after ^{131}I dose for thyroid cancer, warn him to avoid close, prolonged contact with small children (for example, holding children on lap), and instruct him not to sleep in same room with spouse for 7 days after treatment because of increased risk of thyroid cancer in persons exposed to [131]I. Tell patient he may use same bathroom facilities as rest of family.

61

Pituitary hormones

corticotropin (ACTH)
cosyntropin
desmopressin acetate
lypressin
somatrem
vasopressin (antidiuretic
   hormone)
vasopressin tannate

COMBINATION PRODUCTS
None.

---

corticotropin (ACTH)
Acthar♦

Pregnancy Risk Category: C

MECHANISM OF ACTION
By replacing the body's own tropic
hormone, stimulates the adrenal cortex to secrete its entire spectrum of
hormones.

INDICATIONS & DOSAGE
*Diagnostic test of adrenocortical func-
tion—*
Adults: up to 80 units I.M. or S.C. in
divided doses; or a single dose of repository form; or 10 to 25 units
(aqueous form) in 500 ml dextrose 5%
in water I.V. over 8 hours, between
blood samplings.

   Individual dosages generally vary
with adrenal glands' sensitivity to
stimulation as well as with specific
disease. Infants and younger children
require larger doses per kilogram than
do older children and adults.
For therapeutic use—
Adults: 40 units S.C. or I.M. in 4 divided doses (aqueous); 40 units q 12

to 24 hours (gel or repository form).

ADVERSE REACTIONS
CNS: *seizures, dizziness,* papilledema, headache, *euphoria, insomnia,* mood swings, personality
changes, depression, psychosis.
EENT: cataracts, glaucoma.
GI: peptic ulcer with perforation and
hemorrhage, pancreatitis, abdominal
distention, ulcerative esophagitis,
nausea, vomiting.
GU: menstrual irregularities.
Metabolic: *sodium and fluid retention,* calcium and potassium loss, hypokalemic alkalosis, negative nitrogen balance.
Skin: *impaired wound healing,* thin
fragile skin, petechiae, ecchymoses,
facial erythema, increased sweating,
acne, hyperpigmentation, allergic
skin reactions, hirsutism.
Other: muscle weakness, steroid my-
opathy, loss of muscle mass, osteoporosis, vertebral compression fractures, cushingoid state, suppression of
growth in children, *activation of latent diabetes mellitus,* progressive increase in antibodies, loss of ACTH
stimulatory effect, and *hypersensitivity.*

INTERACTIONS
None significant.

NURSING CONSIDERATIONS
• Contraindicated in scleroderma, osteoporosis, systemic fungal infections, ocular herpes simplex, recent
surgery, peptic ulcer, congestive heart
failure, hypertension, sensitivity to

---

pork and pork products, concomitant smallpox vaccination, adrenocortical hyperfunction or primary insufficiency, or Cushing's syndrome. Use with caution in pregnant women or breast-feeding mothers and in women of childbearing age; patients being immunized; latent tuberculosis or tuberculin reactivity; hypothyroidism; cirrhosis; infection (use anti-infective therapy during and after ACTH treatment); acute gouty arthritis (limit ACTH treatment to a few days, and use conventional therapy during and for several days after ACTH treatment); emotional instability or psychotic tendencies; diabetes; abscess; pyogenic infections; renal insufficiency; myasthenia gravis.
• ACTH treatment should be preceded by verification of adrenal responsiveness and test for hypersensitivity and allergic reactions.
• ACTH should be adjunctive; not sole therapy. Oral agents are preferred for long-term therapy.
• Unusual stress may require additional use of rapidly acting corticosteroids. When possible, gradually reduce ACTH dosage to smallest effective dose to minimize induced adrenocortical insufficiency. Reinstitute therapy if stressful situation (trauma, surgery, severe illness) occurs shortly after stopping drug.
• Watch neonates of ACTH-treated mothers for signs of hypoadrenalism.
• Counteract edema by low-sodium, high-potassium intake; nitrogen loss by high-protein diet; and psychotic changes by reducing ACTH dosage or administering sedatives.
• ACTH may mask signs of chronic disease and decrease host resistance and ability to localize infection.
• Note and record weight changes, fluid exchange, and resting blood pressures until minimal effective dose is achieved.
• Refrigerate reconstituted solution and use within 24 hours.

• If administering gel, warm it to room temperature, draw into large needle, and give slowly deep I.M. with 21G or 22G needle. Warn patient that injection is painful.

cosyntropin
Cortrosyn♦

Pregnancy Risk Category: C

MECHANISM OF ACTION
By replacing the body's own tropic hormone, stimulates the adrenal cortex to secrete its entire spectrum of hormones.

INDICATIONS & DOSAGE
Diagnostic test of adrenocortical function—
Adults and children: 0.25 to 1 mg I.M. or I.V. (unless label prohibits I.V. administration) between blood samplings.
Children under 2 years: 0.125 mg I.M. or I.V.

ADVERSE REACTIONS
Skin: pruritus.
Other: flushing, hypersensitivity.

INTERACTIONS
None significant.

NURSING CONSIDERATIONS
• Use cautiously in patients with hypersensitivity to natural corticotropin.
• Drug is synthetic duplication of the biologically active part of the ACTH molecule. It is less likely to produce sensitivity than natural ACTH from animal sources.

desmopressin acetate
DDAVP♦, Stimate

Pregnancy Risk Category: B

MECHANISM OF ACTION
Increases the permeability of the

renal tubular epithelium to adenosine monophosphate and water; the epithelium promotes reabsorption of water and produces a concentrated urine (antidiuretic hormone effect). Desmopressin also increases Factor VIII activity by releasing endogenous Factor VIII from plasma storage sites.

INDICATIONS & DOSAGE
Nonnephrogenic diabetes insipidus, temporary polyuria and polydipsia associated with pituitary trauma—
Adults: 0.1 to 0.4 ml intranasally daily in 1 to 3 doses. Adjust morning and evening doses separately for adequate diurnal rhythm of water turnover. Alternatively, may administer injectable form in dosage of 0.5 to 1 ml I.V. or S.C. daily, usually in two divided doses.
Children 3 months to 12 years: 0.05 to 0.3 ml intranasally daily in 1 or 2 doses.
Treatment of hemophilia A and von Willebrand's disease—
Adults and children: 0.3 mcg/kg diluted in normal saline and infused I.V. slowly over 15 to 30 minutes. May repeat dose if necessary as indicated by laboratory response and the patient's clinical condition.

ADVERSE REACTIONS
CNS: headache.
CV: slight rise in blood pressure at high dosage.
EENT: nasal congestion, rhinitis.
GI: nausea.
GU: vulval pain.
Other: flushing.

INTERACTIONS
None significant.

NURSING CONSIDERATIONS
• Use with caution in coronary artery insufficiency or hypertensive cardiovascular disease.
• Adjust fluid intake to reduce risk of water intoxication and sodium deple-

tion, especially in children or elderly patients.
• Overdose may cause oxytocic or vasopressor activity. Withhold drug until effects subside. Furosemide may be used if fluid retention is excessive.
• Some patients may have difficulty measuring and inhaling drug into nostrils. Teach patient correct method of administration.
• Intranasal use can cause changes in the nasal mucosa resulting in erratic, unreliable absorption. Report any patient's worsening condition to doctor, who may prescribe injectable DDAVP.
• Desmopressin injection should not be used to treat hemophilia A with Factor VIII levels of 0% to 5%, or severe cases of von Willebrand's disease.
• In some patients, use of desmopressin may avoid the hazards of using blood products.
• Has been used successfully to reduce blood loss during cardiac surgery.

---

lypressin
Diapid

Pregnancy Risk Category: B

MECHANISM OF ACTION
Increases the permeability of the renal tubular epithelium to adenosine monophosphate and water; the epithelium promotes reabsorption of water and produces a concentrated urine (antidiuretic hormone effect).

INDICATIONS & DOSAGE
Nonnephrogenic diabetes insipidus—
Adults and children: 1 or 2 sprays (approximately 2 USP posterior pituitary pressor units/spray) in either or both nostrils q.i.d. and an additional dose at bedtime, if needed, to prevent nocturia. If usual dosage is inadequate, increase frequency rather than number of sprays.

ADVERSE REACTIONS
CNS: headache, dizziness.
EENT: nasal congestion or ulceration, irritation, pruritus of nasal passages, rhinorrhea, conjunctivitis.
GI: heartburn due to drip of excess spray into pharynx, abdominal cramps, frequent bowel movements.
GU: possible transient fluid retention from overdose.
Skin: hypersensitivity reaction.

INTERACTIONS
None significant.

NURSING CONSIDERATIONS
• Use with caution in coronary artery disease.
• Particularly useful if diabetes insipidus is unresponsive to other therapy, or if antidiuretic hormones of animal origin cause adverse effects.
• Nasal congestion, allergic rhinitis, or upper respiratory infections may diminish drug absorption and require larger dose or adjunctive therapy.
• Instruct patient to clear nasal passage before inhaling drug.
• Inadvertent inhalation of spray may cause tightness in chest, coughing, and transient dyspnea.
• Test patients sensitive to antidiuretic hormone for sensitivity to lypressin.
• To administer a uniform, well-diffused spray, hold bottle upright with patient in vertical position holding head upright.
• Instruct the patient to carry the medication with him at all times because of its fairly short duration.

---

somatrem
Protropin

Pregnancy Risk Category: C

MECHANISM OF ACTION
Purified growth hormone of recombinant DNA origin that stimulates linear, skeletal muscle, and organ growth.

INDICATIONS & DOSAGE
Long-term treatment of children who have growth failure because of lack of adequate endogenous growth hormone secretion—
Children (pre-puberty): 0.1 mg/kg I.M. or S.C. given three times weekly.

ADVERSE REACTIONS
Endocrine: *hypothyroidism, hyperglycemia.*
Other: *antibodies to growth hormone.*

INTERACTIONS
Glucocorticoids: may inhibit growth-promoting action of somatrem. Glucocorticoid dose may need to be adjusted.

NURSING CONSIDERATIONS
• Contraindicated in patients with closed epiphyses, an active underlying intracranial lesion, or known sensitivity to benzyl alcohol.
• Use cautiously in patients whose growth hormone deficiency results from an intracranial lesion. Patient should be examined frequently for progression or recurrence of the underlying disease.
• Observe patient for signs of glucose intolerance and hyperglycemia.
• Monitor periodic thyroid function tests for hypothyroidism, which may require treatment with a thyroid hormone.
• This drug replaces pituitary-derived human growth hormone, which was removed from the market in 1985 because of an association with a rare but fatal virus infection (Jakob-Creutzfeldt disease). Reassure your patient and his family that somatrem is *pure* and that it is *safe.*
• To prepare the solution, inject the bacteriostatic water for injection (which is supplied) into the vial con-

---

taining the drug. Then swirl the vial with a gentle rotary motion until the contents are completely dissolved. *Don't shake* the vial.

• After reconstitution, vial solution should be clear. Don't inject into the patient if the solution is cloudy or contains any particles.

• Store reconstituted vial in refrigerator. Must use within 7 days.

• Be sure to check this product's expiration date.

---

vasopressin (antidiuretic hormone)
Pitressin ◆

vasopressin tannate
Pitressin Tannate◆

Pregnancy Risk Category: B

MECHANISM OF ACTION
Increases the permeability of the renal tubular epithelium to adenosine monophosphate and water; the epithelium promotes reabsorption of water and produces a concentrated urine (antidiuretic hormone effect).

INDICATIONS & DOSAGE
Nonnephrogenic, nonpsychogenic diabetes insipidus—
Adults: 5 to 10 units I.M. or S.C. b.i.d. to q.i.d., p.r.n.; or intranasally (spray or cotton balls) in individualized doses, based on response. For chronic therapy, inject 2.5 to 5 units Pitressin Tannate in oil suspension I.M. or S.C. q 2 to 3 days.
Children: 2.5 to 10 units I.M. or S.C. b.i.d. to q.i.d., p.r.n.; or intranasally (spray or cotton balls) in individualized doses. For chronic therapy, inject 1.25 to 2.5 units Pitressin Tannate in oil suspension I.M. or S.C. q 2 to 3 days.
Postoperative abdominal distention—
Adults: 5 units (aqueous) I.M. initially, then q 3 to 4 hours, increasing dose to 10 units, if needed. Reduce

dose proportionately for children.
To expel gas before abdominal X-ray—
Adults: inject 10 units S.C. at 2 hours, then again at 30 minutes before X-ray. Enema before first dose may also help to eliminate gas.
Upper GI tract hemorrhage (intraarterial)—
Adults: 0.2 to 0.4 units/minute. Do not use tannate in oil suspension.

ADVERSE REACTIONS
CNS: tremor, dizziness, headache.
CV: *angina in patients with vascular disease,* vasoconstriction. Large doses may cause hypertension, electrocardiographic changes. (With intraarterial infusion: *bradycardia, cardiac dysrhythmias, pulmonary edema.*)
GI: abdominal cramps, nausea, vomiting, diarrhea, intestinal hyperactivity.
GU: uterine cramps, anuria.
Skin: circumoral pallor.
Other: water intoxication (drowsiness, listlessness, headache, confusion, weight gain), hypersensitivity reactions (urticaria, angioneurotic edema, bronchoconstriction, fever, rash, wheezing, dyspnea, *anaphylaxis),* sweating.

INTERACTIONS
Lithium, demeclocycline: reduced antidiuretic activity. Use together cautiously.
Chlorpropamide: increased antidiuretic response. Use together cautiously.

NURSING CONSIDERATIONS
• Contraindicated in chronic nephritis with nitrogen retention. Use cautiously in children, elderly persons, pregnant women, and patients with epilepsy, migraine, asthma, cardiovascular disease, or fluid overload.
• Never inject vasopressin tannate in oil I.V.

- Never inject during first stage of labor; may cause ruptured uterus.
- Monitor specific gravity of urine and intake and output to aid evaluation of drug effectiveness.
- Place tannate in oil in warm water for 10 to 15 minutes. Then shake thoroughly to make suspension uniform before withdrawing I.M. injection dose. Small brown particles must be seen in suspension. Use absolutely dry syringe to avoid dilution.
- Give with 1 to 2 glasses of water to reduce adverse reactions and to improve therapeutic response.
- To prevent possible seizures, coma, and death, observe patient closely for early signs of water intoxication.
- Overhydration more likely with long-acting tannate oil suspension than with aqueous vasopressin solution.
- Use minimum effective dosage to reduce side effects.
- May be used for transient polyuria resulting from antidiuretic hormone deficiency related to neurosurgery or head injury.
- Synthetic desmopressin is sometimes preferred because of longer duration and less frequent side effects.
- Monitor blood pressure of patient on vasopressin twice daily. Watch for excessively elevated blood pressure or lack of response to drug, which may be indicated by hypotension. Also monitor fluid intake and output and daily weights.
- A rectal tube will facilitate gas expulsion following vasopressin injection.

Parathyroid-like agents

calcifediol
calcitonin (human)
calcitonin (salmon)
calcitriol (1,25-
    dihydroxycholecalciferol)
dihydrotachysterol
etidronate disodium

COMBINATION PRODUCTS
None.

---

calcifediol
Calderol

Pregnancy Risk Category: A

MECHANISM OF ACTION
Stimulates calcium absorption from
the GI tract and promotes secretion of
calcium from bone to blood.

INDICATIONS & DOSAGE
*Treatment and management of meta-
bolic bone disease associated with
chronic renal failure—*
Adults: initially, 300 to 350 mcg P.O.
weekly, given on a daily or alternate-
day schedule. Dosage may be increased at 4-week intervals. Optimal
dosage must be carefully determined
for each patient.

ADVERSE REACTIONS
Vitamin D intoxication associated
with hypercalcemia:
CNS: headache, somnolence.
EENT: conjunctivitis, photosensitivity, rhinorrhea.
GI: nausea, vomiting, constipation,
metallic taste, dry mouth, anorexia,
diarrhea.

GU: polyuria.
Other: weakness, bone and muscle
pain.

INTERACTIONS
Cholestyramine: may impair absorption of calcifediol.

NURSING CONSIDERATIONS
• Contraindicated in hypercalcemia
or vitamin D toxicity. Withhold all
preparations containing vitamin D in
patients taking calcifediol. Use cautiously in patients on digitalis because
hypercalcemia may precipitate cardiac dysrhythmias.
• Monitor serum calcium; serum calcium times serum phosphate should
not exceed 70. During titration, serum
calcium should be determined at least
weekly. If hypercalcemia occurs, calcifediol should be discontinued but
resumed after serum calcium returns
to normal.
• Patient should receive adequate
daily intake of calcium.
• Advise patient to adhere to diet and
calcium supplementation and to avoid
nonprescription drugs.
• Teach patient to report signs and
symptoms of hypercalcemia.

---

calcitonin (human)
Cibacalcin

calcitonin (salmon)
Calcimar, Miacalcin

Pregnancy Risk Category: B

MECHANISM OF ACTION
Decreases osteoclastic activity by inhibiting osteocytic osteolysis. Also decreases mineral release and matrix or collagen breakdown in bone.

INDICATIONS & DOSAGE
Paget's disease of bone (osteitis deformans)—
Adults: initially 100 international units (IU) of calcitonin (salmon) daily, S.C. or I.M. Maintenance dosage is 50 to 100 IU daily or every other day. Alternatively, give calcitonin (human) 0.5 mg S.C. daily. If patient obtains sufficient improvement, dosage may be reduced to 0.25 mg. daily 2 or 3 times per week. Some patients may need as much as 1 mg daily.
Hypercalcemia—
Adults: 4 IU/kg I.M. q 12 hours (calcitonin salmon).
Postmenopausal osteoporosis—
Adults: 100 IU I.M. or S.C. daily (calcitonin salmon).

ADVERSE REACTIONS
CNS: headaches.
GI: transient nausea with or without vomiting, diarrhea, anorexia.
GU: transient diuresis.
Metabolic: hyperglycemia.
Local: inflammation at injection site, skin rashes.
Other: *facial flushing;* hypocalcemia; swelling, tingling, and tenderness of hands; unusual taste sensation; *anaphylaxis.*

INTERACTIONS
None significant.

NURSING CONSIDERATIONS
• Contraindicated in allergy to gelatin diluent used to prepare drug. Not recommended for breast-feeding mothers, or women who are or may become pregnant. Safe use in children not established.
• Periodic serum alkaline phosphatase and 24-hour urine hydroxyproline levels should be determined to evaluate drug effect.
• Skin test is usually done before beginning therapy.
• Systemic allergic reactions possible since hormone is protein. Keep epinephrine handy when administering.
• Patients with good initial clinical response to calcitonin who suffer relapse should be evaluated for antibody formation response to the hormone protein.
• Tell patient in whom calcitonin loses its hypocalcemic activity that further medication or increased dosages will be of no value.
• Facial flushing and warmth occur in 20% to 30% of all patients within minutes of injection; usually last about 1 hour. Reassure patient that this is a transient effect.
• Observe patient for signs of hypocalcemic tetany during therapy (muscle twitching, tetanic spasms, and seizures if hypocalcemia is severe).
• Monitor calcium closely. Watch for signs of hypercalcemic relapse: bone pain, renal calculi, polyria, anorexia, nausea, vomiting, thirst, constipation, lethargy, bradycardia, muscle hypotonicity, pathologic fracture, psychosis, and coma.
• Periodic examinations of urine sediment are advisable.
• Calcitonin (human) is indicated especially in patients who have developed resistance to calcitonin (salmon). Calcitonin (human) is associated with risk of diminishing efficacy caused by antibody formation or hypersensitivity reactions.
• Administer the drug at bedtime

Italicized side effects are common or life-threatening.
*Liquid form contains alcohol.   **May contain tartrazine.

when possible to minimize nausea and vomiting.
• Treatment should continue for at least 6 months. Then, if symptoms have been relieved, it may be discontinued until symptoms or radiologic signs recur.
• Be sure to use the freshly reconstituted solution within 2 hours.
• When administered for postmenopausal osteoporosis, remind patient to take adequate calcium and vitamin D supplementation.

calcitriol (1,25-dihydroxycholecalciferol)
Calcijex, Rocaltrol♦

Pregnancy Risk Category: A (D if used in doses > RDA)

MECHANISM OF ACTION
Stimulates calcium absorption from the GI tract and promotes secretion of calcium from bone to blood.

INDICATIONS & DOSAGE
Management of hypocalcemia in patients undergoing chronic dialysis—
Adults: initially, 0.25 mcg P.O. daily. Dosage may be increased by 0.25 mcg daily at 2- to 4-week intervals. Maintenance dosage is 0.25 mcg every other day up to 0.5 to 1.25 mcg daily.
Management of hypoparathyroidism and pseudohypoparathyroidism—
Adults and children over 1 year: initially, 0.25 mcg P.O. daily. Dosage may be increased at 2- to 4-week intervals. Maintenance dosage is 0.25 to 2 mcg daily.

ADVERSE REACTIONS
Vitamin D intoxication associated with hypercalcemia:
CNS: headache, somnolence.
EENT: conjunctivitis, photophobia, rhinorrhea.
GI: nausea, vomiting, constipation, metallic taste, dry mouth, anorexia.
GU: polyuria.
Other: weakness, bone and muscle pain.

INTERACTIONS
None significant.

NURSING CONSIDERATIONS
• Contraindicated in hypercalcemia or vitamin D toxicity. Withhold all preparations containing vitamin D in patients taking calcitriol. Not recommended in breast-feeding mothers. Use cautiously in patients on digitalis; hypercalcemia may precipitate cardiac dysrhythmias.
• Monitor serum calcium; serum calcium times serum phosphate should not exceed 70. During titration, determine serum calcium twice weekly. If hypercalcemia occurs, discontinue, but resume after serum calcium returns to normal. Patient should receive adequate daily intake of calcium—1,000 mg.
• Protect from heat and light.
• Instruct patient to adhere to diet and calcium supplementation and to avoid unapproved nonprescription drugs.
• Patients should not use magnesium-containing antacids while taking this drug.
• Patients should report to doctor immediately any of the following symptoms: weakness, nausea, vomiting, dry mouth, constipation, muscle or bone pain, or metallic taste—early symptoms of vitamin D intoxication.
• Tell patient that although this drug is a vitamin, it must not be taken by anyone for whom it was not prescribed because of its potentially serious toxicities.
• Most potent form of vitamin D available.

dihydrotachysterol
DHT Oral Solution, Hytakerol♦

Pregnancy Risk Category: A (D if used in doses > RDA)

MECHANISM OF ACTION
Stimulates calcium absorption from the GI tract and promotes secretion of calcium from bone to blood.

INDICATIONS & DOSAGE
Familial hypophosphatemia—
Adults and children: 0.5 to 2 mg P.O. daily. Maintenance dosage is 0.3 to 1.5 mg daily.
Hypocalcemia associated with hypo- parathyroidism and pseudohypopara- thyroidism—
Adults: initially, 0.8 to 2.4 mg P.O. daily for several days. Maintenance dosage is 0.2 to 2 mg daily, as re- quired for normal serum calcium. Av- erage dose is 0.6 mg daily.
Children: initially, 1 to 5 mg for sev- eral days. Maintenance dosage is 0.2 to 1 mg daily, as required for normal serum calcium.
Renal osteodystrophy in chronic ure- mia—
Adults: 0.1 to 0.6 mg P.O. daily.
Prophylaxis of hypocalcemic tetany following thyroid surgery—
Adults: 0.25 mg P.O. daily (with cal- cium supplements).

ADVERSE REACTIONS
Vitamin D intoxication associated with hypercalcemia:
CNS: headache, somnolence.
EENT: conjunctivitis, photophobia, rhinorrhea.
GI: nausea, vomiting, constipation, metallic taste, dry mouth, anorexia, diarrhea.
GU: polyuria.
Other: weakness, bone and muscle pain.

INTERACTIONS
Thiazide diuretics: possible hypercal-
cemia in hypoparathyroid patients. Avoid concomitant use.

NURSING CONSIDERATIONS
● Contraindicated in hypercalcemia, hypocalcemia associated with renal insufficiency and hyperphosphatemia, renal stones, hypersensitivity to vita- min D, and in breast-feeding mothers.
● Monitor serum and urine calcium. Watch for signs of hypercalcemia.
● Adequate dietary calcium intake is necessary; usually supplemented with 10 to 15 g oral calcium lactate or glu- conate daily.
● Report hypercalcemia reactions to doctor. Early signs of hypercalcemia include thirst, headache, vertigo, tin- nitus, anorexia.
● 1 mg equal to 120,000 units ergo- calciferol (vitamin D_2).
● Store in tightly closed, light-resis- tant container. Don't refrigerate.

etidronate disodium
Didronel♦

Pregnancy Risk Category: B

MECHANISM OF ACTION
Decreases osteoclastic activity by in- hibiting osteocytic osteolysis. Also decreases mineral release and matrix or collagen breakdown in bone.

INDICATIONS & DOSAGE
Symptomatic Paget's disease—
Adults: 5 mg/kg P.O. daily as a single dose 2 hours before a meal with water or juice. Patient should not eat for 2 hours after dose. May give up to 10 mg/kg daily in severe cases. Maxi- mum dosage is 20 mg/kg daily.
Heterotopic ossification in spinal cord injuries—
Adults: 20 mg/kg daily for 2 weeks, then 10 mg/kg daily for 10 weeks. To- tal treatment period is 12 weeks.
Heterotopic ossification after total hip replacement—
Adults: 20 mg/kg daily for 1 month

Italicized side effects are common or life-threatening.
*Liquid form contains alcohol.   **May contain tartrazine.

before total hip replacement and for 3
months afterward.

ADVERSE REACTIONS
GI: (seen most frequently at 20 mg/
kg daily) diarrhea, increased frequency of bowel movements, nausea.
Other: increased or recurrent bone
pain at pagetic sites, pain at previously asymptomatic sites, increased
risk of fracture, *elevated serum phosphate*.

INTERACTIONS
None significant.

NURSING CONSIDERATIONS
• Use cautiously in enterocolitis, impaired renal function.
• Therapy should not last more than 6
months. After 3 months, resume if
needed. Don't give longer than 3
months at doses above 10 mg/kg
daily.
• Don't give drug with food, milk, or
antacids; may reduce absorption.
• Monitor renal function before and
during therapy.
• Elevated serum phosphate may occur, especially in patients receiving
higher doses. However, serum phosphate usually returns to normal 2 to 4
weeks after drug's discontinued.
• Monitor drug effect by serum alkaline phosphatase and urinary hydroxyproline excretion (both lowered
if therapy effective).
• Tell patient that improvement may
not occur for up to 3 months but may
continue for months after drug is
stopped. Stress importance of good
nutrition, especially diet high in calcium and vitamin D.

63

Diuretics

Thiazide diuretics
bendroflumethiazide
benzthiazide
chlorothiazide
cyclothiazide
hydrochlorothiazide
hydroflumethiazide
methyclothiazide
polythiazide
trichlormethiazide

Thiazide-like diuretics
chlorthalidone
metolazone
quinethazone

Loop diuretics
bumetanide
ethacrynate sodium
ethacrynic acid
furosemide

Carbonic anhydrase inhibitors
acetazolamide
acetazolamide sodium
dichlorphenamide
methazolamide

Miscellaneous diuretics
amiloride hydrochloride
indapamide
mannitol
spironolactone
triamterene
urea (carbamide)

COMBINATION PRODUCTS
ALAZIDE: spironolactone 25 mg and hydrochlorothiazide 25 mg.
ALDACTAZIDE♦: spironolactone 25 mg and hydrochlorothiazide 25 mg.
ALDACTAZIDE 50/50: spironolactone 50 mg and hydrochlorothiazide 50 mg.
ALTEXIDE: spironolactone 25 mg and hydrochlorothiazide 25 mg.
DYAZIDE♦: triamterene 50 mg and hydrochlorothiazide 25 mg.
MAXZIDE: triamterene 75 mg and hydrochlorothiazide 50 mg.
MODURETIC: amiloride hydrochloride 5 mg and hydrochlorothiazide 50 mg.
SPIRONAZIDE: spironolactone 25 mg and hydrochlorothiazide 25 mg.
SPIROZIDE: spironolactone 25 mg and hydrochlorothiazide 25 mg.

acetazolamide
Acetazolam♦♦, Ak-Zol, Apo-Acetazolamide♦♦, Dazamide, Diamox♦, Diamox Sequels♦. Novo-zolamide♦♦

acetazolamide sodium
Diamox Parenteral, Diamox Sodium♦♦

Pregnancy Risk Category: C

MECHANISM OF ACTION
By enzymatic blocking, promotes renal excretion of sodium, potassium, bicarbonate, and water. Bicarbonate ion excretion makes the urine alkaline. Also decreases secretion of aqueous humor in the eye, thereby lowering intraocular pressure. As an anticonvulsant, may inhibit carbonic anhydrase in the CNS and decrease abnormal paroxysmal or excessive neuronal discharge.

INDICATIONS & DOSAGE
Narrow-angle glaucoma—
Adults: 250 mg q 4 hours; or 250 mg
P.O., I.M., or I.V. b.i.d. for short-
term therapy.
Edema in congestive heart failure—
Adults: 250 to 375 mg P.O., I.M., or
I.V. daily in a.m.
Children: 5 mg/kg daily in a.m.
Open-angle glaucoma—
Adults: 250 mg daily to 1 g P.O.,
I.M., or I.V. divided q.i.d.
*Prevention or amelioration of acute
mountain sickness—*
Adults: 250 mg P.O. q 8 to 12 hours.
*Myoclonic, refractory generalized
tonic-clonic (grand mal) or absence
(petit mal), or mixed seizures—*
Adults: 375 mg P.O., I.M., or I.V.
daily up to 250 mg q.i.d. Diamox Se-
quels 250 to 500 mg daily or b.i.d.
Initial dosage when used with other
anticonvulsants usually is 250 mg
daily.
Children: 8 to 30 mg/kg daily, divided t.i.d. or q.i.d. Maximum dosage is 1.5 g daily, or 300 to 900 mg/
m² daily.

ADVERSE REACTIONS
Blood: *aplastic anemia,* hemolytic
anemia, leukopenia.
CNS: drowsiness, paresthesias, con-
fusion.
EENT: transient myopia.
GI: nausea, vomiting, anorexia.
GU: crystalluria, renal calculi, hema-
turia.
Metabolic: *hyperchloremic acidosis,*
hypokalemia, asymptomatic hyper-
uricemia.
Skin: rash.
Local: *pain at injection site,* sterile
abscesses.

INTERACTIONS
None significant.

NURSING CONSIDERATIONS
• Contraindicated in long-term therapy for chronic noncongestive nar-

row-angle glaucoma; also in depressed sodium or potassium serum,
renal or hepatic disease or dysfunction, adrenal gland failure, or hyperchloremic acidosis. Use cautiously in
respiratory acidosis, emphysema,
chronic pulmonary disease, and in
those patients receiving other diuretics.
• Monitor intake/output and electrolytes, especially serum potassium.
When used in diuretic therapy, consult with doctor and dietitian to provide high-potassium diet.
• Weigh patient daily. Rapid weight
loss may cause hypotension.
• Diuretic effect is decreased when
acidosis occurs but can be reestab-
lished by withdrawing drug for several days and then restarting, or by using intermittent administration schedules.
• Reconstitute 500-mg vial with at
least 5 ml sterile water for injection.
Use within 24 hours of reconstitution.
• I.M. injection is painful because of
alkalinity of solution. Direct I.V. administration is preferred (100 to 500
mg/minute).
• Elderly patients are especially susceptible to excessive diuresis.
• Sustained-release form available.
Permits a reduction in dosage frequency.
• May cause false-positive urine protein tests by alkalinizing the urine.
• Oral liquid: soften 1 tablet in 2 teaspoonfuls of very warm water and add
to 2 teaspoonfuls honey or syrup
(chocolate or cherry). Don't use fruit
juice.

amiloride hydrochloride
Midamor♦

Pregnancy Risk Category: B

MECHANISM OF ACTION
Inhibits sodium reabsorption and potassium excretion by direct action on
the distal tubule.

INDICATIONS & DOSAGE
Hypertension; edema associated with congestive heart failure, usually in patients who are also taking thiazide or other potassium-wasting diuretics—
Adults: usual dosage is 5 mg P.O. daily. Dosage may be increased to 10 mg daily, if necessary. As much as 20 mg daily can be given.

ADVERSE REACTIONS
CNS: *headache,* weakness, dizziness.
CV: orthostatic hypotension.
GI: *nausea, anorexia, diarrhea, vomiting,* abdominal pain, constipation.
GU: impotence.
Metabolic: hyperkalemia.

INTERACTIONS
None significant.

NURSING CONSIDERATIONS
• Contraindicated in patients with elevated serum potassium level (greater than 5.5 mEq/liter). Don't administer to patients receiving other potassium-sparing diuretics, such as spironolactone and triamterene. Also contraindicated in anuria.
• Use cautiously in patients with renal impairment, because potassium retention is increased.
• Risk of hyperkalemia is greater when a potassium-wasting drug is not taken concurrently. When amiloride is taken this way, be sure to monitor daily potassium.
• Discontinue immediately if potassium level exceeds 6.5 mEq/liter.
• Warn patient to avoid excessive ingestion of potassium-rich foods or potassium-containing salt substitutes. Concomitant potassium supplement can lead to serious hyperkalemia.
• Administer amiloride with meals to prevent nausea.

bendroflumethiazide
Naturetin♦

Pregnancy Risk Category: B

MECHANISM OF ACTION
Increases urine excretion of sodium and water by inhibiting sodium reabsorption in the cortical diluting site of the ascending loop of Henle.

INDICATIONS & DOSAGE
Edema, hypertension—
Adults: 5 to 20 mg P.O. daily or divided b.i.d.
Children: initially, 0.1 to 0.4 mg/kg (3 to 12 mg/m²) P.O. daily or divided b.i.d.
Maintenance: 0.05 to 0.1 mg/kg (1.5 to 3 mg/m²) P.O. daily or divided b.i.d.

ADVERSE REACTIONS
Blood: *aplastic anemia, agranulocytosis,* leukopenia, thrombocytopenia.
CV: *volume depletion and dehydration,* orthostatic hypotension.
GI: anorexia, nausea, pancreatitis.
Hepatic: hepatic encephalopathy.
Metabolic: *hypokalemia, asymptomatic hyperuricemia, hyperglycemia and impairment of glucose tolerance,* fluid and electrolyte imbalances including dilutional hyponatremia and hypochloremia, metabolic alkalosis, hypercalcemia, gout.
Skin: dermatitis, photosensitivity, rash.
Other: hypersensitivity reactions, such as pneumonitis and vasculitis.

INTERACTIONS
Cholestyramine, colestipol: intestinal absorption of thiazides decreased. Keep doses as separate as possible.
Diazoxide: increased antihypertensive, hyperglycemic, and hyperuricemic effects. Use together cautiously.

NURSING CONSIDERATIONS

• Contraindicated in anuria or hypersensitivity to other thiazides or other sulfonamide-derived drugs. Use cautiously in severe renal disease and impaired hepatic function.

• Monitor intake/output, weight, and serum electrolytes regularly. Monitor serum creatinine and BUN regularly. Not as effective if these are more than twice normal.

• Consult with doctor and dietitian to provide high-potassium diet. Watch for signs of hypokalemia (for example, muscle weakness and cramps). Patients on digitalis have an increased risk of digitalis toxicity from potassium-depleting adverse effect of this diuretic. May be used with potassium-sparing diuretic to prevent potassium loss.

• Foods rich in potassium include citrus fruits, bananas, tomatoes, dates, and apricots.

• Monitor blood sugar. Check insulin requirements in patients with diabetes. May treat severe hyperglycemia with oral antidiabetic agents.

• Monitor blood uric acid, especially in patients with a history of gout.

• Elderly patients are especially susceptible to excessive diuresis.

• Give in a.m. to prevent nocturia.

• In hypertension, therapeutic response may be delayed several days.

• Thiazides and thiazide-like diuretics should be discontinued before tests for parathyroid function are performed.

---

benzthiazide
Aquatag**, Exna**, Hydrex
Pregnancy Risk Category: D

MECHANISM OF ACTION
Increases urine excretion of sodium and water by inhibiting sodium reabsorption in the cortical diluting site of the nephron.

INDICATIONS & DOSAGE
Edema—
Adults: 50 to 200 mg P.O. daily or in divided doses.
Children: 1 to 4 mg/kg P.O. daily in three divided doses.
Hypertension—
Adults: 50 mg P.O. daily b.i.d., t.i.d., or q.i.d., adjusted to patient response.

ADVERSE REACTIONS
Blood: *aplastic anemia, agranulocytosis,* leukopenia, thrombocytopenia.
CV: *volume depletion and dehydration,* orthostatic hypotension.
GI: anorexia, nausea, pancreatitis.
Hepatic: hepatic encephalopathy.
Metabolic: *hypokalemia, asymptomatic hyperuricemia, hyperglycemia and impairment of glucose tolerance,* fluid and electrolyte imbalances including dilutional hyponatremia and hypochloremia, metabolic alkalosis, hypercalcemia, gout.
Skin: dermatitis, photosensitivity, rash.
Other: hypersensitivity reactions, such as pneumonitis and vasculitis.

INTERACTIONS
Cholestyramine, colestipol: intestinal absorption of thiazides decreased. Keep doses as separate as possible.
Diazoxide: increased antihypertensive, hyperglycemic, and hyperuricemic effects. Use together cautiously.

NURSING CONSIDERATIONS
• Contraindicated in anuria or hypersensitivity to other thiazides or other sulfonamide-derived drugs. Use cautiously in severe renal disease and impaired hepatic function.

• Monitor intake/output, weight, and serum electrolytes regularly. Consult with doctor and dietitian to provide high-potassium diet. Watch for signs of hypokalemia (for example, muscle weakness and cramps). Patients on

---

digitalis have an increased risk of digitalis toxicity from the potassium-depleting adverse effect of this diuretic. May use with potassium-sparing diuretic to prevent potassium loss.
• Foods rich in potassium include citrus fruits, bananas, tomatoes, dates, and apricots.
• Monitor serum creatinine and BUN regularly. Not as effective if these levels are more than twice normal.
• Monitor blood sugar. Check insulin requirements in patients with diabetes. May treat severe hyperglycemia with oral antidiabetic agents.
• Monitor blood uric acid level, especially in patients with a history of gout.
• Give in a.m. to prevent nocturia.
• Elderly patients are especially susceptible to excessive diuresis.
• In hypertension, therapeutic response may be delayed several days.
• Thiazides and thiazide-like diuretics should be discontinued before tests for parathyroid function are performed.

bumetanide
Bumex

Pregnancy Risk Category: C

MECHANISM OF ACTION
Inhibits reabsorption of sodium and chloride at the proximal portion of the ascending loop of Henle.

INDICATIONS & DOSAGE
Edema (congestive heart failure, hepatic and renal disease)—
Adults: 0.5 to 2 mg P.O. once daily. If diuretic response not adequate, a second or third dose may be given at 4- to 5-hour intervals. Maximum dosage is 10 mg/day. May be administered parenterally when P.O. not feasible. Usual initial dose is 0.5 to 1 mg I.V. or I.M. If response is not adequate, a second or third dose may be given at 2- to 3-hour intervals. Maxi-

mum dosage is 10 mg/day.

ADVERSE REACTIONS
CNS: dizziness, headache.
CV: *volume depletion and dehydration, orthostatic hypotension,* ECG changes.
EENT: transient deafness.
GI: nausea.
Metabolic: *hypokalemia; hypochloremic alkalosis; asymptomatic hyperuricemia; fluid and electrolyte imbalances, including dilutional hyponatremia, hypocalcemia, hypomagnesemia;* hyperglycemia and impairment of glucose tolerance.
Skin: rash.
Other: muscle pain and tenderness.

INTERACTIONS
Aminoglycoside antibiotics: potentiated ototoxicity. Use together cautiously.
Probenecid, indomethacin: inhibited diuretic response. Use cautiously.

NURSING CONSIDERATIONS
• Contraindicated in anuria, hepatic coma, or in states of severe electrolyte depletion.
• Use cautiously in patients with hepatic cirrhosis and ascites. Supplemental potassium or potassium-sparing diuretics may be used to prevent hypokalemia and metabolic alkalosis in these patients. Use cautiously in patients with depressed renal function.
• Use cautiously in patients allergic to sulfonamides. These patients may show hypersensitivity to bumetanide.
• Potent loop diuretic; can lead to profound water and electrolyte depletion. Monitor blood pressure and pulse rate during rapid diuresis.
• If oliguria or azotemia develops or increases, may require stopping drug.
• Monitor serum electrolytes, BUN, and CO_2 frequently.
• Watch for signs of hypokalemia (for example, muscle weakness and

cramps). Patients also receiving digitalis have an increased risk of digitalis toxicity from the potassium-depleting effect of this diuretic.
• Consult with doctor and dietitian to provide high-potassium diet.
• Foods rich in potassium include citrus fruits, tomatoes, bananas, dates, and apricots.
• Monitor blood sugar in patients with diabetes. May treat severe hyperglycemia with oral antidiabetic agents.
• Monitor blood uric acid, especially in patients with a history of gout.
• Give I.V. doses over 1 to 2 minutes.
• Advise patients taking bumetanide to stand up slowly to prevent dizziness and to limit alcohol intake and strenuous exercise in hot weather since these exacerbate orthostatic hypotension.
• Bumetanide can be safely prescribed in patients allergic to furosemide.
• 1 mg of bumetanide is equal to 40 mg of furosemide.
• May be less ototoxic than furosemide, but the clinical relevance of this has not been determined.
• Give in a.m. to prevent nocturia. If second dose is necessary, give in the early afternoon.
• Intermittent dosage given on alternate days, or for 3 to 4 days with 1 or 2 days intervening, is recommended as the safest and most effective dosage schedule for control of edema.

chlorothiazide
Diuril♦

Pregnancy Risk Category: D

MECHANISM OF ACTION
Increases urine excretion of sodium and water by inhibiting sodium reabsorption in the cortical diluting site of the nephron.

INDICATIONS & DOSAGE
Edema, hypertension—
Adults: 500 mg to 2 g P.O. or I.V. daily or in two divided doses.
Diuresis—
Children over 6 months: 20 mg/kg P.O. or I.V. daily in divided doses.
Children under 6 months: may require 30 mg/kg P.O. or I.V. daily in two divided doses.

ADVERSE REACTIONS
Blood: *aplastic anemia, agranulocytosis,* leukopenia, thrombocytopenia.
CV: *volume depletion and dehydration,* orthostatic hypotension.
GI: anorexia, nausea, pancreatitis.
Hepatic: hepatic encephalopathy.
Metabolic: *hypokalemia, asymptomatic hyperuricemia, hyperglycemia and impairment of glucose tolerance,* fluid and electrolyte imbalances including dilutional hyponatremia and hypochloremia, metabolic alkalosis, hypercalcemia, gout.
Skin: dermatitis, photosensitivity, rash.
Other: hypersensitivity reactions such as pneumonitis and vasculitis.

INTERACTIONS
Cholestyramine, colestipol: intestinal absorption of thiazides decreased. Keep doses as separate as possible.
Diazoxide: increased antihypertensive, hyperglycemic, and hyperuricemic effects. Use together cautiously.

NURSING CONSIDERATIONS
• Contraindicated in anuria; hypersensitivity to other thiazides or other sulfonamide-derived drugs; impaired hepatic function; or progressive hepatic disease. Use cautiously in severe renal disease.
• Monitor intake/output, weight, and serum electrolytes regularly.
• Consult with doctor and dietitian to provide high-potassium diet. Watch for signs of hypokalemia (for exam-

ple, muscle weakness, and cramps). Patients on digitalis have an increased risk of digitalis toxicity from the potassium-depleting effect of the diuretic. May use with potassium-sparing diuretic to prevent potassium loss.
• Foods rich in potassium include citrus fruits, tomatoes, bananas, dates, and apricots.
• Monitor blood sugar. Check insulin requirements in patients with diabetes. May treat severe hyperglycemia with oral antidiabetic agents.
• Monitor serum creatinine and BUN regularly. Not as effective if these levels are more than twice normal.
• Monitor blood uric acid, especially in patients with a history of gout.
• Monitor serum calcium and watch for progressive renal impairment.
• Only injectable thiazide. For I.V. use only—not I.M. or S.C. Reconstitute 500 mg with 18 ml of sterile water for injection. May store reconstituted solutions at room temperature up to 24 hours. Compatible with I.V. dextrose or sodium chloride solutions.
• Avoid I.V. infiltration; can be very painful.
• Give in a.m. to prevent nocturia.
• In hypertension, therapeutic response may be delayed several days.
• Elderly patients are especially susceptible to excessive diuresis.
• The only thiazide available in liquid form.
• Thiazides and thiazide-like diuretics should be stopped before tests for parathyroid function are performed.

chlorthalidone
Apo-Chlorthalidone♦♦, Hygroton♦, Novothalidone♦♦, Thalitone, Uridon♦♦

Pregnancy Risk Category: D

MECHANISM OF ACTION
Increases urine excretion of sodium and water by inhibiting sodium reabsorption in the cortical diluting site of the nephron.

INDICATIONS & DOSAGE
Edema, hypertension—
Adults: 25 to 100 mg P.O. daily, or 100 mg 3 times weekly or on alternate days.
Children: 2 mg/kg P.O. 3 times weekly.

ADVERSE REACTIONS
Blood: *aplastic anemia, agranulocytosis,* leukopenia, thrombocytopenia.
CV: *volume depletion and dehydration,* orthostatic hypotension.
GI: anorexia, nausea, pancreatitis.
GU: impotence.
Hepatic: hepatic encephalopathy.
Metabolic: *hypokalemia, asymptomatic hyperuricemia, hyperglycemia and impairment of glucose tolerance,* fluid and electrolyte imbalances including dilutional hyponatremia and hypochloremia, metabolic alkalosis, hypercalcemia, gout.
Skin: dermatitis, photosensitivity, rash.
Other: hypersensitivity reactions, such as pneumonitis and vasculitis.

INTERACTIONS
Cholestyramine, colestipol: intestinal absorption of thiazides decreased. Keep doses as separate as possible.
Diazoxide: increased antihypertensive, hyperglycemic, and hyperuricemic effects. Use together cautiously.

NURSING CONSIDERATIONS
• Contraindicated in anuria or in hypersensitivity to thiazides or other sulfonamide-derived drugs. Use cautiously in severe renal disease, progressive hepatic disease, and impaired hepatic function.
• Monitor intake/output, weight, and serum electrolytes regularly.
• Consult with doctor and dietitian to provide high-potassium diet. Watch for signs of hypokalemia (for exam-

---

Italicized side effects are common or life-threatening.
*Liquid form contains alcohol.   **May contain tartrazine.

ple, muscle weakness, and cramps). Patients on digitalis have an increased risk of digitalis toxicity from the potassium-depleting effect of this diuretic. May use with potassium-sparing diuretic to prevent potassium loss.
• Foods rich in potassium include citrus fruits, tomatoes, bananas, dates, and apricots.
• Monitor serum creatinine and BUN regularly. Not as effective if these levels are more than twice normal.
• Monitor blood uric acid, especially in patients with a history of gout.
• Monitor blood sugar. Check insulin requirements in patients with diabetes. May treat severe hyperglycemia with oral antidiabetic agents.
• In hypertension, therapeutic response may be delayed several days.
• Give in a.m. to prevent nocturia.
• Elderly patients are especially susceptible to excessive diuresis.
• Thiazides and thiazide-like diuretics should be stopped before tests for parathyroid function are performed.

cyclothiazide
Anhydron, Fluidil

Pregnancy Risk Category: D

MECHANISM OF ACTION
Increases urine excretion of sodium and water by inhibiting sodium reabsorption in the cortical diluting site of the nephron.

INDICATIONS & DOSAGE
Edema—
Adults: 1 to 2 mg P.O. daily. May be used on alternate days as maintenance dosage.
Children: 0.02 to 0.04 mg/kg P.O. daily.
Hypertension—
Adults: 2 mg P.O. daily; up to 2 mg b.i.d. or t.i.d.

ADVERSE REACTIONS
Blood: *aplastic anemia, agranulocy-*

tosis, leukopenia, thrombocytopenia.
CV: *volume depletion and dehydration,* orthostatic hypotension.
GI: anorexia, nausea, pancreatitis.
Hepatic: hepatic encephalopathy.
Metabolic: *hypokalemia, asymptomatic hyperuricemia, hyperglycemia and impairment of glucose tolerance,* fluid and electrolyte imbalances including dilutional hyponatremia and hypochloremia, metabolic alkalosis, hypercalcemia, gout.
Skin: dermatitis, photosensitivity, rash.
Other: hypersensitivity reactions, such as pneumonitis and vasculitis.

INTERACTIONS
Cholestyramine, colestipol: intestinal absorption of thiazides decreased. Keep doses as separate as possible.
Diazoxide: increased antihypertensive, hyperglycemic, and hyperuricemic effects. Use together cautiously.

NURSING CONSIDERATIONS
• Contraindicated in anuria or in hypersensitivity to other thiazides or other sulfonamide-derived drugs. Use cautiously in severe renal disease, impaired hepatic function, and progressive hepatic disease.
• Monitor intake/output, weight, and serum electrolytes regularly.
• Consult with doctor and dietitian to provide high-potassium diet. Watch for signs of hypokalemia (for example, muscle weakness and cramps). Patients on digitalis have an increased risk of digitalis toxicity from the potassium-depleting effect of this diuretic. May use with potassium-sparing diuretic to prevent potassium loss.
• Foods rich in potassium include citrus fruits, tomatoes, bananas, dates, and apricots.
• Monitor blood sugar. Check insulin requirements in patients with diabetes. May treat severe hyperglycemia with oral antidiabetic agents.

- Monitor serum creatinine and BUN regularly. Not as effective if these levels are more than twice normal.
- Monitor blood uric acid, especially in patients with a history of gout.
- In hypertension, therapeutic response may be delayed several days.
- Give in a.m. to prevent nocturia.
- Elderly patients are especially susceptible to excessive diuresis.
- Thiazides and thiazide-like diuretics should be stopped before tests for parathyroid function are performed.

dichlorphenamide
Daranide

Pregnancy Risk Category: C

MECHANISM OF ACTION
Decreases secretion of aqueous humor in the eye, thereby lowering intraocular pressure.

INDICATIONS & DOSAGE
Adjunct in glaucoma—
Adults: initially, 100 to 200 mg P.O., followed by 100 mg q 12 hours until desired response obtained. Maintenance dosage is 25 to 50 mg P.O. daily b.i.d. or t.i.d. Give miotics concomitantly.

ADVERSE REACTIONS
Blood: *aplastic anemia,* hemolytic anemia, leukopenia.
CNS: drowsiness, paresthesias.
EENT: transient myopia.
GI: nausea, vomiting, anorexia.
GU: crystalluria, renal calculi.
Metabolic: *hyperchloremic acidosis,* hypokalemia, asymptomatic hyperuricemia.
Skin: rash.

INTERACTIONS
None significant.

NURSING CONSIDERATIONS
- Contraindicated in hepatic insufficiency, renal failure, adrenocortical insufficiency, hyperchloremic acidosis, depressed sodium or potassium levels, severe pulmonary obstruction with inability to increase alveolar ventilation, or Addison's disease. Long-term use contraindicated in severe, absolute, or chronic noncongestive narrow-angle glaucoma. Use cautiously in respiratory acidosis, monitoring blood pH and blood gases.
- Monitor electrolytes, especially serum potassium in initial treatment. Usually no problem in long-term glaucoma therapy unless risk of hypokalemia from other causes; potassium supplements may be necessary.
- May cause false-positive results in urine protein tests.
- Anticipate that drug will be given every day for glaucoma but intermittently for edema.
- Evaluate patient with glaucoma for eye pain to make sure drug is effective in decreasing intraocular pressure.

ethacrynate sodium
Edecrin Sodium

ethacrynic acid
Edecrin♦

Pregnancy Risk Category: D

MECHANISM OF ACTION
Inhibits reabsorption of sodium and chloride at the proximal portion of the ascending loop of Henle.

INDICATIONS & DOSAGE
Acute pulmonary edema—
Adults: 50 to 100 mg of ethacrynate sodium I.V. slowly over several minutes.
Edema—
Adults: 50 to 200 mg P.O. daily. Refractory cases may require up to 200 mg b.i.d.
Children: initial dose is 25 mg P.O., cautiously, increased in 25-mg increments daily until desired effect is achieved.

Italicized side effects are common or life-threatening.
*Liquid form contains alcohol.   **May contain tartrazine.

ADVERSE REACTIONS

Blood: *agranulocytosis,* neutropenia, thrombocytopenia.
CV: *volume depletion and dehydration,* orthostatic hypotension.
EENT: transient deafness with too-rapid I.V. injection.
GI: abdominal discomfort and pain, diarrhea.
Metabolic: *hypokalemia; hypochloremic alkalosis; asymptomatic hyperuricemia; fluid and electrolyte imbalances including dilutional hyponatremia, hypocalcemia, hypomagnesemia;* hyperglycemia and impairment of glucose tolerance.
Skin: dermatitis.

INTERACTIONS

Aminoglycoside antibiotics: potentiated ototoxic adverse reactions of both ethacrynic acid and aminoglycosides. Use together cautiously.
Warfarin: potentiated anticoagulant effect. Use together cautiously.

NURSING CONSIDERATIONS

• Contraindicated in anuria and in infants. Use cautiously in electrolyte abnormalities. If electrolyte imbalance, azotemia, or oliguria develops, may require stopping drug.
• This drug is a very potent diuretic.
• Monitor intake/output, weight, and serum electrolytes regularly.
• Consult with doctor and dietitian to provide high-potassium diet. Watch for signs of hypokalemia (for example, muscle weakness and cramps).
• Foods rich in potassium include citrus fruits, tomatoes, bananas, dates, and apricots.
• Patients also on digitalis have an increased risk of digitalis toxicity from the potassium-depleting effect.
• I.V. injection painful; may cause thrombophlebitis. Don't give subcutaneously or I.M. Give slowly through tubing of running infusion over several minutes.
• Sodium and potassium chloride supplement may be needed during therapy.
• Reconstitute vacuum vial with 50 ml of dextrose 5% injection or sodium chloride injection. Discard unused solution after 24 hours. Don't use cloudy or opalescent solutions.
• Elderly patients are especially susceptible to excessive diuresis.
• Give P.O. doses in a.m. to prevent nocturia.
• Severe diarrhea may necessitate discontinuing drug.
• Monitor blood uric acid, especially in patients with a history of gout.

furosemide
Agro-Furosemide, Furoside♦♦, Lasix**♦, Myrosemide, Novosemide♦♦, Uritol♦♦

Pregnancy Risk Category: C

MECHANISM OF ACTION
Inhibits reabsorption of sodium and chloride at the proximal portion of the ascending loop of Henle.

INDICATIONS & DOSAGE
Acute pulmonary edema—
Adults: 40 mg I.V. injected slowly; then 40 mg I.V. in 1 to 1½ hours if needed.
Edema—
Adults: 20 to 80 mg P.O. daily in a.m., second dose can be given in 6 to 8 hours; carefully titrated up to 600 mg daily if needed; or 20 to 40 mg I.M. or I.V. Increase by 20 mg q 2 hours until desired response is achieved. I.V. dose should be given slowly over 1 to 2 minutes.
Hypertension—
Adults: 40 mg P.O. b.i.d. Adjust dose according to response.
Infants and children: 2 mg/kg daily; dose increased by 1 to 2 mg/kg in 6 to 8 hours if needed; carefully titrated up to 6 mg/kg daily if needed.
Hypertensive crisis, acute renal failure—

Adults: 100 to 200 mg I.V. over 1 to 2 minutes.
Chronic renal failure—
Adults: initially, 80 mg P.O. daily. Increase by 80 to 120 mg daily until desired response is achieved.

ADVERSE REACTIONS
Blood: *agranulocytosis,* leukopenia, thrombocytopenia.
CV: *volume depletion and dehydration,* orthostatic hypotension.
EENT: transient deafness with too rapid I.V. injection.
GI: abdominal discomfort and pain, diarrhea (with oral solution).
Metabolic: *hypokalemia; hypochloremic alkalosis; asymptomatic hyperuricemia, fluid and electrolyte imbalances including dilutional hyponatremia, hypocalcemia, hypomagnesemia;* hyperglycemia and impairment of glucose tolerance.
Skin: dermatitis.

INTERACTIONS
Aminoglycoside antibiotics: potentiated ototoxicity. Use together cautiously.
Chloral hydrate: sweating, flushing with I.V. furosemide.
Clofibrate: enhanced furosemide effects. Use cautiously.
Indomethacin: inhibited diuretic response. Use cautiously.

NURSING CONSIDERATIONS
• Use cautiously in cardiogenic shock complicated by pulmonary edema, anuria, hepatic coma, or electrolyte imbalances. Drug is not routinely administered to women of childbearing age because its safety in pregnancy hasn't been established.
• Potent loop diuretic; can lead to profound water and electrolyte depletion. Monitor blood pressure and pulse rate during rapid diuresis.
• Sulfonamide-sensitive patients may have allergic reactions to furosemide.
• If oliguria or azotemia develops or

increases, may require stopping drug.
• Monitor serum electrolyte, BUN, and CO_2 frequently.
• Monitor serum potassium level. Watch for signs of hypokalemia (for example, muscle weakness and cramps). Patients also on digitalis have an increased risk of digitalis toxicity from the potassium-depleting effect.
• Consult with doctor and dietitian to provide high-potassium diet.
• Foods rich in potassium include citrus fruits, tomatoes, bananas, dates, and apricots.
• Monitor blood sugar in patients with diabetes. May treat severe hyperglycemia with oral antidiabetic agents.
• Monitor blood uric acid, especially in patients with a history of gout.
• Give I.V. doses over 1 to 2 minutes.
• Don't use parenteral route in infants and children unless oral dosage form is not practical.
• Give P.O. and I.M. preparations in a.m. to prevent nocturia. Give second doses in early afternoon.
• Elderly patients are especially susceptible to excessive diuresis, with potential for circulatory collapse and thromboembolic complications.
• Store tablets in light-resistant container to prevent discoloration (doesn't affect potency). Don't use discolored (yellow) injectable preparation. Oral furosemide solution should be stored in the refrigerator to ensure stability of the drug.
• Promotes calcium excretion. I.V. furosemide often used to treat hypercalcemia.
• Advise patients taking furosemide to stand slowly to prevent dizziness, and to limit alcohol intake and strenuous exercise in hot weather because these exacerbate orthostatic hypotension.
• Advise patients to report immediately ringing in ears, severe abdominal pain, or sore throat and fever; may

Italicized side effects are common or life-threatening.
*Liquid form contains alcohol.   **May contain tartrazine.

indicate furosemide toxicity.

• Discourage patients receiving furosemide therapy at home from storing different types of medication in the same container. This increases the risk of drug errors, especially for patients taking both furosemide and digoxin, since the most popular strengths of these drugs' pills are white tablets approximately equal in size.

• To prepare parenteral furosemide for I.V. infusion, mix drug with dextrose 5% in water, 0.9% sodium chloride solution, or lactated Ringer's solution. Use prepared infusion solution within 24 hours.

hydrochlorothiazide
Apo-Hydro◆◆, Diuchlor H◆◆, Esidrix◆, HydroDIURIL◆, Mictrin, Natrimax◆◆, Novohydrazide◆◆, Oretic, Thiuretic, Urozide◆◆

Pregnancy Risk Category: D

MECHANISM OF ACTION
Increases urine excretion of sodium and water by inhibiting sodium reabsorption in the cortical diluting site of the nephron.

INDICATIONS & DOSAGE
Edema—
Adults: initially, 25 to 100 mg P.O. daily or intermittently for maintenance dosage.
Children over 6 months: 2.2 mg/kg P.O. daily divided b.i.d.
Children under 6 months: up to 3.3 mg/kg P.O. daily divided b.i.d.
Hypertension—
Adults: 25 to 100 mg P.O. daily or divided dosage. Daily dosage increased or decreased according to blood pressure.

ADVERSE REACTIONS
Blood: *aplastic anemia, agranulocytosis,* leukopenia, thrombocytopenia.
CV: *volume depletion and dehydra-*tion, orthostatic hypotension.
GI: anorexia, nausea, pancreatitis.
Hepatic: hepatic encephalopathy.
Metabolic: *hypokalemia, asymptomatic hyperuricemia, hyperglycemia and impairment of glucose tolerance,* fluid and electrolyte imbalances including dilutional hyponatremia and hypochloremia, metabolic alkalosis, hypercalcemia, gout.
Skin: dermatitis, photosensitivity, rash.
Other: hypersensitivity reactions, such as pneumonitis and vasculitis.

INTERACTIONS
Cholestyramine, colestipol: intestinal absorption of thiazides decreased. Keep doses as separate as possible.
Diazoxide: increased antihypertensive, hyperglycemic, and hyperuricemic effects. Use together cautiously.

NURSING CONSIDERATIONS
• Contraindicated in anuria or hypersensitivity to other thiazides or other sulfonamide derivatives. Use cautiously in severe renal disease, impaired hepatic function, and progressive hepatic disease.
• Monitor intake/output, weight, and serum electrolytes regularly.
• Consult with doctor and dietitian to provide high-potassium diet. Watch for hypokalemia (for example, muscle weakness and cramps). Patients also on digitalis have an increased risk of digitalis toxicity from the potassium-depleting effect of this diuretic. May use with potassium-sparing diuretic to prevent potassium loss.
• Foods rich in potassium include citrus fruits, tomatoes, bananas, dates, and apricots.
• Monitor serum creatinine and BUN regularly. Not as effective if these levels are more than twice normal.
• Monitor blood uric acid, especially in patients with a history of gout.
• Check insulin requirements in pa-

tients with diabetes. May treat severe hyperglycemia with oral antidiabetic agents.
• In hypertension, therapeutic response may be delayed several days.
• Give in a.m. to prevent nocturia. Studies have shown that the drug is as effective when administered once daily as it is when given more frequently.
• Elderly patients are especially susceptible to excessive diuresis.
• Thiazides and thiazide-like diuretics should be stopped before tests for parathyroid function are performed.

---

hydroflumethiazide
Diucardin, Saluron

Pregnancy Risk Category: B

MECHANISM OF ACTION
Increases urine excretion of sodium and water by inhibiting sodium reabsorption in the cortical diluting site of the ascending loop of Henle.

INDICATIONS & DOSAGE
Edema—
Adults: 25 to 200 mg P.O. daily in divided doses. Maintenance dosages may be on intermittent or alternate-day schedule.
Children: 1 mg/kg P.O. daily.
Hypertension—
Adults: 50 to 100 mg P.O. daily or b.i.d.

ADVERSE REACTIONS
Blood: *aplastic anemia, agranulocytosis,* leukopenia, thrombocytopenia.
CV: *volume depletion and dehydration,* orthostatic hypotension.
GI: anorexia, nausea, pancreatitis.
Hepatic: hepatic encephalopathy.
Metabolic: *hypokalemia, asymptomatic hyperuricemia, hyperglycemia and impairment of glucose tolerance,* fluid and electrolyte imbalances including dilutional hyponatremia and hypochloremia, metabolic alkalosis,

hypercalcemia, gout.
Skin: dermatitis, photosensitivity, rash.
Other: hypersensitivity reactions, such as pneumonitis and vasculitis.

INTERACTIONS
Cholestyramine, colestipol: intestinal absorption of thiazides decreased. Keep doses as separate as possible.
Diazoxide: increased antihypertensive, hyperglycemic, and hyperuricemic effects. Use together cautiously.

NURSING CONSIDERATIONS
• Contraindicated in anuria or hypersensitivity to other thiazides or other sulfonamide-derived drugs. Use cautiously in severe renal disease, impaired hepatic function, and progressive hepatic disease.
• Monitor intake/output, weight, and serum electrolytes regularly.
• Consult with doctor and dietitian to provide high-potassium diet. Foods rich in potassium include citrus fruits, tomatoes, bananas, dates, and apricots. Watch for hypokalemia (for example, muscle weakness and cramps). May use with potassium-sparing diuretic to prevent potassium loss. Patients also on digitalis have an increased risk of digitalis toxicity from the potassium-depleting effects of this diuretic.
• Monitor serum creatinine and BUN regularly. Not as effective if these levels are more than twice normal.
• Monitor blood uric acid, especially in patients with a history of gout.
• Check insulin requirements in patients with diabetes. May treat severe hyperglycemia with oral antidiabetic agents.
• Give in a.m. to prevent nocturia.
• In hypertension, therapeutic response may be delayed several days.
• Elderly patients are especially susceptible to excessive diuresis.
• Thiazides and thiazide-like diuret-

---

ics should be stopped before tests for parathyroid function are performed.

indapamide
Lozide♦♦, Lozol

Pregnancy Risk Category: B

MECHANISM OF ACTION
Inhibits sodium reabsorption in the cortical diluting site of the nephron. Also has a direct vasodilating effect that may be a result of calcium channel-blocking action.

INDICATIONS & DOSAGE
Edema, hypertension—
Adults: 2.5 mg P.O. as a single daily dose taken in the morning. Dosage may be increased to 5 mg daily.

ADVERSE REACTIONS
CNS: headache, irritability, nervousness.
CV: *volume depletion and dehydration,* orthostatic hypotension.
GI: anorexia, nausea, pancreatitis.
Metabolic: *hypokalemia; asymptomatic hyperuricemia;* fluid and electrolyte imbalances, including dilutional hyponatremia and hypochloremia; metabolic alkalosis; gout.
Skin: dermatitis, photosensitivity, rash.
Other: muscle cramps and spasms.

INTERACTIONS
Diazoxide: increased antihypertensive, hyperglycemic, and hyperuricemic effects. Use together cautiously.

NURSING CONSIDERATIONS
• Contraindicated in anuria or hypersensitivity to other sulfonamide-derived drugs.
• Use cautiously in severe renal disease, impaired hepatic function, and progressive hepatic disease.
• Monitor intake/output, weight, and serum electrolytes regularly.

• Consult with doctor and dietitian to provide high-potassium diet. Foods rich in potassium include citrus fruits, tomatoes, bananas, dates, and apricots. Watch for symptoms of hypokalemia (for example, muscle weakness and cramps). May use with potassium-sparing diuretic to prevent potassium loss. Patients also receiving digitalis have an increased risk of digitalis toxicity from the potassium-depleting effects of this diuretic.
• Monitor serum creatinine and BUN regularly. Not as effective if these levels are more than twice normal.
• Monitor blood uric acid level, especially in patients with a history of gout.
• Check insulin requirements in patients with diabetes. May treat severe hyperglycemia with oral antidiabetic agents.
• Give in a.m. to prevent nocturia.
• In hypertension, therapeutic response may be delayed several days.
• Elderly patients are especially susceptible to excessive diuresis.
• Thiazides and thiazide-like diuretics should be stopped before tests for parathyroid function are performed.

mannitol
Osmitrol♦♦

Pregnancy Risk Category: C

MECHANISM OF ACTION
Increases the osmotic pressure of glomerular filtrate, inhibiting tubular reabsorption of water and electrolytes. Also elevates blood plasma osmolality, resulting in enhanced flow of water into extracellular fluid.

INDICATIONS & DOSAGE
Test dose for marked oliguria or suspected inadequate renal function—
Adults and children over age 12: 200 mg/kg or 12.5 g as a 15% or 20% solution I.V. over 3 to 5 minutes. Response adequate if 30 to 50 ml urine/

hour is excreted over 2 to 3 hours.
Treatment of oliguria—
Adults and children over age 12:
50 to 100 g I.V. as a 15% to 20% solution over 90 minutes to several hours.
Prevention of oliguria or acute renal failure—
Adults and children over age 12:
50 to 100 g I.V. of a concentrated (5% to 25%) solution. Exact concentration is determined by fluid requirements.
Edema—
Adults and children over age 12:
100 g as a 10% to 20% solution over 2- to 6-hour period.
To reduce intraocular pressure or intracranial pressure—
Adults and children over age 12:
1.5 to 2 g/kg as a 15% to 25% solution I.V. over 30 to 60 minutes.
To promote diuresis in drug intoxication—
Adults and children over age 12:
5% to 10% solution continuously up to 200 g I.V., while maintaining 100 to 500 ml urine output/hour and a positive fluid balance.

ADVERSE REACTIONS
CNS: rebound increase in intracranial pressure 8 to 12 hours after diuresis, headache, confusion.
CV: *transient expansion of plasma volume during infusion causing circulatory overload and pulmonary edema,* tachycardia, angina-like chest pain.
EENT: blurred vision, rhinitis.
GI: thirst, nausea, vomiting.
GU: urine retention.
Metabolic: *fluid and electrolyte imbalance, water intoxication, cellular dehydration.*

INTERACTIONS
None significant.

NURSING CONSIDERATIONS
• Contraindicated in anuria, severe pulmonary congestion, frank pulmonary edema, severe congestive heart

disease, severe dehydration, metabolic edema, progressive renal disease or dysfunction, progressive heart failure during administration, or active intracranial bleeding except during craniotomy.
• Monitor vital signs (including central venous pressure) at least hourly; intake/output hourly (report increasing oliguria). Monitor: weight, renal function, fluid balance, serum and urine sodium and potassium levels daily.
• Solution often crystallizes, especially at low temperatures. To redissolve, warm bottle in hot water bath, shake vigorously. Cool to body temperature before giving. Concentrations greater than 15% have greater tendency to crystallize. Do not use solution with undissolved crystals.
• Infusions should always be given I.V. via an in-line filter.
• Avoid infiltration; observe for inflammation, edema, and necrosis.
• For maximum intraocular pressure reduction before surgery, give 1 to 1½ hours preoperatively.
• Can be used to measure glomerular filtration rate.
• Give frequent mouth care or fluids as permitted to relieve thirst.
• Urethral catheter is inserted in comatose or incontinent patients because therapy is based on strict evaluation of intake and output. In patients with urethral catheters, use an hourly urometer collection bag to facilitate accurate evaluation of output.

methazolamide
Neptazane♦

Pregnancy Risk Category: C

MECHANISM OF ACTION
Decreases secretion of aqueous humor in the eye, thereby lowering intraocular pressure.

INDICATIONS & DOSAGE
Glaucoma (open-angle, or preoperatively in obstructive or narrow-angle)—
Adults: 50 to 100 mg b.i.d. or t.i.d.

ADVERSE REACTIONS
Blood: *aplastic anemia,* hemolytic anemia, leukopenia.
CNS: drowsiness, paresthesias.
EENT: transient myopia.
GI: nausea, vomiting, anorexia.
GU: crystalluria, renal calculi.
Metabolic: *hyperchloremic acidosis,* hypokalemia, asymptomatic hyperuricemia.
Skin: rash.

INTERACTIONS
None significant.

NURSING CONSIDERATIONS
• Contraindicated in severe or absolute glaucoma; for long-term use in chronic noncongestive narrow-angle glaucoma; in patients with depressed sodium or potassium serum, renal or hepatic disease or dysfunction, adrenal gland dysfunction, or hyperchloremic acidosis. Use cautiously in respiratory acidosis, emphysema, chronic pulmonary disease.
• Monitor intake/output, weight, and serum electrolytes frequently.
• May cause false-positive urine protein tests by alkalinizing urine.
• A carbonic anhydrase inhibitor.
• Elderly patients are especially susceptible to excessive diuresis.
• Diuretic effect decreases in acidosis.
• Anticipate that drug will be given every day for glaucoma but intermittently for edema. Caution patient to comply with prescribed dosage and schedule to lessen risk of metabolic acidosis.
• Carefully evaluate the patient with glaucoma for eye pain to make sure drug is effective in decreasing intraocular pressure.

methyclothiazide
Aquatensen, Duretic♦♦, Enduron
Pregnancy Risk Category: D

MECHANISM OF ACTION
Increases urine excretion of sodium and water by inhibiting sodium reabsorption in the cortical diluting site of the nephron.

INDICATIONS & DOSAGE
Edema, hypertension—
Adults: 2.5 to 10 mg P.O daily.

ADVERSE REACTIONS
Blood: *aplastic anemia, agranulocytosis,* leukopenia, thrombocytopenia.
CV: *volume depletion and dehydration,* orthostatic hypotension.
GI: anorexia, nausea, pancreatitis.
Hepatic: hepatic encephalopathy.
Metabolic: *hypokalemia, asymptomatic hyperuricemia, hyperglycemia and impairment of glucose tolerance,* fluid and electrolyte imbalances including dilutional hyponatremia and hypochloremia, metabolic alkalosis, hypercalcemia, gout.
Skin: dermatitis, photosensitivity, rash.
Other: hypersensitivity reactions, such as pneumonitis and vasculitis.

INTERACTIONS
Cholestyramine, colestipol: intestinal absorption of thiazides decreased. Keep doses as separate as possible.
Diazoxide: increased antihypertensive, hyperglycemic, and hyperuricemic effects. Use together cautiously.

NURSING CONSIDERATIONS
• Contraindicated in renal decompensation; anuria; or hypersensitivity to other thiazides or other sulfonamide-derived drugs. Use cautiously in potassium depletion, renal disease or dysfunction, impaired hepatic function, and progressive hepatic disease.

• Monitor intake/output, weight, and serum electrolytes regularly.
• Consult with doctor and dietitian to provide high-potassium diet. Foods rich in potassium include citrus fruits, tomatoes, bananas, dates, and apricots. Watch for hypokalemia (for example, muscle weakness and cramps). Patients also on digitalis have an increased risk of digitalis toxicity from the potassium-depleting effect of this diuretic. May use with potassium-sparing diuretic to prevent potassium loss.
• Check insulin requirements in patients with diabetes. May treat severe hyperglycemia with oral antidiabetic agents.
• Monitor serum creatinine and BUN regularly. Not as effective if these level are more than twice normal.
• Monitor blood uric acid, especially in patients with a history of gout.
• In hypertension, therapeutic response may be delayed several days.
• Give in a.m. to prevent nocturia.
• Elderly patients are especially susceptible to excessive diuresis.
• Thiazides and thiazide-like diuretics should be stopped before tests for parathyroid function are performed.

metolazone
Diulo, Microx, Zaroxolyn**◆
Pregnancy Risk Category: D

MECHANISM OF ACTION
Increases urine excretion of sodium and water by inhibiting sodium reabsorption in the cortical diluting site of the ascending loop of Henle.

INDICATIONS & DOSAGE
Edema (heart failure)—
Adults: 5 to 10 mg P.O. daily.
Edema (renal disease)—
Adults: 5 to 20 mg P.O. daily.
Hypertension—
Adults: 2.5 to 5 mg P.O. daily. Maintenance dosage determined by pa-

tient's blood pressure.

ADVERSE REACTIONS
Blood: *aplastic anemia, agranulocytosis,* leukopenia, thrombocytopenia.
CV: *volume depletion and dehydration,* orthostatic hypotension.
GI: anorexia, nausea, pancreatitis.
Hepatic: hepatic encephalopathy.
Metabolic: *hypokalemia, asymptomatic hyperuricemia, hyperglycemia and impairment of glucose tolerance,* fluid and electrolyte imbalances including dilutional hyponatremia and hypochloremia, metabolic alkalosis, hypercalcemia, gout.
Skin: dermatitis, photosensitivity, rash.
Other: hypersensitivity reactions, such as pneumonitis and vasculitis.

INTERACTIONS
Cholestyramine, colestipol: intestinal absorption of thiazides decreased. Keep doses as separate as possible.
Diazoxide: increased antihypertensive, hyperglycemic, and hyperuricemic effects. Use together cautiously.

NURSING CONSIDERATIONS
• Contraindicated in anuria; hepatic coma or precoma; or hypersensitivity to thiazides or other sulfonamide-derived drugs. Use cautiously in hyperuricemia or gout and severely impaired renal function.
• Monitor intake/output, weight, and serum electrolytes regularly.
• Consult with doctor and dietitian to provide high-potassium diet. Foods rich in potassium include citrus fruits, tomatoes, bananas, dates, and apricots. Watch for hypokalemia (for example, muscle weakness and cramps). Patients also on digitalis may have an increased risk of digitalis toxicity from the potassium-depleting effect of this diuretic. May use with potassium-sparing diuretic to prevent potassium loss.

- Check insulin requirements in patients with diabetes. May treat severe hyperglycemia with oral antidiabetic agents.
- Monitor blood uric acid, especially in patients with a history of gout.
- In hypertension, therapeutic response may be delayed several days.
- Give in a.m. to prevent nocturia.
- Elderly patients are especially susceptible to excessive diuresis.
- A thiazide-related diuretic. However, unlike thiazide diuretics, metolazone is effective in patients with decreased renal function.
- Used as an adjunct in furosemide-resistant edema.
- Thiazides and thiazide-like diuretics should be stopped before tests for parathyroid function are performed.

polythiazide
Renese

Pregnancy Risk Category: D

MECHANISM OF ACTION
Increases urine excretion of sodium and water by inhibiting sodium reabsorption in the cortical diluting site of the nephron.

INDICATIONS & DOSAGE
Hypertension—
Adults: 2 to 4 mg P.O. daily.
Edema (heart failure, renal failure)—
Adults: 1 to 4 mg P.O. daily.

ADVERSE REACTIONS
Blood: *aplastic anemia, agranulocytosis,* leukopenia, thrombocytopenia.
CV: *volume depletion and dehydration,* orthostatic hypotension.
GI: anorexia, nausea, pancreatitis.
Hepatic: hepatic encephalopathy.
Metabolic: *hypokalemia, asymptomatic hyperuricemia, hyperglycemia and impairment of glucose tolerance,* fluid and electrolyte imbalances including dilutional hyponatremia and hypochloremia, metabolic alkalosis, hypercalcemia, gout.
Skin: dermatitis, photosensitivity, rash.
Other: hypersensitivity reactions, such as pneumonitis and vasculitis.

INTERACTIONS
Cholestyramine, colestipol: intestinal absorption of thiazides decreased. Keep doses as separate as possible. *Diazoxide:* increased antihypertensive, hyperglycemic, and hyperuricemic effects. Use together cautiously.

NURSING CONSIDERATIONS
- Contraindicated in anuria or hypersensitivity to other thiazides or other sulfonamide-derived drugs. Use cautiously in severe renal disease, impaired hepatic function, and allergies.
- Monitor intake/output, weight, and serum electrolytes regularly.
- Consult with doctor and dietitian to provide high-potassium diet. Foods rich in potassium include citrus fruits, tomatoes, bananas, dates, and apricots. Watch for hypokalemia (for example, muscle weakness and cramps). Patients also on digitalis may have an increased risk of digitalis toxicity from the potassium-depleting effect of this diuretic. May use with potassium-sparing diuretic to prevent potassium loss.
- Monitor blood uric acid, especially in patients with a history of gout.
- Check insulin requirements in patients with diabetes. May treat severe hyperglycemia with oral antidiabetic agents.
- In hypertension, therapeutic response may be delayed several days.
- Give in a.m. to prevent nocturia.
- Elderly patients are especially susceptible to excessive diuresis.
- Thiazides and thiazide-like diuretics should be stopped before tests for parathyroid function are performed.

quinethazone
Hydromox

Pregnancy Risk Category: D

MECHANISM OF ACTION
Increases urine excretion of sodium and water by inhibiting sodium reabsorption in the cortical diluting site of the nephron.

INDICATIONS & DOSAGE
Management of edema or hypertension—
Adults: 50 to 100 mg P.O. daily or 50 mg P.O. b.i.d. Occasionally, up to 150 to 200 mg P.O. daily may be needed.

ADVERSE REACTIONS
Blood: *aplastic anemia, agranulocytosis,* leukopenia, thrombocytopenia.
CV: *volume depletion and dehydration,* orthostatic hypotension.
GI: anorexia, nausea, pancreatitis.
Hepatic: hepatic encephalopathy.
Metabolic: *hypokalemia, asymptomatic hyperuricemia, hyperglycemia and impairment of glucose tolerance,* fluid and electrolyte imbalances including dilutional hyponatremia and hypochloremia, metabolic alkalosis, hypercalcemia, gout.
Skin: dermatitis, photosensitivity, rash.
Other: hypersensitivity reactions, such as pneumonitis and vasculitis.

INTERACTIONS
Cholestyramine, colestipol: intestinal absorption of thiazides decreased. Keep doses as separate as possible.
Diazoxide: increased antihypertensive, hyperglycemic, and hyperuricemic effects. Use together cautiously.

NURSING CONSIDERATIONS
• Contraindicated in anuria or hypersensitivity to quinethazones, thiazides, or other sulfonamide-derived drugs. Use cautiously in severe renal disease, impaired hepatic function, and allergies.
• Monitor intake/output, weight, and serum electrolytes regularly.
• Consult with doctor and dietitian to provide high-potassium diet. Foods rich in potassium include citrus fruits, tomatoes, bananas, dates, and apricots. Watch for hypokalemia (for example, muscle weakness and cramps). Patients also on digitalis have an increased risk of digitalis toxicity from the potassium-depleting effect of this diuretic. May use with potassium-sparing diuretic to prevent potassium loss.
• Monitor serum creatinine and BUN regularly.
• Check insulin requirements in patients with diabetes. May treat severe hyperglycemia with oral hypoglycemics.
• Monitor blood uric acid, especially in patients with a history of gout.
• In hypertension, therapeutic response may be delayed several days.
• Give in a.m. to prevent nocturia.
• Elderly patients are especially susceptible to excessive diuresis.
• Thiazides and thiazide-like diuretics should be stopped before tests for parathyroid function are performed.

spironolactone
Aldactone♦, Novospiroton♦♦, Sincomen♦♦

Pregnancy Risk Category: D

MECHANISM OF ACTION
Antagonizes aldosterone in the distal tubule, increasing excretion of sodium and water but sparing potassium.

INDICATIONS & DOSAGE
Edema—
Adults: 25 to 200 mg P.O. daily in divided doses.
Children: initially, 3.3 mg/kg P.O. daily in divided doses.

Italicized side effects are common or life-threatening.
*Liquid form contains alcohol.   **May contain tartrazine.

Hypertension—
Adults: 50 to 100 mg P.O. daily in divided doses.
Treatment of diuretic-induced hypokalemia—
Adults: 25 to 100 mg P.O. daily when oral potassium supplements are considered inappropriate.
Detection of primary hyperaldosteronism—
Adults: 400 mg P.O. daily for 4 days (short test) or 3 to 4 weeks (long test). If hypokalemia and hypertension are corrected, a presumptive diagnosis of primary hyperaldosteronism is made.

ADVERSE REACTIONS
CNS: headache.
GI: anorexia, nausea, diarrhea.
Metabolic: *hyperkalemia,* dehydration, hyponatremia, transient elevation in BUN, acidosis.
Skin: urticaria.
Other: gynecomastia in men, breast soreness and menstrual disturbances in women.

INTERACTIONS
Aspirin: possible blocked spironolactone effect. Watch for diminished spironolactone response.

NURSING CONSIDERATIONS
• Contraindicated in anuria, acute or progressive renal insufficiency, or hyperkalemia. Use cautiously in fluid or electrolyte imbalances, impaired renal function, and hepatic disease.
• A mild acidosis may occur during therapy. This may be dangerous in patients with hepatic cirrhosis.
• Monitor serum electrolytes, intake/output, weight, and blood pressure regularly.
• Potassium-sparing diuretic; useful as an adjunct to other diuretic therapy. Less potent diuretic than thiazide and loop types. Diuretic effect delayed 2 to 3 days when used alone.
• Maximum antihypertensive response may be delayed up to 2 weeks.

• Warn patient to avoid excessive ingestion of potassium-rich foods or potassium-containing salt substitutes. Concomitant potassium supplement can lead to serious hyperkalemia.
• Elderly patients are more susceptible to excessive diuresis.
• Protect drug from light.
• Breast cancer reported in some patients taking spironolactone, but cause-and-effect relationship not confirmed. Warn against taking drug indiscriminately.
• Give with meals to enhance absorption.
• Because of its antiandrogenic properties, spironolactone has been prescribed to treat hirsutism. The dose for this indication is 200 mg daily.

---

triamterene
Dyrenium♦
Pregnancy Risk Category: D

MECHANISM OF ACTION
Inhibits sodium reabsorption and potassium excretion by direct action on the distal tubule.

INDICATIONS & DOSAGE
Diuresis—
Adults: initially, 100 mg P.O. b.i.d. after meals. Total daily dosage should not exceed 300 mg.

ADVERSE REACTIONS
Blood: megaloblastic anemia related to low folic acid levels.
CNS: dizziness.
CV: hypotension.
EENT: sore throat.
GI: dry mouth, nausea, vomiting.
Metabolic: *hyperkalemia,* dehydration, hyponatremia, transient elevation in BUN, acidosis.
Skin: photosensitivity, rash.
Other: *anaphylaxis,* muscle cramps.

INTERACTIONS
None significant.

NURSING CONSIDERATIONS
• Contraindicated in anuria, severe or progressive renal disease or dysfunction, severe hepatic disease, or hyperkalemia. Use cautiously in impaired hepatic function, diabetes mellitus, pregnancy, or lactation.
• Watch for blood dyscrasias.
• Monitor BUN and serum electrolytes.
• A potassium-sparing diuretic, useful as an adjunct to other diuretic therapy. Less potent than thiazides and loop diuretics. Full diuretic effect delayed 2 to 3 days when used alone.
• Warn patients to avoid excessive ingestion of potassium-rich foods or potassium-containing salt substitutes. Concomitant potassium supplement can lead to serious hyperkalemia.
• Give medication after meals to prevent nausea.
• Withdraw gradually to prevent excessive rebound potassium excretion.

---

trichlormethiazide
Metahydrin**, Naqua
Pregnancy Risk Category: D

MECHANISM OF ACTION
Increases urine excretion of sodium and water by inhibiting sodium reabsorption in the cortical diluting site of the nephron.

INDICATIONS & DOSAGE
Edema—
Adults: 1 to 4 mg P.O. daily or in two divided doses.
Hypertension—
Adults: 2 to 4 mg P.O. daily.

ADVERSE REACTIONS
Blood: *aplastic anemia, agranulocytosis,* leukopenia, thrombocytopenia.
CV: *volume depletion and dehydration,* orthostatic hypotension.
GI: anorexia, nausea, pancreatitis.
Hepatic: hepatic encephalopathy.
Metabolic: *hypokalemia, asymptom-*

atic hyperuricemia, hyperglycemia and impairment of glucose tolerance, fluid and electrolyte imbalances including dilutional hyponatremia and hypochloremia, metabolic alkalosis, hypercalcemia, gout.
Skin: dermatitis, photosensitivity, rash.
Other: hypersensitivity reactions, such as pneumonitis and vasculitis.

INTERACTIONS
Cholestyramine, colestipol: intestinal absorption of thiazides decreased. Keep doses as separate as possible.
Diazoxide: increased antihypertensive, hyperglycemic, and hyperuricemic effects. Use together cautiously.

NURSING CONSIDERATIONS
• Contraindicated in anuria or hypersensitivity to other thiazides or other sulfonamide-derived drugs. Use cautiously in severe renal disease, and impaired hepatic function.
• Monitor intake/output, weight, and serum electrolytes regularly.
• Consult with doctor and dietitian to provide high-potassium diet. Foods rich in potassium include citrus fruits, tomatoes, bananas, dates, and apricots. Watch for hypokalemia (for example, muscle weakness and cramps). Patients also on digitalis have an increased risk of digitalis toxicity from the potassium-depleting effect of this diuretic. May use with potassium-sparing diuretic to prevent hypokalemia.
• Monitor serum creatinine and BUN regularly. Not as effective if these levels are more than twice normal.
• Check insulin requirements in patients with diabetes. May treat severe hyperglycemia with oral antidiabetic agents. Monitor blood sugar.
• Monitor blood uric acid, especially in patients with a history of gout.
• In hypertension, therapeutic response may be delayed several days.

Italicized side effects are common or life-threatening.
*Liquid form contains alcohol.   **May contain tartrazine.

- Give in a.m. to prevent nocturia.
- Elderly patients are especially susceptible to excessive diuresis.
- Thiazides and thiazide-like diuretics should be stopped before tests for parathyroid function are performed.

urea (carbamide)
Ureaphil

Pregnancy Risk Category: C

MECHANISM OF ACTION
Increases the osmotic pressure of glomerular filtrate, inhibiting tubular reabsorption of water and electrolytes. Also elevates blood plasma osmolality, resulting in enhanced flow of water into extracellular fluid.

INDICATIONS & DOSAGE
Intracranial or intraocular pressure—
Adults: 1 to 1.5 g/kg as a 30% solution by slow I.V. infusion over 1 to 2.5 hours.
Children over 2 years: 0.5 to 1.5 g/kg slow I.V. infusion.
Children under 2 years: as little as 0.1 g/kg slow I.V. infusion. Maximum rate is 4 ml/minute.

Maximum adult daily dosage is 120 g. To prepare 135 ml 30% solution, mix contents of 40-g vial of urea with 105 ml dextrose 5% or 10% in water or 10% invert sugar in water. Each ml of 30% solution provides 300 mg urea.

ADVERSE REACTIONS
CNS: *headache.*
CV: tachycardia, congestive heart failure, *pulmonary edema.*
GI: *nausea, vomiting.*
Metabolic: sodium and potassium depletion.
Local: irritation or necrotic sloughing may occur with extravasation.

INTERACTIONS
None significant.

NURSING CONSIDERATIONS
- Contraindicated in severely impaired renal function, marked dehydration, frank hepatic failure, or active intracranial bleeding. Use cautiously in pregnancy, lactation, cardiac disease, hepatic impairment, and sickle cell disease with CNS involvement.
- Avoid rapid I.V. infusion; may cause hemolysis or increased capillary bleeding. Avoid extravasation; may cause reactions ranging from mild irritation to necrosis.
- Don't infuse into leg veins; may cause phlebitis or thrombosis, especially in elderly patients.
- Watch for hyponatremia or hypokalemia (muscle weakness, lethargy); may indicate electrolyte depletion before serum levels are reduced.
- Maintain adequate hydration; monitor intake/output and serum electrolytes.
- In renal disease, monitor BUN frequently.
- Indwelling urethral catheter should be used in comatose patients to ensure bladder emptying. Use an hourly urometer collection bag to facilitate accurate evaluation of diuresis.
- If satisfactory diuresis does not occur in 6 to 12 hours, urea should be discontinued and renal function reevaluated.
- Use freshly reconstituted urea only for I.V. infusion; solution becomes ammonia upon standing.
- Use within minutes of reconstitution.
- Assess breath sounds for crackles, indicating pulmonary edema.

64

Electrolytes and replacement solutions

calcium chloride
calcium gluceptate
calcium gluconate◇
calcium lactate
dextran (low molecular weight)
dextran (high molecular weight)
hetastarch
magnesium sulfate
potassium acetate
potassium bicarbonate
potassium chloride
potassium gluconate
potassium phosphate
Ringer's injection
Ringer's injection, lactated
sodium chloride

COMBINATION PRODUCTS
GRAMCAL♦♦: calcium lactate-gluconate 3,080 mg, calcium carbonate 1,500 mg, and potassium 390 mg; provides 1,000 mg of elemental calcium.
KAOCHLOR-EFF: 20 mEq potassium, 20 mEq chloride (from potassium chloride, potassium citrate, potassium bicarbonate, and betaine hydrochloride).
KLORVESS*: 20 mEq each potassium and chloride (from potassium chloride, potassium bicarbonate, and l-lysine monohydrochloride).
KOLYUM: 20 mEq potassium, 3.4 mEq chloride (from potassium gluconate and potassium chloride).
NEUTRA-PHOS: phosphorus 250 mg, sodium 164 mg, potassium 278 mg (from dibasic and monobasic sodium and potassium phosphate).
TWIN-K-CL: 15 ml supplies 15 mEq of potassium ions as a combination of potassium gluconate, potassium citrate, and ammonium chloride.

---

calcium chloride

calcium gluceptate

calcium gluconate◇

calcium lactate

Pregnancy Risk Category: C

MECHANISM OF ACTION
Replaces and maintains calcium.

INDICATIONS & DOSAGE
Hypocalcemia, hypocalcemic tetany, hypocalcemia during exchange transfusions, cardiac resuscitation for inotropic effect when epinephrine has failed; magnesium intoxication; hypoparathyroidism—
Adults and children: initially 500 mg to 1 g calcium salt I.V., with further dosage based on serum calcium determinations and specific calcium salt. See below for dosages with specific calcium salts.
   Dosage with calcium chloride (1 g [10 ml] yields 13.5 mEq Ca^{++}):
Magnesium intoxication—
Adults and children: initially 500 mg I.V., with further doses based on calcium and magnesium determinations.
Cardiac arrest—
0.5 to 1 g I.V., not to exceed 1 ml/minute; or 200 to 800 mg into the ventricular cavity.
Hypocalcemia—
500 mg to 1 g I.V. at intervals of 1 to 3

Italicized side effects are common or life-threatening.
*Liquid form contains alcohol.   **May contain tartrazine.

days, determined by serum calcium levels.

Dosage with calcium gluconate (1 g [10 ml] yields 4.5 mEq Ca^{++}):
Hypocalcemia—
Adults: 500 mg to 1 g I.V., repeated q 1 to 3 days p.r.n. as determined by serum calcium levels. Further doses depend on serum calcium determinations.
Children: 500 mg/kg I.V. daily. Rate of infusion should not exceed 0.5 ml/minute.

Dosage with calcium gluceptate (1.1 g [5 ml] yields 4.5 mEq Ca^{++}) and calcium salts (18 mg [1 ml] yields 0.898 mEq Ca^{++}):
Hypocalcemia—
Adults: initially 5 to 20 ml I.V., with further doses based on serum calcium determinations. If I.V. injection is impossible, 2 to 5 ml I.M. Average adult oral dose is 1 to 2 g elemental calcium P.O. daily, divided t.i.d. or q.i.d. Average oral dose for children is 45 to 65 mg/kg P.O. daily, divided t.i.d. or q.i.d.
During exchange transfusions—
Adults and children: 0.5 ml I.V. after each 100 ml blood exchanged.

ADVERSE REACTIONS
CNS: from I.V. use, tingling sensations, sense of oppression or heat waves; with rapid I.V. injection, syncope.
CV: mild fall in blood pressure; with rapid I.V. injection, vasodilation, *bradycardia, cardiac dysrhythmias, cardiac arrest.*
GI: with oral ingestion, irritation, hemorrhage, *constipation;* with I.V. administration, chalky taste; with oral calcium chloride, GI hemorrhage, nausea, vomiting, thirst, abdominal pain.
GU: hypercalcemia, polyuria, renal calculi.
Skin: local reaction if calcium salts given I.M., burning, necrosis, tissue sloughing, cellulitis, soft tissue calci-

fication.
Local: with S.C. injection, pain and irritation; *with I.V., vein irritation.*

INTERACTIONS
Cardiac glycosides: increased digitalis toxicity; administer calcium very cautiously (if at all) to digitalized patients.

NURSING CONSIDERATIONS
• Contraindicated in ventricular fibrillation, hypercalcemia, or renal calculi. Use cautiously in patients with sarcoidosis and renal or cardiac disease, and in digitalized patients. Use calcium chloride cautiously in cor pulmonale, respiratory acidosis, and respiratory failure.
• Monitor ECG when giving calcium I.V. Such injections should not exceed 0.7 to 1.5 mEq/minute. Stop if patient complains of discomfort. Following I.V. injection, patient should remain recumbent for a short while.
• I.M. injection should be given in the gluteal region in adults; lateral thigh in infants. I.M. route used only in emergencies when no I.V. route available.
• Monitor blood calcium frequently. Report abnormalities.
• Hypercalcemia may result after large doses in chronic renal failure.
• If possible, administer I.V. into a large vein.
• I.V. route usually recommended in children, but not by scalp vein (can cause tissue necrosis).
• Solutions should be warmed to body temperature before administration.
• Calcium chloride should be given I.V. only. When adding to parenteral solutions that contain other additives, observe closely for precipitate.
• Severe necrosis and tissue sloughing follow extravasation. Calcium gluconate is less irritating to veins and tissues than calcium chloride.

• Following injection, patient should be recumbent for 15 minutes.
• If GI upset occurs, give oral calcium products 1 to 1½ hours after meals.
• Oxalic acid (found in rhubarb and spinach), phytic acid (in bran and whole cereals), and phosphorus (in milk and dairy products) may interfere with absorption of calcium.
• Crash carts usually contain both gluconate and chloride. Make sure doctor specifies form he wants administered.

---

dextran
(low molecular weight)
Dextran 40♦, Gentran 40♦, Rheomacrodex♦

Pregnancy Risk Category: C

MECHANISM OF ACTION
Expands plasma volume and provides fluid replacement.

INDICATIONS & DOSAGE
Plasma volume expansion—
Dosage of 10% solution by I.V. infusion depends on amount of fluid loss.
First 500 ml of Dextran 40 may be infused rapidly with central venous pressure monitoring. Infuse remaining dose slowly. Total daily dosage not to exceed 2 g/kg body weight. If therapy continued past 24 hours, do not exceed 1 g/kg daily. Continue for no longer than 5 days.
Reduction of blood sludging—
500 ml of 10% solution by I.V. infusion.

ADVERSE REACTIONS
Blood: *decreased level of hemoglobin and hematocrit;* with higher doses, increased bleeding time.
GI: nausea, vomiting.
GU: tubular stasis and blocking, increased viscosity of urine.
Hepatic: increased AST (SGOT) and ALT (SGPT) levels.

Skin: hypersensitivity reaction, urticaria.
Other: *anaphylaxis.*

INTERACTIONS
None significant.

NURSING CONSIDERATIONS
• Contraindicated in marked hemostatic defects; marked cardiac decompensation or pulmonary edema; renal disease with severe oliguria or anuria; or extreme dehydration. Use cautiously in active hemorrhage; may cause additional blood loss. Evaluate patient's hydration status before administration.
• Doctor may order dextran 1 (Promit) to protect against dextran-induced anaphylaxis. Administer Promit, 20 ml I.V. over 60 seconds, 1 to 2 minutes before the I.V. infusion of Dextran 40.
• Hazardous when given to patients with heart failure, especially if in saline solution. Use dextrose in water solution instead.
• Works as plasma expander via colloidal osmotic effect, thereby drawing fluid from interstitial to intravascular space. Provides plasma expansion slightly greater than volume infused. Watch for circulatory overload and a rise in central venous pressure readings.
• Monitor urine flow rate during administration. If oliguria or anuria occurs or is not relieved by infusion, stop dextran and give loop diuretic.
• Hydration should be assessed before starting therapy; otherwise, use urine or serum osmolarity because urine specific gravity is affected by urine dextran concentration.
• Check hemoglobin and hematocrit; don't allow to fall below 30% by volume.
• Observe patient closely during early phase of infusion; most anaphylactoid reactions occur during this time.
• May interfere with analyses of

---

blood grouping, cross matching, bilirubin, blood glucose, and protein.
• Store at constant 77° F. (25° C.). May precipitate in storage, but can be heated to dissolve if necessary.

dextran
(high molecular weight)
Dextran 70♦, Dextran 75♦, Gentran 75♦, Macrodex♦

Pregnancy Risk Category: C

MECHANISM OF ACTION
Expands plasma volume and provides fluid replacement.

INDICATIONS & DOSAGE
Plasma expander—
Adults: usual dose 30 g (500 ml of 6% solution) I.V. In emergency situations, may be administered at rate of 1.2 to 2.4 g (20 to 40 ml) per minute. In normovolemic or nearly normovolemic patients, rate of infusion should not exceed 240 mg (4 ml)/minute.

Total dosage during first 24 hours not to exceed 1.2 g/kg; actual dosage depends on amount of fluid loss and resultant hemoconcentration, and must be determined for each patient.

ADVERSE REACTIONS
Blood: *decreased level of hemoglobin and hematocrit;* with doses of 15 ml/kg body weight, prolonged bleeding time and significant suppression of platelet function.
GI: nausea, vomiting.
GU: increased specific gravity and viscosity of urine, tubular stasis and blocking.
Hepatic: increased AST (SGOT) and ALT (SGPT) levels.
Skin: hypersensitivity reaction, urticaria.
Other: fever, arthralgia, nasal congestion, *anaphylaxis.*

INTERACTIONS
None significant.

NURSING CONSIDERATIONS
• Contraindicated in marked hemostatic defects; marked cardiac decompensation or pulmonary edema; renal disease with severe oliguria or anuria; or extreme dehydration. Use cautiously in active hemorrhage; may cause additional blood loss.
• Doctor may order dextran 1 (Promit) to protect against dextran-induced anaphylaxis. Administer Promit, 20 ml I.V. over 60 seconds, 1 to 2 minutes before the I.V. infusion of Dextran 70.
• Hazardous when given to patients with heart failure, especially if in saline solution. Use dextrose in water solution instead.
• Works as plasma expander via colloidal osmotic effect, thereby drawing fluid from interstitial to intravascular space. Provides plasma expansion slightly greater than volume infused. Watch for circulatory overload.
• Monitor urine flow rate during administration. If oliguria or anuria occurs or is not relieved by infusion, stop dextran and give loop diuretic.
• Hydration should be assessed before starting therapy; otherwise, use urine or serum osmolarity because urine specific gravity is affected by the urine dextran concentration.
• Check hemoglobin and hematocrit; don't allow to fall below 30% by volume.
• Draw blood samples *before* starting infusion.
• Observe patient closely during early phase of infusion; most anaphylactoid reactions occur during this time.
• May interfere with analyses of blood grouping, cross matching, bilirubin, blood glucose, and protein.
• May precipitate in storage, but can be heated to dissolve if necessary.

hetastarch
Hespan
Pregnancy Risk Category: C

MECHANISM OF ACTION
Expands plasma volume and provides fluid replacement.

INDICATIONS & DOSAGE
Plasma expander—
Adults: 500 to 1,000 ml I.V. depending on amount of blood lost and resultant hemoconcentration. Total dosage usually not to exceed 1,500 ml/day. Up to 20 ml/kg hourly may be used in hemorrhagic shock.

ADVERSE REACTIONS
CNS: headaches.
CV: peripheral edema of lower extremities.
EENT: periorbital edema.
GI: nausea, vomiting.
Skin: urticaria.
Other: wheezing, mild fever.

INTERACTIONS
None significant.

NURSING CONSIDERATIONS
• Contraindicated in severe bleeding disorders, with severe congestive heart failure, or renal failure with oliguria and anuria.
• To avoid circulatory overload, monitor patients with impaired renal function carefully.
• Discontinue if allergic or sensitivity reactions occur. If necessary, administer an antihistamine.
• When used in continuous-flow centrifugation, leukapheresis ratio is usually 1 part hetastarch to 8 parts venous whole blood.
• Hetastarch is *not* a substitute for blood or plasma.
• Available in 500-ml I.V. infusion bottles.
• Discard partially used bottles.

magnesium sulfate
Pregnancy Risk Category: B

MECHANISM OF ACTION
Replaces and maintains magnesium levels. As an anticonvulsant, reduces muscle contractions by interfering with the release of acetylcholine at the myoneural junction.

INDICATIONS & DOSAGE
Hypomagnesemia—
Adults: 1 g, or 8.12 mEq, of 50% solution (2 ml) I.M. q 6 hours for 4 doses, depending on serum magnesium level.
Severe hypomagnesemia (serum magnesium 0.8 mEq/liter or less, with symptoms)—
6 g, or 50 mEq, of 50% solution I.V. in 1 liter of solution over 4 hours.
   Subsequent doses depend on serum magnesium levels.
Magnesium supplementation in hyperalimentation—
Adults: 8 to 24 mEq daily added to hyperalimentation solution.
Children over 6 years: 2 to 10 mEq daily added to hyperalimentation solution.
   Each 2 ml of 50% solution contains 1 g, or 8.12 mEq, magnesium sulfate.
Acute treatment of preeclampsia and eclampsia—
Adults: loading dose: 2 to 4 g (4 to 8 ml of 50% solution) given by slow I.V. bolus (over 5 minutes).
Maintenance dosage: 1 to 2 g hourly as a constant infusion. Prepare by adding 8 ml of 50% solution to 250 ml dextrose 5% in water.
Hypomagnesemic seizures—
Adults: 1 to 2 g (as 10% solution) I.V. over 15 minutes, then 1 g I.M. q 4 to 6 hours, based on patient response and magnesium blood level.
Seizures secondary to hypomagnesemia in acute nephritis—
Adults: 0.2 ml/kg of 50% solution I.M. q 4 to 6 hours, p.r.n. or 100 mg/

Italicized side effects are common or life-threatening.
*Liquid form contains alcohol.   **May contain tartrazine.

kg of 10% solution I.V. very slowly. Titrate dosage according to magnesium blood level and seizure response.

ADVERSE REACTIONS
CNS: toxicity: *weak or absent deep tendon reflexes,* flaccid paralysis, hypothermia, drowsiness, hypocalcemia (perioral paresthesias, twitching carpopedal spasm, tetany, and seizures). **CV:** slow, weak pulse; cardiac dysrhythmias (hypocalcemia); *hypotension.*
Skin: flushing, sweating.
Other: *respiratory paralysis,* hypocalcemia.

INTERACTIONS
Neuromuscular blocking agents: may cause increased neuromuscular blockage. Use cautiously.

NURSING CONSIDERATIONS
• Contraindicated in impaired renal function, myocardial damage, or heart block, and in actively progressing labor. Use parenteral magnesium with extreme caution in patients receiving digitalis preparations. Treating magnesium toxicity with calcium in such patients could cause serious alterations in cardiac conduction; heart block may result.
• I.V. bolus dose *must* be injected slowly in order to avoid respiratory or cardiac arrest.
• If available, use a continual infusion pump when administering infusion.
• Maximum infusion rate is 150 mg/minute. Rapid drip causes feeling of heat.
• Keep I.V. calcium available to reverse magnesium intoxication.
• Monitor vital signs every 15 minutes when giving I.V. for severe hypomagnesemia. Watch for respiratory depression and signs of heart block. Respirations should be more than 16/minute before dose is given.
• Monitor intake/output. Output

should be 100 ml or more during 4-hour period before dose.
• Test knee-jerk and patellar reflexes before each additional dose. If absent, give no more magnesium until reflexes return; otherwise, patient may develop temporary respiratory failure and need cardiopulmonary resuscitation or I.V. administration of calcium.
• Check magnesium level after repeated doses.
• After giving to toxemic mothers within 24 hours before delivery, watch neonate for signs of magnesium toxicity, including neuromuscular and respiratory depression.

---

potassium acetate
Pregnancy Risk Category: C

MECHANISM OF ACTION
Replaces and maintains potassium level.

INDICATIONS & DOSAGE
Potassium replacement—
I.V. should be used for life-threatening hypokalemia or when oral replacement not feasible. Give no more than 20 mEq hourly in concentration of 40 mEq/liter or less. Total 24-hour dosage should not exceed 150 mEq (3 mEq/kg in children). Potassium replacement should be done with ECG monitoring and frequent serum potassium determinations.
Prevention of hypokalemia—
Adults and children: 20 mEq P.O. daily, in divided doses b.i.d., t.i.d., or q.i.d.
Potassium depletion—
Adults and children: usual dose 40 to 100 mEq P.O. daily, in divided doses b.i.d., t.i.d., or q.i.d.

ADVERSE REACTIONS
Signs of hyperkalemia:
CNS: paresthesias of the extremities, listlessness, mental confusion, weakness or heaviness of legs, flaccid pa-

ralysis.
CV: *peripheral vascular collapse with fall in blood pressure, cardiac dysrhythmias,* heart block, possible cardiac arrest, ECG changes (prolonged P-R intervals; wide QRS complex; ST segment depression; tall, tented T waves).
GI: nausea, vomiting, abdominal pain, diarrhea, bowel ulceration.
GU: oliguria.
Skin: cold skin, gray pallor.

INTERACTIONS
None significant.

NURSING CONSIDERATIONS
• Contraindicated in severe renal impairment with oliguria, anuria, azotemia; untreated Addison's disease; or in acute dehydration, hyperkalemia, hyperkalemic form of familial periodic paralysis, and conditions associated with extensive tissue breakdown. Use cautiously in patients with cardiac disease, patients receiving potassium-sparing diuretics, and those with renal impairment.
• During therapy, monitor ECG, renal function, intake/output, and serum potassium, serum creatinine, and BUN. Never give potassium postoperatively until urine flow is established.
• Give slowly as diluted solution; potentially fatal hyperkalemia may result from too-rapid infusion.
• Parenteral potassium given by infusion only; never I.V. push or I.M.
• Observe for pain and redness at infusion site. Large-bore needle reduces local irritation.
• Watch for signs of GI ulceration: obstruction, hemorrhage, pain, distention, severe vomiting, and bleeding.
• Reconstitute potassium acetate powder with liquids; give after meals with a full glass of water or fruit juice to minimize GI irritation.
• To prevent serious hyperkalemia,

potassium deficits must be replaced gradually.

potassium bicarbonate
K-Lyte, K-Lyte DS
Pregnancy Risk Category: A

MECHANISM OF ACTION
Replaces and maintains potassium.

INDICATIONS & DOSAGE
Hypokalemia—
25 mEq or 50 mEq tablet P.O., dissolved in water 1 to 4 times a day.

ADVERSE REACTIONS
CNS: paresthesias of the extremities, listlessness, mental confusion, weakness or heaviness of legs, flaccid paralysis.
CV: *cardiac dysrhythmias,* ECG changes (prolonged P-R interval; wide QRS complex; ST segment depression; tall, tented T waves).
GI: *nausea, vomiting, abdominal pain,* diarrhea, ulcerations, hemorrhage, obstruction, perforation.

INTERACTIONS
None significant.

NURSING CONSIDERATIONS
• Contraindicated in severe renal impairment with oliguria, anuria, azotemia, and untreated Addison's disease; also in acute dehydration, hyperkalemia, hyperkalemic form of familial periodic paralysis, and conditions associated with extensive tissue breakdown. Use with caution in cardiac disease and patients receiving potassium-sparing diuretics.
• Monitor serum potassium, BUN, serum creatinine, and intake/output.
• Never switch potassium products without a doctor's order.
• Dissolve potassium bicarbonate tablets in 6 to 8 ounces of cold water. Dissolve completely to minimize GI irritation.

• Have patient take with meals and sip slowly over a 5- to 10-minute period.
• Potassium bicarbonate cannot be given instead of potassium chloride.
• Potassium bicarbonate does not correct hypochloremic alkalosis.
• Available in lime and orange flavors. Check for patient's flavor preference.

potassium chloride
K-Lor, K-Lyte/Cl♦, Kaochlor 10%*♦, Kaochlor S-F 10%*, Kaon-Cl, Kaon-Cl 20%*, Kato Powder, Kay Ciel*♦, Klor-10%*, Klor-Con, Kloride***, Klorvess, Klotrix, K-Tab, Micro-K Extencaps♦, SK-Potassium Chloride, Slow-K♦, Ten-K

Pregnancy Risk Category: A

MECHANISM OF ACTION
Replaces and maintains potassium level.

INDICATIONS & DOSAGE
Hypokalemia—
40 to 100 mEq P.O. daily in three or four divided doses for treatment; 20 mEq for prevention. Further dosage based on serum potassium.

I.V. route when oral replacement not feasible or when hypokalemia life-threatening. Usual dose 20 mEq hourly in concentration of 40 mEq/liter or less. Total daily dosage not to exceed 150 mEq (3 mEq/kg in children). Potassium replacement should be done only with ECG monitoring and frequent serum potassium determinations.

ADVERSE REACTIONS
Signs of hyperkalemia:
CNS: paresthesias of the extremities, listlessness, mental confusion, weakness or heaviness of limbs, flaccid paralysis.
CV: *peripheral vascular collapse with fall in blood pressure, cardiac dys-*
rhythmias, heart block, possible cardiac arrest, ECG changes (prolonged P-R interval; wide QRS; ST segment depression; tall, tented T waves).
GI: *nausea, vomiting, abdominal pain,* diarrhea, GI ulcerations (possible stenosis, hemorrhage, obstruction, perforation).
GU: oliguria.
Skin: cold skin, gray pallor.
Local: *postinfusion phlebitis.*

INTERACTIONS
None significant.

NURSING CONSIDERATIONS
• Contraindicated in severe renal impairment with oliguria, anuria, azotemia, and untreated Addison's disease; also in acute dehydration, hyperkalemia, hyperkalemic form of familial periodic paralysis, and conditions associated with extensive tissue breakdown. Use with caution in cardiac disease, and those patients receiving potassium-sparing diuretics.
• Potassium should not be given during immediate postoperative period until urine flow is established.
• Parenteral potassium given by infusion only; never I.V. push or I.M.
• Small amounts of lidocaine injection (1 to 3 ml of the 1% strength) may be added directly to the potassium chloride solution. This will help reverse postinfusion phlebitis.
• Give slowly as dilute solution; potentially fatal hyperkalemia may result from too rapid infusion.
• Give oral potassium supplements with extreme caution because its many forms deliver varying amounts of potassium. Never switch products without a doctor's order. Tell the doctor if patient tolerates one product better than another.
• Sugar-free liquid available (Kaochlor S-F 10%).
• Use a liquid preparation for potassium supplement if tablet or capsule passage is likely to be delayed, such

as in GI obstruction.
- Have patient sip liquid potassium slowly to minimize GI irritation.
- Give with or after meals with full glass of water or fruit juice to lessen GI distress.
- Make sure powders are completely dissolved before giving.
- Enteric-coated tablets not recommended due to potential for GI bleeding and small-bowel ulcerations.
- Tablets in wax matrix sometimes lodge in esophagus and cause ulceration in cardiac patients who have esophageal compression from enlarged left atrium. In such patients and in those with esophageal stasis or obstruction, use liquid form.
- Microencapsulated form (Micro-K) has been shown in one study to cause less GI bleeding than the wax matrix tablets. However, this hasn't been completely confirmed.
- Often used orally with diuretics that cause potassium excretion. Potassium chloride most useful since diuretics waste chloride ion. Hypokalemic alkalosis treated best with potassium chloride.
- Monitor ECG and serum electrolytes during therapy.
- Don't crush sustained-release potassium products.

---

potassium gluconate
Kaon Liquid*, Kaon Tablets♦,
Potassium Rougier♦♦

Pregnancy Risk Category: A

MECHANISM OF ACTION
Replaces and maintains potassium.

INDICATIONS & DOSAGE
Hypokalemia—
40 to 100 mEq P.O. daily in three or four divided doses for treatment; 20 mEq daily for prevention. Further dosage based on serum potassium determinations.

ADVERSE REACTIONS
CNS: paresthesias of the extremities, listlessness, mental confusion, weakness or heaviness of legs, flaccid paralysis.
CV: cardiac dysrhythmias, ECG changes (prolonged P-R interval; wide QRS complex; ST segment depression; tall, tented T waves).
GI: *nausea, vomiting, abdominal pain,* diarrhea, GI ulcerations with oral products (especially enteric-coated tablets); ulcerations may be accompanied by stenosis, hemorrhage, obstruction, perforation.

INTERACTIONS
None significant.

NURSING CONSIDERATIONS
- Contraindicated in severe renal impairment with oliguria, anuria, azotemia, and untreated Addison's disease; also in acute dehydration, hyperkalemia, hyperkalemic form of familial periodic paralysis, and conditions associated with extensive tissue breakdown. Use with caution in patients with cardiac disease and in those receiving potassium-sparing diuretics.
- Monitor serum potassium, BUN, serum creatinine, and intake/output.
- Give oral potassium supplements with extreme caution because their many forms deliver varying amounts of potassium. Never switch products without a doctor's order. If one product is tolerated better than another, tell the doctor so dosage can be changed.
- Have patient sip liquid potassium slowly to minimize GI irritation.
- Give with or after meals with full glass of water or fruit juice to lessen GI distress.
- Potassium gluconate does not correct hypokalemic hypochloremic alkalosis.
- Enteric-coated tablets not recommended because of potential for GI

Italicized side effects are common or life-threatening.
*Liquid form contains alcohol.   **May contain tartrazine.

bleeding and small-bowel ulcerations.
• Monitor ECG and serum electrolytes during therapy.

potassium phosphate

Pregnancy Risk Category: C

MECHANISM OF ACTION
Replaces and maintains potassium.

INDICATIONS & DOSAGE
Hypokalemia—
I.V. should be used when oral replacement not feasible or when hypokalemia life-threatening. Dosage up to 20 mEq hourly in concentration of 60 mEq/liter or less. Total daily dosage not to exceed 150 mEq. Should be done only with ECG monitoring and frequent serum potassium determinations.
   Average P.O. dose: 40 to 100 mEq.
Hypophosphatemia—
0.32 to 0.45 mM/kg of phosphate administered I.V. over 12 hours after diluting in a larger volume of fluid.
   Dosage is adjusted according to individual needs of patient.

ADVERSE REACTIONS
Signs of hyperkalemia:
CNS: paresthesias of the extremities, listlessness, mental confusion, weakness or heaviness of legs, flaccid paralysis; hypocalcemia—perioral paresthesias, twitching, carpopedal spasm, tetany, and seizures.
CV: *peripheral vascular collapse with fall in blood pressure, cardiac dysrhythmias, heart block, possible cardiac arrest,* ECG changes (prolonged P-R interval; wide QRS complex; ST segment depression; tall, tented T waves).
GI: nausea, vomiting, abdominal pain, diarrhea.
GU: oliguria.
Skin: cold skin, gray pallor.
Other: soft tissue calcification.

INTERACTIONS
None significant.

NURSING CONSIDERATIONS
• Contraindicated in severe renal impairment with oliguria, anuria, azotemia, and untreated Addison's disease; also in acute dehydration, hyperkalemia, hyperkalemic form of familial periodic paralysis, extensive tissue damage, or hypocalcemia. Use with caution in patients with cardiac disease, and in those receiving potassium-sparing diuretics.
• Never give potassium postoperatively until urine flow is established.
• Monitor ECG for indications of tissue potassium; serum potassium and calcium as well as BUN and creatinine for renal function; inorganic phosphorus; and intake/output.
• Give slowly as dilute solution; potentially fatal hyperkalemia may result from too-rapid infusion.
• Parenteral potassium given by infusion only; never I.V. push or I.M.
• Reconstitute powder in juice. Give after meals.

Ringer's injection

Pregnancy Risk Category: C

MECHANISM OF ACTION
Replaces fluids and electrolytes.

INDICATIONS & DOSAGE
Fluid and electrolyte replacement—
Adults and children: dose highly individualized, but usually 1.5 to 3 liters (2% to 6% body weight) infused I.V. over 18 to 24 hours.

ADVERSE REACTIONS
CV: fluid overload.

INTERACTIONS
None significant.

NURSING CONSIDERATIONS
• Contraindicated in renal failure, ex-

cept as emergency volume expander. Use cautiously in congestive heart failure, circulatory insufficiency, renal dysfunction, hypoproteinemia, and pulmonary edema.
• Ringer's injection contains sodium, 147 mEq/liter; potassium, 4 mEq/liter; calcium, 4.5 mEq/liter; and chloride, 155.5 mEq/liter. This electrolyte content is insufficient for treating severe electrolyte deficiencies, although it does provide electrolytes in levels approximately equal to those of the blood.

Ringer's injection, lactated
(Hartmann's solution, Ringer's lactate solution)
Pregnancy Risk Category: C

MECHANISM OF ACTION
Replaces fluids and electrolytes.

INDICATIONS & DOSAGE
Fluid and electrolyte replacement—
Adults and children: dosage highly individualized, but usually 1.5 to 3 liters (2% to 6% body weight) infused I.V. over 18 to 24 hours.

ADVERSE REACTIONS
CV: fluid overload.

INTERACTIONS
None significant.

NURSING CONSIDERATIONS
• Contraindicated in renal failure, except as emergency volume expander. Use cautiously in congestive heart failure, circulatory insufficiency, renal dysfunction, hypoproteinemia, and pulmonary edema.
• Ringer's injection, lactated, contains sodium, 130 mEq/liter; potassium, 4 mEq/liter; calcium, 3 mEq/liter; chloride, 109.7 mEq/liter; and lactate, 28 mEq/liter.
• Approximates more closely the electrolyte concentration in blood

plasma than Ringer's injection.

sodium chloride
Pregnancy Risk Category: C

MECHANISM OF ACTION
Replaces and maintains sodium and chloride levels.

INDICATIONS & DOSAGE
Highly individualized fluid and electrolyte replacement in hyponatremia caused by electrolyte loss or in severe salt depletion—
400 ml of 3% or 5% solutions only with frequent electrolyte determination and only if given slow I.V.; *with 0.45% solution:* 3% to 8% of body weight, according to deficiencies, over 18 to 24 hours; *with 0.9% solution:* 2% to 6% of body weight, according to deficiencies, over 18 to 24 hours.
Management of "heat cramp" caused by excessive perspiration—
Adults: 1 g P.O. with every glass of water.

ADVERSE REACTIONS
CV: aggravation of congestive heart failure; edema and pulmonary edema if too much given or given too rapidly.
Metabolic: hypernatremia and aggravation of existing acidosis with excessive infusion; serious electrolyte disturbance, loss of potassium.

INTERACTIONS
None significant.

NURSING CONSIDERATIONS
• Use with caution in congestive heart failure, circulatory insufficiency, renal dysfunction, and hypoproteinemia.
• Infuse 3% and 5% solutions very slowly and with caution to avoid pulmonary edema. Use only for critical situations. Observe patient continually.

• Concentrates available for addition to parenteral nutrient solutions. Don't confuse these small volumes of parenterals with normal saline injection. *Read label carefully.*
• Monitor serum electrolytes.

65

Potassium-removing resin

sodium polystyrene sulfonate

COMBINATION PRODUCTS
None.

sodium polystyrene sulfonate
Kayexalate♦, SPS
Pregnancy Risk Category: C

MECHANISM OF ACTION
The potassium-removing resin exchanges sodium ions for potassium ions in the intestine: 1 g of sodium polystyrene sulfonate is exchanged for 0.5 to 1 mEq of potassium. The resin is then eliminated. Much of the exchange capacity is used for cations other than potassium (calcium and magnesium) and possibly for fats and proteins.

INDICATIONS & DOSAGE
Hyperkalemia—
Adults: 15 g P.O. daily to q.i.d. in water or sorbitol (3 to 4 ml/g of resin).
Children: 1 g of resin P.O. for each mEq of potassium to be removed.

Oral administration preferred since drug should remain in intestine for at least 6 hours; otherwise, consider nasogastric administration.

Nasogastric administration: mix dose with appropriate medium: aqueous suspension or diet appropriate for renal failure; instill in plastic tube.
Rectal administration:
Adults: 30 to 50 g/100 ml of sorbitol q 6 hours as warm emulsion deep into sigmoid colon (20 cm). In persistent vomiting or paralytic ileus, high retention enema of sodium polystyrene sulfonate (30 g) suspended in 200 ml of 10% methylcellulose, 10% dextrose, or 25% sorbitol solution.

ADVERSE REACTIONS
GI: *constipation,* fecal impaction (in elderly patients), anorexia, gastric irritation, nausea, vomiting, *diarrhea (with sorbitol emulsions).*
Other: *hypokalemia,* hypocalcemia, hypomagnesemia, sodium retention.

INTERACTIONS
Antacids and laxatives (nonabsorbable cation-donating type, including magnesium hydroxide): systemic alkalosis, reduced potassium exchange capability. Don't use together.

NURSING CONSIDERATIONS
• Use with caution in elderly patients and those on digitalis therapy, with severe congestive heart failure, severe hypertension, and marked edema.
• Treatment may result in potassium deficiency. Monitor serum potassium at least once daily. Usually stopped when potassium is reduced to 4 or 5 mEq/liter. Watch for other signs of hypokalemia: irritability, confusion, cardiac dysrhythmias, ECG changes, severe muscle weakness and sometimes paralysis, and digitalis toxicity in digitalized patients.
• Monitor for symptoms of other electrolyte deficiencies (magnesium, calcium) since drug is nonselective.

Italicized side effects are common or life-threatening.
*Liquid form contains alcohol.   **May contain tartrazine.

Monitor serum calcium in patients receiving sodium polystyrene therapy for more than 3 days. Supplementary calcium may be needed.

• Watch for sodium overload. About ⅓ of resin's sodium is retained.

• Premixed forms are available (SPS and others).

• Do not heat resin. This will impair effectiveness of drug. Mix resin only with water or sorbitol for P.O. administration. Above all, *never* mix with orange juice (high potassium content) to disguise taste.

• Chill oral suspension for greater palatability.

• If sorbitol is given, it may be mixed with resin suspension.

• Consider solid form. Resin cookie and candy recipes are available; perhaps pharmacist or dietitian can supply.

• Watch for constipation in oral or nasogastric administration. Use sorbitol (10 to 20 ml of 70% syrup every 2 hours as needed) to produce one or two watery stools daily.

• If preparing manually, mix polystyrene resin only with water and sorbitol for rectal use. Do not use other vehicles (that is, mineral oil) for rectal administration to prevent impactions. Ion exchange requires aqueous medium. Sorbitol content prevents impaction.

• Prevent fecal impaction in elderly by administering resin rectally. Give cleansing enema before rectal administration. Explain necessity of retaining enema to patient. Retention for 6 to 10 hours is ideal, but 30 to 60 minutes is acceptable.

• Prepare rectal dose at room temperature. Stir emulsion gently during administration.

• Use #28 French rubber tube for rectal dose; insert 20 cm into sigmoid colon. Tape tube in place. Alternatively, consider a Foley catheter with a 30-ml balloon inflated distal to anal sphincter to aid in retention. This is especially helpful for patients with poor sphincter control (for example, after cerebrovascular accident). Use gravity flow. Drain returns constantly through Y-tube connection. When giving rectally, place patient in knee-chest position or with hips on pillow for a while if back-leakage occurs.

• After rectal administration, flush tubing with 50 to 100 ml of nonsodium fluid to ensure delivery of all medication.

• Flush rectum to remove the resin.

• If hyperkalemia is severe, more drastic modalities should be added; for example, dextrose 50% with regular insulin I.V. push. Do not depend solely on polystyrene resin to lower serum potassium in severe hyperkalemia.

Unmarked trade names available in the United States only.
♦ Also available in Canada.   ♦♦ Available in Canada only.   ◊ Also available OTC.

66

Hematinics

ferrous fumarate◇
ferrous gluconate◇
ferrous sulfate◇
iron dextran

COMBINATION PRODUCTS
FERMALOX◇: ferrous sulfate 200 mg, and magnesium hydroxide and dried aluminum hydroxide gel 200 mg.
FEROCYL◇: iron (as fumarate) 50 mg and docusate sodium 100 mg.
FERRO-SEQUELS◇: iron (as fumarate) 50 mg and docusate sodium 100 mg.
SIMRON◇: iron (as gluconate) 10 mg and polysorbate 20, 400 mg.

---

ferrous fumarate◇
Eldofe, Feostat, Ferranol, Fersamal♦♦, Fumasorb, Fumerin, Hemocyte, Ircon♦, Maniron, Novofumar♦♦, Palafer♦♦, Span-FF

Pregnancy Risk Category: A

MECHANISM OF ACTION
Provides elemental iron, an essential component in the formation of hemoglobin. Each 100 mg of ferrous fumarate provides 33 mg of elemental iron.

INDICATIONS & DOSAGE
Iron deficiency
Adults: 200 mg P.O. t.i.d. or q.i.d.
Children: 3 mg/kg P.O. t.i.d., increased to 6 mg/kg P.O. t.i.d. as needed and tolerated.

ADVERSE REACTIONS
GI: *nausea,* vomiting, *constipation, black stools.*

Other: elixir may stain teeth.

INTERACTIONS
Antacids, cholestyramine resin, pancreatic extracts, vitamin E: decreased iron absorption. Separate doses if possible.
Chloramphenicol: watch for delayed response to iron therapy.
Vitamin C: concurrent administration may increase iron absorption. Beneficial drug interaction.

NURSING CONSIDERATIONS
• Contraindicated in hemosiderosis and hemochromatosis. Use cautiously in peptic ulcer, regional enteritis, and ulcerative colitis. Also use cautiously on long-term basis.
• GI upset related to dose. Between-meal dosing preferable, but can be given with some foods although absorption may be decreased. Enteric-coated products reduce GI upset but also reduce amount of iron absorbed.
• Iron is toxic; parents should be aware of iron poisoning in children.
• Tablets may be given with juice or water, but not in milk or antacids. Give with orange juice to promote iron absorption.
• To avoid staining teeth, give elixir iron preparations with straw; patient may take with water or fruit juice.
• Check for constipation; record color and amount of stool. Teach dietary measures for preventing constipation.
• Oral iron may turn stools black. This unabsorbed iron is harmless; however, it could mask the presence

---

Italicized side effects are common or life-threatening.
*Liquid form contains alcohol.   **May contain tartrazine.

of melena.
• Monitor hemoglobin and reticulocyte counts during therapy.
• Combination products—Simron, Ferro-Sequels, Ferocyl, Fer-Regules—contain stool softeners to help prevent constipation. Fermalox contains antacids to help relieve GI upset, if present; don't use this product unless absolutely necessary because of decreased iron absorption. Usually, combination iron products should be avoided.

ferrous gluconate◇
Fergon*♦, Ferralet, Fertinic♦♦, Novoferrogluc♦♦

Pregnancy Risk Category: A

MECHANISM OF ACTION
Provides elemental iron, an essential component in the formation of hemoglobin. Each 100 mg of ferrous gluconate provides 11.6 mg of elemental iron.

INDICATIONS & DOSAGE
Iron deficiency—
Adults: 300 to 325 mg P.O. q.i.d., increased to 650 mg q.i.d. as needed and tolerated.
Children 2 years or older: 8 mg/kg P.O. daily in divided doses.

ADVERSE REACTIONS
GI: *nausea*, vomiting, *constipation, black stools.*
Other: elixir may stain teeth.

INTERACTIONS
Antacids, cholestyramine resin, pancreatic extracts, vitamin E: decreased iron absorption. Separate doses if possible.
Chloramphenicol: watch for delayed response to iron therapy.
Vitamin C: may increase iron absorption. Beneficial drug interaction.

NURSING CONSIDERATIONS
• Contraindicated in peptic ulcer, regional enteritis, ulcerative colitis, hemosiderosis, and hemochromatosis. Use cautiously on long-term basis and in patients with anemia.
• GI upset related to dose. Between-meal dosing preferable, but can be given with some foods although absorption may be decreased. Enteric-coated products reduce GI upset but also reduce amount of iron absorbed.
• Tell patient to continue regular dosing schedule if he misses a dose. Patient shouldn't double the dose.
• Iron is toxic; parents should be aware of iron poisoning in children.
• Dilute liquid preparations in juice (preferably orange juice) or water, but not in milk or antacids. Give tablets with orange juice to promote absorption.
• To avoid staining teeth, give elixir iron preparations with straw; patient may take with water or fruit juice.
• Check for constipation; record color and amount of stool. Teach dietary measures for preventing constipation.
• Oral iron may turn stools black. This unabsorbed iron is harmless; however, it could mask melena.
• Monitor hemoglobin and reticulocyte counts during therapy.

ferrous sulfate◇
Feosol*, Fer-In-Sol*♦, Fero-Grad♦♦, Fero-Gradumet, Ferolix*, Ferospace, Ferralyn, Irospan, Mol-Iron*, Novoferrosulfa♦♦, Slow-Fe♦, Telefon

Pregnancy Risk Category: A

MECHANISM OF ACTION
Provides elemental iron, an essential component in the formation of hemoglobin. Each 100 mg of ferrous sulfate provides 20 mg of elemental iron.

INDICATIONS & DOSAGE
Iron deficiency—
Adults: 325 mg P.O. t.i.d. or q.i.d. Alternatively, give 1 delayed release capsule (160 or 525 mg) P.O. once or twice daily.
Children: 5 mg/kg P.O. daily, increased to 10 mg/kg P.O. t.i.d. as needed and tolerated.
Prophylaxis for iron deficiency anemia—
Pregnant women: 150 to 300 mg P.O. daily in divided doses.
Premature or undernourished infants: 1 to 2 mg/kg P.O. daily (as elemental iron) in divided doses.

ADVERSE REACTIONS
GI: *nausea,* vomiting, *constipation, black stools.*
Other: elixir may stain teeth.

INTERACTIONS
Antacids, cholestyramine resin, pancreatic extracts, vitamin E: decreased iron absorption. Separate doses if possible.
Chloramphenicol: watch for delayed response to iron therapy.
Vitamin C: may increase iron absorption. Beneficial drug interaction.

NURSING CONSIDERATIONS
• Contraindicated in hemosiderosis and hemochromatosis. Use cautiously in peptic ulcer, ulcerative colitis, and regional enteritis. Also use cautiously on long-term basis.
• GI upset related to dose. Between-meal dosing preferable, but can be given with some foods although absorption may be decreased. Enteric-coated products reduce GI upset but also reduce amount of iron absorbed.
• Tell patient to continue regular dosing schedule if he misses a dose. Patient shouldn't double the dose.
• Iron is toxic; parents should be aware of iron poisoning in children.
• Dilute liquid preparations in juice or water, but not in milk or antacids.

Dilute liquids in orange juice; give tablets with orange juice to promote iron absorption.
• To avoid staining teeth, give elixir iron preparations with straw.
• Check for constipation; record color and amount of stool. Teach dietary measures for preventing constipation.
• Oral iron may turn stools black. This unabsorbed iron is harmless; however, it could mask melena.
• Monitor hemoglobin and reticulocyte counts during therapy.

---

iron dextran
Hydextran, Imferon♦, K-FeRON
Pregnancy Risk Category: C

MECHANISM OF ACTION
Provides elemental iron, an essential component in the formation of hemoglobin; 1 ml iron dextran provides 50 mg elemental iron.

INDICATIONS & DOSAGE
Iron deficiency anemia—
Adults: I.M. or I.V. injections of iron are advisable only for patients for whom oral administration is impossible or ineffective. Test dose (0.5 ml) required before administration.
I.M. (by Z-track): inject 0.5 ml test dose. If no reactions next daily dose should ordinarily not exceed 0.5 ml (25 mg) for infants under 5 kg; 1 ml (50 mg) for children under 9 kg; 2 ml (100 mg) for patients under 50 kg; 5 ml (250 mg) for patients over 50 kg.
I.V. push: inject 0.5 ml test dose. If no reaction, within 2 to 3 days the dosage may be raised to 2 ml daily I.V., 1 ml/minute undiluted and infused slowly until total dose is achieved. No single dose should exceed 100 mg.
I.V. infusion: dosages are expressed in terms of elemental iron. Dilute in 250 to 1,000 ml of normal saline solution; dextrose increases local vein irritation. Infuse test dose of 25 mg slowly

---

Italicized side effects are common or life-threatening.
*Liquid form contains alcohol.   **May contain tartrazine.

over 5 minutes. If no reaction occurs in 5 minutes, infusion may be started. Infuse total dose slowly over approximately 6 to 12 hours.

ADVERSE REACTIONS
CNS: headache, transitory paresthesias, arthralgia, myalgia, dizziness, malaise, syncope.
CV: *hypotensive reaction, peripheral vascular flushing with overly rapid I.V. administration, tachycardia.*
GI: nausea, vomiting, metallic taste, transient loss of taste perception.
Local: *soreness and inflammation at injection site (I.M.); brown skin discoloration at injection site (I.M.); local phlebitis at injection site (I.V.).*
Skin: rash, urticaria.
Other: *anaphylaxis.*

INTERACTIONS
None significant.

NURSING CONSIDERATIONS
• Contraindicated in all anemias other than iron deficiency anemia. Use with extreme caution in patients with impaired hepatic function and rheumatoid arthritis.
• Monitor vital signs for drug reaction. Reactions are varied, ranging from pain, inflammation, and myalgia to hypotension, shock, and death.
• Inject deeply into upper outer quadrant of buttock—never into arm or other exposed area—with a 2- to 3-inch, 19G or 20G needle. Use Z-track technique to avoid leakage into subcutaneous tissue and staining of skin.
• Skin staining may be minimized by using a separate needle to withdraw the drug from its container.
• Monitor hemoglobin concentration, hematocrit, and reticulocyte count.
• Use I.V. in these situations: insufficient muscle mass for deep intramuscular injection; impaired absorption from muscle due to stasis or edema; possibility of uncontrolled intramuscular bleeding from trauma (as may

occur in hemophilia); and with massive and prolonged parenteral therapy (as may be necessary in cases of chronic substantial blood loss).
• Upon completion of I.V. iron dextran infusion, flush the vein with 10 ml of 0.9% sodium chloride solution.
• Patient should rest 15 to 30 minutes after I.V. administration.
• Check hospital policy before administering I.V. Some do not permit infusion method because its safety is controversial.
• Not removed by hemodialysis.

67

Anticoagulants and heparin antagonist

dicumarol
heparin calcium
heparin sodium
protamine sulfate
warfarin sodium

COMBINATION PRODUCTS
None.

---

dicumarol
Dicumarol Pulvules

Pregnancy Risk Category: D

MECHANISM OF ACTION
Inhibits vitamin K-dependent activation of clotting factors II, VII, IX, and X, which are formed in the liver.

INDICATIONS & DOSAGE
Treatment of pulmonary emboli; prevention and treatment of deep vein thrombosis, myocardial infarction, rheumatic heart disease with heart valve damage, atrial dysrhythmias—
Adults: 200 to 300 mg P.O. on first day, 25 to 200 mg P.O. daily thereafter, based on prothrombin times.

ADVERSE REACTIONS
Blood: *hemorrhage with excessive dosage,* leukopenia, *agranulocytosis.*
GI: anorexia, nausea, vomiting, cramps, *diarrhea,* mouth ulcers.
GU: hematuria.
Skin: dermatitis, urticaria, alopecia, *rash.*
Other: *fever.*

INTERACTIONS
Acetaminophen: increased bleeding possible with chronic (greater than 2 weeks) therapy with acetaminophen. Monitor very carefully.
Allopurinol, amiodarone, chloramphenicol, clofibrate, diflunisal, thyroid drugs, heparin, anabolic steroids, cimetidine, disulfiram, glucagon, inhalation anesthetics, metronidazole, quinidine, influenza vaccine, sulindac, sulfinpyrazone, sulfonamides, tricyclic antidepressants: increased prothrombin time. Monitor patient carefully for bleeding. Consider anticoagulant dosage reduction.
Barbiturates: inhibition of hypoprothrombinemic effect of anticoagulants. If barbiturates are withdrawn, reduce anticoagulant dosage; inhibition may last weeks after barbiturate is withdrawn, but fatal hemorrhage can occur when inhibiting effect disappears.
Cholestyramine: decreased response when administered too close together. Administer 6 hours after oral anticoagulants.
Ethacrynic acid, indomethacin, mefenamic acid, oxyphenbutazone, phenylbutazone, salicylates: increased prothrombin time; ulcerogenic effects. Don't use together.
Glutethimide, chloral hydrate, sulfinpyrazone, triclofos sodium: increased or decreased prothrombin time. Avoid use if possible, or monitor patient carefully.
Griseofulvin, haloperidol, ethchlorvynol, carbamazepine, rifampin: decreased prothrombin time with reduced anticoagulant effect. Monitor patient carefully.

Italicized side effects are common or life-threatening.
*Liquid form contains alcohol.   **May contain tartrazine.

NURSING CONSIDERATIONS

• Contraindicated in hemophilia, thrombocytopenic purpura, leukemia with pronounced bleeding tendency, open wounds or ulcers, impaired hepatic or renal function, severe hypertension, acute nephritis, subacute bacterial endocarditis. Use cautiously during menses, during use of any drainage tube, and in any patient in whom slight bleeding is dangerous. Use with extreme caution (if at all) in psychiatric patients, debilitated patients, or cachectic patients.

• Use caution when adding or stopping any drug for patient receiving anticoagulants. May change the clotting status and result in hemorrhage.

• Fever and skin rash signal severe adverse reactions. Withhold drug and call doctor.

• Give drug at same time daily. Stress importance of complying with recommended dosage and keeping follow-up appointments. Patient should carry a card that identifies him as a potential bleeder.

• Regularly inspect patient for bleeding gums, bruises on arms or legs, petechiae, nosebleeds, melena, tarry stools, hematuria, hematemesis. Tell patient and family to watch for these signs and notify doctor immediately.

• Warn patient to avoid over-the-counter products containing aspirin, other salicylates, or drugs that may interact with dicumarol.

• Because onset of action is delayed, heparin sodium is often given during first few days of treatment. When heparin is being given simultaneously, don't draw blood for prothrombin time within 5 hours of intermittent I.V. heparin administration. However, prothrombin time may be drawn at any time during continuous heparin infusion.

• Dose given depends on prothrombin time (PT). Doctors usually try to maintain PT at 1.5 to 2 times normal. PT values depend on procedure and reagents used in individual laboratory.

• Tell patient to notify doctor if menses is heavier than usual.

• Tell patient to use electric razor when shaving to avoid scratching skin and to brush teeth with a soft toothbrush.

• May turn alkaline urine red-orange.

• Duration of action 2 to 6 days.

• Light to moderate alcohol intake does not significantly affect prothrombin times.

• Tell patient to eat a consistent amount of leafy green vegetables every day. These contain vitamin K, and eating different amounts daily may alter anticoagulant effect.

heparin calcium
Calcilean♦♦, Calciparine♦

heparin sodium
Hepalean♦♦, Heparin Lock Flush Solution (Tubex), Hep Lock, Liquaemin Sodium

Pregnancy Risk Category: C

MECHANISM OF ACTION

Accelerates formation of an antithrombin III–thrombin complex. It inactivates thrombin and prevents conversion of fibrinogen to fibrin.

INDICATIONS & DOSAGE

Treatment of deep vein thrombosis, myocardial infarction—
Adults: initially, 5,000 to 7,500 units I.V. push, then adjust dose according to PTT results and give dose I.V. q 4 hours (usually 4,000 to 5,000 units); or 5,000 to 7,500 units I.V. bolus, then 1,000 units/hour by I.V. infusion pump. Wait 8 hours following bolus dose, and adjust hourly rate according to PTT.

Treatment of pulmonary embolism—
Adults: initially, 7,500 to 10,000 units I.V. push, then adjust dose according to PTT results and give dose

I.V. q 4 hours (usually 4,000 to 5,000 units); or 7,500 to 10,000 units I.V. bolus, then 1,000 units hourly by I.V. infusion pump. Wait 8 hours following bolus dose, and adjust hourly rate according to PTT.

Prophylaxis of embolism—
Adults: 5,000 units S.C. q 12 hours.
Open heart surgery—
Adults: (total body perfusion) 150 to 300 units/kg continuous I.V infusion.
Treatment of pulmonary emboli; prevention and treatment of deep vein thrombosis—
Children: initially, 50 units/kg I.V. drip. Maintenance dose is 100 units/ kg I.V. drip q 4 hours. Constant infusion: 20,000 units/m² daily. Dosages adjusted according to PTT.
As an I.V. flush to maintain patency of I.V. indwelling catheters—
10 to 100 units as an I.V. flush. Not intended for therapeutic use.

Heparin dosing is highly individualized, depending upon disease state, age, renal and hepatic status.

ADVERSE REACTIONS
Blood: *hemorrhage with excessive dosage, overly prolonged clotting time, thrombocytopenia.*
Local: irritation, mild pain.
Other: *"white clot" syndrome,* hypersensitivity reactions including chills, fever, pruritus, rhinitis, burning of feet, conjunctivitis, lacrimation, arthralgia, urticaria.

INTERACTIONS
Anticoagulants, oral: additive anticoagulation. Monitor prothrombin time and partial thromboplastin time.
Salicylates: increased anticoagulant effect. Don't use together.

NURSING CONSIDERATIONS
• Conditionally contraindicated in active bleeding; blood dyscrasias; or bleeding tendencies such as hemophilia, thrombocytopenia, or hepatic disease with hypoprothrombinemia; suspected intracranial hemorrhage; suppurative thrombophlebitis; inaccessible ulcerative lesions (especially of GI tract); open ulcerative wounds; extensive denudation of skin; ascorbic acid deficiency and other conditions causing increased capillary permeability; during or after brain, eye, or spinal cord surgery; during continuous tube drainage of stomach or small intestine; in subacute bacterial endocarditis; shock; advanced renal disease; threatened abortion; severe hypertension. Although the use of heparin is clearly hazardous in these conditions, a decision to use it depends on the comparative risk in failure to treat the coexisting thromboembolic disorder.
• Use cautiously during menses; in mild hepatic or renal disease; alcoholism; in patients in occupations with the risk of physical injury; immediately postpartum; and in patients with history of allergies, asthma, or GI ulcers.
• Monitor platelet counts regularly. Thrombocytopenia caused by heparin may be associated with a type of arterial thrombosis known as "white clot" syndrome.
• Measure partial thromboplastin time (PTT) carefully and regularly. Anticoagulation present when PTT values are 1.5 to 2 times control values.
• Drug requirements are higher in early phases of thrombogenic diseases and febrile states; lower when patient becomes stabilized.
• Regularly inspect patient for bleeding gums, bruises on arms or legs, petechiae, nosebleeds, melena, tarry stools, hematuria, hematemesis. Tell patient and family to watch for these signs and notify doctor immediately.
• Tell patient to avoid over-the-counter medications containing aspirin, other salicylates, or drugs that may interact with heparin.
• Heparin comes in various concen-

Italicized side effects are common or life-threatening.
*Liquid form contains alcohol.   **May contain tartrazine.

trations. Check order and vial carefully.
• Low-dose injections given sequentially between iliac crests in lower abdomen deep into subcutaneous fat. Inject drug slowly subcutaneously into fat pad. Leave needle in place for 10 seconds after injection; then withdraw needle. Alternate site every 12 hours—right for a.m., left for p.m.
• Don't massage after subcutaneous injection. Watch for signs of bleeding at injection site. Rotate sites and keep accurate record.
• Check constant I.V. infusions regularly, even when pumps are in good working order, to prevent overdosage or underdosage.
• I.M. administration not recommended.
• I.V. administration preferred because of long-term effect and irregular absorption when given subcutaneously. Whenever possible, administer I.V. heparin using infusion pump to provide maximum safety.
• Concentrated heparin solutions (greater than 100 units/ml) can irritate blood vessels.
• Place notice above patient's bed to inform I.V. team or lab personnel to apply pressure dressings after taking blood.
• Avoid excessive I.M. injections of other drugs to prevent or minimize hematomas. If possible, don't give I.M. injections at all.
• Elderly patients should usually start at lower doses.
• When intermittent I.V. therapy is utilized, always draw blood ½ hour before next scheduled dose to avoid falsely elevated PTT.
• Blood for PTT can be drawn any time after 8 hours of initiation of continuous I.V. heparin therapy. Never draw blood for PTT from the I.V. tubing of the heparin infusion, or from vein of infusion. Falsely elevated PTT will result. Always draw blood from opposite arm.

• Give on time; try not to skip a dose or "catch up" with an I.V. containing heparin. If I.V. is out, get it restarted as soon as possible, and reschedule bolus dose immediately.
• Never piggyback other drugs into an infusion line while heparin infusion is running. Many antibiotics and other drugs inactivate heparin. Never mix any drug with heparin in syringe when bolus therapy is used.
• Abrupt withdrawal may cause increased coagulability. Usually, heparin therapy is followed by oral anticoagulants for prophylaxis.

protamine sulfate
Pregnancy Risk Category: C

MECHANISM OF ACTION
Forms a physiologically inert complex with heparin sodium.

INDICATIONS & DOSAGE
Heparin overdose—
Adults: dosage based on venous blood coagulation studies, usually 1 mg for each 78 to 95 units of heparin. Give diluted to 1% (10 mg/ml) slow I.V. injection over 1 to 3 minutes. Maximum dose is 50 mg/10 minutes.

ADVERSE REACTIONS
CV: fall in blood pressure, bradycardia.
Other: transitory flushing, feeling of warmth, dyspnea.

INTERACTIONS
None significant.

NURSING CONSIDERATIONS
• Use cautiously after cardiac surgery.
• Should be given slowly to reduce adverse reactions. Have equipment available to treat shock.
• Monitor patient continually. Check vital signs frequently.
• Watch for spontaneous bleeding

(heparin "rebound"), especially in patients undergoing dialysis and those who have had cardiac surgery.
• Protamine sulfate may act as anticoagulant in very high doses.
• 1 mg of protamine neutralizes 78 to 95 units of heparin.
• Heparin antagonist.

warfarin sodium
Coumadin♦, Panwarfin, Warfilone Sodium♦♦

Pregnancy Risk Category: D

MECHANISM OF ACTION
Inhibits vitamin K–dependent activation of clotting factors II, VII, IX, and X, which are formed in the liver.

INDICATIONS & DOSAGE
Treatment of pulmonary emboli; prevention and treatment of deep vein thrombosis, myocardial infarction, rheumatic heart disease with heart valve damage, atrial dysrhythmias—
Adults: 10 to 15 mg P.O. for 3 days, then dosage based on daily prothrombin (PT) times. Usual maintenance dosage is 2 to 10 mg P.O. daily. Alternate regimen: initially, 40 to 60 mg P.O. daily; then 2 to 10 mg daily based on PT determinations.
   Warfarin sodium also available for I.V. use (50 mg/vial). Reconstitute with sterile water for injection. I.V. form rarely used and may be in periodic short supply.

ADVERSE REACTIONS
Blood: *hemorrhage with excessive dosage,* leukopenia.
GI: paralytic ileus, intestinal obstruction (both resulting from hemorrhage), diarrhea, vomiting, cramps, nausea.
GU: excessive uterine bleeding.
Skin: dermatitis, urticaria, *rash,* necrosis, alopecia.
Other: *fever.*

INTERACTIONS
Acetaminophen: increased bleeding possible with chronic (greater than 2 weeks) therapy with acetaminophen. Monitor very carefully.
Amiodarone, chloramphenicol, clofibrate, diflunisal, thyroid drugs, heparin, anabolic steroids, cimetidine, disulfiram, glucagon, inhalation anesthetics, metronidazole, quinidine, influenza vaccine, sulindac, sulfinpyrazone, sulfonamides: increased prothrombin time. Monitor patient carefully for bleeding. Consider anticoagulant dosage reduction.
Barbiturates: inhibition of hypoprothrombinemic effect of anticoagulants. If barbiturates are withdrawn, reduce anticoagulant dose; inhibition may last weeks after barbiturate is withdrawn, but fatal hemorrhage can occur when inhibiting effect disappears.
Cholestyramine: decreased response when administered too close together. Administer 6 hours after oral anticoagulants.
Ethacrynic acid, indomethacin, mefenamic acid, oxyphenbutazone, phenylbutazone, salicylates: increased prothrombin time; ulcerogenic effects. Don't use together.
Glutethimide, chloral hydrate, triclofos sodium: increased or decreased prothrombin time. Avoid use if possible, or monitor patient carefully.
Griseofulvin, haloperidol, ethchlorvynol, carbamazepine, paraldehyde, rifampin: decreased prothrombin time with reduced anticoagulant effect. Monitor patient carefully.

NURSING CONSIDERATIONS
• Contraindicated in bleeding or hemorrhagic tendencies resulting from open wounds, visceral cancer, GI ulcers, severe hepatic or renal disease, severe uncontrolled hypertension, subacute bacterial endocarditis, vitamin K deficiency; after recent operations in eye, brain, or spinal cord. Use

---

Italicized side effects are common or life-threatening.
*Liquid form contains alcohol.   **May contain tartrazine.

cautiously in diverticulitis, colitis, mild or moderate hypertension, mild or moderate hepatic or renal disease, lactation; with drainage tubes in any orifice; with regional or lumbar block anesthesia; or in any condition increasing risk of hemorrhage.

• Observe nursing infants of mothers on drug for unexpected bleeding.

• PT determinations essential for proper control. High incidence of bleeding when PT exceeds 2.5 times control values. Doctors usually try to maintain PT at 1.5 to 2 times normal.

• Give at same time daily. Stress importance of complying with recommended dosage and keeping follow-up appointments. Patient should carry a card that identifies him as a potential bleeder.

• Elderly patients and patients with renal or hepatic failure are especially sensitive to warfarin effect.

• Half-life of warfarin's anticoagulant effect is 36 to 44 hours.

• Warfarin effect can be neutralized by vitamin K injections.

• Regularly inspect patient for bleeding gums, bruises on arms or legs, petechiae, nosebleeds, melena, tarry stools, hematuria, hematemesis. Tell patient and family to watch for these signs and notify doctor immediately.

• Warn patient to avoid over-the-counter products containing aspirin, other salicylates, or drugs that may interact with warfarin sodium.

• Food and enteral feedings that contain vitamin K may cause inadequate anticoagulation. Warn patient to read labels.

• Because onset of action is delayed, heparin sodium is often given during first few days of treatment. When heparin is being given simultaneously, don't draw blood for prothrombin time within 5 hours of intermittent I.V. heparin administration. However, blood for prothrombin time may be drawn at any time during continuous heparin infusion.

• Fever and skin rash signal severe adverse reactions. Withhold drug and call doctor immediately.

• Tell patient to notify doctor if menses is heavier than usual. May require dosage adjustment.

• Tell patient to use electric razor when shaving to avoid scratching skin and to brush teeth with a soft toothbrush.

• Best oral anticoagulant when patient must receive antacids or phenytoin.

• Light to moderate alcohol intake does not significantly affect prothrombin time.

• Possibly effective in treatment of transient cerebral ischemic attacks.

• Tell patient to eat a consistent amount of leafy green vegetables every day. These contain vitamin K, and eating different amounts daily may alter anticoagulant effects.

68

Hemostatics

absorbable gelatin sponge
aminocaproic acid
antihemophilic factor (AHF)
dicresulene polymer
Factor IX complex
microfibrillar collagen hemostat
oxidized cellulose
thrombin

COMBINATION PRODUCTS
None.

absorbable gelatin sponge
Gelfoam

MECHANISM OF ACTION
Absorbs and holds many times its
weight in blood. Also provides a
framework for growth of granulation
tissue.

INDICATIONS & DOSAGE
Decubitus ulcers—
Adults: place aseptically deep into ulcer. Don't disturb or remove; may add
extra p.r.n.
*To provide hemostasis in surgery (ad-
junct)—*
Adults: apply saturated with isotonic
sodium chloride injection or thrombin
solution. Hold in place for 10 to 15
seconds. When oozing is controlled,
allow material to remain in place.

ADVERSE REACTIONS
None reported.

INTERACTIONS
None significant.

NURSING CONSIDERATIONS
• Contraindicated in frank infection,
or postpartum bleeding or hemorrhage; also for use as a sole hemostatic agent in abnormal bleeding.
• Avoid overpacking when placed
into body cavities or closed tissue
spaces.
• Systemically absorbed within 4 to 6
weeks; no need to remove.

aminocaproic acid
Amicar♦

Pregnancy Risk Category: C

MECHANISM OF ACTION
Inhibits plasminogen activator substances. To a lesser degree, it blocks
antiplasmin activity by inhibiting fibrinolysis.

INDICATIONS & DOSAGE
*Excessive bleeding resulting from hy-
perfibrinolysis—*
Adults: initially, 5 g P.O. or slow I.V.
infusion, followed by 1 to 1.25 g
hourly until bleeding is controlled.
Maximum dosage is 30 g daily.

ADVERSE REACTIONS
Blood: generalized thrombosis.
CNS: dizziness, malaise, headache.
CV: hypotension, bradycardia, dys-
rhythmias (with rapid I.V. infusion).
EENT: tinnitus, nasal stuffiness, con-
junctival suffusion.
GI: nausea, cramps, diarrhea.
Skin: rash.
Other: malaise.

Italicized side effects are common or life-threatening.
*Liquid form contains alcohol.   **May contain tartrazine.

INTERACTIONS
Oral contraceptives, estrogens: increased probability of hypercoagulability. Use together cautiously.

NURSING CONSIDERATIONS
• Contraindicated in active intravascular clotting. Use cautiously in thrombophlebitis and cardiac, hepatic, or renal disease.
• Monitor coagulation studies, heart rhythm, and blood pressure. Notify doctor of any change immediately.
• Also used as antidote for streptokinase or urokinase toxicity; not beneficial in treating thrombocytopenia.
• Dilute solution with sterile water for injection, normal saline injection, dextrose 5% in water, or Ringer's injection.
• Available in liquid form.
• Drug is sometimes helpful as an adjunct in treating hemophilia.

---

antihemophilic factor (AHF)
Antihemophilic Globulin (AHG)♦, Hemofil, Hemofil T, Koate, Profilate

Pregnancy Risk Category: C

MECHANISM OF ACTION
Directly replaces deficient clotting factor.

INDICATIONS & DOSAGE
Hemophilia A (Factor VIII deficiency)—
Adults and children: 10 to 20 units/kg I.V. push or infusion q 8 to 24 hours. Maintenance dosages may be less. Infusion rate usually 10 to 20 ml reconstituted solution per 3 minutes. Dosage varies with individual needs.

ADVERSE REACTIONS
CNS: headache, paresthesias, clouding or loss of consciousness.
CV: tachycardia, hypotension, possible intravascular hemolysis in patients with blood type A, B, or AB.
EENT: visual disturbances.
GI: nausea, vomiting.
Skin: erythema, *urticaria*.
Other: *chills, fever, backache, flushing,* chest constriction; hypersensitivity.

INTERACTIONS
None significant.

NURSING CONSIDERATIONS
• Use cautiously in neonates, infants, and patients with hepatic disease because of susceptibility to hepatitis, which may be transmitted in antihemophilic factor.
• Monitor vital signs regularly. Take baseline pulse rate before I.V. administration. If pulse rate increases significantly, flow rate should be reduced or administration stopped.
• Monitor patient for allergic reactions.
• For I.V. use only. Use plastic syringe; drug may interact with glass syringe, causing binding of ground-glass surface.
• Refrigerate concentrate until ready to use, but not after reconstituted. Refrigeration after reconstitution may cause the active ingredient to precipitate. Before reconstituting, concentrate and diluent bottles should be warmed to room temperature. To mix drug, gently roll vial between hands. Reconstituted solution unstable; use within 3 hours. Store away from heat. Don't shake or mix with other I.V. solutions.
• As ordered, administer hepatitis B vaccine before administering antihemophilic factor.
• Monitor coagulation studies before and during therapy.

---

dicresulene polymer
Negatan

MECHANISM OF ACTION
An astringent and protein denaturant.

INDICATIONS & DOSAGE
Cervical bleeding—
Women: apply 1-inch gauze dipped in 1:10 dilution of drug; insert in cervical canal. If tolerated, may increase to full-strength solution. Remove pack after 24 hours; give 2-quart douche of dilute negatol or vinegar.
Oral ulcers—
Adults and children: apply to dried lesion with applicator, leave for 1 minute, then neutralize with large amounts of water.

ADVERSE REACTIONS
Local: *burning sensation.*
Skin: erythema, superficial desquamation when applied to skin.

INTERACTIONS
None significant.

NURSING CONSIDERATIONS
• Vaginal membrane turns grayish after vaginal use.
• When used in vagina, patient should wear a perineal pad to prevent soiling of clothing.
• When used for oral ulcers, may apply topical anesthetic first to prevent burning sensation.
• Always clean and dry area to be treated.
• Astringent, styptic, and protein denaturant; highly acidic.

Factor IX complex
Konyne, Profilnine, Proplex
Pregnancy Risk Category: C

MECHANISM OF ACTION
Directly replaces deficient clotting factor.

INDICATIONS & DOSAGE
Factor IX deficiency (hemophilia B or Christmas disease), anticoagulant overdosage—
Adults and children: units required equal 0.8 to 1 × body weight in kg × percentage of desired increase of Factor IX level, by slow I.V. infusion or I.V. push. Dosage is highly individualized, depending on degree of deficiency, level of Factor IX desired, weight of patient, and severity of bleeding.

ADVERSE REACTIONS
CNS: headache.
CV: *thromboembolic reactions,* possible intravascular hemolysis in patients with blood type A, B, or AB.
Other: *transient fever, chills, flushing, tingling,* hypersensitivity.

INTERACTIONS
None significant.

NURSING CONSIDERATIONS
• Contraindicated in hepatic disease, intravascular coagulation, or fibrinolysis. Use cautiously in neonates and infants because of susceptibility to hepatitis, which may be transmitted with Factor IX complex.
• Observe patient for allergic reactions, and monitor vital signs regularly.
• As ordered, administer hepatitis B vaccine before administering Factor IX complex.
• Avoid rapid infusion. If tingling sensation, fever, chills, or headache develops during I.V. infusion, decrease flow rate and notify the doctor.
• Reconstitute with 20 ml sterile water for injection for each vial of lyophilized drug. Keep refrigerated until ready to use; warm to room temperature before reconstituting. Use within 3 hours of reconstitution. Unstable in solution. Don't shake, refrigerate, or mix reconstituted solution with other I.V. solutions. Store away from heat.

Italicized side effects are common or life-threatening.
*Liquid form contains alcohol.   **May contain tartrazine.

microfibrillar collagen hemostat
Avitene

Pregnancy Risk Category: C

MECHANISM OF ACTION
Attracts and aggregates platelets.

INDICATIONS & DOSAGE
To provide hemostasis in surgery (adjunct)—
Adults and children: amount depends on severity of bleeding. Compress area with dry sponges. Apply drug directly to bleeding site for 1 to 5 minutes. Gently remove excess. Reapply if needed.

ADVERSE REACTIONS
Blood: hematoma.
Local: exacerbation of wound dehiscence, abscess formation, foreign body reaction, adhesion formation.
Other: enhanced infection in contaminated wounds, mediastinitis, hypersensitivity.

INTERACTIONS
None significant.

NURSING CONSIDERATIONS
• Contraindicated in closure of skin incisions; it may interfere with healing.
• Not for injection.
• Don't spill on nonbleeding surfaces.
• Don't dilute. Always apply dry.
• Adheres to wet gloves, instruments, or tissue surfaces. Handle and apply with smooth, dry forceps. Apply directly to source of bleeding.

oxidized cellulose
Oxycel♦, Surgicel♦

MECHANISM OF ACTION
Absorbs and holds many times its weight in blood.

INDICATIONS & DOSAGE
To provide hemostasis in surgery (adjunct); external bleeding at tumor sites—
Adults and children: apply with sterile technique, p.r.n. Remove after hemostasis, if possible, with dry sterile forceps. Leave in place if necessary.

ADVERSE REACTIONS
CNS: headache when used as packing for epistaxis, or after rhinologic procedures or application to surface wounds.
EENT: sneezing, epistaxis, stinging, or burning when used as packing for rhinologic procedures; nasal membrane necrosis or septal perforation.
Local: encapsulation of fluid, foreign body reaction, burning or stinging after application to surface wounds.
Other: possible prolongation of drainage in cholecystectomies.

INTERACTIONS
Thrombin: may decrease blood clotting effectiveness.

NURSING CONSIDERATIONS
• Contraindicated in controlling hemorrhage from large arteries; for use on nonhemorrhagic, serous, oozing surfaces; in implantation in bone defects.
• Don't pack or wad unless it will be removed after hemostasis. Don't apply too tightly when used as wrap sheet in vascular surgery. Apply loosely against bleeding surface.
• Always remove after hemostasis when used in laminectomies or near optic nerve chain.
• Don't autoclave this product.
• Use only amount needed to produce hemostasis. Remove excess before surgical closure.
• Use minimal amounts in urologic procedures.
• In large wounds, don't overlap skin edges.
• Use sterile technique to remove from open wounds after hemostasis.

Don't remove without irrigating material first; otherwise, fresh bleeding may occur.
• Don't moisten. Hemostatic effect is greater when applied dry.
• Should not be used for permanent packing in fractures because it may result in cyst formation.

---

thrombin
Thrombinar♦

Pregnancy Risk Category: C

MECHANISM OF ACTION
Clots to form fibrin in the presence of fibrinogen.

INDICATIONS & DOSAGE
Bleeding from parenchymatous tissue, cancellous bone, dental sockets, nasal and laryngeal surgery, and in plastic surgery and skin-grafting procedures—
Adults: apply 100 units per ml of sterile isotonic sodium chloride solution or sterile distilled water to area where clotting needed (or may apply dry powder in bone surgery); in major bleeding, apply 1,000 to 2,000 units/ml sterile isotonic sodium chloride solution. Sponge blood from area before application, but avoid sponging area after application.
GI hemorrhage—
Adults: give 60 ml (2 oz) of milk, followed by 60 ml of milk containing 10,000 to 20,000 units thrombin. Repeat t.i.d. for 4 to 5 days or until bleeding is controlled.

ADVERSE REACTIONS
Systemic: hypersensitivity and fever.

INTERACTIONS
None significant.

NURSING CONSIDERATIONS
• Contraindicated in patients with hypersensitivity to thrombin or bovine products.
• Obtain patient history of reactions to thrombin or bovine products.
• Observe patient for allergic reactions, and monitor vital signs regularly.
• Have blood typed and cross matched to treat possible hemorrhage.
• Don't inject topical thrombin or allow it to enter large blood vessels. I.V. injection may cause death because of severe intravascular clotting.
• May be used with absorbable gelatin sponge but not with oxidized cellulose. Check sponge labeling before use.
• Neutralize stomach acids before oral use in GI hemorrhage.
• Keep refrigerated, preferably frozen, until ready to use. Unstable in solution. Use within 24 hours of reconstitution; discard after 48 hours. Store away from heat.
• Broken down by diluted acid, alkali, and salts of heavy metals.

69

Blood derivatives

normal serum albumin 5%
normal serum albumin 25%
plasma protein fraction

COMBINATION PRODUCTS
None.

normal serum albumin 5%
Albuminar 5%, Albutein 5%,
Buminate 5%, Plasbumin 5%

normal serum albumin 25%
Albuminar 25%, Albumisol 25%,
Buminate 25%, Plasbumin 25%

Pregnancy Risk Category: C

MECHANISM OF ACTION
Normal serum albumin 25% provides
intravascular oncotic pressure in a 5:1
ratio, which causes a shift of fluid
from interstitial spaces to the circulation and slightly increases plasma protein concentration. Normal serum albumin 5% supplies colloid to the
blood and expands plasma volume.

INDICATIONS & DOSAGE
Shock—
Adults: initially, 500 ml (5% solution) by I.V. infusion, repeat q 30
minutes, p.r.n. Dosage varies with patient's condition and response.
Children: 25% to 50% adult dose in
nonemergency.
Hypoproteinemia—
Adults: 1,000 to 1,500 ml 5% solution by I.V. infusion daily, maximum
rate 5 to 10 ml/minute; or 25 to 100 g
25% solution by I.V. infusion daily,
maximum rate 3 ml/minute. Dosage

varies with patient's condition and response.
Burns—dosage varies according to extent of burn and patient's condition.
Usually maintain plasma albumin at 2
to 3 g/100 ml.
Hyperbilirubinemia—
Infants: 1 g albumin (4 ml 25%)/kg
before transfusion.

ADVERSE REACTIONS
CV: *vascular overload after rapid infusion,* hypotension, altered pulse
rate.
GI: increased salivation, nausea,
vomiting.
Skin: urticaria.
Other: chills, fever, altered respiration.

INTERACTIONS
None significant.

NURSING CONSIDERATIONS
• Contraindicated in severe anemia or
heart failure. Use cautiously in low
cardiac reserve, absence of albumin
deficiency, and restricted sodium intake.
• Do not give more than 250 g in 48
hours.
• Watch for hemorrhage or shock if
used after surgery or injury.
• Monitor vital signs carefully.
• Watch for signs of vascular overload (heart failure or pulmonary
edema).
• Patient should be properly hydrated
before infusion of solution.
• Avoid rapid I.V. infusion. Specific
rate is individualized according to pa-

tient's age, condition, and diagnosis.
• Dilute with sterile water for injection, 0.9% sodium chloride solution, or dextrose 5% in water injection. Use solution promptly; contains no preservatives. Discard unused solution.
• Don't use cloudy solutions or those containing sediment. Solution should be clear amber color.
• Freezing may cause bottle to break. Follow storage instructions on bottle.
• One volume of 25% albumin is equivalent to five volumes of 5% albumin in producing hemodilution and relative anemia.
• This product is very expensive, and random supply shortages occur often.
• Monitor intake/output, hemoglobin, hematocrit, and serum protein and electrolytes during therapy.

plasma protein fraction
Plasmanate, Plasma-Plex, Plasmatein, Protenate

Pregnancy Risk Category: C

MECHANISM OF ACTION
Supplies colloid to the blood and expands plasma volume.

INDICATIONS & DOSAGE
Shock—
Adults: varies with patient's condition and response, but usual dose is 250 to 500 ml (12.5 to 25 g protein), usually no faster than 10 ml/minute.
Children: 22 to 33 ml/kg I.V. infused at rate of 5 to 10 ml/minute.
Hypoproteinemia—
Adults: 1,000 to 1,500 ml I.V. daily. Maximum infusion rate 8 ml/minute.

ADVERSE REACTIONS
CNS: headache.
CV: variable effects on blood pressure after rapid infusion or intraarterial administration; *vascular overload after rapid infusion.*
GI: nausea, vomiting, hypersalivation.

Skin: erythema, urticaria.
Other: flushing, chills, fever, back pain, dyspnea.

INTERACTIONS
None significant.

NURSING CONSIDERATIONS
• Contraindicated in patients with severe anemia or heart failure, and those patients undergoing cardiac bypass. Use cautiously in hepatic or renal failure, low cardiac reserve, and restricted sodium intake.
• Monitor blood pressure. Infusion should be slowed or stopped if hypotension suddenly occurs.
• Vital signs should return to normal gradually; monitor hourly.
• Watch for signs of vascular overload (heart failure or pulmonary edema).
• Monitor intake/output. Watch for decreased urine output. Notify doctor if this occurs.
• Check expiration date on container before using. Discard solutions in containers that have been opened for more than 4 hours. Solution contains no preservatives.
• Don't use solutions that are cloudy, contain sediment, or have been frozen.
• If patient is dehydrated, give additional fluids either P.O. or I.V.
• Do not give more than 250 g (5,000 ml 5%) in 48 hours.
• Contains 130 to 160 mEq sodium/liter.

70

Thrombolytic enzymes

alteplase
streptokinase
urokinase

COMBINATION PRODUCTS
None.

---

alteplase
Activase

Pregnancy Risk Category: C

MECHANISM OF ACTION
Binds to fibrin in a thrombus, and locally converts plasminogen to plasmin, which initiates local fibrinolysis.

INDICATIONS & DOSAGE
Lysis of thrombi obstructing coronary arteries in acute myocardial infarction—
Adults: 100 mg I.V. infusion over 3 hours as follows: 60 mg in the first hour, of which 6 to 10 mg is given as a bolus over the first 1 to 2 minutes. Then 20 mg/hr infusion for 2 hours. Smaller adults (<65 kg) should receive a dose of 1.25 mg/kg in a similar fashion (60% in the first hour, with 10% as a bolus; then 20% of the total dose per hour for 2 hours).

ADVERSE REACTIONS
Blood: bleeding.
CNS: *cerebral hemorrhage,* fever.
CV: hypotension, dysrhythmias.
GI: bleeding, nausea, vomiting.
Other: hypersensitivity, urticaria.

INTERACTIONS
Aspirin, dipyridamole, heparin, coumarin anticoagulants: increased risk of bleeding. Monitor patient carefully.

NURSING CONSIDERATIONS
• Contraindicated in active internal bleeding, intracranial neoplasm, arteriovenous malformation, aneurysm, and severe uncontrolled hypertension. Also contraindicated in a history of cardiovascular accident, recent (within 2 months) intraspinal or intracranial trauma or surgery, or known bleeding diathesis.
• Do not exceed dose of 100 mg. Higher doses are associated with an increased incidence of intracranial bleeding.
• Coronary thrombolysis is associated with dysrhythmias induced by reperfusion of ischemic myocardium. Such dysrhythmias are not different from those commonly associated with myocardial infarction. Have antiarrhythmic agents readily available and carefully monitor the ECG.
• Successful recanalization of occluded coronary arteries and improvement of heart function are time-dependent phenomena and require initiation of treatment with alteplase as soon as possible after the onset of symptoms.
• Bleeding is the most common adverse effect and may occur internally and at external puncture sites. Carefully monitor patient.
• Heparin therapy is frequently initiated after treatment with alteplase to decrease the risk of rethrombosis.
• Reconstitute drug with sterile water for injection (without preservatives)

only. Do not use vial if the vacuum is not present. Reconstitute with a large bore (18G) needle, directing the stream of sterile water at the lyophilized cake. Slight foaming is common, and the resulting solution should be clear to pale yellow. Avoid excess agitation of solution.

• Drug may be administered as reconstituted (1 mg/ml) or diluted with an equal volume of normal saline or dextrose 5% in water to make a 0.5 mg/ml solution. Adding other to the infusion is not recommended.

• Reconstitute alteplase solution immediately before use, and administer it within 8 hours. The drug may be temporarily stored at 35° to 86° F. (2° to 30° C.), but it is stable for 8 hours at room temperature. Discard any solution unused after that time because it contains no preservatives.

---

streptokinase
Kabikinase, Streptase♦

Pregnancy Risk Category: C

MECHANISM OF ACTION
Activates plasminogen in two steps. Plasminogen and streptokinase form a complex that exposes the plasminogen-activating site. Plasminogen is converted to plasmin by cleavage of the peptide bond.

INDICATIONS & DOSAGE
Arteriovenous cannula occlusion—
Adults: 250,000 IU in 2 ml I.V. solution by I.V. pump infusion into each occluded limb of the cannula over 25 to 35 minutes. Clamp off cannula for 2 hours. Then aspirate contents of cannula; flush with saline solution and reconnect.
Venous thrombosis, pulmonary embolism, and arterial thrombosis and embolism—
Adults: loading dose is 250,000 IU I.V. infusion over 30 minutes. Sustaining dose is 100,000 IU/hour I.V.

infusion for 72 hours for deep vein thrombosis and 100,000 IU/hour over 24 to 72 hours by I.V. infusion pump for pulmonary embolism.
Lysis of coronary artery thrombi following acute myocardial infarction—
Adults: loading dose is 20,000 IU via coronary catheter, followed by a maintenance dose. Maintenance dose is 2,000 IU/minute for 60 minutes as an infusion. Alternatively, may be administered as an I.V. infusion. Usual adult dose is 1.5 million units infused over 60 minutes.

ADVERSE REACTIONS
Blood: bleeding, low hematocrit.
CV: transient lowering or elevation of blood pressure.
EENT: periorbital edema.
Skin: urticaria.
Local: phlebitis at injection site.
Other: *hypersensitivity to drug, fever, anaphylaxis,* musculoskeletal pain, minor breathing difficulty, bronchospasms, angioneurotic edema.

INTERACTIONS
Anticoagulants: concurrent use with streptokinase is not recommended. Reversing the effects of oral anticoagulants must be considered before beginning therapy; heparin must be stopped and its effect allowed to diminish.
Aspirin, indomethacin, phenylbutazone, drugs affecting platelet activity: increased risk of bleeding. Do not use together.

NURSING CONSIDERATIONS
• Contraindicated in ulcerative wounds, active internal bleeding, and recent cerebrovascular accident; recent trauma with possible internal injuries; visceral or intracranial malignancy; ulcerative colitis; diverticulitis; severe hypertension; acute or chronic hepatic or renal insufficiency; uncontrolled hypocoagulation; chronic pulmonary disease with cavi-

tation; subacute bacterial endocarditis or rheumatic valvular disease; recent cerebral embolism, thrombosis, or hemorrhage. Also contraindicated within 10 days after intraarterial diagnostic procedure or any surgery, including liver or kidney biopsy, lumbar puncture, thoracentesis, paracentesis, or extensive or multiple cutdowns.

• Use cautiously when treating arterial emboli that originate from left side of heart because of danger of cerebral infarction.

• I.M. injections are contraindicated during streptokinase therapy.

• Before initiating therapy, draw blood to determine PTT and PT. Rate of I.V. infusion depends on thrombin time and streptokinase resistance.

• If the patient has had either a recent streptococcal infection or recent treatment with streptokinase, a higher loading dose may be necessary.

• Preparation of I.V. solution: reconstitute each vial with 5 ml normal saline solution for injection. Further dilute to 45 ml. Don't shake; roll gently to mix. Use within 24 hours. Store at room temperature in powder form; refrigerate after reconstitution.

• Monitor patient for excessive bleeding every 15 minutes for the first hour, every 30 minutes for the second through eighth hours, then once every shift. If bleeding is evident, stop therapy. Pretreatment with heparin or drugs affecting platelets causes high risk of bleeding.

• Monitor pulses, color, and sensity of extremities every hour.

• Have typed and crossmatched packed red cells and whole blood ready to treat possible hemorrhage.

• Keep aminocaproic acid available to treat bleeding. Corticosteroids are used to treat allergic reactions.

• Before using streptokinase to clear an occluded arteriovenous cannula, try flushing with heparinized saline.

• Bruising more likely during therapy; avoid unnecessary handling of patient. Side rails should be padded.

• Maintain the involved extremity in straight alignment to prevent bleeding from the infusion site.

• Keep venipuncture sites to a minimum; use pressure dressing on puncture sites for at least 15 minutes.

• Keep a laboratory flow sheet on patient's chart to monitor partial thromboplastin time, prothrombin time, hemoglobin, and hematocrit.

• Monitor vital signs frequently.

• Watch for signs of hypersensitivity. Notify doctor immediately.

• Heparin by continuous infusion is usually started within an hour after stopping streptokinase. Use infusion pump to administer heparin.

• Should be used only by doctors with wide experience in thrombotic disease management where clinical and laboratory monitoring can be performed.

• Thrombolytic therapy in patients with acute myocardial infarction is associated with decreased infarct size, improved ventricular function, and decreased incidence of congestive heart failure. Streptokinase must be administered within 6 hours of the onset of symptoms for optimal effect.

urokinase

Abbokinase, Win-Kinase

Pregnancy Risk Category: B

MECHANISM OF ACTION

Activates plasminogen by directly cleaving peptide bonds at two different sites.

INDICATIONS & DOSAGE

Lysis of acute massive pulmonary emboli and lysis of pulmonary emboli accompanied by unstable hemodynamics—

Adults: for I.V. infusion only by constant infusion pump that will deliver a total volume of 195 ml.
Priming dose: 4,400 IU/kg of urokinase–normal saline solution admix-

---

ture given over 10 minutes. Follow with 4,400 IU/kg hourly for 12 to 24 hours. Total volume should not exceed 200 ml. Follow therapy with continuous I.V. infusion of heparin, then oral anticoagulants.

Coronary artery thrombosis—
Adults: following a bolus dose of heparin ranging from 2,500 to 10,000 units, infuse 6,000 IU/minute of urokinase into the occluded artery for up to 12 hours. Average total dosage is 500,000 IU.

Venous catheter occlusion—
Instill 5,000 IU into occluded line, wait 5 minutes, then aspirate. Repeat aspiration attempts q 5 minutes for 30 minutes. If not patent after 30 minutes, cap line and let urokinase work for 30 to 60 minutes before aspirating. May require second instillation.

ADVERSE REACTIONS
Blood: bleeding, low hematocrit.
Local: phlebitis at injection site.
Other: hypersensitivity (not as frequent as streptokinase), musculoskeletal pain, bronchospasm, *anaphylaxis.*

INTERACTIONS
Anticoagulants: concurrent use with urokinase is not recommended. Consider reversing the effects of oral anticoagulants before beginning therapy; heparin must be stopped and its effect allowed to diminish.
Aspirin, indomethacin, phenylbutazone, other drugs affecting platelet activity: increased risk of bleeding. Do not use together.

NURSING CONSIDERATIONS
• Contraindicated in ulcerative wounds, active internal bleeding, and cerebrovascular accident; recent trauma with possible internal injuries; visceral or intracranial malignancy; pregnancy and first 10 days postpartum; ulcerative colitis; diverticulitis; severe hypertension; acute or chronic hepatic or renal insufficiency; uncontrolled hypocoagulation; chronic pulmonary disease with cavitation; subacute bacterial endocarditis or rheumatic valvular disease; and recent cerebral embolism, thrombosis, or hemorrhage. Also contraindicated within 10 days after intraarterial diagnostic procedure or any surgery, including liver or kidney biopsy, lumbar puncture, thoracentesis, paracentesis, or extensive or multiple cutdowns.
• I.M. injections are contraindicated during urokinase therapy.
• Maintain the involved extremity in straight alignment to prevent bleeding from the infusion site.
• To prepare I.V. solution: add 5.2 ml sterile water for injection to vial. Dilute further with 0.9% normal saline solution before infusion. Don't use bacteriostatic water for injection to reconstitute; it contains preservatives.
• Monitor patient for bleeding every 15 minutes for the first hour; every 30 minutes for the second through eighth hours; then once every shift. Pretreatment with drugs affecting platelets places patient at high risk of bleeding.
• Monitor pulses, color, and sensitivity of extremities every hour.
• Have typed and crossmatched red cells, whole blood, and aminocaproic acid available to treat bleeding. Corticosteroids are used to treat allergic reactions.
• Keep a laboratory flow sheet on patient's chart to monitor partial thromboplastin time, prothrombin time, hemoglobin, and hematocrit.
• Watch for signs of hypersensitivity.
• Monitor vital signs.
• Keep venipuncture sites to a minimum; use pressure dressing on puncture sites for at least 15 minutes.
• Heparin by continuous infusion is usually started within an hour after urokinase has been stopped.
• Bruising is more likely during therapy; avoid unnecessary handling of patient. Side rails should be padded.

Italicized side effects are common or life-threatening.
*Liquid form contains alcohol.   **May contain tartrazine.

71

Alkylating agents

busulfan
carmustine (BCNU)
chlorambucil
cisplatin (cis-platinum)
cyclophosphamide
dacarbazine (DTIC)
ifosfamide
lomustine (CCNU)
mechlorethamine hydrochloride
  (nitrogen mustard)
melphalan
streptozocin
thiotepa
uracil mustard

COMBINATION PRODUCTS
None.

busulfan
Myleran♦

Pregnancy Risk Category: D

MECHANISM OF ACTION
Cross-links strands of cellular DNA and interferes with RNA transcription, causing an imbalance of growth that leads to cell death. Cell cycle-nonspecific.

INDICATIONS & DOSAGE
Chronic myelocytic (granulocytic) leukemia—
Adults: 4 to 8 mg P.O. daily up to 12 mg P.O. daily until WBC falls to 15,000/mm³; stop drug until WBC rises to 50,000/mm³, then resume treatment as before; or 4 to 8 mg P.O. daily until WBC falls to 10,000 to 20,000/mm³, then reduce daily dosage as needed to maintain WBC at this level (usually 2 mg daily).
Children: 0.06 to 0.12 mg/kg or 2.3 to 4.6 mg/m²/day P.O.; adjust dosage to maintain WBC at 20,000/mm³, but never less than 10,000/mm³.

ADVERSE REACTIONS
Blood: WBC falling after about 10 days and continuing to fall for 2 weeks after stopping drug; *thrombocytopenia,* leukopenia, anemia.
GI: nausea, vomiting, diarrhea, cheilosis, glossitis.
GU: amenorrhea, testicular atrophy, impotence.
Metabolic: Addison-like wasting syndrome, profound hyperuricemia due to increased cell lysis.
Skin: transient hyperpigmentation, anhidrosis.
Other: gynecomastia; alopecia; *irreversible pulmonary fibrosis, commonly termed "busulfan lung."*

INTERACTIONS
None significant.

NURSING CONSIDERATIONS
• Use cautiously in patients recently given other myelosuppressive drugs or radiation treatment, and in those with depressed neutrophil or platelet count.
• Warn patient to watch for signs of infection (fever, sore throat, fatigue) and bleeding (easy bruising, nosebleeds, bleeding gums, melena). Take temperature daily.
• Pulmonary fibrosis may occur as late as 4 to 6 months after treatment with busulfan.

• Persistent cough and progressive dyspnea with alveolar exudate may result from drug toxicity, not pneumonia. Instruct patient to report symptoms so dosage adjustments can be made.

• To prevent hyperuricemia with resulting uric acid nephropathy, allopurinol may be used with adequate hydration. Monitor serum uric acid.

• Patient response usually begins within 1 to 2 weeks (increased appetite, sense of well-being, decreased total leukocyte count, reduction in size of spleen).

• Anticoagulants and aspirin products should be used cautiously. Watch closely for signs of bleeding. Instruct patient to avoid any OTC product containing aspirin.

• Avoid all I.M. injections when platelets are below 100,000/mm³.

• Therapeutic effects are often accompanied by toxicity.

carmustine (BCNU)
BiCNU♦

Pregnancy Risk Category: D

MECHANISM OF ACTION
Cross-links strands of cellular DNA and interferes with RNA transcription, causing an imbalance of growth that leads to cell death. Cell cycle-nonspecific.

INDICATIONS & DOSAGE
Brain, colon, and stomach cancer; Hodgkin's disease; non-Hodgkin's lymphomas; melanomas; multiple myeloma; and hepatoma—
Adults: 75 to 100 mg/m² I.V. by slow infusion daily for 2 days; repeat q 6 weeks if platelets are above 100,000/mm³ and WBC is above 4,000/mm³. Dosage is reduced 50% when WBC is less than 2,000/mm³ and platelets are less than 25,000/mm³.

Alternate therapy: 200 mg/m² I.V. slow infusion as a single dose, re-

peated q 6 to 8 weeks; or 40 mg/m² I.V. slow infusion for 5 consecutive days, repeated q 6 weeks.

ADVERSE REACTIONS
Blood: *cumulative bone marrow depression, delayed 4 to 6 weeks, lasting 1 to 2 weeks; leukopenia; thrombocytopenia.*
CNS: ataxia, drowsiness.
GI: *nausea, which begins in 2 to 6 hours (can be severe); vomiting.*
GU: nephrotoxicity.
Hepatic: hepatotoxicity.
Metabolic: possible hyperuricemia in lymphoma patients when rapid cell lysis occurs.
Skin: facial flushing.
Local: *intense pain at infusion site from venous spasm.*
Other: pulmonary fibrosis.

INTERACTIONS
Cimetidine: may increase carmustine's bone marrow toxicity. Avoid combination if possible.

NURSING CONSIDERATIONS
• To reduce pain on infusion, dilute further or slow infusion rate.

• Warn patient to watch for signs of infection (fever, sore throat, fatigue) and bleeding (easy bruising, nosebleeds, bleeding gums, melena). Take temperature daily.

• Monitor CBC.

• To reduce nausea, give antiemetic before administering.

• Don't mix with other drugs during administration.

• To reconstitute, dissolve 100 mg carmustine in 3 ml absolute alcohol provided by manufacturer. Dilute solution with 27 ml sterile water for injection. Resultant solution contains 3.3 mg carmustine/ml in 10% alcohol. Dilute in normal saline solution or dextrose 5% in water for I.V. infusion. Give at least 250 ml over 1 to 2 hours.

• May store reconstituted solution in

---

refrigerator for 24 hours.
• May decompose at temperatures above 80° F. (26.6° C.).
• Solution is unstable in plastic I.V. bags. Administer only in glass containers.
• If powder liquefies or appears oily, it is a sign of decomposition. Discard.
• To prevent hyperuricemia with resulting uric acid nephropathy, allopurinol may be used with adequate hydration. Monitor serum uric acid.
• Avoid contact with skin, as carmustine will cause a brown stain. If drug comes into contact with skin, wash off thoroughly.
• Anticoagulants and aspirin products should be used cautiously. Watch closely for signs of bleeding. Instruct patient to avoid any OTC product containing aspirin.
• Avoid all I.M. injections when platelets are below 100,000/mm³.
• Since carmustine crosses the blood/brain barrier, it may be used to treat primary brain tumors.
• Preparation of parenteral form is associated with carcinogenic, mutagenic, and teratogenic risks for personnel. Follow institutional policy to reduce risks.
• Therapeutic effects are often accompanied by toxicity.

chlorambucil
Leukeran◆

Pregnancy Risk Category: D

MECHANISM OF ACTION
Cross-links strands of cellular DNA and interferes with RNA transcription, causing an imbalance of growth that leads to cell death. Cell cycle-nonspecific.

INDICATIONS & DOSAGE
Chronic lymphocytic leukemia, diffuse lymphocytic lymphoma, nodular lymphocytic lymphoma, Hodgkin's disease, ovarian carcinoma, mycosis fungoides—
Adults: 0.1 to 0.2 mg/kg P.O. daily for 3 to 6 weeks, then adjust for maintenance (usually 2 mg daily).
Children: 0.1 to 0.2 mg/kg/day or 4.5 mg/m² P.O. daily as a single dose or in divided doses.

ADVERSE REACTIONS
Blood: leukopenia, delayed up to 3 weeks, lasting up to 10 days after last dose; thrombocytopenia; anemia; myelosuppression (usually moderate, gradual, and rapidly reversible).
GI: *nausea, vomiting.*
GU: *azoospermia, infertility.*
Metabolic: hyperuricemia.
Skin: *exfoliative dermatitis,* rashes.
Other: allergic febrile reactions.

INTERACTIONS
None significant.

NURSING CONSIDERATIONS
• Place patient on neutropenia precautions if WBC falls below 2,000/mm³ or granulocytes fall below 1,000/mm³.
• Severe neutropenia reversible up to cumulative dosage of 6.5 mg/kg in a single course.
• Warn patient to watch for signs of infection (fever, sore throat, fatigue) and bleeding (easy bruising, nosebleeds, bleeding gums, melena). Take temperature daily.
• Monitor CBC.
• To prevent hyperuricemia with resulting uric acid nephropathy, allopurinol may be used with adequate hydration. Monitor serum uric acid.
• Avoid all I.M. injections when platelets are below 100,000/mm³.
• Anticoagulants and aspirin products should be used cautiously. Watch closely for signs of bleeding. Instruct patient to avoid OTC products containing aspirin.
• Therapeutic effects are often accompanied by toxicity.

cisplatin (cis-platinum)
Platinol♦

Pregnancy Risk Category: D

MECHANISM OF ACTION
Cross-links strands of cellular DNA and interferes with RNA transcription, causing an imbalance of growth that leads to cell death. Cell cycle-nonspecific.

INDICATIONS & DOSAGE
Adjunctive therapy in metastatic testicular cancer—
Adults: 20 mg/m^2 I.V. daily for 5 days. Repeat every 3 weeks for 3 cycles or longer.
Adjunctive therapy in metastatic ovarian cancer—
100 mg/m^2 I.V. Repeat every 4 weeks; or 50 mg/m^2 I.V. every 3 weeks with concurrent doxorubicin HCl therapy. Give as I.V. infusion in 2 liters normal saline solution with 37.5 g mannitol over 6 to 8 hours.
Treatment of advanced bladder cancer—
Adults: 50 to 70 mg/m^2 I.V. once every 3 to 4 weeks. Patients who have received other antineoplastics or radiation therapy should receive 50 mg/m^2 every 4 weeks.
Note: Prehydration and mannitol diuresis may reduce renal toxicity and ototoxicity significantly.

ADVERSE REACTIONS
Blood: *mild myelosuppression in 25% to 30% of patients, leukopenia, thrombocytopenia,* anemia; nadirs in circulating platelets and leukocytes on days 18 to 23, with recovery by day 39.
CNS: peripheral neuritis, loss of taste, seizures.
EENT: *tinnitus, hearing loss.*
GI: *nausea, vomiting, beginning 1 to 4 hours after dose and lasting 24 hours; diarrhea;* metallic taste.
GU: *more prolonged and severe renal toxicity with repeated courses of therapy.*
Other: *anaphylactoid reaction.*

INTERACTIONS
Aminoglycoside antibiotics: additive nephrotoxicity. Monitor renal function studies very carefully.

NURSING CONSIDERATIONS
• Dosage modification may be required in preexisting renal impairment, myelosuppression, or hearing impairment.
• Hydrate patient with normal saline solution before giving drug. Maintain urine output of 100 ml/hour for 4 consecutive hours before therapy and for 24 hours after therapy.
• Mannitol may be given as 12.5 g I.V. bolus before starting cisplatin infusion. Follow, if ordered, by infusion of mannitol at rate of up to 10 g/hour p.r.n. to maintain urine output during and 6 to 24 hours after cisplatin infusion.
• Do not repeat dosage unless platelets are over 100,000/mm^3, WBC is over 4,000/mm^3, creatinine is under 1.5 mg/dl, or BUN is under 25 mg/dl.
• Warn patient to watch for signs of infection (fever, sore throat, fatigue) and bleeding (easy bruising, nosebleeds, bleeding gums, melena). Take temperature daily.
• Monitor CBC, electrolytes (especially potassium and magnesium), platelets, and renal function studies before initial and subsequent dosages.
• Tell patient to report tinnitus immediately to prevent permanent hearing loss. Do audiometry prior to initial dosage and subsequent courses.
• Nausea and vomiting may be severe and protracted (up to 24 hours). Antiemetics can be started 24 hours before therapy. Monitor intake/output. Continue I.V. hydration until patient can tolerate adequate oral intake.
• Delayed-onset vomiting (3 to 5 days after treatment) has been reported.

Italicized side effects are common or life-threatening.
*Liquid form contains alcohol.   **May contain tartrazine.

Patients may need prolonged anti-emetic treatment.
- Reconstitute with sterile water for injection. Stable for 24 hours in normal saline solution at room temperature. Don't refrigerate.
- Infusions are most stable in chloride-containing solutions (such as normal saline, 0.45% normal saline, and 0.22% normal saline).
- Given with bleomycin and vinblastine for testicular cancer and with doxorubicin for ovarian cancer.
- Renal toxicity is cumulative. Renal function must return to normal before next dose can be given.
- Avoid all I.M. injections when platelets are below 100,000/mm³.
- Metoclopramide has been used very effectively to treat and prevent nausea and vomiting.
- Anaphylactoid reaction usually responds to immediate treatment with epinephrine, corticosteroids, or antihistamines.
- Preparation of parenteral form is associated with carcinogenic, mutagenic, and teratogenic risks for personnel. Follow institutional policy to reduce risks.
- Therapeutic effects are often accompanied by toxicity.

cyclophosphamide
Cytoxan**♦, Neosar, Procytox♦♦
Pregnancy Risk Category: D

MECHANISM OF ACTION
Cross-links strands of cellular DNA and interferes with RNA transcription, causing an imbalance of growth that leads to cell death. Cell cycle-nonspecific.

INDICATIONS & DOSAGE
Breast, head, neck, lung, and ovarian cancer; Hodgkin's disease; chronic lymphocytic leukemia; chronic myelocytic leukemia; acute lymphoblastic leukemia; neuroblastoma; retinoblas- *toma; non-Hodgkin's lymphomas; multiple myeloma; mycosis fungoides; sarcomas—*

Adults: initially, 40 to 50 mg/kg I.V. in divided doses over 2 to 5 days; then adjust for maintenance. Or 1 to 5 mg/kg P.O. daily, depending upon patient tolerance. Maintenance dosage is 1 to 5 mg/kg P.O. daily; or 10 to 15 mg/kg q 7 to 10 days I.V.; or 3 to 5 mg/kg I.V. twice weekly.

Children: 2 to 8 mg/kg daily or 60 to 250 mg/m² daily P.O. or I.V. for 6 days (dosage depends on susceptibility of neoplasm). Maintenance dosage 2 to 5 mg/kg or 50 to 150 mg/m² P.O. twice weekly.

ADVERSE REACTIONS
Blood: *leukopenia,* nadir between days 8 to 15, recovery in 17 to 28 days; thrombocytopenia; anemia.
CV: *cardiotoxicity* (with very high doses and in combination with doxorubicin).
GI: anorexia; *nausea and vomiting beginning within 6 hours, lasting 4 hours;* stomatitis; mucositis.
GU: gonadal suppression (may be irreversible), *hemorrhagic cystitis,* bladder fibrosis, nephrotoxicity.
Metabolic: hyperuricemia; syndrome of inappropriate antidiuretic hormone secretion (with high doses).
Other: *reversible alopecia in 50% of patients, especially with high doses;* secondary malignancies, *pulmonary fibrosis (high doses).*

INTERACTIONS
Corticosteroids, chloramphenicol: reduced activity of cyclophosphamide. Use cautiously.
Succinylcholine: may cause apnea. Don't use together.

NURSING CONSIDERATIONS
- Dosage modification may be required in severe leukopenia, thrombocytopenia, malignant cell infiltration of bone marrow, recent radiation ther-

apy or chemotherapy, or hepatic or renal disease.

• Advise both male and female patients to practice contraception while taking this drug and for 4 months after; drug is potentially teratogenic.

• Monitor CBC and renal and hepatic functions.

• Encourage fluid intake (3 liters daily) to prevent hemorrhagic cystitis. Don't give drug at bedtime, because voiding is too infrequent to avoid cystitis. If hemorrhagic cystitis occurs, discontinue drug. Cystitis can occur months after therapy has been stopped.

• Encourage patients to void every 1 to 2 hours while awake to minimize risk of hemorrhagic cystitis.

• Lyophilized preparation is much easier to reconstitute. Request this form from the pharmacy when preparing I.V.

• Reconstituted solution is stable 6 days refrigerated or 24 hours at room temperature.

• Avoid all I.M. injections when platelets are below 100,000/mm³.

• Can be given by direct I.V. push into a running I.V. line or by infusion in normal saline solution or dextrose 5% in water.

• To prevent hyperuricemia with resulting uric acid nephropathy, allopurinol may be used with adequate hydration. Monitor serum uric acid.

• Warn patient that alopecia is likely to occur, but that it is reversible.

• Monitor for cyclophosphamide toxicity if patient's corticosteroid therapy is discontinued.

• Preparation of parenteral form is associated with carcinogenic, mutagenic, and teratogenic risks for personnel. Follow institutional policy to reduce risks.

• Therapeutic effects are often accompanied by toxicity.

dacarbazine (DTIC)
DTIC-Dome♦

Pregnancy Risk Category: C

MECHANISM OF ACTION
Cross-links strands of cellular DNA and interferes with RNA transcription, causing an imbalance of growth that leads to cell death. Cell cycle-nonspecific.

INDICATIONS & DOSAGE
Metastatic malignant melanoma—
Adults: 2 to 4.5 mg/kg or 70 to 160 mg/m² I.V. daily for 10 days, then repeat q 4 weeks as tolerated; or 250 mg/m² I.V. daily for 5 days, repeated at 3-week intervals.
Hodgkin's disease—
Adults: 150 mg/m² daily (in combination with other agents) daily for 5 days, repeated q 4 weeks; or 375 mg/m² on the first day of a combination regimen, repeated q 15 days.

ADVERSE REACTIONS
Blood: *leukopenia and thrombocytopenia,* nadir between 3 and 4 weeks.
GI: *severe nausea and vomiting begin within 1 to 3 hours in 90% of patients, last 1 to 12 hours; anorexia.*
Skin: phototoxicity.
Local: severe pain if I.V. infiltrates or if solution is too concentrated; tissue damage.
Other: *flulike syndrome* (fever, malaise, myalgia beginning 7 days after treatment stopped and possibly lasting 7 to 21 days), alopecia, *anaphylaxis.*

INTERACTIONS
None significant.

NURSING CONSIDERATIONS
• Contraindicated in patients with hypersensitivity to the drug.
• Use lower dosage if renal or bone marrow function is impaired. Stop drug if WBC falls to 3,000/mm³ or platelets drop to 100,000/mm³. Moni-

---

Italicized side effects are common or life-threatening.
*Liquid form contains alcohol.   **May contain tartrazine.

tor CBC.
• Warn patient to watch for signs of infection (fever, sore throat, fatigue) and bleeding (easy bruising, nosebleeds, bleeding gums, melena). Take temperature daily.
• Discard refrigerated solution after 72 hours and room temperature solution after 8 hours.
• Avoid all I.M. injections when platelets are below 100,000/mm³.
• Give I.V. infusion in 50 to 100 ml dextrose 5% in water over 30 minutes. May dilute further or slow infusion to decrease pain at infusion site. Make sure drug does not infiltrate.
• If I.V. infiltrates, discontinue immediately and apply ice to area for 24 to 48 hours.
• During infusion, protect bag from direct sunlight to avoid possible drug breakdown.
• For Hodgkin's disease, usually given with bleomycin, vinblastine, and doxorubicin.
• Advise patient to avoid sunlight and sunlamps for first 2 days after treatment.
• Anticoagulants and aspirin products should be used cautiously. Watch closely for signs of bleeding. Instruct patient to avoid OTC products containing aspirin.
• Administering antiemetics before giving dacarbazine may help decrease nausea. Nausea and vomiting may sometimes subside after several doses.
• Reassure patient that flulike syndrome may be treated with mild antipyretics, such as acetaminophen.
• Preparation of parenteral form is associated with carcinogenic, mutagenic, and teratogenic risks for personnel. Follow institutional policy to reduce risks.
• Therapeutic effects are often accompanied by toxicity.

ifosfamide
Ifex

Pregnancy Risk Category: D

MECHANISM OF ACTION
Cross-links strands of cellular DNA, and interferes with RNA transcription causing an imbalance of growth that leads to cell death. Cell cycle-nonspecific.

INDICATIONS & DOSAGE
Testicular cancer—
Adults: 1.2 g/m²/day for 5 consecutive days. Treatment is repeated every 3 weeks or after the patient recovers from hematologic toxicity.

ADVERSE REACTIONS
Blood: leukopenia, thrombocytopenia, *myelosuppression.*
CNS: *lethargy, somnolescence, confusion, depressive psychosis,* coma.
GI: *nausea, vomiting.*
GU: *hemorrhagic cystitis (dose-limiting adverse reaction occurring in up to 50% of patients), hematuria,* nephrotoxicity.
Hepatic: elevated liver enzymes.
Other: *alopecia.*

INTERACTIONS
Allopurinol: may produce excessive ifosfamide effect by prolonging half-life. Monitor for enhanced toxicity.
Barbiturates: induce hepatic enzymes, hastening the formation of toxic metabolites. Ifosfamide toxicity may be increased.
Corticosteroids: may inhibit hepatic enzymes, reducing ifosfamide's effect. Monitor for enhanced ifosfamide toxicity if concurrent steroid dosage is suddenly reduced or discontinued.
Myelosuppressants: enhanced hematologic toxicity. Dosage adjustment may be necessary.

NURSING CONSIDERATIONS
• Use cautiously in renal or hepatic

impairment.

• Ifosfamide should be administered with a protecting agent (like mesna) to prevent hemorrhagic cystitis. Adequate fluid intake (2 liters/day, either P.O. or I.V.) is essential.

• Obtain a urinalysis prior to each dose. If microscopic hematuria is present, drug should be witheld until it resolves.

• Bladder irrigation with normal saline solution may decrease the possibility of cystitis.

• Avoid giving the drug at bedtime, because infrequent voiding during the night may increase the possibility of cystitis. Stop the drug if patient develops cystitis.

• Warn patient to watch for signs of infection (fever, sore throat, fatigue) and bleeding (easy bruising, nosebleeds, bleeding gums, melena). Take temperature daily.

• Avoid all I.M. injections when platelets are below 100,000/mm³.

• Anticoagulants and aspirin products should be used cautiously. Watch closely for signs of bleeding. Instruct patient to avoid OTC products containing aspirin.

• Administering antiemetics before giving ifosfamide may help decrease nausea.

• Assess patient for changes in mental status and cerebellar dysfunction. Dosage may have to be decreased.

• Prepare I.V. solution by reconstituting 1 gram vial with 20 ml sterile water for injection or bacteriostatic water for injection to yield a solution of 50 mg/ml. It may then be further diluted with sterile water, dextrose 2.5% or 5% in water, 0.45% or 0.9% sodium chloride injection, 5% dextrose and 9% sodium chloride injection, or Ringer's lactated injection.

• Reconstituted solution is stable 1 week at room temperature or 3 weeks refrigerated. However, use solution within 6 hours if drug was reconstituted with sterile water without a preservative (such as benzyl alcohol or parabens).

• Infusing each dose slowly (over at least 30 minutes)will decrease possibility of cystitis.

• Monitor CBC and renal and liver function tests.

• Monitor patient for CNS changes.

• Preparation of parenteral form is associated with carcinogenic, mutagenic, and teratogenic risks for personnel. Follow institutional policy to reduce risks.

lomustine (CCNU)
CeeNU♦

Pregnancy Risk Category: D

MECHANISM OF ACTION
Cross-links strands of cellular DNA and interferes with RNA transcription, causing an imbalance of growth that leads to cell death. Cell cycle-nonspecific.

INDICATIONS & DOSAGE
Brain tumors, Hodgkin's disease—
Adults and children: 130 mg/m² P.O. as a single dose q 6 weeks. Reduce dosage according to degree of bone marrow suppression. Repeat doses should not be given until WBC is more than 4,000/mm³ and platelet count is more than 100,000/mm³.

ADVERSE REACTIONS
Blood: *leukopenia, delayed up to 6 weeks, lasting 1 to 2 weeks; thrombocytopenia, delayed up to 4 weeks, lasting 1 to 2 weeks.*
GI: *nausea and vomiting beginning within 4 to 5 hours, lasting 24 hours;* stomatitis.
GU: nephrotoxicity, progressive azotemia.

INTERACTIONS
None significant.

Italicized side effects are common or life-threatening.
*Liquid form contains alcohol.   **May contain tartrazine.

NURSING CONSIDERATIONS

• Dosage modification may be required in patients with decreased platelets, leukocytes, or erythrocytes, and in patients receiving other myelosuppressive drugs.

• Give 2 to 4 hours after meals. Lomustine will be more completely absorbed if taken when the stomach is empty. To avoid nausea, give antiemetic before administering.

• May be useful in cancer involving CNS, since cerebrospinal fluid level equals 30% to 50% of plasma level 1 hour after administration.

• Monitor CBC weekly. Usually not administered more often than every 6 weeks; bone marrow toxicity is cumulative and delayed.

• Warn patient to watch for signs of infection (fever, sore throat, fatigue) and bleeding (easy bruising, nosebleeds, bleeding gums, melena). Take temperature daily.

• Monitor serum uric acid.

• Periodically monitor liver function.

• Avoid all I.M. injections when platelets are below 100,000/mm³.

• Anticoagulants and aspirin products should be used cautiously. Watch closely for signs of bleeding. Instruct patient to avoid OTC products containing aspirin.

• Since lomustine crosses the blood/brain barrier, it may be used to treat primary brain tumors.

• Therapeutic effects are often accompanied by toxicity.

---

mechlorethamine hydrochloride (nitrogen mustard)
Mustargen♦

Pregnancy Risk Category: D

MECHANISM OF ACTION
Cross-links strands of cellular DNA and interferes with RNA transcription, causing an imbalance of growth that leads to cell death. Cell cycle-nonspecific.

INDICATIONS & DOSAGE
Breast, lung, and ovarian cancer; Hodgkin's disease; non-Hodgkin's lymphomas; diffuse lymphocytic lymphoma—
Adults: 0.4 mg/kg or 10 mg/m² I.V. as a single dose or in divided doses q 3 to 6 weeks. Give through running I.V. infusion. Dosage reduced in prior radiation or chemotherapy to 0.2 to 0.4 mg/kg. Dosage based on ideal or actual body weight, whichever is less.
Neoplastic effusions—
Adults: 0.4 mg/kg intracavitarily.

ADVERSE REACTIONS
Blood: *nadir of myelosuppression occurring by days 4 to 10, lasting 10 to 21 days;* mild anemia begins in 2 to 3 weeks, possibly lasting 7 weeks.
EENT: tinnitus; *metallic taste* (immediately after dose); deafness with high doses.
GI: *nausea, vomiting, and anorexia* begin within minutes, last 8 to 24 hours.
Metabolic: hyperuricemia.
Local: *thrombophlebitis, sloughing, severe irritation if drug extravasates or touches skin.*
Other: *alopecia,* may precipitate herpes zoster.

INTERACTIONS
None significant.

NURSING CONSIDERATIONS
• Dosage modification may be required in severe anemia, depressed neutrophil or platelet count, or in patients recently treated with radiation or chemotherapy. Monitor CBC.

• Avoid contact with skin or mucous membranes. Wear gloves when preparing solution to prevent accidental skin contact. If contact occurs, wash with copious amounts of water.

• Mechlorethamine is a potent vesicant. Be sure I.V. doesn't infiltrate. If

---

drug extravasates, apply cold compresses and infiltrate the area with isotonic sodium thiosulfate.

• When given intracavitarily for sclerosing effect, turn patient from side to side every 15 minutes to 1 hour to distribute drug.

• Very unstable solution. Prepare immediately before infusion. Use within 15 minutes. Discard unused solution.

• To prevent hyperuricemia with resulting uric acid nephropathy, mechlorethamine may be used with adequate hydration. Monitor serum uric acid.

• Avoid all I.M. injections when platelets are below 100,000/mm³.

• Warn patient to watch for signs of infection (fever, sore throat, fatigue) and bleeding (easy bruising, nosebleeds, bleeding gums, melena). Take temperature daily.

• Anticoagulants and aspirin products should be used cautiously. Watch closely for signs of bleeding. Instruct patient to avoid OTC products containing aspirin.

• Any equipment used in the preparation and administration of mechlorethamine should be disposed of properly and according to institutional policy. Unused solution should be neutralized with an equal volume of 5% sodium bicarbonate and 5% sodium thiosulfate.

• Preparation of parenteral form is associated with carcinogenic, mutagenic, and teratogenic risks for personnel. Follow institutional policy to reduce risks.

• Therapeutic effects are often accompanied by toxicity.

melphalan
Alkeran♦

Pregnancy Risk Category: D

MECHANISM OF ACTION
Cross-links strands of cellular DNA and interferes with RNA transcription, causing an imbalance of growth that leads to cell death. Cell cycle-nonspecific.

INDICATIONS & DOSAGE
Multiple myeloma—
Adults: initially, 6 mg P.O. daily for 2 to 3 weeks, then stop drug for up to 4 weeks or until WBC and platelets stop dropping and begin to rise again; resume with maintenance dosage of 2 mg daily. Stop drug if WBC is below 3,000/mm³ or platelets are below 100,000/mm³. Alternate therapy: 0.15 mg/kg P.O. daily for 7 days, or 0.25 mg/kg for 4 days; repeat q 4 to 6 weeks.
Nonresectable advanced ovarian cancer—
Adults: 0.2 mg/kg daily, P.O. for 5 days. Repeat every 4 to 5 weeks, depending on bone marrow recovery.

ADVERSE REACTIONS
Blood: *thrombocytopenia, leukopenia, agranulocytosis.*
Other: *pneumonitis and pulmonary fibrosis.*

INTERACTIONS
None significant.

NURSING CONSIDERATIONS
• Not recommended in severe leukopenia, thrombocytopenia, or anemia; or in chronic lymphocytic leukemia.

• Monitor serum uric acid and CBC.

• Avoid all I.M. injections when platelets are below 100,000/mm³.

• May need dosage reduction in renal impairment.

• Therapeutic effects are often accompanied by toxicity.

• Drug of choice in multiple myeloma in combination with prednisone.

• Anticoagulants and aspirin products should be used cautiously. Watch closely for signs of bleeding. Instruct patient to avoid OTC products containing aspirin.

• Administer on empty stomach, because absorption is decreased by food.

streptozocin
Zanosar♦

Pregnancy Risk Category: C

MECHANISM OF ACTION
Cross-links strands of cellular DNA and interferes with RNA transcription, causing an imbalance of growth that leads to cell death. Cell cycle-nonspecific.

INDICATIONS & DOSAGE
Treatment of metastatic islet cell carcinoma of the pancreas; colon cancer; exocrine pancreatic tumors; and carcinoid tumors—
Adults and children: 500 mg/m^2 I.V. for 5 consecutive days q 6 weeks until maximum benefit or until toxicity is observed. Alternatively, 1,000 mg/m^2 at weekly intervals for the first 2 weeks. Don't exceed a single dose of 1,500 mg/m^2.

ADVERSE REACTIONS
Blood: *leukopenia, thrombocytopenia.*
GI: *nausea, vomiting,* diarrhea.
Hepatic: elevated liver enzymes.
Metabolic: hyperglycemia and hypoglycemia.
Renal: *renal toxicity (evidenced by azotemia, glycosuria, and renal tubular acidosis),* mild proteinuria.

INTERACTIONS
Other potentially nephrotoxic drugs such as aminoglycosides: increased risk of renal toxicity. Use cautiously. *Phenytoin:* may decrease the effects of streptozocin. Monitor carefully.

NURSING CONSIDERATIONS
• Dosage modification may be required in patients with preexisting renal or hepatic disease.
• Renal toxicity resulting from streptozocin therapy is dose-related and cumulative. Monitor renal function before and after each course of therapy. Urinalysis, BUN, creatinine, serum electrolytes, and creatinine clearance should be obtained before, and at least weekly during, drug administration. Weekly monitoring should continue for 4 weeks after each course.
• Mild proteinuria is one of the first signs of renal toxicity. Make sure doctor is aware if and when this occurs. The dosage of the drug may have to be reduced.
• Test urine for protein and glucose each nursing shift.
• Monitor CBC and liver function studies at least weekly.
• Warn patient to watch for signs of infection (fever, sore throat, fatigue) and bleeding (easy bruising, nosebleeds, bleeding gums, melena). Take temperature daily.
• Nausea and vomiting occurs in almost *all* patients. Make sure patient is being treated with an antiemetic.
• Reconstitute the streptozocin powder with 0.9% sodium chloride injection. This will produce a pale gold solution.
• Best to use within 12 hours of reconstitution. However, drug will remain stable for at least 48 hours, especially if kept refrigerated.
• The product contains no preservatives and is not intended as a multiple-dose vial.
• When preparing the solution, wear gloves to protect the skin from contact. If contact occurs, wash with copious amounts of water.
• Unopened and unreconstituted vials of streptozocin should be stored in the refrigerator.
• Preparation of parenteral form is associated with carcinogenic, mutagenic, and teratogenic risks for personnel. Follow institutional policy to reduce risks.
• Therapeutic effects are often ac-

companied by toxicity.

thiotepa
Thiotepa♦

Pregnancy Risk Category: D

MECHANISM OF ACTION
Cross-links strands of cellular DNA and interferes with RNA transcription, causing an imbalance of growth that leads to cell death. Cell cycle-nonspecific.

INDICATIONS & DOSAGE
Adults and children over 12 years:
Breast and ovarian cancer; lymphomas and bronchogenic carcinomas—
0.2 mg/kg I.V. daily for 4 to 5 days at intervals of 2 to 4 weeks.
Bladder tumor—
60 mg in 60 ml water instilled in bladder for 2 hours once weekly for 4 weeks.
Neoplastic effusions—
0.6 to 0.8 mg/kg intracavitarily, p.r.n. Stop drug or decrease dosage if WBC is below 4,000/mm³ or if platelets are below 150,000/mm³.

ADVERSE REACTIONS
Blood: *leukopenia begins within 5 to 30 days; thrombocytopenia; neutropenia.*
GI: *nausea, vomiting.*
GU: amenorrhea, decreased spermatogenesis.
Metabolic: hyperuricemia.
Skin: hives, rash.
Local: intense pain at administration site.
Other: headache, fever, tightness of throat, dizziness.

INTERACTIONS
None significant.

NURSING CONSIDERATIONS
• Use cautiously in bone marrow suppression and renal or hepatic dysfunction.

• Monitor CBC weekly for at least 3 weeks after last dosage. Warn patient to report even mild infections.
• GU adverse reactions reversible in 6 to 8 months.
• May require use of local anesthetic at injection site if intense pain occurs.
• For bladder instillation: Dehydrate patient 8 to 10 hours before therapy. Instill drug into bladder by catheter; ask patient to retain solution for 2 hours. Volume may be reduced to 30 ml if discomfort is too great with 60 ml. Reposition patient every 15 minutes for maximum area contact.
• Toxicity delayed and prolonged because drug binds to tissues and stays in body several hours.
• Refrigerate dry powder; protect from light.
• Use only sterile water for injection to reconstitute. Refrigerated solution is stable for 5 days.
• To prevent hyperuricemia with resulting uric acid nephropathy, allopurinol may be used with adequate hydration. Monitor serum uric acid.
• Avoid all I.M. injections when platelets are below 100,000/mm³.
• Warn patient to watch for signs of infection (fever, sore throat, fatigue) and bleeding (easy bruising, nosebleeds, bleeding gums, melena). Take temperature daily.
• Can be given by all parenteral routes, including direct injection into the tumor.
• Anticoagulants and aspirin products should be used cautiously. Watch closely for signs of bleeding. Instruct patient to avoid OTC products containing aspirin.
• Preparation of parenteral form is associated with carcinogenic, mutagenic, and teratogenic risks for personnel. Follow institutional policy to reduce risks.
• Therapeutic effects are often accompanied by toxicity.

Italicized side effects are common or life-threatening.
*Liquid form contains alcohol.   **May contain tartrazine.

uracil mustard
Uracil Mustard Capsules**

Pregnancy Risk Category: X

MECHANISM OF ACTION
Cross-links strands of cellular DNA and interferes with RNA transcription, causing an imbalance of growth that leads to cell death. Cell cycle-nonspecific.

INDICATIONS & DOSAGE
Chronic lymphocytic and myelocytic leukemia; Hodgkin's disease; non-Hodgkin's lymphomas of the histiocytic and lymphocytic types; reticulum cell sarcoma; lymphomas; mycosis fungoides; polycythemia vera; cancer of ovaries, cervix, and lungs—
Adults: 1 to 2 mg P.O. daily for 3 months or until desired response or toxicity; maintenance dosage is 1 mg daily for 3 out of 4 weeks until optimum response or relapse; or 3 to 5 mg P.O. for 7 days not to exceed total dosage of 0.5 mg/kg, then 1 mg daily until response, then 1 mg daily 3 out of 4 weeks.

ADVERSE REACTIONS
Blood: bone marrow suppression, delayed 2 to 4 weeks; *thrombocytopenia; leukopenia;* anemia.
CNS: irritability, nervousness, mental cloudiness, and depression.
GI: *nausea, vomiting, diarrhea, epigastric distress,* abdominal pain, anorexia.
Metabolic: hyperuricemia.
Skin: pruritus, dermatitis, hyperpigmentation, alopecia.

INTERACTIONS
None significant.

NURSING CONSIDERATIONS
• Dosage modification may be required in severe thrombocytopenia, aplastic anemia, leukopenia, or acute leukemia.
• Give at bedtime to reduce nausea.
• Warn patient to watch for signs of infection (fever, sore throat, fatigue) and bleeding (easy bruising, nosebleeds, bleeding gums, melena). Take temperature daily.
• Monitor platelet count. Check CBC once or twice weekly for 4 weeks; then 4 weeks after stopping drug.
• To prevent hyperuricemia and resulting uric acid nephropathy, allopurinol may be used with adequate hydration. Monitor serum uric acid.
• Avoid all I.M. injections when platelets are below 100,000/mm³.
• Warn patient to watch for signs of infection (fever, sore throat, fatigue) and bleeding (easy bruising, nosebleeds, bleeding gums, melena). Take temperature daily.
• Anticoagulants and aspirin products should be used cautiously. Watch closely for signs of bleeding. Instruct patient to avoid OTC products containing aspirin.
• Therapeutic effects are often accompanied by toxicity.

Antimetabolites

cytarabine (ara-C, cytosine
  arabinoside)
floxuridine
fluorouracil (5-fluorouracil, 5-FU)
hydroxyurea
mercaptopurine (6-MP, 6-
  mercaptopurine)
methotrexate
methotrexate sodium
thioguanine (6-thioguanine, 6-
  TG)
trimetrexate gluconate

COMBINATION PRODUCTS
None.

---

cytarabine (ara-C, cytosine arabinoside)
Cytosar-U♦

Pregnancy Risk Category: D

MECHANISM OF ACTION
Inhibits DNA synthesis.

INDICATIONS & DOSAGE
Acute myelocytic and other acute leukemias—
Adults and children: 200 mg/m² daily by continuous I.V. infusion for 5 days.
Meningeal leukemias and meningeal neoplasms—
Adults and children: 10 to 30 mg/m² intrathecally once every 4 days.

ADVERSE REACTIONS
Blood: WBC nadir 5 to 7 days after drug stopped; *leukopenia,* anemia, *thrombocytopenia,* reticulocytopenia; platelet nadir occurring on day 10; *megaloblastosis.*
CNS: neurotoxicity with high doses.
EENT: *keratitis.*
GI: *nausea, vomiting,* diarrhea, dysphagia; reddened area at juncture of lips, followed by sore mouth, oral ulcers in 5 to 10 days; high dose given via rapid I.V. may cause projectile vomiting.
Hepatic: hepatotoxicity (usually mild and reversible).
Metabolic: hyperuricemia.
Skin: rash.
Other: flulike syndrome.

INTERACTIONS
None significant.

NURSING CONSIDERATIONS
• Dosage modification may be required in thrombocytopenia, leukopenia, renal or hepatic disease, and after other chemotherapy or radiation therapy.
• Watch for signs of infection (cough, fever, sore throat) and bleeding (easy bruising, nosebleeds, bleeding gums). Monitor CBC.
• Excellent mouth care can help prevent stomatitis.
• Nausea and vomiting more frequent when large doses are administered rapidly by I.V. push. These reactions are less frequent with infusion. To reduce nausea, give antiemetic before administering.
• Steroid eye drops are prescribed to prevent drug-induced keratitis.
• Monitor intake/output carefully. Maintain high fluid intake and give allopurinol, if ordered, to avoid urate

---

Italicized side effects are common or life-threatening.
*Liquid form contains alcohol.   **May contain tartrazine.

nephropathy in leukemia induction therapy. Monitor serum uric acid.
• Monitor hepatic function.
• Use preservative-free normal saline or Elliot's B solution for intrathecal use.
• Reconstituted solution is stable for 48 hours. Discard cloudy reconstituted solution.
• Avoid I.M. injections of any drugs in patients with severely depressed platelet count (thrombocytopenia) to prevent bleeding.
• Warn patient to watch for signs of infection (fever, sore throat, fatigue) and bleeding (easy bruising, nosebleeds, bleeding gums, melena). Take temperature daily.
• Modify or discontinue therapy if polymorphonuclear granulocyte count is below 1,000/mm³ or if platelet count is below 50,000/mm³.
• Assess patients receiving high doses for neurotoxicity. May first appear as nystagmus, but can progress to ataxia and cerebellar dysfunction.
• Preparation of parenteral form is associated with carcinogenic, mutagenic, and teratogenic risks for personnel. Follow institutional policy to reduce risks.

floxuridine
FUDR

Pregnancy Risk Category: D

MECHANISM OF ACTION
Inhibits DNA synthesis.

INDICATIONS & DOSAGE
Brain, breast, head, neck, liver, gallbladder, and bile duct cancer—
Adults: 0.1 to 0.6 mg/kg daily by intraarterial infusion (use pump for continuous, uniform rate); or 0.4 to 0.6 mg/kg daily into hepatic artery.

ADVERSE REACTIONS
Blood: *leukopenia, anemia,* thrombocytopenia.

CNS: cerebellar ataxia, vertigo, nystagmus, seizures, depression, hemiplegia, hiccups, lethargy.
EENT: blurred vision.
GI: *stomatitis, cramps, nausea, vomiting, diarrhea, bleeding, enteritis.*
Hepatic: cholangitis, jaundice, elevated liver enzymes.
Skin: *erythema,* dermatitis, pruritus, rash.

INTERACTIONS
None significant.

NURSING CONSIDERATIONS
• Dosage modification may be required in poor nutritional state, bone marrow suppression, or serious infection. Use cautiously following high-dose pelvic irradiation or use of alkylating agent, and in impaired hepatic or renal function.
• Severe skin and GI adverse reactions require stopping drug. Use of antacid eases but probably won't prevent GI distress.
• Excellent mouth care can help prevent stomatitis.
• Monitor intake/output, CBC, and renal and hepatic function.
• Discontinue if WBC falls below 3,500/mm³ or if platelet count below 100,000/mm³.
• Therapeutic effect may be delayed 1 to 6 weeks. Make sure patient is aware of time it may take for improvement to be noted.
• Reconstitute with sterile water for injection. Dilute further in dextrose 5% in water or normal saline solution for actual infusion.
• Avoid I.M. injections of any drugs in patients with thrombocytopenia to prevent bleeding.
• Refrigerated solution is stable for no more than 2 weeks.
• Observe perfused arterial area. Check line for bleeding, blockage, displacement, or leakage.
• Often administered via hepatic arterial infusion in treatment of hepatic

metastases.
• Preparation of parenteral form is associated with carcinogenic, mutagenic, and teratogenic risks for personnel. Follow institutional policy to reduce risks.

fluorouracil
(5-fluorouracil, 5-FU)
Adrucil♦

Pregnancy Risk Category: D

MECHANISM OF ACTION
Inhibits DNA synthesis.

INDICATIONS & DOSAGE
Colon, rectal, breast, ovarian, cervical, bladder, liver, and pancreatic cancer—
Adults: 12.5 mg/kg I.V. daily for 3 to 5 days q 4 weeks; or 15 mg/kg weekly for 6 weeks. (Dosages recommended based on lean body weight.) Maximum single recommended dose is 800 mg, although higher single doses (up to 1.5 g) have been used. The injectable form has been given orally but is not recommended.

ADVERSE REACTIONS
Blood: *leukopenia,* thrombocytopenia, anemia; WBC nadir 9 to 14 days after first dose; platelet nadir in 7 to 14 days.
CNS: acute cerebellar syndrome.
GI: *stomatitis, GI ulcer may precede leukopenia, nausea, vomiting in 30% to 50% of patients;* diarrhea.
Skin: *dermatitis,* hyperpigmentation (especially in blacks), nail changes, pigmented palmar creases.
Other: *reversible alopecia in 5% to 20% of patients, weakness, malaise.*

INTERACTIONS
None significant.

NURSING CONSIDERATIONS
• Use cautiously following major surgery; when patient is in poor nutri-

tional state; and with serious infections and bone marrow suppression. Use cautiously following high-dose pelvic irradiation or use of alkylating agents, in impaired hepatic or renal function, and in widespread neoplastic infiltration of bone marrow.
• Watch for stomatitis or diarrhea (signs of toxicity). May use topical oral anesthetic to soothe lesions. Discontinue if diarrhea occurs.
• Encourage good and frequent oral hygiene to prevent superinfection of denuded mucosa.
• Give antiemetic before administering drug to reduce nausea.
• Do WBC and platelet counts daily. Drug should be stopped when WBC is less than 3,500/mm³. Watch for ecchymoses, petechiae, easy bruising, and anemia. Drug should be stopped if platelet count is less than 100,000/mm³.
• Dermatologic side effects reversible when drug is stopped. Patient should use highly protective sun blockers to avoid inflammatory erythematous dermatitis.
• Therapeutic concentrations are not reached in cerebrospinal fluid.
• Slowing infusion rate so it takes from 2 to 8 hours lessens toxicity.
• Monitor intake/output, CBC, and renal and hepatic functions.
• Don't refrigerate fluorouracil.
• Don't use cloudy solution. If crystals form, redissolve by warming.
• Solution is more stable in plastic I.V. bags than in glass bottles. Use plastic I.V. containers for administering continuous infusions.
• Sometimes ordered as 5-fluorouracil or 5-FU. The numeral 5 is part of the drug name and should not be confused with dosage units.
• Sometimes administered via hepatic arterial infusion in treatment of hepatic metastases.
• Warn patient that alopecia may occur but is reversible.
• To prevent bleeding, avoid I.M. in-

jections of any drugs in patients with thrombocytopenia.
• Fluorouracil toxicity may be delayed for 1 to 3 weeks.
• Preparation of parenteral form is associated with carcinogenic, mutagenic, and teratogenic risks for personnel. Follow institutional policy to reduce risks.

hydroxyurea
Hydrea**♦

Pregnancy Risk Category: D

MECHANISM OF ACTION
Inhibits DNA synthesis.

INDICATIONS & DOSAGE
Melanoma; resistant chronic myelocytic leukemia; recurrent, metastatic, or inoperable ovarian cancer—
Adults: 80 mg/kg P.O. as single dose q 3 days; or 20 to 30 mg/kg P.O. daily.

ADVERSE REACTIONS
Blood: *leukopenia,* thrombocytopenia, anemia, *megaloblastosis; dose-limiting and dose-related bone marrow suppression, with rapid recovery.*
CNS: drowsiness, hallucinations.
GI: *anorexia, nausea, vomiting, diarrhea,* stomatitis.
GU: increased BUN and serum creatinine levels.
Metabolic: hyperuricemia.
Skin: rash, pruritus.

INTERACTIONS
None significant.

NURSING CONSIDERATIONS
• Dosage modification may be required following other chemotherapy or radiation therapy.
• Use with caution in renal dysfunction. Discontinue if WBC is less than 3,500/mm³ or if platelet count is less than 100,000/mm³.
• Warn patient to watch for signs of infection (fever, sore throat, fatigue)

and bleeding (easy bruising, nosebleeds, bleeding gums, melena). Take temperature daily.
• If patient can't swallow capsule, he may empty contents into water and take immediately.
• Monitor intake/output; keep patient hydrated.
• Routinely measure BUN, uric acid, and serum creatinine.
• Drug crosses blood/brain barrier.
• Auditory and visual hallucinations and blood toxicity increase when decreased renal function exists.
• May exacerbate postirradiation erythema.
• Avoid all I.M. injections when platelets are below 100,000/mm³.

mercaptopurine (6-MP, 6-mercaptopurine)
Purinethol♦

Pregnancy Risk Category: D

MECHANISM OF ACTION
Inhibits RNA and DNA synthesis.

INDICATIONS & DOSAGE
Acute lymphoblastic leukemia (in children), acute myeloblastic leukemia, chronic myelocytic leukemia—
Adults: 80 to 100 mg/m² P.O. daily as a single dose up to 5 mg/kg daily.
Children: 70 mg/m² P.O. daily.
    Usual maintenance for adults and children: 1.5 to 2.5 mg/kg daily.

ADVERSE REACTIONS
Blood: *decreased RBC; leukopenia, thrombocytopenia, and anemia; all may persist several days after drug is stopped.*
GI: *nausea, vomiting, and anorexia in 25% of patients;* painful oral ulcers.
Hepatic: *jaundice, hepatic necrosis.*
Metabolic: hyperuricemia.

INTERACTIONS
Allopurinol: slowed inactivation of mercaptopurine. Decrease mercapto-

purine to ¼ or ⅓ normal dose.

NURSING CONSIDERATIONS
• Dosage modifications may be required following chemotherapy or radiation therapy, in depressed neutrophil or platelet count, and in impaired hepatic or renal function.
• Observe for signs of bleeding and infection.
• Hepatic dysfunction is reversible when drug is stopped. Watch for jaundice, clay-colored stools, and frothy dark urine. Drug should be stopped if hepatic tenderness occurs.
• Do weekly blood counts; watch for precipitous fall.
• Warn patient to watch for signs of infection (fever, sore throat, fatigue) and bleeding (easy bruising, nosebleeds, bleeding gums, melena). Take temperature daily.
• Monitor intake/output. Encourage fluid intake (3 liters daily).
• Sometimes ordered as 6-mercaptopurine or 6-MP. The numeral 6 is part of drug name and does not signify number of dosage units.
• Warn patient that improvement may take 2 to 4 weeks or longer.
• GI adverse reactions less common in children than in adults.
• Avoid all I.M. injections when platelets are below 100,000/mm³.
• Monitor serum uric acid. If allopurinol is necessary, use cautiously.
• Preparation of parenteral form is associated with carcinogenic, mutagenic, and teratogenic risks for personnel. Follow institutional policy to reduce risks.

---

methotrexate

methotrexate sodium
Folex, Mexate, Rheumatrex
Pregnancy Risk Category: D

MECHANISM OF ACTION
Prevents reduction of folic acid to tetrahydrofolate by binding to dihydrofolate reductase.

INDICATIONS & DOSAGE
Trophoblastic tumors (choriocarcinoma, hydatidiform mole)—
Adults: 15 to 30 mg P.O. or I.M. daily for 5 days. Repeat after 1 or more weeks, according to response or toxicity.
Acute lymphoblastic and lymphatic leukemia—
Adults and children: 3.3 mg/m² P.O., I.M., or I.V. daily for 4 to 6 weeks or until remission occurs; then 20 to 30 mg/m² P.O. or I.M. twice weekly.
Meningeal leukemia—
Adults and children: 10 to 15 mg/m² intrathecally q 2 to 5 days until cerebrospinal fluid is normal. Use only 20-, 50-, or 100-mg vials of powder with no preservatives; dilute using 0.9% sodium chloride injection *without* preservatives or Elliot's B solution. Use only new vials of drug and diluent. Use immediately.
Burkitt's lymphoma (Stage I or Stage II)—
Adults: 10 to 25 mg P.O. daily for 4 to 8 days with 1-week rest intervals.
Lymphosarcoma (Stage III)—
Adults: 0.625 to 2.5 mg/kg daily P.O., I.M., or I.V.
Mycosis fungoides—
Adults: 2.5 to 10 mg P.O. daily or 50 mg I.M. weekly; or 25 mg I.M. twice weekly.
Psoriasis—
Adults: 10 to 25 mg P.O., I.M., or I.V. as single weekly dose.
Rheumatoid arthritis—
Adults: Initially 7.5 mg P.O. weekly, either in a single dose or divided as 2.5 mg P.O. every 12 hours for 3 doses once a week. Dosage may be gradually increased to a maximum of 20 mg weekly.

ADVERSE REACTIONS
Blood: WBC and platelet nadir occur-

Italicized side effects are common or life-threatening.
*Liquid form contains alcohol.   **May contain tartrazine.

ring on day 7; anemia, *leukopenia, thrombocytopenia* (all dose-related).

CNS: *arachnoiditis within hours of intrathecal use;* subacute neurotoxicity which may begin a few weeks later; necrotizing demyelinating leukoencephalopathy a few years later.

GI: *stomatitis; diarrhea leading to hemorrhagic enteritis and intestinal perforation; nausea; vomiting.*

GU: *tubular necrosis.*

Hepatic: hepatic dysfunction leading to cirrhosis or hepatic fibrosis.

Metabolic: hyperuricemia.

Skin: exposure to sun may aggravate psoriatic lesions, rash, photosensitivity.

Other: alopecia; *pulmonary interstitial infiltrates;* long-term use in children may cause osteoporosis.

INTERACTIONS

Probenecid, phenylbutazone, salicylates, sulfonamides: increased methotrexate toxicity; don't use together if possible.

NURSING CONSIDERATIONS

• Dosage modification may be required in impaired hepatic or renal function, bone marrow suppression, aplasia, leukopenia, thrombocytopenia, or anemia. Use cautiously in infection, peptic ulcer, ulcerative colitis, and in very young, elderly, or debilitated patients.

• Warn patient to avoid conception during and immediately after therapy because of possible abortion or congenital anomalies.

• GI adverse reactions may require stopping drug.

• Rash, redness, or ulcerations in mouth or pulmonary adverse reactions may signal serious complications.

• Monitor serum uric acid.

• Monitor intake/output daily. Encourage fluid intake (2 to 3 liters daily).

• Alkalinize urine by giving sodium bicarbonate tablets to prevent precipitation of drug, especially with high doses. Maintain urine pH at more than 6.5. Reduce dosage if BUN 20 to 30 mg% or creatinine 1.2 to 2 mg%. Stop drug if BUN more than 30 mg% or creatinine more than 2 mg%.

• Watch for increases in AST (SGOT), ALT (SGPT), alkaline phosphatase; may signal hepatic dysfunction.

• Watch for bleeding (especially GI) and infection.

• Warn patient to use highly protective sun screening agent when exposed to sunlight.

• Take temperature daily, and watch for cough, dyspnea, and cyanosis.

• Leucovorin rescue is necessary with high dose protocols (greater than 100-mg doses). Don't confuse with folic acid. This rescue technique is effective against systemic toxicity but does not interfere with the tumor cells' absorption of the methotrexate.

• Avoid all I.M. injections in patients with thrombocytopenia.

• Advise patient not to discontinue leucovorin rescue if he experiences severe nausea and vomiting. Parenteral therapy may be necessary.

• Teach patient good oral care to prevent superinfection of oral cavity.

• Preparation of parenteral form is associated with carcinogenic, mutagenic, and teratogenic risks for personnel. Follow institutional policy to reduce risks.

thioguanine (6-thioguanine, 6-TG)
Lanvis◆◆

Pregnancy Risk Category: D

MECHANISM OF ACTION
Inhibits purine synthesis.

INDICATIONS & DOSAGE
Acute leukemia, chronic granulocytic leukemia—

Adults and children: initially, 2 mg/kg daily P.O. (usually calculated to nearest 20 mg); then increased gradually to 3 mg/kg daily if no toxic effects occur.

ADVERSE REACTIONS
Blood: *leukopenia,* anemia, *thrombocytopenia* (occurs slowly over 2 to 4 weeks).
GI: nausea, vomiting, stomatitis, diarrhea, anorexia.
Hepatic: hepatotoxicity, jaundice.
Metabolic: hyperuricemia.

INTERACTIONS
None significant.

NURSING CONSIDERATIONS
• Dosage modification may be required in renal or hepatic dysfunction.
• Stop drug if hepatotoxicity or hepatic tenderness occurs. Watch for jaundice; may be reversible if drug is stopped promptly.
• Do CBC daily during induction, then weekly during maintenance therapy.
• Monitor serum uric acid.
• Sometimes ordered as 6-thioguanine. The numeral 6 is part of drug name and does not signify dosage units.
• Avoid all I.M. injections when platelets are below 100,000/mm^3.

---

trimetrexate gluconate
Pregnancy Risk Category: C

MECHANISM OF ACTION
Prevents reduction of folic acid to tetrahydrofolate by binding to dihydrofolate reductase.

INDICATIONS & DOSAGE
Neoplastic disorders—
Adults: Dosage and indication will vary with protocol.
Treatment of Pneumocystis carinii *pneumonia in patients with AIDS (ap-* proved as a treatment—IND [Investigational New Drug])—
Adults: Dosage may vary with protocol. 30 mg/m^2 I.V. bolus daily for 21 days, administered with leucovorin (20 mg/m^2 I.V. or P.O. daily).

ADVERSE REACTIONS
Blood: *neutropenia, thrombocytopenia.*
Skin: rash.
Other: *hepatotoxicity, peripheral neuropathy.*

INTERACTIONS
None reported.

NURSING CONSIDERATIONS
• Avoid I.M. injections in patients with thrombocytopenia.
• Warn patient to watch for signs of infection (fever, sore throat, fatigue) and bleeding (easy bruising, nosebleeds, bleeding gums, melena). Take temperature daily.
• Store intact vials in refrigerator.
• Reconstitute 50-mg vial with 1.9 ml sterile water for injection to yield a solution of 25 mg/ml.
• Incompatible with chloride-containing solutions (including normal saline solution).
• Preparation of parenteral form is associated with carcinogenic, mutagenic, and teratogenic risks for personnel. Follow institutional policy to reduce risks.

Italicized side effects are common or life-threatening.
*Liquid form contains alcohol.   **May contain tartrazine.

73

Antibiotic antineoplastic agents

bleomycin sulfate
dactinomycin (actinomycin D)
daunorubicin hydrochloride
doxorubicin hydrochloride
mitomycin
plicamycin (mithramycin)
procarbazine hydrochloride

COMBINATION PRODUCTS
None.

bleomycin sulfate
Blenoxane♦

Pregnancy Risk Category: D

MECHANISM OF ACTION
Inhibits DNA synthesis and causes scission of single- and double-stranded DNA.

INDICATIONS & DOSAGE
Dosage and indications may vary. Check patient's protocol with doctor.
Cervical, esophageal, head, neck, and testicular cancer—
Adults: 10 to 20 units/m^2 I.V., I.M., or S.C. 1 or 2 times weekly to total 300 to 400 units.
Hodgkin's disease—
Adults: 10 to 20 units/m^2 I.V., I.M., or S.C. 1 or 2 times weekly. After 50% response, maintenance 1 unit I.M. or I.V. daily or 5 units I.M. or I.V. weekly.
Lymphomas—
Adults: first 2 doses should be 2 units or less, and patient should be monitored for any allergic reaction. If no reaction occurs, then follow above dosing schedule.

ADVERSE REACTIONS
CNS: hyperesthesia of scalp and fingers, headache.
GI: *stomatitis, prolonged anorexia in 13% of patients,* nausea, vomiting, diarrhea.
Skin: *erythema, vesiculation, and hardening and discoloration of palmar and plantar skin in 8% of patients;* desquamation of hands, feet, and pressure areas; *hyperpigmentation; acne.*
Other: *reversible alopecia,* swelling of interphalangeal joints, *pulmonary fibrosis in 10% of patients, pulmonary adverse reactions (fine crackles, fever, dyspnea), leukocytosis and nonproductive cough, allergic reaction (fever up to 106° F. [41.1° C.] with chills up to 5 hours after injection; anaphylaxis in 1% to 6% of patients).*

INTERACTIONS
None significant.

NURSING CONSIDERATIONS
• Use cautiously in renal or pulmonary impairment.
• Pulmonary adverse reactions common in patients over 70 years. Fatal pulmonary fibrosis occurs in 1% of patients, especially when cumulative dose exceeds 400 units.
• Pulmonary function tests should be performed to establish pre-treatment baseline. Drug should be stopped if pulmonary function test shows a marked decline.
• Monitor chest X-ray and listen to lungs.
• Monitor injection site for signs of

irritation.
• Drug concentrates in keratin of squamous epithelium. To prevent linear streaking, don't use adhesive dressings on skin.
• Allergic reactions may be delayed for several hours, especially in lymphoma.
• Advise patient that alopecia may occur, but is usually reversible.
• Refrigerated, reconstituted solution is stable for 4 weeks; at room temperature, it's stable for 2 weeks.
• Bleomycin-induced fever is common and may be treated with antipyretics. This reaction usually occurs within 3 to 6 hours of administration.
• Refrigerate unopened vials containing dry powder.
• Preparation of parenteral form is associated with carcinogenic, mutagenic, and teratogenic risks for personnel. Follow institutional policy to reduce risks.

---

dactinomycin (actinomycin D)
Cosmegen♦

Pregnancy Risk Category: C

MECHANISM OF ACTION
Interferes with DNA-dependent RNA synthesis by intercalation.

INDICATIONS & DOSAGE
Dosage and indications may vary. Check patient's protocol with doctor.
Melanomas, sarcomas, trophoblastic tumors in women, testicular cancer—
Adults: 500 mcg I.V. daily for 5 days not to exceed 15 mg/kg or 400 to 600 mg/m² daily; wait 2 to 4 weeks and repeat. Or 2 mg I.V. single weekly dose for 3 weeks; wait for bone marrow recovery, then repeat in 3 to 4 weeks.
Wilms' tumor, rhabdomyosarcoma, Ewing's sarcoma—
Children: 15 mcg/kg I.V. daily for 5 days. Maximum dosage 500 mcg daily. Wait for bone marrow recovery.

ADVERSE REACTIONS
Blood: anemia, *leukopenia, thrombocytopenia, pancytopenia.*
GI: *anorexia, nausea, vomiting,* abdominal pain, diarrhea, *stomatitis.*
Skin: *erythema;* desquamation; *hyperpigmentation of skin, especially in previously irradiated areas; acne-like eruptions (reversible).*
Local: phlebitis, severe damage to soft tissue.
Other: reversible alopecia.

INTERACTIONS
None significant.

NURSING CONSIDERATIONS
• Contraindicated in renal, hepatic, or bone marrow impairment.
• Stomatitis, diarrhea, leukopenia, thrombocytopenia may require modifying dosage and schedule.
• Give antiemetic before administering to reduce nausea.
• Monitor renal and hepatic functions.
• Monitor CBC daily and platelet counts frequently.
• Warn patient to watch for signs of infection (fever, sore throat, fatigue) and bleeding (easy bruising, nosebleeds, bleeding gums, melena). Take temperature daily.
• Warn patient that alopecia may occur but is usually reversible.
• Use only sterile water (without preservatives) as diluent for injection. Discard unused solutions since they do not contain a preservative.
• Dactinomycin is a vesicant. Administer through a running I.V. with good blood return. If infiltration occurs, apply cold compresses to area.
• Preparation of parenteral form is associated with carcinogenic, mutagenic, and teratogenic risks for personnel. Follow institutional policy to reduce risks.

Italicized side effects are common or life-threatening.
*Liquid form contains alcohol.   **May contain tartrazine.

daunorubicin hydrochloride
Cerubidine♦

Pregnancy Risk Category: D

MECHANISM OF ACTION
Interferes with DNA-dependent RNA synthesis by intercalation.

INDICATIONS & DOSAGE
Dosage and indications may vary. Check patient's protocol with doctor.
Remission induction in acute nonlymphocytic leukemia (myelogenous, monocytic, erythroid) in adults—
As a single agent: 60 mg/m² daily I.V. on days 1, 2, and 3 q 3 to 4 weeks.
In combination: 45 mg/m² daily I.V. on days 1, 2, and 3 of the first course and on days 1 and 2 of subsequent courses with cytosine arabinoside infusions.
Note: Dose should be reduced if hepatic function is impaired.

ADVERSE REACTIONS
Blood: *bone marrow suppression* (lowest blood counts 10 to 14 days after administration).
CV: *irreversible cardiomyopathy (dose-related), ECG changes, dysrhythmias,* pericarditis, myocarditis.
GI: *nausea, vomiting, stomatitis, esophagitis,* anorexia, diarrhea.
GU: nephrotoxicity, transient red urine.
Hepatic: hepatotoxicity.
Skin: rash.
Local: *severe cellulitis or tissue sloughing if drug extravasates.*
Other: *generalized alopecia,* fever, chills.

INTERACTIONS
Heparin: don't mix. May form a precipitate.

NURSING CONSIDERATIONS
• Use cautiously in myelosuppression and impaired cardiac, renal, and liver function.

• Stop drug immediately in signs of CHF or cardiomyopathy. Prevent by limiting cumulative dose to 550 mg/m²; 450 mg/m² when patient has been receiving radiation therapy that encompasses the heart or any other cardiotoxic agent, such as cyclophosphamide.
• Monitor ECG before treatment, monthly during therapy.
• Note if resting pulse rate is high (a sign of cardiac adverse reactions).
• *Avoid extravasation;* inject into tubing of freely flowing I.V. *Never* give I.M. or S.C. If extravasation occurs, discontinue I.V. immediately and apply ice to area for 24 to 48 hours. Local infiltration with hydrocortisone sodium succinate injection (50 to 100 mg) and/or sodium bicarbonate (5 ml of 8.4% injection) may be ordered.
• Monitor CBC and hepatic function.
• Warn patient that urine may be red for 1 to 2 days and that it's a normal side effect, not hematuria.
• Advise patient that alopecia may occur but is usually reversible.
• Nausea and vomiting may be very severe and last 24 to 48 hours.
• Reconstituted solution is stable for 24 hours at room temperature or 48 hours refrigerated. Optimally, use within 8 hours of preparation.
• Reddish color looks very similar to doxorubicin (Adriamycin). *Do not confuse the two drugs.*
• Preparation of parenteral form is associated with carcinogenic, mutagenic, and teratogenic risks for personnel. Follow institutional policy to reduce risks.

doxorubicin hydrochloride
Adriamycin RDF♦

Pregnancy Risk Category: D

MECHANISM OF ACTION
Interferes with DNA-dependent RNA synthesis by intercalation.

INDICATIONS & DOSAGE

Dosage and indications may vary. Check patient's protocol with doctor. *Bladder, breast, cervical, head, neck, liver, lung, ovarian, prostatic, stomach, testicular, and thyroid cancer; Hodgkin's disease; acute lymphoblastic and myeloblastic leukemia; Wilms' tumor; neuroblastomas; lymphomas; sarcomas—*

Adults: 60 to 75 mg/m² I.V. as single dose q 3 weeks; or 30 mg/m² I.V. in single daily dose, days 1 to 3 of 4-week cycle. Alternatively, 20 mg/m² I.V. once weekly or 30 mg/m² I.V. on 3 successive days, repeated every 4 weeks. Maximum cumulative dose 550 mg/m².

ADVERSE REACTIONS

Blood: *leukopenia, especially agranulocytosis, during days 10 to 15, with recovery by day 21; thrombocytopenia.*

CV: *cardiac depression, seen in such ECG changes as sinus tachycardia, T wave flattening, ST segment depression, voltage reduction; dysrhythmias in 11% of patients; irreversible cardiomyopathy (sometimes with pulmonary edema) with mortality of 30% to 75%.*

GI: *nausea, vomiting,* diarrhea, *stomatitis,* esophagitis.

GU: enhancement of cyclophosphamide-induced bladder injury, transient red urine.

Skin: *hyperpigmentation of skin, especially in previously irradiated areas.*

Local: *severe cellulitis or tissue sloughing if drug extravasates.*

Other: hyperpigmentation of nails and dermal creases, *complete alopecia within 3 to 4 weeks;* hair may regrow 2 to 5 months after drug is stopped.

INTERACTIONS

Streptozocin: increased and prolonged blood levels. Dosage may have to be adjusted.

Heparin: don't mix together. May form a precipitate.

NURSING CONSIDERATIONS

• Dosage modification may be required in myelosuppression and in impaired cardiac or hepatic function.
• Stop drug or slow rate of infusion if tachycardia develops.
• Stop drug immediately in signs of CHF. Prevent by limiting cumulative dose to 550 mg/m²; 450 mg/m² when patient is also receiving cyclophosphamide or irradiation to cardiac area.
• Monitor ECG before treatment, monthly during therapy.
• *Avoid extravasation;* inject slowly by I.V. push into tubing of freely flowing I.V. *Never* give I.M. or S.C. If extravasation occurs, discontinue I.V. immediately and apply ice to area for 24 to 48 hours.
• If vein streaking occurs, slow administration rate. However, if welts occur, stop administration and report to doctor.
• Monitor CBC and hepatic function.
• Warn patient to watch for signs of infection (fever, sore throat, fatigue) and bleeding (easy bruising, nosebleeds, bleeding gums, melena). Take temperature daily.
• Warn patient urine will be red for 1 to 2 days.
• Dosage should be reduced in hepatic dysfunction.
• Warn patient that alopecia will occur but is usually reversible.
• Refrigerated, reconstituted solution is stable for 48 hours; at room temperature, it's stable for 24 hours.
• If cumulative dose exceeds 550 mg/m² body surface area, 30% of patients develop cardiac adverse reactions, which begin 2 weeks to 6 months after stopping drug.
• The alternative dosage schedule (once-weekly dosing) has been found to cause a lower incidence of cardiomyopathy.

Italicized side effects are common or life-threatening.
*Liquid form contains alcohol.   **May contain tartrazine.

• Decrease dosage if serum bilirubin is increased: 50% dosage when bilirubin is 1.2 to 3 mg/100 ml; 25% dosage when bilirubin is greater than 3 mg/100 ml.

• Esophagitis is very common in patients who have also received radiation therapy.

• Premedicate with antiemetic to reduce nausea.

• Reddish color looks very similar to daunorubicin (cerubidine). *Do not confuse the two drugs.*

• Preparation of parenteral form is associated with carcinogenic, mutagenic, and teratogenic risks for personnel. Follow institutional policy to reduce risks.

mitomycin
Mutamycin♦

Pregnancy Risk Category: D

MECHANISM OF ACTION
Acts like an alkylating agent, cross-linking strands of DNA. This causes an imbalance of cell growth, leading to cell death.

INDICATIONS & DOSAGE
Dosage and indications may vary. Check patient's protocol with doctor. *Breast, colon, head, neck, lung, pancreatic, and stomach cancer; malignant melanoma—*
Adults: 2 mg/m² I.V. daily for 5 days. Stop drug for 2 days, then repeat dosage for 5 more days; or 20 mg/m² as a single dose. Repeat cycle 6 to 8 weeks. Stop drug if WBC less than 4,000/mm³ or platelets less than 75,000/mm³.

ADVERSE REACTIONS
Blood: *thrombocytopenia, leukopenia (may be delayed up to 8 weeks and may be cumulative with successive doses).*
CNS: paresthesias.
GI: *nausea, vomiting,* anorexia, stomatitis.
Local: desquamation, induration, pruritus, *pain at injection site.* Extravasation causes cellulitis, ulceration, sloughing.
Other: *reversible alopecia; purple coloration of nail beds;* fever; *microangiopathic hemolytic anemia, syndrome characterized by thrombocytopenia, renal failure, and hypertension; interstitial pneumonitis.*

INTERACTIONS
None significant.

NURSING CONSIDERATIONS
• Dosage modification is required when platelet count is below 75,000/mm³, WBC is less than 4,000/mm³; in coagulation or bleeding disorders, serious infections, and impaired renal function.

• Continue CBC and blood studies at least 7 weeks after therapy is stopped.

• Warn patient to watch for signs of infection (fever, sore throat, fatigue) and bleeding (easy bruising, nosebleeds, bleeding gums, melena). Take temperature daily.

• Advise patient that alopecia may occur, but that it's usually reversible.

• Reconstituted solution stable 1 week at room temperature, 2 weeks refrigerated.

• Has been administered topically by bladder instillation and has been given intraarterially through the hepatic artery.

• Monitor renal function.

• Avoid all I.M. injections in patients with thrombocytopenia.

• Preparation of parenteral form is associated with carcinogenic, mutagenic, and teratogenic risks for personnel. Follow institutional policy to reduce risks.

plicamycin (mithramycin)
Mithracin

Pregnancy Risk Category: C

MECHANISM OF ACTION
Forms a complex with DNA, thus inhibiting RNA synthesis. Also inhibits osteocytic activity, blocking calcium and phosphorus resorption from bone.

INDICATIONS & DOSAGE
Dosage and indications may vary. Check patient's protocol with doctor.
Hypercalcemia associated with advanced malignancy—
Adults: 25 mcg/kg I.V. daily for 1 to 4 days.
Testicular cancer—
Adults: 25 to 30 mcg/kg I.V. daily for up to 10 days (based on ideal body weight or actual weight, whichever is less).

ADVERSE REACTIONS
Blood: *thrombocytopenia; bleeding syndrome, from epistaxis to generalized hemorrhage; facial flushing.*
GI: *nausea, vomiting,* anorexia, diarrhea, stomatitis, metallic taste.
GU: proteinuria; increased BUN, serum creatinine.
Metabolic: *decreased serum calcium,* potassium, and phosphorus.
Skin: periorbital pallor, usually the day before toxic symptoms occur.
Local: extravasation causes irritation, cellulitis.

INTERACTIONS
None significant.

NURSING CONSIDERATIONS
• Contraindicated in thrombocytopenia and in coagulation and bleeding disorders. Dosage modification may be required in renal, hepatic, or bone marrow impairment.
• Slow infusion reduces nausea that develops with I.V. push.
• Monitor LDH, AST (SGOT), ALT (SGPT), alkaline phosphatase, BUN, creatinine, potassium, calcium, and phosphorus levels.
• Monitor platelet count and prothrombin time before and during therapy.
• Warn patient to watch for signs of infection (fever, sore throat, fatigue) and bleeding (easy bruising, nosebleeds, bleeding gums, melena). Take temperature daily.
• Facial flushing is an early indicator of bleeding.
• Give antiemetic before administering to reduce nausea.
• Avoid extravasation. Plicamycin is a vesicant. If I.V. infiltrates, stop immediately; use ice packs. Restart I.V.
• Avoid contact with skin or mucous membranes.
• Therapeutic effect in hypercalcemia may not be seen for 24 to 48 hours; may last 3 to 15 days.
• Precipitous drop in calcium possible. Monitor patient for tetany, carpopedal spasm, Chvostek's sign, muscle cramps; check serum calcium.
• Store lyophilized powder in refrigerator. Remains stable after reconstitution for 24 hours; 48 hours in refrigerator.
• Preparation of parenteral form is associated with carcinogenic, mutagenic, and teratogenic risks for personnel. Follow institutional policy to reduce risks.

procarbazine hydrochloride
Matulane, Natulan♦♦

Pregnancy Risk Category: D

MECHANISM OF ACTION
Inhibits DNA, RNA, and protein synthesis.

INDICATIONS & DOSAGE
Dosage and indications may vary. Check patient's protocol with doctor.
Hodgkin's disease, lymphomas, brain and lung cancer—

Italicized side effects are common or life-threatening.
*Liquid form contains alcohol.   **May contain tartrazine.

Adults: 2 to 4 mg/kg P.O. daily in a single dose or divided doses for the first week. Then, 4 to 6 mg/kg daily until WBC falls below 4,000/mm^3 or platelets fall below 100,000/mm^3. After bone marrow recovers, resume maintenance dosage of 1 to 2 mg/kg/day.

Children: 50 mg/m^2 P.O. daily for first week, then 100 mg/m^2 until response or toxicity occurs. Maintenance dosage is 50 mg/m^2 P.O. daily after bone marrow recovery.

ADVERSE REACTIONS
Blood: bleeding tendency, *thrombocytopenia, leukopenia,* anemia.
CNS: nervousness, depression, insomnia, nightmares, *hallucinations,* confusion.
EENT: retinal hemorrhage, nystagmus, photophobia.
GI: *nausea, vomiting, anorexia,* stomatitis, dry mouth, dysphagia, diarrhea, constipation.
Skin: dermatitis.
Other: reversible alopecia, pleural effusion.

INTERACTIONS
Alcohol: mild disulfiram-like reaction. Warn patient not to drink alcohol.
Meperidine: may cause severe hypotension and possible death. Don't give together.

NURSING CONSIDERATIONS
• Use cautiously in inadequate bone marrow reserve, leukopenia, thrombocytopenia, anemia, and impaired hepatic or renal function.
• Warn patient to watch for signs of infection (fever, sore throat, fatigue) and bleeding (easy bruising, nosebleeds, bleeding gums, melena). Take temperature daily.
• Nausea and vomiting may be decreased if taken at bedtime and in divided doses.
• Warn patient not to drink alcoholic beverages while taking this drug.
• Procarbazine inhibits MAO and can cause disulfiram-like reaction if taken with other MAO inhibitors, tricyclic antidepressants, or foods with a high tyramine content.
• Instruct patient to stop medication and check with doctor immediately if disulfiram-like reaction occurs (chest pains, rapid or irregular heartbeat, severe headache, stiff neck).
• Monitor CBC and platelet counts.
• Avoid all I.M. injections in patients with thrombocytopenia.
• Preparation of parenteral form is associated with carcinogenic, mutagenic, and teratogenic risks for personnel. Follow institutional policy to reduce risks.

74

Antineoplastics altering hormone balance

aminoglutethimide
estramustine phosphate sodium
flutamide
leuprolide acetate
megestrol acetate
mitotane
tamoxifen citrate
testolactone
trilostane

COMBINATION PRODUCTS
None.

---

aminoglutethimide
Cytadren♦

Pregnancy Risk Category: D

MECHANISM OF ACTION
Blocks conversion of cholesterol to
delta-5-pregnenolone in the adrenal
cortex, inhibiting the synthesis of glucocorticoids, mineralocorticoids, and
other steroids.

INDICATIONS & DOSAGE
*Suppression of adrenal function in
Cushing's syndrome and adrenal cancer; metastatic breast cancer—*
Adults: 250 mg P.O. q.i.d. at 6-hour
intervals. Dosage may be increased in
increments of 250 mg daily every 1 to
2 weeks to a maximum daily dosage
of 2 g.

ADVERSE REACTIONS
Blood: transient leukopenia, *severe
pancytopenia.*
CNS: *drowsiness,* headache, dizzi-
ness.
CV: hypotension, tachycardia.

Endocrine: adrenal insufficiency,
masculinization, hirsutism.
GI: nausea, anorexia.
Skin: *morbilliform skin rash,* pruri-
tus, urticaria.
Other: fever, myalgia.

INTERACTIONS
None significant.

NURSING CONSIDERATIONS
• May cause adrenal hypofunction,
especially under stressful conditions,
such as surgery, trauma, or acute illness. Patients may need hydrocortisone and mineralocorticoid supplements in these situations. Monitor
such patients carefully.
• Monitor blood pressure frequently.
Advise patient to stand up slowly in
order to minimize orthostatic hypotension.
• May cause a decrease in thyroid
hormone production. Monitor thyroid
function studies.
• Perform baseline hematologic studies and monitor CBC periodically.
• Warn patient to watch for signs of
infection (fever, sore throat, fatigue)
and bleeding (easy bruising, nosebleeds, bleeding gums, melena). Take
temperature daily.
• Warn patient that drug can cause
drowsiness and dizziness. Advise him
to avoid activities that require alertness and good psychomotor coordination until CNS effects of the drug are
known.
• Tell patient to report if skin rash
persists for more than 8 days. Reassure patient that drowsiness, nausea,

---

Italicized side effects are common or life-threatening.
*Liquid form contains alcohol.   **May contain tartrazine.

and loss of appetite will diminish within 2 weeks after start of aminoglutethimide therapy. However, if these symptoms persist, tell patient to notify doctor.

estramustine phosphate sodium
Emcyt♦

Pregnancy Risk Category: D

MECHANISM OF ACTION
A combination of estrogen and an alkylating agent; acts by its ability to bind selectively to a protein present in the human prostate.

INDICATIONS & DOSAGE
Palliative treatment of metastatic or progressive cancer of the prostate—
Adults: 10 to 16 mg/kg P.O. in 3 to 4 divided doses. Usual dosage is 14 mg/kg daily. Therapy should continue for up to 3 months and, if successful, be maintained as long as the patient responds.

ADVERSE REACTIONS
Blood: leukopenia, thrombocytopenia.
CV: *myocardial infarction, CVA, edema, pulmonary emboli,* thrombophlebitis, CHF, hypertension.
GI: *nausea, vomiting,* diarrhea.
Skin: rash, pruritus.
Other: *painful gynecomastia and breast tenderness,* thinning of hair, hyperglycemia.

INTERACTIONS
None significant.

NURSING CONSIDERATIONS
• Contraindicated in patients hypersensitive to estradiol and nitrogen mustard. Also contraindicated in active thrombophlebitis or thromboembolic disorders, except in those cases where the actual tumor mass is the cause of the thromboembolic phenomenon.
• Use cautiously in patients with history of thrombophlebitis or thromboembolic disorders and cerebrovascular or coronary artery disease.
• Estramustine may exaggerate preexisting peripheral edema or CHF. Weight gain should be monitored regularly in these patients.
• Monitor blood pressure and glucose tolerance periodically throughout therapy.
• Each 140 mg capsule contains 12.5 mg sodium.
• Because of the possibility of mutagenic effects, advise patient and spouse to use contraceptive measures if woman is of childbearing age.
• Estramustine is a combination of the estrogen estradiol and a nitrogen mustard. Shown to be effective in patients refractory to estrogen therapy alone.
• Patient may continue estramustine as long as he's responding favorably. Some patients have taken the drug for more than 3 years.
• Store capsules in refrigerator.

flutamide
Eulexin

Pregnancy Risk Category: D

MECHANISM OF ACTION
Inhibits androgen uptake or prevents binding of androgens in nucleus of cells within target tissues.

INDICATIONS & DOSAGE
Treatment of metastatic prostatic carcinoma (stage D_2) in combination with leutinizing hormone-releasing hormone analogs such as leuprolide acetate—
Adults: 250 mg P.O. q. 8 hours.

ADVERSE REACTIONS
CNS: *loss of libido.*
CV: edema, hypertension.
GI: *diarrhea, nausea, vomiting.*

GU: *impotence*.
Metabolic: gynecomastia, elevated of hepatic enzymes, hepatitis.
Skin: rash, photosensitivity.
Other: *hot flashes*.

INTERACTIONS
None reported.

NURSING CONSIDERATIONS
• Contraindicated in patients with hypersensitivity to flutamide.
• Periodic liver tests should be performed in patients receiving chronic therapy with flutamide.
• Patients should understand that flutamide must be taken continuously with the agent used for medical castration (such as leuprolide acetate) to allow the full benefit of therapy. Leuprolide suppresses testosterone production, while flutamide inhibits testosterone action at the cellular level. Together they can impair the growth of androgen-responsive tumors. Patients should not discontinue either drug without consulting the doctor.

---

leuprolide acetate
Lupron
Pregnancy Risk Category: B

MECHANISM OF ACTION
Initially stimulates but then inhibits the release of follicle-stimulating and luteinizing hormone. This results in testosterone suppression.

INDICATIONS & DOSAGE
Management of advanced prostate cancer—
Adults: 1 mg S.C. daily.

ADVERSE REACTIONS
Endocrine: *hot flashes*.
GI: nausea, vomiting.
Local: skin reactions at injection site.
Other: pulmonary embolus, peripheral edema, decreased libido, transient bone pain during first week of treatment.

INTERACTIONS
None significant.

NURSING CONSIDERATIONS
• Be sure to administer S.C. Don't give I.M. or I.V.
• Leuprolide is a nonsurgical alternative to orchiectomy for prostate cancer.
• Studies show leuprolide is therapeutically equivalent to diethylstilbestrol in "medical castration" palliation treatment but has significantly milder and fewer adverse reactions.
• Reassure your patient who has had undesirable effects from other endocrine therapies that leuprolide is much easier to tolerate.
• Reassure patient that bone pain is transient and will disappear after about 1 week.
• Patients may be maintained on this drug for long-term treatment.
• Patients should be carefully instructed about proper administration techniques, and they should be advised to use only the syringes provided by the manufacturer.
• If another syringe must be substituted, a low dose insulin syringe (U-100, 0.5 ml) may be an appropriate choice.
• Advise patients to store the drug at room temperature, protected from light and sources of heat.

---

megestrol acetate
Megace♦
Pregnancy Risk Category: X

MECHANISM OF ACTION
Changes the tumor's hormonal environment and alters the neoplastic process.

INDICATIONS & DOSAGE
Breast cancer—

Women: 40 mg P.O. q.i.d.
Endometrial cancer—
Women: 40 to 320 mg P.O. daily in divided doses.

ADVERSE REACTIONS
GU: dysfunctional uterine bleeding when drug is discontinued.
Other: carpal tunnel syndrome, thrombophlebitis, alopecia.

INTERACTIONS
None significant.

NURSING CONSIDERATIONS
• Use cautiously in patients with history of thrombophlebitis.
• Adequate trial is 2 months. Reassure patient that therapeutic response isn't immediate.

---

mitotane
Lysodren♦

Pregnancy Risk Category: C

MECHANISM OF ACTION
Selectively destroys adrenocortical tissue and hinders extraadrenal metabolism of cortisol.

INDICATIONS & DOSAGE
Inoperable adrenocortical cancer—
Adults: initially, 1 to 6 g daily divided t.i.d. or q.i.d.; increased to 9 to 10 g P.O. daily, divided t.i.d. or q.i.d. Dosage is adjusted until maximum tolerated dosage is achieved (varies from 2 to 16 g daily but is usually 8 to 10 g daily).
Children: initially, 0.5 to 1 g P.O. daily in divided doses. Increase dosage based upon patient tolerance and response.

ADVERSE REACTIONS
CNS: *depression, somnolence, vertigo;* brain damage and dysfunction in long-term, high-dose therapy.
GI: *severe nausea, vomiting,* diarrhea, anorexia.

Metabolic: adrenal insufficiency.
Skin: dermatitis.

INTERACTIONS
None significant.

NURSING CONSIDERATIONS
• Dosage modification may be required in hepatic disease.
• Drug should not be used in a patient with shock or trauma. Use of corticosteroids may avoid acute adrenocorticoid insufficiency.
• Assess and record behavioral and neurologic signs for baseline data daily throughout therapy.
• Give antiemetic before administering to reduce nausea.
• Dosage may be reduced if GI or skin adverse reactions are severe.
• Obese patients may need higher dosage and may have longer-lasting adverse reactions, since drug distributes mostly to body fat.
• Warn ambulatory patient of CNS adverse reactions; advise him to avoid hazardous tasks requiring mental alertness or physical coordination.
• Monitor effectiveness by reduction in pain, weakness, anorexia.
• Adequate trial is at least 3 months, but therapy can continue if clinical benefits are observed.

---

tamoxifen citrate
Nolvadex♦

Pregnancy Risk Category: C

MECHANISM OF ACTION
Acts as an estrogen antagonist.

INDICATIONS & DOSAGE
Advanced premenopausal and postmenopausal breast cancer—
Women: 10 mg P.O. b.i.d.

ADVERSE REACTIONS
Blood: transient fall in WBC or platelets.
GI: nausea in 10% of patients, vomit-

ing, anorexia.
GU: vaginal discharge and bleeding.
Metabolic: hypercalcemia.
Skin: rash.
Other: temporary bone or tumor pain, hot flashes in 7% of patients. Brief exacerbation of pain from osseous metastases.

INTERACTIONS
None significant.

NURSING CONSIDERATIONS
• Monitor CBC closely in patients with preexisting leukopenia or thrombocytopenia.
• Acts as an "antiestrogen." Best results have been reported in patients with positive estrogen receptors.
• Adverse reactions are usually minor and well tolerated.
• Reassure patient that acute exacerbation of bone pain during tamoxifen therapy usually indicates drug will produce good response. Use analgesic to relieve pain.
• Short-term therapy induces ovulation in premenopausal women. *Mechanical* contraceptive recommended.
• Monitor serum calcium. Drug may compound hypercalcemia related to bone metastases.
• Also used to treat breast cancer in men and advanced ovarian cancer in women. Has been used to stimulate ovulation in women with oligomenorrhea or amenorrhea who previously used oral contraceptives.

testolactone
Teslac

Pregnancy Risk Category: C

MECHANISM OF ACTION
Changes the tumor's hormonal environment and alters the neoplastic process.

INDICATIONS & DOSAGE
Advanced postmenopausal breast cancer—
Women: 250 mg P.O. q.i.d.

ADVERSE REACTIONS
CV: increased blood pressure, edema.
GI: nausea, vomiting, diarrhea.
Metabolic: hypercalcemia.
Other: alopecia.

INTERACTIONS
None significant.

NURSING CONSIDERATIONS
• Contraindicated in male breast cancer and not recommended for premenopausal women.
• Adequate trial is 3 months. Reassure patient that therapeutic response isn't immediate.
• Monitor fluids and electrolytes, especially calcium.
• Immobilized patients are prone to hypercalcemia. Exercise may prevent it. Force fluids to aid calcium excretion.
• Drug causes less virilization than testosterone.
• Higher-than-recommended doses do not increase incidence of remission.
• Testolactone is an androgen.

trilostane
Modrastane

Pregnancy Risk Category: X

MECHANISM OF ACTION
Reversibly lowers elevated circulating levels of glucocorticoids by inhibiting the enzyme system essential for their production in the adrenal gland.

INDICATIONS & DOSAGE
Adrenal cortical hyperfunction in Cushing's syndrome—
Adults: 30 mg P.O. q.i.d. initially. May be increased at intervals of 3 to 4 days to maximum of 480 mg daily.

ADVERSE REACTIONS
CNS: headache.
CV: *orthostatic hypotension.*
EENT: burning of oral and nasal membranes.
GI: *diarrhea, upset stomach,* nausea, flatulence, bloating.
Metabolic: hyperkalemia.
Skin: flushing, rash.
Other: fever, fatigue.

INTERACTIONS
Aminoglutethimide, mitotane: may cause severe adrenocortical hypofunction.

NURSING CONSIDERATIONS
• Contraindicated in patients with severe renal or hepatic disease.
• Use cautiously in patients who are receiving other drugs that suppress adrenal function.
• Trilostane may prevent normal response to physiologic stressful situation. Therefore, patients who develop a severe illness or need surgery may need to have this drug temporarily discontinued.
• Because the drug may cause orthostatic hypotension by suppressing aldosterone production, monitor blood pressure regularly in all patients.
• Patient should show therapeutic response within 2 weeks. If no response has occurred, the doctor may discontinue the drug.
• Most patients show a therapeutic response at doses below 360 mg/day.
• Trilostane is prescribed when surgery or pituitary radiation is inappropriate or must be delayed. Explain to patient that the drug does not cure the underlying disease.

75

Miscellaneous antineoplastic agents

amsacrine (m-AMSA)
asparaginase (L-asparaginase)
Erwinia asparaginase
etoposide (VP-16)
interferon alfa-2a
interferon alfa-2b
teniposide (VM-26)
vinblastine sulfate (VLB)
vincristine sulfate

COMBINATION PRODUCTS
None.

amsacrine (m-AMSA)

Pregnancy Risk Category: C

MECHANISM OF ACTION
Intercalates DNA and inhibits DNA synthesis, producing a cytotoxic effect.

INDICATIONS & DOSAGE
Ovarian carcinoma, lymphomas—
Adults: 30 to 50 mg/m²/day I.V. for 3 days, or 90 to 180 mg/m² as a single dose.
Acute myelogenous leukemia—
Adults: 75 to 120 mg/m²/day for 5 days given by I.V. or intraarterial infusion.

ADVERSE REACTIONS
Blood: *leukopenia (usually dose-limiting adverse reaction),* mild thrombocytopenia.
CNS: *seizures at dosages as low as 40 mg/m²/day.*
CV: rare ventricular dysrhythmias and cardiac arrests, possibly caused by the diluent.

GI: infrequent and mild nausea and vomiting, stomatitis at higher doses.
Other: *local irritation and mild phlebitis,* abnormal liver function tests.

INTERACTIONS
Heparin: don't mix. May form a precipitate.

NURSING CONSIDERATIONS
• Use cautiously in impaired hepatic function.
• To prepare solution for administration, two sterile liquids are combined. Add 1.5 ml from the amsacrine ampule (50 mg/ml) to the vial containing 13.5 ml of lactic acid. The combined solution will contain 5 mg/ml of amsacrine and is stable for at least 48 hours at room temperature.
• Use glass syringes for combining the amsacrine and lactic acid. The diluent in the amsacrine may dissolve plastic syringes.
• The solution may be further diluted for infusion with dextrose 5% in water (D₅W) to minimize vein irritation. Administer doses of less than 100 mg in at least 100 ml of D₅W, doses from 100 to 199 mg in 250 ml D₅W, and doses 200 mg or greater in a minimum of 500 ml D₅W. Solutions for infusion are stable at least 48 hours at room temperature.
• Solutions should be infused slowly over several hours to minimize vein irritation.
• Do not add amsacrine to normal saline or other chloride-containing solution. Precipitation may occur.
• Do not administer amsacrine

Italicized side effects are common or life-threatening.
*Liquid form contains alcohol.   **May contain tartrazine.

through membrane-type in-line filters. The diluent may dissolve the filter.
- Inform the patient that the drug may turn the urine orange.
- Monitor CBC and liver function tests.
- Monitor patient closely for CNS and cardiac toxicity during administration.
- Avoid direct contact of amsacrine with skin due to possible sensitization.

asparaginase
(L-asparaginase)
Elspar, Kidrolase♦♦

Pregnancy Risk Category: C

MECHANISM OF ACTION
Destroys the amino acid asparagine, which is needed for protein synthesis in acute lymphocytic leukemia. This leads to death of the leukemic cell.

INDICATIONS & DOSAGE
Acute lymphocytic leukemia (when used along with other drugs)—
Adults and children: 1,000 IU/kg I.V. daily for 10 days, injected over 30 minutes or by slow I.V. push; or 6,000 IU/m² I.M. at intervals specified in protocol.
Sole induction agent for acute lymphocytic leukemia—
200 IU/kg I.V. daily for 28 days.

ADVERSE REACTIONS
Blood: *hypofibrinogenemia* and depression of other clotting factors, thrombocytopenia, *leukopenia*, depression of serum albumin.
CNS: lethargy, somnolence.
GI: *vomiting (may last up to 24 hours)*, anorexia, nausea, cramps, weight loss.
GU: *azotemia*, renal failure, uric acid nephropathy, glycosuria, polyuria.
Hepatic: elevated AST (SGOT), ALT (SGPT), *hepatotoxicity*.

Metabolic: elevated alkaline phosphatase and bilirubin (direct and indirect); increase or decrease in total lipids; *hyperglycemia; increased blood ammonia*.
Skin: *rash, urticaria*.
Other: *hemorrhagic pancreatitis and anaphylaxis (relatively common)*.

INTERACTIONS
Methotrexate: decreased methotrexate effectiveness.
Vincristine, prednisone: concurrent use is associated with increased toxicity.

NURSING CONSIDERATIONS
- Contraindicated in pancreatitis and previous hypersensitivity unless desensitized. Use cautiously in preexisting hepatic dysfunction.
- Should be administered in hospital setting with close supervision.
- Keep epinephrine, diphenhydramine, and I.V. corticosteroids available for treatment of anaphylaxis.
- Don't use as sole agent to induce remission unless combination therapy is inappropriate. Not recommended for maintenance therapy.
- Risk of hypersensitivity increases with repeated dosages. Patient may be desensitized, but this doesn't rule out risk of allergic reactions. Routine administration of 2 IU I.V. test dose may identify high-risk patients.
- Give I.V. injection over 30-minute period through a running infusion of sodium chloride injection or dextrose 5% injection.
- For I.M. injection, limit dose at single injection site to 2 ml.
- Because of vomiting, patient may need parenteral fluids for 24 hours or until oral fluids are tolerated.
- Monitor CBC and bone marrow function. Bone marrow regeneration may take 5 to 6 weeks.
- Obtain frequent serum amylase determinations to check pancreatic status. If elevated, asparaginase should

be discontinued.
• Tumor lysis can result in uric acid nephropathy. Prevent occurrence by increasing fluid intake. Allopurinol should be started before therapy begins.
• Warn patient to watch for signs of infection (fever, sore throat, fatigue) and bleeding (easy bruising, nosebleeds, bleeding gums, melena). Take temperature daily.
• Monitor blood and urine glucose before and during therapy. Watch for signs of hyperglycemia, such as glycosuria and polyuria.
• Reconstitute with either 2 to 5 ml sterile water for injection or sodium chloride injection.
• Don't shake vial; may cause loss of potency. Don't use cloudy solutions.
• Refrigerate unopened dry powder. Reconstituted solution is stable for 6 hours at room temperature, 24 hours refrigerated.
• Preparation of parenteral form is associated with carcinogenic, mutagenic, and teratogenic risks for personnel. Follow institutional policy to reduce risks.

Erwinia asparaginase
Pregnancy Risk Category: C

MECHANISM OF ACTION
Destroys the amino acid asparagine, which is needed for protein synthesis.

INDICATIONS & DOSAGE
Acute lymphocytic leukemia (in combination with other drugs)—
Adults: 5,000 to 10,000 IU/m²/day for 7 days every 3 weeks or 10,000 to 40,000 IU/m² every 2 to 3 weeks.
  Doses may be given I.V. over 15 to 30 minutes or by I.M. injection.
Children: 6,000 to 10,000 IU/m² I.V. or I.M. daily for 14 days; or 60,000 IU/m² every other day for a total of 12 doses; or 1,000 IU/kg for 10 days.

ADVERSE REACTIONS
Blood: *hypofibrinogenemia and depression of other clotting factors,* leukopenia (rare), and thrombocytopenia.
CNS: *lethargy,* somnolence.
GI: mild nausea and vomiting, anorexia, weight loss.
GU: (rare) azotemia and renal failure.
Hepatic: hepatotoxicity, elevated liver function tests, hypoalbuminemia.
Metabolic: *hyperglycemia.*
Skin: rash, urticaria.
Other: *acute pancreatitis, anaphylaxis* (relatively common), *fever.*

INTERACTIONS
None significant.

NURSING CONSIDERATIONS
• Contraindicated in pancreatitis.
• *Erwinia* strain of asparaginase is usually reserved for those patients with previous reactions to *Escherichia coli* asparaginase. The two forms of the drug are not cross-reactive.
• Use cautiously in preexisting hepatic dysfunction.
• Monitor vital signs closely.
• Should be administered in a hospital setting with close supervision.
• Risk of hypersensitivity increases with repeated dosages.
• Keep epinephrine, diphenhydramine, and I.V. corticosteroids available for treatment of anaphylaxis.
• Don't use as sole agent to induce remission unless combination therapy is inappropriate. Not recommended for maintenance therapy.
• Give I.V. infusion or I.V. push over 30 minutes through a running infusion of normal saline solution or dextrose 5% in water.
• For I.M. injection, limit dose at single injection site to 2 ml.
• Reconstitute with 2 to 5 ml sterile water for injection or sodium chloride injection. For I.M. use, each 10,000 I.V. vial may be dissolved in 1 ml of

diluent.
- Don't shake vial; may cause loss of potency. Don't use cloudy solutions.
- Reconstituted solutions are stable for 3 weeks at either room temperature or refrigerated. Solutions further diluted for infusion are stable at room temperature or refrigerated for at least 4 days.
- The reconstituted solution should be withdrawn from the vial within 15 minutes to minimize protein denaturation resulting from contact with the stopper.
- Monitor CBC and renal and liver function tests.
- Watch for signs of bleeding, such as petechiae and ecchymoses.
- Monitor blood sugar, and test urine for glycosuria before and during therapy.
- Obtain frequent serum amylase and lipase determinations to check pancreatic status. If serum levels are elevated, asparaginase should be discontinued.
- Preparation of parenteral form is associated with carcinogenic, mutagenic, and teratogenic risks for personnel. Follow institutional policy to reduce risks.

---

etoposide (VP-16)
VePesid♦

Pregnancy Risk Category: D

MECHANISM OF ACTION
A semi-synthetic derivative of podophyllotoxin that arrests cell mitosis.

INDICATIONS & DOSAGE
Small-cell carcinoma of the lung, acute nonlymphocytic leukemia, lymphosarcoma, Hodgkin's disease, testicular carcinoma—
Adults: 45 to 75 mg/m^2 daily I.V. or P.O. for 3 to 5 days repeated q 3 to 5 weeks; or 200 to 250 mg/m^2 I.V. or P.O. weekly; or 125 to 140 mg/m^2 daily I.V. or P.O. three times a week q

5 weeks.

ADVERSE REACTIONS
Blood: *myelosuppression (dose-limiting), leukopenia,* thrombocytopenia.
CV: hypotension from rapid infusion.
GI: nausea and vomiting.
Local: infrequent phlebitis.
Other: occasional headache and fever, *reversible alopecia, anaphylaxis* (rare).

INTERACTIONS
Warfarin: etoposide may further increase prothrombin time.

NURSING CONSIDERATIONS
- Intrapleural and intrathecal administration of this drug is contraindicated.
- Give drug by slow I.V. infusion (over at least 30 minutes) to prevent severe hypotension.
- The oral form is now available.
- Blood pressure should be monitored before infusion and at 30-minute intervals during infusion. If systolic blood pressure falls below 90 mm Hg, infusion should be stopped and doctor notified.
- Have diphenhydramine, hydrocortisone, epinephrine, and airway available in case of an anaphylactic reaction.
- Monitor CBC. Observe patient for signs of bone marrow suppression.
- The drug may be diluted for infusion in either dextrose 5% in water or normal saline solution to a concentration of 0.2 or 0.4 mg/ml. Higher concentrations may crystallize.
- Solutions diluted to 0.2 mg/ml are stable for 96 hours at room temperature in plastic or glass unprotected from light; solutions diluted to 0.4 mg/ml are stable for 48 hours under the same conditions.
- Do not administer through membrane-type in-line filters because the diluent may dissolve the filter.
- Etoposide has produced complete

---

remissions in small-cell lung cancer and testicular cancer.
• Preparation of parenteral form is associated with carcinogenic, mutagenic, and teratogenic risks for personnel. Follow institutional policy to reduce risks.

interferon alfa-2a
Roferon-A

interferon alfa-2b
Intron A

Pregnancy Risk Category: C

MECHANISM OF ACTION
Interferons bind to specific membrane receptors on the cell surface. Then, interferon initiates a complex sequence of immunologic events that inhibit virus replication and suppress cell proliferation.

INDICATIONS & DOSAGE
Treatment of hairy cell leukemia—
For alfa-2a:
Adults: for induction, give 3 million units S.C. or I.M. daily for 16 to 24 weeks. For maintenance, 3 million units S.C. or I.M. three times a week.
For alfa-2b:
Adults: 2 million units/m² I.M. or S.C. three times a week (for both induction and maintenance).

ADVERSE REACTIONS
Blood: *leukemia.*
CNS: *fatigue,* headache, *dizziness, confusion,* nervousness, depression, paresthesias.
CV: hypotension, edema, palpitations.
GI: nausea, vomiting, diarrhea, *anorexia.*
Skin: *rash, dry or inflamed oropharynx, dry skin, pruritus,* alopecia.
Other: *flulike symptoms (fever, myalgias, chills).*

INTERACTIONS
None reported.

NURSING CONSIDERATIONS
• Dosage modification may be required in cardiac disease or history of cardiac illness, severe renal or hepatic disease, seizure disorders, compromised CNS function, and bone marrow suppression.
• Monitor for CNS adverse reactions, such as decreased mental status and dizziness. Periodic neuropsychiatric monitoring is recommended.
• If patient does not respond within 6 weeks, treatment should be discontinued for reevaluation of therapy.
• Almost all patients experience flulike symptoms at the beginning of therapy. These effects tend to diminish with continued therapy.
• Analgesics and antipyretics, such as acetaminophen, may help to relieve flulike symptoms. Bedtime administration may also help to lessen these effects.
• Warn patients against changing brands of interferon. The 2a and 2b forms have different dosages.
• Teach patients correct home administration technique. Advise them to read enclosed patient package insert carefully.
• Patients should be well hydrated during treatment. Encourage adequate fluid intake.
• S.C. administration route should be used in patients whose platelets are below 50,000/mm³.

teniposide (VM-26)
Pregnancy Risk Category: D

MECHANISM OF ACTION
A semi-synthetic derivative of podophyllotoxin that arrests cell mitosis.

INDICATIONS & DOSAGE
Hodgkin's and non-Hodgkin's lymphomas, acute lymphocytic leukemia,

---

Italicized side effects are common or life-threatening.
*Liquid form contains alcohol.   **May contain tartrazine.

bladder carcinoma—
Adults: 50 to 100 mg/m² I.V. once or twice weekly for 4 to 6 weeks, or 40 to 50 mg/m² daily I.V. for 5 days repeated every 3 to 4 weeks.

ADVERSE REACTIONS
Blood: *myelosuppression (dose-limiting), leukopenia,* some thrombocytopenia.
CV: hypotension from rapid infusion.
GI: nausea and vomiting.
Local: *phlebitis,* extravasation.
Other: alopecia (rare), *anaphylaxis* (rare).

INTERACTIONS
None significant.

NURSING CONSIDERATIONS
• May be diluted for infusion in either dextrose 5% in water or normal saline solution, but cloudy solutions should be discarded.
• Infuse over 45 to 90 minutes to prevent hypotension.
• Don't administer through a membrane-type in-line filter because the diluent may dissolve the filter.
• Solutions containing 0.5 to 2 mg/ml are stable for 4 hours. Solutions containing 0.1 to 0.2 mg/ml are stable for 6 hours.
• Monitor blood pressure before infusion and at 30-minute intervals during infusion. If systolic blood pressure falls below 90 mm Hg, stop infusion and notify doctor.
• Have diphenhydramine, hydrocortisone, epinephrine, and airway available in case of anaphylaxis.
• Monitor CBC. Observe patient for signs of bone marrow suppression.
• Avoid extravasation.
• Drug may be given by local bladder instillation as a treatment for bladder cancer.
• Preparation of parenteral form is associated with carcinogenic, mutagenic, and teratogenic risks for personnel. Follow institutional policy to

reduce risks.

---

vinblastine sulfate (VLB)
Velban, Velbe♦♦
Pregnancy Risk Category: D

MECHANISM OF ACTION
Arrests mitosis in metaphase, blocking cell division.

INDICATIONS & DOSAGE
Breast or testicular cancer, Hodgkin's and non-Hodgkin's lymphomas, choriocarcinoma, lymphosarcoma, neuroblastoma, mycosis fungoides, histiocytosis—
Adults and children: 0.1 mg/kg or 3.7 mg/m² I.V. weekly or q 2 weeks. May be increased to maximum dosage (adults) of 0.5 mg/kg or 18.5 mg/m² I.V. weekly according to response. Dosage should not be repeated if WBC less than 4,000/mm³.

ADVERSE REACTIONS
Blood: *leukopenia* (nadir days 4 to 10 and lasts another 7 to 14 days), *thrombocytopenia.*
CNS: depression, *paresthesias, peripheral neuropathy and neuritis, numbness, loss of deep tendon reflexes, muscle pain and weakness.*
EENT: pharyngitis.
GI: *nausea, vomiting, stomatitis,* ulcer and bleeding, *constipation, ileus, anorexia, weight loss,* abdominal pain.
GU: oligospermia, aspermia, urine retention.
Skin: dermatitis, vesiculation.
Local: *irritation, phlebitis,* cellulitis, necrosis if I.V. extravasates.
Other: *acute bronchospasm,* reversible alopecia in 5% to 10% of patients, *pain in tumor site,* low fever.

INTERACTIONS
None significant.

NURSING CONSIDERATIONS
• Contraindicated in severe leukopenia or bacterial infection. Use cautiously in jaundice or hepatic dysfunction.
• After administering, monitor for life-threatening acute bronchospasm reaction. If this occurs, notify doctor immediately. Reaction most likely to occur in patient who is also receiving mitomycin.
• Give antiemetic before administering to reduce nausea.
• Drug should be stopped if stomatitis occurs.
• Assess bowel activity. Give laxatives as needed. May use stool softeners prophylactically.
• Don't repeat dosage more frequently than every 7 days or severe leukopenia will develop.
• Less neurotoxic than vincristine.
• Assess for numbness and tingling in hands and feet. Assess gait for early evidence of footdrop.
• Should be injected directly into vein or tubing of running I.V. over 1 minute. May also be given in a 50-ml dextrose 5% in water or normal saline solution and infused over 15 minutes. If extravasation occurs, stop infusion. The manufacturer recommends that moderate heat be applied to the area of leakage. Local injection of hyaluronidase may help disperse the drug. Some clinicians prefer to apply ice packs on and off every 2 hours for 24 hours, with local injection of hydrocortisone or 0.9% sodium chloride.
• Warn patient that alopecia may occur but is usually reversible.
• Adequate trial 12 weeks; reassure patient that therapeutic response isn't immediate.
• Reconstitute 10-mg vial with 10 ml of sodium chloride injection or sterile water. This yields 1 mg/ml.
• Refrigerate reconstituted solution. Discard after 30 days.
• Don't confuse vinblastine with vincristine or the investigational agent vindesine.
• Preparation of parenteral form is associated with carcinogenic, mutagenic, and teratogenic risks for personnel. Follow institutional policy to reduce risks.

vincristine sulfate
Oncovin♦
Pregnancy Risk Category: D

MECHANISM OF ACTION
Arrests mitosis in metaphase, blocking cell division.

INDICATIONS & DOSAGE
Acute lymphoblastic and other leukemias, Hodgkin's disease, lymphosarcoma, reticulum cell sarcoma, neuroblastoma, rhabdomyosarcoma, Wilms' tumor, osteogenic and other sarcomas, lung and breast cancer—
Adults: 1 to 2 mg/m² I.V. weekly.
Children: 1.5 to 2 mg/m² I.V. weekly. Maximum single dosage (adults and children) is 2 mg.

ADVERSE REACTIONS
Blood: rapidly reversible mild anemia and leukopenia.
CNS: *peripheral neuropathy,* sensory loss, *loss of deep tendon reflexes, paresthesias, wristdrop and footdrop,* ataxia, cranial nerve palsies (headache, *jaw pain,* hoarseness, vocal cord paralysis, visual disturbances), *muscle weakness and cramps,* depression, agitation, insomnia; some neurotoxicities may be permanent.
EENT: diplopia, optic and extraocular neuropathy, ptosis.
GI: *constipation, cramps,* ileus that mimics surgical abdomen, *nausea, vomiting,* anorexia, *stomatitis,* weight loss, dysphagia.
GU: urine retention.
Local: severe local reaction when extravasated, *phlebitis,* cellulitis.
Other: *acute bronchospasm, reversible alopecia (up to 71% of patients).*

Italicized side effects are common or life-threatening.
*Liquid form contains alcohol.   **May contain tartrazine.

INTERACTIONS
Mitomycin: possibly increased frequency of bronchospasm and acute pulmonary reactions.
Asperaginase: decreased hepatic clearance of vincristine.
Digoxin: decreased digoxin effects. Monitor serum digoxin.
Calcium channel blockers: enhanced vincristine accumulation in cells.

NURSING CONSIDERATIONS
• Use cautiously in jaundice or hepatic dysfunction, neuromuscular disease, infection, and with other neurotoxic drugs.
• After administering, monitor for life-threatening acute bronchospasm reaction. If this occurs, notify doctor immediately. Reaction most likely to occur in patient who is also receiving mitomycin.
• Because of neurotoxicity, don't give drug more than once a week. Children more resistant to neurotoxicity than adults. Neurotoxicity is dose-related and usually reversible.
• Should be given directly into vein or tubing of running I.V. slowly over 1 minute. May also be given in a 50-ml dextrose 5% in water or normal saline solution and infused over 15 minutes. If drug infiltrates, apply ice packs on and off every 2 hours for 24 hours.
• Check for depression of Achilles tendon reflex, numbness, tingling, footdrop or wristdrop, difficulty in walking, ataxia, and slapping gait. Also check ability to walk on heels. Support patient when walking.
• Monitor bowel function. Give stool softener, laxative, or water before dosing. Constipation may be an early sign of neurotoxicity.
• Warn patient that alopecia may occur but is usually reversible.
• Be extremely careful about doses. Don't confuse vincristine with vinblastine or the investigational agent vindesine.
• 5-mg vials are for multiple-dose use only. Don't administer entire vial to one patient as a single dose.
• All vials (1-mg, 2-mg, 5-mg) contain 1 mg/ml solution and should be refrigerated.
• Preparation of parenteral form is associated with carcinogenic, mutagenic, and teratogenic risks for personnel. Follow institutional policy to reduce risks.

76

Immunosuppressants

azathioprine
cyclosporine
lymphocyte immune globulin
    (antithymocyte globulin
    [equine], ATG)
muromonab-CD3

COMBINATION PRODUCTS
None.

---

azathioprine
Imuran♦

Pregnancy Risk Category: D

MECHANISM OF ACTION
Inhibits purine synthesis.

INDICATIONS & DOSAGE
Immunosuppression in renal transplants—
Adults and children: initially, 3 to 5 mg/kg P.O. daily usually beginning on the day of transplantation. Maintain at 1 to 3 mg/kg daily (dosage varies considerably according to patient response).
Treatment of severe, refractory rheumatoid arthritis—
Adults: initially, 1 mg/kg taken as a single dose or as two doses. If patient response is not satisfactory after 6 to 8 weeks, dosage may be increased by 0.5 mg/kg daily (up to a maximum of 2.5 mg/kg daily) at 4-week intervals.

ADVERSE REACTIONS
Blood: *leukopenia, bone marrow suppression,* anemia, pancytopenia, thrombocytopenia.

GI: nausea, vomiting, anorexia, *pancreatitis,* steatorrhea, mouth ulceration, esophagitis.
Hepatic: hepatotoxicity, jaundice.
Skin: rash.
Other: *immunosuppression (possibly profound),* arthralgia, muscle wasting, alopecia.

INTERACTIONS
Allopurinol: impaired inactivation of azathioprine. Decrease azathioprine dose to ¼ or ⅓ normal dose.

NURSING CONSIDERATIONS
• Use cautiously in hepatic or renal dysfunction.
• Watch for clay-colored stools, dark urine, pruritus, and yellow skin and sclera; and for increased alkaline phosphatase, bilirubin, AST (SGOT), and ALT (SGPT).
• In renal homotransplants, start drug 1 to 5 days before surgery.
• Hemoglobin, WBC, and platelet count should be done at least once monthly; more often at beginning of treatment. Drug should be stopped immediately when WBC is less than 3,000/mm³ to prevent irreversible bone marrow suppression.
• This is a potent immunosuppressive. Warn patient to report even mild infections (colds, fever, sore throat, and malaise).
• Patient should avoid conception during therapy and 4 months after stopping therapy.
• Warn patient that some thinning of hair is possible.
• Avoid I.M. injections of any drugs

Italicized side effects are common or life-threatening.
*Liquid form contains alcohol.   **May contain tartrazine.

in patients with severely depressed platelet counts (thrombocytopenia) to prevent bleeding.
• When used for refractory rheumatoid arthritis, inform patient that it may take up to 12 weeks to be effective.

---

cyclosporine
Sandimmune

Pregnancy Risk Category: C

MECHANISM OF ACTION
Inhibits the action of T lymphocytes.

INDICATIONS & DOSAGE
Prophylaxis of organ rejection in kidney, liver, bone marrow, and heart transplants—
Adults and children: 15 mg/kg P.O. (oral solution) 4 to 12 hours before transplantation. Continue this daily dosage postoperatively for 1 to 2 weeks. Then, gradually reduce dosage by 5%/week to maintenance level of 5 to 10 mg/kg/day. Alternatively, administer I.V. concentrate 4 to 5 mg/kg 4 to 12 hours before transplantation. Postoperatively, repeat this dosage daily until patient can tolerate oral solution.

ADVERSE REACTIONS
CNS: *tremor,* headache.
CV: hypertension.
GI: *gum hyperplasia,* nausea, vomiting, diarrhea, oral thrush.
GU: *nephrotoxicity.*
Hepatic: hepatotoxicity.
Skin: *hirsutism,* acne.
Other: sinusitis, flushing.

INTERACTIONS
Ketoconazole, amphotericin B, cimetidine: may increase blood levels of cyclosporine. Monitor for increased toxicity.
Phenytoin, rifampin: possible decreased immunosuppressant effect. May need to increase cyclosporine dosage.

NURSING CONSIDERATIONS
• Cyclosporine may cause nephrotoxicity. Monitor BUN and serum creatinine levels. Nephrotoxicity may develop 2 to 3 months after transplant surgery. Report these findings to doctor. He may reduce the dosage.
• Differentiation between transplanted kidney rejection and cyclosporine-induced nephrotoxicity must be made.
• Monitor liver function tests for hepatotoxicity, which usually occurs during first month post–organ transplant.
• Cyclosporine should always be given concomitantly with adrenal corticosteroids.
• Absorption of cyclosporine oral solution can be erratic. Monitor cyclosporine blood levels at regular intervals.
• Measure oral doses carefully in an oral syringe. To increase palatability, mix with whole milk, chocolate milk, or fruit juice. Use a glass container to minimize adherence to container walls.
• Dosage should be given once daily in the morning. Encourage patient to take drug at the same time each day.
• Patient may take with meals if drug causes nausea.
• Stress to patient that therapy should not be stopped without doctor's approval.
• To prevent thrush, patient should swish and swallow nystatin four times daily.
• If hirsutism occurs, tell patient she may use a depilatory.

---

lymphocyte immune globulin (antithymocyte globulin [equine], ATG)
Atgam

Pregnancy Risk Category: C

MECHANISM OF ACTION
Inhibits cell-mediated immune responses by either altering T cell function or eliminating antigen-reactive T cells.

INDICATIONS & DOSAGE
Prevention of acute renal allograft rejection—
Adults and children: 15 mg/kg I.V. daily for 14 days followed by alternate-day dosing for 14 days; the first dose should be given within 24 hours of transplantation.
Treatment of acute renal allograft rejection—
Adults and children: 10 to 15 mg/kg I.V. daily for 14 days followed by alternate-day dosing for 14 days. Therapy should be initiated when rejection is diagnosed.

ADVERSE REACTIONS
Blood: leukopenia, thrombocytopenia, *hemolysis,* hyperglycemia, elevated serum hepatic enzymes.
CNS: malaise, seizures.
CV: *hypotension, chest pain,* thrombophlebitis, tachycardia, edema, *pulmonary edema,* iliac vein obstruction, renal artery stenosis.
EENT: *dyspnea, laryngospasm.*
GI: *nausea, vomiting,* diarrhea, stomatitis, hiccups, epigastric pain, abdominal distension.
Other: febrile reactions, serum sickness, *anaphylaxis,* rash, infections, arthralgia, night sweats, lymphadenopathy.

INTERACTIONS
None reported.

NURSING CONSIDERATIONS
• Use cautiously in patients receiving additional immunosuppressive therapy (e.g., corticosteroids, azathioprine) because of the increased potential for infection. ATG concentrate should not be diluted with dextrose solutions or solutions with a low salt concentration since a precipitate may form. The proteins in ATG can be denatured by air. ATG is unstable in acidic solutions.
• An intradermal skin test is recommended at least 1 hour before the first dose. Marked local swelling or erythema larger than 10 mm indicates an increased potential for severe systemic reaction (e.g., anaphylaxis).
• Monitor patient for signs of infection.
• ATG solutions must be filtered during administration; filters with pore sizes of 0.2 to 5 microns have been used.
• ATG concentrate is very heat-sensitive; refrigerate at 2° to 8° C. (do not freeze).
• Do not use solutions that are more than 12 hours old.

muromonab-CD3
Orthoclone OKT3

Pregnancy Risk Category: C

MECHANISM OF ACTION
Muromonab-CD3 is an IgG antibody that reacts in the T-lymphocyte membrane with a molecule (CD3) needed for antigen recognition. This drug depletes the blood of CD3-positive T cells, which leads to restoration of allograft function and reversal of rejection.

INDICATIONS & DOSAGE
Treatment of acute allograft rejection in renal transplant patients—
Adults: 5 mg I.V. bolus once daily for 10 to 14 days.
Children: 2.5 mg I.V. bolus once

Italicized side effects are common or life-threatening.
*Liquid form contains alcohol.   **May contain tartrazine.

daily for 10 to 14 days.

ADVERSE REACTIONS
CV: *chest pain.*
GI: *nausea, vomiting,* diarrhea.
Other: *severe pulmonary edema, fever, chills, tremors, dyspnea, infection.*

INTERACTIONS
None reported.

NURSING CONSIDERATIONS
• Contraindicated in patients with fluid overload, as evidenced by chest X-ray or a weight gain greater than 3% within the week before treatment.
• Muromonab-CD3 is a monoclonal antibody preparation. Patients develop antibodies to this preparation that can lead to loss of effectiveness and more severe adverse reactions if a second course of therapy is attempted. Therefore, experts believe that this drug should be used for only a single course of treatment.
• Most adverse reactions develop within ½ hour to 6 hours after the first dose.
• Treatment should begin in a facility where the patient can be monitored closely and that is equipped and staffed for cardiopulmonary resuscitation.
• Assess patient for signs of fluid overload before treatment.
• Chest X-ray must be taken within 24 hours before starting drug treatment.
• Inform patient of expected adverse reactions. Reassure him that they will be less severe as treatment progresses.
• Administering an antipyretic before giving the drug may help lower incidence of expected pyrexia and chills. Corticosteroids may also be administered before first injection to help decrease incidence of adverse reactions. Methylprednisolone sodium succinate (1mg/kg) preinjection, followed by hydrocortisone sodium succinate (100 mg) 30 minutes postinjection, have been recommended to alleviate the severity of the first dose reaction.

77

Vaccines and toxoids

BCG vaccine
cholera vaccine
diphtheria and tetanus toxoids, adsorbed
diphtheria and tetanus toxoids and pertussis vaccine (DPT)
diphtheria toxoid, adsorbed
Haemophilus b conjugate vaccine
Haemophilus b polysaccharide vaccine (HIB)
hepatitis B vaccine
hepatitis B vaccine (recombinant)
influenza virus vaccine, 1989-1990 trivalent types A & B (sub virion)
influenza virus vaccine, 1989-1990 trivalent types A & B (whole virion)
measles, mumps, and rubella virus vaccine, live
measles (rubeola) and rubella virus vaccine, live attenuated
measles (rubeola) virus vaccine, live attenuated
meningitis vaccines
mumps virus vaccine, live
plague vaccine
pneumococcal vaccine, polyvalent
poliovirus vaccine, live, oral, trivalent
rabies vaccine, human diploid cell (HDCV)
rubella and mumps virus vaccine, live
rubella virus vaccine, live attenuated (RA 27/3)
tetanus toxoid, adsorbed
tetanus toxoid fluid

typhoid vaccine
yellow fever vaccine

COMBINATION PRODUCTS
None.

BCG vaccine

Pregnancy Risk Category: C

MECHANISM OF ACTION
Promotes active immunity to tuberculosis.

INDICATIONS & DOSAGE
Tuberculosis exposure, cancer immunotherapy—
Adults and children: 0.1 ml intradermally.
Neonates: 0.05 ml intradermally.

ADVERSE REACTIONS
Local: lymphangitis, lymph node and skin abscess, ulceration at site of injection (2 to 3 weeks after injection), lupus reaction.
Other: urticaria of trunk and limbs, lymphadenitis, osteomyelitis, *anaphylaxis.*

INTERACTIONS
Isoniazid (INH): inhibited multiplication of BCG. Avoid using together.
Immunosuppressive therapy: may reduce response to BCG vaccine. Avoid if possible.

NURSING CONSIDERATIONS
● Contraindicated in hypogammaglobulinemia, positive tuberculin reaction (when meant for use as immu-

---

Italicized side effects are common or life-threatening.
*Liquid form contains alcohol.   **May contain tartrazine.

noprophylactic after exposure to tuberculosis), immunosuppression, fresh smallpox vaccination, burns, and in patients receiving corticosteroid therapy. Use cautiously in chronic skin disease. Inject in area of healthy skin only.
• Obtain history of allergies and reaction to immunization.
• Vaccine is of no value as immunoprophylactic in patients with positive tuberculin test.
• Keep epinephrine 1:1,000 available to treat anaphylaxis.
• Recommended injection site is over insertion of deltoid muscle.
• Do not shake vial following reconstitution.
• Expected lesion forms in 7 to 10 days.
• Allow an interval of at least 3 weeks between BCG and rubella vaccination.
• Don't administer to children with febrile illness.
• Live vaccine; destroy by autoclaving or formaldehyde solution before disposal.
• Patient should have tuberculin skin test 2 to 3 months after BCG vaccination to determine success of vaccine.
• Use of BCG has shown some value in treatment of various cancers, such as leukemia, some lung cancers, malignant melanoma, multiple myeloma, and some breast tumors. Currently, researchers are trying to find ways of augmenting the immune system's response to cancer. They hope to stimulate the body to destroy tumor cells.

cholera vaccine
Pregnancy Risk Category: C

MECHANISM OF ACTION
Promotes active immunity to cholera.

INDICATIONS & DOSAGE
Primary immunization—
Adults and children over 10 years:
two doses of 0.5 ml I.M. or 1 ml S.C., 1 week to 1 month apart, before traveling in cholera area. Booster is 0.5 ml q 6 months as long as protection is needed.
Children 5 to 10 years: 0.3 ml I.M. or S.C.
Children 6 months to 4 years: 0.2 ml I.M. or S.C. Boosters of same dose should be given q 6 months as long as protection is needed.

ADVERSE REACTIONS
Systemic: malaise, fever, flushing, urticaria, tachycardia, hypotension, diarrhea, headache, *anaphylaxis*.
Local: erythema, swelling, pain, induration.

INTERACTIONS
Yellow fever vaccine: simultaneous administration may interfere with immune response to cholera vaccine and yellow fever vaccine. Administer 3 weeks apart.

NURSING CONSIDERATIONS
• Contraindicated in corticosteroid therapy or in immunosuppression. Defer in acute illness.
• Obtain history of allergies and reaction to immunization.
• Keep epinephrine 1:1,000 available.
• May be given intradermally, but I.M. and S.C. routes give higher levels of protection.
• Administer I.M. in deltoid muscle in adults and children over 3 years.

diphtheria and tetanus toxoids, adsorbed
Pregnancy Risk Category: C

MECHANISM OF ACTION
Promotes immunity to diphtheria and tetanus by inducing production of antitoxins.

INDICATIONS & DOSAGE
Primary immunization—
Adults and children over 7 years: use adult strength; 0.5 ml I.M. 4 to 6 weeks apart for two doses and a third dose 1 year later. Booster is 0.5 ml I.M. q 10 years.
Children 1 to 6 years: use pediatric strength; 0.5 ml I.M. at least 4 weeks apart for two doses. Give booster dosage 6 to 12 months after the second injection. If the final immunizing dose is given after the 7th birthday, use the adult strength.
Infants 6 weeks to 1 year: use pediatric strength; 0.5 ml I.M. at least 4 weeks apart for three doses. Give booster dose 6 to 12 months after third injection.

ADVERSE REACTIONS
Systemic: chills, fever, malaise, *anaphylaxis.*
Local: stinging, edema, erythema, pain, induration.

INTERACTIONS
None significant.

NURSING CONSIDERATIONS
• Contraindicated in immunosuppression, radiation, or corticosteroid therapy. Defer in respiratory illness or polio outbreaks, or acute illness except in emergency. Use single antigen during polio risks. In children under 6 years, use only when diphtheria, tetanus, and pertussis combination is contraindicated because of pertussis component.
• Verify strength (pediatric or adult) of toxoid used.
• Obtain history of allergies and reaction to immunization.
• Keep epinephrine 1:1,000 available.
• Give in site not previously used for vaccines or toxoids.

diphtheria and tetanus toxoids and pertussis vaccine (DPT)
Tri-Immunol

MECHANISM OF ACTION
Promotes active immunity to diphtheria, tetanus, and pertussis by inducing production of antitoxins and antibodies.

INDICATIONS & DOSAGE
Primary immunization—
Children 6 weeks to 6 years: 0.5 ml I.M. 2 months apart for three doses and a fourth dose 1 year later. Booster is 0.5 ml I.M. when starting school.
  Not advised for adults or children over 6 years.

ADVERSE REACTIONS
Systemic: slight fever, chills, malaise, *seizures, encephalopathy, anaphylaxis.*
Local: *soreness, redness,* expected nodule remaining several weeks.

INTERACTIONS
Immunosuppressive therapy: may reduce response to DPT vaccine. Avoid if possible.

NURSING CONSIDERATIONS
• Contraindicated in corticosteroid therapy, immunosuppression, and history of seizures. Defer in acute febrile illness.
• Children with preexisting neurologic disorders should not receive pertussis component. Also, children who react to any DPT injection by exhibiting neurologic signs shouldn't receive pertussis component in any succeeding injections. Diphtheria and tetanus toxoids (DT) should be given instead.
• DPT injection may be given at same time as trivalent oral polio vaccine.
• Obtain history of allergies and reaction to immunization.
• Keep epinephrine 1:1,000 avail-

---

able.
• Not to be used for active infection.
• Don't give subcutaneously.
• Shake before using. Refrigerate.
• Administer only by deep I.M. injection, preferably in thigh or deltoid muscle.

diphtheria toxoid, adsorbed

MECHANISM OF ACTION
Promotes immunity to diphtheria by inducing production of antitoxin.

INDICATIONS & DOSAGE
Diphtheria immunization—
Children under 6 years: 0.5 ml I.M. 6 to 8 weeks apart for two doses and a third dose 1 year later. Booster is 0.5 ml I.M. at 5- to 10-year intervals. Not advised for adults or for children over 6 years; instead, use adult strength of diphtheria toxoid (usually combined with tetanus toxoid).

ADVERSE REACTIONS
Systemic: fever, malaise, urticaria, tachycardia, flushing, pruritus, hypotension, aches and pains, *anaphylaxis*.
Local: erythema, pain, induration, expected nodule persistent for several weeks.

INTERACTIONS
None significant.

NURSING CONSIDERATIONS
• Contraindicated in immunosuppression, radiation or corticosteroid therapy, and in children under 12 months with cerebral damage. Defer in acute illness or polio outbreak, except in emergency.
• Obtain history of allergies and reaction to immunization.
• Keep epinephrine 1:1,000 available to treat anaphylaxis.
• Shake vial well before using. Store in refrigerator.

Haemophilus b conjugate vaccine
Hibivax

Haemophilus b polysaccharide vaccine (HIB)
b-Capsa I, Hib-Imune

MECHANISM OF ACTION
Promotes active immunity to *Haemophilus influenzae* type b.

INDICATIONS & DOSAGE
Immunization—
Conjugate vaccine:
Infants up to 2 years: 0.5 ml I.M. as a single dose. A booster dose is not required.
Polysaccharide vaccine:
Children 2 to 6 years: 0.5 ml S.C. Single administration only.

ADVERSE REACTIONS
Local: *erythema and pain at injection site.*
Systemic: fever, *anaphylaxis*.

INTERACTIONS
None significant.

NURSING CONSIDERATIONS
• Contraindicated in immunosuppression. Defer immunization in acute illness.
• The conjugate vaccine is formed when HIB is chemically bound to diphtheria toxoid. It produces a stronger immune response in most patients, but does not replace routine diphtheria immunization.
• Don't administer intradermally or I.V. Must administer S.C. or I.M., depending on the type of vaccine.
• All children should receive the vaccine by 24 months of age, but preferably *at* 24 months.
• Polysaccharide vaccine is not generally recommended for infants under 18 months because vaccine will not

protect very young children against *H. influenzae* type b. However, vaccine may be given to children 18 to 23 months old if they're at high risk for disease (for example, if attending day care). Warn parent, however, that vaccine may not be completely effective.

• This vaccine will *not* protect children against any other microorganisms that cause meningitis. Will protect against *H. influenzae* type b only.

• This vaccine and DPT can be given simultaneously, but should be administered at different sites.

• Don't administer to children with febrile illness.

• Reconstitute polysaccharide vaccine vial with diluent provided in package. Inject 6 ml diluent into one vial of vaccine; mix to dissolve contents. The vial will provide 10 doses. Record the date of reconstitution on the label of the vaccine vial. Store in refrigerator and protect from light. Vaccine is stable for 30 days. Don't freeze.

• Keep epinephrine 1:1,000 available in case of a severe allergic reaction.

• *H. influenzae* type b is an important cause of meningitis in infants and preschool children.

---

hepatitis B vaccine
Heptavax-B♦

Pregnancy Risk Category: C

MECHANISM OF ACTION
Promotes active immunity to hepatitis B.

INDICATIONS & DOSAGE
Immunization against infection caused by all known subtypes of hepatitis B virus. Recommended for immunization of selected populations who are considered to be at increased risk of contracting hepatitis B infection—
Adults and children over 10 years: initial dose of 1 ml I.M. followed by

another dose of 1 ml 1 month later. This is followed by a third dose of 1 ml 6 months after the first dose.
Children 3 months to 10 years: initial dose of 0.5 ml I.M. followed by another dose of 0.5 ml 1 month later. This is followed by a third dose of 0.5 ml 6 months after the first dose.
Dialysis and immunocompromised patients: initial dose of 2 ml I.M. followed by another dose of 2 ml 1 month later. This is followed by a third dose of 2 ml 6 months after the first dose. (The 2-ml doses should be divided into two 1-ml doses and administered at different sites.)

ADVERSE REACTIONS
Local: discomfort at injection site, local inflammation.
Systemic: slight fever, transient malaise, headache, dizziness, nausea, vomiting.

INTERACTIONS
None reported.

NURSING CONSIDERATIONS
• Use cautiously in any serious, active infections; compromised cardiac or pulmonary status; and in those for whom a febrile or systemic reaction could pose a serious risk.

• Hepatitis B vaccine has *not* been associated with an increased incidence of AIDS (acquired immunodeficiency syndrome).

• The Centers for Disease Control reports that response to hepatitis B vaccine is significantly better when administered in the arm rather than the buttock.

• May be administered S.C., but only to persons, such as hemophiliacs, who are at risk of hemorrhage.

• Although anaphylaxis has not been reported, epinephrine should always be available when administering this drug to counteract any possible reaction.

• The recommended dosage regimen

Italicized side effects are common or life-threatening.
*Liquid form contains alcohol.   **May contain tartrazine.

provides immunity for at least 5 years.

• The following persons are at increased risk of infection and should be considered for the vaccine: certain health care personnel (especially those working with dialysis patients, in blood banks, and in emergency medicine); selected patients and patient contacts; certain endemic populations (Alaskan Eskimos, Indo-Chinese and Haitian refugees); certain military personnel; morticians and embalmers; sexually active homosexuals; prostitutes; prisoners; and users of illicit injectable drugs.

• Thoroughly agitate vial just before administration to restore suspension.

• Store both opened and unopened vials in the refrigerator. Don't freeze.

---

hepatitis B vaccine (recombinant)
Recombivax-HB

Pregnancy Risk Category: C

MECHANISM OF ACTION
Provides active immunity to hepatitis B.

INDICATIONS & DOSAGE
Immunization against infection caused by all known subtypes of hepatitis B virus. Recommended for immunization of selected populations considered at increased risk for hepatitis B infection—
Adults and children over 10 years: initial dose of 1 ml I.M., followed by another 1-ml dose 1 month later and a third 1-ml dose 6 months after the first dose.
Children birth to 10 years: initial dose of 0.5 ml I.M., followed by another 0.5-ml dose 1 month later and a third 0.5-ml dose 6 months after the first dose.

ADVERSE REACTIONS
Local: discomfort at injection site,
local inflammation.
Systemic: fatigue, headache, fever, malaise, nausea, diarrhea, pharyngitis, hypersensitivity.

INTERACTIONS
None reported.

NURSING CONSIDERATIONS
• Don't administer the second or third dose to any patient who develops symptoms of hypersensitivity after the first dose. Ask patients to report any reaction they experience after the first dose.

• Use cautiously in any serious active infections; compromised cardiac or pulmonary status; and in those patients for whom a febrile or systemic reaction could pose a serious risk.

• Although anaphylaxis has not been reported, epinephrine should always be available when administering this drug to counteract any possible reaction.

• The Centers for Disease Control reports that response to hepatitis B vaccine is significantly better when vaccine is administered in the arm rather than the buttock.

• May be administered S.C., but only to persons who are at risk for hemorrhage, such as hemophiliacs.

• The following persons are at increased risk for infection and should be considered for the vaccine: certain health care personnel (especially those working with dialysis patients, in blood banks, and in emergency medicine); selected patients and patient contacts; certain endemic populations (Alaskan Eskimos, Indo-Chinese and Haitian refugees); certain military personnel; morticians and embalmers; sexually active homosexuals; prostitutes; prisoners; and users of illicit injectable drugs.

• Thoroughly agitate vial just before administration to restore suspension.

• Store both opened and unopened vials in the refrigerator. Don't freeze.

• Recombivax is manufactured by recombinant DNA technology. It is not a product of human plasma.

---

influenza virus vaccine, 1989-1990 trivalent types A & B (sub virion)
Fluogen, Fluzone

influenza virus vaccine, 1989-1990 trivalent types A & B (whole virion)
Fluzone

Pregnancy Risk Category: C

MECHANISM OF ACTION
Promotes immunity to influenza by inducing production of antibodies.

INDICATIONS & DOSAGE
Influenza prophylaxis with the following antigens: A/Taiwan/1/86 (H1N1), A/Shanghai/11/87 (H3N2), and B/Yamagata/16/88—
Adults and children over 12 years: 0.5 ml whole or split virus I.M. Only one dose is required.
Children 3 to 12 years: 0.5 ml split virus I.M. Repeat dose in 4 weeks unless child received 1978-79 to 1988-89 vaccine.
Children 6 to 35 months: 0.25 ml split virus I.M. Repeat dose in 4 weeks unless child has been previously vaccinated.

ADVERSE REACTIONS
Systemic: fever, malaise, myalgia, *Guillain-Barré syndrome* (rare), *anaphylaxis*.
Local: erythema, induration.
Fever and malaise reactions occur most often in children and in others not exposed to influenza viruses. Severe reactions in adults are rare.

INTERACTIONS
None significant.

NURSING CONSIDERATIONS
• Contraindicated in egg allergy. Defer in acute respiratory or other active infection.
• Obtain history of allergies, especially to eggs, and reaction to immunization.
• Ideally, vaccinations should be performed in November, since outbreaks of influenza generally don't occur until December. Try to avoid administering the vaccine too early in the season because antibody titers may begin to decline prior to the flu season.
• Children 12 years and under should receive their second dose in December, if possible.
• Vaccines could be given to both children and adults throughout the flu season, even as late as April.
• Give injections for adults and older children in deltoid muscle; in anterolateral aspect of thigh for infants and children under 3 years.
• Keep epinephrine 1:1,000 available.
• Strongly recommended for anyone over 6 months, and patients with chronic disease, metabolic disorders, or medical conditions that put them at risk of complications from influenza. Also strongly recommended for health care workers and household members that may come in contact with persons at high risk of medical complications of influenza.
• Influenza vaccine available as whole virus and split virus preparations. Split virus vaccines cause somewhat fewer adverse reactions than whole virus in children.
• Fever, malaise, and myalgia may begin 6 to 12 hours after vaccination and persist 1 to 2 days.
• Allergic reactions, which occur immediately, are extremely rare.
• Paralysis associated with Guillain-Barré syndrome is rare, and has only been associated with the 1976 vaccine.
• Patient should be made aware of

Italicized side effects are common or life-threatening.
*Liquid form contains alcohol.   **May contain tartrazine.

risk as compared with risk of influenza and its complications.
• Pneumococcal vaccine may be given at the same time but at a different injection site.

measles, mumps, and rubella virus vaccine, live
M-M-R-II♦

Pregnancy Risk Category: X

MECHANISM OF ACTION
Promotes immunity to measles, mumps, and rubella virus by inducing production of antibodies.

INDICATIONS & DOSAGE
Immunization—
Children 12 months to puberty: 1 vial (1,000 units) S.C.

ADVERSE REACTIONS
Systemic: fever, rash, regional lymphadenopathy, urticaria, *anaphylaxis.*
Local: erythema.

INTERACTIONS
Immune serum globulin, whole blood, plasma: antibodies in serum may interfere with immune response. Don't use vaccine within 3 months of transfusion.

NURSING CONSIDERATIONS
• Contraindicated in immunosuppression; cancer; blood dyscrasias; corticosteroid or radiation therapy; gamma globulin disorders; fever; or active, untreated tuberculosis. Use cautiously in patients with hypersensitivity to neomycin, chickens, ducks, eggs, or feathers. Defer immunization in acute illness.
• Presence of maternal antibodies may prevent response in children under 12 months.
• Treat fever with antipyretics.
• Store in refrigerator; protect from light. Solution may be used if red,

pink, or yellow, but must be clear.
• Use only diluent supplied. Discard 8 hours after reconstituting.
• Obtain history of allergies, especially to ducks, rabbits, antibiotics, and reaction to immunization.
• Inject in outer aspect of upper arm. Don't give I.V.
• Keep epinephrine 1:1,000 available.

measles (rubeola) and rubella virus vaccine, live attenuated
M-R-Vax-II

Pregnancy Risk Category: X

MECHANISM OF ACTION
Promotes immunity to measles and rubella virus by inducing production of antibodies.

INDICATIONS & DOSAGE
Immunization—
Children 15 months to puberty: 1 vial (1,000 units) S.C.

ADVERSE REACTIONS
Systemic: fever, rash, lymphadenopathy, *anaphylaxis.*

INTERACTIONS
Immune serum globulin, whole blood, plasma: antibodies in serum may interfere with immune response. Don't use vaccine within 3 months of transfusion.
Tuberculin skin test: may temporarily decrease response to test. Defer skin testing.

NURSING CONSIDERATIONS
• Contraindicated in immunosuppression; cancer; blood dyscrasias; corticosteroid or radiation therapy; gamma globulin disorders; fever; or active, untreated tuberculosis. Use cautiously in patients with hypersensitivity to neomycin, chickens, ducks, eggs, or feathers; when there is a history of fe-

brile seizures; or in cerebral injury. Defer immunization in acute illness.
• Do not give within 1 month of other live virus vaccines, except oral poliovirus vaccine.
• Allow an interval of at least 3 weeks between BCG and rubella vaccines.
• Store in refrigerator and protect from light. Solution may be used if red, pink, or yellow, but must be clear (with no precipitation).
• Use only diluent supplied. Discard 8 hours after reconstituting.
• Inject in outer aspect of upper arm. Don't inject I.V.
• Keep epinephrine 1:1,000 available.

---

measles (rubeola) virus vaccine, live attenuated
Attenuvax♦

Pregnancy Risk Category: X

MECHANISM OF ACTION
Promotes immunity to measles virus by inducing production of antibodies.

INDICATIONS & DOSAGE
Immunization—
Adults and children 15 months or over: 0.5 ml (1,000 units) S.C.

ADVERSE REACTIONS
Systemic: fever, rash, lymphadenopathy, *anaphylaxis,* febrile seizures in susceptible children, anorexia, leukopenia.
Local: erythema, swelling, tenderness.

INTERACTIONS
Immune serum globulin, whole blood, plasma: antibodies in serum may interfere with immune response. Don't use vaccine within 3 months of transfusion.
Tuberculin skin test: may temporarily decrease response to test. Defer skin testing.

NURSING CONSIDERATIONS
• Contraindicated in immunosuppression; cancer; blood dyscrasias; corticosteroid or radiation therapy; gamma globulin disorders; or active, untreated tuberculosis; fever. Use with caution in patients with hypersensitivity to neomycin, chickens, eggs, or feathers. Defer in acute illness or after administration of blood or plasma.
• Ideally, should be given during second year of life.
• Warn patient to avoid pregnancy for 3 months after vaccination.
• Do not give I.V.
• Obtain history of allergies, especially to eggs, and reaction to immunization.
• Keep epinephrine 1:1,000 available.
• Store in refrigerator and protect from light. Solution may be used if red, pink, or yellow, but must be clear (with no precipitation).
• Use only diluent supplied. Discard 8 hours after reconstituting.
• May be given with oral poliovirus vaccine.

---

meningitis vaccines
Menomune-A/C, Menomune-A/C/Y/W-135

Pregnancy Risk Category: C

MECHANISM OF ACTION
Promotes active immunity to meningitis.

INDICATIONS & DOSAGE
Meningococcal meningitis prophylaxis—
Adults and children over 2 years: 0.5 ml S.C.

ADVERSE REACTIONS
Systemic: headache, malaise, chills, fever, cramps, *anaphylaxis.*
Local: pain, erythema, induration.

INTERACTIONS
None significant.

NURSING CONSIDERATIONS
• Contraindicated in immunosuppression. Defer in acute illness.
• Tell patient to avoid pregnancy for 3 months after vaccination.
• Obtain history of allergies and reaction to immunization.
• Do not give I.V.
• Keep epinephrine 1:1,000 available.

mumps virus vaccine, live
Mumpsvax♦

Pregnancy Risk Category: X

MECHANISM OF ACTION
Promotes active immunity to mumps.

INDICATIONS & DOSAGE
Immunization—
Adults and children over 1 year: 1 vial (5,000 units) S.C.

ADVERSE REACTIONS
Systemic: *slight fever,* rash, malaise, mild allergic reactions.

INTERACTIONS
Immune serum globulin, whole blood, plasma: antibodies in serum may interfere with immune response. Don't use vaccine within 3 months of transfusion.
Tuberculin skin test: may temporarily decrease response to test. Defer skin testing.

NURSING CONSIDERATIONS
• Contraindicated in immunosuppression; cancer; blood dyscrasias; corticosteroid or radiation therapy; gamma globulin disorders; active, untreated tuberculosis; or pregnancy. Use cautiously in patients with hypersensitivity to neomycin, chickens, ducks, eggs, or feathers. Defer in acute or febrile illness and for 3 months following transfusions or treatment with immune serum globulin.
• Keep epinephrine 1:1,000 available.
• Mumpsvax should not be given less than 1 month before or after immunization with other live virus vaccines, with the exception of Attenuvax, Meruvax, and/or monovalent or trivalent live, oral poliovirus vaccine, which may be administered simultaneously.
• The vaccine will not protect if given after exposure to natural mumps.
• Not recommended for infants under 12 months because retained maternal mumps antibodies may interfere with the immune response.
• Stress importance of avoiding pregnancy for 3 months after immunization. If necessary, provide contraceptive information.
• Treat fever with antipyretics.
• Do not give I.V.
• Store in refrigerator and protect from light. Solution may be used if red, pink, or yellow (but must be clear).
• Use only diluent supplied. Discard 8 hours after reconstituting.
• Obtain history of allergies, especially to antibiotics, and reaction to immunization.

plague vaccine
Pregnancy Risk Category: C

MECHANISM OF ACTION
Promotes active immunity to plague.

INDICATIONS & DOSAGE
Primary immunization and booster—
Adults and children over 10 years: 1 ml I.M. followed by 0.2 ml in 4 weeks, then 0.2 ml 6 months after the first dose. Booster is 0.1 to 0.2 ml q 6 months while in plague area.
Children 5 to 10 years: ⅗ adult primary or booster dose.
Children 1 to 4 years: ⅖ adult primary or booster dose.

Children under 1 year: ⅕ adult primary or booster dose.

ADVERSE REACTIONS
Systemic: malaise, headache, slight fever, lymphadenopathy, *anaphylaxis*.
Local: swelling, *induration, erythema*.

INTERACTIONS
None significant.

NURSING CONSIDERATIONS
• Contraindicated in immunosuppression. Defer in respiratory infection.
• Deltoid area is the preferred injection site.
• Obtain history of allergies and reaction to immunization.
• Keep epinephrine 1:1,000 available.

pneumococcal vaccine, polyvalent
Pneumovax 23♦, Pnu-Imune 23

Pregnancy Risk Category: C

MECHANISM OF ACTION
Promotes active immunity to infections caused by *Streptococcus pneumoniae*.

INDICATIONS & DOSAGE
Pneumococcal immunization—
Adults and children over 2 years:
0.5 ml I.M. or S.C.
Not recommended for children under 2 years.

ADVERSE REACTIONS
Systemic: *slight fever, anaphylaxis*.
Local: soreness, severe, local reaction can occur when revaccination takes place within 3 years.

INTERACTIONS
None significant.

NURSING CONSIDERATIONS
• Check immunization history carefully to avoid revaccination within 3 years.
• Inject in deltoid or midlateral thigh. Don't inject I.V.
• Keep refrigerated. Reconstitution or dilution not necessary.
• Treat fever with mild antipyretics.
• Protects against 23 pneumococcal types, which account for 90% of pneumococcal disease.
• Also may be administered to children to prevent pneumococcal otitis media.
• Obtain history of allergies and reaction to immunization.
• Keep epinephrine 1:1,000 available.

poliovirus vaccine, live, oral, trivalent
Orimune

Pregnancy Risk Category: C

MECHANISM OF ACTION
Promotes immunity to poliomyelitis by inducing humoral antibodies and antibodies in the lymphatic tissue.

INDICATIONS & DOSAGE
Poliovirus immunization—
Children and non-immunized adults: two 0.5-ml doses should be administered 8 weeks apart. Give third 0.5-ml dose 6 to 12 months after second dose. A reinforcing dose of 0.5 ml should be given before entry to school.
Infants: administer 0.5-ml dose at age 2 months, 4 months, and 18 months. Optional dose may be given at 6 months.

ADVERSE REACTIONS
Systemic: *paralytic poliomyelitis*.

INTERACTIONS
Immune serum globulin, whole blood, plasma: antibodies in serum may interfere with immune response. Don't use vaccine within 3 months of trans-

---

Italicized side effects are common or life-threatening.
*Liquid form contains alcohol.   **May contain tartrazine.

fusion.

Tuberculin skin test: skin test may be suppressed. Don't test for 6 weeks.

NURSING CONSIDERATIONS
• Contraindicated in immunosuppression, cancer, immunoglobulin abnormalities and in radiation, antimetabolite, alkylating agent, or corticosteroid therapy. Defer in acute illness, vomiting, or diarrhea.
• Should not be administered to newborns younger than 6 weeks.
• Use with caution in siblings of child with known immunodeficiency syndrome.
• This vaccine is not effective in modifying or preventing existing or incubating poliomyelitis.
• Check the parents' immunization history when they bring in child for vaccine; this is an excellent time for parents to receive booster immunizations.
• Keep frozen until used. Once thawed, if unopened, may store refrigerated up to 30 days. Opened vials may be refrigerated up to 7 days. Thaw before administration.
• Color change from pink to yellow has no effect on the efficacy of the vaccine. Yellow color results from vaccine being stored at low temperatures.
• Obtain history of allergies and reaction to immunization.
• Not for parenteral use.

---

rabies vaccine, human diploid cell (HDCV)
Imovax

Pregnancy Risk Category: C

MECHANISM OF ACTION
Promotes active immunity to rabies.

INDICATIONS & DOSAGE
Postexposure antirabies immunization—
Adults and children: five 1-ml doses

of HDCV I.M. (for example, in the deltoid region). Give first dose as soon as possible after exposure; give an additional dose on each of days 3, 7, 14, and 28 after first dose.
Preexposure prophylaxis immunization for persons in high-risk groups—
Adults and children: three 1-ml injections administered I. M. Give first dose on day 0 (the first day of therapy), second dose on day 7, and third dose on either day 21 or 28. Alternatively, give 0.1 ml intradermally on the same dosage schedule.

ADVERSE REACTIONS
Systemic: headache, nausea, abdominal pain, muscle aches, dizziness, fever, diarrhea, *anaphylaxis, serum sickness.*
Local: *pain, erythema, swelling or itching at injection site.*

INTERACTIONS
Corticosteroids and immunosuppressive agents: Decreased response to rabies vaccine. Avoid concomitant use.

NURSING CONSIDERATIONS
• Stop corticosteroids during immunizing period.
• When postexposure immunization is indicated, pregnancy is not a contraindication.
• Persons with a history of hypersensitivity should be given rabies vaccine with caution.
• Some patients who receive booster doses experience serum sickness–like allergic reactions. These reactions usually respond to antihistamines.
• Keep epinephrine 1:1,000 available.
• The Centers for Disease Control recommends a booster dose with Imovax for all persons who have been potentially exposed to rabies since October 15, 1984, and who have received postexposure prophylaxis with Wyvac unless acceptable titers were proven.
• The alternative regimen of 0.1-ml

---

doses is only for *preexposure* prophylaxis. For postexposure prophylaxis, only the 1-ml doses should be used.

rubella and mumps virus vaccine, live
Biavax II

Pregnancy Risk Category: X

MECHANISM OF ACTION
Promotes immunity to rubella and mumps by inducing production of antibodies.

INDICATIONS & DOSAGE
Measles and mumps immunization—
Adults and children over 1 year: 1 vial (1,000 units) S.C.

ADVERSE REACTIONS
Systemic: fever, rash, thrombocytopenic purpura, urticaria, arthritis, arthralgia, polyneuritis, *anaphylaxis*.
Local: pain, erythema, induration, lymphadenopathy.

INTERACTIONS
Immune serum globulin, whole blood, plasma: antibodies in serum may interfere with immune response. Don't give vaccine within 3 months of transfusion.
Tuberculin skin test: may temporarily decrease response to test. Defer skin testing.

NURSING CONSIDERATIONS
• Contraindicated in immunosuppression; cancer; blood dyscrasias; corticosteroid or radiation therapy; gamma globulin disorders; active, untreated tuberculosis; fever; or pregnancy. Use with caution in patients with hypersensitivity to neomycin, chickens, ducks, eggs, or feathers. Defer in acute illness and after administration of immune serum globulin, blood, or plasma.
• Stress importance of avoiding pregnancy for 3 months after immuniza-

tion. If necessary, provide contraceptive information.
• Store in refrigerator and protect from light. Solution may be used if red, pink, or yellow (but must be clear).
• Use only diluent supplied. Discard 8 hours after reconstituting.
• Obtain history of allergies, especially to ducks, rabbits, and antibiotics, and reaction to immunization.
• Inject into outer aspect of upper arm. Don't inject I.V.
• Keep epinephrine 1:1,000 available.
• Allow an interval of at least 3 weeks between BCG and rubella vaccines.

rubella virus vaccine, live attenuated (RA 27/3)
Meruvax II♦

Pregnancy Risk Category: X

MECHANISM OF ACTION
Promotes immunity to rubella by inducing production of antibodies.

INDICATIONS & DOSAGE
Measles immunization—
Adults and children over 1 year: 1 vial (1,000 units) S.C.

ADVERSE REACTIONS
Systemic: *joint pain,* fever, rash, thrombocytopenic purpura, urticaria, arthritis, arthralgia, polyneuritis, *anaphylaxis*.
Local: pain, erythema, induration, lymphadenopathy.

INTERACTIONS
Immune serum globulin, whole blood, plasma: antibodies in serum may interfere with immune response. Don't use vaccine within 3 months of transfusion.
Tuberculin skin test: may temporarily decrease response to test. Defer skin

testing.

NURSING CONSIDERATIONS
• Contraindicated in immunosuppression; cancer; blood dyscrasias; corticosteroid or radiation therapy; gamma globulin disorders; active, untreated tuberculosis; or fever. Use cautiously in patients with hypersensitivity to neomycin, chickens, ducks, eggs, or feathers. Defer in acute illness and after administration of human immune serum globulin, blood, or plasma.
• Stress importance of avoiding pregnancy for 3 months after immunization. If necessary, provide contraceptive information.
• Store in refrigerator and protect from light. Solution may be used if red, pink, or yellow (but must be clear).
• Use only diluent supplied. Discard 8 hours after reconstituting.
• Obtain history of allergies, especially to ducks and rabbits, and reaction to immunization.
• Inject into outer aspect of upper arm. Don't inject I.V.
• Keep epinephrine 1:1,000 available.
• Allow an interval of at least 3 weeks between BCG and rubella vaccines.

---

tetanus toxoid, adsorbed

tetanus toxoid fluid
Pregnancy Risk Category: C

MECHANISM OF ACTION
Promotes immunity to tetanus by inducing production of antitoxin.

INDICATIONS & DOSAGE
Primary immunization—
Adults and children: 0.5 ml (adsorbed) I.M. 4 to 6 weeks apart for two doses, then third dose 1 year after the second.
Primary immunization—

Adults and children: 0.5 ml (fluid) I.M. or S.C. 4 to 8 weeks apart for three doses, then fourth dose of 0.5 ml 6 to 12 months after third dose. Booster is 0.5 ml I.M. at 10-year intervals.

ADVERSE REACTIONS
Systemic: slight fever, chills, malaise, aches and pains, flushing, urticaria, pruritus, tachycardia, hypotension, *anaphylaxis*.
Local: erythema, induration, nodule.

INTERACTIONS
None significant.

NURSING CONSIDERATIONS
• Contraindicated in immunosuppression and immunoglobulin abnormalities. Defer in acute illness and polio outbreaks, except in emergencies.
• For prevention, not treatment, of tetanus infections.
• Determine date of last tetanus immunization.
• Don't use hot or cold compresses; may increase severity of local reaction.
• Obtain history of allergies and reaction to immunization.
• Keep epinephrine 1:1,000 available.
• Adsorbed form produces longer duration of immunity. Fluid form provides quicker booster effect in patients actively immunized previously.
• Do not confuse this drug with tetanus immune globulin, human.

---

typhoid vaccine
Pregnancy Risk Category: C

MECHANISM OF ACTION
Provides active immunity to typhoid fever.

INDICATIONS & DOSAGE
Primary immunization—
Adults and children over 10 years:

VACCINES AND TOXOIDS **697**

0.5 ml S.C.; repeat in 4 weeks.
Booster is the same dose as primary immunization q 3 years.
Children 6 months to 10 years: 0.25 ml S.C.; repeat in 4 weeks. Booster is the same dose as primary immunization q 3 years.

ADVERSE REACTIONS
Systemic: *fever,* malaise, headache, nausea, *anaphylaxis.*
Local: swelling, pain, inflammation.

INTERACTIONS
None significant.

NURSING CONSIDERATIONS
• Contraindicated in corticosteroid therapy. Defer in acute illness.
• Treat fever with antipyretics.
• Do not give intradermally.
• Obtain history of allergies and reaction to immunization.
• Keep epinephrine 1:1,000 available.
• Store at 35.6° to 50° F. (2° to 10° C.).
• Shake thoroughly before withdrawing from vial.

yellow fever vaccine
YF-Vax

Pregnancy Risk Category: D

MECHANISM OF ACTION
Provides active immunity to yellow fever.

INDICATIONS & DOSAGE
Primary vaccination—
Adults and children over 6 months: 0.5 ml deep S.C. Booster is 0.5 ml S.C. q 10 years.

ADVERSE REACTIONS
Systemic: fever, malaise, *anaphylaxis.*
Local: mild swelling, pain.

INTERACTIONS
Cholera vaccine: concurrent administration may interfere with immune response to both yellow fever vaccine and cholera vaccine. Administer 3 weeks apart.

NURSING CONSIDERATIONS
• Contraindicated in gamma globulin deficiency, immunosuppression, cancer, corticosteroid or radiation therapy, allergies to chickens or eggs, or in pregnancy. Also contraindicated in infants under 9 months except in high-risk areas.
• Reconstitute with sodium chloride injection that contains no preservatives (preservatives decrease potency).
• Must be kept frozen. Don't use unless shipping case contains some dry ice upon arrival. Avoid vigorous shaking; carefully swirl mixture until suspension is uniform. Use within 1 hour after reconstitution. Discard remainder.
• Obtain history of allergies, especially to eggs, and reaction to immunization.
• Don't give within 1 month of other live virus vaccines.
• Keep epinephrine 1:1,000 available.

Italicized side effects are common or life-threatening.
*Liquid form contains alcohol.   **May contain tartrazine.

78

Antitoxins and antivenins

black widow spider antivenin
botulism antitoxin, bivalent
   equine
crotaline antivenin, polyvalent
diphtheria antitoxin, equine
Micrurus fulvius antivenin
tetanus antitoxin (TAT), equine

COMBINATION PRODUCTS
None.

black widow spider antivenin

Antivenin *(Latrodectus mactans)*♦

Pregnancy Risk Category: D

MECHANISM OF ACTION
Neutralizes and binds venom.

INDICATIONS & DOSAGE
Black widow spider bite—
Adults and children: 2.5 ml I.M. in deltoid. Second dose may be needed.

ADVERSE REACTIONS
Systemic: hypersensitivity, *anaphylaxis, neurotoxicity*.

INTERACTIONS
None significant.

NURSING CONSIDERATIONS
• If possible, hospitalize patient.
• Immobilize patient; splint the bitten limb to prevent spread of venom.
• Test for sensitivity before giving. Use 0.2 ml of a 1:10 dilution in normal saline solution.
• Epinephrine 1:1,000 should be available in case of adverse reaction.

• Venom is neurotoxic and may cause respiratory paralysis and convulsions. Watch patient carefully for 2 to 3 days.
• Obtain accurate patient history of allergies, especially to horses, and reaction to immunization.
• Earliest possible use of antivenin recommended for best results.
• Antivenin may be given I.V. in severe cases (when patient is in shock), in 10 to 50 ml of saline solution over 15 minutes.

botulism antitoxin, bivalent equine

Pregnancy Risk Category: D

MECHANISM OF ACTION
Neutralizes and binds toxin.

INDICATIONS & DOSAGE
Botulism—
Adults and children: 1 vial I.V. stat and q 4 hours, p.r.n., until patient's condition improves. Dilute antitoxin 1:10 in dextrose 5% or 10% in water or normal saline solution before giving. Give first 10 ml of dilution over 5 minutes; after 15 minutes, rate may be increased.

ADVERSE REACTIONS
Systemic: hypersensitivity, *anaphylaxis,* serum sickness (urticaria, pruritus, fever, malaise, arthralgia) may occur in 5 to 13 days.

INTERACTIONS
None significant.

NURSING CONSIDERATIONS
- Test for sensitivity before giving.
- Epinephrine 1:1,000 should be available in case of adverse reaction. Bivalent antitoxin contains antibodies against types A and B *Clostridium botulinum*. Antitoxins against all other types available only from Centers for Disease Control in Atlanta: Monday to Friday, 8 a.m. to 4:30 p.m. (E.S.T.), (404) 329-3670; nights, weekends, and holidays (emergencies only), (404) 329-2888.
- Obtain accurate patient history of allergies, especially to horses, and reaction to immunization.
- Earliest possible use of antitoxin is recommended for best results.

crotaline antivenin, polyvalent
Pregnancy Risk Category: D

MECHANISM OF ACTION
Neutralizes and binds venom.

INDICATIONS & DOSAGE
Crotalid (rattlesnake) bites—
Adults and children: initially, 10 to 50 ml or more I.M. or S.C., depending on severity of bite and patient response. If large amount of venom, 70 to 100 ml I.V. directly into superficial vein. Subsequent doses based on patient's response; may give 10 ml q ½ to 2 hours, p.r.n. If bite is in extremity, inject part of initial dose at various sites around limb above swelling; don't inject in finger or toe. The smaller the patient, the larger the initial dose.

ADVERSE REACTIONS
Systemic: hypersensitivity, *anaphylaxis, neurotoxicity, serum sickness.*

INTERACTIONS
Antihistamines: enhanced toxicity of crotaline venoms. Don't use together.

NURSING CONSIDERATIONS
- Test for sensitivity before giving. Give 0.02 to 0.03 ml of a 1:10 dilution in 0.9% normal saline solution intradermally. Read results after 5 to 10 minutes.
- Immobilize patient immediately. Splint the bitten extremity.
- Epinephrine 1:1,000 should be available in case of adverse reaction.
- Type and cross match blood as soon as possible since hemolysis from venom prevents accurate cross matching.
- Early use of antivenin is recommended for best results.
- Watch patient carefully for delayed allergic reaction or relapse.
- Children, who have less resistance and less body fluid to dilute venom, may need twice the adult dose.
- Obtain accurate patient history of allergies, especially to horses, and reaction to immunization.
- Discard unused reconstituted drug.

diphtheria antitoxin, equine
Pregnancy Risk Category: D

MECHANISM OF ACTION
Neutralizes and binds toxin.

INDICATIONS & DOSAGE
Diphtheria prevention—
Adults and children: 1,000 to 5,000 units I.M.
Diphtheria treatment—
Adults and children: 20,000 to 80,000 units or more slow I.V. Additional doses may be given in 24 hours. I.M. route may be used in mild cases.

ADVERSE REACTIONS
Systemic: hypersensitivity, *anaphylaxis,* serum sickness (urticaria, pruritus, fever, malaise, arthralgia) may occur in 7 to 12 days.

INTERACTIONS
None significant.

Italicized side effects are common or life-threatening.
*Liquid form contains alcohol.   **May contain tartrazine.

NURSING CONSIDERATIONS

- Test for sensitivity before giving.
- Epinephrine 1:1,000 should be available in case of adverse reaction.
- Obtain accurate patient history of allergies, especially to horses, and reaction to immunization.
- Therapy should begin immediately, without delay for culture reports, if patient has symptoms of diphtheria (sore throat, fever, tonsillar membrane.
- Refrigerate antitoxin at 35.6° to 50° F. (2° to 10° C.). Warm to 90° to 95° F. (32.2° to 35° C.), never higher.

Micrurus fulvius antivenin

Pregnancy Risk Category: D

MECHANISM OF ACTION
Neutralizes and binds venom.

INDICATIONS & DOSAGE
Eastern and Texas coral snake bite—
Adults and children: 3 to 5 vials slow I.V. through running I.V. of 0.9% normal saline solution. Give first 1 to 2 ml over 3 to 5 minutes, and watch for signs of allergic reaction. If no signs develop, continue injection. Up to 10 vials may be needed. Not effective for Sonoran or Arizona coral snake bites.

ADVERSE REACTIONS
Systemic: hypersensitivity, *anaphylaxis.*

INTERACTIONS
None significant.

NURSING CONSIDERATIONS
- Test for sensitivity before giving.
- Immobilize patient or splint bitten limb to prevent spread of venom.
- If possible, hospitalize patient.
- Early use of antivenin recommended for best results.
- Venom is neurotoxic and may cause respiratory paralysis. Watch patient carefully for 24 hours. Have epineph-

rine 1:1,000 available in case of adverse reaction.
- Obtain accurate patient history of allergies, especially to horses, and reaction to immunization.

---

tetanus antitoxin (TAT), equine

Pregnancy Risk Category: D

MECHANISM OF ACTION
Neutralizes and binds toxin.

INDICATIONS & DOSAGE
Tetanus prophylaxis—
Patients over 30 kg: 3,000 to 5,000 units I.M. or S.C.
Patients under 30 kg: 1,500 to 3,000 units I.M. or S.C.
Tetanus treatment—
All patients: 10,000 to 20,000 units injected into wound. Give additional 40,000 to 100,000 units I.V. Start tetanus toxoid at same time but at different site and with a different syringe.

ADVERSE REACTIONS
Local: pain, numbness, skin rash.
Systemic: joint pain, hypersensitivity, *anaphylaxis, serum sickness.*

INTERACTIONS
None significant.

NURSING CONSIDERATIONS
- Test for sensitivity before giving. Give 0.1 ml as a 1:1,000 dilution in normal saline solution intradermally.
- Use only when tetanus immune globulin (human) not available.
- Obtain accurate patient history of allergies, especially to horses, and reaction to immunization. If respiratory difficulty develops, give 0.4 ml of 1:1,000 solution epinephrine.
- Give preventive dose to those who have had two or fewer injections of tetanus toxoid and who have tetanus-prone injuries more than 24 hours old.

79

Biological response modifiers

**erythropoietin, recombinant
    human (r-HuEPO)**
interferon alfa-2a, recombinant
interferon alfa-2b, recombinant
interleukin-2, recombinant

COMBINATION PRODUCTS
None.

---

erythropoietin, recombinant human (r-HuEPO)
Epogen

MECHANISM OF ACTION
A naturally occurring hormone, produced by recombinant DNA techniques. Erythropoietin is one of the factors controlling the rate of red cell production. It acts on the erythroid tissues in the bone marrow stimulating the mitotic activity of erythroid progenitor cells and early precursor cells. It functions as a growth factor and as a differentiating factor.

INDICATIONS & DOSAGE
Available only through investigational protocol.
Anemia due to reduced production of endogenous erythropoietin, end-stage renal disease—
Adults: 5 to 500 units/kg I.V. (S.C. in some patients) three times weekly postdialysis (predialysis in some patients). Maintenance dosage may be ½ or ⅓ of the starting dose.

ADVERSE REACTIONS
Blood: iron deficiency, elevated plate-let count.
CV: hypertension.
Other: increased clotting of arterio-venous grafts.

INTERACTIONS
None reported.

NURSING CONSIDERATIONS
• Information based upon current literature. Dosage, indications, and adverse effects profile may change with additional clinical experience.
• After injection (usually within 2 hours), some patients complain of pain or discomfort in their limbs (long bones) and pelvis. Coldness and sweating may also occur. These symptoms may persist up to 12 hours and then disappear.
• Patients with end-stage renal disease may experience an improved appetite and enhanced well-being as a result of increased hematocrit.
• Indicators of effective treatment include increased reticulocyte count, erythron transfer in uptake, and hematocrit with decreased transfusion requirements.
• Erythropoietin has also been used to correct the hemostatic defect associated with uremia.
• Additional clinical trials are investigating r-HuEPO for treatment of the anemia of AIDS patients receiving zidovudine, of cancer patients undergoing chemotherapy, and of patients with rheumatoid arthritis. It is also being investigated for facilitating autologous transfusion by helping to produce more units of blood before

---

Italicized side effects are common or life-threatening.
*Liquid form contains alcohol.   **May contain tartrazine.

surgery.
• Advise the patient that blood specimens will be drawn weekly for blood counts and, depending on their results, dosage adjustments may be necessary.
• Blood count should be monitored during therapy. Hematocrit may rise and cause excessive clotting.

interferon alfa-2a, recombinant
Referon-A

Pregnancy Risk Category: C

MECHANISM OF ACTION
Interferon alfa-2a is a sterile protein product produced by recombinant DNA techniques. Its exact mechanism of action is unknown, but appears to involve direct antiproliferative action against tumor cells or viral cells to inhibit replication, and modulation of host immune response by enhancing the phagocytic activity of macrophages and by augmenting specific cytotoxicity of lymphocytes for target cells.

INDICATIONS & DOSAGE
Treatment of hairy-cell leukemia—
Adults: for induction, give 3 million units S.C. or I.M. daily for 16 to 24 weeks. For maintenance, 3 million units S.C. or I.M. three times a week.
Treatment of AIDS-related Kaposi's sarcoma—
Adults: for induction, give 36 million units S.C. or I.M. daily for 10 to 12 weeks. For maintenance, 36 million units S.C. or I.M. three times a week.

ADVERSE REACTIONS
Blood: leukemia, mild thrombocytopenia.
CNS: dizziness, confusion, paresthesias, numbness, lethargy, depression, nervousness, difficulty in thinking or concentrating, insomnia, sedation, apathy, anxiety, irritability, fatigue, vertigo, gait disturbances, poor coordination.
CV: hypotension, chest pain, dysrhythmias, palpitations, syncope, CHF, hypertension, edema.
EENT: visual disturbances, dryness or inflammation of the oropharynx, rhinorrhea, sinusitis, conjunctivitis, earache, eye irritation, rhinitis.
GI: anorexia, nausea, diarrhea, vomiting, abdominal fullness, abdominal pain, flatulence and constipation, hypermotility, gastric distress, dysgeusia.
GU: transient impotence.
Hepatic: hepatitis.
Respiratory: bronchospasm, coughing, dyspnea, tachypnea.
Skin: rash, dryness, pruritus, partial alopecia, urticaria, flushing.
Local: inflammation at injection site (rare).
Other: flu-like syndrome (fever, fatigue, myalgias, headache, chills, arthralgia), diaphoresis, hot flashes, excessive salivation, cyanosis.

INTERACTIONS
Aminophylline: may reduce the clearance of aminophylline.
CNS depressants: enhanced CNS effects.

NURSING IMPLICATIONS
• Information based on current literature. Dosage, indications, and adverse effects profile may change with additional clinical experience.
• Use cautiously in severe hepatic or renal function impairment, seizure disorders, compromised CNS function, cardiac disease, and myelosuppression.
• S.C. administration route should be used in patients whose platelet count is below 50,000/mm³.
• Different brands of interferon may not be equivalent and may require different dosage.
• Almost all patients experience flu-like symptoms at the beginning of

---

Unmarked trade names available in the United States only.
♦Also available in Canada.   ♦♦Available in Canada only.   ◇Also available OTC.

therapy. These effects tend to diminish with continued therapy. Premedication with acetaminophen minimizes flu-like symptoms.

• Patients should be well hydrated, especially during initial stages of treatment.

• Administer at bedtime to minimize daytime drowsiness.

• Severe adverse reactions may require reduction of dosage to one-half or discontinuation of therapy until reactions subside.

• Advise patient that laboratory tests will be performed before and periodically during therapy. Such tests will include a complete blood cell count with differential, platelet count, blood chemistry and electrolyte studies, liver function tests, and if the patient has a preexisting cardiac disorder or advanced stages of cancer, ECGs.

• Interferons may decrease hemoglobin, hemotocrit, leukocytes, platelets, and neutrophils; increase prothrombin and partial thromboplastin time; and increase serum levels of AST (SGOT), ALT (SGPT), LDH, alkaline phosphatase calcium, phosphorus, and fasting glucose. These effects are dose-related and reversible; recovery occurs within several days or weeks after withdrawal of interferon.

• Monitor for CNS adverse reactions, such as decreased mental status and dizziness. Periodic neuropsychiatric monitoring is recommended during therapy.

• Special precautions required for patients who develop thrombocytopenia: exercise extreme care in performing invasive procedures; inspect injection site and skin frequently for signs of bruising; limit frequency of I.M. injections; test urine, emesis fluid, stool, and secretions for occult blood.

• Instruct patient in proper oral hygiene during treatment, because the bone marrow suppressant effects of interferon may lead to microbial infection, delayed healing, and gingival bleeding. Interferon may also decrease salivary flow.

• Advise patient to check with doctor for further instructions after missing a dose.

• If patient is to self-administer drug, teach patient how to prepare and administer the injection and how to use disposable syringe. Give information on drug stability.

• Store drug in refrigerator.

• Emphasize need to follow doctor's instructions about taking and recording temperature, and how and when to take acetaminophen.

• Concurrent use with a live virus vaccine may potentiate replication of vaccine virus, increase adverse effects, and decrease patient's antibody response.

• Warn patient not to have any immunization without doctor's approval and to avoid contact with persons who have taken oral polio vaccine. Because interferon may decrease antibody response and potentiate replication of vaccine viruses, the patient is at special risk for infection during therapy.

• Tell patient drug may cause temporary loss of some hair. Normal hair growth should return when drug is withdrawn.

• Neurotoxicity and cardiotoxicity are more common in elderly patients, especially those with underlying CNS or cardiac impairment.

• Use with blood dyscrasia-causing medications, bone marrow suppressant therapy, or radiation therapy may increase bone marrow suppressant effects. Dosage reduction may be required.

Italicized side effects are common or life-threatening.
*Liquid form contains alcohol.   **May contain tartrazine.

interferon alfa-2b, recombinant

Intron A

Pregnancy Risk Category: C

MECHANISM OF ACTION

Interferon alfa-2b is a sterile protein product produced by recombinant DNA techniques. Its exact mechanism of action is unknown, but appears to involve direct antiproliferative action against tumor cells or viral cells to inhibit replication, and modulation of host immune response by enhancing the phagocytic activity of macrophages and by augmenting specific cytotoxicity of lymphocytes for target cells.

INDICATIONS & DOSAGE

Treatment of hairy-cell leukemia—
Adults: 2 million units/m^2 I.M. or S.C. three times a week.
Treatment of condylomata acuminata (genital or venereal warts)—
Adults: 1 million units per lesion intralesionally three times per week for 3 weeks.
Treatment of AIDS-related Kaposi's sarcoma—
Adults: 30 million units/m^2 S.C. or I.M. three times a week.

ADVERSE REACTIONS

Blood: leukemia, mild thrombocytopenia.
CNS: dizziness, confusion, paresthesias, lethargy, depression, difficulty in thinking or concentrating, insomnia, sedation, anxiety, fatigue, hypoesthesia, amnesia, agitation, weakness.
CV: hypotension, chest pain.
EENT: visual disturbances, hearing disorders, stye, pharyngitis, nasal congestion, sinusitis, rhinitis.
GI: anorexia, nausea, diarrhea, vomiting, abdominal pain, dyspepsia, constipation, loose stools, eructation, dry mouth, dysgeusia.
GU: transient impotence, gynecomastia.
Respiratory: dyspnea, coughing.
Skin: rash, dryness, pruritus, partial alopecia, urticaria, moniliasis, flushing, dermatitis.
Other: flu-like symptoms (fever, fatigue, headache, chills, muscle aches), arthralgia, asthenia, rigors, leg cramps, arthrosis, bone disorders, back pain, increased sweating, stomatitis, gingivitis, decreased libido, hypertonia, migraine, thirst.

INTERACTIONS

CNS depressants: CNS effects enhanced.

NURSING IMPLICATIONS

• Information based upon current literature. Dosage, indications, and adverse effects profile may change with additional clinical experience.
• Use cautiously in history of cardiovascular disease, pulmonary disease, diabetes mellitus, coagulation disorders, and severe myelosuppresion.
• Concurrent use with a live virus vaccine may potentiate replication of vaccine virus, increase adverse effects, and decrease patient's antibody response.
• Use with blood dyscrasia-causing medications, bone marrow suppressant therapy, or radiation therapy may increase bone marrow supressant effects. Dosage reduction may be required.
• S.C. administration route should be used in patients whose platelet count is below 50,000/mm^3.
• Different brands of interferon may not be equivalent and may require different dosage.
• Almost all patients experience flu-like symptoms at the beginning of therapy. These effects tend to diminish with continued therapy. Premedicate with acetaminophen to minimize flu-like symptoms.
• Patients should be well hydrated,

especially during initial stages of treatment.

• Administer at bedtime to minimize daytime drowsiness.

• Severe adverse reactions may require reduction of dosage to one-half or discontinuation of therapy until reactions subside.

• Advise patient that laboratory tests will be performed before and periodically during therapy. Such tests will include a complete blood cell count with differential, platelet count, blood chemistry and electrolyte studies, liver function tests, and if the patient has a preexisting cardiac disorder or advanced stages of cancer, ECGs.

• When administering interferon for condylomata acuminata, use only 10 million IU vial since dilution of other strengths required for intralesional use results in a hypertonic solution. Do not reconstitute 10 million IU vial with more than 1 ml diluent. Use tuberculin or similar syringe and 25 to 30 gauge needle. Do not inject too deeply beneath lesion or too superficially. As many as five lesions can be treated at one time. To ease discomfort, administer in evening with acetaminophen.

• Maximum response usually occurs 4 to 8 weeks after initiation of therapy. If results are not satisfactory after 12 to 16 weeks, a second course may be instituted. Patients with six to ten condylomata may receive a second course of treatment; patients with more than ten condylomata may receive additional courses.

• Interferons may decrease hemoglobin, hemotocrit, leukocytes, platelets, and neutrophils; increase prothrombin and partial thromboplastin time; and increase serum levels of AST (SGOT), ALT (SGPT), LDH, alkaline phosphatase calcium, phosphorus, and fasting glucose. These effects are dose-related and reversible; recovery occurs within several days or weeks after withdrawal of interferon.

• Monitor for adverse CNS reactions, such as decreased mental status and dizziness. Periodic neuropsychiatric monitoring is recommended during therapy.

• Special precautions required for patients who develop thrombocytopenia: exercise extreme care in performing invasive procedures; inspect injection site and skin frequently for signs of bruising; limit frequency of I.M. injections; test urine, emesis fluid, stool, and secretions for occult blood.

• Instruct patient in proper oral hygiene during treatment, because the bone marrow suppressant effects of interferon may lead to microbial infection, delayed healing, and gingival bleeding. Interferon may also decrease salivary flow.

• Advise patient to check with doctor for further instructions after missing a dose.

• If patient is to self-administer drug, teach patient how to prepare the injection and how to use disposable syringe. Give information on drug stability.

• Store drug in refrigerator.

• Emphasize need to follow doctor's instructions about taking and recording temperature, and how and when to take acetaminophen.

• Warn patient not to have any immunization without doctor's approval, and to avoid contact with persons who have taken oral polio vaccine. Because interferon may decrease antibody response and potentiate replication of vaccine viruses, the patient is at risk for infection during therapy.

• Tell patient drug may cause temporary loss of some hair. Normal hair growth should return when drug is withdrawn.

• Neurotoxicity and cardiotoxicity are more common in elderly patients, especially those with underlying CNS or cardiac impairment.

Italicized side effects are common or life-threatening.
*Liquid form contains alcohol.   **May contain tartrazine.

interleukin-2, recombinant

MECHANISM OF ACTION
Interleukin-2 is a lymphokine that stimulates proliferation of T-lymphocytes and thus amplifies immune response to an antigen; it also acts on B-lymphocytes and induces production of interferon-gamma and the activation of natural killer cells.

INDICATIONS & DOSAGE
Available only through investigational protocol.
Adoptive immunotherapy of malignant neoplasms, such as renal cell carcinoma, melanoma, and non-Hodgkin's lymphoma—
Adults: administer with lymphokine-activated killer (LAK) cells. Dilute interleukin-2 in 50 ml of 0.9% sodium chloride solution containing 5% human serum albumin. Give 10,000, 30,000, or 100,000 units I.V. q 8 hours, and continue for several days, depending on tolerance.
To restore immune response in patients with acquired immunodeficiency syndrome (AIDS)—
Adults: up to 2.5 million units daily by continuous 24 hour I.V. infusion, for 5 days per week over 4 to 8 weeks.

ADVERSE REACTIONS
Blood: anemia, thrombocytopenia, eosinophila.
CNS: headache, confusion, disorientation, drowsiness, restlessness, parathesias, coma, psychosis, hallucinations.
CV: hypotension, decreased vascular resistance and increased capillary permeability, myocardial infarction, dysrhythmias, CHF, edema.
GI: nausea, vomiting, diarrhea, stomatitis.
GU: uremia, oliguria, decreased urine output, elevated serum creatinine.
Hepatic: elevated transaminase and bilirubin.
Skin: rashes, itching.
Other: fluid retention, weight gain, fever, fatigue, chills, dyspnea.

INTERACTIONS
None reported.

NURSING CONSIDERATIONS
• Information based upon current literature. Dosage, indications, and adverse effects profile may change with additional clinical experience.
• Advise patient that adverse reactions usually subside after completion of therapy.
• If chills occur, I.V. meperidine may be administered. Nausea may be controlled with antiemetics such as prochlorperazine; headache may be treated with acetaminophen.
• Advise patients that laboratory tests will be performed before and periodically during therapy. Such tests will include complete blod count and liver function studies. Monitor results of these tests and notify the doctor of abnormalities.
• In various clinical trials, interleukin-2 has been given by I.V. bolus, by continuous I.V. infusion, by subcutaneous injection, and by intrahepatic or peritoneal infusion. It has also been administered I.V. piggyback three times daily, by 24 hour infusions twice a week, by weekly I.V. bolus injection, or by continuous I.V. infusion over 5 to 6 days.

Ophthalmic anti-infectives

bacitracin
boric acid
chloramphenicol
erythromycin
gentamicin sulfate
idoxuridine (IDU)
natamycin
polymyxin B sulfate
silver nitrate 1%
sulfacetamide sodium 10%
sulfacetamide sodium 15%
sulfacetamide sodium 30%
tetracycline hydrochloride
tobramycin
trifluridine
vidarabine

COMBINATION PRODUCTS

BLEPHAMIDE S.O.P. STERILE OPHTHALMIC OINTMENT: sodium sulfacetamide 10% and prednisolone acetate 0.2%.

CETAPRED OINTMENT♦: sodium sulfacetamide 10% and prednisolone acetate 0.25%.

CHLOROMYCETIN-HYDROCORTISONE OPHTHALMIC♦: chloramphenicol 0.25% and hydrocortisone acetate 0.5% (as the prepared solution).

CORTISPORIN OPHTHALMIC OINTMENT♦: polymyxin B sulfate 10,000 units, bacitracin zinc 400 units, neomycin sulfate 0.35%, and hydrocortisone 1%.

CORTISPORIN OPHTHALMIC SUSPENSION♦: polymyxin B sulfate 10,000 units, neomycin sulfate 0.35%, and hydrocortisone 1%.

ISOPTO CETAPRED: sulfacetamide sodium 10% and prednisolone acetate 0.25%.

MAXITROL OINTMENT/OPHTHALMIC SUSPENSION♦: dexamethasone 0.1%, neomycin sulfate 0.35%, and polymyxin B sulfate 10,000 units.

METIMYD OPHTHALMIC OINTMENT/SUSPENSION: sodium sulfacetamide 10% and prednisolone acetate 0.5%.

MYCITRACIN OPHTHALMIC OINTMENT: polymyxin B sulfate 5,000 units, neomycin sulfate 3.5 mg, and bacitracin 500 units.

NEODECADRON OPHTHALMIC OINTMENT♦: dexamethasone phosphate 0.1% and neomycin sulfate 0.35%.

NEOSPORIN OPHTHALMIC: polymyxin B sulfate 10,000 units, neomycin sulfate 1.75 mg, and gramicidin 0.025 mg.

NEOSPORIN OPHTHALMIC OINTMENT♦: polymyxin B sulfate 10,000 units, neomycin sulfate 3.5 mg, and bacitracin zinc 400 units/g.

NEOTAL: polymyxin B sulfate 5,000 units, neomycin sulfate 5 mg, and bacitracin zinc 400 units.

OPHTHA P/S OPHTHALMIC SUSPENSION: prednisolone acetate 0.5%, sodium sulfacetamide 10%.

OPHTHOCORT: chloramphenicol 1.0%, polymyxin B sulfate 10,000 units, and hydrocortisone acetate 0.5%.

OPTIMYD: prednisolone phosphate 0.5% and sodium sulfacetamide 10%.

POLYSPORIN OPHTHALMIC OINTMENT: polymyxin B sulfate 10,000 units, and bacitracin zinc 500 units.

STATROL: neomycin sulfate 3.5 mg and polymyxin B sulfate 10,000 units.

SULFAPRED: sodium sulfacetamide 10%, prednisolone acetate 0.25%,

---

Italicized side effects are common or life-threatening.
*Liquid form contains alcohol.   **May contain tartrazine.

and phenylephrine HCl 0.125%.
VASOCIDIN OPHTHALMIC OINTMENT:
sodium sulfacetamide 10%, predniso-
lone acetate 0.5%, and phenylephrine
HCl 0.125%.
VASOCIDIN OPHTHALMIC SOLU-
TION♦: sodium sulfacetamide 10%,
prednisolone phosphate 0.25%.
VASOSULF♦: sodium sulfacetamide
15% and phenylephrine HCl 0.125%.

bacitracin

Pregnancy Risk Category: C

MECHANISM OF ACTION
Inhibits protein synthesis. Bactericidal or bacteriostatic, depending on
concentration and infection.

INDICATIONS & DOSAGE
Ocular infections—
Adults and children: apply small
amount into conjunctival sac several
times daily or p.r.n. until favorable response is observed.

ADVERSE REACTIONS
Eye: slowed corneal wound healing,
temporary visual haze.
Other: overgrowth of nonsusceptible
organisms.

INTERACTIONS
Heavy metals (e.g., silver nitrate): inactivate bacitracin. Don't use together.

NURSING CONSIDERATIONS
• Use cautiously in patients with hereditary predisposition to antibiotic
hypersensitivity.
• Warn patient to avoid sharing washcloths and towels with family members during infection.
• Always wash hands before and after
applying ointment.
• Cleanse eye area of excessive exudate before application.
• Tell patient to watch for signs of
sensitivity, such as itching lids, swell-

ing, or constant burning. Patient who
develops such signs should stop drug
and notify doctor immediately.
• Teach patient how to apply. Advise
him to wash his hands before and after administering and not to touch tip
of tube or dropper to eye or surrounding tissue.
• Stress importance of compliance
with recommended therapy.
• Warn patient that ointment may
cause blurred vision.
• Solution not commercially available
but may be prepared by pharmacy.
May be stored up to 3 weeks in refrigerator.
• Store in tightly closed, light-resistant container.
• Tell patient not to share eye medications with family members. If a family
member develops the same symptoms,
instruct him to contact the doctor.

boric acid
Blinx, Collyrium, Neo-Flo
Pregnancy Risk Category: C

MECHANISM OF ACTION
Unknown. However, drug has fungistatic and bacteriostatic properties.

INDICATIONS & DOSAGE
*For irrigation following tonometry,
gonioscopy, foreign body removal, or
use of fluorescein; used to soothe and
cleanse the eye; used in conjunction
with contact lens—*
Adults: irrigate eye with 2% solution
or apply 5% or 10% ointment, p.r.n.

ADVERSE REACTIONS
Note: toxic if absorbed from abraded
skin areas, granulating wounds, or
ingestion.

INTERACTIONS
Polyvinyl alcohol (Liquifilm): may
form insoluble complex. Check with
pharmacy on contents in other eye
drugs and contact lens wetting solu-

Unmarked trade names available in the United States only.
♦Also available in Canada.   ♦♦Available in Canada only.   ◇Also available OTC.

tions.

NURSING CONSIDERATIONS
• Contraindicated in eye lacerations.
• Don't apply to abraded cornea or skin.
• Always wash hands before and after instilling solution or ointment.
• Not for use with soft contact lenses.
• Tell patient not to share eye solution with family members.
• Avoid contaminating solution container.

---

chloramphenicol
Antibiopto, Chloromycetin Ophthalmic♦, Chloroptic♦, Chloroptic S.O.P., Fenicol♦♦, Isopto Fenicol♦♦, Ophthoclor Ophthalmic, Pentamycetin♦♦

Pregnancy Risk Category: C

MECHANISM OF ACTION
Inhibits protein synthesis.

INDICATIONS & DOSAGE
Surface bacterial infection involving conjunctiva or cornea—
Adults and children: instill 2 drops of solution in eye q hour until condition improves, or instill q.i.d., depending on severity of infection. Apply small amount of ointment to lower conjunctival sac at bedtime as supplement to drops. May use ointment alone by applying a small amount of ointment to lower conjunctival sac q 3 to 6 hours or more frequently, if necessary. Continue until condition improves.

ADVERSE REACTIONS
Note: systemic adverse reactions have not been reported with short-term topical use.
Blood: *bone marrow hypoplasia with prolonged use, aplastic anemia.*
Eye: optic atrophy in children, stinging or burning of eye after instillation.
Other: overgrowth of nonsusceptible

organisms; hypersensitivity, including itching and burning eye, dermatitis, angioedema.

INTERACTIONS
None significant.

NURSING CONSIDERATIONS
• Not for long-term use. Notify doctor if no improvement in 3 days.
• If patient has more than a superficial infection, systemic therapy should also be used.
• One of the safest topical ocular antibiotics, especially for endophthalmitis.
• Warn patient to avoid sharing washcloths and towels with family members during infection.
• Cleanse eye area of excessive exudate before application.
• Tell patient to watch for signs of sensitivity, such as itching lids, swelling, or constant burning. Patient who develops such signs should stop drug and notify doctor immediately.
• Teach patient how to instill. Advise him to wash hands before and after administering ointment or solution, and warn him not to touch tip of applicator to eye or surrounding tissue. Tell him to apply light finger-pressure on lacrimal sac for 1 minute after drops are instilled. Stress importance of compliance with recommended therapy.
• If chloramphenicol drops are to be given q 1 hour, then tapered, follow order closely to ensure adequate anterior chamber levels.
• Store in tightly closed, light-resistant container.
• Tell patient not to share eye medications with family members. If a family member develops the same symptoms, instruct him to contact the doctor.

Italicized side effects are common or life-threatening.
*Liquid form contains alcohol.   **May contain tartrazine.

erythromycin
Ilotycin Ophthalmic♦

Pregnancy Risk Category: C

MECHANISM OF ACTION
Inhibits protein synthesis. Bacteriostatic, but may be bactericidal in high concentrations or against highly susceptible organisms.

INDICATIONS & DOSAGE
Acute and chronic conjunctivitis, trachoma, other eye infections—
Adults and children: apply 0.5% ointment 1 or more times daily, depending upon severity of infection.
Prophylaxis of ophthalmia neonatorum—
Neonates: a ribbon of ointment approximately 0.5 to 1 cm long placed in the lower conjunctival sacs shortly after birth.

ADVERSE REACTIONS
Eye: slowed corneal wound healing.
Other: overgrowth of nonsusceptible organisms with long-term use; hypersensitivity, including itching and burning eyes; urticaria; dermatitis; angioedema.

INTERACTIONS
None significant.

NURSING CONSIDERATIONS
• Has a limited antibacterial spectrum. Use only when sensitivity studies show it is effective against infecting organisms. Don't use in infections of unknown etiology.
• For prophylaxis of ophthalmia neonatorum, apply ointment no later than 1 hour after birth.
• Warn patient to avoid sharing washcloths and towels with family members during infection.
• Cleanse eye area of excessive exudate before application.
• Tell patient to watch for signs of sensitivity, such as itching lids, swelling, or constant burning. Patient who develops such signs should stop drug and notify doctor immediately.
• Teach patient how to apply. Advise him to wash hands before and after administering ointment and warn patient not to touch tip of applicator to eye or surrounding tissue. Tell him to apply light finger-pressure on lacrimal sac for one minute after administering. Stress importance of compliance with recommended therapy.
• Warn patient that ointment may cause blurred vision.
• Store at room temperature in tightly closed, light-resistant container.
• Tell patient not to share eye medications with family members. If a family member develops the same symptoms, instruct him to contact the doctor.

gentamicin sulfate
Garamycin Ophthalmic♦, Genoptic

Pregnancy Risk Category: C

MECHANISM OF ACTION
Inhibits protein synthesis.

INDICATIONS & DOSAGE
External ocular infections (conjunctivitis, keratoconjunctivitis, corneal ulcers, blepharitis, blepharoconjunctivitis, meibomianitis, and dacryocystitis) caused by susceptible organisms, especially Pseudomonas aeruginosa, Proteus, Klebsiella pneumoniae, Escherichia coli, *and other gram-negative organisms—*
Adults and children: instill 1 to 2 drops in eye q 4 hours. In severe infections, may use up to 2 drops q 1 hour. Apply ointment to lower conjunctival sac b.i.d. or t.i.d.

ADVERSE REACTIONS
Note: systemic absorption from excessive use may cause systemic toxicities.
Eye: burning or stinging with oint-

ment, transient irritation from solution.

Other: hypersensitivity, overgrowth of nonsusceptible organisms with long-term use.

INTERACTIONS
None significant.

NURSING CONSIDERATIONS
• Contraindicated in aminoglycoside hypersensitivity. Use cautiously in impaired renal function.
• Have culture taken before giving drug.
• If topical ocular gentamicin is administered concomitantly with systemic gentamicin, be sure to carefully monitor serum gentamicin.
• Stress importance of following recommended therapy. *Pseudomonas* infections can cause complete vision loss within 24 hours if infection is not controlled.
• Warn patient to avoid sharing washcloths and towels with family members during infection.
• Always wash hands before and after applying ointment or solution.
• Cleanse eye area of excessive exudate before application.
• Tell patient to watch for signs of sensitivity, such as itching lids, swelling, or constant burning. Patient who develops such signs should stop drug and notify doctor immediately.
• Teach patient how to instill. Advise him to wash hands before and after administering ointment or solution, and not to touch tip of tube or dropper to eye or surrounding tissue. Tell him to apply light finger-pressure on lacrimal sac for 1 minute after drops are instilled. Stress importance of compliance with recommended therapy.
• Store away from heat.
• Tell patient not to share eye medications with family members. If a family member develops the same symptoms, instruct him to contact the doctor.

idoxuridine (IDU)
Herplex♦, Stoxil♦

Pregnancy Risk Category: C

MECHANISM OF ACTION
Interferes with DNA synthesis.

INDICATIONS & DOSAGE
Herpes simplex keratitis—
Adults and children: instill 1 drop of solution into conjunctival sac q 1 hour during day and q 2 hours at night, or apply ointment to conjunctival sac q 4 hours or 5 times daily, with last dose at bedtime. A response should be seen in 7 days; if not, discontinue and begin alternate therapy. Therapy should not be continued longer than 21 days.

ADVERSE REACTIONS
Eye: temporary visual haze; irritation, pain, burning, or inflammation of eye; mild edema of eyelid or cornea; photosensitivity; small punctate defects in corneal epithelium, corneal ulceration; slowed corneal wound healing with ointment.
Other: hypersensitivity.

INTERACTIONS
None significant.

NURSING CONSIDERATIONS
• Contraindicated in deep ulceration.
• Not for long-term use.
• Idoxuridine should not be mixed with other topical eye medications.
• Don't use old solution; causes ocular burning and has no antiviral activity.
• Warn patient to avoid sharing washcloths and towels with family members during infection.
• Tell patient to watch for signs of sensitivity, such as itching lids, swelling, or constant burning. Patient who develops such signs should stop drug and notify doctor immediately.
• Teach patient how to instill. Advise him to wash hands before and after

---

Italicized side effects are common or life-threatening.
*Liquid form contains alcohol.   **May contain tartrazine.

administering and warn him not to touch dropper or tip to eye or surrounding tissue. Tell him to apply light finger-pressure on lacrimal sac for 1 minute after drops are instilled.
• Cleanse eye area of excessive exudate before application. Stress importance of compliance with recommended therapy.
• Refrigerate idoxuridine 0.1% solution. Store in tightly closed, light-resistant container.
• Tell patient not to share eye medications with family members. If a family member develops the same symptoms, instruct him to contact the doctor.
• If photophobia develops, patient should wear sunglasses.

natamycin
Natacyn
Pregnancy Risk Category: C

MECHANISM OF ACTION
Increases fungal cell-membrane permeability.

INDICATIONS & DOSAGE
Treatment of fungal keratitis—
Adults: initial dosage is 1 drop instilled in conjunctival sac q 1 to 2 hours. After 3 to 4 days, reduce dosage to 1 drop 6 to 8 times daily.

ADVERSE REACTIONS
Eye: ocular edema, hyperemia.

INTERACTIONS
None significant.

NURSING CONSIDERATIONS
• Only antifungal available as ophthalmic preparation.
• Treatment of choice for fungal keratitis. May also be used to treat fungal blepharitis and conjunctivitis.
• Therapy should be continued for 14 to 21 days, or until active disease subsides.
• Reduce dosage gradually at 4- to 7-

day intervals to ensure that organism has been eliminated.
• If infection does not improve with 7 to 10 days of therapy, clinical and laboratory reevaluation is recommended.
• Warn patient to avoid sharing washcloths and towels with family members during infection.
• Cleanse eye area of excessive exudate before application.
• Teach patient how to instill. Advise him to wash hands before and after administering ointment or solution, to apply light finger-pressure on lacrimal sac for 1 minute after drops are instilled, and not to touch tip of dropper to eye or surrounding tissue. Stress importance of compliance with recommended therapy.
• Tell patient not to share eye medications with family members. If a family member develops the same symptoms, instruct him to contact the doctor.
• Shake well before use. May be kept in refrigerator or at room temperature.

polymyxin B sulfate
Pregnancy Risk Category: C

MECHANISM OF ACTION
Inhibits protein synthesis.

INDICATIONS & DOSAGE
Used alone or in combination with other agents for treating corneal ulcers resulting from Pseudomonas *infection or other gram-negative organism infections—*
Adults and children: instill 1 to 3 drops of 0.1% to 0.25% (10,000 to 25,000 units/ml) q 1 hour. Increase interval according to patient response; or up to 10,000 units subconjunctivally daily by doctor.

ADVERSE REACTIONS
Eye: eye irritation, conjunctivitis.
Other: overgrowth of nonsusceptible organisms, hypersensitivity (local

burning, itching).

INTERACTIONS
None significant.

NURSING CONSIDERATIONS
• One of the most effective antibiotics against gram-negative organisms, especially *Pseudomonas*.
• Often used in combination with neomycin sulfate.
• In severe, life-threatening *Pseudomonas* infections, polymyxin B may be used as an ocular irrigant.
• Warn patient to avoid sharing washcloths and towels with family members during infection.
• Tell patient to watch for signs of sensitivity, such as itching lids, swelling, or constant burning. Patient who develops such signs should stop drug and notify doctor immediately.
• Cleanse eye area of excessive exudate before application.
• Teach patient how to instill. Advise him to wash hands before and after administering ointment or solution, and warn patient not to touch tip of dropper to eye or surrounding tissue. Apply light finger-pressure on lacrimal sac for 1 minute after drops are instilled. Stress importance of compliance with recommended therapy.
• Reconstitute carefully to ensure correct drug concentration in solution.
• Tell patient not to share eye medications with family members. If a family member develops the same symptoms, instruct him to contact the doctor.

---

silver nitrate 1%

Pregnancy Risk Category: C

MECHANISM OF ACTION
Causes protein denaturation, which prevents gonorrheal ophthalmia neonatorum. Bacteriostatic, germicidal, and astringent.

INDICATIONS & DOSAGE
Prevention of gonorrheal ophthalmia neonatorum—
Neonates: cleanse lids thoroughly; instill 1 drop of 1% solution into each eye.

ADVERSE REACTIONS
Eye: periorbital edema, temporary staining of lids and surrounding tissue, conjunctivitis (with concentrations of 1% or greater).

INTERACTIONS
Bacitracin: inactivates silver nitrate. Don't use together.

NURSING CONSIDERATIONS
• Legally required for neonates in most states.
• Don't use repeatedly.
• If 2% solution is accidentally used in eye, prompt irrigation with normal saline solution is advised to prevent eye irritation.
• Solution may stain skin and utensils. Handle carefully.
• May delay instillation slightly to allow neonate to bond with mother.
• Always wash hands before instilling solution.
• Store wax ampules away from light and heat.
• Don't irrigate eyes after instillation.

Italicized side effects are common or life-threatening.
*Liquid form contains alcohol.   **May contain tartrazine.

sulfacetamide sodium 10%
Bleph-10 Liquifilm Ophthalmic◆,
Cetamide Ophthalmic◆, Sodium
Sulamyd 10% Ophthalmic◆, Sulf-10
Ophthalmic◆

sulfacetamide sodium 15%
Isopto Cetamide Ophthalmic◆,
Sulfacel-15 Ophthalmic

sulfacetamide sodium 30%
Sodium Sulamyd 30% Ophthalmic◆

Pregnancy Risk Category: C

MECHANISM OF ACTION
Prevents uptake of para-aminobenzoic
acid, a metabolite of bacterial folic-
acid synthesis.

INDICATIONS & DOSAGE
*Inclusion conjunctivitis, corneal ul-
cers, trachoma, prophylaxis to ocular
infection—*
Adults and children: instill 1 to 2
drops of 10% solution into lower conjunctival sac q 2 to 3 hours during
day, less often at night; or instill 1 to 2
drops of 15% solution into lower conjunctival sac q 1 to 2 hours initially,
increasing interval as condition responds; or instill 1 drop of 30% solution into lower conjunctival sac q 2
hours. Instill ½" to 1" of 10% ointment into conjunctival sac q.i.d. and
h.s. May use ointment at night along
with drops during the day.

ADVERSE REACTIONS
Eye: slowed corneal wound healing
(ointment), *pain on instilling eyedrop,* headache or brow pain.
Other: hypersensitivity (including
itching or burning), overgrowth of
nonsusceptible organisms, *Stevens-
Johnson syndrome,* sensitivity to
light.

INTERACTIONS
*Local anesthetics (procaine, tetra-
caine), para-aminobenzoic acid deriv-*
atives: decreased sulfacetamide sodium action. Wait ½ to 1 hour after
instilling anesthetic or para-aminobenzoic acid derivative before instilling sulfacetamide.

NURSING CONSIDERATIONS
• Contraindicated in sulfonamide hypersensitivity.
• Often used with systemic tetracycline in treating trachoma and inclusion conjunctivitis.
• Replaced by other antibiotics in
treating major ocular infections; still
used in minor ocular infections.
• Purulent exudate interferes with
sulfacetamide action. Remove as
much exudate as possible from lids
before instilling sulfacetamide.
• Incompatible with silver preparations.
• Warn patient eyedrop burns
slightly.
• Warn patient to avoid sharing washcloths and towels with family members during infection.
• Tell patient to watch for signs of
sensitivity, such as itching lids, swelling, or constant burning. Patient who
develops such signs should stop drug
and notify doctor immediately.
• Teach patient how to instill. Advise
him to wash hands before and after
administering ointment or solution,
not to touch tip of dropper to eye or
surrounding tissues, and to apply light
finger-pressure on lacrimal sac for 1
minute after drops are instilled. Stress
importance of compliance with recommended therapy.
• Wait at least 5 minutes before administering other eyedrops.
• Warn patient not to touch tip of tube
or dropper to eye or surrounding tissue.
• Warn patient that solution may stain
clothing.
• Store in tightly closed, light-resistant container away from heat.
• Don't use discolored (dark brown)
solution.

• Tell patient not to share eye medications with family members. If a family member develops the same symptoms, instruct him to contact the doctor.
• May minimize photophobia by wearing sunglasses.

tetracycline hydrochloride
Achromycin Ophthalmic♦

Pregnancy Risk Category: D

MECHANISM OF ACTION
Inhibits protein synthesis.

INDICATIONS & DOSAGE
Superficial ocular infections and inclusion conjunctivitis—
Adults and children: instill 1 to 2 drops in eye b.i.d., q.i.d., or more often, depending on severity of infection.
Trachoma—
Adults and children: instill 2 drops in each eye b.i.d., t.i.d., or q.i.d. Continue for 1 to 2 months or longer, or use 1% ointment t.i.d. or q.i.d. for 30 days.
Prophylaxis of ophthalmia neonatorum—
Neonates: 1 to 2 drops into each eye shortly after delivery.

ADVERSE REACTIONS
Eye: itching.
Other: hypersensitivity (eye itching and dermatitis), overgrowth of nonsusceptible organisms with long-term use.

INTERACTIONS
None significant.

NURSING CONSIDERATIONS
• Tell patient or family that trachoma therapy should continue for 1 to 2 months or longer. Trachoma may cause blindness if left untreated or if not treated properly.
• Tell patient that gnats and flies are vectors of the trachoma organism.

Warn patient with trachoma not to let them settle around eye area. Also explain that infection is spread by direct contact, so handwashing is essential to prevent spread.
• For prophylaxis of ophthalmia neonatorum, apply ointment no later than 1 hour after birth.
• Warn patient to avoid sharing washcloths and towels with family members during infection.
• Tell patient to watch for signs of sensitivity, such as itching lids, swelling, or constant burning. Patient who develops such signs should stop drug and notify doctor immediately.
• Cleanse eye area of excessive exudate before application.
• Teach patient how to instill. Advise him to wash hands before and after administering ointment or solution and not to touch tip of dropper to eye or surrounding tissue. Apply light finger-pressure on lacrimal sac for 1 minute after drops are instilled. Stress importance of compliance with recommended therapy.
• Store in tightly closed, light-resistant container.
• Tell patient not to share eye medications with family members. If a family member develops the same symptoms, instruct him to contact the doctor.

tobramycin
Tobrex♦

Pregnancy Risk Category: D

MECHANISM OF ACTION
Inhibits protein synthesis.

INDICATIONS & DOSAGE
Treatment of external ocular infections caused by susceptible gram-negative bacteria—
Adults and children: In mild to moderate infections, instill 1 or 2 drops into the affected eye q 4 hours. In severe infections, instill 2 drops into the infected eye hourly.

ADVERSE REACTIONS
Eye: burning or stinging upon instillation, lid itching, lid swelling.
Other: hypersensitivity.

INTERACTIONS
Tetracycline-containing eye preparations: incompatible with tyloxapol, an ingredient in Tobrex. Don't use together.

NURSING CONSIDERATIONS
• Prolonged use may result in overgrowth of nonsusceptible organisms, including fungi.
• If topical ocular tobramycin is administered concomitantly with systemic tobramycin, be sure to carefully monitor serum levels.
• Clinical symptoms of tobramycin overdose include keratitis, erythema, increased lacrimation, edema, and lid itching. Stop drug and notify doctor if any of these occur.
• Always wash hands before and after instilling solution.
• Warn patient to avoid sharing washcloths and towels with family members during infection.
• Tell patient to watch for signs of sensitivity, such as itching lids, swelling, or constant burning. Patient who develops such signs should discontinue drug and notify doctor immediately.
• Cleanse eye area of excessive exudate before application.
• Teach patient how to instill. Advise him to wash hands before and after administering ointment or solution and warn patient not to touch tip of dropper to eye or surrounding tissue. Apply light finger-pressure on lacrimal sac for 1 minute after drops are instilled. Stress importance of compliance with recommended therapy.
• Often used to combat gram-negative organisms that are resistant to gentamicin.

trifluridine
Viroptic Ophthalmic Solution 1%♦
Pregnancy Risk Category: C

MECHANISM OF ACTION
Interferes with DNA synthesis.

INDICATIONS & DOSAGE
Primary keratoconjunctivitis and recurrent epithelial keratitis caused by herpes simplex virus, types I and II—
Adults: 1 drop of solution q 2 hours while patient is awake, to a maximum of 9 drops daily until re-epithelialization of the corneal ulcer occurs; then 1 drop q 4 hours (minimum 5 drops daily) for an additional 7 days.

ADVERSE REACTIONS
Eye: *stinging upon instillation,* edema of eyelids, increased intraocular pressure.

INTERACTIONS
None significant.

NURSING CONSIDERATIONS
• Should be prescribed only for those patients with clinical diagnosis of herpetic keratitis.
• Consider another form of therapy if improvement doesn't occur after 7 days' treatment or complete re-epithelialization after 14 days' treatment. Trifluridine shouldn't be used more than 21 days continuously due to potential ocular toxicity.
• Watch for signs of increased intraocular pressure.
• Reassure patient that mild local irritation of the conjunctiva and cornea that occurs when solution is instilled is usually temporary.
• More effective drug than vidarabine or idoxuridine with fewer adverse reactions.
• Warn patient to avoid sharing washcloths and towels with family members during infection.
• Cleanse eye area of excessive exu-

date before application.
• Teach patient how to instill. Advise him to wash hands before and after administering solution. Warn patient not to touch tip of dropper to eye or surrounding tissue. Apply light finger-pressure on lacrimal sac for 1 minute after drops are instilled. Stress importance of complying with recommended therapy.
• Tell patient not to share eye medications with family members. If a family member develops the same disease symptoms, instruct him to contact the doctor.

---

vidarabine
Vira-A Ophthalmic◆

Pregnancy Risk Category: C

MECHANISM OF ACTION
Interferes with DNA synthesis.

INDICATIONS & DOSAGE
Acute keratoconjunctivitis, superficial keratitis, and recurrent epithelial keratitis resulting from herpes simplex types I and II—
Adults and children: instill ½" ointment into lower conjunctival sac 5 times daily at 3-hour intervals.

ADVERSE REACTIONS
Eye: temporary burning, itching, mild irritation of eye, lacrimation, foreign body sensation, conjunctival injection, superficial punctate keratitis, eye pain, photophobia.
Other: hypersensitivity.

INTERACTIONS
None significant.

NURSING CONSIDERATIONS
• Not for long-term use.
• Warn patient not to exceed recommended frequency or duration of dosage.
• Not effective against RNA virus, adenoviral ocular infections, or bacte-

rial, fungal, or chlamydial infections.
• Warn patient to avoid sharing washcloths and towels with family members during infection.
• Tell patient to watch for signs of sensitivity, such as itching lids, swelling, or constant burning. Patient who develops such signs should stop drug and notify doctor immediately.
• Cleanse eye area of excessive exudate before application.
• Teach patient how to instill. Advise him to wash hands before and after administering ointment and warn him not to touch tip of tube to eye or surrounding tissue. Apply light finger-pressure on lacrimal sac for 1 minute after drops are instilled. Stress importance of compliance with recommended therapy.
• Store in tightly closed, light-resistant container.
• Tell patient not to share eye medications with family members. If a family member develops the same symptoms, instruct him to contact the doctor.
• Explain to patient that the ointment may produce a temporary visual haze.
• If photophobia develops, patient should wear sunglasses.

Ophthalmic anti-inflammatory agents

dexamethasone
dexamethasone sodium phosphate
fluorometholone
flurbiprofen sodium
medrysone
prednisolone acetate (suspension)
prednisolone sodium phosphate (solution)

COMBINATION PRODUCTS
Corticosteroids for ophthalmic use are commonly combined with antibiotics and sulfonamides. See Chapter 80, OPHTHALMIC ANTI-INFECTIVES.

---

dexamethasone
Maxidex Ophthalmic Suspension♦

dexamethasone sodium phosphate
Decadron Phosphate Ophthalmic♦, Maxidex Ophthalmic♦

Pregnancy Risk Category: C

MECHANISM OF ACTION
Decreases the infiltration of leukocytes at the site of inflammation.

INDICATIONS & DOSAGE
Uveitis; iridocyclitis; inflammatory conditions of eyelids, conjunctiva, cornea, anterior segment of globe; corneal injury from chemical or thermal burns, or penetration of foreign bodies; allergic conjunctivitis—
Adults and children: instill 1 to 2 drops into conjunctival sac. In severe disease, drops may be used hourly, ta-

pering to discontinuation as condition improves. In mild conditions, drops may be used up to 4 to 6 times daily. Treatment may extend from a few days to several weeks.

ADVERSE REACTIONS
Eye: increased intraocular pressure; thinning of cornea, interference with corneal wound healing, increased susceptibility to viral or fungal corneal infection, corneal ulceration; with excessive or long-term use, glaucoma exacerbations, cataracts, defects in visual acuity and visual field, optic nerve damage.
Other: systemic effects and adrenal suppression with excessive or long-term use.

INTERACTIONS
None significant.

NURSING CONSIDERATIONS
• Contraindicated in acute superficial herpes simplex (dendritic keratitis), vaccinia, varicella, or other fungal or viral diseases of cornea and conjunctiva; ocular tuberculosis, or any acute, purulent, untreated infection of the eye. Use cautiously in corneal abrasions, since these may be infected (especially with herpes); in glaucoma (any form), because of possibility of increasing intraocular pressure (glaucoma medications may need to be increased to compensate).
• Viral and fungal infections of the cornea may be exacerbated by the application of steroids.
• Warn patient to call doctor immedi-

---

ately and to stop drug if visual acuity changes or visual field diminishes.
• Not for long-term use.
• May use eye pad with ointment.
• Teach patient how to instill. Advise him to wash hands before and after administering and warn him not to touch dropper tip to eye or surrounding tissue. Apply light finger-pressure on lacrimal sac for 1 minute following instillation.
• Watch for corneal ulceration; may require stopping drug.
• Dexamethasone has greater anti-inflammatory effect than dexamethasone sodium phosphate.
• Warn patient not to use leftover medication for a new eye inflammation; may cause serious problems.
• Tell patient not to share eye medications with family members. If a family member develops similar symptoms, instruct him to contact the doctor.

---

fluorometholone
FML Liquifilm Ophthalmic♦

Pregnancy Risk Category: C

MECHANISM OF ACTION
Decreases the infiltration of leukocytes at the site of inflammation.

INDICATIONS & DOSAGE
Inflammatory and allergic conditions of cornea, conjunctiva, sclera, anterior uvea—
Adults and children: instill 1 to 2 drops in conjunctival sac b.i.d. to q.i.d. May use q hour during first 1 to 2 days if needed.

ADVERSE REACTIONS
Eye: increased intraocular pressure, thinning of cornea, interference with corneal wound healing, corneal ulceration, increased susceptibility to viral or fungal corneal infections; with excessive or long-term use, glaucoma exacerbations, cataracts, decreased

visual acuity, diminished visual field, optic nerve damage.
Other: systemic effects and adrenal suppression in excessive or long-term use.

INTERACTIONS
None significant.

NURSING CONSIDERATIONS
• Contraindicated in vaccinia, varicella, acute superficial herpes simplex (dendritic keratitis), or other fungal or viral eye diseases; ocular tuberculosis; or any acute, purulent, untreated eye infection. Use cautiously in corneal abrasions since these may be contaminated (especially with herpes).
• Not for long-term use.
• Less likely to cause increased intraocular pressure with long-term use than other ophthalmic anti-inflammatory drugs (except medrysone).
• Store in tightly covered, light-resistant container.
• Warn patient to call doctor immediately and to stop drug if visual acuity decreases or visual field diminishes.
• Shake well before using.
• Teach patient how to instill. Advise him to wash hands before and after administering ointment or solution, and warn him not to touch dropper or tip to eye or surrounding tissue. Apply light finger-pressure on lacrimal sac for 1 minute following instillation.
• Warn patient not to use leftover medication for a new eye inflammation; may cause serious problems.
• Tell patient not to share eye medications with family members. If a family member develops similar symptoms, instruct him to contact the doctor.

Italicized side effects are common or life-threatening.
*Liquid form contains alcohol.   **May contain tartrazine.

flurbiprofen sodium
Ocufen

Pregnancy Risk Category: C

MECHANISM OF ACTION
Constricts the iris sphincter, thereby inhibiting miosis. The mechanism is independent of cholinergic action.

INDICATIONS & DOSAGE
Inhibition of intraoperative miosis—
Adults: instill 1 drop approximately every ½ hour, beginning 2 hours before surgery. Give a total of 4 drops.

ADVERSE REACTIONS
Eye: transient burning and stinging upon instillation, ocular irritation.

INTERACTIONS
None reported.

NURSING CONSIDERATIONS
• Contraindicated in epithelial herpes simplex keratitis.
• This is an NSAID. Use cautiously in patients who may be allergic to aspirin and other NSAIDs.
• Use cautiously in patients with bleeding tendencies and those who are receiving medications that may prolong clotting times.
• Wound healing may be delayed.

medrysone
HMS Liquifilm Ophthalmic♦

Pregnancy Risk Category: C

MECHANISM OF ACTION
Decreases the infiltration of leukocytes at the site of inflammation.

INDICATIONS & DOSAGE
Allergic conjunctivitis, vernal conjunctivitis, episcleritis, ophthalmic epinephrine sensitivity reaction—
Adults and children: instill 1 drop in conjunctival sac b.i.d. to q.i.d. May use q hour during first 1 to 2 days if needed.

ADVERSE REACTIONS
Eye: thinning of cornea, interference with corneal wound healing, increased susceptibility to viral or fungal corneal infection, corneal ulceration; with excessive or long-term use, glaucoma exacerbations, cataracts, visual acuity and visual field defects, optic nerve damage.
Other: systemic effects and adrenal suppression with excessive or long-term use.

INTERACTIONS
None significant.

NURSING CONSIDERATIONS
• Contraindicated in vaccinia, varicella, acute superficial herpes simplex (dendritic keratitis), viral diseases of conjunctiva and cornea, ocular tuberculosis, fungal or viral eye diseases, iritis, uveitis, or any acute, purulent, untreated eye infection. Use cautiously in corneal abrasions since these may be contaminated (especially with herpes).
• Shake well before using. Don't freeze.
• Teach patient how to instill. Advise him to wash hands before and after applying ointment or solution, and warn him not to touch dropper or tip to eye or surrounding tissue. Apply light finger-pressure on lacrimal sac for 1 minute following instillation.
• Warn patient not to use leftover medication for a new eye inflammation; may cause serious problems.
• Tell patient not to share eye medications with family members. If a family member develops similar symptoms, instruct him to contact the doctor.

prednisolone acetate (suspension)
Econopred Ophthalmic,
Econopred Plus Ophthalmic, Pred-
Forte♦, Pred Mild Ophthalmic♦,
Predulose Ophthalmic

prednisolone sodium phosphate (solution)
Alto-Pred, Hydeltrasol Ophthalmic,
Inflamase Forte♦, Inflamase
Ophthalmic♦

Pregnancy Risk Category: C

MECHANISM OF ACTION
Decreases the infiltration of leukocytes at the site of inflammation.

INDICATIONS & DOSAGE
*Inflammation of palpebral and bulbar
conjunctiva, cornea, and anterior segment of globe—*
Adults and children: instill 1 to 2
drops in eye. In severe conditions,
may be used hourly, tapering to discontinuation as inflammation subsides. In mild conditions, may be used
up to 4 to 6 times daily.

ADVERSE REACTIONS
Eye: increased intraocular pressure;
thinning of cornea, interference with
corneal wound healing, increased susceptibility to viral or fungal corneal
infection, corneal ulceration; with excessive or long-term use, glaucoma
exacerbations, cataracts, visual acuity
and visual field defects, optic nerve
damage.
Other: systemic effects and adrenal
suppression with excessive or long-
term use.

INTERACTIONS
None significant.

NURSING CONSIDERATIONS
• Contraindicated in acute, untreated, purulent, ocular infections;
acute superficial herpes simplex (dendritic keratitis); vaccinia, varicella, or
other viral or fungal eye diseases; or
ocular tuberculosis. Use cautiously in
corneal abrasions since these may be
contaminated (especially with
herpes).
• Tell patient on long-term therapy to
have frequent tonometric examinations.
• Shake suspensions before using,
and store in tightly covered container.
• Teach patient how to instill. Advise
patient to wash hands before and after
applying ointment or solution, and
warn him not to touch dropper or tip
to eye or surrounding area. Apply
light finger-pressure on lacrimal sac
for 1 minute following instillation.
• Warn patient not to use leftover
medication for a new eye inflammation; may cause serious problems.
• Tell patient not to share eye medications with family members. If a family member develops similar symptoms, instruct him to contact the doctor.
• Check dosage before administering
to ensure using the correct strength.

Italicized side effects are common or life-threatening.
*Liquid form contains alcohol.   **May contain tartrazine.

82

Miotics

acetylcholine chloride
carbachol (intraocular)
carbachol (topical)
echothiophate iodide
pilocarpine hydrochloride
pilocarpine nitrate

COMBINATION PRODUCTS
E-PILO♦: epinephrine bitartrate 1%
and pilocarpine hydrochloride 1%,
2%, 3%, 4%, or 6%.
ISOPTO P-ES: pilocarpine hydrochloride 2% and physostigmine salicylate
0.25%.
P_1E_1, P_2E_1, P_3E_1, P_4E_1, P_6E_1: epinephrine bitartrate 1% and pilocarpine hydrochloride 1%, 2%, 3%, 4%, or 6%.

acetylcholine chloride
Miochol♦

Pregnancy Risk Category: C

MECHANISM OF ACTION
A cholinergic drug that causes contraction of the sphincter muscles of the iris, resulting in miosis. Also produces ciliary spasm, deepening of the anterior chamber, and vasodilation of conjunctival vessels of the outflow tract.

INDICATIONS & DOSAGE
Anterior segment surgery—
Adults and children: doctor instills 0.5 to 2 ml of 1% solution gently in anterior chamber of eye.

ADVERSE REACTIONS
None reported with 1% concentration. Iris atrophy possible with higher concentrations.

INTERACTIONS
None significant.

NURSING CONSIDERATIONS
• Reconstitute immediately before using.
• Shake vial gently until clear solution is obtained.
• Discard any unused solution.
• Complete miosis within seconds.
• Don't gas-sterilize vial. Ethylene oxide may produce formic acid.

carbachol (intraocular)
Miostat♦

carbachol (topical)
Carbacel, Isopto Carbachol♦

Pregnancy Risk Category: C

MECHANISM OF ACTION
A cholinergic drug that causes contraction of the sphincter muscles of the iris, resulting in miosis. Also produces ciliary spasm, deepening of the anterior chamber, and vasodilation of conjunctival vessels of the outflow tract.

INDICATIONS & DOSAGE
Ocular surgery (to produce pupillary miosis)—
Adults: doctor gently instills 0.5 ml (intraocular form) into the anterior chamber for production of satisfactory miosis. It may be instilled before or after securing sutures.
Open-angle glaucoma—

Adults: instill 1 drop (topical form) into eye daily, b.i.d., t.i.d., or q.i.d.

ADVERSE REACTIONS
CNS: headache.
Eye: accommodative spasm, blurred vision, conjunctival vasodilation, eye and brow pain.
GI: abdominal cramps, diarrhea.
Other: sweating, flushing, asthma.

INTERACTIONS
None significant.

NURSING CONSIDERATIONS
• Contraindicated in acute iritis, corneal abrasion. Use cautiously in acute heart failure, bronchial asthma, peptic ulcer, hyperthyroidism, GI spasm, urinary tract obstruction, Parkinson's disease.
• Used in open-angle glaucoma, especially when patient is resistant or allergic to pilocarpine HCl or nitrate.
• Teach patient how to instill. Advise him to wash hands before and after administering ointment or solution, and to apply light finger-pressure on lacrimal sac for 1 minute after drops are instilled. Warn him not to exceed recommended dosage.
• For single-dose intraocular use only. Premixed; discard unused portions.
• Tell glaucoma patient that long-term use may be necessary. Stress compliance. Tell him to remain under medical supervision for periodic tonometric readings.
• In case of toxicity, atropine should be given parenterally.
• Caution patient not to drive for 1 or 2 hours after administration until effect on vision is determined.
• Reassure patient that blurred vision usually diminishes with prolonged use.

echothiophate iodide
Phospholine Iodide♦

Pregnancy Risk Category: C

MECHANISM OF ACTION
An anticholinesterase drug that inhibits the enzymatic destruction of acetylcholine by inactivating cholinesterase. This leaves acetylcholine free to act on the effector cells of the iridic sphincter and ciliary muscles, causing pupillary constriction and accommodation spasm.

INDICATIONS & DOSAGE
Primary open-angle glaucoma, conditions obstructing aqueous outflow, accommodative esotropia—
Adults and children: instill 1 drop 0.03% to 0.125% solution into conjunctival sac daily. Maximum 1 drop b.i.d. Use lowest possible dosage to continuously control intraocular pressure.

ADVERSE REACTIONS
CNS: fatigue, muscle weakness, paresthesias, headache.
CV: bradycardia, hypotension.
Eye: ciliary or accommodative spasm, ciliary or conjunctival injection, nonreversible cataract formation (time- and dose-related), reversible iris cysts, pupillary block, blurred or dimmed vision, eye or brow pain, lid twitching, hyperemia, photosensitivity, lens opacities, lacrimation, retinal detachment.
GI: diarrhea, nausea, vomiting, abdominal pain, intestinal cramps, salivation.
GU: frequent urination.
Other: flushing, sweating, bronchial constriction.

INTERACTIONS
Organophosphorus insecticides (parathion, malathion): may have an additive effect that could cause systemic effects. Warn patient exposed to

---

Italicized side effects are common or life-threatening.
*Liquid form contains alcohol.   **May contain tartrazine.

insecticides of this danger.
Succinylcholine: respiratory and cardiovascular collapse. Don't use together.
Systemic anticholinesterase for myasthenia gravis: effects may be additive. Monitor patient for signs of toxicity.

NURSING CONSIDERATIONS
• Contraindicated in narrow-angle glaucoma, epilepsy, vasomotor instability, parkinsonism, iodide hypersensitivity, active uveal inflammation, bronchial asthma spastic GI conditions, urinary tract obstruction, peptic ulcer, severe bradycardia or hypotension, vascular hypertension, myocardial infarction, history of retinal detachment. Use cautiously in patients routinely exposed to organophosphorus insecticides. May cause nausea, vomiting, and diarrhea, progressing to muscle weakness and respiratory difficulty. Use cautiously in patients with myasthenia gravis receiving anticholinesterase therapy.
• Toxicity is cumulative. Toxic systemic symptoms don't appear for weeks or months after initiating therapy.
• Reconstitute powder carefully to avoid contamination. Use only diluent provided. Discard refrigerated, reconstituted solution after 6 months; discard solution at room temperature after 1 month.
• Warn patient that transient brow pain or dimmed or blurred vision is common at first but usually disappears within 5 to 10 days.
• Instill at bedtime since drug causes transient blurred vision.
• Tell patient to remain under constant medical supervision. Warn him not to exceed recommended dosage.
• Report salivation, diarrhea, profuse sweating, urinary incontinence, or muscle weakness.
• Stop drug at least 2 weeks preoperatively if succinylcholine is to be used in surgery.

• Atropine sulfate (subcutaneous, I.M., or I.V.) is antidote of choice.
• A potent, long-acting, irreversible drug.
• Teach patient how to instill. Advise him to wash hands before and after administering ointment or solution, and to apply light finger-pressure on lacrimal sac for 1 minute following instillation. Warn him not to touch tip of dropper to eye or surrounding tissue.

---

pilocarpine hydrochloride
Adsorbocarpine, Isopto Carpine♦, Miocarpine♦♦, Ocusert Pilo♦, Pilocar, Pilocel, Pilomiotin♦, Pilopine HS

pilocarpine nitrate
P.V. Carpine Liquifilm♦
Pregnancy Risk Category: C

MECHANISM OF ACTION
A cholinergic drug that causes contraction of the sphincter muscles of the iris, resulting in miosis. Also produces ciliary spasm, deepening of the anterior chamber, and vasodilation of conjunctival vessels of the outflow tract.

INDICATIONS & DOSAGE
Primary open-angle glaucoma—
Adults and children: instill 1 to 2 drops in eye daily b.i.d., t.i.d., q.i.d., or as directed by doctor. Or, may apply ointment (Pilopine HS) once daily.
   Alternatively, apply one Ocusert Pilo system (20 or 40 mcg/hour) every 7 days.
Emergency treatment of acute narrow-angle glaucoma—
Adults and children: 1 drop of a 2% solution every 5 minutes for three to six doses, followed by 1 drop every 1 to 3 hours until pressure is controlled.

ADVERSE REACTIONS
Eye: suborbital headache, *myopia,* ciliary spasm, *blurred vision,* conjunctival irritation, lacrimation, changes in visual field, *brow pain.*
GI: nausea, vomiting, abdominal cramps, diarrhea, salivation.
Other: bronchiolar spasm, pulmonary edema, hypersensitivity.

INTERACTIONS
Carbachol, echothiophate: additive effect. Don't use together.
Phenylephrine HCl: decreased dilation by phenylephrine HCl. Don't use together.

NURSING CONSIDERATIONS
• Contraindicated in acute iritis, acute inflammatory disease of anterior segment of eye, secondary glaucoma. Use cautiously in bronchial asthma and hypertension.
• Warn patient that vision will be temporarily blurred. Warn patient to avoid hazardous activities until this effect subsides.
• Transient brow pain and myopia are common at first; usually disappear in 10 to 14 days.
• Teach patient how to instill. Advise him to wash hands before and after administering ointment or solution, and to apply light finger-pressure on lacrimal sac for 1 minute following instillation of drops. Warn him not to touch dropper to eye or surrounding tissue.
• Widely used drug to treat primary open-angle glaucoma.
• Used to counteract effects of mydriatics and cycloplegics after surgery or ophthalmoscopic examination.
• May be used alternately with atropine to break adhesions.
• In acute narrow-angle glaucoma before surgery, may be used alone or with mannitol, urea, glycerol, or acetazolamide.
• If the Ocusert Pilo system falls out of the eye during sleep, patient should wash hands, rinse the system in cool tap water, and reposition it in the eye. Tell patient not to use it if deformed.
• If the ointment is prescribed, instruct patient to apply at bedtime, as it will blur vision.

Italicized side effects are common or life-threatening.
*Liquid form contains alcohol.   **May contain tartrazine.

83

Mydriatics

atropine sulfate
cyclopentolate hydrochloride
epinephrine bitartrate
epinephrine hydrochloride
epinephryl borate
homatropine hydrobromide
phenylephrine hydrochloride
scopolamine hydrobromide
tropicamide

COMBINATION PRODUCTS

CYCLOMYDRIL OPHTHALMIC: cyclopertolate HCl 0.2% and phenylephrine HCl 1%.
MUROCOLL-2: scopolamine HBr 0.3% and phenylephrine HCl 10%.

---

atropine sulfate
Atropisol, BufOpto Atropine, Isopto Atropine♦

Pregnancy Risk Category: C

MECHANISM OF ACTION
Anticholinergic action leaves the pupil under unopposed adrenergic influence, causing it to dilate.

INDICATIONS & DOSAGE
Acute iris inflammation (iritis)—
Adults: 1 to 2 drops of 1% solution or small amount of ointment b.i.d. to t.i.d.
Children: instill 1 to 2 drops of 0.5% solution daily b.i.d. or t.i.d.
Cycloplegic refraction—
Adults: instill 1 to 2 drops of 1% solution 1 hour before refracting.
Children: instill 1 to 2 drops of 0.5% solution to each eye b.i.d. for 1 to 3 days before eye examination and 1 hour before refraction, or instill small amount of ointment daily or b.i.d. 2 to 3 days before examination.

ADVERSE REACTIONS
Eye: ocular congestion in long-term use, conjunctivitis, contact dermatitis, edema, *blurred vision,* eye dryness, *photophobia.*
Systemic: flushing, dry skin and mouth, fever, tachycardia, abdominal distention in infants, ataxia, irritability, confusion, somnolence.

INTERACTIONS
None significant.

NURSING CONSIDERATIONS
• Contraindicated in angle closure glaucoma (narrow-angle). Use cautiously in infants, children, and elderly or debilitated patients.
• Warn patient vision will be temporarily blurred. Dark glasses ease discomfort of photophobia.
• Not for internal use. Treat drops and ointment as poison. Keep physostigmine available as antidote for poisoning. Signs of poisoning are disorientation and confusion.
• Watch for signs of glaucoma: increased intraocular pressure, ocular pain, headache, progressive blurring of vision.
• Most potent mydriatic and cycloplegic available; long duration.
• Systemic adverse reactions most commonly occur in children and elderly patients.
• Warn patient to avoid hazardous activities such as operating machinery

---

or driving a car until the temporary visual impairment caused by this drug wears off.
• Teach patient how to instill. Advise him to wash hands before and after administering solution, and to apply light finger-pressure on lacrimal sac for 1 minute following instillation. Warn patient not to touch dropper or tip of tube to eye or surrounding tissue.
• Advise patient to use sugarless hard candy or gum if dry mouth is a problem.

cyclopentolate hydrochloride
AK-Pentolate, Cyclogyl♦
Pregnancy Risk Category: C

MECHANISM OF ACTION
Anticholinergic action leaves the pupil under unopposed adrenergic influence, causing it to dilate.

INDICATIONS & DOSAGE
Diagnostic procedures requiring mydriasis and cycloplegia—
Adults: instill 1 drop 1% solution in eye, followed by 1 more drop in 5 minutes. Use 2% solution in heavily pigmented irises.
Children: instill 1 drop of 0.5%, 1%, or 2% solution in each eye, followed in 5 minutes with 1 drop 0.5% or 1% solution, if necessary.

ADVERSE REACTIONS
Eye: burning sensation on instillation, blurred vision, eye dryness, *photophobia,* ocular congestion, contact dermatitis, conjunctivitis.
Systemic: flushing, tachycardia, urine retention, dry skin, fever, ataxia, irritability, confusion, somnolence, hallucinations, seizures, behavioral disturbances in children.

INTERACTIONS
None significant.

NURSING CONSIDERATIONS
• Contraindicated in narrow-angle glaucoma. Use cautiously in elderly patients.
• Potent drug with mydriatic and cycloplegic effect; superior to homatropine hydrobromide and has shorter duration of action.
• Instruct patient to wear dark glasses to ease discomfort of photophobia.
• Warn patient drug will burn when instilled.
• Warn patient to avoid hazardous activities such as operating machinery or driving until the temporary visual impairment caused by this drug subsides.
• Teach patient how to instill. Advise him to wash hands before and after administering, and to apply light finger-pressure on lacrimal sac for 1 minute following instillation. Warn patient not to touch tip of dropper to eye or surrounding tissue.

epinephrine bitartrate
Epitrate♦, Mytrate

epinephrine hydrochloride
Epifrin♦, Glaucon♦

epinephryl borate
Epinal♦, Eppy/N♦
Pregnancy Risk Category: C

MECHANISM OF ACTION
An adrenergic that dilates the pupil by contracting the dilator muscle.

INDICATIONS & DOSAGE
Open-angle glaucoma—
Adults: instill 1 to 2 drops of 1% or 2% bitartrate solution in eye with frequency determined by tonometric readings (once q 2 to 4 days up to q.i.d.), or instill 1 drop 0.5%, 1%, or 2% HCl solution (or 0.5% or 1% epinephryl borate solution) in eye b.i.d.
During surgery—
Adults: 1 or more drops of 0.1% epi-

nephrine HCl up to 3 times.

ADVERSE REACTIONS
Eye: corneal or conjunctival pigmentation or corneal edema in long-term use; follicular hypertrophy; chemosis; conjunctivitis; iritis; hyperemic conjunctiva; maculopapular rash; severe stinging, burning, and tearing upon instillation; browache.
Systemic: palpitations, tachycardia.

INTERACTIONS
Cyclopropane or halogenated hydrocarbons: dysrhythmias, tachycardia. Use together cautiously, if at all.
Tricyclic antidepressants, antihistamines (diphenhydramine, dexchlorpheniramine): potentiated cardiac effects of epinephrine.

NURSING CONSIDERATIONS
• Contraindicated in shallow anterior chamber or narrow-angle glaucoma.
• Use cautiously in diabetes mellitus, hypertension, Parkinson's disease, hyperthyroidism, aphakia (eye without lens), cardiac disease, or cerebral arteriosclerosis; in elderly patients or pregnant women.
• May stain soft contact lenses.
• Use with pilocarpine: additive effect in lowering intraocular pressure.
• Monitor blood pressure and other systemic effects.
• Don't use darkened solution.
• Also used during surgery to control local bleeding, or injected into the anterior chamber to produce rapid mydriasis during cataract removal.
• Teach patient how to instill. Advise him to wash hands before and after administering and to apply light finger-pressure on lacrimal sac for 1 minute following instillation. Warn patient not to touch dropper to eye or surrounding tissue.
• Epinephrine salts are not interchangeable. Don't substitute one salt if another one is ordered.

homatropine hydrobromide
Homatrine, Homatropine♦, Isopto
Pregnancy Risk Category: C

MECHANISM OF ACTION
Anticholinergic action leaves the pupil under unopposed adrenergic influence, causing it to dilate.

INDICATIONS & DOSAGE
Cycloplegic refraction—
Adults and children: instill 1 to 2 drops 2% or 5% solution in eye; repeat in 5 to 10 minutes.
Uveitis—
Adults and children: instill 1 to 2 drops 2% or 5% solution in eye up to every 3 to 4 hours.

ADVERSE REACTIONS
Eye: irritation, *blurred vision, photophobia.*
Systemic: flushing, dry skin and mouth, fever, tachycardia, ataxia, irritability, confusion, somnolence.

INTERACTIONS
None significant.

NURSING CONSIDERATIONS
• Contraindicated in angle closure glaucoma (narrow-angle). Use cautiously in infants, elderly or debilitated patients; patients with cardiac disease; or patients with increased intraocular pressure.
• Patients who are hypersensitive to atropine will also be hypersensitive to homatropine.
• Warn patient that vision will be temporarily blurred after instillation. Tell patient to avoid hazardous activities such as operating machinery or driving a car until blurring subsides. Patient should wear dark glasses to ease discomfort of photophobia.
• May produce symptoms of atropine SO_4 poisoning, such as severe dryness of mouth, tachycardia.
• Not for internal use. Treat as poi-

son. Keep physostigmine available as antidote for poisoning.

• Teach patient how to instill. Advise him to wash hands before and after administering and to apply light finger-pressure on lacrimal sac for 1 minute following instillation. Warn patient not to touch dropper tip to eye or surrounding tissue.

• Similar to atropine SO_4 but weaker, with a shorter duration of action.

• Advise patient to use sugarless hard candy or gum if dry mouth is a problem.

---

phenylephrine hydrochloride
Mydfrin♦, Neo-Synephrine♦

Pregnancy Risk Category: C

MECHANISM OF ACTION
An adrenergic that dilates the pupil by contracting the dilator muscle of the pupil.

INDICATIONS & DOSAGE
Mydriasis (without cycloplegia)—
Adults and children: instill 1 drop 2.5% or 10% solution in eye before examination.
Posterior synechia (adhesion of iris)—
Adults and children: instill 1 drop 10% solution in eye.

Do not use 10% concentration in infants; use cautiously in elderly patients.

ADVERSE REACTIONS
CNS: headache, browache.
CV: *hypertension* (with 10% solution), tachycardia, palpitations, premature ventricular contractions.
Eye: transient burning or stinging on instillation, blurred vision, reactive hyperemia, allergic conjunctivitis, iris floaters, narrow-angle glaucoma, rebound miosis, dermatitis.
Other: pallor, trembling, sweating.

INTERACTIONS
Guanethidine: increased mydriatic and pressor effects of phenylephrine HCl. Use together cautiously.
Levodopa (systemic): reduced mydriatic effect of phenylephrine HCl. Use together cautiously.
MAO inhibitors and beta blockers: may cause dysrhythmias due to increased pressor effect. Use together cautiously.
Tricyclic antidepressants: potentiated cardiac effects of epinephrine. Use together cautiously.

NURSING CONSIDERATIONS
• Contraindicated in narrow-angle glaucoma, soft contact lens use. Avoid 10% solution and use cautiously in marked hypertension, cardiac disorders, and in children of low body weight.

• Should be avoided in patients with idiopathic orthostatic hypotension. May produce high blood pressure.

• Protect from light and heat.

• Warn patient not to exceed recommended dosage. Systemic effects can result. Monitor blood pressure and pulse rate.

• Potential for systemic adverse reactions less severe with 2.5% solution. Adverse reactions and toxicity much more likely with 10% solution.

• Teach patient how to instill. Advise him to wash hands before and after administering and to apply light finger-pressure on lacrimal sac for 1 minute following instillation. Warn patient not to touch dropper tip to eye or surrounding tissue.

• May cause blurred vision. Warn patient to avoid driving a car or operating machinery until this effect subsides.

Italicized side effects are common or life-threatening.
*Liquid form contains alcohol.   **May contain tartrazine.

scopolamine hydrobromide
Isopto Hyoscine

Pregnancy Risk Category: C

MECHANISM OF ACTION
Anticholinergic action leaves the pupil under unopposed adrenergic influence, causing it to dilate.

INDICATIONS & DOSAGE
Cycloplegic refraction—
Adults: instill 1 to 2 drops 0.25% solution in eye 1 hour before refraction.
Children: instill 1 drop 0.25% solution or ointment b.i.d. for 2 days before refraction.
Iritis, uveitis—
Adults: 1 to 2 drops of 0.25% solution daily b.i.d. or t.i.d.

ADVERSE REACTIONS
Eye: ocular congestion with prolonged use, conjunctivitis, *blurred vision,* eye dryness, increased intraocular pressure, *photophobia,* contact dermatitis.
Systemic: flushing, fever, dry skin and mouth, tachycardia, hallucinations, ataxia, irritability, confusion, delirium, somnolence, acute psychotic reactions.

INTERACTIONS
None significant.

NURSING CONSIDERATIONS
• Contraindicated in angle closure glaucoma (shallow anterior chamber or narrow-angle). Use cautiously in cardiac disease, increased intraocular pressure, and in elderly patients.
• Observe patient closely for systemic effects (disorientation, delirium).
• Warn patient that vision will be temporarily blurred; tell patient to avoid hazardous activities such as driving or operating machinery until this effect subsides.
• Instruct patient to wear dark glasses to ease discomfort of photophobia.

• May be used when patient is sensitive to atropine. Faster acting and has shorter duration of action and fewer adverse effects.
• Teach patient how to instill. Advise him to wash hands before and after administering and to apply light finger-pressure on lacrimal sac for 1 minute following instillation. Warn him not to touch dropper tip to eye or surrounding tissue.

tropicamide
Mydriacyl♦

Pregnancy Risk Category: C

MECHANISM OF ACTION
Anticholinergic action leaves the pupil under unopposed adrenergic influence, causing it to dilate.

INDICATIONS & DOSAGE
Adults and children:
Cycloplegic refractions—
instill 1 to 2 drops of 1% solution in each eye; repeat in 5 minutes. Additional drop may be instilled in 20 to 30 minutes.
Fundus examinations—
instill 1 to 2 drops 0.5% solution in each eye 15 to 20 minutes before examination.

ADVERSE REACTIONS
Eye: *transient stinging on instillation,* increased intraocular pressure (less than with other mydriatic agents because of shorter duration of action), *blurred vision, photophobia.*
Systemic: flushing, fever, dry skin, dry mouth and throat, ataxia, irritability, confusion, somnolence, hallucinations, behavioral disturbances in children.

INTERACTIONS
None significant.

NURSING CONSIDERATIONS
• Contraindicated in narrow-angle

and shallow anterior chamber glaucoma. Use cautiously in elderly patients.

• Shortest acting cycloplegic, but mydriatic effect greater than cycloplegic effect.

• Causes transient stinging; vision temporarily blurred. Warn patient to avoid driving and other hazardous activities that require good vision.

• Instruct patient to wear dark glasses if photophobia occurs (lasts about 2 hours).

• Teach patient how to instill. Advise him to wash hands before and after administering and to apply light finger-pressure on lacrimal sac for 1 minute following instillation. Warn him not to touch dropper to eye or surrounding tissue.

84

Ophthalmic vasoconstrictors

naphazoline hydrochloride
  0.012%, 0.02%, 0.1%◊
phenylephrine hydrochloride
  0.12%, 2.5%, 10%◊
tetrahydrozoline hydrochloride
  (0.05%)◊
zinc sulfate◊

COMBINATION PRODUCTS
ALBALON-A LIQUIFILM♦: naphazoline hydrochloride 0.05% and antazoline phosphate 0.5%.
BLEPHAMIDE LIQUIFILM SUSPENSION♦: phenylephrine hydrochloride 0.12%, sulfacetamide sodium 10%, and prednisolone acetate 0.2%.
EDTA, 1.4% polyvinyl alcohol, polysorbate 80, sodium thiosulfate, and benzalkonium chloride.
PHENYLZIN◊: zinc sulfate 0.25% and phenylephrine hydrochloride 0.12%.
PREFRIN-A♦: phenylephrine hydrochloride 0.12%, pyrilamine maleate 0.1%, and antipyrine 0.1%.
VASOCIDIN OPHTHALMIC OINTMENT♦: phenylephrine HCl 0.125%, sodium sulfacetamide 10%, and prednisolone acetate 0.5%.
VASOCIDIN OPHTHALMIC SOLUTION♦: phenylephrine HCl 0.125%, sodium sulfacetamide 10%, and prednisolone sodium phosphate 0.25%.
VASOCON-A OPHTHALMIC SOLUTION♦: naphazoline hydrochloride 0.05% and antazoline phosphate 0.5%.
ZINCFRIN♦◊: phenylephrine hydrochloride 0.12% and zinc sulfate 0.25%.

naphazoline hydrochloride
0.012%, 0.02%, 0.1%◊
AK-Con, Albalon Liquifilm♦, Clear Eyes, Naphcon, Naphcon Forte♦, Vasoclear, Vasocon Regular♦

Pregnancy Risk Category: C

MECHANISM OF ACTION
Produces vasoconstriction by local adrenergic action on the blood vessels of the conjunctiva.

INDICATIONS & DOSAGE
Ocular congestion, irritation, itching—
Adults: instill 1 to 2 drops in eye q 3 to 4 hours.

ADVERSE REACTIONS
Eye: transient stinging, pupillary dilation, irritation.

INTERACTIONS
MAO inhibitors: hypertensive crisis if naphazoline HCl is systemically absorbed. Use together cautiously.

NURSING CONSIDERATIONS
• Contraindicated in narrow-angle glaucoma, hypersensitivity to any ingredients. Use cautiously in patients with hyperthyroidism, cardiac disease, hypertension, and diabetes mellitus, and in elderly patients.
• Can produce marked sedation and coma if ingested by child.
• Advise patient that photophobia may follow pupil dilation if he is sensitive to drug. Tell patient to report this to the doctor if it occurs.

Unmarked trade names available in the United States only.
♦Also available in Canada.   ♦♦Available in Canada only.   ◊Also available OTC.

- Warn patient not to exceed recommended dosage. Rebound congestion and conjunctivitis may occur with frequent or prolonged use.
- Notify doctor if blurred vision, pain, or lid edema develops.
- Store in tightly closed container.
- Most widely used ocular decongestant.
- Teach patient how to instill. Advise him to wash hands before and after administering, and to apply light finger-pressure on lacrimal sac for 1 minute after instillation. Warn him not to touch tip of dropper to eye or surrounding tissues.

phenylephrine hydrochloride 0.12%, 2.5%, 10%◊
AK-Dilate, Isopto Frin, Prefrin Liquifilm♦

Pregnancy Risk Category: C

MECHANISM OF ACTION
Produces vasoconstriction by local adrenergic action on the blood vessels of the conjunctiva.

INDICATIONS & DOSAGE
Decongestant, minor eye irritations—
Adults and children: 2 drops of 0.12% in affected eye. May repeat in 3 to 4 hours, p.r.n.

ADVERSE REACTIONS
CNS: headache.
Eye: transient stinging, iris floaters, narrow-angle glaucoma, blurred vision, reactive hyperemia, browache.

INTERACTIONS
MAO inhibitors: may cause hypertensive crisis. Don't use together.

NURSING CONSIDERATIONS
- Contraindicated in narrow-angle glaucoma, in patients taking tricyclic antidepressants or MAO inhibitors, and in patients with hypersensitivity to any ingredient.
- May exacerbate hypertension in hypertensive patients.
- Do not use butacaine drops as local anesthetic, since phenylephrine and butacaine are incompatible.
- Do not exceed prescribed dose.
- Monitor blood pressure and pulse rate; watch for overdosage.
- Do not use if solution is dark brown or contains precipitate.
- Keep container tightly sealed and away from light.
- Teach patient how to instill. Advise him to wash hands before and after administering, and to apply light finger-pressure on lacrimal sac for 1 minute after installation. Warn him not to touch tip of dropper to eye or surrounding tissues.
- Caution patient not to share eye medications with others.

tetrahydrozoline hydrochloride (0.05%)◊
Murine Plus, Optigene, Soothe, Tetrasine, Visine

Pregnancy Risk Category: C

MECHANISM OF ACTION
Produces vasoconstriction by local adrenergic action on the blood vessels of the conjunctiva.

INDICATIONS & DOSAGE
Ocular congestion, irritation, and allergic conditions—
Adults and children over 2 years: instill 1 to 2 drops in eye b.i.d. or t.i.d., or as directed by doctor.

ADVERSE REACTIONS
Eye: transient stinging, pupillary dilation, increased intraocular pressure, irritation, iris floaters in elderly.
Systemic: drowsiness, CNS depression, cardiac irregularities, headache, dizziness, tremors, insomnia.

Italicized side effects are common or life-threatening.
*Liquid form contains alcohol.   **May contain tartrazine.

INTERACTIONS
MAO inhibitors: hypertensive crisis if tetrahydrozoline HCl is systemically absorbed. Don't use together.

NURSING CONSIDERATIONS
• Contraindicated in patients receiving MAO inhibitors, and in those with hypersensitivity to any ingredients or narrow-angle glaucoma. Use cautiously in patients with hyperthyroidism, heart disease, hypertension, and diabetes mellitus and in the elderly.
• Do not exceed recommended dosage. Rebound congestion may occur with frequent or prolonged use.
• Warn patient to stop drug and notify doctor if relief is not obtained within 48 hours, or if redness or irritation persists or increases.
• Available without prescription.
• Teach patient how to instill. Advise him to wash hands before and after administering, and to apply light finger-pressure on lacrimal sac for 1 minute after instillation. Warn patient not to touch dropper tip to eye or surrounding tissues.
• Caution patient not to share eye medications with others.

zinc sulfate◊
Bufopto Zinc Sulfate, Eye-Sed Ophthalmic, Op-Thal-Zin

Pregnancy Risk Category: C

MECHANISM OF ACTION
Produces astringent action on the conjunctiva.

INDICATIONS & DOSAGE
Ocular congestion, irritation—
Adults and children: solution 0.2%—instill 1 to 2 drops in eye b.i.d. or t.i.d.

ADVERSE REACTIONS
Eye: irritation.

INTERACTIONS
None significant.

NURSING CONSIDERATIONS
• Use cautiously in patients with a shallow anterior chamber, predisposition to narrow-angle glaucoma.
• A decongestant astringent.
• Store in tightly closed container.
• Teach patient how to instill. Advise him to wash hands before and after administering, and to apply light finger-pressure on lacrimal sac for 1 minute after instillation. Warn patient not to touch dropper tip to eye or surrounding tissues.

85

Topical ophthalmic anesthetics

proparacaine hydrochloride
tetracaine hydrochloride

COMBINATION PRODUCTS
None.

proparacaine hydrochloride
Alcaine♦, Ophthaine♦, Ophthetic♦

Pregnancy Risk Category: C

MECHANISM OF ACTION
Produces anesthesia by preventing initiation and transmission of impulses at the nerve-cell membrane.

INDICATIONS & DOSAGE
Anesthesia for tonometry, gonioscopy; suture removal from cornea, removal of corneal foreign bodies—
Adults and children: instill 1 to 2 drops 0.5% solution in eye just before procedure.
Anesthesia for cataract extraction, glaucoma surgery—
Adults and children: instill 1 drop 0.5% solution in eye every 5 to 10 minutes for 5 to 7 doses.

ADVERSE REACTIONS
Eye: occasional conjunctival redness, transient pain.
Other: hypersensitivity.

INTERACTIONS
None significant.

NURSING CONSIDERATIONS
• Use cautiously in patients with cardiac disease and hyperthyroidism.
• *Not* for long-term use; may delay wound healing.
• Warn patient not to rub or touch eye while cornea is anesthetized, since this may cause corneal abrasion and greater discomfort when anesthesia wears off.
• Protective eyepatch recommended following procedure.
• Warn patient that corneal pain is relieved only temporarily in abrasion.
• Systemic reactions unlikely when used in recommended doses.
• Topical ophthalmic anesthetic of choice in diagnostic and minor surgical procedures.
• Don't use discolored solution.
• Store in tightly closed container.
• Ophthaine brand packaged in bottle that looks similar in size and shape to Hemoccult. When taking bottle from shelf, check label carefully.

tetracaine hydrochloride
Anacel, Pontocaine♦

Pregnancy Risk Category: C

MECHANISM OF ACTION
Produces anesthesia by preventing initiation and transmission of impulses at the nerve-cell membrane.

INDICATIONS & DOSAGE
Anesthesia for tonometry, gonioscopy; removal of corneal foreign bodies, suture removal from cornea; other diagnostic and minor surgical procedures—
Adults and children: instill 1 to 2 drops 0.5% solution in eye just before procedure.

Italicized side effects are common or life-threatening.
*Liquid form contains alcohol.   **May contain tartrazine.

ADVERSE REACTIONS

Eye: transient stinging in eye 30 seconds after initial instillation, epithelial damage in excessive or long-term use.

Other: sensitization in repeated use (allergic skin rash, urticaria).

INTERACTIONS

Sulfonamides: interference with sulfonamide antibacterial activity. Wait ½ hour after anesthesia before instilling sulfonamide.

NURSING CONSIDERATIONS

• Systemic absorption unlikely in recommended doses.
• Avoid repeated use.
• Does not dilate the pupil, paralyze accommodation, or increase intraocular pressure.
• Protective eyepatch recommended following procedure.
• Don't use discolored solution. Keep container tightly closed.
• Warn patient not to touch or rub the eye while the cornea is anesthetized. This may cause corneal abrasion and greater discomfort when the anesthetic wears off.

Artificial tears

artificial tears◇
eye irrigation solutions◇

COMBINATION PRODUCTS
None.

artificial tears◇
Adsorbotear♦, Hypotears, Isopto
Alkaline, Isopto Plain, Isopto
Tears♦, Lacril♦, Lacrisert, Liquifilm
Forte, Liquifilm Tears, Lyteers,
Methulose, Neo-Tears, Tearisol,
Tears Naturale♦, Tears Plus, Ultra
Tears, Visculose

Pregnancy Risk Category: C

MECHANISM OF ACTION
Augments insufficient tear production.

INDICATIONS & DOSAGE
Insufficient tear production—
Adults and children: instill 1 to 2
drops in eye t.i.d., q.i.d., or p.r.n.
*Moderate to severe dry eye syndromes,
including keratoconjunctivitis sicca—*
Adults: insert 1 Lacrisert rod daily
into inferior cul-de-sac. Some patients may require twice daily use.

ADVERSE REACTIONS
Eye: discomfort; burning, pain on instillation; blurred vision (especially
with Lacrisert); crust formation on
eyelids and eyelashes in products with
high viscosity, such as Adsorbotear,
Isopto Tears, and Tearisol.

INTERACTIONS
Borate external irrigation solutions:

may form gummy deposits on the lid
when used with artificial tear products containing polyvinyl alcohol (Liquifilm Forte, Liquifilm Tears). Keep
patient's eyelids clean.

NURSING CONSIDERATIONS
• Contraindicated in patients with hypersensitivity to active product or preservatives.
• Teach patient how to instill. Warn
him not to touch dropper to eye or surrounding tissue. Advise him to wash
hands before and after administration.
• To avoid contamination of solution,
warn patient not to touch tip of container to eye, surrounding tissue, or
other surface.
• Instruct patient that product should
be used by one person only.
• Lacrisert rod should be inserted
with special applicator that is included in the package. Familiarize patient with illustrated instructions that
are also included.

eye irrigation solutions◇
Blinx, Collyrium♦, Dacriose, Eye-
Stream, I-Lite Eye Drops, Lauro Eye
Wash, Lavoptik Eye Wash, Murine
Eye Drops, Neo-Flo, Sterile Normal
Saline (0.9%)

MECHANISM OF ACTION
Cleans the eye.

INDICATIONS & DOSAGE
Eye irrigation—
Adults and children: flush eye with 1
to 2 drops t.i.d., q.i.d., or p.r.n.

Italicized side effects are common or life-threatening.
*Liquid form contains alcohol.   **May contain tartrazine.

ADVERSE REACTIONS
None reported.

INTERACTIONS
Products containing polyvinyl alcohol: may form gel and gummy deposits on the eye. Keep eyelids clean.

NURSING CONSIDERATIONS
• Contraindicated in patients with hypersensitivity to active ingredient or preservatives.
• To avoid contamination, don't touch tip of container to eye, surrounding tissue, or other surface.
• Check date of expiration to make sure solution is potent.
• Store in tightly closed, light-resistant container.
• Teach patient how to instill. Advise him to wash hands before and after administration.
• Should be used by one person only.
• When irrigating, have patient turn his head to side and irrigate from inner to outer canthus. Have tissues handy.

87

Miscellaneous ophthalmics

apraclonidine hydrochloride
betaxolol hydrochloride
cromolyn sodium
dipivefrin 0.1%
fluorescein sodium
glycerin, anhydrous
isosorbide
levobunolol hydrochloride
sodium chloride, hypertonic
timolol maleate

COMBINATION PRODUCTS
FLURESS: sodium fluorescein 0.25%
and benoxinate HCl 0.4%.

---

apraclonidine hydrochloride
Iopidine

Pregnancy Risk Category: C

MECHANISM OF ACTION
An alpha-adrenergic agonist that reduces intraocular pressure, possibly
by decreasing production of aqueous
humor.

INDICATIONS & DOSAGE
Prevention or control of intraocular
pressure elevations after argon laser
trabeculoplasty or iridotomy—
Adults: instill 1 drop in the eye 1 hour
before initiation of laser surgery on
the anterior segment, followed by 1
drop immediately after completion of
surgery.

ADVERSE REACTIONS
CNS: insomnia, irritability, dream
disturbances, headache.
CV: bradycardia, vasovagal attack,

palpitations, hypotension, orthostatic
hypotension.
EENT: upper eyelid elevation, conjunctival blanching, mydriasis, burning, discomfort, foreign body sensation, eye dryness and itching, blurred
vision, allergic response, conjunctival
microhemorrhage, taste disturbances,
dry mouth, nasal burning or dryness,
increased pharyngeal secretions.
GI: abdominal pain, discomfort,
diarrhea, vomiting.
Skin: pruritus not associated with
rash.
Other: sweaty palms, body heat sensation, decreased libido, extremity
pain or numbness.

INTERACTIONS
None reported.

NURSING CONSIDERATIONS
• Contraindicated in patients with hypersensitivity to apraclonidine or
clonidine.
• Patients who tend to develop exaggerated decreases in intraocular pressure after drug therapy should be
monitored closely.
• Onset of action is usually less than
1 hour, and drug effects usually peak
within 4 to 5 hours.
• Systemic effects of the drug (altered
heart rate and blood pressure) are uncommon after usual dose, but patients
with severe systemic disease, including hypertension, should be monitored closely.
• Observe patient closely for vasovagal attack during laser surgery.

Italicized side effects are common or life-threatening.
*Liquid form contains alcohol.   **May contain tartrazine.

betaxolol hydrochloride
Betoptic

Pregnancy Risk Category: C

MECHANISM OF ACTION
Reduces formation and possibly increases outflow of aqueous humor. A cardioselective beta-blocker.

INDICATIONS & DOSAGE
Chronic open-angle glaucoma and ocular hypertension—
Adults: instill 1 drop in eyes b.i.d.

ADVERSE REACTIONS
CNS: insomnia.
Eye: *stinging upon instillation*, occasional tearing.

INTERACTIONS
None significant.

NURSING CONSIDERATIONS
• Contraindicated in sinus bradycardia, greater than first-degree AV block, cardiogenic shock, or patients with overt heart failure.
• Use cautiously in patients with a history of heart failure; patients with restricted pulmonary function; patients with diabetes mellitus.
• Betaxolol differs from timolol and levobunolol in that it is a cardioselective beta-adrenergic blocker. Therefore, this drug does not significantly affect the heart rate. Its pulmonary systemic effects are considerably milder than those of timolol and levobunolol.
• Betaxolol is intended for twice-daily dosage. Encourage your patient to comply with this regimen.
• In some patients, a few weeks' treatment may be required to stabilize pressure-lowering response. Determine intraocular pressure after 4 weeks of treatment.
• Teach patient how to instill. Advise him to wash hands before and after administering and to apply light finger-pressure on lacrimal sac for 1 minute following instillation. Warn patient not to touch dropper to eye or surrounding tissue.

cromolyn sodium
Opticrom 4% ophthalmic solution

Pregnancy Risk Category: B

MECHANISM OF ACTION
Inhibits degranulation of sensitized mast cells that follows exposure to specific antigens. Also inhibits release of histamine and slow-reacting substance of anaphylaxis (SRS-A).

INDICATIONS & DOSAGE
Treatment and prevention of allergic ocular disorders such as vernal keratoconjunctivitis and conjunctivitis, giant papillary conjunctivitis, vernal keratitis, and allergic keratoconjunctivitis—
Adults and children: 1 to 2 drops in each eye 4 to 6 times a day at regular intervals.

ADVERSE REACTIONS
Eye: transient stinging or burning upon instillation.

INTERACTIONS
None significant.

NURSING CONSIDERATIONS
• Because preparation contains benzalkonium chloride as a preservative, advise patient not to wear soft contact lenses during treatment period. Patient may resume wearing them a few hours after the drug's discontinued.
• Advise patient to instill medication at regular intervals.
• Tell patient that relief of symptoms may take several days to a week.
• Cromolyn is a safe treatment for some types of allergic conjunctivitis and keratitis and may be as effective as steroids.
• Teach patient how to instill. Advise

him to wash hands before and after administering and to apply light finger-pressure on lacrimal sac for 1 minute following instillation. Warn patient not to touch dropper to eye or surrounding tissue.

---

dipivefrin 0.1%
Propine♦

Pregnancy Risk Category: B

MECHANISM OF ACTION
A prodrug of epinephrine (in the eye, dipivefrin is converted to epinephrine). The liberated epinephrine appears to decrease aqueous production and increase aqueous outflow.

INDICATIONS & DOSAGE
To reduce intraocular pressure in chronic open-angle glaucoma—
Adults: for initial glaucoma therapy, 1 drop in eye q 12 hours.

ADVERSE REACTIONS
CV: tachycardia, hypertension.
Eye: burning, stinging.

INTERACTIONS
None significant.

NURSING CONSIDERATIONS
• Contraindicated in narrow-angle glaucoma.
• Use cautiously in patients with aphakia.
• Dipivefrin is a prodrug of epinephrine: It's converted to epinephrine when it enters the eye.
• May have fewer adverse reactions than conventional epinephrine therapy.
• Often used concomitantly with other antiglaucoma drugs.
• Available as a 0.1% solution in 5-, 10-, and 15-ml dropper bottles.
• Teach patient how to instill. Advise him to wash hands before and after administration. Warn him not to touch dropper to eye or surrounding tissue.

---

fluorescein sodium
Fluorescite, Fluor-I-Strip, Fluor-I-Strip A.T.♦, Ful-Glo♦, Funduscein Injections♦

Pregnancy Risk Category: C

MECHANISM OF ACTION
Produces an intense green fluorescence in alkaline solution (pH 5.0 or less) or a bright yellow if viewed under cobalt blue illumination.

INDICATIONS & DOSAGE
Diagnostic in corneal abrasions and foreign bodies; fitting hard contact lenses; lacrimal patency; fundus photography; applanation tonometry—
Topical solution: instill 1 drop of 2% solution followed by irrigation, or moisten strip with sterile water. Touch conjunctiva or fornix with moistened tip. Flush eye with irrigating solution. Patient should blink several times after application.
Indicated in retinal angiography—
Intravenous:
Adults: 5 ml of 10% solution (500 mg) or 3 ml of 25% solution (750 mg) injected rapidly into antecubital vein, by doctor or a specially trained nurse.
Children: 0.077 ml of 10% solution (7.7 mg/kg body weight) or 0.044 ml of 25% solution (11 mg/kg body weight) injected rapidly into antecubital vein by doctor.

ADVERSE REACTIONS
Topical use:
Eye: stinging, burning, yellow streaks from tears.
Intravenous use:
CNS: headache persisting for 24 to 36 hours.
GI: nausea, vomiting.
GU: bright yellow urine (persists for 24 to 36 hours).
Skin: yellow skin discoloration (fades in 6 to 12 hours).
Local: extravasation at injection site, thrombophlebitis.

Italicized side effects are common or life-threatening.
*Liquid form contains alcohol.   **May contain tartrazine.

Other: hypersensitivity, including urticaria and *anaphylaxis*.

INTERACTIONS
None significant.

NURSING CONSIDERATIONS
• Use with caution in patients with history of allergy or bronchial asthma.
• Never instill while patient is wearing soft contact lens. Drug will ruin it.
• Use topical anesthetic before instilling to partially relieve burning and irritation.
• Always use aseptic technique. Easily contaminated by *Pseudomonas*.
• Yellow skin discoloration may persist 6 to 12 hours.
• Warn patient that urine will be bright yellow after I.V. injection.
• Routine urinalysis will be abnormal within 1 hour after I.V. injection.
• A water-soluble dye.
• Don't freeze; store below 80° F. (26.7° C.).
• Defects appear green under normal light, or bright yellow under cobalt blue illumination. Foreign bodies are surrounded by a green ring. Similar lesions of the conjunctiva are delineated in orange-yellow.
• Always keep an emergency tray with antihistamine, epinephrine, and oxygen available when giving parenterally.

glycerin, anhydrous
Ophthalgan
Pregnancy Risk Category: C

MECHANISM OF ACTION
Removes excess fluid from the cornea.

INDICATIONS & DOSAGE
Corneal edema before ophthalmoscopy or gonioscopy in acute glaucoma and bullous keratitis—
Adults and children: instill 1 to 2 drops glycerin, anhydrous after instilling a local anesthetic.

ADVERSE REACTIONS
Eye: pain if instilled without topical anesthetic.

INTERACTIONS
None significant.

NURSING CONSIDERATIONS
• Use topical tetracaine HCl or proparacaine HCl before instilling to prevent discomfort.
• Don't touch tip of dropper to eye, surrounding tissues, or tear-film; glycerin will absorb moisture.
• Used to temporarily restore corneal transparency when cornea is too edematous to permit diagnosis.
• Store in tightly closed container.

isosorbide
Ismotic
Pregnancy Risk Category: C

MECHANISM OF ACTION
Acts as an osmotic agent by promoting redistribution of water and thereby producing diuresis.

INDICATIONS & DOSAGE
Short-term reduction of intraocular pressure due to glaucoma—
Adults: initially, 1.5 g/kg P.O. Usual dosage range is 1 to 3 g/kg.

ADVERSE REACTIONS
CNS: vertigo, light-headedness, lethargy.
GI: gastric discomfort, diarrhea, anorexia.
Metabolic: hypernatremia, hyperosmolality, thirst.

INTERACTIONS
None significant.

NURSING CONSIDERATIONS
• Contraindicated in anuria due to se-

vere renal disease, severe dehydration, frank or impending acute pulmonary edema, and hemorrhagic glaucoma.
• Repetitive doses should be used cautiously, especially in patients with diseases associated with salt retention, such as congestive heart failure. Carefully monitor patient's fluid and electrolyte balance.
• Pour over cracked ice, and tell patient to sip the medication. This procedure improves palatability.
• Especially useful for rapid reduction in intraocular pressure.

levobunolol hydrochloride
Betagan

Pregnancy Risk Category: C

MECHANISM OF ACTION
Reduces formation and possibly increases outflow of aqueous humor. A nonselective beta-blocker.

INDICATIONS & DOSAGE
Chronic open-angle glaucoma and ocular hypertension—
Adults: instill 1 drop in eyes once or twice daily.

ADVERSE REACTIONS
CNS: headache, dizziness, depression.
CV: slight reduction in resting heart rate.
Eye: *transient stinging and burning.* Long-term use may decrease corneal sensitivity.
GI: nausea.
Skin: urticaria.
Other: evidence of beta blockade and systemic absorption *(hypotension, bradycardia, syncope, exacerbation of asthma,* and *congestive heart failure).*

INTERACTIONS
Propranolol, metoprolol, and other oral beta-adrenergic blocking agents: increased ocular and systemic effect.

Use together cautiously.

NURSING CONSIDERATIONS
• Contraindicated in bronchial asthma, a history of bronchial asthma or severe chronic obstructive pulmonary disease; sinus bradycardia; second-degree and third-degree AV block; cardiac failure; cardiogenic shock.
• Use cautiously in patients with chronic bronchitis and emphysema, diabetes mellitus, and hyperthyroidism.
• Levobunolol is faster acting than timolol. The onset of action occurs within 1 hour; maximum effect is between 2 and 6 hours.
• Teach patient how to instill. Advise him to wash hands before and after administering and to apply light finger-pressure on lacrimal sac for 1 minute after instillation. Warn patient not to touch dropper to eye or surrounding tissue.

sodium chloride, hypertonic
Adsorbonac Ophthalmic Solution, Muro-128 Ointment, Sodium Chloride Ointment 5%

Pregnancy Risk Category: C

MECHANISM OF ACTION
Removes excess fluid from the cornea.

INDICATIONS & DOSAGE
Corneal edema (postoperative) after cataract extraction or corneal transplantation; also in trauma or bullous keratopathy—
Adults and children: instill 1 to 2 drops q 3 to 4 hours, or apply ointment at bedtime.

ADVERSE REACTIONS
Eye: slight stinging.
Other: hypersensitivity.

Italicized side effects are common or life-threatening.
*Liquid form contains alcohol.   **May contain tartrazine.

INTERACTIONS
None significant.

NURSING CONSIDERATIONS
• An osmotic agent used to reduce corneal edema when repeated instillation is indicated.
• May use a few drops of sterile irrigation solution inside bottle cap to prevent caking on dropper bottle tip.
• Store in tightly closed container.
• Ointment may cause blurred vision.
• Teach patient how to instill. Advise him to wash hands before and after administering and to apply light finger-pressure on lacrimal sac for 1 minute after drops are instilled. Warn patient not to touch dropper to eye or surrounding tissue.

timolol maleate
Timoptic Solution

Pregnancy Risk Category: C

MECHANISM OF ACTION
Reduces aqueous formation and possibly increases aqueous outflow. A beta-blocker.

INDICATIONS & DOSAGE
Chronic open-angle glaucoma, secondary glaucoma, aphakic glaucoma, ocular hypertension—
Adults: initially, instill 1 drop 0.25% solution in each eye b.i.d.; reduce to 1 drop daily for maintenance. If patient doesn't respond, instill 1 drop 0.5% solution in each eye b.i.d. If intraocular pressure is controlled, dosage may be reduced to 1 drop in each eye daily.

ADVERSE REACTIONS
CNS: headache, depression, fatigue.
CV: slight reduction in resting heart rate.
Eye: minor irritation. Long-term use may decrease corneal sensitivity.
GI: anorexia.
Other: apnea in infants, *evidence of beta blockade and systemic absorption (hypotension, bradycardia, syncope, exacerbation of asthma, and congestive heart failure).*

INTERACTIONS
Propranolol HCl, metoprolol tartrate, other oral beta-adrenergic blocking agents: increased ocular and systemic effect. Use together cautiously.

NURSING CONSIDERATIONS
• Use cautiously in bronchial asthma, sinus bradycardia, second- and third-degree heart block, cardiogenic shock, right ventricular failure resulting from pulmonary hypertension, congestive heart failure, severe cardiac disease, and in infants with congenital glaucoma.
• In some patients, a few weeks may be required to stabilize pressure-lowering response. Determine intraocular pressure after 4 weeks of treatment.
• Warn patient not to touch dropper to eye or surrounding tissue.
• Can be used safely in patients with glaucoma who wear conventional (PMMA) hard contact lenses.
• Teach patient how to instill. Advise him to wash hands before and after administering and to apply light finger-pressure on lacrimal sac for 1 minute following instillation. Warn him not to touch dropper to eye or surrounding tissue.

Otics

acetic acid○
benzocaine○
boric acid○
carbamide peroxide○
chloramphenicol
hydrocortisone
hydrocortisone acetate
methylprednisolone disodium phosphate
neomycin sulfate
triethanolamine polypeptide oleate-condensate

COMBINATION PRODUCTS
COLY-MYCIN S OTIC: Each ml contains neomycin SO_4 3.3 mg, colistin SO_4 3 mg, hydrocortisone acetate 10 mg, and thonzonium bromide 0.05%.
CORTISPORIN OTIC♦: Each ml contains neomycin SO_4 5 mg, polymyxin B 10,000 units, and hydrocortisone 1%.

---

acetic acid○
Domeboro Otic♦, VoSol Otic♦

Pregnancy Risk Category: C

MECHANISM OF ACTION
Inhibits or destroys bacteria present in the ear canal.

INDICATIONS & DOSAGE
External ear canal infection—
Adults and children: 4 to 6 drops into ear canal t.i.d. or q.i.d., or insert saturated wick for first 24 hours, then continue with instillations.
Prophylaxis of swimmer's ear—
Adults and children: 2 drops in each ear b.i.d.

ADVERSE REACTIONS
Ear: irritation or itching.
Skin: urticaria.
Other: overgrowth of nonsusceptible organisms.

INTERACTIONS
None significant.

NURSING CONSIDERATIONS
• Use cautiously in perforated eardrum.
• Has anti-infective, anti-inflammatory, and antipruritic effects.
• *Pseudomonas aeruginosa* particularly sensitive to drug.
• Reculture persistent drainage.
• Avoid touching ear with dropper.

---

benzocaine○
Americaine-Otic♦, Auralgan♦, Eardro, Myringacaine, Tympagesic

Pregnancy Risk Category: C

MECHANISM OF ACTION
Produces analgesic effects. A local anesthetic.

INDICATIONS & DOSAGE
Cerumen removal—
Adults and children: fill ear canal t.i.d. for 2 days.
Pain from otitis media—
Adults and children: fill ear canal with solution and plug with cotton. May repeat q 1 to 2 hours, p.r.n.

ADVERSE REACTIONS
Ear: irritation or itching.
Skin: urticaria.

Italicized side effects are common or life-threatening.
*Liquid form contains alcohol.   **May contain tartrazine.

Other: edema.

INTERACTIONS
None significant.

NURSING CONSIDERATIONS
• Contraindicated in perforated eardrum.
• Local anesthetic effect only.
• Use with antibiotic to treat underlying cause of pain, because use alone may mask more serious condition.
• Tell patient to call doctor if pain lasts longer than 48 hours.
• Avoid touching ear with dropper. Do not rinse dropper.
• Irrigate ear gently to remove impacted cerumen.
• Keep in dark, tightly closed container, away from moisture and light.

boric acid◊
Ear-Dry, Swim Ear
Pregnancy Risk Category: C

MECHANISM OF ACTION
Inhibits or destroys bacteria present in the ear canal. Weak bacteriostatic action; also fungistatic agent.

INDICATIONS & DOSAGE
External ear canal infection—
Adults and children: fill ear canal with solution and plug with cotton. Repeat t.i.d. or q.i.d.

ADVERSE REACTIONS
Ear: irritation or itching.
Skin: urticaria.
Other: overgrowth of nonsusceptible organisms.

INTERACTIONS
None significant.

NURSING CONSIDERATIONS
• Contraindicated in perforated eardrum or excoriated membranes in ear.
• Watch for signs of superinfection (continual pain, inflammation, fever).

• If cotton plug used, always moisten with medication.
• Avoid touching ear with dropper.

carbamide peroxide◊
Debrox
Pregnancy Risk Category: C

MECHANISM OF ACTION
Emulsifies and disperses accumulated cerumen. A ceruminolytic.

INDICATIONS & DOSAGE
Impacted cerumen—
Adults and children: 5 to 10 drops into ear canal b.i.d. for 3 to 4 days.

ADVERSE REACTIONS
None reported.

INTERACTIONS
None significant.

NURSING CONSIDERATIONS
• Contraindicated in perforated eardrum.
• Tell patient to call doctor if redness, pain, or swelling persists.
• Irrigation of ear may be necessary to aid in removal of cerumen.
• Avoid touching ear with dropper.

chloramphenicol
Chloromycetin Otic♦,
Sopamycetin♦♦
Pregnancy Risk Category: C

MECHANISM OF ACTION
Inhibits or destroys bacteria present in the ear canal.

INDICATIONS & DOSAGE
External ear canal infection—
Adults and children: 2 to 3 drops into ear canal t.i.d. or q.i.d.

ADVERSE REACTIONS
Ear: itching or burning.
Local: pruritus, burning, urticaria,

vesicular or maculopapular dermatitis.
Systemic: sore throat, angioedema.
Other: overgrowth of nonsusceptible organisms.

INTERACTIONS
None significant.

NURSING CONSIDERATIONS
• Avoid prolonged use.
• Obtain history of use and reaction to drug.
• Watch for signs of superinfection (continued pain, inflammation, fever).
• Reculture persistent drainage.
• Watch for signs of sore throat (early sign of toxicity).
• Avoid touching ear with dropper.

hydrocortisone

hydrocortisone acetate
Cortamed◆◆

Pregnancy Risk Category: C

MECHANISM OF ACTION
Controls inflammation, edema, and pruritus.

INDICATIONS & DOSAGE
Inflammation of external ear canal—
Adults and children: 3 to 5 drops into ear canal t.i.d. or q.i.d.
Available in 0.25%, 0.5%, and 1% concentrations.

ADVERSE REACTIONS
Systemic: adrenal suppression with long-term use.
Other: may mask or exacerbate underlying infection.

INTERACTIONS
None reported.

NURSING CONSIDERATIONS
• Contraindicated in perforated eardrum, fungal infections, herpes or

other viral infections.
• Use with antibiotic to treat inflammation caused by infection.
• Use alone in allergic otitis externa.
• Avoid touching ear with dropper.

methylprednisolone disodium phosphate
Medrol◆◆

Pregnancy Risk Category: C

MECHANISM OF ACTION
Controls inflammation, edema, and pruritus.

INDICATIONS & DOSAGE
Inflammation of external ear canal—
Adults and children: 2 to 3 drops into ear canal t.i.d. or q.i.d.

ADVERSE REACTIONS
Systemic: adrenal suppression with long-term use.
Other: may mask or exacerbate underlying infection.

INTERACTIONS
None significant.

NURSING CONSIDERATIONS
• Contraindicated in perforated eardrum, fungal infection, herpes, or other viral infections.
• Use with antibiotic to treat inflammation caused by infection.
• Use alone to treat seborrheic, contact, or uninfected eczematoid dermatitis.
• Avoid touching ear with dropper.

neomycin sulfate
Otobiotic

Pregnancy Risk Category: C

MECHANISM OF ACTION
Inhibits or destroys bacteria present in the ear canal.

INDICATIONS & DOSAGE

External ear canal infection—
Adults and children: 2 to 5 drops into ear canal t.i.d. or q.i.d.

ADVERSE REACTIONS

Ear: ototoxicity (in patients undergoing tympanoplasty).
Local: burning, erythema, vesicular dermatitis, urticaria.
Other: overgrowth of nonsusceptible organisms.

INTERACTIONS

None significant.

NURSING CONSIDERATIONS

• Contraindicated in perforated eardrum.
• Obtain history of use and reaction to neomycin.
• Observe for signs of hearing loss.
• Watch for signs of superinfection (continued pain, inflammation, fever).
• Reculture persistent drainage.
• Best used in combination with other antibiotics.
• Avoid touching ear with dropper.

triethanolamine polypeptide oleate-condensate

Cerumenex♦

Pregnancy Risk Category: C

MECHANISM OF ACTION

Emulsifies and disperses accumulated cerumen. A ceruminolytic.

INDICATIONS & DOSAGE

Impacted cerumen—
Adults and children: fill ear canal with solution and insert cotton plug. After 15 to 30 minutes, flush ear with warm water.

ADVERSE REACTIONS

Ear: erythema, pruritus.
Skin: severe eczema.

INTERACTIONS

None significant.

NURSING CONSIDERATIONS

• Contraindicated in perforated eardrum, otitis media, and allergies. Do patch test by placing 1 drop of drug on inner forearm; cover with small bandage. Read in 24 hours. If any reaction (redness, swelling) occurs, don't use drug.
• Tell patient not to use drops more often than prescribed. Flush ear gently with warm water, using soft rubber bulb ear syringe, within 30 minutes after instillation.
• Moisten cotton plug with medication before insertion.
• Keep container tightly closed and away from moisture.
• Avoid touching ear with dropper.

Nasal agents

beclomethasone dipropionate
dexamethasone sodium
  phosphate
ephedrine sulfate◇
epinephrine hydrochloride◇
flunisolide
naphazoline hydrochloride◇
oxymetazoline hydrochloride◇
phenylephrine hydrochloride◇
tetrahydrozoline hydrochloride
xylometazoline hydrochloride◇

COMBINATION PRODUCTS
4-WAY NASAL SPRAY◇: phenylephrine hydrochloride 0.5%, naphazoline
hydrochloride 0.05%, and pyrilamine
maleate 0.2%.

---

beclomethasone dipropionate
Beconase Nasal Inhaler♦,
Vancenase Nasal Inhaler♦

Pregnancy Risk Category: C

MECHANISM OF ACTION
Unknown.

INDICATIONS & DOSAGE
*Relief of symptoms of seasonal or pe-
rennial rhinitis; prevention of recurrence of nasal polyps after surgical removal—*
Adults and children over 12 years:
Usual dosage is one spray (42 mcg) in
each nostril 2 to 4 times daily (total
dosage 168 to 336 mcg daily). Most
patients require one spray in each nostril t.i.d. (252 mcg daily).
  Not recommended for children under age 12.

ADVERSE REACTIONS
CNS: headache.
EENT: *mild transient nasal burning
and stinging,* nasal congestion, sneez-
ing, epistaxis, watery eyes.
GI: nausea and vomiting.
Other: development of nasopharyn-
geal fungal infections.

INTERACTIONS
None reported.

NURSING CONSIDERATIONS
• Use cautiously, if at all, in patients
with active or quiescent respiratory
tract tubercular infections or in untreated fungal, bacterial, or systemic
viral or ocular herpes simplex infections.
• Use cautiously in patients who have
recently had nasal septal ulcers or nasal surgery or trauma.
• Recommended dosages will not
suppress hypothalamic-pituitary-adrenal (HPA) function. Warn patient
not to exceed this dosage.
• Indicated when conventional treatment (antihistamines, decongestants)
fails.
• Beclomethasone is not effective for
active exacerbations. Nasal decongestants or oral antihistamines may be
needed instead.
• Advise patients to use drug regularly, as prescribed; its effectiveness
depends on regular use.
• Explain that the therapeutic effects
of this corticosteroid, unlike those of
decongestants, are not immediate.
Most patients achieve benefit within a
few days, but some may need 2 to 3

Italicized side effects are common or life-threatening.
*Liquid form contains alcohol.   **May contain tartrazine.

weeks for maximum benefit.
• If symptoms don't improve within 3 weeks or if nasal irritation persists, patient should stop drug and notify doctor.
• Observe for fungal infections.
• Teach patient good nasal and oral hygiene.
• Teach patient how to use. Shake container and invert. After clearing nasal passages, tilt head back, insert nozzle into nostril pointing away from septum. While holding other nostril closed, inspire and spray. Shake container again and repeat in other nostril.

dexamethasone sodium phosphate
Decadron Phosphate♦, Turbinaire

Pregnancy Risk Category: C

MECHANISM OF ACTION
Unknown.

INDICATIONS & DOSAGE
Allergic or inflammatory conditions, nasal polyps—
Adults: 2 sprays in each nostril b.i.d. or t.i.d. Maximum 12 sprays daily.
Children 6 to 12 years: 1 or 2 sprays in each nostril b.i.d. Maximum 8 sprays daily.
    Each spray delivers 0.1 mg dexamethasone sodium phosphate equal to 0.084 mg dexamethasone.

ADVERSE REACTIONS
EENT: nasal irritation, dryness, rebound nasal congestion.
Other: hypersensitivity, systemic side effects with prolonged use (pituitary-adrenal suppression, sodium retention, congestive heart failure, hypertension, hypokalemia, headaches, convulsions, peptic ulcer, ecchymoses, petechiae, masking of infection).

INTERACTIONS
None significant.

NURSING CONSIDERATIONS
• Contraindicated in cutaneous tuberculosis, fungal and herpetic lesions. Use cautiously in diabetes mellitus, peptic ulcer, or tuberculosis, as systemic absorption can activate disease.
• Mothers should not breast-feed, as systemic absorption can occur.
• Control underlying bacterial infection with anti-infectives.
• Irritation or sensitivity may require stopping drug.
• Don't break, incinerate, or store in extreme heat; contents under pressure.
• Gradually reduce dose as nasal condition improves.
• Fluid retention can occur as a result of systemic absorption.
• Teach patient how to use according to directions in package. Patient should shake container and invert. After cleaning nasal passages, should tilt head back, insert nozzle into nostril pointing away from septum. While holding other nostril closed, inspire and spray. Shake container again and repeat in other nostril.
• Only one person should use nasal spray.
• Hypertension and hypokalemia can occur with systemic absorption. Monitor blood pressure, serum potassium frequently.
• Should not be used for prolonged periods.
• Teach patient good nasal and oral hygiene.

ephedrine sulfate◊
Efedron Nasal Jelly, Va-tro-nol Nose Drops

Pregnancy Risk Category: C

MECHANISM OF ACTION
Produces local vasoconstriction of dilated arterioles to reduce blood flow

---

Unmarked trade names available in the United States only.
♦Also available in Canada.　　　♦♦Available in Canada only.　　　◊Also available OTC.

and nasal congestion.

INDICATIONS & DOSAGE
Nasal congestion—
Adults and children: apply 3 to 4 drops 0.5% solution or apply a small amount of jelly to nasal mucosa. Use no more frequently than q 4 hours.

ADVERSE REACTIONS
CNS: nervousness, excitation.
CV: *tachycardia.*
EENT: rebound nasal congestion with long-term or excessive use.
Local: mucosal irritation.

INTERACTIONS
MAO inhibitors: hypertensive crisis if ephedrine is absorbed. Don't use together.

NURSING CONSIDERATIONS
• Use cautiously in hyperthyroidism, coronary artery disease, hypertension, or diabetes mellitus, as systemic absorption can occur.
• Tell patient not to exceed recommended dose. Use only when needed.
• Teach patient how to apply. Only one person should use dropper bottle.

epinephrine hydrochloride∘
Adrenalin Chloride♦

Pregnancy Risk Category: C

MECHANISM OF ACTION
Produces local vasoconstriction of dilated arterioles to reduce blood flow and nasal congestion.

INDICATIONS & DOSAGE
Nasal congestion, local superficial bleeding—
Adults and children: apply 0.1% solution to oral or nasal mucosa.

ADVERSE REACTIONS
CNS: nervousness, excitation.
CV: *tachycardia.*
EENT: rebound nasal congestion,

slight sting upon application.

INTERACTIONS
None significant.

NURSING CONSIDERATIONS
• Use cautiously in hyperthyroidism, coronary artery disease, hypertension, or diabetes mellitus, as systemic absorption can occur.
• Tell patient not to exceed recommended dose. Use only when needed.
• Teach patient how to apply. Only one person should use dropper bottle.

flunisolide
Nasalide Spray

Pregnancy Risk Category: C

MECHANISM OF ACTION
Unknown.

INDICATIONS & DOSAGE
Relief of symptoms of seasonal or perennial rhinitis—
Adults: starting dose is 2 sprays (50 mcg) in each nostril b.i.d. Total daily dosage is 200 mcg. If necessary, dose may be increased to 2 sprays in each nostril t.i.d. Maximum total daily dosage is 8 sprays in each nostril (400 mcg daily).
Children 6 to 14 years: starting dose is 1 spray (25 mcg) in each nostril t.i.d. or 2 sprays (50 mcg) in each nostril b.i.d. Total daily dosage is 150 to 200 mcg. Maximum total daily dosage is 4 sprays in each nostril (200 mcg daily).
Not recommended for children under age 6.

ADVERSE REACTIONS
CNS: headache.
EENT: *mild, transient nasal burning and stinging,* nasal congestion, sneezing, epistaxis, watery eyes.
GI: nausea, vomiting.
Other: development of nasopharyngeal fungal infections.

Italicized side effects are common or life-threatening.
*Liquid form contains alcohol.   **May contain tartrazine.

INTERACTIONS
None reported.

NURSING CONSIDERATIONS
• Use cautiously, if at all, in patients with active or quiescent respiratory tract tubercular infections or in untreated fungal, bacterial, or systemic viral or ocular herpes simplex infections.
• Use cautiously in patients who have recently had nasal septal ulcers or nasal surgery or trauma.
• Recommended dosages will not suppress hypothalamic-pituitary-adrenal (HPA) function. Warn patient not to exceed this dosage.
• Indicated when conventional treatment (antihistamines, decongestants) fails.
• Flunisolide is not effective for acute exacerbations. Nasal decongestants or oral antihistamines may be needed instead.
• Advise patient to use drug regularly, as prescribed; its effectiveness depends on regular use.
• Explain that the therapeutic effects of this corticosteroid, unlike those of decongestants, are not immediate. Most patients achieve benefit within a few days, but some may need 2 to 3 weeks for maximum benefit.
• Patients with dryness and crusting of the nasal mucosa may prefer the liquid spray of flunisolide to the aerosolized powder of beclomethasone.
• If symptoms don't improve within 3 weeks or if nasal irritation persists, patient should stop drug and notify doctor.
• Teach patient how to apply. Clear nasal passages. After priming inhaler, tilt head slightly forward, insert spray tip into nostril pointing away from septum. While holding other nostril closed, inspire and spray. Repeat in other nostril.

naphazoline hydrochloride◇
Privine♦

Pregnancy Risk Category: C

MECHANISM OF ACTION
Produces local vasoconstriction of dilated arterioles to reduce blood flow and nasal congestion.

INDICATIONS & DOSAGE
Nasal congestion—
Adults: apply 2 drops or sprays of 0.05% solution to nasal mucosa q 3 to 4 hours.
Children 6 to 12 years: 1 to 2 drops or sprays of 0.05% solution. Repeat q 3 to 6 hours, p.r.n. Use no longer than 3 to 5 days.

ADVERSE REACTIONS
EENT: rebound nasal congestion with excessive or long-term use, sneezing, stinging, dryness of mucosa.
Other: systemic side effects in children after excessive or long-term use; marked sedation.

INTERACTIONS
None significant.

NURSING CONSIDERATIONS
• Contraindicated in narrow-angle glaucoma. Use cautiously in hyperthyroidism, heart disease, hypertension, or diabetes mellitus, as systemic absorption can occur.
• Warn patient not to exceed recommended dosage.
• Tell patient to notify doctor if nasal congestion persists after 5 days.
• Teach patient how to apply. Hold spray container and head upright. Only one person should use dropper bottle or nasal spray.
• Do not shake container.

oxymetazoline hydrochloride◇
Afrin, Duration

Pregnancy Risk Category: C

MECHANISM OF ACTION
Produces local vasoconstriction of dilated arterioles to reduce blood flow and nasal congestion.

INDICATIONS & DOSAGE
Nasal congestion—
Adults and children over 6 years: apply 2 to 4 drops or sprays 0.05% solution to nasal mucosa b.i.d.
Children 2 to 6 years: apply 2 to 3 drops 0.025% solution to nasal mucosa b.i.d. Use no longer than 3 to 5 days. Dosage for younger children has not been established.

ADVERSE REACTIONS
CNS: headache, drowsiness, dizziness, insomnia.
CV: palpitations, *hypotension with cardiovascular collapse,* hypertension.
EENT: rebound nasal congestion or irritation with excessive or long-term use, dryness of nose and throat, increased nasal discharge, stinging, sneezing.
Other: systemic side effects in children with excessive or long-term use; possible sedation.

INTERACTIONS
None significant.

NURSING CONSIDERATIONS
• Use cautiously in hyperthyroidism, cardiac disease, hypertension, or diabetes mellitus, as systemic absorption can occur.
• Tell patient not to exceed recommended dose. Use only when needed.
• Warn patient that excessive use may cause bradycardia, hypotension, dizziness, and weakness.
• Teach patient how to apply. Have patient hold head upright and sniff spray briskly. Only one person should use dropper bottle or nasal spray.

phenylephrine hydrochloride◇
Alconefrin, Coricidin Nasal Mist, Coryzine, Ephrine, Neo-Synephrine♦, Sinarest Nasal Spray, Sinophen Intranasal, SuperAnahist Nasal Spray

Pregnancy Risk Category: C

MECHANISM OF ACTION
Produces local vasoconstriction of dilated arterioles to reduce blood flow and nasal congestion.

INDICATIONS & DOSAGE
Nasal congestion—
Adults: 1 to 2 drops or sprays of 0.25% to 1% solution; apply jelly or spray to nasal mucosa.
Children 6 to 12 years: apply 1 to 2 drops or sprays of 0.25% solution.
Children under 6 years: apply 2 to 3 drops or sprays of 0.125% solution.
  Drops, spray, or jelly can be given q 4 hours, p.r.n.

ADVERSE REACTIONS
CNS: headache, tremors, dizziness, nervousness.
CV: *palpitations, tachycardia,* premature ventricular contractions, hypertension, pallor.
EENT: transient burning, stinging; dryness of nasal mucosa; rebound nasal congestion may occur with continued use.
GI: nausea.

INTERACTIONS
None significant.

NURSING CONSIDERATIONS
• Contraindicated in narrow-angle glaucoma. Use cautiously in hyperthyroidism, hypertension, diabetes mellitus, or ischemic cardiac disease,

---

Italicized side effects are common or life-threatening.
*Liquid form contains alcohol.   **May contain tartrazine.

as systemic absorption may occur.
• Tell patient not to exceed recommended dose. Use only when needed.
• Teach patient how to apply. Have patient hold head erect to minimize swallowing of medication. Only one person should use dropper bottle or nasal spray.

tetrahydrozoline hydrochloride
Tyzine HCl, Tyzine Pediatric

Pregnancy Risk Category: C

MECHANISM OF ACTION
Produces local vasoconstriction of dilated arterioles to reduce blood flow and nasal congestion.

INDICATIONS & DOSAGE
Nasal congestion—
Adults and children over 6 years: apply 2 to 4 drops 0.1% solution or spray to nasal mucosa q 4 to 6 hours, p.r.n.
Children 2 to 6 years: apply 2 to 3 drops 0.05% solution to nasal mucosa q 4 to 6 hours, p.r.n.

ADVERSE REACTIONS
EENT: transient burning, stinging; sneezing, rebound nasal congestion in excessive or long-term use.

INTERACTIONS
None significant.

NURSING CONSIDERATIONS
• Contraindicated in narrow-angle glaucoma. Use cautiously in hyperthyroidism, hypertension, diabetes mellitus.
• Don't use 0.1% solution in children under 6 years.
• Tell patient not to exceed recommended dose. Use only as needed.
• Show patient how to apply. Only one person should use dropper or nasal spray.

xylometazoline hydrochloride◊
4-Way Long Acting, Neo-Synephrine II, Otrivin♦, Sine-Off Nasal Spray, Sinex-L.A.

Pregnancy Risk Category: C

MECHANISM OF ACTION
Produces local vasoconstriction of dilated arterioles to reduce blood flow and nasal congestion.

INDICATIONS & DOSAGE
Nasal congestion—
Adults and children over 12 years: apply 2 to 3 drops or 1 to 2 sprays of 0.1% solution to nasal mucosa q 8 to 10 hours.
Children under 12 years: apply 2 to 3 drops or 1 spray of 0.05% solution to nasal mucosa q 8 to 10 hours.

ADVERSE REACTIONS
EENT: rebound nasal congestion or irritation with excessive or long-term use; transient burning, stinging; dryness or ulceration of nasal mucosa; sneezing.

INTERACTIONS
None significant.

NURSING CONSIDERATIONS
• Contraindicated in narrow-angle glaucoma. Use cautiously in hyperthyroidism, cardiac disease, hypertension, diabetes mellitus, and advanced arteriosclerosis, as systemic absorption can occur.
• Tell patient not to exceed recommended dose.
• Teach patient how to apply. Have patient hold head upright and sniff spray briskly. Only one person should use dropper bottle or nasal spray.

Unmarked trade names available in the United States only.
♦ Also available in Canada.   ♦♦ Available in Canada only.   ◊ Also available OTC.

Local anti-infectives

acyclovir
amphotericin B
bacitracin
butoconazole nitrate
carbol-fuchsin solution
chloramphenicol
chlortetracycline hydrochloride
ciclopirox olamine
clotrimazole
econazole nitrate
erythromycin
gentamicin sulfate
gentian violet (methylrosaniline
  chloride)◇
haloprogin
iodochlorhydroxyquin
  (clioquinol)◇
ketoconazole
mafenide acetate
metronidazole 0.75% (topical)
miconazole nitrate 2%
mupirocin
naftifine
neomycin sulfate
nitrofurazone
nystatin
oxiconazole nitrate
silver sulfadiazine
tetracycline hydrochloride
tolnaftate
undecylenic acid (zinc
  undecylenate)

COMBINATION PRODUCTS
CORDRAN-N CREAM, OINTMENT:
flurandrenolide 0.05% and neomycin
sulfate 0.5%.
LANABIOTIC◇: polymyxin B sulfate
5,000 units, neomycin sulfate 5 mg,
bacitracin 500 units, and lidocaine 40
mg/g.

LOTRISONE CREAM: clotrimazole 1%
and betamethasone dipropionate
0.05%.
MYCITRACIN OINTMENT◇: polymyxin
B sulfate 5,000 units, bacitracin 500
units, and neomycin sulfate 3.5 mg/g.
MYCOLOG II CREAM, OINTMENT: triamcinolone acetonide 0.1%, and nystatin 100,000 units/g.
NEO-CORTEF OINTMENT♦: hydrocortisone acetate 1% and neomycin sulfate 0.5%.
NEODECADRON CREAM: dexamethasone phosphate 0.1% and neomycin
sulfate 0.5%.
NEO-POLYCIN OINTMENT◇: polymyxin B sulfate 5,000 units, neomycin sulfate 5 mg, and zinc bacitracin
400 units/g.
NEOSPORIN CREAM♦ ♦ ◇: polymyxin B
sulfate 10,000 units, neomycin sulfate
5 mg.
NEOSPORIN OINTMENT◇: polymyxin
B sulfate 5,000 units, bacitracin zinc
400 units, and neomycin sulfate 5 mg/
g.
POLYSPORIN OINTMENT♦: polymyxin
B sulfate 10,000 units and zinc bacitracin 500 units/g.

---

acyclovir
Zovirax♦

Pregnancy Risk Category: C

MECHANISM OF ACTION
Inhibits herpes virus DNA synthesis
by interfering with the action of viral
DNA polymerase.

INDICATIONS & DOSAGE
Initial herpes genitalis; limited, non-life-threatening mucocutaneous herpes simplex virus infections in immunocompromised patients—
Adults and children: apply sufficient quantity to adequately cover all lesions q 3 hours six times daily for 7 days.

ADVERSE REACTIONS
Skin: transient burning and stinging, rash, pruritus.

INTERACTIONS
None reported.

NURSING CONSIDERATIONS
• For cutaneous use only. Don't apply to the eye.
• Although the dose size for each application will vary depending upon the total lesion area, use approximately a ½″ ribbon of ointment on each 4-inch square of surface area.
• Ointment must thoroughly cover all lesions.
• Apply with a finger cot or rubber glove to prevent autoinoculation of other body sites and transmission of infection to other persons.
• Therapy should be initiated as early as possible following onset of signs and symptoms of herpes.
• Most studies show that acyclovir is not effective when used to treat *recurrent* genital herpes.
• Emphasize importance of compliance for successful therapy.
• Teach patient that he may transmit the virus even during treatment.

---

amphotericin B
Fungizone Cream, Lotion, Ointment (3% amphotericin B)♦
Pregnancy Risk Category: B

MECHANISM OF ACTION
Alters the permeability of the cell membrane of fungi. Fungistatic.

INDICATIONS & DOSAGE
Cutaneous or mucocutaneous candidal infections—
Adults and children: apply liberally b.i.d., t.i.d., or q.i.d. for 1 to 3 weeks; up to several months for interdigital lesions and paronychias.

ADVERSE REACTIONS
Skin: possible drying, contact sensitivity, erythema, burning, pruritus.

INTERACTIONS
None significant.

NURSING CONSIDERATIONS
• Cream or lotion preferred for such areas as folds of groin, armpit, and neck creases.
• Cream discolors skin slightly when rubbed in; lotion or ointment doesn't. Lotion may stain nail lesions.
• Watch for and report signs of local irritation.
• Avoid occlusive dressings.
• Store at room temperature; avoid freezing.
• Well tolerated, even by infants, for long periods.
• Tell patient to continue using medication for full length of time prescribed, even if condition has improved.

---

bacitracin
Baciguent♦, Bacitin♦♦
Pregnancy Risk Category: C

MECHANISM OF ACTION
Inhibits bacterial cell-wall synthesis.

INDICATIONS & DOSAGE
Topical infections, impetigo, abrasions, cuts, and minor wounds—
Adults and children: apply thin film b.i.d. or t.i.d. or more often, depending on severity of condition.

ADVERSE REACTIONS
Skin: stinging, rashes, and other al-

lergic reactions; itching, burning, swelling of lips or face.
Other: *possible systemic adverse reactions when used over large areas for prolonged periods: potentially nephrotoxic and ototoxic; allergic reactions;* tightness in chest, hypotension.

INTERACTIONS
None significant.

NURSING CONSIDERATIONS
• Contraindicated for application in the external ear canal if the eardrum is perforated.
• Patients allergic to neomycin may also be allergic to bacitracin.
• Consider alternative treatment for burns that cover more than 20% of body surface, especially if patient suffers impaired renal function.
• If no improvement or if condition worsens, stop using and notify doctor.
• Prolonged use may result in overgrowth of nonsusceptible organisms.

---

butoconazole nitrate
Femstat

Pregnancy Risk Category: C

MECHANISM OF ACTION
Controls or destroys fungus by disrupting cell membrane permeability and reducing osmotic resistance.

INDICATIONS & DOSAGE
Local treatment of vulvovaginal mycotic infections caused by Candida *species—*
Adults (nonpregnant): one applicatorful intravaginally at bedtime for 3 days.
Adults (pregnant): one applicatorful intravaginally at bedtime for 6 days. Use only during 2nd and 3rd trimester.

ADVERSE REACTIONS
Skin: vulvar itching, soreness, and swelling; itching of the fingers.

INTERACTIONS
None significant.

NURSING CONSIDERATIONS
• Caution your patient not to use during first trimester of pregnancy.
• Butoconazole may be used with oral contraceptive and antibiotic therapy.
• Diagnosis of *Candida* vulvovaginal infection should be confirmed by smears or cultures.
• Symptom resolution comparable to 7-day miconazole cream therapy. Antifungal effect of butoconazole therapy is apparent after only 3 days of therapy.
• Teach patient how to apply. Tell patient not to use tampons during treatment.
• The patient's sexual partner should wear a condom during intercourse until treatment is complete. He should consult his doctor if he experiences penile itching, redness, or discomfort.
• Advise patient to do the following to prevent reinfection: Keep cool and dry, wear loose-fitting cotton clothing, avoid feminine hygiene sprays, wash daily with unscented soap, dry thoroughly with clean towel, and maintain proper bowel hygiene by wiping from front to back.

---

carbol-fuchsin solution
Castaderm, Castellani's Paint

Pregnancy Risk Category: C

MECHANISM OF ACTION
Disrupts protein synthesis. A fungicidal and bactericidal agent.

INDICATIONS & DOSAGE
Tinea, dermatophytosis, skin infections—
Adults and children: apply liberally one or two times daily.

ADVERSE REACTIONS
Blood: possibility of bone marrow hypoplasia with use over long periods

---

Italicized side effects are common or life-threatening.
*Liquid form contains alcohol.   **May contain tartrazine.

or at frequent intervals.
Skin: *contact dermatitis.*

INTERACTIONS
None significant.

NURSING CONSIDERATIONS
• Warn patient to expect a stinging sensation.
• An initial test application over a small area is recommended. If contact dermatitis or sensitivity occurs, discontinue use.
• Discontinue use after 1 week if no improvement shown; consult doctor. Toxicities may develop in long-term use.
• Poisonous; warn against swallowing. Store in tight, light-resistant container.
• Instruct patient to continue using for full treatment period prescribed, even if condition has improved.
• Don't apply to eroded skin or over extensive areas.
• Will stain clothing.
• Clean skin with soap and water before application.

---

chloramphenicol
Chloromycetin♦ (1% chloramphenicol)

Pregnancy Risk Category: C

MECHANISM OF ACTION
Disrupts protein synthesis.

INDICATIONS & DOSAGE
Superficial skin infections caused by susceptible bacteria—
Adults and children: after thorough cleansing, apply t.i.d. or q.i.d.

ADVERSE REACTIONS
Skin: possible contact sensitivity; itching, burning, urticaria, angioneurotic edema in patients hypersensitive to any of the components.
Other: *blood dyscrasias.*

INTERACTIONS
None significant.

NURSING CONSIDERATIONS
• If no improvement or if condition worsens, stop using and report to doctor.
• Prolonged use may result in overgrowth of nonsusceptible organisms.
• For all but very superficial infections, topical use of this drug should be supplemented by appropriate systemic medication.
• Discontinue if signs of hypersensitivity develop.
• Tell patient to continue using for full treatment period prescribed, even if condition has improved.

---

chlortetracycline hydrochloride
Aureomycin 3%♦

Pregnancy Risk Category: D

MECHANISM OF ACTION
Disrupts protein synthesis.

INDICATIONS & DOSAGE
Superficial infections of the skin caused by susceptible bacteria—
Adults and children: rub into affected area b.i.d. or t.i.d.

ADVERSE REACTIONS
Skin: *dermatitis,* drying.

INTERACTIONS
None significant.

NURSING CONSIDERATIONS
• Drug has lanolin base. Don't use in persons allergic to wool.
• Prolonged use may result in overgrowth of nonsusceptible organisms.
• If no improvement or if condition worsens, stop using and report to doctor.
• Treated skin fluoresces under ultraviolet light.

---

ciclopirox olamine
Loprox◆

Pregnancy Risk Category: B

MECHANISM OF ACTION
Depletes essential intracellular substrates of fungi.

INDICATIONS & DOSAGE
Treatment of tinea pedis, tinea cruris, tinea corporis, and tinea versicolor; cutaneous candidiasis—
Adults and children over 10 years: massage gently into the affected and surrounding areas b.i.d., in the morning and evening.

ADVERSE REACTIONS
Local: pruritus, burning.

INTERACTIONS
None reported.

NURSING CONSIDERATIONS
• If sensitivity or chemical irritation occurs, discontinue treatment.
• Use the drug for the full treatment period even though symptoms may have improved. Notify doctor if there's no improvement after 4 weeks.
• Available as a 1% cream in a water-soluble base.
• Don't use occlusive dressings.
• Hypopigmentation from *tinea versicolor* will resolve gradually.

clotrimazole
Canesten◆◆, Gyne-Lotrimin, Lotrimin (1% clotrimazole), Mycelex, Mycelex-G

Pregnancy Risk Category: B

MECHANISM OF ACTION
Alters fungal cell wall permeability.

INDICATIONS & DOSAGE
Superficial fungal infections (tinea pedis, tinea cruris, tinea corporis, tinea versicolor, candidiasis)—

Adults and children: apply thinly and massage into affected and surrounding area, morning and evening, 1 to 8 weeks.
Candidal vulvovaginitis—
Adults: insert 1 applicatorful or 1 tablet intravaginally daily for 7 to 14 days at bedtime. Alternatively, insert two 100-mg tablets once daily for 3 consecutive days or one 500-mg tablet one time only at bedtime.
Oropharyngeal candidiasis—
Adults and children: dissolve lozenge in mouth 5 times daily for 14 consecutive days.

ADVERSE REACTIONS
GI: nausea and vomiting (with lozenges).
GU: (with vaginal use) *mild vaginal burning, irritation.*
Hepatic: elevated AST (SGOT) levels (from lozenges).
Skin: blistering, *erythema,* edema, pruritus, burning, stinging, peeling, urticaria, skin fissures, general irritation.

INTERACTIONS
None significant.

NURSING CONSIDERATIONS
• Not for ophthalmic use.
• Watch for and report irritation or sensitivity. Discontinue use.
• Improvement usually within a week; if no improvement in 4 weeks, diagnosis should be reviewed.
• Emphasize the need to continue treatment for full course even if symptoms have improved.
• Warn patients not to use occlusive wrappings or dressings.
• Shortened dosage schedule with tablets may be used when compliance is a problem.
• Lozenges are indicated in treating oral candidiasis.
• Hypopigmentation from *tinea versicolor* will resolve gradually.

Italicized side effects are common or life-threatening.
*Liquid form contains alcohol.   **May contain tartrazine.

econazole nitrate
Ecostatin♦, Spectazole

Pregnancy Risk Category: C

MECHANISM OF ACTION
Alters fungal cell wall permeability.

INDICATIONS & DOSAGE
Treatment of tinea pedis, tinea cruris, and tinea corporis; cutaneous candidiasis—
Adults and children: apply sufficient quantity to cover affected areas b.i.d. in the morning and evening.
Tinea versicolor—
Adults and children: apply once daily.

ADVERSE REACTIONS
Local: burning, itching, stinging, erythema.

INTERACTIONS
Topical corticosteroids: may inhibit antifungal effect.

NURSING CONSIDERATIONS
• If condition persists or worsens or if irritation (burning, itching, stinging, redness) occurs, discontinue use and report this to doctor.
• Use medication for entire treatment period, even though symptoms may have improved. Notify doctor if there is no improvement; after 2 weeks (tinea cruris, corporis and versicolor) or 4 weeks (tinea pedis).
• Cleanse affected area before applying.
• Available as a 1% cream in a water-soluble base.
• Don't use occlusive dressings.
• Hypopigmentation from *tinea versicolor* will resolve gradually.

erythromycin
A/T/S, EryDerm, Staticin ♦

Pregnancy Risk Category: B

MECHANISM OF ACTION
Disrupts protein synthesis.

INDICATIONS & DOSAGE
Superficial skin infections due to susceptible organisms, acne vulgaris—
Adults and children: clean affected area; apply t.i.d. or q.i.d.

ADVERSE REACTIONS
Skin: sensitivity reactions, erythema, burning, *dryness, pruritus.*

INTERACTIONS
None significant.

NURSING CONSIDERATIONS
• Prolonged use may result in overgrowth of nonsusceptible organisms.
• If no improvement or if condition worsens, stop using and notify doctor.
• Wash, rinse, and dry affected areas before application.
• Don't use near eyes, nose, mouth, or other mucous membranes.

gentamicin sulfate
Garamycin♦

Pregnancy Risk Category: C

MECHANISM OF ACTION
Disrupts protein synthesis.

INDICATIONS & DOSAGE
Primary and secondary bacterial infections, superficial burns, skin ulcers, infected insect bites and stings, infected lacerations and abrasions, wounds from minor surgery—
Adults and children over 1 year: rub in small amount gently t.i.d. or q.i.d., with or without gauze dressing.

ADVERSE REACTIONS
Skin: minor skin irritation; possible

photosensitivity; allergic contact dermatitis.

INTERACTIONS
None significant.

NURSING CONSIDERATIONS
• If no improvement or if condition worsens, stop using and report to doctor.
• Should be used in selected patients. Widespread use may lead to resistant organisms.
• Avoid use on large skin lesions or over a wide area because of possible systemic toxic effects.
• Prolonged use may result in overgrowth of nonsusceptible organisms.
• May treat bacterial infections that have not responded to other antibacterial agents.
• Store in cool place.
• Remove crusts before application of gentamicin in impetigo contagiosa.

---

gentian violet (methylrosaniline chloride)◊
Bismuth Violet Solution (1% and 2%), Crystal Violet

Pregnancy Risk Category: C

MECHANISM OF ACTION
Fungistatic and antibacterial activity.

INDICATIONS & DOSAGE
Superficial infections of skin; lesions, except ulcerative lesions of face, particularly Candida albicans—
Adults and children: apply with swab b.i.d. or t.i.d. Keep affected area clean, dry, and exposed to air to prevent spread of infection.

ADVERSE REACTIONS
Skin: *permanent discoloration if applied to granulation tissue;* irritation or ulceration of mucous membranes.

INTERACTIONS
None significant.

NURSING CONSIDERATIONS
• Do not use on ulcerative lesions of the face.
• Apply carefully to avoid undue staining. Will stain skin and clothing.
• Do not use occlusive dressings.
• Tattooing of the skin may occur if applied to granulation tissue.

---

haloprogin
Halotex♦

Pregnancy Risk Category: B

MECHANISM OF ACTION
Fungistatic and fungicidal activity.

INDICATIONS & DOSAGE
Superficial fungal infections (tinea pedis, tinea cruris, tinea corporis, tinea manuum, and tinea versicolor)—
Adults and children: apply liberally b.i.d. for 2 to 3 weeks.

ADVERSE REACTIONS
Skin: burning sensation, irritation, vesicle formation, increased maceration, *pruritus or exacerbation of preexisting lesions.*

INTERACTIONS
None significant.

NURSING CONSIDERATIONS
• Diagnosis should be reconsidered if no improvement in 4 weeks.
• Tell patient to continue using for full treatment period prescribed, even if condition has improved.
• Tell patient to notify doctor if increased irritation occurs.
• Don't allow drug to come in contact with the eyes.

Italicized side effects are common or life-threatening.
*Liquid form contains alcohol.   **May contain tartrazine.

iodochlorhydroxyquin (clioquinol)◇
Quinoform, Vioform♦

Pregnancy Risk Category: C

MECHANISM OF ACTION
Fungistatic and fungicidal activity.

INDICATIONS & DOSAGE
Inflamed skin conditions, including eczema, athlete's foot, and other fungal infections; cutaneous or mucocutaneous mycotic infections caused by Candida *species (monilia)—*
Adults and children over age 2: apply a thin layer b.i.d. or t.i.d., or as directed. Continue for 1 week after cessation of symptoms.

ADVERSE REACTIONS
Skin: *possible burning, itching, acneiform eruptions,* allergic contact dermatitis.

INTERACTIONS
Systemic corticosteroids: possible increased absorption. Use together cautiously.

NURSING CONSIDERATIONS
• Contraindicated in patients with hypersensitivity to iodine or iodine-containing preparations. Contraindicated in tuberculosis, vaccinia, and varicella.
• Don't use to treat diaper rash.
• Note all adverse reactions and precautions of each component in the combination antifungals.
• Presence in urine may cause false-positive result for phenylketonuria (PKU) or inaccurate thyroid function tests. Discontinue at least 1 month before thyroid function tests.
• Drug will stain fabric and hair.

ketoconazole
Nizoral

Pregnancy Risk Category: C

MECHANISM OF ACTION
Inhibits yeast growth by altering the permeability of the cell membrane.

INDICATIONS & DOSAGE
Treatment of tinea corporis, tinea cruris, and tinea versicolor caused by susceptible organisms—
Adults: apply once daily to cover the affected and immediate surrounding area. Apply twice daily, if necessary, in the more resistant cases.

ADVERSE REACTIONS
Skin: severe irritation, pruritus, stinging.
Systemic: localized allergic reaction.

INTERACTIONS
None reported.

NURSING CONSIDERATIONS
• Discontinue if sensitivity or chemical irritation occurs.
• Most patients show improvement soon after treatment begins. However, treatment of tinea cruris or tinea corporis should continue for at least 2 weeks to reduce the possibility of recurrence.
• Check with doctor if condition worsens. The drug may have to be discontinued and diagnosis redetermined.

mafenide acetate
Sulfamylon♦

Pregnancy Risk Category: C

MECHANISM OF ACTION
Interferes with bacterial cellular metabolism.

INDICATIONS & DOSAGE
Adjunctive treatment of second- and

third-degree burns—
Adults and children: apply 1/16″ thickness of cream daily or b.i.d. to cleansed, debrided wounds. Reapply p.r.n. to keep burned area covered.

ADVERSE REACTIONS
Blood: eosinophilia.
Skin: pain, *burning sensation,* rash, itching, swelling, hives, blisters, erythema, facial edema.
Other: *metabolic acidosis.*

INTERACTIONS
None significant.

NURSING CONSIDERATIONS
• Use with caution in acute renal failure and in patients with known hypersensitivity to sulfonamides.
• Closely monitor acid-base balance, especially in the presence of pulmonary and renal dysfunction.
• If acidosis occurs, discontinue use for 24 to 48 hours.
• Can cause pain and burning at application site; if they occur, notify doctor. Severe and prolonged pain may indicate allergy. If other allergic reactions occur, treatment may have to be temporarily discontinued.
• Sometimes difficult to distinguish between adverse reactions and effects of severe burn.
• Cleanse area before applying. Mafenide washes off with water.
• Keep burn areas medicated at all times.
• Bathe patient daily, if possible.
• For burns, using reverse isolation technique with sterile gloves and instruments to apply cream minimizes risk of further wound contamination.

metronidazole 0.75% (topical)
MetroGel

Pregnancy Risk Category: B

MECHANISM OF ACTION
Exact mechanism of action is unknown. Probably exerts an antiinflammatory effect through its antibacterial and antiprotozoal actions.

INDICATIONS AND DOSAGE
Topical treatment of acne rosacea—
Adults: Apply a thin film twice daily to affected area during the morning and evening. Significant results should appear within 3 weeks and continue for the first 9 weeks of therapy.

ADVERSE REACTIONS
EENT: lacrimation (if drug applied in area around the eyes).

INTERACTIONS
Oral anticoagulants: May potentiate anticoagulant effect. Monitor patient for potential adverse effects.

NURSING CONSIDERATIONS
• Contraindicated in patients with hypersensitivity to metronidazole or its other ingredients (such as parabens).
• Instruct patient to avoid use of the drug around the eyes.
• If local reactions occur, advise patient to apply less frequently or to discontinue and contact doctor.
• Use cautiously in patients with history or evidence of blood dyscrasias because chemically-related compounds are associated with blood dyscrasias.
• Topical metronidazole therapy has not been associated with the adverse effects observed with parenteral or oral metronidazole therapy (including disulfiram-like reactions after alcohol ingestion). However, some of the drug can be absorbed following topical use.

Italicized side effects are common or life-threatening.
*Liquid form contains alcohol.   **May contain tartrazine.

Limited clinical experience hasn't shown any of these adverse effects.
• Advise patient to cleanse area thoroughly before use. Patient may use cosmetics after applying the drug.

miconazole nitrate 2%
Micatin, Monistat-Derm Cream and Lotion♦, Monistat 7 Vaginal Cream♦, Monistat 7 Vaginal Suppository♦, Monistat 3 Vaginal Suppository

Pregnancy Risk Category: C

MECHANISM OF ACTION
Controls or destroys fungus by disrupting fungal cell membrane permeability.

INDICATIONS & DOSAGE
Tinea pedis, tinea cruris, tinea corporis, tinea versicolor, cutaneous candidiasis (moniliasis), infections from common dermatophytes—
Adults and children: apply or spray sparingly b.i.d. for 2 to 4 weeks.
Vulvovaginal candidiasis—
Adults: insert 1 applicatorful or suppository (Monistat 7) intravaginally for 7 days at bedtime; repeat course if necessary. Alternatively, insert suppository (Monistat 3) intravaginally for 3 days at bedtime.

ADVERSE REACTIONS
Skin: isolated reports of irritation, burning, maceration.
Other: (with vaginal cream) vulvovaginal burning, itching, or irritation.

INTERACTIONS
None significant.

NURSING CONSIDERATIONS
• For external or intravaginal use only. Keep out of eyes.
• Discontinue if sensitivity or chemical irritation occurs.
• Tell patient to continue using for full treatment period prescribed, even if condition has improved.
• Do not use occlusive dressings.
• When using intravaginal forms, tell patient to cautiously insert high into the vagina with applicator provided.
• Concurrent use of intravaginal forms and certain latex products, such as vaginal contraceptive diaphragms are not recommended because of possible interaction.

mupirocin
Bactroban

Pregnancy Risk Category: C

MECHANISM OF ACTION
Inhibits bacterial protein and RNA synthesis.

INDICATIONS & DOSAGE
Treatment of common bacterial skin infections caused by susceptible bacteria—
Adults and children: apply to affected areas b.i.d. to t.i.d.

ADVERSE REACTIONS
Local: burning, itching, stinging, rash.

INTERACTIONS
None reported.

NURSING CONSIDERATIONS
• Mupirocin has proven especially useful in the treatment of impetigo in early clinical trials.
• Local reactions appear to be from the polyethylene glycol vehicle.
• If no improvement or condition worsens, notify doctor immediately.
• Prolonged use may cause overgrowth of nonsusceptible bacteria and fungi.
• Not intended for use on burns.
• Do not use in eye.

naftifine
Naftin

Pregnancy Risk Category: B

MECHANISM OF ACTION
Inhibits sterol biosynthesis in susceptible fungi by blocking the actions of the enzyme squalene 2,3 epoxidase. A broad spectrum fungicidal agent.

INDICATIONS & DOSAGE
Treatment of tinea corporis and tinea cruris—
Adults: Apply to affected area b.i.d.

ADVERSE REACTIONS
Local: burning, dryness, itching, stinging, local irritation.

INTERACTIONS
None significant.

NURSING CONSIDERATIONS
• Not for opthalmic use. Instruct patient to keep cream away from mucous membranes (eyes, nose, and mouth).
• Instruct patient to wash hands after application.
• Therapy should be reevaluated if there is not improvement after 4 weeks.
• Instruct patient to discontinue therapy and notify doctor if irritation or sensitivity develops.
• Cultures should be done to confirm diagnosis before therapy.

neomycin sulfate
Mycifradin♦♦, Myciguent♦

Pregnancy Risk Category: C

MECHANISM OF ACTION
Disrupts protein synthesis.

INDICATIONS & DOSAGE
Topical bacterial infections, burns, wounds, skin grafts, following surgical procedure, primary pyodermas,
pruritus, trophic ulcerations, otitis externa—
Adults and children: rub in small quantity gently b.i.d., t.i.d., or as directed.

ADVERSE REACTIONS
Skin: *rashes, contact dermatitis,* urticaria.
Other: *possible nephrotoxicity, ototoxicity, and neuromuscular blockade; possible systemic absorption when used on extensive areas of the body.*

INTERACTIONS
None significant.

NURSING CONSIDERATIONS
• If no improvement or if condition worsens, stop using and report to doctor.
• Don't use on more than 20% of the body surface and on patient with impaired renal function unless risk/benefit ratio has been assessed.
• Prolonged use may result in overgrowth of nonsusceptible organisms.
• In those combination products that contain corticosteroids, use of occlusive dressings increases corticosteroid absorption and the likelihood of systemic effects.
• Enhanced systemic absorption occurs on denuded or abraded areas.
• Watch for signs of hypersensitivity and contact dermatitis.
• Evaluate patient for signs of ototoxicity with prolonged or extended use.

nitrofurazone
Furacin♦

Pregnancy Risk Category: C

MECHANISM OF ACTION
Inhibits bacterial enzymes.

INDICATIONS & DOSAGE
Adjunctive treatment of second- and third-degree burns (especially when

---

Italicized side effects are common or life-threatening.
*Liquid form contains alcohol.   **May contain tartrazine.

resistance to other antibiotics and sulfonamides occurs); prevention of skin allograft rejection—
Adults and children: apply directly to lesion daily or every few days, depending on severity of burn.

ADVERSE REACTIONS
GU: possible renal toxicity.
Skin: *erythema, pruritus,* burning, edema, severe reactions (vesiculation, denudation, ulceration), *allergic contact dermatitis.*

INTERACTIONS
None significant.

NURSING CONSIDERATIONS
• Use cautiously in patients with known or suspected renal impairment. Monitor serum creatinine regularly.
• If irritation, sensitization, or infection occurs, discontinue use.
• When using wet dressing, protect skin around wound with zinc oxide ointment.
• Cleanse wound as indicated by doctor before each dressing change.
• Solution should be stored in tight, light-resistant containers (brown bottles). Avoid exposure of solution at all times to direct light, prolonged heat, and alkaline materials.
• Drug may discolor in light but is still usable because it retains its potency.
• Discard cloudy solutions if warming to 55° to 60° C. (131° to 140° F.) does not restore clarity.
• Use reverse isolation and/or sterile application technique to prevent further wound contamination.

---

nystatin
Mycostatin♦, Nadostine♦♦, Nilstat
Pregnancy Risk Category: B

MECHANISM OF ACTION
Alters the permeability of the cell membrane of fungi.

INDICATIONS & DOSAGE
Infant eczema, pruritus ani and vulvae, localized forms of candidiasis—
Adults and children: apply to affected area b.i.d. for 2 weeks.
Vulvovaginal candidiasis—
Adults: one vaginal tablet daily or b.i.d. for 14 days.

ADVERSE REACTIONS
Skin: occasional contact dermatitis from preservatives present in some formulations.

INTERACTIONS
None significant.

NURSING CONSIDERATIONS
• Generally well tolerated by all age-groups, including debilitated infants.
• Preparation does not stain skin or mucous membranes.
• Cream is recommended for intertriginous areas; powder, for very moist areas; ointment, for dry areas.
• Tell patient to continue using for full treatment period prescribed, even if condition has improved. Immuno-suppressed patients may use the drug chronically.
• Do not use occlusive dressings.
• Store vaginal tablets in the refrigerator.

---

oxiconazole nitrate
Oxistat
Pregnancy Risk Category: B

MECHANISM OF ACTION
Inhibits ergosterol synthesis in susceptible fungal organisms, thereby weakening cytoplasmic membrane integrity.

INDICATIONS AND DOSAGE
Topical treatment of dermal infections caused by tinea rubrum and tinea mentagrophytes (tinea pedis, tinea

---

cruris, and tinea corporis)—
Adults: Apply to affected area once
daily (in the evening) for 2 weeks (1
month for tinea pedis).

ADVERSE REACTIONS
Skin: itching, burning, irritation,
maceration, erythema, fissuring.

INTERACTIONS
None reported.

NURSING CONSIDERATIONS
• Contraindicated in patients with hypersensitivity to oxiconazole nitrate.
• Be sure patient understands that
drug is for external use only. Instruct
him to avoid using it near the eyes.
• Animal studies have shown that oxiconazole is excreted in breast milk.
Drug should be used with caution in
breast-feeding women.

---

silver sulfadiazine
Flamazine♦♦, Silvadene
Pregnancy Risk Category: C

MECHANISM OF ACTION
Acts upon cell membrane and cell
wall.

INDICATIONS & DOSAGE
*Prevention and treatment of wound in-
fection especially for second- and
third-degree burns—*
Adults and children: apply ¹⁄₁₆″
thickness of ointment to cleansed and
debrided burn wound, then apply
daily or b.i.d.

ADVERSE REACTIONS
Blood: *neutropenia (in 3% to 5%) of
those receiving extensive applications.*
Skin: pain, burning, rashes, itching.

INTERACTIONS
Topical proteolytic enzymes: inactivity
of enzymes when used together. Do
not use together.

NURSING CONSIDERATIONS
• Contraindicated in premature and
newborn infants during first month of
life. (Drug may increase possibility of
kernicterus.) Use with caution in hypersensitivity to sulfonamides.
• If hepatic or renal dysfunction occurs, consider discontinuing drug.
• Inspect patient's skin daily, and note
any changes. Notify doctor if burning
or excessive pain develops.
• Use only on affected areas. Keep
medicated at all times.
• For patients with extensive burns,
monitor serum sulfadiazine concentrations and renal function, and check
urine for sulfa crystals.
• Bathe patient daily, if possible.
• Discard darkened cream.
• Reverse isolation and/or sterile application technique recommended to
prevent wound contamination.

---

tetracycline hydrochloride
Topicycline
Pregnancy Risk Category: D

MECHANISM OF ACTION
Disrupts protein synthesis.

INDICATIONS & DOSAGE
Acne vulgaris—
Adults and children over 12 years:
apply generously to affected areas
b.i.d. until skin is thoroughly wet.

ADVERSE REACTIONS
Skin: temporary stinging or burning
on application; slight yellowing of
treated skin, especially in patients
with light complexions; severe dermatitis; treated skin areas fluoresce under black lights.

INTERACTIONS
None significant.

NURSING CONSIDERATIONS
• If no improvement or if condition
worsens, stop using and notify doctor.

Italicized side effects are common or life-threatening.
*Liquid form contains alcohol.   **May contain tartrazine.

• Prolonged use may result in over-growth of nonsusceptible organisms.
• Patient may continue normal use of cosmetics.
• Store at room temperature, away from excessive heat.
• Medication to be used by one person only. Tell patient not to share with family members.
• Apply in morning and evening. Warn that drug should be used or discarded within 2 months.
• Explain that floating plug in bottle of Topicycline—an inert and harmless result of proper reconstitution of the preparation—shouldn't be removed.
• Serum levels with topical tetracycline HCl are much lower than those for orally administered drug, so significant systemic effects are unlikely.
• To control flow rate of solution, increase or decrease pressure of the applicator against the skin.

---

tolnaftate
Aftate, Pitrex♦♦, Tinactin♦

Pregnancy Risk Category: C

MECHANISM OF ACTION
Fungistatic and fungicidal activity.

INDICATIONS & DOSAGE
Superficial fungal infections of the skin, infections due to common pathogenic fungi, tinea pedis, tinea cruris, tinea corporis, tinea manuum, tinea versicolor—
Adults and children: ¼″ to ½″ ribbon of cream or 3 drops of lotion to cover about the size of one hand; same amount of cream or 3 drops of lotion to cover the toes and interdigital webs of one foot. Apply and massage gently into skin b.i.d. for 2 weeks, up to 6 weeks.

ADVERSE REACTIONS
None significant.

INTERACTIONS
None significant.

NURSING CONSIDERATIONS
• Discontinue if condition worsens. Check with doctor.
• Odorless, greaseless. Won't stain or discolor skin, hair, nails, or clothing.
• Only a small quantity of cream or lotion is needed; area should not be wet with solution when application is completed.
• Commonly available product used to treat athlete's foot (tinea pedis). If no improvement after 10 days, consult doctor.
• Tell patient to continue using for full treatment period prescribed, even if condition has improved.
• Don't use as a side agent to treat hair or nail infections. Will not eradicate fungus from these structures.
• Powder or aerosol may continue to be used inside socks and shoes of persons susceptible to tinea infections.

---

undecylenic acid (zinc undecylenate)
Cruex, Desenex♦, NP-27, Ting

Pregnancy Risk Category: C

MECHANISM OF ACTION
Fungistatic and fungicidal activity.

INDICATIONS & DOSAGE
Athlete's foot and ringworm of the body exclusive of nails and hairy areas—
Adults and children: apply b.i.d. to thoroughly cleansed area.

ADVERSE REACTIONS
Skin: possible irritation in hypersensitive person.

INTERACTIONS
None significant.

NURSING CONSIDERATIONS
• Tell patient to continue using for

---

full treatment period prescribed, even if condition has improved.
• Apply for at least 2 weeks to minimize risk of relapse.
• Liquids are preferable for hairy areas while powders are preferable in moist areas, for example, between skin folds.

Scabicides and pediculicides

benzyl benzoate lotion
copper oleate solution
   (with tetrahydronaphthalene)◊
crotamiton
lindane
permethrin
pyrethrins◊

COMBINATION PRODUCTS
None.

benzyl benzoate lotion
Scabanca◆◆

Pregnancy Risk Category: C

MECHANISM OF ACTION
Unknown.

INDICATIONS & DOSAGE
Parasitic infestation (scabies, Phthirus pubis)—
Adults and children: first, scrub entire body with soap and water. Remove scales or crusts. Then apply the 28% lotion undiluted over entire body, except the face, while still damp. Be sure to apply around nails. Let dry. Apply second coat on the most involved areas. Bathe after 48 hours. Adults require 30 ml. Children require 20 ml.
Pediculosis capitis—
Adults and children: apply to scalp and leave on overnight; shampoo out in morning. Repeat next night if necessary.

ADVERSE REACTIONS
Skin: *irritation, itching; contact dermatitis with repeated applications.*

INTERACTIONS
None significant.

NURSING CONSIDERATIONS
• Contraindicated when skin is raw or inflamed. Notify doctor immediately if skin irritation or hypersensitivity develops; tell patient to discontinue drug and to wash it off skin.
• If live mites or new lesions occur, retreatment may be indicated in 7 to 10 days.
• Preferred over lindane for treatment of infants, young children, and pregnant or breast-feeding women.
• Do not apply to face, eyes, mucous membranes, or urethral meatus. If accidental contact with eyes does occur, flush with water and notify doctor.
• Instruct patient to change and sterilize (boil, launder, dry clean, or apply very hot iron) all clothing and bed linen after drug is washed off.
• Itching may continue for several weeks; this does not indicate that therapy is ineffective. Reassure patient that itching will cease.
• Topical corticosteroids may be needed if dermatitis develops from scratching.
• After application for lice infestation, use a fine comb dipped in white vinegar on hair to remove nits from hairy areas.
• Instruct patient to reapply if drug is washed off during treatment time.
• Don't apply to infant's or small children's hands because they will put hands in their mouths.
• Hospitalized patients should be placed in isolation with linen-han-

---

dling precautions until treatment is completed.
• Store drug in light-resistant container; avoid exposure to excessive heat.

copper oleate solution (with tetrahydro-naphthalene)◊
Cuprex

Pregnancy Risk Category: C

MECHANISM OF ACTION
Unknown.

INDICATIONS & DOSAGE
Parasitic infestation (pediculoses capitis and pubis)—
Adults and children: first, scrub entire body with soap and water. Apply gently and sparingly 3 to 4 tablespoonfuls onto affected areas; after 15 minutes wash off with soap and water.

ADVERSE REACTIONS
Skin: *irritation with repeated use, or if used on raw or inflamed skin.*

INTERACTIONS
None significant.

NURSING CONSIDERATIONS
• Contraindicated when skin is raw or inflamed, or when there is a severe infection. Notify doctor immediately if skin irritation or hypersensitivity develops; tell patient to discontinue drug and to wash it off skin.
• Preferred to lindane in treatment of infants, young children, pregnant or breast-feeding women.
• Do not apply more than twice within 48 hours.
• Do not apply to face, eyes, mucous membranes, or urethral meatus. If accidental contact with eyes does occur, flush with water and notify doctor.
• Instruct patient to change and sterilize (boil, launder, dry clean, or apply very hot iron) all clothing and bed

linen after application.
• After application, use a fine comb dipped in white vinegar on hair to remove nits.
• Tendency for overuse of pediculicides. Estimate amount needed.
• Hospitalized patients should be placed in isolation with linen-handling precautions until treatment is completed.
• Solution is flammable. Store away from direct sunlight or open flame.
• If necessary, may retreat in 7 to 10 days.

crotamiton
Eurax◆

Pregnancy Risk Category: C

MECHANISM OF ACTION
Unknown.

INDICATIONS & DOSAGE
Parasitic infestation (scabies)—
Adults and children: scrub entire body with soap and water. Then, apply a thin layer of cream over entire body, from chin down (with special attention to folds, creases, interdigital spaces, and genital area). Apply second coat in 24 hours. Wait additional 48 hours, then wash off.
General itching—
apply locally b.i.d. or t.i.d.

ADVERSE REACTIONS
Skin: *irritation.*

INTERACTIONS
None significant.

NURSING CONSIDERATIONS
• Contraindicated when skin is raw or inflamed. Notify doctor immediately if skin irritation or hypersensitivity develops; tell patient to discontinue drug and to wash it off skin.
• Do not apply to face, eyes, mucous membranes, or urethral meatus. If accidental contact with eyes does occur,

---

Italicized side effects are common or life-threatening.
*Liquid form contains alcohol.   **May contain tartrazine.

flush with water and notify doctor.
• Instruct patient to change and sterilize (boil, launder, dry clean, or apply very hot iron) all clothing and bed linen after drug is washed off.
• Topical corticosteroids may be needed if dermatitis develops from scratching.
• Tendency to overuse scabicides. Estimate amount needed.
• Question other family members and sexual contacts about infestation.
• Instruct patient to reapply if drug is washed off during treatment time.
• Hospitalized patients should be placed in isolation with special linen-handling precautions until treatment is completed.

lindane
gBh♦♦, Kwell, Kwellada♦♦, Scabene

Pregnancy Risk Category: C

MECHANISM OF ACTION
Appears to inhibit neuronal membrane function in arthropods.

INDICATIONS & DOSAGE
Parasitic infestation (scabies, pediculosis)—
Adults and children: scrub entire body with soap and water.
Cream or lotion—apply thin layer over entire skin surface (with special attention to folds, creases, interdigital spaces, and genital area) for scabies, or to hairy areas for pediculosis. After 12 hours, wash off drug. If second application is needed, wait 1 week before repeating, but never more than twice in a week.
Shampoo—apply 30 ml undiluted to affected area and work into lather for 4 to 5 minutes. Rinse thoroughly and rub with dry towel.

ADVERSE REACTIONS
CNS: dizziness, seizures.
Skin: irritation with repeated use.

INTERACTIONS
None significant.

NURSING CONSIDERATIONS
• Contraindicated when skin is raw or inflamed. Notify doctor immediately if skin irritation or hypersensitivity develops; tell patient to discontinue drug and to wash it off skin.
• Use cautiously in infants and young children as there's a greater risk for CNS toxicity in this group.
• Do not apply to open areas or acutely inflamed skin, or to face, eyes, mucous membranes, or urethral meatus. If accidental contact with eyes does occur, flush with water and notify doctor. Avoid inhaling vapors.
• Discourage repeated use, which can lead to skin irritation and systemic toxicity. Repeat use only if live lice or nits are found after 1 week.
• Warn patient that itching may continue for several weeks after effective treatment, especially in scabies.
• Topical corticosteroids or oral antihistamines may be needed for itching.
• Instruct patient to change and sterilize (boil, launder, dry clean, or apply very hot iron) all clothing and bed linen after drug is washed off.
• After application, use a fine comb dipped in white vinegar on hair to remove nits.
• Lindane shampoo can be used to clean combs or brushes; wash them thoroughly afterward. Warn patient not to use routinely.
• Instruct patient to reapply if drug is washed off during treatment time.
• Hospitalized patients should be placed in isolation with special linen-handling precautions until treatment is completed.
• Extremely toxic to CNS if accidentally swallowed.

permethrin
Nix

Pregnancy Risk Category: B

MECHANISM OF ACTION
Acts on the parasites' nerve cells to disrupt the sodium channel current, causing paralysis of the parasite.

INDICATIONS & DOSAGE
Treatment of infestation with Pediculus humanus capitis (head lice) and its nits—
Adults and children: use after hair has been washed with shampoo, rinsed with water, and towel-dried. Apply a sufficient amount (25 to 50 ml) of liquid to saturate the hair and scalp. Allow to remain on hair for 10 minutes before rinsing off with water.

ADVERSE REACTIONS
Skin: itching, burning, stinging, tingling, numbness or scalp discomfort, mild erythema, rash on the scalp.

INTERACTIONS
None reported.

NURSING CONSIDERATIONS
• Contraindicated in patients hypersensitive to pyrethrins or chrysanthemums.
• Don't use in infants because their skin is more permeable than that of children or adults.
• A single treatment is usually all that is necessary. Combing of nits is not required for effectiveness, but drug package supplies a fine-tooth comb for cosmetic use as desired.
• A second application may be necessary if lice are observed 7 days after the initial application.
• Head lice infestation is frequently accompanied by pruritus, erythema, and edema. Reassure patient that treatment with permethrin may temporarily worsen these symptoms.
• Permethrin has been shown to be at least as effective as lindane (Kwell) in treating head lice.
• Not indicated to treat scabies.

pyrethrins◇
A-200 Pyrinate, Barc, Pyrinyl, RID, TISIT, Triple X

Pregnancy Risk Category: C

MECHANISM OF ACTION
Acts as contact poison that disrupts the parasite's nervous system, causing the parasite's paralysis and death.

INDICATIONS & DOSAGE
Treatment of infestations of head, body, and pubic (crab) lice and their eggs—
Adults and children: apply to hair, scalp, or other infested area until entirely wet. Allow to remain for 10 minutes, but no longer. Wash thoroughly with warm water and soap, or shampoo. Remove dead lice and eggs with fine-toothed comb. Treatment may be repeated, if necessary, but don't exceed two applications within 24 hours. May repeat in 7 to 10 days to kill newly hatched lice.

ADVERSE REACTIONS
Skin: *irritation with repeated use.*

INTERACTIONS
None significant.

NURSING CONSIDERATIONS
• Contraindicated when skin is raw or inflamed. Notify doctor immediately if skin irritation develops; tell patient to discontinue drug and to wash it off skin. Also contraindicated in patients allergic to ragweed. Use cautiously in infants and small children.
• Do not apply to open areas or acutely inflamed skin, or to face, eyes, mucous membranes, or urethral meatus. If accidental contact with eyes does occur, flush with water and notify doctor.

Italicized side effects are common or life-threatening.
*Liquid form contains alcohol.   **May contain tartrazine.

• Discourage repeated use, which can lead to skin irritation and possible systemic toxicity.

• Topical corticosteroids or oral antihistamines may be needed if dermatitis develops from scratching.

• Instruct patient to change and sterilize (boil, launder, dry clean, or apply very hot iron) all clothing and bed linen after drug is washed off.

• Products containing pyrethrins are available without prescription. Some authorities believe pyrethrins and lindane (Kwell) are equally effective for lice infestation and that pyrethins are less hazardous.

• Not effective against scabies.

92

Topical corticosteroids

alclometasone dipropionate
amcinonide
betamethasone benzoate
betamethasone dipropionate
betamethasone valerate
clobetasol propionate
clocortolone pivalate
desonide
desoximetasone
dexamethasone
dexamethasone sodium
  phosphate
diflorasone diacetate
fluocinolone acetonide
fluocinonide
flurandrenolide
halcinonide
hydrocortisone◇
hydrocortisone acetate◇
hydrocortisone valerate
methylprednisolone acetate
mometasone furoate
triamcinolone acetonide

COMBINATION PRODUCTS
Corticosteroids for topical use are
commonly combined with antibiotics,
antifungals, and sulfonamides. (See
also Chapter 14, SULFONAMIDES, and
Chapter 72, ANTIBIOTIC ANTINEO-
PLASTIC AGENTS.)

---

alclometasone dipropionate
Aclovate

Pregnancy Risk Category: C

MECHANISM OF ACTION
Diffuses across cell membranes to
form complexes with specific cytoplasmic receptors.

INDICATIONS & DOSAGE
*Inflammation of corticosteroid-respon-
sive dermatoses—*
Adults: apply a thin film to affected
areas b.i.d. or t.i.d. Gently massage
until the medication disappears.

ADVERSE REACTIONS
Skin: burning, itching, irritation, dryness, folliculitis, striae, acneiform
eruptions, perioral dermatitis, hypopigmentation, hypertrichosis, allergic
contact dermatitis. With occlusive
dressings: *secondary infection, maceration, atrophy, striae, miliaria.*

INTERACTIONS
None significant.

NURSING CONSIDERATIONS
• Use cautiously in viral skin diseases, such as varicella, vaccinia, and
herpes simplex; in fungal infections;
and in bacterial skin infections.
• Avoid application near eyes or mucous membranes. Do not apply to
face, armpits, groin, or under breasts
unless specifically ordered.
• Systemic absorption especially
likely with occlusive dressings, prolonged treatment, or application to extensive body surface.
• Stop drug and notify doctor if patient develops signs of systemic absorption, skin irritation or ulceration,
hypersensitivity, or infection. (If antifungals or antibiotics are being used
concurrently, and infection does not
respond immediately, corticosteroids
should be discontinued until infection
is controlled.)

Italicized side effects are common or life-threatening.
*Liquid form contains alcohol.   **May contain tartrazine.

• Before applying, wash skin gently. To prevent damage to skin, rub medication in gently, leaving a thin coat. When treating hairy sites, part hair and apply directly to lesion.

• Occlusive dressing (if ordered): Apply cream, then cover with a thin, pliable, nonflammable plastic film; seal to adjacent normal skin with hypoallergenic tape. Minimize adverse reactions by using occlusive dressing intermittently. Don't leave in place longer than 16 hours each day. Occlusive dressings should not be used in presence of infections or with weeping or exudative lesions.

• Notify doctor and remove occlusive dressing if fever develops.

• Change dressings as ordered by doctor. Inspect skin for infection, striae, and atrophy. Discontinue drug and notify doctor if these occur.

• Treatment should be continued for a few days after clearing of lesions to prevent recurrence.

---

amcinonide
Cyclocort♦

Pregnancy Risk Category: C

MECHANISM OF ACTION
Diffuses across cell membranes and complexes with specific cytoplasmic receptors.

INDICATIONS & DOSAGE
Inflammation of corticosteroid-responsive dermatoses—
Adults and children: apply a light film to affected areas b.i.d. or t.i.d. Cream should be rubbed in gently and thoroughly until it disappears.

ADVERSE REACTIONS
Skin: burning, itching, irritation, dryness, folliculitis, striae, acneiform eruptions, perioral dermatitis, hypopigmentation, hypertrichosis, allergic contact dermatitis. With occlusive dressings: *secondary infection, macer-ation, atrophy, striae, miliaria.*

INTERACTIONS
None significant.

NURSING CONSIDERATIONS
• Use cautiously in viral diseases of skin, such as varicella, vaccinia, herpes simplex; fungal infections; bacterial skin infections.

• Avoid application near eyes or mucous membranes. Do not use on face, armpits, groin, in ear canal, or under breasts unless specifically ordered.

• Systemic absorption especially likely with occlusive dressings, prolonged treatment, or extensive body-surface treatment.

• When used in young children, avoid the use of plastic pants or tight-fitting diapers in treated areas.

• Stop drug and notify doctor if patient develops signs of systemic absorption, skin irritation or ulceration, hypersensitivity, or infection. (If antifungals or antibiotics are being used with corticosteroids and infection does not respond immediately, corticosteroids should be stopped until infection is controlled.)

• Before applying, gently wash skin. To prevent damage to skin, rub medication in gently, leaving a thin coat. When treating hairy sites, part hair and apply directly to lesion.

• Occlusive dressing (if ordered): apply cream, then cover with a thin, pliable, nonflammable plastic film; seal to adjacent normal skin with hypoallergenic tape. Minimize adverse reactions by using occlusive dressing intermittently. Don't leave in place longer than 16 hours each day. Occlusive dressings should not be used in presence of infections or with weeping or exudative lesions.

• For patient with eczematous dermatitis who may develop irritation with adhesive material, hold dressing in place with gauze, elastic bandages, stockings, or stockinette.

• Notify doctor and remove occlusive dressing if fever develops.
• Change dressings as ordered by doctor. Inspect skin for infection, striae, and atrophy. Discontinue drug and notify doctor if these occur.
• Treatment should be continued for a few days after clearing of lesions to prevent recurrence.

---

betamethasone benzoate
Beben♦, Benisone, Uticort

Pregnancy Risk Category: C

MECHANISM OF ACTION
Diffuses across cell membranes and complexes with specific cytoplasmic receptors.

INDICATIONS & DOSAGE
Inflammation of corticosteroid-responsive dermatoses—
Adults and children: clean area; apply cream, lotion, or gel sparingly daily to q.i.d.

ADVERSE REACTIONS
Skin: burning, itching, irritation, dryness, folliculitis, striae, acneiform eruptions, perioral dermatitis, hypopigmentation, hypertrichosis, allergic contact dermatitis. With occlusive dressings: *secondary infection, maceration, atrophy, striae, miliaria.*

INTERACTIONS
None significant.

NURSING CONSIDERATIONS
• Use cautiously in viral diseases of skin, such as varicella, vaccinia, herpes simplex; fungal infections; bacterial skin infections.
• Avoid application near eyes, mucous membranes, or in ear canal.
• Due to alcohol content of vehicle, gel preparations may cause mild, transient stinging, especially if used on or near excoriated skin.
• Systemic absorption especially likely with occlusive dressings, prolonged treatment, or extensive body-surface treatment.
• When used in young children, avoid the use of plastic pants or tight-fitting diapers in treated areas.
• Stop drug and notify doctor if patient develops signs of systemic absorption, skin irritation or ulceration, hypersensitivity, or infection. (If antifungals or antibiotics are being used with corticosteroids and infection does not respond immediately, corticosteroids should be stopped until infection is controlled.)
• Before applying, gently wash skin. To prevent damage to skin, rub medication in gently, leaving a thin coat. When treating hairy sites, part hair and apply directly to lesion.
• Occlusive dressing (if ordered): Apply cream, then cover with a thin, pliable, nonflammable plastic film; seal to adjacent normal skin with hypoallergenic tape. Minimize adverse reactions by using occlusive dressing intermittently. Don't leave in place longer than 16 hours each day. Occlusive dressings should not be used in presence of infections or with weeping or exudative lesions.
• For patient with eczematous dermatitis who may develop irritation with adhesive material, hold dressing in place with gauze, elastic bandages, stockings, or stockinette.
• Notify doctor and remove occlusive dressing if fever develops.
• Change dressings as ordered by doctor. Inspect skin for infection, striae, and atrophy. Discontinue drug and notify doctor if these occur.
• Treatment should be continued for a few days after clearing of lesions to prevent recurrence.

Italicized side effects are common or life-threatening.
*Liquid form contains alcohol.   **May contain tartrazine.

betamethasone dipropionate
Alphatrex, Diprolene, Diprosone♦, Maxivate, Valnac

Pregnancy Risk Category: C

MECHANISM OF ACTION
Diffuses across cell membranes and complexes with specific cytoplasmic receptors.

INDICATIONS & DOSAGE
Inflammation of corticosteroid-responsive dermatoses—
Adults and children over age 12: clean area; apply cream, lotion, or ointment sparingly b.i.d.
Aerosol—Direct spray onto affected area from a distance of 6″ (15 cm) for 3 seconds t.i.d. to q.i.d. Maximum dosage is 45 g/week.

ADVERSE REACTIONS
Skin: burning, itching, irritation, dryness, folliculitis, perioral dermatitis, allergic contact dermatitis, hypopigmentation, hypertrichosis, acneiform eruptions, *maceration of skin, secondary infection, atrophy, striae, miliaria.*

INTERACTIONS
None significant.

NURSING CONSIDERATIONS
• Use cautiously in viral diseases of skin, such as varicella, vaccinia, herpes simplex; fungal infections; bacterial skin infections.
• Avoid application near eyes, mucous membranes, or in ear canal.
• Systemic absorption especially likely with occlusive dressings, prolonged treatment, or extensive body-surface treatment.
• Betamethasone dipropionate should not be used with occlusive dressings. Treated areas of skin should not be bandaged, covered, or wrapped.
• Stop drug and notify doctor if patient develops signs of systemic absorption, skin irritation or ulceration, hypersensitivity, or infection. (If antifungals or antibiotics are being used with corticosteroids and infection does not respond immediately, corticosteroids should be stopped until infection is controlled.)
• Before applying, gently wash skin. To prevent damage to skin, rub medication in gently, leaving a thin coat. When treating hairy sites, part hair and apply directly to lesion.
• Aerosol preparation contains alcohol and may produce irritation or burning in open lesions. When using about the face, cover patient's eyes and warn against inhalation of spray. To avoid freezing tissues, do not spray longer than 3 seconds or closer than 6″.
• Change dressing as ordered by doctor. Inspect skin for infection, striae, and atrophy. Discontinue drug and notify doctor if these occur.

betamethasone valerate
Betatrex, Beta-Val, Betnovate♦♦, Betnovate 1/2♦♦, Celestoderm-V♦♦, Celestoderm-V/2♦♦, Valisone♦

Pregnancy Risk Category: C

MECHANISM OF ACTION
Diffuses across cell membranes and complexes with specific cytoplasmic receptors.

INDICATIONS & DOSAGE
Inflammation of corticosteroid-responsive dermatoses—
Adults and children: clean area; apply cream, lotion, ointment, or aerosol sparingly daily to q.i.d.
Betnovate 1/2 and Celestoderm-V/2 contain less betamethasone.

ADVERSE REACTIONS
Skin: burning, itching, irritation, dryness, folliculitis, hypertrichosis, hypopigmentation, acneiform eruptions,

---

perioral dermatitis, allergic contact dermatitis.With occlusive dressings: *maceration of skin, secondary infection, atrophy, striae, miliaria.*

INTERACTIONS
None significant.

NURSING CONSIDERATIONS
• Use cautiously in viral diseases of skin, such as varicella, vaccinia, herpes simplex; fungal infections; bacterial skin infections.
• Avoid application near eyes, mucous membranes, or in ear canal.
• Systemic absorption especially likely with occlusive dressings, prolonged treatment, or extensive body-surface treatment.
• When used in children, avoid the use of plastic pants or tight-fitting diapers in treated areas.
• Stop drug and notify doctor if patient develops signs of systemic absorption, skin irritation or ulceration, hypersensitivity, or infection. (If antifungals or antibiotics are being used with corticosteroids and infection does not respond immediately, corticosteroids should be stopped until infection is controlled.)
• Before applying, gently wash skin. To prevent damage to skin, rub medication in gently, leaving a thin coat. When treating hairy sites, part hair and apply directly to lesions.
• Occlusive dressing (if ordered): Apply cream or ointment, then cover with a thin, pliable, nonflammable plastic film; seal to adjacent normal skin with hypoallergenic tape. Minimize adverse reactions by using occlusive dressing intermittently. Don't leave in place longer than 16 hours each day. Occlusive dressings should not be used in presence of infection or with weeping or exudative lesions.
• For patient with eczematous dermatitis who may develop irritation with adhesive material, hold dressing in place with gauze, elastic bandages, stockings, or stockinette.
• Notify doctor and remove occlusive dressing if fever develops.
• Change dressing as ordered by doctor. Inspect skin for infection, striae, and atrophy. Discontinue drug and notify doctor if these occur.
• Treatment should be continued for a few days after clearing of lesions to prevent recurrence.

clobetasol propionate
Temovate

Pregnancy Risk Category: C

MECHANISM OF ACTION
Diffuses across cell membranes and forms complexes with specific cytoplasmic receptors.

INDICATIONS & DOSAGE
Inflammation of corticosteroid-responsive dermatoses—
Adults: apply a thin layer to affected skin areas b.i.d., once in the morning and once at night. Do not use more than 50 g of cream or ointment per week. Therapy should be limited to a maximum of 14 days.

ADVERSE REACTIONS
Skin: burning, itching, irritation, dryness, folliculitis, perioral dermatitis, allergic contact dermatitis, hypopigmentation, hypertrichosis, acneiform eruptions.

INTERACTIONS
None significant.

NURSING CONSIDERATIONS
• Use cautiously in viral skin diseases, such as varicella, vaccinia, herpes simplex; fungal infections; bacterial skin infections.
• Clobetasol is a potent, fluoridated corticosteroid. Warn patient not to use for longer than 14 consecutive days.
• Avoid application near eyes, mu-

cous membranes, or in ear canal.
• Occlusive dressings should not be used. Treated areas of skin should not be bandaged, covered, or wrapped.
• Stop drug and notify doctor if patient develops signs of systemic absorption, skin irritation or ulceration, hypersensitivity, or infection. (If antifungals or antibiotics are being used with corticosteroids and infection does not respond immediately, corticosteroids should be stopped until infection is controlled.)
• Before applying, gently wash skin. To prevent damage to skin, rub medication in gently, leaving a thin coat. When treating hairy sites, part hair and apply directly to lesions.
• Inspect skin for infection, striae, and atrophy. Discontinue drug and notify doctor if these occur.
• Do not refrigerate.

clocortolone pivalate
Cloderm

Pregnancy Risk Category: C

MECHANISM OF ACTION
Diffuses across cell membranes and complexes with specific cytoplasmic receptors.

INDICATIONS & DOSAGE
Inflammation of corticosteroid-responsive dermatoses, such as atopic dermatitis, contact dermatitis, seborrheic dermatitis—
Adults and children: apply cream sparingly to affected areas one to four times daily and rub in gently.

ADVERSE REACTIONS
Skin: burning, itching, irritation, dryness, folliculitis, striae, acneiform eruptions, perioral dermatitis, hypertrichosis, hypopigmentation, allergic contact dermatitis. With occlusive dressings: *secondary infection, maceration, atrophy, striae, miliaria.*

INTERACTIONS
None significant.

NURSING CONSIDERATIONS
• Use cautiously in viral diseases of skin, such as varicella, vaccinia, herpes simplex; fungal infections; bacterial skin infections.
• Avoid application near eyes or mucous membranes.
• Systemic absorption especially likely with occlusive dressings, prolonged treatment, or extensive body-surface treatment.
• When used in young children, avoid the use of plastic pants or tight-fitting diapers in treated areas.
• Stop drug and notify doctor if patient develops signs of systemic absorption, skin irritation or ulceration, hypersensitivity, or infection. (If antifungals or antibiotics are being used with corticosteroids and infection does not respond immediately, corticosteroids should be stopped until infection is controlled.)
• Before applying, gently wash skin. To prevent damage to skin, rub medication in gently, leaving a thin coat. When treating hairy sites, part hair and apply directly to lesion.
• Occlusive dressing (if ordered): Apply cream, then cover with a thin, pliable, nonflammable plastic film; seal to adjacent normal skin with hypoallergenic tape. Minimize adverse reactions by using occlusive dressing intermittently. Don't leave in place longer than 16 hours each day. Occlusive dressings should not be used in presence of infections or with weeping or exudative lesions.
• For patient with eczematous dermatitis who may develop irritation with adhesive material, hold dressing in place with gauze, elastic bandages, or stockinette.
• Notify doctor and remove occlusive dressing if fever develops.
• Change dressings as ordered by doctor. Inspect skin for infection,

striae, and atrophy. Discontinue drug and notify doctor if these occur.
• Treatment should be continued for a few days after clearing of lesions to prevent recurrence.

desonide
DesOwen, Tridesilon♦
Pregnancy Risk Category: C

MECHANISM OF ACTION
Diffuses across cell membranes and complexes with specific cytoplasmic receptors.

INDICATIONS & DOSAGE
Adjunctive therapy for inflammation in acute and chronic corticosteroid-responsive dermatoses—
Adults and children: clean area; apply cream, lotion, or gel sparingly b.i.d. to q.i.d.

ADVERSE REACTIONS
Skin: burning, itching, irritation, dryness, folliculitis, perioral dermatitis, allergic contact dermatitis, hypertrichosis, hypopigmentation, acneiform eruptions. With occlusive dressings: *maceration of skin, secondary infection, atrophy, striae, miliaria.*

INTERACTIONS
None significant.

NURSING CONSIDERATIONS
• Use cautiously in viral diseases of skin, such as varicella, vaccinia, herpes simplex; fungal infections; bacterial skin infections.
• Avoid application near eyes, mucous membranes, or in ear canal.
• Systemic absorption especially likely with occlusive dressings, prolonged treatment, or extensive body-surface treatment.
• When used in young children, avoid the use of plastic pants or tight-fitting diapers in treated areas.
• Stop drug and notify doctor if patient develops signs of systemic absorption, skin irritation or ulceration, hypersensitivity, or infection. (If antifungals or antibiotics are being used with corticosteroids and infection does not respond immediately, corticosteroids should be stopped until infection is controlled.)
• Before applying, gently wash skin. To prevent damage to skin, rub medication in gently, leaving a thin coat. When treating hairy sites, part hair and apply directly to lesion.
• Occlusive dressing (if ordered): Apply cream or ointment, then cover with a thin, pliable, nonflammable plastic film; seal to adjacent normal skin with hypoallergenic tape. Minimize adverse reactions by using occlusive dressing intermittently. Don't leave in place longer than 16 hours each day. Occlusive dressings should not be used in presence of infection or with weeping or exudative lesions.
• For patient with eczematous dermatitis who may develop irritation with adhesive material, hold dressing in place with gauze, elastic bandages, stockings, or stockinette.
• Notify doctor and remove occlusive dressing if fever develops.
• Change dressing as ordered by doctor. Inspect skin for infection, striae, and atrophy. Discontinue drug and notify doctor if these occur.
• Treatment should be continued for a few days after clearing of lesions to prevent recurrence.

desoximetasone
Topicort♦
Pregnancy Risk Category: C

MECHANISM OF ACTION
Diffuses across cell membranes and complexes with specific cytoplasmic receptors.

INDICATIONS & DOSAGE
Inflammation of corticosteroid-

Italicized side effects are common or life-threatening.
*Liquid form contains alcohol.   **May contain tartrazine.

responsive dermatoses—
Adults and children: clean area; apply cream sparingly b.i.d. to t.i.d.

ADVERSE REACTIONS
Skin: burning, itching, irritation, dryness, folliculitis, hypertrichosis, acneiform eruptions, perioral dermatitis, hypopigmentation, allergic contact dermatitis. With occlusive dressings: *maceration of skin, secondary infection, atrophy, striae, miliaria.*

INTERACTIONS
None significant.

NURSING CONSIDERATIONS
• Use cautiously in viral diseases of skin, such as varicella, vaccinia, herpes simplex; fungal infections; bacterial skin infections.
• Avoid application near eyes, mucous membranes, or in ear canal.
• Systemic absorption especially likely with occlusive dressings, prolonged treatment, or extensive body-surface treatment.
• When used in young children, avoid the use of plastic pants or tight-fitting diapers in treated areas.
• Stop drug and notify doctor if patient develops signs of systemic absorption, skin irritation or ulceration, hypersensitivity, or infection. (If antifungals or antibiotics are being used with corticosteroids and infection does not respond immediately, corticosteroids should be stopped until infection is controlled.)
• Before applying, gently wash skin. To prevent damage to skin, rub medication in gently, leaving a thin coat. When treating hairy sites, part hair and apply directly to lesions.
• Occlusive dressing (if ordered): Apply cream, then cover with a thin, pliable, nonflammable plastic film; seal to adjacent normal skin with hypoallergenic tape. To minimize adverse reactions, use occlusive dressing intermittently. Don't leave in place longer

than 16 hours each day. Occlusive dressings should not be used in presence of infection or with weeping or exudative lesions.
• For patient with eczematous dermatitis who may develop irritation with adhesive material, hold dressing in place with gauze, elastic bandages, stockings, or stockinette.
• Notify doctor and remove occlusive dressing if fever develops.
• Change dressing as ordered by doctor. Inspect skin for infection, striae, and atrophy. Discontinue drug and notify doctor if these occur.
• Treatment should be continued for a few days after clearing of lesions to prevent recurrence.
• Gel contains alcohol and may cause burning or irritation in open lesions.
• Store in tightly sealed containers.

---

dexamethasone
Aeroseb-Dex, Decaderm, Decaspray

Pregnancy Risk Category: C

MECHANISM OF ACTION
Diffuses across cell membranes and complexes with specific cytoplasmic receptors.

INDICATIONS & DOSAGE
Inflammation of corticosteroid-responsive dermatoses—
Adults and children: clean area; apply gel or aerosol sparingly b.i.d. to q.i.d.

Aerosol use on scalp—shake can well and apply to dry scalp after shampooing. Hold can upright. Slide applicator tube under hair so that it touches scalp. Spray while moving tube to all affected areas, keeping tube under hair and in contact with scalp throughout spraying, which should take about 2 seconds. Inadequately covered areas may be spot sprayed. Slide applicator tube through hair to touch scalp, press and immediately release spray button. Don't massage medication into scalp or spray forehead or eyes.

ADVERSE REACTIONS
Skin: burning, itching, irritation, dryness, folliculitis, hypertrichosis, acneiform eruptions, perioral dermatitis, hypopigmentation, allergic contact dermatitis. With occlusive dressings: *maceration of skin, secondary infection, atrophy, striae, miliaria.*

INTERACTIONS
None significant.

NURSING CONSIDERATIONS
• Use cautiously in viral diseases of skin, such as varicella, vaccinia, herpes simplex; fungal infections; bacterial skin infections.
• Avoid application near eyes, mucous membranes, or in ear canal.
• Systemic absorption especially likely with occlusive dressings, prolonged treatment, or extensive body-surface treatment.
• When used in young children, avoid the use of plastic pants or tight-fitting diapers in treated areas.
• Stop drug and notify doctor if patient develops signs of systemic absorption, skin irritation or ulceration, hypersensitivity, or infection. (If antifungals or antibiotics are being used with corticosteroids and infection does not respond immediately, corticosteroids should be stopped until infection is controlled.)
• Before applying, gently wash skin. To prevent damage to skin, rub medication in gently, leaving a thin coat. When treating hairy sites, part hair and apply directly to lesions.
• For patient with eczematous dermatitis who may develop irritation with adhesive material, hold dressing in place with gauze, elastic bandages, stockings, or stockinette.
• Notify doctor and remove occlusive dressing if fever develops.

• Change dressing as ordered by doctor. Inspect skin for infection, striae, and atrophy. Discontinue drug and notify doctor if these occur.
• Occlusive dressings should not be used in presence of infection or with weeping or exudative lesions.
• Aerosol preparation contains alcohol and may produce irritation or burning in open lesions. When using about the face, cover patient's eyes and warn against inhalation of the spray. To avoid freezing tissues, do not spray longer than 3 seconds or closer than 6″ (15 cm).
• Treatment should be continued for a few days after clearing of lesions to prevent recurrence.

---

dexamethasone sodium phosphate
Decadron Phosphate♦

Pregnancy Risk Category: C

MECHANISM OF ACTION
Diffuses across cell membranes and complexes with specific cytoplasmic receptors.

INDICATIONS & DOSAGE
Inflammation of corticosteroid-responsive dermatoses—
Adults and children: clean area; apply cream sparingly t.i.d. or q.i.d.

ADVERSE REACTIONS
Skin: burning, itching, irritation, dryness, folliculitis, hypertrichosis, hypopigmentation, acneiform eruptions, perioral dermatitis, allergic contact dermatitis. With occlusive dressings: *maceration of skin, secondary infection, atrophy, striae, miliaria.*

INTERACTIONS
None significant.

NURSING CONSIDERATIONS
• Use cautiously in viral diseases of skin, such as varicella, vaccinia,

---

Italicized side effects are common or life-threatening.
*Liquid form contains alcohol.   **May contain tartrazine.

herpes simplex; fungal infections; bacterial skin infections.
- Avoid application near eyes, mucous membranes, or in ear canal.
- Systemic absorption especially likely with occlusive dressings, prolonged treatment, or extensive body-surface treatment.
- When used in young children, avoid the use of plastic pants or tight-fitting diapers in treated areas.
- Stop drug and notify doctor if patient develops signs of systemic absorption, skin irritation or ulceration, hypersensitivity, or infection. (If antifungals or antibiotics are being used along with corticosteroids and infection does not respond immediately, corticosteroids should be stopped until infection is controlled.)
- Before applying, gently wash skin. To prevent damage to skin, rub medication in gently, leaving a thin coat. When treating hairy sites, part hair and apply directly to lesions.
- Occlusive dressing (if ordered): Apply cream heavily, then cover with a thin, pliable, nonflammable plastic film; seal to adjacent normal skin with hypoallergenic tape. To minimize adverse reactions, use occlusive dressing intermittently. Don't leave in place longer than 16 hours each day. Occlusive dressings should not be used in presence of infection or with weeping or exudative lesions.
- For patient with eczematous dermatitis who may develop irritation with adhesive material, hold dressing in place with gauze, elastic bandages, stockings, or stockinette.
- Notify doctor and remove occlusive dressing if fever develops.
- Change dressing as ordered by doctor. Inspect skin for infection, striae, and atrophy. Discontinue drug and notify doctor if these occur.
- Treatment should be continued for a few days after clearing of lesions to prevent recurrence.

diflorasone diacetate
Florone♦, Flutone, Maxiflor, psorcon

Pregnancy Risk Category: C

MECHANISM OF ACTION
Diffuses across cell membranes and complexes with specific cytoplasmic receptors.

INDICATIONS & DOSAGE
Inflammation of corticosteroid-responsive dermatoses—
Adults and children: clean area; apply ointment daily to t.i.d.; apply cream b.i.d. to q.i.d. Apply sparingly in a thin film.

ADVERSE REACTIONS
Skin: burning, itching, irritation, dryness, folliculitis, perioral dermatitis, hypertrichosis, hypopigmentation, acneiform eruptions. With occlusive dressings: *maceration, secondary infection, atrophy, striae, miliaria.*

INTERACTIONS
None significant.

NURSING CONSIDERATIONS
- Use cautiously in viral diseases of skin, such as varicella, vaccinia, herpes simplex; fungal infections; bacterial skin infections.
- Use very cautiously in young children. A high-potency corticosteroid.
- Avoid application near eyes, mucous membranes, or in ear canal.
- Systemic absorption especially likely with occlusive dressings, prolonged treatment, or extensive body-surface treatment.
- When used in young children, avoid the use of plastic pants or tight-fitting diapers in treated areas.
- Stop drug and notify doctor if patient develops signs of systemic absorption, skin irritation or ulceration, hypersensitivity, or infection. (If antifungals or antibiotics are being used

---

Unmarked trade names available in the United States only.
♦ Also available in Canada.   ♦♦ Available in Canada only.   ◊ Also available OTC.

concomitantly, corticosteroids should be stopped until infection is controlled.)

• Before applying, gently wash skin. To prevent damage to skin, rub medication in gently, leaving a thin coat. When treating hairy sites, part hair and apply directly to lesion.

• Occlusive dressing (if ordered): Apply cream or ointment, then cover with a thin, pliable, nonflammable plastic film; seal to adjacent normal skin with hypoallergenic tape. Minimize adverse reactions by using occlusive dressing intermittently. Don't leave in place longer than 16 hours each day. Occlusive dressings should not be used in presence of infection or with weeping or exudative lesions.

• For patient with eczematous dermatitis who may develop irritation with adhesive material, hold dressing in place with gauze, elastic bandages, stockings, or stockinette.

• Notify doctor and remove occlusive dressing if fever develops.

• Change dressing as ordered by doctor. Inspect skin for infection, striae, and atrophy. Discontinue drug and notify doctor if these occur.

• Occlusive dressings should not be used with psorcon.

• Diflorasone is often effective with once-daily application.

---

fluocinolone acetonide
Fluocet, Fluonid, Flurosyn, Synalar♦, Synemol

Pregnancy Risk Category: C

MECHANISM OF ACTION
Diffuses across cell membranes and complexes with specific cytoplasmic receptors.

INDICATIONS & DOSAGE
Inflammation of corticosteroid-responsive dermatoses—
Adults and children over 2 years: clean area; apply cream, ointment, or solution sparingly b.i.d. to q.i.d. Treat multiple or extensive lesions sequentially, applying to only small areas at any one time.

ADVERSE REACTIONS
Skin: burning, itching, irritation, dryness, folliculitis, hypertrichosis, hypopigmentation, acneiform eruptions, perioral dermatitis, allergic contact dermatitis. With occlusive dressings: *maceration of skin, secondary infection, atrophy, striae, miliaria.*

INTERACTIONS
None significant.

NURSING CONSIDERATIONS
• Use cautiously in viral diseases of skin, such as varicella, vaccinia, herpes simplex; fungal infections; bacterial skin infections.

• Avoid application near eyes, mucous membranes, or in ear canal.

• Systemic absorption especially likely with occlusive dressings, prolonged treatment, or extensive body-surface treatment.

• When used in young children, avoid the use of plastic pants or tight-fitting diapers in treated areas.

• Stop drug and notify doctor if patient develops signs of systemic absorption, skin irritation or ulceration, hypersensitivity, or infection. (If antifungals or antibiotics are being used with corticosteroids and infection does not respond immediately, corticosteroids should be stopped until infection is controlled.)

• Before applying, gently wash skin. To prevent damage to skin, rub medication in gently, leaving a thin coat. When treating hairy sites, part hair and apply directly to lesion.

• Occlusive dressing (if ordered): Apply gently and sparingly to the lesion until cream disappears. Then reapply, leaving a thin coat. Cover with a thin, pliable, nonflammable plastic film; seal to adjacent normal skin with hy-

poallergenic tape. To minimize adverse reactions, use occlusive dressing intermittently. Don't leave in place longer than 16 hours each day. Occlusive dressings should not be used in presence of infection or with weeping or exudative lesions.
• For patient with eczematous dermatitis who may develop irritation with adhesive material, hold dressing in place with gauze, elastic bandages, stockings, or stockinette.
• Notify doctor and remove occlusive dressing if fever develops.
• Change dressing as ordered by doctor. Inspect skin for infection, striae, and atrophy. Discontinue drug and notify doctor if these occur.
• Fluonid solution on dry lesions may increase dryness, scaling, or itching; on denuded or fissured areas, may produce burning or stinging. If burning or stinging persists and dermatitis has not improved, solution should be discontinued.

fluocinonide
Lidemol♦♦, Lidex♦, Lidex-E, Topsyn♦

Pregnancy Risk Category: C

MECHANISM OF ACTION
Diffuses across cell membranes and complexes with specific cytoplasmic receptors.

INDICATIONS & DOSAGE
Inflammation of corticosteroid-responsive dermatoses—
Adults and children: clean area; apply cream, ointment, or gel sparingly t.i.d. or q.i.d.

ADVERSE REACTIONS
Skin: burning, itching, irritation, dryness, folliculitis, hypertrichosis, hypopigmentation, acneiform eruptions, perioral dermatitis, allergic contact dermatitis. With occlusive dressings: *maceration of skin, secondary infec-*

tion, atrophy, striae, miliaria.

INTERACTIONS
None significant.

NURSING CONSIDERATIONS
• Use cautiously in viral diseases of skin, such as varicella, vaccinia, and herpes simplex; untreated purulent bacterial skin infections; fungal infections; bacterial skin infections.
• Avoid application near eyes, mucous membranes, or in ear canal.
• Systemic absorption especially likely with occlusive dressings, prolonged treatment, or extensive body-surface treatment.
• When used in young children, avoid the use of plastic pants or tight-fitting diapers in treated areas.
• Stop drug and notify doctor if patient develops signs of systemic absorption, skin irritation or ulceration, hypersensitivity, or infection. (If antifungals or antibiotics are being used with corticosteroids and infection does not respond immediately, corticosteroids should be stopped until infection is controlled.)
• Before applying, gently wash skin. To prevent damage to skin, rub medication in gently, leaving a thin coat. When treating hairy sites, part hair and apply directly to lesion.
• Occlusive dressing (if ordered): Apply cream or ointment heavily, then cover with a thin, pliable, nonflammable plastic film; seal to adjacent normal skin with hypoallergenic tape. To minimize adverse reactions, use occlusive dressing intermittently. Don't leave in place longer than 16 hours each day. Occlusive dressings should not be used in presence of infection or with weeping or exudative lesions.
• For patient with eczematous dermatitis who may develop irritation with adhesive material, hold dressing in place with gauze, elastic bandages, stockings, or stockinette.
• Notify doctor and remove occlusive

dressing if fever develops.
• Change dressing as ordered by doctor. Inspect skin for infection, striae, and atrophy. Discontinue drug and notify doctor if these occur.
• Treatment should be continued for a few days after clearing of lesions to prevent recurrence.

---

flurandrenolide
Cordran, Cordran SP, Cordran Tape, Drenison♦♦, Drenison 1/4♦♦, Drenison Tape♦♦

Pregnancy Risk Category: C

MECHANISM OF ACTION
Diffuses across cell membranes and complexes with specific cytoplasmic receptors.

INDICATIONS & DOSAGE
Inflammation of corticosteroid-responsive dermatoses—
Adults and children: clean area; apply cream, lotion, or ointment sparingly b.i.d. or t.i.d. Apply tape q 12 to 24 hours. Before applying tape, cleanse skin carefully, removing scales, crust, and dried exudates. Allow skin to dry for 1 hour before applying new tape. Shave or clip hair to allow good contact with skin and comfortable removal. If tape ends loosen prematurely, trim off and replace with fresh tape. Lowest incidence of adverse reactions if tape is replaced q 12 hours, but may be left in place for 24 hours if well tolerated and adheres satisfactorily.
Drenison 1/4—for maintenance therapy of widespread or chronic lesions.

ADVERSE REACTIONS
Skin: burning, itching, irritation, dryness, folliculitis, hypertrichosis, hypopigmentation, acneiform eruptions, allergic contact dermatitis. With occlusive dressings: *maceration of skin, secondary infection, atrophy, striae, miliaria.* With tape: purpura, stripping of epidermis, furunculosis.

INTERACTIONS
None significant.

NURSING CONSIDERATIONS
• Use cautiously in viral diseases of skin, such as varicella, vaccinia, herpes simplex; fungal infections; bacterial skin infections.
• Tape not advised for exudative lesions or those in intertriginous areas.
• Tape should be cut with scissors. Don't tear.
• Avoid application near eyes, mucous membranes, or in ear canal.
• Systemic absorption especially likely with occlusive dressings, prolonged treatment, or extensive body-surface treatment.
• When used in young children, avoid the use of plastic pants or tight-fitting diapers in treated areas.
• Stop drug and notify doctor if patient develops signs of systemic absorption, skin irritation or ulceration, hypersensitivity, or infection. (If antifungals or antibiotics are being used with corticosteroids and infection does not respond immediately, corticosteroids should be stopped until infection is controlled.)
• Before applying, gently wash skin. To prevent damage to skin, rub medication in gently, leaving a thin coat. When treating hairy sites, part hair and apply directly to lesion.
• Occlusive dressing (if ordered): Apply cream heavily, then cover with a thin, pliable, nonflammable plastic film; seal to adjacent normal skin with hypoallergenic tape. To minimize adverse reactions, use occlusive dressing intermittently. Don't leave in place longer than 16 hours each day. Occlusive dressings should not be used in presence of infection or with weeping or exudative lesions.
• For patient with eczematous dermatitis who may develop irritation with adhesive material, hold dressing in

---

place with gauze, elastic bandages, stockings, or stockinette.
• Notify doctor and remove occlusive dressing if fever develops.
• Inspect skin for infection, striae, and atrophy. Discontinue drug and notify doctor if these occur.
• Treatment should be continued for a few days after clearing of lesions to prevent recurrence.

halcinonide
Halciderm, Halog♦

Pregnancy Risk Category: C

MECHANISM OF ACTION
Diffuses across cell membranes and complexes with specific cytoplasmic receptors.

INDICATIONS & DOSAGE
Inflammation of acute and chronic corticosteroid-responsive dermatoses—
Adults and children: clean area; apply cream, ointment, or solution sparingly b.i.d. or t.i.d.

ADVERSE REACTIONS
Skin: burning, itching, irritation, dryness, folliculitis, hypertrichosis, hypopigmentation, acneiform eruptions, allergic contact dermatitis. With occlusive dressings: *maceration of skin, secondary infection, atrophy, striae, miliaria.*

INTERACTIONS
None significant.

NURSING CONSIDERATIONS
• Use cautiously in viral diseases of skin, such as varicella, vaccinia, herpes simplex; fungal infections; bacterial skin infections.
• Avoid application near eyes, mucous membranes, or in ear canal.
• Systemic absorption especially likely with occlusive dressings, prolonged treatment, or extensive body-

surface treatment.
• When used in young children, avoid the use of plastic pants or tight-fitting diapers in treated areas.
• Stop drug and notify doctor if patient develops signs of systemic absorption, skin irritation or ulceration, hypersensitivity, or infection. (If antifungals or antibiotics are being used with corticosteroids and infection does not respond immediately, corticosteroids should be stopped until infection is controlled.)
• Before applying, gently wash skin. To prevent damage to skin, rub medication in gently, leaving a thin coat. When treating hairy sites, part hair and apply directly to lesion.
• Occlusive dressing with cream: Gently rub small amount into lesion until it disappears. Reapply, leaving a thin coating on lesion, and cover with occlusive dressing. With ointment: Apply to lesion and cover with occlusive dressing. Cover with a thin, pliable, nonflammable plastic film; seal to adjacent normal skin with hypoallergenic tape. To minimize adverse reactions, use occlusive dressing intermittently. Don't leave in place longer than 16 hours each day.
• Good results have been obtained by applying occlusive dressings in the evening and removing them in the morning (that is, 12-hour occlusion). Medication should then be reapplied in the morning, without using the occlusive dressings during the day.
• For patient with eczematous dermatitis who may develop irritation with adhesive material, hold dressing in place with gauze, elastic bandages, stockings, or stockinette.
• Notify doctor and remove occlusive dressing if fever develops.
• Occlusive dressings should not be used in presence of infection or with weeping or exudative lesions.
• Change dressing as ordered by doctor. Inspect skin for infection, striae, and atrophy. Discontinue drug and no-

tify doctor if these occur.
• Treatment should be continued for a few days after clearing of lesions to prevent recurrence.

---

hydrocortisone◦
Acticort, Aeroseb-HC♦, Carmol HC, Cetacort, Cort-Dome, Cortinal, Cortizone 5, Cortril, Cremesone, Delacort, Dermacort, Dermolate, Durel-Cort, Ecosone, HC Cream, HI-Cor-2.5, Hycortole, Hydrocortex, Hytone, Ivocort, Maso-Cort, Microcort♦, Penecort, Proctocort, Rhus Tox HC, Rocort, Unicort♦

hydrocortisone acetate◦
Cortaid, Cortamed♦♦, Cortef, Corticreme♦♦, Cortifoam, Epifoam, Hydrocortisone Acetate, MyCort Lotion, Proctofoam-HC

hydrocortisone valerate
Westcort Cream♦

Pregnancy Risk Category: C

MECHANISM OF ACTION
Diffuses across cell membranes and complexes with specific cytoplasmic receptors.

INDICATIONS & DOSAGE
Inflammation of corticosteroid-responsive dermatoses; adjunctive typical management of seborrheic dermatitis of scalp; may be safely used on face, groin, armpits, and under breasts—
Adults and children: clean area; apply cream, lotion, ointment, foam, or aerosol sparingly daily to q.i.d. Aerosol—shake can well. Direct spray onto affected area from a distance of 6″ (15 cm). Apply for only 3 seconds (to avoid freezing tissues). Apply to dry scalp after shampooing; no need to massage or rub medication into scalp after spraying. Apply daily until acute phase is controlled, then

reduce dosage to 1 to 3 times a week as needed to maintain control.
For rectal administration: shake can well. One applicatorful daily to b.i.d. for 2 to 3 weeks, then every other day as necessary.

ADVERSE REACTIONS
Skin: burning, itching, irritation, dryness, folliculitis, hypertrichosis, hypopigmentation, acneiform eruptions, allergic contact dermatitis. With occlusive dressings: *maceration of skin, secondary infection, atrophy, striae, miliaria.*

INTERACTIONS
None significant.

NURSING CONSIDERATIONS
• Use cautiously in viral diseases of skin, such as varicella, vaccinia, herpes simplex; fungal infections; bacterial skin infections.
• Avoid application near eyes, mucous membranes, or in ear canal.
• Systemic absorption especially likely with occlusive dressings, prolonged treatment, or extensive body-surface treatment.
• When used in young children, avoid the use of plastic pants or tight-fitting diapers in treated areas.
• Stop drug and notify doctor if patient develops signs of systemic absorption, skin irritation or ulceration, hypersensitivity, or infection. (If antifungals or antibiotics are being used with corticosteroids and infection does not respond immediately, corticosteroids should be stopped until infection is controlled.)
• Before applying, gently wash skin. To prevent damage to skin, rub medication in gently, leaving a thin coat. When treating hairy sites, part hair and apply directly to lesion.
• Occlusive dressing (if ordered): Apply cream heavily, then cover with a thin, pliable, nonflammable plastic film; seal to adjacent normal skin

---

with hypoallergenic tape. To minimize adverse reactions, use occlusive dressing intermittently. Don't leave in place longer than 16 hours each day. Occlusive dressings should not be used in presence of infection or with weeping or exudative lesions.
• For patient with eczematous dermatitis who may develop irritation with adhesive material, it may be helpful to hold dressing in place with gauze, elastic bandages, stockings, or stockinette.
• Notify doctor and remove occlusive dressing if fever develops.
• Aerosol preparation contains alcohol and may produce irritation or burning in open lesions. When using about the face, cover patient's eyes and warn against inhalation of the spray. To avoid freezing tissues, do not spray longer than 3 seconds or closer than 6″ (15 cm).
• Change dressing as ordered by doctor. Inspect skin for infection, striae, and atrophy. Discontinue drug and notify doctor if these occur.
• Treatment should be continued for a few days following clearing of lesions to prevent recurrence.
• The 0.5% strength is available without prescription. Urge patients not to self-medicate for longer than 7 days in a row.

---

methylprednisolone acetate
Medrol♦

Pregnancy Risk Category: C

MECHANISM OF ACTION
Diffuses across cell membranes and complexes with specific cytoplasmic receptors.

INDICATIONS & DOSAGE
Inflammation of corticosteroid-responsive dermatoses—
Adults and children: clean area; apply ointment daily to q.i.d.

ADVERSE REACTIONS
Skin: burning, itching, irritation, dryness, folliculitis, hypertrichosis, hypopigmentation, acneiform eruptions, allergic contact dermatitis. With occlusive dressings: *maceration of skin, secondary infection, atrophy, striae, miliaria.*

INTERACTIONS
None significant.

NURSING CONSIDERATIONS
• Use cautiously in viral diseases of skin, such as varicella, vaccinia, herpes simplex; fungal infections; bacterial skin infections.
• Avoid application near eyes, mucous membranes, or in ear canal.
• Systemic absorption especially likely with occlusive dressings, prolonged treatment, or extensive body-surface treatment.
• When used in young children, avoid the use of plastic pants or tight-fitting diapers in treated areas.
• Stop drug and notify doctor if patient develops signs of systemic absorption, skin irritation or ulceration, hypersensitivity, or infection. (If antifungals or antibiotics are being used with corticosteroids and infection does not respond immediately, corticosteroids should be stopped until infection is controlled.)
• Before applying, gently wash skin. To prevent damage to skin, rub medication in gently, leaving a thin coat. When treating hairy sites, part hair and apply directly to lesion.
• Occlusive dressing (if ordered): Apply ointment heavily, then cover with a thin, pliable, nonflammable plastic film; seal to adjacent normal skin with hypoallergenic tape. To minimize adverse effects, use occlusive dressing intermittently. Don't leave in place longer than 16 hours each day. Occlusive dressings should not be used in presence of infection or with weeping or exudative lesions.

• For patient with eczematous dermatitis who may develop irritation with adhesive material, hold dressing in place with gauze, elastic bandages, stockings, or stockinette.
• Notify doctor and remove occlusive dressing if fever develops.
• Change dressing as ordered by doctor. Inspect skin for infection, striae, and atrophy. Discontinue drug and notify doctor if these occur.
• Treatment should be continued for a few days after clearing of lesions to prevent recurrence.

mometasone furoate
Elocon

Pregnancy Risk Category: C

MECHANISM OF ACTION
Diffuses across cell membranes and complexes with specific cytoplasmic receptors.

INDICATIONS & DOSAGE
Inflammatory and pruritic manifestations of corticosteroid-responsive dermatoses—
Adults: apply cream or ointment to affected areas once daily. Do not use occlusive dressings.

ADVERSE REACTIONS
Skin: burning, pruritus, atrophy, irritation, acneiform eruptions, hypopigmentation, allergic contact dermatitis.
Other: HPA axis suppression, Cushing's syndrome.

INTERACTIONS
None reported.

NURSING CONSIDERATIONS
• Use cautiously in viral diseases of skin, such as varicella, vaccinia, herpes simplex; fungal infections; bacterial skin infections.
• Use very cautiously in young children. A high-potency corticosteroid.
• Avoid application near eyes, mucous membranes, or in ear canal.
• Systemic absorption especially likely with occlusive dressings, prolonged treatment, or extensive body-surface treatment.
• Stop drug and notify doctor if patient develops signs of systemic absorption, skin irritation or ulceration, hypersensitivity, or infection. (If antifungals or antibiotics are being used concomitantly, corticosteroids should be stopped until infection is controlled.)
• Before applying, gently wash skin. To prevent damage to skin, rub medication in gently, leaving a thin coat. When treating hairy sites, part hair and apply directly to lesion.

triamcinolone acetonide
Aristocort♦, Kenalog♦

Pregnancy Risk Category: C

MECHANISM OF ACTION
Diffuses across cell membranes and complexes with specific cytoplasmic receptors.

INDICATIONS & DOSAGE
Inflammation of corticosteroid-responsive dermatoses—
Adults and children: clean area; apply cream, ointment, lotion, foam, or aerosol sparingly b.i.d. to q.i.d.
Aerosol—shake can well. Direct spray onto affected area from a distance of approximately 6″ (15 cm) and apply for only 3 seconds.
Paste (for oral lesions)—press small amount into lesion without rubbing until thin film develops. Apply after meals and at bedtime.

ADVERSE REACTIONS
Skin: burning, itching, irritation, dryness, folliculitis, hypertrichosis, hypopigmentation, acneiform eruptions, perioral dermatitis, allergic contact dermatitis. With occlusive dressings: *maceration of skin, secondary infec-*

Italicized side effects are common or life-threatening.
*Liquid form contains alcohol.   **May contain tartrazine.

tion, atrophy, striae, miliaria.

INTERACTIONS
None significant.

NURSING CONSIDERATIONS
• Use cautiously in viral diseases of skin, such as varicella, vaccinia, herpes simplex; fungal infections; bacterial skin infections.
• Avoid application near eyes, mucous membranes, or in ear canal.
• Systemic absorption especially likely with occlusive dressings, prolonged treatment, or extensive body-surface treatment.
• When used in young children, avoid the use of plastic pants or tight-fitting diapers in treated areas.
• Stop drug and notify doctor if patient develops signs of systemic absorption, skin irritation or ulceration, hypersensitivity, or infection. (If antifungals or antibiotics are being used with corticosteroids and infection does not respond immediately, corticosteroids should be stopped until infection is controlled.)
• Before applying, gently wash skin. To prevent damage to skin, rub medication in gently, leaving a thin coat. When treating hairy sites, part hair and apply directly to lesion.
• Aerosol preparation contains alcohol and may produce irritation or burning in open lesions. When using about the face, cover patient's eyes and warn against inhalation of the spray. To avoid freezing tissues, do not spray longer than 3 seconds or closer than 6″ (15 cm).
• Occlusive dressing (if ordered): Apply cream or ointment heavily, then cover with a thin, pliable, nonflammable plastic film; seal to adjacent normal skin with hypoallergenic tape. To minimize adverse reactions, use occlusive dressing intermittently. Don't leave in place longer than 16 hours each day.
• Change dressing as ordered by doctor. Inspect skin for infection, striae, and atrophy.
• Treatment should be continued for a few days after clearing of lesions to prevent recurrence.

93

Antipruritics and topical anesthetics

benzocaine◇
carbamide peroxide◇
dibucaine hydrochloride◇
dyclonine hydrochloride
ethyl chloride
lidocaine◇
lidocaine hydrochloride
pramoxine hydrochloride◇
tetracaine
tetracaine hydrochloride◇
triamcinolone acetonide

COMBINATION PRODUCTS
BALNETAR♦: water-dispersible emollient tar 2.5% in lanolin fraction, mineral oil, and nonionic emulsifiers.
CARMOL HC: urea 10% and hydrocortisone acetate 1%.
CETACAINE LIQUID: benzocaine 14%, tetracaine HCl 2%, benzalkonium chloride 0.5%, butyl aminobenzoate 2%, and cetyl dimethyl ethyl ammonium bromide in a bland water-soluble base.
DERMOPLAST SPRAY◇: benzocaine 20% and menthol 0.5%.
ESTAR GEL♦: coal tar 5% and alcohol 29%.
LAVATAR♦: tar distillate 33.3% in water-miscible emulsion base.
MEDICONE DRESSING (CREAM): benzocaine 0.5%, 8-hydroxyquinoline sulfate 0.05%, cod liver oil 12.5%, zinc oxide 12.5%, and menthol 0.18% with petrolatum, lanolin, talcum, and paraffin.
POLYTAR BATH◇: polytar 25% (juniper, pine, and coal tars, vegetable oil and solubilized crude coal tar) in water-miscible emulsion base.
pSORIGEL◇: coal tar solution 7.5% and alcohol 1%.
SEBUTONE♦◇: tar (equivalent to 0.5% coal tar) in surface-active soapless cleansers and wetting agents, sulfur 2%, and salicylic acid 2%.
TAR DOAK LOTION♦: tar distillate 5% and nonionic emulsifiers.
ZETAR EMULSION♦: 30% colloidal whole coal tar in polysorbates.
ZETAR SHAMPOO♦◇: whole coal tar 1% and parachlorometaxylenol 0.5% in foam shampoo base.

---

benzocaine◇
Americaine♦, Benzocol, Dermoplast, Hurricaine♦, Orabase with Benzocaine, Oracin, Ora-Jel, Rhulicream, Solarcaine♦, Spec-T Anesthetic, Trocaine

Pregnancy Risk Category: C

MECHANISM OF ACTION
Blocks conduction of impulses at the sensory nerve endings.

INDICATIONS & DOSAGE
Pain from toothache, cold sore, canker sore, oral irritation, minor sore throat—
Adults and children: apply syrup or jelly to affected area, or suck lozenges.
Local anesthetic for pruritic dermatoses, localized idiopathic pruritus, and sunburn—
Adults and children: apply locally b.i.d. or t.i.d.
Hemorrhoids or rectal irritation—
Adults and children: apply ointment b.i.d. or t.i.d.

Italicized side effects are common or life-threatening.
*Liquid form contains alcohol.   **May contain tartrazine.

ADVERSE REACTIONS
Blood: methemoglobinemia (infants).
Local: sensitization, rash.
Other: possible tolerance.

INTERACTIONS
None significant.

NURSING CONSIDERATIONS
• Contraindicated in hypersensitivity to procaine or other para-aminobenzoic acid derivatives (often used in topical sun-blocking agents).
• Contraindicated in infants under 1 year. Use cautiously in children under 6 years and in severe oral trauma or sepsis.
• Discontinue if rash or irritation develops.
• Avoid contact with eyes.
• If spray preparation used, hold can 6″ to 12″ (15 to 30 cm) from affected area and spray liberally. Avoid inhalation.
• If using rectally, cleanse and thoroughly dry rectal area before applying.
• Has a short duration of action.
• Not intended for use in infection.
• Obtain history of reactions to local anesthetics.
• Watch for allergic reactions, such as reddening or swelling. If condition persists, drug should be stopped and doctor notified.
• Teach patient how to apply.

carbamide peroxide◇
Cankaid, Gly-Oxide, Proxigel

Pregnancy Risk Category: C

MECHANISM OF ACTION
Serves as a source of hydrogen peroxide to produce nascent oxygen, which aids in cleaning and debriding.

INDICATIONS & DOSAGE
Canker sores, herpetic and other lesions, gingivitis, denture irritation, traumatic or surgical wounds—

Adults and children over 3 years: apply, undiluted, to oral mucosa q.i.d. or p.r.n., leave for several minutes, then expectorate. Don't rinse mouth.

ADVERSE REACTIONS
None reported.

INTERACTIONS
None significant.

NURSING CONSIDERATIONS
• Use only as adjunct to regular professional care.
• Don't dilute. Gently massage affected area with medication. Teach patient how to apply. Tell him not to drink or rinse his mouth for 5 minutes after use.
• Warn patient that drug foams in mouth when mixed with saliva.
• Use after meals and at bedtime for best results.
• If severe or persistent inflammation continues, patient should notify doctor or dentist.
• Provides chemomechanical cleansing and debriding action and has nonselective microbial activity.
• Store in cool place.
• Only one person should use dropper bottle or tube.

dibucaine hydrochloride◇
Nupercainal Cream♦, Nupercainal Ointment♦, Nupercainal Suppositories

Pregnancy Risk Category: C

MECHANISM OF ACTION
Blocks conduction of impulses at the sensory nerve endings.

INDICATIONS & DOSAGE
Abrasions, sunburn, minor burns, hemorrhoids, and other painful skin conditions—
Adults and children: 0.5% to 1% lotion, cream, or ointment applied lo-

---

Unmarked trade names available in the United States only.
♦Also available in Canada.   ♦♦Available in Canada only.   ◇Also available OTC.

cally several times a day. Insert suppositories rectally in morning, evening, and after every bowel movement.

ADVERSE REACTIONS
Local: sensitization, rash.

INTERACTIONS
None significant.

NURSING CONSIDERATIONS
• Contraindicated in patients allergic to amide-type anesthetics, such as lidocaine.
• Avoid contact with eyes.
• Before applying cream or ointment rectally or inserting suppository, cleanse and thoroughly dry rectal area.
• Ointment should be applied rectally using rectal applicator.
• Discontinue use if rash develops.
• Poisoning can occur if these preparations are swallowed. Keep out of children's reach.

dyclonine hydrochloride
Dyclone

Pregnancy Risk Category: C

MECHANISM OF ACTION
Blocks conduction of impulses at the sensory nerve endings.

INDICATIONS & DOSAGE
To relieve surface pain and itching caused by minor burns or trauma, surgical wounds, pruritus ani or vulvae, aphthous stomatitis, insect bites, and pruritic dermatoses. Also, to anesthetize mucous membranes before endoscopic procedures—
Adults and children: 0.5% solution or 1% ointment applied t.i.d. or q.i.d.
Urethral dilation or cystourethroscopy—
Adults: 10 ml of 0.5% solution may be instilled into the urethra.

ADVERSE REACTIONS
Local: *irritation at site of application may occur.*

INTERACTIONS
None significant.

NURSING CONSIDERATIONS
• Avoid prolonged use in patients with chronic conditions.
• May be useful in patients hypersensitive to other local anesthetics because it is a ketone.
• Contraindicated in cystoscopic examinations following an I.V. pyelogram. Iodine-containing contrast material will cause precipitate to form with dyclonine.
• Can be combined with diphenhydramine elixir to provide an effective treatment for stomatitis.
• Avoid accidental contact with drug; it produces temporary numbness.
• Effect lasts 30 to 60 minutes.

ethyl chloride
Ethyl Chloride Spray

Pregnancy Risk Category: C

MECHANISM OF ACTION
Produces local anesthesia by producing the sensation of coldness.

INDICATIONS & DOSAGE
For irritation—
Adults and children: hold container about 24″ (60 cm) from skin and spray rhythmically to cover area evenly once or twice. Application may be repeated.
As a local anesthetic in minor operative procedures and to relieve pain caused by insect stings and burns and irritation caused by myofascial and visceral pain syndromes—
Adults and children: dosage varies with different procedures. Use smallest dosage needed to produce desired effect. For local anesthesia, hold container about 12″ (30 cm) from area to

---

Italicized side effects are common or life-threatening.
*Liquid form contains alcohol.   **May contain tartrazine.

produce a fine spray.
Infants: hold a cotton ball saturated with ethyl chloride to injection site, and give injection when site dries.

ADVERSE REACTIONS
Skin: sensitization; *frostbite and tissue necrosis may occur with prolonged spraying.*
Other: excessive cooling may increase pain and muscle spasms.

INTERACTIONS
None significant.

NURSING CONSIDERATIONS
• Do not apply to broken skin or mucous membranes.
• Protect skin adjacent to treated area with petrolatum to avoid tissue sloughing.
• Avoid use near eyes.
• Avoid inhalation when spraying.
• Highly flammable; do not use in areas where open flames or sparks are possible.
• Avoid accidental contact with drug; it produces temporary numbness.
• Duration of action is less than 1 minute.

lidocaine◇

lidocaine hydrochloride
Stanacaine, Xylocaine Jelly (2%)♦, Xylocaine Ointment (5%)♦, Xylocaine Solution (4%)♦, Xylocaine Viscous Solution (2%)♦

Pregnancy Risk Category: C

MECHANISM OF ACTION
Blocks conduction of impulses at the sensory nerve endings.

INDICATIONS & DOSAGE
Local anesthesia of skin or mucous membranes, pain from dental extractions, stomatitis—
Adults and children: apply 2% to 5% solution, ointment, or 15 ml of Xylocaine Viscous q 3 to 4 hours to oral or nasal mucosa.
In procedures involving the male or female urethra—
Adults: instill about 15 ml (male) or 3 to 5 ml (female) into urethra.
Pain, burning, or itching caused by burns, sunburn, or skin irritation—
Adults and children: apply liberally.

ADVERSE REACTIONS
Local: sensitization, rash.

INTERACTIONS
None significant.

NURSING CONSIDERATIONS
• Use with caution on severely traumatized mucosa, where sepsis is present, or for anesthesia of oropharyngeal mucosa, since gag reflex may be suppressed by lidocaine and aspiration may occur.
• Use cautiously in cardiac disease, hyperthyroidism, or severe oral or nasal trauma or sepsis, as systemic absorption can occur. Don't use in infants.
• The 4% solution can be sprayed or poured onto abrasions to facilitate cleansing and removal of foreign substances (gravel, glass, etc.).
• Discontinue use if rash or irritation develops.
• Apply Xylocaine Ointment carefully to prevent contact with skin in other than the affected area; it produces numbness.
• Duration of action is up to 1 hour. When used for oropharyngeal anesthesia, advise patient to delay eating for 1 hour to avoid aspiration.
• Chronic, prolonged use for oropharynx anesthesia can lead to systemic absorption and toxicity.
• Because of risk of systemic absorption, should be applied to lesions with an oral swab.
• Teach patient how to use. Xylocaine Viscous should be swished around in mouth. Elderly or debilitated patients

shouldn't swallow it.
• Obtain history of reactions to local anesthetics.
• Taste can be improved by adding a drop of oil of peppermint.

pramoxine hydrochloride◇
ProctoFoam, Tronolane, Tronothane♦

Pregnancy Risk Category: C

MECHANISM OF ACTION
Blocks conduction of impulses at the sensory nerve endings.

INDICATIONS & DOSAGE
Pain and itching caused by dermatoses, minor burns, surgical wounds, and insect bites—
Adults and children: apply every 3 to 4 hours.
Hemorrhoids—
Adults: one applicatorful of aerosol foam b.i.d. to t.i.d. and after bowel movements.

ADVERSE REACTIONS
Local: stinging or burning, sensitization.

INTERACTIONS
None significant.

NURSING CONSIDERATIONS
• Can be safely used in those allergic to other local anesthetics.
• May be applied with gauze or sprayed directly on skin. Avoid contact with eyes.
• Cleanse and thoroughly dry rectal area before applying ointment or cream or inserting suppository.
• Not for prolonged use. Consult doctor after 4 consecutive weeks of use.

tetracaine

tetracaine hydrochloride◇
Pontocaine♦

Pregnancy Risk Category: C

MECHANISM OF ACTION
Blocks conduction of impulses at the sensory nerve endings.

INDICATIONS & DOSAGE
Pain in hemorrhoids, minor burns, ulcers, sunburn, and poison ivy—
Adults and children: apply 5% ointment or 1% cream—no more than 1 oz for adults or ¼ oz for children daily.

ADVERSE REACTIONS
Local: sensitization, rash.

INTERACTIONS
None significant.

NURSING CONSIDERATIONS
• Contraindicated in hypersensitivity to procaine or other para-aminobenzoic acid derivatives.
• Before applying rectally, cleanse and thoroughly dry rectal area.
• Discontinue use if rash develops.

triamcinolone acetonide
Kenalog in Orabase♦

Pregnancy Risk Category: C

MECHANISM OF ACTION
Reduces inflammation and helps heal oral ulcers and lesions by interfering with the protein synthesis of various enzymes.

INDICATIONS & DOSAGE
Stomatitis; erosive lichen planus; traumatic oral lesions, including sore denture spots—
Adults and children: press ¼" of 0.1% emollient dental paste onto affected area until thin film develops.

Repeat b.i.d. or t.i.d. Don't rub in or protection of film will be lost.

ADVERSE REACTIONS
Systemic: with prolonged use, adrenal insufficiency, altered glucose metabolism, peptic ulcer activation.

INTERACTIONS
None significant.

NURSING CONSIDERATIONS
• Contraindicated in oral herpetic or viral lesions. Use cautiously in diabetes mellitus, peptic ulcer, and tuberculosis, as systemic absorption can occur.
• Apply after meals and at bedtime for best results.
• Lesions should be as dry as possible before application.

94

Astringents

acetic acid lotion◊
aluminum acetate (Burow's solution)◊
aluminum sulfate and calcium acetate (modified Burow's solution)◊
hamamelis water (witch hazel)◊

COMBINATION PRODUCTS

ASTRINGENTS WITH ANESTHETICS, for example, Nupercainal Suppositories.
ASTRINGENTS WITH ANTIPRURITIC/ ANTIHISTAMINE, for example, Caladryl, Ziradryl.
ASTRINGENTS WITH ANTIPRURITIC/ ANTIHISTAMINE AND ANESTHETIC, for example, Rhulicream, Rhulihist, Rhulispray.
ASTRINGENTS WITH ANTISEPTICS, for example, Lavoris, Tanac, Tucks Pads.
ASTRINGENTS WITH ANTISEPTICS AND ANESTHETICS, for example, Pazo Hemorrhoid Suppositories and Ointment, Rectal Medicone Suppositories and Unguent, Tanicaine Suppositories and Ointment, Wyanoid Ointment.
ASTRINGENTS WITH DEODORANTS, for example, most antiperspirant/deodorants commonly available.

acetic acid lotion◊
(0.1% glacial acetic acid in alcohol)

MECHANISM OF ACTION
Precipitates protein, causing tissue to contract.

INDICATIONS & DOSAGE
Superficial fungal or bacterial infection to toughen skin and prevent bedsores—
Adults and children: apply and work into area p.r.n.

ADVERSE REACTIONS
Skin: burning and irritation of denuded skin and mucous membranes.

INTERACTIONS
Heavy metals: causes precipitation of the metal acetate.

NURSING CONSIDERATIONS
• Contraindicated under occlusive dressings.
• Never confuse acetic acid solutions with *glacial* acetic acid solutions. Glacial form is a concentrate.
• Keep away from eyes and mucous membranes.
• Always apply to freshly cleansed area, free of other medications.
• Especially useful for treating superficial gram-negative infections.

aluminum acetate (Burow's solution)◊
Acid Mantle Creme♦, Buro-sol

aluminum sulfate and calcium acetate (modified Burow's solution)◊
Bluboro Powder, Domeboro Powder♦ and Tablets♦

MECHANISM OF ACTION
Precipitates protein, causing tissue to contract.

INDICATIONS & DOSAGE
Mild skin irritation from exposure to soaps, detergents, chemicals, diaper rash, acne, scaly skin, eczema—
Adults and children: apply p.r.n.
Skin inflammation, insect bites, poison ivy or other contact dermatoses, swelling, athlete's foot—
Adults and children: mix powder or tablet with 1 pint of lukewarm tap water and apply for 15 to 30 minutes every 4 to 8 hours; bandage loosely.

ADVERSE REACTIONS
Skin: irritation; extension of inflammation possible.

INTERACTIONS
None significant.

NURSING CONSIDERATIONS
- Contraindicated under occlusive dressings; use open wet dressings only.
- When solution is prepared, immediately decant clear portion. Discard precipitate. Use only clear solution, *not* precipitate, for soaks. Never strain or filter solutions. Decanted portion may be stored at room temperature for up to 7 days.
- In general, no more than a third of the body should be treated at any one time, since excessive wet dressings may cause chilling and hypothermia.
- Keep away from eyes and mucous membranes.
- Discontinue if irritation develops.
- Prolonged or excessive use may produce necrosis.

hamamelis water (witch hazel)◇

Mediconet (wipes), Tucks (Cream, Ointment, Pads)

MECHANISM OF ACTION
Precipitates protein, causing tissue to contract.

INDICATIONS & DOSAGE
Anal discomfort, itching, burning, minor external hemorrhoidal or outer vaginal discomfort, diaper rash—
Adults and children: apply t.i.d. or q.i.d.

ADVERSE REACTIONS
Skin: hypersensitivity.

INTERACTIONS
None significant.

NURSING CONSIDERATIONS
- Discontinue if irritation or itching does not improve.
- Use pads or wipes after bowel movement instead of toilet tissue to help prevent pruritus ani or vulvae.
- Cream can be used by breast-feeding mother for nipple care, but wash area clean before breast-feeding baby.

95

Antiseptics and disinfectants

alcohol, ethyl◦
alcohol, isopropyl◦
benzalkonium chloride◦
boric acid◦
chlorhexidine gluconate◦
formaldehyde◦
hexachlorophene
hydrogen peroxide◦
iodine◦
merbromin◦
potassium permanganate◦
povidone-iodine◦
silver protein, mild◦
sodium hypochlorite◦
thimerosal◦

COMBINATION PRODUCTS
ZEASORB POWDER◦: parachlorometaxylenol 0.5%, aluminum dihydroxy
allantoinate 0.2%, and microporous
cellulose 45%.

alcohol, ethyl◦
Alcohol, Ethanol

Pregnancy Risk Category: C

MECHANISM OF ACTION
Destroys or inhibits the growth of microorganisms.

INDICATIONS & DOSAGE
*To disinfect skin, instruments, and
ampules—*
disinfect as needed.

ADVERSE REACTIONS
Skin: dryness, irritation.

INTERACTIONS
None significant.

NURSING CONSIDERATIONS
• Effective as fat-solvent germicidal;
ineffective against spore-forming organisms, tubercle bacilli, and viruses.
• Alcohol used as 70% solution
known commonly as "rubbing alcohol."
• Should be left on the skin for at
least 2 minutes.
• Don't use in open wounds.

alcohol, isopropyl◦
isopropyl alcohol 99%, isopropyl
aqueous alcohol 75%, isopropyl
rubbing alcohol 70%

Pregnancy Risk Category: C

MECHANISM OF ACTION
Destroys or inhibits the growth of microorganisms.

INDICATIONS & DOSAGE
*To disinfect skin, instruments, and
ampules—*
disinfect as needed.

ADVERSE REACTIONS
Skin: dryness, irritation.

INTERACTIONS
None significant.

NURSING CONSIDERATIONS
• Isopropyl alcohol is slightly more
effective than ethyl alcohol as an antibacterial agent, but it also tends to
cause more dryness.
• Should be left on the skin for at
least 2 minutes.
• 75% solution for disinfection and

Italicized side effects are common or life-threatening.
*Liquid form contains alcohol.   **May contain tartrazine.

storage of thermometers.
• Not effective against spore-forming organisms, tubercle bacilli, or viruses.
• Combined with formaldehyde, makes effective germicide.
• Don't use in open wounds.

benzalkonium chloride◇
Benzachlor-50♦♦, Benz-All, Ionax Scrub♦♦, Mercurochrome II, Sabol Shampoo♦♦, Zalkon, Zephiran♦

Pregnancy Risk Category: C

MECHANISM OF ACTION
Destroys or inhibits the growth of microorganisms.

INDICATIONS & DOSAGE
Preoperative disinfection of unbroken skin—
apply 1:750 to 1:1,000 tincture or spray.
Disinfection of mucous membranes and denuded skin—
apply 1:10,000 to 1:5,000 aqueous solution.
Irrigation of vagina—
instill 1:5,000 to 1:2,000 aqueous solution.
Irrigation of bladder or urethra—
instill 1:20,000 to 1:5,000 aqueous solution.
Irrigation of infected deep wounds—
instill 1:20,000 to 1:3,000 aqueous solution.
Preservation of metallic instruments, ampules, thermometers, and rubber articles—
wipe with or soak objects in 1:5,000 to 1:750 solution.
Disinfection of operating room equipment—
wipe with 1:5,000 solution.

ADVERSE REACTIONS
Skin: hypersensitivity, allergic contact dermatitis.

INTERACTIONS
Soaps: inactivate benzalkonium chloride. Remove soap traces with alcohol.

NURSING CONSIDERATIONS
• Germicidal for some nonspore-forming organisms and fungi. *Pseudomonas aeruginosa* strains are resistant; no effect on tubercle bacilli. Limited viricidal use.
• Used as preservative in some ophthalmic solutions.
• Before applying to skin, remove all traces of soap with water, and apply 70% alcohol.
• Don't store cotton, wool gauze, or sponges in solution. They absorb benzalkonium chloride and reduce the strength of the solution.
• Don't use with occlusive dressings or vaginal packs.
• Store in bottles with screw caps.
• Incompatible with iodine, silver nitrate, fluorescein, nitrates, peroxide, lanolin, potassium permanganate, aluminum, caramel, kaolin, pine oil, zinc sulfate, zinc oxide, and yellow oxide of mercury.
• To prevent rust of metallic instruments stored in benzalkonium chloride, add sodium nitrite to final solution. Change solution weekly.
• Available also as 17% concentrate (Zephiran). Even after dilution, this form of Zephiran should be used only on inanimate objects.
• Mercurochrome II, a brand of benzalkonium chloride, *does not* contain merbromin. Don't confuse with Mercurochrome.

boric acid◇
Bluboro, boric acid solution 5%, Borofax, Ting

Pregnancy Risk Category: C

MECHANISM OF ACTION
Destroys or inhibits the growth of microorganisms. A mild antiseptic and

astringent.

INDICATIONS & DOSAGE
Skin conditions (athlete's foot) as a compress, powder, or ointment (2% to 5%)—
Adults and children (not infants): apply as directed.

ADVERSE REACTIONS
Signs of systemic absorption:
CNS: delirium, seizures, restlessness, headache.
CV: *circulatory collapse,* tachycardia.
GI: irritation, nausea, vomiting, diarrhea.
GU: renal damage.
Other: hypothermia.

INTERACTIONS
None significant.

NURSING CONSIDERATIONS
• Do not use in children under 2 years unless directed by doctor.
• May be significantly absorbed through abraded skin or granulating wounds.
• Avoid long-term use.
• Ingestion of 5 g (infants) or 20 g (adults) may be fatal.

chlorhexidine gluconate◇
Exidine, Hibiclens Liquid, Hibistat, Peridex

Pregnancy Risk Category: C

MECHANISM OF ACTION
Destroys or inhibits the growth of microorganisms. Bactericidal; broad spectrum of activity.

INDICATIONS & DOSAGE
Surgical hand scrub, hand wash, hand rinse, skin wound cleanser—
use p.r.n.
Gingivitis—
use 0.12% strength (Peridex oral rinse) p.r.n.

ADVERSE REACTIONS
EENT: irritating to eyes. Causes deafness if instilled into middle ear through perforated eardrum.

INTERACTIONS
None significant.

NURSING CONSIDERATIONS
• Can be used several times a day without causing excessive irritation or dryness.
• Low potential for producing skin reactions.
• Keep out of eyes and ears.
• Action is residual. Do not cleanse skin with alcohol after application.
• Can be left on skin as an antibacterial lotion.
• Antibacterial effect is not lessened by blood, pus, or soap.
• Action begins 10 seconds after application.

formaldehyde◇
Formalin (37% solution of formaldehyde)

MECHANISM OF ACTION
Destroys or inhibits the growth of microorganisms.

INDICATIONS & DOSAGE
Cold sterilization of equipment—
disinfect as needed.
Tissue preservative—
cover tissue.

ADVERSE REACTIONS
EENT: fumes cause eye, nose, and throat irritation.
Skin: irritation, allergic contact dermatitis.
Other: pungent odor.

INTERACTIONS
None significant.

NURSING CONSIDERATIONS
• 0.5% solution germicidal against

Italicized side effects are common or life-threatening.
*Liquid form contains alcohol.   **May contain tartrazine.

all forms of microorganisms, including spores, in 6 to 12 hours; 10% solution used to disinfect inanimate objects.
• Use the 0.12% strength only as an oral rinse.
• Not affected by organic matter.
• Used with alcohol and sodium nitrite to disinfect instruments and articles that can't tolerate heat (cold sterilization).
• Avoid skin or mucous membrane contact with solutions greater than 0.5%.
• Always dilute 37% solution.

hexachlorophene
pHisoHex♦, pHisoScrub, SeptiSoft, WescoHEX♦

Pregnancy Risk Category: C

MECHANISM OF ACTION
Destroys or inhibits the growth of microorganisms. A bacteriostatic agent.

INDICATIONS & DOSAGE
Surgical scrub, bacteriostatic skin cleanser—
use as directed in 0.25% to 3% concentrations.

ADVERSE REACTIONS
Note: systemic absorption can cause neurotoxic effects, including irritability, generalized clonic muscular contractions, decerebrate rigidity, seizures, optic atrophy. (Systemic absorption is especially significant when used on mucous membranes and broken skin and burns.)
Skin: dermatitis, mild scaling, dryness (especially when combined with excessive scrubbing).

INTERACTIONS
None significant.

NURSING CONSIDERATIONS
• Don't use on infants (especially premature infants). Use cautiously on

burn patients. These patients tend to absorb significant amounts of hexachlorophene through the skin and may develop neurotoxic effects.
• Spectrum of activity limited to gram-positive organisms, especially staphylococcus.
• Must be used preoperatively for at least 3 days for maximum effectiveness.
• After cleansing area, rinse thoroughly (especially the scrotum and perineum). Do not apply alcohol or organic solvents to cleansed area.

hydrogen peroxide◊
3% to 6% solution

Pregnancy Risk Category: C

MECHANISM OF ACTION
Destroys or inhibits the growth of microorganisms. Germicidal, particularly against anaerobic organisms.

INDICATIONS & DOSAGE
Cleansing wound—
use 1.5% to 3% solution.
Mouth wash for necrotizing ulcerative gingivitis—
gargle with 3% solution.
Cleansing douche—
use 2% solution.

ADVERSE REACTIONS
EENT: excessive use as mouthwash may cause "hairy tongue."

INTERACTIONS
None significant.

NURSING CONSIDERATIONS
• Don't inject into closed body cavities or abscesses; generated gas can't escape.
• Use to remove mucus from inner cannula of tracheostomy tube.
• Store tightly capped in cool, dry place. Protect from light and heat.
• Do not shake bottle. This causes decomposition.

• 6% solution will bleach hair.

iodine◇

Sepp Antiseptic Applicators (2% mild iodine tincture), solution (2% iodine and 2.4% sodium and iodide in water)∗, strong iodine tincture (7% iodine and 5% potassium iodide in diluted alcohol), tincture (2% iodine and 2.4% sodium iodide in diluted alcohol)

Pregnancy Risk Category: D

MECHANISM OF ACTION
Destroys or inhibits the growth of microorganisms. A microbicidal agent effective against bacteria, fungi, viruses, protozoa, and yeasts.

INDICATIONS & DOSAGE
Preoperative disinfection of skin (small wounds and abraded areas)—
apply p.r.n.

ADVERSE REACTIONS
Skin: irritation, redness, swelling (sign of hypersensitivity), allergic contact dermatitis.

INTERACTIONS
None significant.

NURSING CONSIDERATIONS
• If skin reaction develops, remove iodine residue from skin and stop use.
• To prevent skin irritation, do not cover areas treated with iodine.
• Aqueous solution less irritating.
• Sodium thiosulfate renders iodine colorless and is used to remove stains. It is also the antidote of choice for accidental ingestion.

merbromin◇

Mercurochrome (2% aqueous solution)

Pregnancy Risk Category: C

MECHANISM OF ACTION
Destroys or inhibits the growth of microorganisms. Bacteriostatic.

INDICATIONS & DOSAGE
General antiseptic and first-aid prophylactic—
Adults and children: apply p.r.n. as 1% to 2% solution or tincture.

ADVERSE REACTIONS
Skin: sensitization, allergic contact dermatitis.

INTERACTIONS
None significant.

NURSING CONSIDERATIONS
• Don't use on large areas of abraded skin, because mercury may be absorbed and produce systemic toxicity.
• Least effective mercurial antiseptic. Its activity is decreased in presence of organic matter.
• Cleanse injury with soap and water and let dry before applying.
• Stains may be removed with 2% permanganate solution, followed by 5% oxalic acid solution.
• Never heat solution.
• To prepare 1% solution, dilute with equal parts of water.
• Note that Mercurochrome II does *not* contain merbromin, but contains benzalkonium chloride.

potassium permanganate◇

Pregnancy Risk Category: C

MECHANISM OF ACTION
Destroys or inhibits the growth of microorganisms. An antiseptic astringent with fungicidal properties.

Italicized side effects are common or life-threatening.
*Liquid form contains alcohol.   **May contain tartrazine.

INDICATIONS & DOSAGE

Topical antiseptic—
apply 1:10,000 to 1:500 solution.
Vaginal douche—
instill 1:5,000 to 1:1,000 solution as directed.

ADVERSE REACTIONS

Skin: solutions greater than 1:5,000 are irritating to skin.

INTERACTIONS

Iodine: precipitates iodine salt. Do not use together.

NURSING CONSIDERATIONS

• Germicidal effects reduced by organic matter.
• Stains caused by potassium permanganate can be removed with dilute acids (lemon juice, oxalic acid, or diluted hydrochloric acid).
• Undissolved crystals may cause chemical burn.
• Never mix with charcoal or give charcoal as antidote; may explode.

---

povidone-iodine◇
ACU-dyne♦, Aerodine, Betadine♦, Bridine♦♦, Efo-Dine, Mallisol, Polydine, Proviodine♦♦, Sepp

Pregnancy Risk Category: D

MECHANISM OF ACTION

Destroys or inhibits the growth of microorganisms.

INDICATIONS & DOSAGE

Many uses, including preoperative skin preparation and scrub, germicide for surface wounds, postoperative application to incisions, prophylactic application to urinary meatus of catheterized patients, miscellaneous disinfection—
Adults: apply p.r.n.

ADVERSE REACTIONS

Skin: local hypersensitivity reactions, allergic contact dermatitis.

INTERACTIONS

None significant.

NURSING CONSIDERATIONS

• Should not be used as a vaginal antiseptic during pregnancy.
• Germicidal activity of iodine with minimal irritation to skin and mucous membranes.
• Thought to be superior to soap as a disinfectant; less effective than aqueous or alcoholic solutions of iodine.
• Treated areas may be bandaged or taped.
• Germicidal activity reduced if area cleansed with alcohol or other organic solvents after application of povidone-iodine.
• Prolonged, excessive use may lead to systemic absorption and toxicity.
• Betadine vaginal gel should not be used in patients hypersensitive to iodine.
• Don't combine with alcohol or hydrogen peroxide.

---

silver protein, mild◇
Argyrol S.S., Solargentum

Pregnancy Risk Category: C

MECHANISM OF ACTION

Destroys or inhibits the growth of microorganisms.

INDICATIONS & DOSAGE

Topical application for inflammation of eye, nose, throat—
Adults and children: apply p.r.n. as a 5% to 25% solution.

ADVERSE REACTIONS

Skin: argyria in long-term use.

INTERACTIONS

None significant.

NURSING CONSIDERATIONS

• Store in amber glass bottles; protect from light.

Unmarked trade names available in the United States only.
♦Also available in Canada.   ♦♦Available in Canada only.   ◇Also available OTC.

• Should not be used long-term.

sodium hypochlorite◦

5% solution (instruments, swimming pools), Modified Dakin's solution, 0.5% aqueous solution for wounds

Pregnancy Risk Category: C

MECHANISM OF ACTION
Destroys or inhibits the growth of microorganisms. Germicidal and weakly fungicidal.

INDICATIONS & DOSAGE
Athlete's foot, wound irrigation, disinfection of walls and floors—
apply as directed.

ADVERSE REACTIONS
Skin: irritation, bleeding.

INTERACTIONS
None significant.

NURSING CONSIDERATIONS
• Interferes locally with thrombin formation, delaying blood clotting. Dissolves necrotic tissue.
• Unstable in solution. Make fresh solution and use immediately.
• Avoid contact with hair due to its bleaching properties.

thimerosal◦

Aeroaid Thimerosal, Merthiolate♦

Pregnancy Risk Category: C

MECHANISM OF ACTION
Destroys or inhibits the growth of microorganisms.

INDICATIONS & DOSAGE
Preoperative disinfection of skin; antiseptic for open wounds—
apply or instill to affected area daily b.i.d. or t.i.d. as a 0.1% solution or tincture.

ADVERSE REACTIONS
Skin: erythematous, vesicular, papular eruptions (indicate hypersensitivity); irritation with tincture; allergic contact dermatitis.

INTERACTIONS
None significant.

NURSING CONSIDERATIONS
• Contraindicated in hypersensitivity to mercury-containing compounds.
• Should not be instilled into external ears. May cause mercury toxicity.
• Do not use when aluminum salts may come in contact with skin.
• Incompatible with permanganate, strong acids, and heavy metals.
• Cleanse wound thoroughly before applying tincture. Allow tincture to dry completely before applying dressing.

Italicized side effects are common or life-threatening.
*Liquid form contains alcohol.   **May contain tartrazine.

Emollients, demulcents, and protectants

aluminum paste◇
calamine◇
collodion, flexible◇
collodion, USP◇
compound benzoin tincture◇
dexpanthenol◇
glycerin◇
liquid petrolatum◇
methyl salicylate◇
oatmeal◇
para-aminobenzoic acid (PABA)◇
petrolatum◇
starch◇
talc (magnesium silicate)◇
vitamins A and D ointment◇
zinc gelatin◇

COMBINATION PRODUCTS
CALADRYL LOTION◇: diphenhydramine hydrochloride 1%, calamine, camphor, and alcohol 2%.

---

aluminum paste◇
(10% aluminum in zinc oxide ointment with liquid petrolatum)

Pregnancy Risk Category: C

MECHANISM OF ACTION
Softens dry skin by preventing evaporation of perspiration. Also promotes healing by reducing irritation and friction.

INDICATIONS & DOSAGE
Emollient and protectant for colostomy area or other surgical sites—
apply p.r.n.

ADVERSE REACTIONS
None.

INTERACTIONS
Topical enzymes: aluminum may inactivate preparations used to debride wounds. Don't use together.

NURSING CONSIDERATIONS
• Zinc oxide paste can be used as an alternative.
• Observe for inflammation or infection since protectants are occlusive layers that retain moisture, exclude air, and trap cutaneous bacteria.
• Don't use in weeping wounds.
• Skin should be cleaned daily or more often as needed.
• Emollients and protectants may be used alone, as vehicles for medications, or with other topical medications. Check with doctor.
• Apply evenly with tongue depressor or finger, and remove with cloth soaked in mineral or vegetable oil.

---

calamine◇
liniment (15% calamine), lotion (8% calamine), ointment (17% calamine), Rhulispray (1% calamine)

Pregnancy Risk Category: C

MECHANISM OF ACTION
Promotes healing by reducing irritation and friction.

INDICATIONS & DOSAGE
Topical astringent and protectant for itching, poison ivy and poison oak, nonpoisonous insect bites, mild sunburn, minor skin irritations—
apply p.r.n.

Unmarked trade names available in the United States only.
♦Also available in Canada.   ♦♦Available in Canada only.   ◇Also available OTC.

ADVERSE REACTIONS
Skin: transient, light stinging; irritation; dry skin.

INTERACTIONS
None significant.

NURSING CONSIDERATIONS
• Contraindicated in hypersensitivity to any of the drug's components.
• Watch for sensitivity reactions to calamine. Preparations containing antihistamines may cause sensitivity.
• Always shake well before use.
• Don't use cotton to apply; it will absorb the solute. Use gauze sponge.
• Do not apply to blistered, raw, or oozing areas of the skin.
• Toxic if taken internally.
• Observe for inflammation or infection since protectants are occlusive layers that retain moisture, exclude air, and trap skin bacteria.
• Skin should be cleaned daily or more often as needed.
• Emollients, demulcents, and protectants may be used alone, as vehicles for medications, or with other topical medications. Check with doctor.
• May irritate and dry skin.
• Keep away from eyes and mucous membranes.
• Keep container tightly closed so solvent won't evaporate.

---

collodion, flexible◇
(5% pyroxylin in 1 part alcohol, 3 parts ether plus 20% camphor, 30% castor oil)

collodion, USP◇
(5% pyroxylin in 1 part alcohol, 3 parts ether)

Pregnancy Risk Category: C

MECHANISM OF ACTION
Promotes healing by reducing irritation and friction.

INDICATIONS & DOSAGE
Protectant; vehicle for other medicinal agents; and sealant for small wounds—
apply to dry skin p.r.n., or use flexible collodion when a flexible noncontracting film is desired.

ADVERSE REACTIONS
None.

INTERACTIONS
None significant.

NURSING CONSIDERATIONS
• Observe for inflammation or infection since protectants are occlusive layers that retain moisture, exclude air, and trap cutaneous bacteria.
• Skin should be cleaned daily or more often as needed.
• Protectants may be used alone, as vehicles for medications, or with other topical medications. Check with doctor.
• Camphor in flexible collodion is weakly antiseptic and antipruritic; may irritate and dry skin.
• Highly flammable; never use near flame or cigarettes.
• Keep container tightly closed so solvent won't evaporate.
• Toxic if taken internally.
• Avoid excessive inhalation of vapors.

---

compound benzoin tincture◇
(10% benzoin in alcohol mixed with glycerin and water)
Benzoin Spray♦

Pregnancy Risk Category: C

MECHANISM OF ACTION
Promotes healing by reducing irritation and friction. Also cools and soothes.

INDICATIONS & DOSAGE
Demulcent and protectant for cuta-

Italicized side effects are common or life-threatening.
*Liquid form contains alcohol.   **May contain tartrazine.

neous ulcers, bedsores, cracked nipples, fissures of lips and anus—
apply locally once daily or b.i.d.

ADVERSE REACTIONS
Skin: contact dermatitis.

INTERACTIONS
None significant.

NURSING CONSIDERATIONS
• Do not apply to acutely inflamed areas.
• Observe for inflammation or infection since protectants are occlusive layers that retain moisture, exclude air, and trap cutaneous bacteria.
• Skin should be cleaned daily or more often as needed.
• Protectants may be used alone, as vehicles for medications, or with other topical medications.
• For demulcent and expectorant action in laryngitis or croup, use in boiling water and have patient inhale vapors.
• Spray is not intended for use as inhalant.
• Can be mixed with magnesium-aluminum hydroxide and applied on bedsores.

dexpanthenol◊
Panthoderm♦ (dexpanthenol 2% in a water-miscible cream base)

Pregnancy Risk Category: C

MECHANISM OF ACTION
Softens dry skin by preventing evaporation of perspiration.

INDICATIONS & DOSAGE
Epithelial-bed stimulator in emollient base: itching, wounds, insect bites, poison ivy, poison oak, diaper rash, chafing, mild eczema, decubitus ulcers, dry lesions—
apply topically, p.r.n.

ADVERSE REACTIONS
None.

INTERACTIONS
None significant.

NURSING CONSIDERATIONS
• Contraindicated in wounds of hemophilia patients.
• Before each new application *always* thoroughly cleanse affected area, removing all traces of previously applied medication. Observe for inflammation or infection.
• Dry lesions respond better than oozing lesions.

glycerin◊
Corn Huskers Lotion (tragacanth 1 g, glycerin 30 ml, propylene glycol 10 ml)

Pregnancy Risk Category: C

MECHANISM OF ACTION
Softens dry skin by preventing evaporation of perspiration.

INDICATIONS & DOSAGE
Emollient and lubricant: rectal tubes and catheters; dry skin, hands—
apply p.r.n.

ADVERSE REACTIONS
None.

INTERACTIONS
None significant.

NURSING CONSIDERATIONS
• Applied undiluted to inflamed, dehydrated skin. Paradoxically, excessive use may dry the skin.
• Diluted with rose water, glycerin is useful for irritated or dry lips.

liquid petrolatum◇

Light Liquid Petrolatum, NF; Liquid
Petrolatum, USP; Mineral Oil

Pregnancy Risk Category: C

MECHANISM OF ACTION
Softens dry skin by preventing evaporation of perspiration. Also promotes healing by reducing irritation and friction.

INDICATIONS & DOSAGE
Protectant and emollient—
apply locally, full strength, or diluted.

ADVERSE REACTIONS
None.

INTERACTIONS
None significant.

NURSING CONSIDERATIONS
• Occasionally used with other drugs.
• Available in two forms: light mineral oil and heavy mineral oil.
• Heavy mineral oil can be used internally as a laxative. Never use light mineral oil as a laxative. Mineral oil used as nose drops can cause lipid pneumonia.
• Observe for inflammation or infection since protectants are occlusive layers that retain moisture, exclude air, and trap skin bacteria.
• Skin should be cleaned daily or more often as needed.
• Difficult to wash off.
• Emollients and protectants may be used alone, as vehicles for medications, or with other topical medications.

methyl salicylate◇

(betula oil, gaultheria oil, sweet
birch oil, wintergreen oil)
Banalg, Baumodyne Gel and
Ointment

Pregnancy Risk Category: C

MECHANISM OF ACTION
A counterirritant that increases circulation to the area of application.

INDICATIONS & DOSAGE
Counterirritant for minor pains of osteoarthritis, rheumatism, sprains, muscle and tendon soreness and tightness, lumbago, sciatica—
Adults: apply with gentle massage several times daily.
 Not recommended for children.

ADVERSE REACTIONS
Skin: rash, irritation, burning, blistering.

INTERACTIONS
None significant.

NURSING CONSIDERATIONS
• Use cautiously in patients with aspirin hypersensitivity.
• Never apply directly, undiluted to skin.
• Warning: As little as 4 ml ingested by children can cause fatal toxicity; in adults as little as 30 ml. Since GI absorption may be delayed, treat such ingestion with emetic lavage, then a saline cathartic. Continue lavage until no odor of methyl salicylate can be detected in the washings.
• Absorbed through skin; prolonged increased application can cause toxicity. Toxic effects include hyperpnea leading to respiratory alkalosis, nausea, vomiting, tinnitus, hyperpyrexia, and seizures.
• Discontinue if rash or redness occurs. Consult doctor if pain or redness persists more than 10 days.
• Avoid getting near eyes, open

Italicized side effects are common or life-threatening.
*Liquid form contains alcohol.   **May contain tartrazine.

wounds, or mucous membranes.
• Do not apply to broken or irritated skin.
• Do not wrap or bandage treated area.
• Store in tightly closed container.

oatmeal◇
Aveeno Colloidal♦, Aveeno Oilated Bath (with liquid petrolatum and hypoallergenic lanolin)♦

MECHANISM OF ACTION
Softens dry skin by preventing evaporation of perspiration. Also soothes and cools.

INDICATIONS & DOSAGE
Emollient and demulcent for local irritation—
use as a lotion; 1 level tablespoon to a cup of warm water.
Skin irritation, pruritus, common dermatoses, sunburn, dry skin—
Adults: 1 packet in tub of warm water.
Children: 1 to 2 rounded tablespoons in 3″ to 4″ (8 to 10 cm) of bath water.
Infants: 2 or 3 level teaspoons, depending on size of bath.

ADVERSE REACTIONS
None.

INTERACTIONS
None significant.

NURSING CONSIDERATIONS
• Not to be ingested.
• Instruct patient to exercise caution to avoid slipping in tub.
• Avoid getting in eyes.
• Disperse well by adding to water under running faucet, if possible.

para-aminobenzoic acid (PABA)◇
Pabanol♦, Pre-Sun♦, PreSun Gel♦, RVPaba Lipstick♦

Pregnancy Risk Category: C

MECHANISM OF ACTION
Promotes healing by reducing irritation and friction.

INDICATIONS & DOSAGE
Topical protectant for sunburn protection, sun-sensitive skin, slow tanning—
Adults: apply evenly to skin indoors before exposure to sun. Don't apply to wet skin. Follow directions on various products for number and time of applications; reapply after swimming.
   Not recommended for infants.

ADVERSE REACTIONS
Skin: photosensitivity dermatitis.
Local: allergic contact dermatitis, irritation, sensitization.

INTERACTIONS
None significant.

NURSING CONSIDERATIONS
• Contraindicated in hypersensitivity to any of the drug's components and for persons with damaged or diseased skin.
• Discontinue if skin rash occurs.
• Encourage slow tanning and short exposure to sun.
• Always apply to thoroughly dried skin. Will not protect if applied to wet skin.
• Avoid contact with eyes and lids.
• Avoid contact with open flame.
• May stain clothing and other fabrics, such as towels and washcloths.
• Follow product directions for correct application.
• Observe for inflammation and infection since protectants produce an occlusive layer that retains perspiration, excludes air, and traps cutaneous

bacteria, producing sites for anaerobic infections.

petrolatum◊
Vaseline♦

Pregnancy Risk Category: C

MECHANISM OF ACTION
Promotes healing by reducing irritation and friction. Also softens dry skin by preventing evaporation of perspiration.

INDICATIONS & DOSAGE
Topical protectant and emollient—
use alone or with other drugs, as directed.

ADVERSE REACTIONS
Skin: folliculitis.

INTERACTIONS
None significant.

NURSING CONSIDERATIONS
• Stable, does not become rancid.
• Observe for inflammation or infection since protectants are occlusive layers that retain moisture, exclude air, and trap skin bacteria.
• Skin should be cleaned daily or more often as needed.
• Emollients and protectants may be used alone, as vehicles for medications, or with other topical medications.

starch◊

MECHANISM OF ACTION
Absorbs moisture to relieve dry skin.

INDICATIONS & DOSAGE
Demulcent for minor skin irritations, pruritus associated with common dermatoses—
mix 2 cups of starch with 4 cups of water, add to tub of water, and soak affected area for 30 minutes.

ADVERSE REACTIONS
None.

INTERACTIONS
None significant.

NURSING CONSIDERATIONS
• Instruct patient to exercise caution to avoid slipping in tub.
• Use of cornstarch in intertriginous areas may promote or accelerate a yeast infection since yeast can feed on the sugar.

talc
(magnesium silicate)◊

MECHANISM OF ACTION
Promotes healing by reducing irritation and friction.

INDICATIONS & DOSAGE
Topical lubricant, protectant, drying agent, absorbent dusting powder: irritation, such as intertrigo prickly heat—
sprinkle on affected areas p.r.n. for soothing and lubrication.

ADVERSE REACTIONS
None.

INTERACTIONS
None significant.

NURSING CONSIDERATIONS
• Don't use on surgical gloves; causes granulation and adhesions in open wounds.
• Avoid dust entering eyes or inhalation of talc dust.
• Should not be used on open, weeping surfaces; it cakes and crusts.

vitamins A and D ointment◇
A&D, Balmex, Caldesene
Medicated, Clocream, Comfortine,
Desitin, Primaderm

Pregnancy Risk Category: A

MECHANISM OF ACTION
Soothes irritation and cools inflammation. Also softens dry skin by preventing evaporation of perspiration.

INDICATIONS & DOSAGE
*Emollient, demulcent, and epithelial-
bed stimulant for superficial burns,
sunburn, abrasions, slow-healing lesions, chapped skin, diaper rash, skin
care of infants or bedridden patients—*
apply several times daily p.r.n.

ADVERSE REACTIONS
Skin: irritation.

INTERACTIONS
None significant.

NURSING CONSIDERATIONS
• Discontinue if skin condition persists or irritation develops.
• Observe for inflammation or infection since emollients and demulcents
are occlusive layers that retain moisture, exclude air, and trap cutaneous
bacteria.
• Skin should be cleaned daily or
more often as needed.
• Emollients and demulcents may be
used alone, as vehicles for medications, or with other topical medications. Check with doctor.

zinc gelatin◇
Dome-Paste, Unna's Boot

Pregnancy Risk Category: C

MECHANISM OF ACTION
Promotes healing by reducing irritation and friction.

INDICATIONS & DOSAGE
*Protectant for lesions or injuries of
lower legs or arms—*
Wrap the wet bandage in place, and
retain for about 1 week. Dome-Paste,
in 3″ and 4″ (8 to 10 cm) bandages,
can be applied directly to arm or leg.

ADVERSE REACTIONS
None.

INTERACTIONS
None significant.

NURSING CONSIDERATIONS
• Observe for inflammation and infection since protectants produce an
occlusive layer that retains perspiration, excludes air, and traps cutaneous
bacteria, producing sites for anaerobic infections. Before each new application, *always* thoroughly cleanse affected area, removing all traces of
previously applied medication.
• Don't apply too tightly. Check for
vasoconstriction.
• Zinc gelatin boot can be removed by
unwinding outer bandage and soaking
leg or arm in warm water until dressing floats off. Tell patient not to
shower or take tub bath with zinc gelatin boot on leg.
• When applying topical medications
to the skin before application of the
bandage, apply the medication in the
direction of the hair follicle to prevent
folliculitis.

ethanolamine oleate
podophyllum resin
resorcinol
resorcinol monoacetate
salicylic acid◊
silver nitrate
sulfur◊
sulfurated lime solution◊

COMBINATION PRODUCTS
ACNE-AID CREAM◊: sulfur 2.5%, resorcinol 1.25%, and parachlorometaxylenol 0.375% in a microporous cellulose base.
ACNOMEL CREAM♦◊: sulfur 8%, resorcinol 2%, and alcohol 11% in a greaseless base.
CLEARASIL CREAM◊: benzoyl peroxide 10% and bentonite.
COMPOUND W WART REMOVER◊: salicylic acid 14%, acetic acid 11%, in castor oil, alcohol, ether, and collodion.

---

ethanolamine oleate
Ethamolin

Pregnancy Risk Category: C

MECHANISM OF ACTION
A mild sclerosing agent that produces a local inflammatory response and scarring which prevents bleeding.

INDICATIONS & DOSAGE
Treatment of bleeding esophageal varices—

Adults: Local injection of 1.5 to 5 ml. per varix. Maximum total dosage per treatment should not exceed 20 ml or about 0.4 ml/kg. Injections are administered by doctors familiar with the technique.

ADVERSE REACTIONS
GI: esophageal ulcer, esophageal stricture, esophagitis, esophageal tearing, local mucosal sloughing or necrosis, periesophageal abcess and perforation.
GU: acute renal failure.
Respiratory: pleural effusion or infiltration, pneumonia, aspiration pneumonia.
Other: fever, retrosternal pain, *anaphylaxis*.

INTERACTIONS
None reported.

NURSING CONSIDERATIONS
• Contraindicated in patients with hypersensitivity to ethanolamine, oleic acid, or ethanolamine oleate.
• Ethanolamine oleate will not correct portal hypertension, the cause of esophageal varices. Vascular recanalization and collateral formation may occur, and patients may need further treatment.
• Sclerotherapy is not indicated for asymptomatic esophageal varices or varicosities of the leg.
• Be prepared to treat anaphylaxis in patients undergoing sclerotherapy with ethanolamine oleate. It is rare but has been fatal. Have epinephrine 1:1,000 available, and control allergic reactions with antihistamines.
• Severe necrosis may occur with injection. Monitor breath sounds. Tell patient to report chest pain immedi-

---

Italicized side effects are common or life-threatening.
*Liquid form contains alcohol.   **May contain tartrazine.

ately.

• Patients with concomitant cardiopulmonary disease should receive smaller doses of sclerosing agents to minimize adverse effects.

• Submucosal injections are not recommended because they are more likely to cause mucosal ulceration.

• Therapy is usually initiated at the first bleeding episode, with follow-up sclerotherapy after 1 week, 6 weeks, 3 months, and 6 months if needed.

podophyllum resin
Podoben

Pregnancy Risk Category: X

MECHANISM OF ACTION
Inhibits cell division and other cellular processes, leading to cell death.

INDICATIONS & DOSAGE
Venereal warts—
Adults: apply podophyllum resin preparation to the lesion, cover with waxed paper, and bandage. Leave covered for 4 to 6 hours, then wash lesion to remove medication. Repeat at weekly intervals, if indicated.
Multiple superficial epitheliomatoses and keratoses—
Adults: apply daily with applicator and allow to dry. Remove necrotic tissue before each reapplication.

ADVERSE REACTIONS
Blood: thrombocytopenia, leukopenia when systemically absorbed.
Local: irritation of normal skin.
Other: peripheral neuropathy when systemically absorbed.

INTERACTIONS
Other keratolytics: may cause extensive damage to the skin. Do not use together.

NURSING CONSIDERATIONS
• Contraindicated in pregnancy; may be harmful to fetus.

• Resin is irritating and cytotoxic, and should not be applied to normal skin. Petrolatum can be applied to adjacent areas for protection during treatment.

• Should be applied only by a doctor because of toxicity.

• Do not use on extensive areas or for prolonged therapy; drug is absorbed systemically.

• Warn patient that soreness from local irritation may develop 12 to 48 hours after treatment.

• Should not be used without medical supervision.

• Don't use adjacent to mucous membrane areas.

• Will not remove large venereal warts; surgery is another option.

• Don't use on recently biopsied warts.

resorcinol

resorcinol monoacetate
Euresol, Resorcin

Pregnancy Risk Category: C

MECHANISM OF ACTION
Softens keratin and loosens cornified epithelium.

INDICATIONS & DOSAGE
Acute eczema, urticaria, and other inflammatory skin diseases (1% or 2% concentration in alcohol); acne or seborrhea (5% lotion or 10% soap liniment for scalp); chronic eczema, psoriasis (2% to 10% ointment); acne scarring (45% peeling paste)—
Adults and children: apply as directed.

ADVERSE REACTIONS
Skin: irritation, moderate erythema or scaling.
Other: darkening of light hair (resorcinol only).

INTERACTIONS
None significant.

NURSING CONSIDERATIONS
- Do not use preparations on or near eyes.
- Not for use on broken, inflamed, or ulcerated areas.
- If skin irritation persists, discontinue medication.
- Apply lotion with cotton ball to affected area.
- When applying the peeling paste, closely observe the patient and site of application until paste is removed.
- Use carefully with topical acne preparations because of local irritation.

---

salicylic acid◇
Calicylic, Keralyt♦, Salactic Liquifilm, Salonil, Tran-Ver-Sal

Pregnancy Risk Category: C

MECHANISM OF ACTION
Softens keratin and loosens cornified epithelium.

INDICATIONS & DOSAGE
Superficial fungal infections, acne, psoriasis, seborrheic dermatitis, other scaling dermatoses, hyperkeratosis, calluses, warts—
Adults and children: apply to affected area and place under occlusion at night.

ADVERSE REACTIONS
Skin: irritation, drying.
Other: salicylism with percutaneous absorption.

INTERACTIONS
Iodine, iron salts, and oxidizing substances: incompatible. Don't use together.

NURSING CONSIDERATIONS
- Use with caution in patients with diabetes or peripheral vascular disease. The skin inflammation that may result is difficult to treat. Limit use for children under 12 years. (Do not exceed 1 oz in 24 hours.)
- Avoid contact with eyes and mucous membranes.
- If excessive skin drying or irritation occurs, apply a bland cream or lotion.
- Rinse hands after application (unless they are being treated).
- Transdermal patch (Tran-Sal) now available for removal of warts.
- Skin should be hydrated for at least 5 minutes before treatment and washed the morning after treatment.
- Most preparations are occlusive, which increases percutaneous absorption. Therefore, do not use on large surface areas for prolonged periods.
- Not for use on broken, inflamed, or ulcerated areas.
- Also has bacteriostatic and fungistatic properties.

---

silver nitrate

Pregnancy Risk Category: C

MECHANISM OF ACTION
Denatures protein producing a caustic or corrosive effect.

INDICATIONS & DOSAGE
Cauterization of mucous membranes, fissures, aphthous lesions (5% to 10% solution); cauterization of granulomatous tissues and warts (solid form)—
Adults and children: applied only by doctor at his discretion.

ADVERSE REACTIONS
Local: *argyria (permanent silver discoloration of skin).*

INTERACTIONS
None significant.

NURSING CONSIDERATIONS
- May cause burns. Avoid accidental contact with skin and eyes. If accidental contact with skin occurs, flush

---

Italicized side effects are common or life-threatening.
*Liquid form contains alcohol.   **May contain tartrazine.

with water for at least 15 minutes; if accidental contact with eyes, call doctor at once.
- Warn that silver nitrate stains skin and clothing.
- Silver nitrate pencils must be moistened with water before use.
- Silver nitrate is used as a wet dressing in low concentrations (0.125% to 0.5%) as a local anti-infective for treatment of burns, wounds, or ulcers.
- May be painful in higher concentrations.

sulfur◇
Acnophill, Bensulfoid, Liquimat, Transact, Xerac

Pregnancy Risk Category: C

MECHANISM OF ACTION
Softens keratin and loosens cornified epithelium.

INDICATIONS & DOSAGE
Acne, ringworm, psoriasis, seborrheic dermatitis, chigger infestation, scabies, favus, staphylococcal folliculitis—
Adults and children: apply preparation to affected areas b.i.d., t.i.d., or as directed.

ADVERSE REACTIONS
Local: excessive drying of skin, blackheads, contact dermatitis.

INTERACTIONS
None significant.

NURSING CONSIDERATIONS
- Prolonged use may cause severe contact dermatitis.
- When initiating therapy, use sparingly for patients with sensitive skin.
- Avoid contact with eyes. If accidental contact occurs, flush with water.
- Wash skin thoroughly before application. Tell patient that tingling sensation may be felt upon application.
- Skin is more reactive to drug in

cold, dry climates, so decrease frequency of application. In hot, humid climates, increase frequency of application.
- Do not use on same area with topical acne preparation or preparations containing a peeling agent (for example, benzoyl peroxide); may cause severe irritation.
- The 10% ointment is used for scabies. Don't use on children or infants.
- Do not use on same area with any mercury-containing preparation; may cause a foul odor, irritate the skin, or stain skin black.
- Also has antiseptic and parasiticide properties.

sulfurated lime solution◇
Vlemasque, Vleminckx's solution

Pregnancy Risk Category: C

MECHANISM OF ACTION
Softens keratin and loosens cornified epithelium.

INDICATIONS & DOSAGE
Acne vulgaris, seborrhea—
Adults and children: dilute 1 packet in 1 pint hot water and apply as hot dressing for 15 to 20 minutes daily. Or apply as a mask to affected, dry areas, and rinse away with warm water after 15 to 20 minutes once daily.
Generalized furunculosis—
Adults and children: add 30 to 60 ml solution to bath water.

ADVERSE REACTIONS
Local: may cause excessive drying of skin.

INTERACTIONS
None significant.

NURSING CONSIDERATIONS
- Discontinue use if excessive drying or skin irritation develops.
- Avoid contact with jewelry, metallic objects, or clothing.

- Avoid getting solution in eyes, nose, or mouth.
- Fumes are irritating and malodorous (rotten eggs). Ventilate adequately. Odors are minimized with Vlemasque.
- Do not use in same area with topical acne preparations; may cause severe irritation.
- Do not use in same area with mercury-containing preparations; may cause a foul odor, irritate skin, or stain skin black.

Miscellaneous dermatomucosal agents

anthralin◇
benzoyl peroxide◇
collagenase
dextranomer◇
etretinate
fluorouracil
hydroquinone
isotretinoin
methoxsalen
minoxidil (topical)
selenium sulfide◇
sutilains
tretinoin (vitamin A acid, retinoic acid)

COMBINATION PRODUCTS
SULFOXYL REGULAR: benzoyl peroxide 5% and sulfur 2%.
SULFOXYL STRONG: benzoyl peroxide 10% and sulfur 5%.
VANOXIDE♦◇: benzoyl peroxide 5% and chlorhydroxyquinoline 0.25%.
VANOXIDE-HC♦: benzoyl peroxide 5%, chlorhydroxyquinoline 0.25%, and hydrocortisone 0.5%.

---

anthralin◇
Anthra-Derm

Pregnancy Risk Category: C

MECHANISM OF ACTION
Acts as a local antieczematous and antipsoriatic agent. Restores normal rate of keratinization and epidermal cell proliferation.

INDICATIONS & DOSAGE
Psoriasis, chronic dermatitis—
Adults and children: apply thinly daily or b.i.d. Concentrations range from 0.1% to 1%; start with lowest and increase, if necessary.

ADVERSE REACTIONS
GU: possible renal toxicity.
Skin: erythema on healthy skin.

INTERACTIONS
None significant.

NURSING CONSIDERATIONS
• Contraindicated in renal damage. Should not be used on acute or inflammatory eruptions.
• Partial excretion in urine may cause renal irritation, casts, and albuminuria. Check urine weekly.
• Discontinue if allergic reaction, pustular folliculitis, or renal irritation occurs.
• Don't get in eyes. May cause conjunctivitis, keratitis, or corneal opacity.
• Wear plastic gloves to apply anthralin; wash hands thoroughly after using.
• Cover with gauze dressing to protect clothing. May stain clothing.
• May cause alkaline urine and a temporary yellow-brown discoloration to gray or white hair and skin. Anthralin stain may be removed from skin by applying 3% to 6% salicylic acid cream or ointment.
• Avoid applying medication to normal skin by coating the area surrounding the lesion with petrolatum.
• Remove with light application of mineral oil before bathing.

---

benzoyl peroxide○
Benoxyl♦, Benzac♦, Benzagel♦,
Clear by Design, Desquam-X♦♦,
Dry and Clear♦, Oxy-5♦, Oxy-10,
OxyCover♦, Panoxyl♦, Persadox
HP, Persa-Gel♦, Xerac BP♦

Pregnancy Risk Category: C

MECHANISM OF ACTION
Antimicrobial and comedolytic.

INDICATIONS & DOSAGE
Acne—
Adults and children: apply once
daily to q.i.d., depending on tolerance
and effect.

ADVERSE REACTIONS
Skin: stinging on application,
warmth, painful irritation, pruritus,
vesicles, allergic contact dermatitis.

INTERACTIONS
None significant.

NURSING CONSIDERATIONS
• Contraindicated in sensitivity to
any of the drug's ingredients.
• Patient should wash face thoroughly 20 to 30 minutes before applying.
• Don't use near the eyes, on mucous
membranes, or on denuded or highly
inflamed skin.
• Dryness, redness, and peeling
should occur 3 to 4 days after starting
treatment. If these common reactions
cause considerable discomfort, discontinue temporarily.
• If painful irritation or vesicles develop, discontinue use.
• May bleach hair or clothing.

collagenase
Santyl

Pregnancy Risk Category: C

MECHANISM OF ACTION
An enzymatic debriding agent that digests undenatured collagen fibers in

necrotic tissue and removes substrates
for bacterial proliferation.

INDICATIONS & DOSAGE
*Debridement of dermal ulcers and se-
verely burned areas—*
Adults and children: apply ointment
(250 units/g) to lesion daily or every
other day.

ADVERSE REACTIONS
Skin: slight erythema of surrounding
area, especially if ointment is not confined to lesion.
Other: hypersensitivity reactions.

INTERACTIONS
*Detergents; hexachlorophene; antisep-
tics, soaks, or acidic solutions (especially those containing heavy metal
ions):* decreased enzymatic activity.
Do not use together.

NURSING CONSIDERATIONS
• Use with caution in debilitated patients and in leukopenia, because debriding enzymes may increase risk of
bacteremia; watch for signs of septicemia.
• Before application, cleanse lesion
with gauze saturated in normal saline
solution, neutral buffer solution, or
hydrogen peroxide; use topical antibacterial agent (such as neomycin-
bacitracin-polymyxin B) if infection
is present. Apply to lesion in powder
form before using collagenase. If infection persists, discontinue collagenase until infection is healed. Confine
collagenase ointment to area of lesion
(Lassar's paste may protect surrounding skin). Apply ointment in thin layers to ensure contact with necrotic tissue and complete wound coverage;
apply collagenase ointment with
tongue depressor on deep wounds;
with gauze on shallow wounds. Remove any debris that comes off easily.
Remove excess ointment, and cover
wound with sterile gauze pad.
• Discontinue when sufficient de-

Italicized side effects are common or life-threatening.
*Liquid form contains alcohol.   **May contain tartrazine.

bridement has occurred.
• Observe wound to monitor therapy. Appearance of granulation may indicate effectiveness. Notify doctor if signs of inflammation occur.
• If enzymatic action must be stopped, apply Burow's solution.
• Avoid getting ointment in eyes. If this occurs, flush with water at once.
• Protect drug from heat.

dextranomer◊
Debrisan♦

Pregnancy Risk Category: C

MECHANISM OF ACTION
A synthetic polymer that aids in granulation by absorbing exudate, bacteria, and contaminants.

INDICATIONS & DOSAGE
To clean secreting wounds, such as venous stasis and decubitus ulcers, infected surgical wounds, and burns—
Adults and children: apply to affected area daily, b.i.d., or more often, p.r.n. Apply to ⅛″ or ¼″ thickness, and cover with sterile gauze.

ADVERSE REACTIONS
Skin: temporary pain.

INTERACTIONS
Ointment bases, such as Vaseline: negate action of dextranomer. Don't mix together.

NURSING CONSIDERATIONS
• Before application, cleanse wound with sterile water, saline solution, or other appropriate solution. Don't dry.
• Don't use in body cavities or deep fistulas.
• Pack cratered wounds with beads, allowing room for expansion of beads. Cover with dressing to hold beads in place.
• When saturated, medication turns gray-yellow and should be removed with sterile water, saline solution, or other cleansing solution.
• Dextranomer beads are not effective in cleaning nonsecreting wounds. Discontinue use when the wound has stopped secreting.
• Dextranomer beads are hydrophilic; each gram can absorb 4 ml of exudate.
• Keep drug away from moisture; store in tightly closed container.
• Avoid contact with eyes. Wash hands thoroughly after application.
• To prevent falls, be careful not to spill beads onto floor.
• Dextranomer reduces tissue edema so wound may appear larger after use.
• Beads must be thoroughly removed before any surgical procedure.

etretinate
Tegison

Pregnancy Risk Category: X

MECHANISM OF ACTION
Unknown.

INDICATIONS & DOSAGE
Treatment of severe recalcitrant psoriasis, including the erythrodermic and generalized pustular types in patients unresponsive to standard therapy (topical tar plus UVB light, psoralens plus UVA light, systemic corticosteroids, and methotrexate)—
Adults: initially, 0.75 to 1 mg/kg daily in divided doses. Don't exceed maximum initial dose of 1.5 mg/kg daily. After initial response, begin maintenance dosage of 0.5 to 0.75 mg/kg daily.

ADVERSE REACTIONS
Blood: *blood dyscrasias,* anemia, altered prothrombin time.
CNS: *benign intracranial hypertension (pseudotumor cerebri), fatigue, headache,* dizziness, lethargy.
CV: thrombosis, edema.
EENT: *eye pain, sore tongue, chapped lips.*
GI: *appetite change, nausea.*

Hepatic: *hepatitis, elevated liver enzymes.*
GU: *white blood cells in urine,* proteinuria, hematuria.
Metabolic: *hypokalemia or hyperkalemia, hyperlipidemia.*
Skin: *skin peeling, itching.*
Other: *bone pain,* dyspnea.

INTERACTIONS
Milk: increases etretinate's absorption. Avoid concomitant consumption of milk.
Vitamin A: additive toxic effects. Avoid concomitant use.

NURSING CONSIDERATIONS
• Contraindicated in patients who are pregnant, who intend to become pregnant, or who may not use reliable contraception during and after treatment because drug causes severe birth defects.
• Significant residual blood levels of etretinate have been reported as long as 2.9 years after discontinuation of treatment. Consequently, the period of time after treatment during which pregnancy must be avoided to prevent teratogenicity is unknown.
• Women of childbearing age must not receive etretinate unless pregnancy is excluded by a pregnancy test within 2 weeks before initiating therapy. Therapy may begin on the 2nd or 3rd day of the next normal menstrual period.
• Patient should use effective contraception for 1 month before therapy begins, during treatment, and for an indefinite time after treatment is discontinued.
• Monitor liver function tests at 1- to 2-week intervals for the first 1 to 2 months of therapy, and thereafter at intervals of 1 to 3 months. Suspected hepatotoxicity requires discontinuation of etretinate.
• Monitor blood lipids every 1 to 2 weeks during treatment.
• Tell patient to promptly report

headache, nausea and vomiting, and visual disturbances (possible early signs of pseudotumor cerebri). These reactions require immediate check for papilledema. If present, discontinue drug immediately.
• Advise patient not to take vitamin A supplements to avoid possible additive adverse reactions.
• Reassure patient that transient exacerbation of psoriasis is common during the beginning of therapy.
• Advise patient to expect dry skin and possible difficulty tolerating contact lenses during treatment.
• Advise patient to take this drug with meals, but to avoid taking it with milk or milk products.

fluorouracil
Efudex♦, Fluoroplex♦
Pregnancy Risk Category: D

MECHANISM OF ACTION
Interferes with DNA synthesis by inhibiting thymidylate synthetase.

INDICATIONS & DOSAGE
Multiple actinic or solar keratoses; superficial basal cell carcinoma—
Adults and children: apply cream (5%) or solution (1%, 2%, or 5%) b.i.d.

ADVERSE REACTIONS
Skin: erythema, pain, burning, scaling, pruritus, hyperpigmentation, contact dermatitis, soreness, suppuration, swelling.

INTERACTIONS
None significant.

NURSING CONSIDERATIONS
• Wash hands immediately after handling medication.
• Patient should avoid prolonged exposure to sunlight or ultraviolet light.
• Apply with caution near eyes, nose, and mouth.

Italicized side effects are common or life-threatening.
*Liquid form contains alcohol.   **May contain tartrazine.

• Warn patient that treated area may be unsightly during therapy and for several weeks after therapy. Complete healing may take 1 or 2 months.
• Ingestion and systemic absorption may cause leukopenia, thrombocytopenia, stomatitis, diarrhea, or GI ulceration, bleeding, and hemorrhage.
• Application to large ulcerated areas may cause systemic toxicity.
• Use 1% concentration on the face. Reserve higher concentrations for thicker-skinned areas or resistant lesions.
• For superficial basal cell carcinoma confirmed by biopsy, use 5% strength.
• Lesions resistant to fluorouracil should be biopsied.
• Avoid occlusive dressings as they increase the risk of inflammatory reactions in adjacent normal skin.

hydroquinone
Artra Skin Tone Cream, Derma-Blanch, Eldopaque♦, Eldopaque-Forte♦, Eldoquin♦, Eldoquin Forte♦, Esoterica Medicated Cream♦, Melanex, Quinnone

Pregnancy Risk Category: C

MECHANISM OF ACTION
Inhibits tyrosinase, preventing the conversion of tyrosine to melanin.

INDICATIONS & DOSAGE
Bleaching of blemished skin, lentigo, chloasma, freckles, old-age spots, and other skin conditions due to increased melanin—
Adults and children over 12 years: apply 2% to 4% concentration daily or b.i.d.

ADVERSE REACTIONS
Skin: mild irritation, sensitization, rash.

INTERACTIONS
None significant.

NURSING CONSIDERATIONS
• Contraindicated in prickly heat, sunburn, or irritated skin.
• Don't use near eyes.
• Test for sensitivity by applying a small amount of low-concentration medication on skin before treatment. Allergic reactions should appear within 24 hours.
• If rash or irritation develops, discontinue therapy. Topical steroids can reduce irritation and sensitization.
• Depigmentation is not permanent.
• Advise patient to use opaque sunscreen when outdoors since sun can darken lesions faster than hydroquinone can lighten them.

isotretinoin
Accutane♦

Pregnancy Risk Category: X

MECHANISM OF ACTION
Normalizes keratinization, reversibly decreases the size of sebaceous glands, and alters the composition of sebum to a less viscous form that's less likely to cause follicular plugging.

INDICATIONS & DOSAGE
Severe cystic acne unresponsive to conventional therapy—
Adults and adolescents: 0.5 to 2 mg/kg daily P.O. given in 2 divided doses and continued for 15 to 20 weeks.

ADVERSE REACTIONS
Blood: anemia, elevated platelet count.
CNS: headache, fatigue, *pseudotumor cerebri* (benign intracranial hypertension).
EENT: *conjunctivitis,* corneal deposits, dry eyes.
Endocrine: hyperglycemia.
GI: nonspecific GI symptoms, gum bleeding and inflammation.
Hepatic: elevated AST (SGOT), ALT (SPGT), and alkaline phosphatase.
Skin: *cheilosis, rash, dry skin,* peel-

ing of palms and toes, skin infection, photosensitivity.
Other: *hypertriglyceridemia, musculoskeletal pain (skeletal hyperostosis),* thinning of hair.

INTERACTIONS
Vitamin A and vitamin supplements containing vitamin A: increase in isotretinoin's toxic effects. Don't use together without doctor's permission.

NURSING CONSIDERATIONS
• Isotretinoin is contraindicated in women of childbearing age unless the patient has had a negative serum pregnancy test within 2 weeks before beginning therapy; will begin drug therapy on the 2nd or 3rd day of the next menstrual period; and will comply with stringent contraception measures for 1 month before therapy, during therapy, and for at least 1 month after therapy. *Severe fetal abnormalities may occur if used during pregnancy.*
• Contraindicated in patients hypersensitive to parabens, which are used as preservatives.
• Tell patient to immediately report any visual disturbances and bone or skeletal pain.
• Patients who experience headache, nausea and vomiting, or visual disturbances should be screened for papilledema. Signs and symptoms of pseudotumor cerebri require immediate discontinuation of therapy and prompt neurologic intervention.
• Perform serum lipid studies and liver function tests before therapy begins and then at regular intervals until response to drug is established, usually about 4 weeks.
• Monitor blood glucose regularly.
• Monitor creatine phosphokinase levels in patients who undergo vigorous physical activity.
• Warn patient that contact lenses may feel uncomfortable during isotretinoin therapy.
• If a second course of therapy is

needed, it shouldn't be started until at least 8 weeks after the completion of the first course because improvement may continue after withdrawal of the drug.
• Most adverse reactions appear to be dose-related, occurring at dosages greater than 1 mg/kg daily. They are generally reversible when therapy is discontinued or dosage is reduced.
• Advise patient to take drug with or shortly after meals to ensure adequate absorption.

methoxsalen
Oxsoralen♦
Pregnancy Risk Category: C

MECHANISM OF ACTION
A potent photosensitizer of the skin that promotes melanin formation by facilitating the action of ultraviolet light.

INDICATIONS & DOSAGE
Protect against sunburn, enhance pigmentation, and induce repigmentation in vitiligo—
Adults and children over 12 years: for small, well-defined lesions, apply topically weekly or less often and expose to ultraviolet A light gradually, as directed.
Psoriasis—
Adults: oral dosage is based on weight and administered 2 hours before exposure to ultraviolet A light. May repeat 2 to 3 times weekly, at least 48 hours apart.

ADVERSE REACTIONS
CNS: nervousness, insomnia, mental depression.
GI: discomfort, nausea, diarrhea.
Skin: edema, erythema, blistering, burning, peeling, *photosensitivity.*
Other: leg cramps.

INTERACTIONS
Photosensitizing agents: do not use to-

gether.

NURSING CONSIDERATIONS
• Contraindicated in hepatic insufficiency, porphyria, acute systemic lupus erythematosus, or hydromorphic, polymorphic light eruptions; and in patients who are aphakic (or who have cataracts). Use with caution in familial history of sunlight allergy, GI diseases, chronic infection, and history of basal cell carcinoma.
• Regulate therapy carefully. Overexposure to light can cause serious burning or blistering.
• Topical treatment should be directly supervised by a doctor.
• When applied topically to face or hands, patient should protect area from light (except during treatment exposure) for 24 hours before and after therapy.
• Protect eyes and lips during light exposure treatments.
• Significant changes require 6 to 9 months of therapy.
• During the next 24 hours after oral therapy, patient should wear wraparound sunglasses that absorb longwave ultraviolet light in daylight, apply a sunscreen, and avoid outdoor activities as much as possible.

minoxidil (topical)
Rogaine

Pregnancy Risk Category: C

MECHANISM OF ACTION
Stimulation of hair growth may be related to dilation of arterial microcapillaries around hair follicles.

INDICATIONS AND DOSAGE
Treatment of male pattern baldness (alopecia androgenetica) of the vertex and scalp—
Adults: Apply 1 ml of 2% solution to affected area twice daily. Total daily dosage should not exceed 2 ml.

ADVERSE REACTIONS
CNS: headache, dizziness, faintness, light-headedness.
CV: edema, chest pain, increased or decreased blood pressure, palpitations, increased or decreased pulse rate.
EENT: sinusitis.
GU: urinary tract infections, renal calculi, urethritis.
Metabolic: edema, weight gain.
Respiratory: bronchitis, upper respiratory infection.
Skin: irritant dermatitis, allergic contact dermatitis, eczema, hypertrichosis, local erythema, pruritus, dry skin or scalp, flaking, alopecia, exacerbation of hair loss.
Other: back pain, tendonitis.

INTERACTIONS
Topical corticosteroids, petrolatum, topical retinoids, or other drugs that may enhance skin absorption: increased risk of systemic effects of minoxidil. Do not apply minoxidil with other drugs.

NURSING CONSIDERATIONS
• Contraindicated in patients with hypersensitivity to any component of the topical solution. Adverse effects are uncommon.
• Tell patient to avoid inhalation of any spray or mist from the drug. Avoid spraying around the eyes, because the solution contains alcohol and may be irritating.
• Patient needs to have a normal, healthy scalp before beginning therapy, because absorption of the drug through irritated skin may cause adverse systemic effects.
• Treatment with topical minoxidil is most likely to be successful in patients with balding area smaller than 4″ (10 cm) within the last 10 years.
• Patients with a history of heart disease should be aware that this drug may exacerbate their illness.
• Teach patient to monitor pulse rate

and body weight.
• Patients need medical follow-ups 1 month after initiation of therapy and every 6 months thereafter.
• Teach patient how to correctly apply topical minoxidil. Hair and scalp should be thoroughly dry before application, and the drug should not be applied to any other areas of the body. Patient should not use the drug on irritated or sunburned scalp, or with any other medication on the scalp. Tell patient to thoroughly wash his hands after application.
• Advise patient that therapy will be prolonged and will continue for at least 4 months before clinical effects appear. About 40% of patients will see moderate to dense hair growth.
• Discontinuing the drug may result in the loss of new hair growth. New hair growth is usually fine and may be colorless, but will resemble existing hair after continued treatment.

selenium sulfide◇
Exsel◆, Selsun◆, Selsun Blue
Pregnancy Risk Category: C

MECHANISM OF ACTION
Has irritant, antibacterial, and antifungal properties.

INDICATIONS & DOSAGE
Dandruff, seborrheic scalp dermatitis—
Adults and children: massage 1 to 2 teaspoonfuls into wet scalp. Leave on for 2 to 3 minutes. Rinse thoroughly, and repeat application. Apply twice weekly for 2 weeks, then 2 to 3 times a week, or as often as needed.

ADVERSE REACTIONS
Skin: oily or dry scalp and hair, hair discoloration or loss, sensitivity reactions.

INTERACTIONS
None significant.

NURSING CONSIDERATIONS
• Contraindicated in sulfur hypersensitivity.
• Use with caution around areas of acute inflammation or exudation to avoid undue irritation.
• If sensitivity reactions occur, discontinue use.
• Reduce hair discoloration by thorough rinsing after treatment.
• Avoid contact with eyes.
• Highly toxic if ingested.

sutilains
Travase◆
Pregnancy Risk Category: C

MECHANISM OF ACTION
A proteolytic enzyme that selectively digests necrotic tissue.

INDICATIONS & DOSAGE
Debridement of second- and third-degree burns, adjunctive debridement of decubitus ulcers, pyogenic wounds, or ulcers resulting from peripheral vascular disease—
Adults and children: apply thinly to area extending ¼″ to ½″ beyond area to be debrided. Cover with loose, wet dressing t.i.d. or q.i.d.

ADVERSE REACTIONS
CNS: local paresthesias.
Skin: mild pain, bleeding, transient dermatitis.

INTERACTIONS
Detergents, anti-infectives, and compounds containing metallic ions: adversely affects enzymatic activity. Don't use together.

NURSING CONSIDERATIONS
• Contraindicated in wounds involving major body cavities or containing exposed nerves or nerve tissue, fungating neoplastic ulcers, wounds in women of childbearing age, or in patients who have limited cardiac or

---

Italicized side effects are common or life-threatening.
*Liquid form contains alcohol.   **May contain tartrazine.

pulmonary reserves.
• Should be used only on 10% to 15% of the burned area at a time.
• Use cautiously near eyes. If accidental contact occurs, flush eyes repeatedly with large amounts of normal saline solution or sterile water.
• Before application, cleanse and irrigate affected area with normal saline solution or sterile water to remove antibacterial agents.
• May give mild analgesic to reduce painful reactions, but discontinue if pain is severe; also discontinue if bleeding or dermatitis occurs.
• For best response, keep affected area moist.
• In concomitant use of topical antimicrobial agent, apply sutilains first.
• Store in refrigerator at 35.6° to 50° F. (2° to 10° C.).

---

tretinoin (vitamin A acid, retinoic acid)
Retin-A

Pregnancy Risk Category: B

MECHANISM OF ACTION
Inhibits comedones by increasing epidermal cell mitosis and turnover.

INDICATIONS & DOSAGE
Acne vulgaris (especially grades I, II, and III), treatment of fine wrinkles from photodamaged skin—
Adults and children: cleanse affected area and lightly apply solution once daily h.s.

ADVERSE REACTIONS
Skin: *feeling of warmth, slight stinging, local erythema, peeling,* chapping, swelling, blistering, crusting, temporary hyper- or hypopigmentation.

INTERACTIONS
None significant.

NURSING CONSIDERATIONS
• Contraindicated in hypersensitivity to any tretinoin component. Use with caution in eczema.
• If severe local irritation develops, discontinue temporarily and readjust dosage when application is resumed.
• Some redness and scaling are normal reactions.
• Beneficial effects should be seen within 6 weeks of treatment.
• Relapses generally occur within 3 to 6 weeks after treatment.
• Patient should wash face with a mild soap no more than two or three times a day. Warn against using strong or medicated cosmetics, soaps, or other skin cleansers. Patient should also avoid topical products containing alcohol, astringents, spices, and lime since these may interfere with drug.
• Exposure to sunlight or ultraviolet rays should be minimal during treatment. If patient is sunburned, delay therapy until sunburn subsides.
• Patient who can't avoid exposure to sunlight should use a SPF 15 sunscreen and protective clothing.
• Avoid contact with eyes, mouth, and mucous membranes.

Local anesthetics

bupivacaine hydrochloride
chloroprocaine hydrochloride
etidocaine hydrochloride
lidocaine hydrochloride
mepivacaine hydrochloride
procaine hydrochloride
tetracaine hydrochloride

COMBINATION PRODUCTS
None, although epinephrine is added
to some solutions to prolong effect.

---

bupivacaine hydrochloride
Marcaine♦, Sensorcaine

Pregnancy Risk Category: C

MECHANISM OF ACTION
A local anesthetic of the amide type.
Blocks depolarization by interfering
with sodium-potassium exchange
across the nerve cell membrane, preventing generation and conduction of
the nerve impulse. When combined
with epinephrine, action is prolonged.

INDICATIONS & DOSAGE
*Available with or without epinephrine.
Dosages given are for drug* without
epinephrine.
Epidural:

Sol.	Vol. (ml)	Dose (mg)
0.50%	10 to 20	50 to 100
0.25%	10 to 20	25 to 50

Caudal:

Sol.	Vol. (ml)	Dose (mg)
0.50%	15 to 30	75 to 150
0.25%	15 to 30	37.5 to 75

Peripheral nerve block:

Sol.	Vol. (ml)	Dose (mg)
0.50%	5 to 80	25 to 400 (max.)

May repeat dose q 3 hours. Dosage
and interval may be increased with
epinephrine. Maximum 400 mg daily.

ADVERSE REACTIONS
Skin: dermatologic reactions.
Other: edema, status asthmaticus,
anaphylaxis, anaphylactoid reactions.
   The following systemic effects may
result from high blood levels of the
drug:
CNS: anxiety, nervousness, seizures
followed by drowsiness, unconsciousness, tremors, twitches, shivering, *respiratory arrest.*
CV: myocardial depression, *dysrhythmias, cardiac arrest.*
EENT: blurred vision, tinnitus.
GI: nausea, vomiting.

INTERACTIONS
*Enflurane, halothane, and related
drugs:* cardiac dysrhythmias when
used with bupivacaine *with* epinephrine. Use with extreme caution.
*MAO inhibitors, cyclic antidepres-
sants:* severe, sustained hypertension
when used with bupivacaine *with* epinephrine. Use with extreme caution.
Chloroprocaine: may lessen bupivacaine's action. Don't use together.

NURSING CONSIDERATIONS
• Contraindicated in children under
12 years and for spinal, paracervical
block, or topical anesthesia. Use cautiously in debilitated, elderly, or

---

Italicized side effects are common or life-threatening.
*Liquid form contains alcohol.   **May contain tartrazine.

acutely ill patients; and in patients with severe hepatic disease or drug allergies.

• Although the 0.75% solution is still available, it is not to be used for obstetrical surgery. According to the FDA, lower concentrations are effective and much less hazardous.

• Use solutions with epinephrine cautiously in cardiovascular disorders and in body areas with limited blood supply (ears, nose, fingers, toes).

• Keep resuscitative equipment and drugs available.

• Don't use solution with preservatives for caudal or epidural block.

• Onset in 4 to 17 minutes; duration is 3 to 6 hours.

• Discard partially used vials without preservatives.

• Check solution for particles.

chloroprocaine hydrochloride

Nesacaine (for infiltration and regional anesthesia), Nesacaine-CE (for caudal and epidural anesthesia)

Pregnancy Risk Category: C

MECHANISM OF ACTION
A local anesthetic of the ester type. Blocks depolarization by interfering with sodium-potassium exchange across the nerve cell membrane, preventing generation and conduction of the nerve impulse.

INDICATIONS & DOSAGE
Available only without epinephrine.
Infiltration and nerve block:
Adults: Dosage limit is 11 mg/kg (14 mg/kg when used with epinephrine).

Sol.	Vol. (ml)	Dose (mg)
1%	3 to 20	30 to 200
2%	2 to 40	40 to 800

Caudal and epidural:

Sol.	Vol. (ml)	Dose (mg)
2% to 3%	15 to 25	300 to 750

May repeat with smaller doses q 40 to 50 minutes. Dose and interval may be increased with epinephrine. Maximum adult dosage is 800 mg, or 1 g when mixed with epinephrine.

ADVERSE REACTIONS
Skin: dermatologic reactions.
Other: edema, status asthmaticus, *anaphylaxis,* anaphylactoid reactions. The following systemic effects may result from high blood levels of the drug:
CNS: anxiety, nervousness, seizures followed by drowsiness, unconsciousness, tremors, twitches, shivering, *respiratory arrest.*
CV: myocardial depression, *dysrhythmias, cardiac arrest.*
EENT: blurred vision, tinnitus.
GI: nausea, vomiting.

INTERACTIONS
None significant.

NURSING CONSIDERATIONS
• Contraindicated in hypersensitivity to procaine, tetracaine, or other para-aminobenzoic acid derivatives, and for spinal or topical anesthesia. Epidural and caudal blocks are contraindicated in CNS disease. Use cautiously in debilitated, elderly, or acutely ill patients; in children; and in patients with drug allergies, paracervical block, or cardiovascular disease.

• With epidural use, a 3-ml test dose should be injected at least 10 minutes before giving total dose to check for intravascular or subarachnoid injection. Motor paralysis and extensive sensory anesthesia indicate subarachnoid injection.

• Repeat the test dose if patient is moved in a way that might displace the epidural catheter.

• At least 5 minutes should elapse after each test before proceeding further.

• Don't use solution with preservatives for caudal or epidural block.

• Don't use discolored solution.

- Keep resuscitative equipment and drugs available.
- Duration is 30 to 60 minutes.
- Discard partially used vials without preservatives.
- Check solution for particles.

etidocaine hydrochloride
Duranest

Pregnancy Risk Category: B

MECHANISM OF ACTION
A local anesthetic of the amide type. Blocks depolarization by interfering with sodium-potassium exchange across the nerve cell membrane, preventing generation and conduction of the nerve impulse. When combined with epinephrine, action is prolonged.

INDICATIONS & DOSAGE
Available with or without epinephrine. Doses cited are for drug with *epinephrine. Dose and interval are decreased without epinephrine.*
Adults: Dose limit is 4 mg/kg or 300 mg per injection. When combined with epinephrine, dose limit is 5.5 mg/kg or 400 mg/injection.
Peripheral nerve block:

Sol.	Vol. (ml)	Dose (mg)
0.5%	5 to 40	25 to 200
1%	5 to 40	50 to 400

Central neural block:
Lower limbs, cesarean section, lumbar peridural

Sol.	Vol. (ml)	Dose (mg)
1%	10 to 30	100 to 300
1.5%	10 to 20	150 to 300

Vaginal:

Sol.	Vol. (ml)	Dose (mg)
1%	5 to 20	50 to 200

Caudal:

Sol.	Vol. (ml)	Dose (mg)
1%	10 to 30	100 to 300

ADVERSE REACTIONS
Skin: dermatologic reactions.
Other: edema, status asthmaticus, *anaphylaxis,* anaphylactoid reactions.

The following systemic effects may result from high blood levels of the drug:
CNS: anxiety, apprehension, nervousness, seizures followed by drowsiness, unconsciousness, tremors, twitches, shivering, and *respiratory arrest.*
CV: myocardial depression, *dysrhythmias, cardiac arrest.*
EENT: blurred vision, tinnitus.
GI: nausea, vomiting.

INTERACTIONS
Enflurane, halothane, and related drugs: cardiac dysrhythmias when used with etidocaine *with* epinephrine. Use with extreme caution.
MAO inhibitors, cyclic antidepressants, phenothiazines: severe, sustained hypertension or hypotension when used with etidocaine solution *with* epinephrine. Use with extreme caution.

NURSING CONSIDERATIONS
- Contraindicated in inflammation or infection in puncture region, children under 14 years, septicemia, severe hypertension, spinal deformities, neurologic disorders, and spinal block. Use cautiously in debilitated, elderly, or acutely ill patients; severe shock; heart block; epidural block in obstetrics; general drug allergies; and hepatic and renal disease.
- Use solutions with epinephrine cautiously in cardiovascular disease and in body areas with limited blood supply (ears, nose, fingers, toes).
- Don't use solution with preservatives for caudal or epidural block.
- Keep resuscitative equipment and drugs available.
- Onset in 2 to 8 minutes; duration is 3 to 6 hours.
- Check solution for particles.

lidocaine hydrochloride
Ardecaine, Dilocaine, Dolicaine, L-
Caine, Nervocaine, Norocaine,
Rocaine, Stanacaine, Ultracaine,
Xylocaine Hydrochloride♦

Pregnancy Risk Category: B

MECHANISM OF ACTION
A local anesthetic of the amide type.
Blocks depolarization by interfering
with sodium-potassium exchange
across the nerve cell membrane, preventing generation and conduction of
the nerve impulse. When combined
with epinephrine, action is prolonged.

INDICATIONS & DOSAGE
Available with or without epinephrine.
Doses cited are for drug without *epinephrine except where indicated.*
For anesthesia other than spinal—
maximum single adult dose is 4.5 mg/
kg or 300 mg.
*With epinephrine for anesthesia other
than spinal—*
maximum single adult dose is 7 mg/
kg or 500 mg. Don't repeat dose more
often than q 2 hours.
Caudal (obstetrics) *or epidural* (thoracic):

Sol.	Vol. (ml)	Dose (mg)
1%	20 to 30	200 to 300

Caudal (surgery):

Sol.	Vol. (ml)	Dose (mg)
1.5%	15 to 20	225 to 300

Epidural (lumbar anesthesia):

Sol.	Vol. (ml)	Dose (mg)
1.5%	15 to 20	225 to 300
2%	10 to 15	200 to 300

Maximum dose 200 to 300 mg/hour.
Spinal surgical anesthesia:

Sol.	Vol. (ml)	Dose (mg)
5% with	1.5 to 2	75 to 100
7.5%		

dextrose
    Dosage and interval are increased
with epinephrine.
For anesthesia other than spinal—
maximum single adult dose is 4.5 mg/
kg or 300 mg.

*With epinephrine for anesthesia other
than spinal—*
maximum single adult dose is 7 mg/
kg or 500 mg. Don't repeat dose more
often than q 2 hours.

ADVERSE REACTIONS
Skin: dermatologic reactions.
Other: edema, status asthmaticus,
anaphylaxis, anaphylactoid reactions.
    The following systemic effects may
result from high blood levels of the
drug:
CNS: anxiety, nervousness, seizures
followed by drowsiness, unconsciousness, tremors, twitches, shivering, *respiratory arrest.*
CV: myocardial depression, *dysrhythmias, cardiac arrest.*
EENT: blurred vision, tinnitus.
GI: nausea, vomiting.

INTERACTIONS
*Enflurane, halothane, and related
drugs:* cardiac dysrhythmias when
used with lidocaine *with* epinephrine.
Use with extreme caution.
*MAO inhibitors, cyclic antidepres-
sants:* severe, sustained hypertension
when used with lidocaine *with* epinephrine. Use with extreme caution.

NURSING CONSIDERATIONS
• Contraindicated in inflammation or
infection in puncture region, septicemia, severe hypertension, spinal
deformities, and neurologic disorders.
Use cautiously in debilitated, elderly,
or acutely ill patients; severe shock;
heart block; obstetrics; general drug
allergies; and paracervical block.
• Use solutions with epinephrine cautiously in cardiovascular disorders
and in body areas with limited blood
supply (ears, nose, fingers, toes).
• Keep resuscitative equipment and
drugs available.
• With epidural use, a 2- to 5-ml test
dose should be injected at least 5 minutes before giving total dosage to
check for intravascular or subarach-

noid injection. Motor paralysis and extensive sensory anesthesia indicate subarachnoid injection. Sudden onset of tachycardia, hypotension, or adverse CNS effects may indicate intravascular injection.

• Solutions containing preservatives should not be used for spinal, epidural, or caudal block.

• Discard partially used vials without preservatives.

• Check solution for particles.

---

mepivacaine hydrochloride
Carbocaine♦, Cavacaine, Isocaine♦

Pregnancy Risk Category: C

MECHANISM OF ACTION
A local anesthetic of the amide type. Blocks depolarization by interfering with sodium-potassium exchange across the nerve cell membrane, preventing generation and conduction of the nerve impulse. When combined with levonordefrin, action is prolonged.

INDICATIONS & DOSAGE
Available with or without levonordefrin (vasoconstrictor). Doses cited are for drug without levonordefrin.
Nerve block:

Sol.	Vol. (ml)	Dose (mg)
1%	5 to 20	50 to 200
2%	5 to 20	100 to 400

Transvaginal block or infiltration (maximum dose):

Sol.	Vol. (ml)	Dose (mg)
1%	40	400

Paracervical block (obstetrics):

Sol.	Vol. (ml)	Dose (mg)
1%	10	100

Give on each side (200 mg total) per 90-minute block.
Caudal and epidural:

Sol.	Vol. (ml)	Dose (mg)
1%	15 to 30	150 to 300
1.5%	10 to 25	150 to 375
2%	10 to 20	200 to 400

Therapeutic block (pain management):

Sol.	Vol. (ml)	Dose (mg)
1%	1 to 5	10 to 50
2%	1 to 5	20 to 100

Adults: maximum single dose 7 mg/ kg up to 550 mg. Don't repeat more often than q 90 minutes. Maximum dosage 1,000 mg daily.
Children: maximum dose 5 to 6 mg/ kg. In children under 3 years or weighing less than 14 kg, use 0.5% or 1.5% solution only. Dose and interval may be increased with levonordefrin.

ADVERSE REACTIONS
Skin: dermatologic reactions.
Other: edema, status asthmaticus, *anaphylaxis,* anaphylactoid reactions.
The following systemic effects may result from high blood levels of the drug:
CNS: anxiety, nervousness, seizures followed by drowsiness, unconsciousness, tremors, twitches, shivering, *respiratory arrest.*
CV: myocardial depression, *dysrhythmias, cardiac arrest.*
EENT: blurred vision, tinnitus.
GI: nausea, vomiting.

INTERACTIONS
Enflurane, halothane, and related drugs: cardiac dysrhythmias when used with mepivacaine *with* levonordefrin. Use with extreme caution.
MAO inhibitors, cyclic antidepressants: severe, sustained hypertension when used with mepivacaine *with* levonordefrin. Use with extreme caution.

NURSING CONSIDERATIONS
• Contraindicated in sensitivity to methylparaben, in heart block, or for spinal anesthesia. Use cautiously in debilitated, elderly, or acutely ill patients, and for paracervical block.
• Use solutions with levonordefrin cautiously in cardiovascular disease and in body areas with limited blood

---

Italicized side effects are common or life-threatening.
*Liquid form contains alcohol.   **May contain tartrazine.

supply (ears, nose, fingers, toes).
• Monitor fetal heart rate when paracervical block is used in delivery.
• Keep resuscitative equipment and drugs available.
• Don't use solutions with preservatives for caudal or epidural block.
• Onset in 15 minutes; duration is 3 hours.
• Discard partially used vials without preservatives.
• Check solution for particles.

---

procaine hydrochloride
Novocain♦, Unicaine

Pregnancy Risk Category: C

MECHANISM OF ACTION
A local anesthetic of the ester type. Blocks depolarization by interfering with sodium-potassium exchange across the nerve cell membrane, preventing generation and conduction of the nerve impulse.

INDICATIONS & DOSAGE
Spinal anesthesia—
Maximum dose is 11 mg/kg (14 mg/kg when mixed with epinephrine).
Before using, dilute 10% solution with 0.9% sodium chloride injection, sterile distilled water, or cerebrospinal fluid.
For hyperbaric technique, use dextrose solution.
Perineum: use 0.5 ml 10% solution and 0.5 ml diluent injected at fourth lumbar interspace.
Perineum and lower extremities: use 1 ml 10% solution and 1 ml diluent injected at third or fourth lumbar interspace.
Up to costal margin: use 2 ml 10% solution and 1 ml diluent injected at second, third, or fourth lumbar interspace.
Epidural block:

Sol.	Vol. (ml)	Dose (mg)
1.5%	25	375

Peripheral nerve block:

Sol.	Vol. (ml)	Dose (mg)
1%	50	500
2%	25	500

Infiltration: use 250 to 600 mg 0.25% to 0.5% solution. Maximum initial dose 1 g. Dose and interval may be increased with epinephrine. Maximum dosage 11 mg/kg to 14 mg/kg or epinephrine.

ADVERSE REACTIONS
Skin: dermatologic reactions.
Other: edema, status asthmaticus, *anaphylaxis,* anaphylactoid reactions.
The following systemic effects may result from high blood levels of the drug:
CNS: anxiety, nervousness, seizures followed by drowsiness, unconsciousness, tremors, twitches, shivering, *respiratory arrest*.
CV: myocardial depression, *dysrhythmias, cardiac arrest*.
EENT: blurred vision, tinnitus.
GI: nausea, vomiting.

INTERACTIONS
Echothiophate iodide: reduced hydrolysis of procaine. Use together cautiously.

NURSING CONSIDERATIONS
• Contraindicated in traumatized urethra and in hypersensitivity to chloroprocaine, tetracaine, or other paraaminobenzoic acid derivatives. Use cautiously in hyperexcitable patients and in CNS diseases, infection at puncture site, shock, profound anemia, cachexia, sepsis, hypertension, hypotension, GI hemorrhage, bowel perforation or strangulation, peritonitis, cardiac decompensation, massive pleural effusions, and increased intraabdominal pressure.
• Contraindications in obstetric use are pelvic disproportion, placenta previa, abruptio placentae, floating fetal head, and intrauterine manipulation.

• Keep resuscitative equipment and drugs available.

• A 1- to 5-ml test dose should be given 5 to 15 minutes before total epidural dose. Motor paralysis and extensive sensory anesthesia indicate subarachnoid injection. Sudden onset of tachycardia, hypotension, or adverse CNS effects may indicate intravascular injection.

• Use solution without preservatives for epidural block.

• Onset in 2 to 5 minutes; duration 60 minutes.

• Discard partially used vials without preservatives.

• Check solution for particles.

---

tetracaine hydrochloride
Pontocaine♦

Pregnancy Risk Category: C

MECHANISM OF ACTION
A local anesthetic of the ester type. Blocks depolarization by interfering with sodium-potassium exchange across the nerve cell membrane, preventing generation and conduction of the nerve impulse.

INDICATIONS & DOSAGE
Low spinal (saddle block) in vaginal delivery—
give 2 to 5 mg as hyperbaric solution (in 10% dextrose).
Perineum and lower extremities: give 5 to 10 mg.
Up to costal margin: give 15 to 20 mg.

ADVERSE REACTIONS
Skin: dermatologic reactions.
Other: edema, status asthmaticus, *anaphylaxis,* anaphylactoid reactions.
   The following systemic effects may result from high blood levels of the drug:
CNS: anxiety, nervousness, seizures followed by drowsiness, unconsciousness, tremors, twitches, shivering, and *respiratory arrest*.

CV: myocardial depression, *dysrhythmias, cardiac arrest*.
EENT: blurred vision, tinnitus.
GI: nausea, vomiting.

INTERACTIONS
None significant.

NURSING CONSIDERATIONS
• Contraindicated in infection at injection site, serious CNS diseases, and in hypersensitivity to procaine, chloroprocaine, tetracaine, or other para-aminobenzoic acid derivatives. Use cautiously in shock, profound anemia, cachexia, hypertension, hypotension, peritonitis, cardiac decompensation, massive pleural effusion, increased intracranial pressure, infection, and in highly nervous patients.

• Saddle block contraindicated in cephalopelvic disproportion, placenta previa, abruptio placentae, intrauterine manipulation, and floating fetal head.

• Don't use cloudy, discolored, or crystallized solutions.

• Keep resuscitative equipment and drugs available.

• 10 times as strong as procaine hydrochloride.

• Onset in 15 minutes; duration up to 3 hours.

• When cerebrospinal fluid is added to powdered drug or drug solution during spinal anesthesia, solution may be cloudy.

• If administering by topical spray, advise patient not to inhale solution.

• Protect from light; store in refrigerator.

Italicized side effects are common or life-threatening.
*Liquid form contains alcohol.   **May contain tartrazine.

100

General anesthetics

droperidol
etomidate
fentanyl citrate with droperidol
ketamine hydrochloride
methohexital sodium
thiopental sodium

COMBINATION PRODUCTS
None.

---

droperidol
Inapsine♦

Pregnancy Risk Category: C

MECHANISM OF ACTION
Acts at subcortical levels to produce sedation.

INDICATIONS & DOSAGE
Premedication—
Adults: 2.5 to 10 mg (1 to 4 ml) I.M. 30 to 60 minutes preoperatively.
Children 2 to 12 years: 1 to 1.5 mg (0.4 to 0.6 ml) per 20 to 25 lbs of body weight I.M.
As an induction agent—
Adults: 2.5 mg (1 ml) per 20 to 25 lbs I.V. with analgesic and/or general anesthetic.
Children 2 to 12 years: 1 to 1.5 mg (0.4 to 0.6 ml) per 20 to 25 lbs I.V. Dosage should be titrated.
Elderly and debilitated patients: initial dose should be decreased.
*Maintenance dosage in general anesthesia—*1.25 to 2.5 mg (0.5 to 1 ml) I.V.

ADVERSE REACTIONS
Blood: *agranulocytosis.*

CNS: extrapyramidal reactions (dystonia, akathisia), upward rotation of eyes and oculogyric crises, extended neck, flexed arms, fine tremor of limbs, dizziness, chills or shivering, facial sweating, restlessness, decreased seizure threshold.
CV: hypotension, tachycardia.

INTERACTIONS
None significant.

NURSING CONSIDERATIONS
• Use cautiously in elderly or debilitated patients and in patients with hypotension or other cardiovascular disease, impaired hepatic or renal function, and Parkinson's disease.
• Watch for extrapyramidal reactions. Call doctor at once if any occur.
• Approved by FDA *only* for use preoperatively and during induction and maintenance of anesthesia.
• A butyrophenone compound, related to haloperiodol; has greater tendency to cause extrapyramidal reactions than other antipsychotics.
• Keep I.V. fluids and vasopressors handy for hypotension.
• Monitor vital signs frequently; notify doctor of any changes immediately.
• Give I.V. injections slowly.
• Do not place patient in Trendelenburg's position (that is, shock position); severe hypotension and deeper anesthesia may result, causing respiratory arrest.

---

etomidate
Amidate, Hypnomidate

Pregnancy Risk Category: C

MECHANISM OF ACTION
Inhibits the firing rate of neurons within the ascending reticular-activating system.

INDICATIONS & DOSAGE
Induction of general anesthesia—
Adults and children over 10 years: 0.2 to 0.6 mg/kg I.V. over a period of 30 to 60 seconds.

ADVERSE REACTIONS
CNS: *myoclonic movements, averting movements, tonic movements, transient apnea, hyperventilation, hypoventilation.*
CV: hypertension, hypotension, tachycardia, bradycardia.
EENT: *eye movements,* laryngospasms.
GI: nausea or vomiting following induction of anesthesia.
Skin: inhibition of adrenal steroid production.
Local: *transient venous pain.*
Other: hiccups, snoring.

INTERACTIONS
None significant.

NURSING CONSIDERATIONS
• Should not be used during labor and delivery, including cesarean sections.
• Smaller increments of I.V. etomidate may be administered to adults during short operations to supplement subpotent anesthetic agents, such as nitrous oxide.
• Other commonly used preanesthesia drugs may be given before etomidate is used.
• Etomidate has a rapid onset of action (about 1 minute). Duration of effect is short (3 to 5 minutes).
• Transient muscle movements can be decreased by first administering 0.1

mg of fentanyl.
• Muscle movements seem more common in patients who feel transient venous pain after injection.
• Monitor vital signs before, during, and after anesthesia.
• Have resuscitative equipment and drugs ready. Maintain airway.
• Corticosteroid supplementation may be ordered to counteract reported inhibition of adrenal steroid production.
• Etomidate has a much lower incidence of cardiovascular and respiratory effects; therefore advantageous for inducing anesthesia in high-risk surgical patients.

fentanyl citrate with droperidol
Innovar (Each ml contains [in a 1:50 ratio] fentanyl 0.05 mg as a citrate and droperidol 2.5 mg.)
Controlled Substance Schedule II

Pregnancy Risk Category: C

MECHANISM OF ACTION
Acts as a CNS depressant to produce a general calming effect, reduced motor activity, and analgesia.

INDICATIONS & DOSAGE
Dosages vary depending on application; use of other agents; and patient's age, body weight, and clinical status.
Anesthesia—
Adults:
*Premedication—*0.5 to 2 ml I.M. 45 to 60 minutes before surgery.
*Adjunct to general anesthesia—*Induction: 1 ml/20 to 25 lb body weight by slow I.V. to produce neuroleptanalgesia.
Maintenance: not indicated as sole agent for maintenance of surgical anesthesia. Used in combination with other agents. To prevent excessive accumulation of the relatively long-acting droperidol component, fentanyl alone should be used in increments of

0.025 to 0.05 mg (0.5 to 1 ml) for maintenance of analgesia. However, during prolonged surgery, additional 0.5- to 1-ml amounts of Innovar may be given with caution.
Diagnostic procedures—0.5 to 2 ml I.M. 45 to 60 minutes before procedure. In prolonged procedure, give 0.5 to 1 ml I.V. with caution and without a general anesthetic.
Adjunct in regional anesthesia—1 to 2 ml I.M. or slow I.V.
Children:
Premedication—0.25 ml/20 lb body weight I.M. 45 to 60 minutes before surgery.
Adjunct to general anesthesia—0.5 ml/20 lb body weight (total combined dose for induction and maintenance). Following induction with Innovar, fentanyl alone in a dose of ¼ to ⅓ of adult dosage should be used to avoid accumulation of droperidol. However, during prolonged surgery, additional amounts of Innovar may be administered with caution. Safety of use in children under 2 years has not been established.

ADVERSE REACTIONS
CNS: emergence delirium and hallucinations, postoperative drowsiness.
CV: vasodilation, *hypotension,* decreased pulmonary arterial pressure, bradycardia, or tachycardia.
EENT: blurred vision, *laryngospasms.*
GI: *nausea, vomiting.*
Respiratory: *respiratory depression, apnea,* or *arrest.*
Other: drug dependence, muscle rigidity, chills, *shivering,* diaphoresis.

INTERACTIONS
CNS depressants (such as barbiturates, tranquilizers, narcotics, and general anesthetics): additive or potentiating effect. Dosage should be reduced.
MAO inhibitors: severe and unpredictable potentiation of Innovar. Do not use together or within 2 weeks of MAO inhibitor therapy.

NURSING CONSIDERATIONS
• Contraindicated in intolerance to either component. Use with caution in patients with head injuries and increased intracranial pressure, chronic obstructive pulmonary disease, hepatic and renal dysfunction, bradyarrhythmias, and in elderly or debilitated patients.
• Hypotension is a common side effect. However, if blood pressure drops, also consider hypovolemia as a possible cause. Use appropriate parenteral fluids to help restore blood pressure.
• Vital signs should be monitored frequently.
• Be aware that respiratory depression, rigidity of respiratory muscles, and respiratory arrest can occur. Have narcotic antagonist and resuscitative equipment on hand.
• Maintain airway.
• Postoperative EEG pattern may return to normal slowly.
• If narcotic analgesics are required postoperatively, use initially in reduced doses, as low as ¼ to ⅓ those usually recommended.
• When Innovar is given for anesthesia induction, fentanyl (Sublimaze) should be used for maintenance analgesia during procedure.
• Premedication with Innovar has sometimes been associated with patient agitation and refusal of surgery. Administration of diazepam may relieve this.

---

ketamine hydrochloride
Ketalar♦

Pregnancy Risk Category: C

MECHANISM OF ACTION
Interrupts association pathways in the brain, causing dissociative anesthesia, a feeling of dissociation from the en-

---

vironment.

INDICATIONS & DOSAGE
Induce anesthesia for procedures, especially short-term diagnostic or surgical, not requiring skeletal muscle relaxation; before giving other general anesthetics or to supplement low-potency agents, such as nitrous oxide—
Adults and children: 1 to 4.5 mg/kg I.V., administered over 60 seconds; or 6.5 to 13 mg/kg I.M. To maintain anesthesia, repeat in increments of half to full initial dose.

ADVERSE REACTIONS
CNS: *tonic and clonic movements resembling seizures, respiratory depression, apnea when administered too rapidly.*
CV: *increased blood pressure and pulse rate,* hypotension, bradycardia.
EENT: diplopia, nystagmus, slight increase in intraocular pressure, *laryngospasms, salivation.*
GI: mild anorexia, nausea, vomiting.
Skin: transient erythema, measles-like rash.
Other: *dream-like states, hallucinations, confusion, excitement,* irrational behavior, psychic abnormalities.

INTERACTIONS
Thyroid hormones: may elevate blood pressure and cause tachycardia. Give cautiously.

NURSING CONSIDERATIONS
• Contraindicated in patients with history of CVA; patients who would be endangered by a significant rise in blood pressure; and in severe hypertension, severe cardiac decompensation, or surgery of the pharynx, larynx, or bronchial tree (unless used with muscle relaxants). Use with caution in chronic alcoholism, alcohol-intoxicated patients, and in patients with cerebrospinal fluid pressure elevated before anesthesia.
• Because of rapid induction, patient should be physically supported during administration.
• Do not inject barbiturates and ketamine from same syringe, as they are chemically incompatible.
• Monitor vital signs before, during, and after anesthesia.
• Check cardiac function in patients with hypertension or cardiac depression.
• Maintain airway.
• Resuscitative equipment should be available and ready for use.
• Start supportive respiration if respiratory depression occurs. Use mechanical support if possible rather than administering analeptics.
• Keep verbal, tactile, and visual stimulation at a minimum during recovery phase to reduce incidence of emergent reactions.
• Hallucinations and excitement can occur on emergence from anesthesia; they can be abated by administering diazepam.
• A potent hallucinogen that can readily produce dissociative anesthesia (patient feels detached from environment). Dissociative effect and hallucinatory side effects have made this a popular drug of abuse among young people.

---

methohexital sodium
Brevital Sodium, Brietal Sodium♦♦
Controlled Substance Schedule IV

Pregnancy Risk Category: D

MECHANISM OF ACTION
Inhibits the firing rate of neurons within the ascending reticular-activating system.

INDICATIONS & DOSAGE
General anesthetic for short-term procedures (oral surgery, gynecologic and genitourinary examinations); reduction of fractures; before electro-

---

Italicized side effects are common or life-threatening.
*Liquid form contains alcohol.   **May contain tartrazine.

convulsive therapy; for prolonged anesthesia when used with gaseous anesthetics—
Adults and children: 5 to 12 ml 1% solution (50 to 120 mg) I.V. at 1 ml/5 seconds. Dose required for induction may vary from 50 to 120 mg or more; average about 70 mg. Induction dose provides anesthesia for 5 to 7 minutes.
Maintenance—
Intermittent injection: 2 to 4 ml 1% solution (20 to 40 mg) q 4 to 7 minutes.
Continuous I.V. drip: administer 0.2% solution (1 drop/second).

ADVERSE REACTIONS
CNS: *muscular twitching,* headache, emergence delirium.
CV: *transient hypotension, tachycardia,* circulatory depression, *peripheral vascular collapse.*
GI: excessive salivation, *nausea, vomiting.*
Respiratory: *laryngospasm, bronchospasm, respiratory depression, apnea.*
Skin: tissue necrosis with extravasation.
Local: thrombophlebitis, pain at injection site, injury to nerves adjacent to injection site.
Other: hiccups, coughing, acute allergic reactions. Extended use may cause cumulative effect.

INTERACTIONS
None significant.

NURSING CONSIDERATIONS
• Contraindicated in severe hepatic dysfunction, hypersensitivity to barbiturates, or porphyria; in shock or impending shock; and in patients for whom general anesthetics would be hazardous. Use with caution in debilitated patients; in asthma, respiratory obstruction, severe hypertension or hypotension, myocardial disease, CHF, severe anemia, and extreme obesity.
• Maintain pulmonary ventilation.
• Avoid extravascular or intraarterial injections.
• Monitor vital signs before, during, and after anesthesia.
• Have resuscitative equipment and drugs ready.
• Reduce postoperative nausea by having patient fast before administration.
• Incompatible with silicone; avoid contact with rubber stoppers or parts of syringes that have been treated with silicone.
• Incompatible with lactated Ringer's solution.
• Do not mix with acid solutions, such as atropine sulfate.
• Solvents recommended are 5% glucose solution or normal saline solution instead of distilled water.
• Rate of flow must be individualized for each patient.
• Solutions may be stored and used as long as they remain clear and colorless. Solutions cannot be heated for sterilization.
• Has potential for abuse.

thiopental sodium
Pentothal Sodium♦
(injection and rectal suspension)
Controlled Substance Schedule III
Pregnancy Risk Category: C

MECHANISM OF ACTION
Inhibits the firing rate of neurons within the ascending reticular-activating system.

INDICATIONS & DOSAGE
Induce anesthesia before administering other anesthetics—
210 to 280 mg (3 to 4 ml/kg) usually required for average adult (70 kg).
General anesthetic for short-term procedures—
Adults: 2 to 3 ml 2.5% solution (50 to 75 mg) administered I.V. only at in-

---

tervals of 20 to 40 seconds, depending on reaction. Dose may be repeated with caution, if necessary.

Convulsive states following anesthesia—
75 to 125 mg (3 to 5 ml of 2.5% solution) immediately.

Psychiatric disorders (narcoanalysis, narcosynthesis)—
100 mg/minute (4 ml/minute 2.5% solution) until confusion occurs and before sleep.

Basal anesthesia by rectal administration—
Adults and children: administer up to 1 g/22.5 kg (50 lb) body weight, or 0.5 ml 10% solution/kg body weight. Maximum 1 to 1.5 g (children weighing 34 kg or more) and 3 to 4 g (adults weighing 91 kg or more).

Note: Thiopental is rarely administered rectally for basal sedation or anesthesia because of variable absorption from the rectum.

ADVERSE REACTIONS
CNS: *prolonged somnolence,* retrograde amnesia.
CV: *myocardial depression, dysrhythmias.*
Skin: tissue necrosis with extravasation.
Respiratory: *respiratory depression (momentary apnea following each injection is typical), bronchospasm, laryngospasm.*
Local: pain at injection site.
Other: sneezing, coughing, *shivering.*

INTERACTIONS
None significant.

NURSING CONSIDERATIONS
• Contraindicated in absence of suitable veins for I.V. administration, hypersensitivity to barbiturates, status asthmaticus, porphyria, respiratory depression or obstruction, decompensated cardiac disease, severe anemia, hepatic cirrhosis, shock, renal dysfunction, myxedema.

• Give test dose (1 to 3 ml 2.5% solution) to assess reaction to drug.
• When used as general anesthetic, give atropine sulfate as premedication to diminish laryngeal reflexes and to prevent laryngeal spasm.
• Have resuscitative equipment and oxygen ready. Maintain airway.
• Avoid extravasation.
• Monitor vital signs before, during, and after anesthesia.
• Solutions of atropine sulfate, *d*-tubocurarine, or succinylcholine may be given concurrently.
• Do not heat solutions for sterilization. Solutions should be used within 24 hours.
• Has potential for abuse.

Italicized side effects are common or life-threatening.
*Liquid form contains alcohol.   **May contain tartrazine.

101

Vitamins and minerals

vitamin A◊
vitamin B complex◊
  cyanocobalamin (vitamin B$_{12}$)◊
  folic acid (vitamin B$_9$)◊
  hydroxocobalamin (vitamin
    B$_{12a}$)
  leucovorin calcium
    (citrovorum factor or folinic
    acid)
  niacin (vitamin B$_3$, nicotinic
    acid)◊
  niacinamide (nicotinamide)◊
  pyridoxine hydrochloride
    (vitamin B$_6$)◊
  riboflavin (vitamin B$_2$)◊
  thiamine hydrochloride
    (vitamin B$_1$)◊
vitamin C (ascorbic acid)◊
vitamin D◊
  cholecalciferol (D$_3$)◊
  ergocalciferol (D$_2$)◊
vitamin E◊
vitamin K analogs
  menadione/menadiol sodium
    diphosphate (vitamin K$_3$)
  phytonadione (vitamin K$_1$)
multivitamins◊
sodium fluoride◊
trace elements
zinc sulfate◊

COMBINATION PRODUCTS
B complex vitamins◊
B complex vitamins with iron◊
B complex with vitamin C◊
B vitamin combinations◊
Calcium and vitamin products◊
Fluoride with vitamins
Geriatric supplements with multivitamins and minerals◊
Miscellaneous vitamins and minerals◊

Multivitamins◊
Multivitamins and minerals with hormones◊
Multivitamins with B$_{12}$◊
Vitamin A and D combinations◊

---

vitamin A◊
Acon, Aquasol A♦

*Pregnancy Risk Category: A (X if >
RDA)*

MECHANISM OF ACTION
Coenzyme necessary for retinal function, bone growth, and differentiation of epithelial tissues.

INDICATIONS & DOSAGE
*Severe vitamin A deficiency with
xerophthalmia—*
Adults and children over 8 years:
500,000 IU P.O. daily for 3 days, then
50,000 IU P.O. daily for 14 days, then
maintenance with 10,000 to 20,000
IU P.O. daily for 2 months, followed
by adequate dietary nutrition and
RDA vitamin A supplements.
Severe vitamin A deficiency—
Adults and children over 8 years:
100,000 IU P.O. or I.M. daily for 3
days, then 50,000 IU P.O. or I.M.
daily for 14 days, then maintenance
with 10,000 to 20,000 IU P.O. daily
for 2 months, followed by adequate
dietary nutrition and RDA vitamin A
supplements.
Children 1 to 8 years: 17,500 to
35,000 IU I.M. daily for 10 days.
Infants under 1 year: 7,500 to
15,000 IU I.M. daily for 10 days.
Maintenance only—

Children 4 to 8 years: 15,000 IU I.M. daily for 2 months, then adequate dietary nutrition and RDA vitamin A supplements.
Children under 4 years: 10,000 IU I.M. daily for 2 months, then adequate dietary nutrition and RDA vitamin A supplements.

ADVERSE REACTIONS

Adverse effects are usually seen only with toxicity (hypervitaminosis A).
Blood: hypoplastic anemia, leukopenia.
CNS: irritability, headache, increased intracranial pressure, fatigue, lethargy, malaise.
EENT: miosis, papilledema, exophthalmos.
GI: anorexia, epigastric pain, diarrhea.
GU: hypomenorrhea.
Hepatic: jaundice, hepatomegaly.
Skin: alopecia; drying, cracking, scaling of skin; pruritus; lip fissures; massive desquamation; increased pigmentation; night sweating.
Other: skeletal—slow growth, decalcification of bone, fractures, hyperostosis, painful periostitis, premature closure of epiphyses, migratory arthralgia, cortical thickening over the radius and tibia, bulging fontanelles; splenomegaly.

INTERACTIONS

Mineral oil, cholestyramine resin: reduced GI absorption of fat-soluble vitamins. If needed, give mineral oil at bedtime.

NURSING CONSIDERATIONS

• Oral administration contraindicated in malabsorption syndrome; if malabsorption is from inadequate bile secretion, oral route may be used with concurrent administration of bile salts (dehydrocholic acid). Also contraindicated in hypervitaminosis A. I.V. administration contraindicated except for special water-miscible forms intended for infusion with large parenteral volumes. I.V. push of vitamin A of any type is also contraindicated (anaphylaxis or anaphylactoid reactions and death have resulted).
• Evaluate patient's vitamin A intake from fortified foods, dietary supplements, self-administered drugs, and prescription drug sources.
• In pregnant women, avoid doses exceeding RDA.
• To avoid toxicity, discourage patient self-administration of megavitamin doses without specific indications. Also stress that the patient should not share prescribed vitamins with family members or others. If family member feels vitamin therapy may be of value, have him contact his doctor.
• Watch for adverse effects if dosage is high.
• Acute toxicity has resulted from single doses of 25,000 IU/kg of body weight; 350,000 IU in infants and over 2,000,000 IU in adults have also proved acutely toxic.
• Chronic toxicity in infants (3 to 6 months) has resulted from doses of 18,500 IU daily for 1 to 3 months. In adults, chronic toxicity has resulted from doses of 50,000 IU daily for over 8 months; 500,000 IU daily for 2 months; and 1,000,000 IU daily for 3 days.
• Monitor patient closely during vitamin A therapy for skin disorders since high dosages may induce chronic toxicity.
• Liquid preparations available if nasogastric administration is necessary. May be mixed with cereal or fruit juice.
• Record eating and bowel habits. Report abnormalities to doctor.
• Adequate vitamin A absorption requires suitable protein intake, bile (give supplemental salts if necessary), concurrent RDA doses of vitamin E, and zinc (multivitamins usually supply zinc, but supplements may be necessary in long-term total parenteral

---

Italicized side effects are common or life-threatening.
*Liquid form contains alcohol.   **May contain tartrazine.

nutrition).
- Absorption is fastest and most complete with water-miscible preparations, intermediate with emulsions, and slowest with oil suspensions.
- In severe hepatic dysfunction, diabetes, and hypothyroidism, use vitamin A rather than carotenes for vitamin A therapy because the vitamin itself is more easily absorbed and the diseases adversely affect conversion of carotenes into vitamin A. If carotenes are prescribed, dosage should be doubled.
- Because of the potential for additive toxicity, vitamin supplements containing vitamin A should be used cautiously in patients taking isotretinoin (Accutane).
- Protect from light and heat.

cyanocobalamin (vitamin B₁₂)◊
Anacobin◆◆, Bedoce, Bedoz◆◆, Betalin 12, Crystamine, Cyanabin◆◆, Cyanocobalamin, Cyano-Gel, Dodex, Kaybovite, Poyamin, Redisol, Rubesol-1000, Rubion◆◆, Rubramin◆, Sigamine

hydroxocobalamin (vitamin B₁₂ₐ)◊
Alpha-Ruvite, Codroxomin, Droxomin, Rubesol-L.A.

Pregnancy Risk Category: A (C if > RDA)

MECHANISM OF ACTION
Coenzyme for various metabolic functions. Necessary for cell replication and hematopoiesis.

INDICATIONS & DOSAGE
Vitamin B₁₂ deficiency caused by inadequate diet, subtotal gastrectomy, or any other condition, disorder, or disease except malabsorption related to pernicious anemia or other GI disease—
Adults: 25 mcg P.O. daily as dietary supplement, or 30 to 100 mcg S.C. or I.M. daily for 5 to 10 days, depending on severity of deficiency. Maintenance dosage is 100 to 200 mcg I.M. once monthly. For subsequent prophylaxis, advise adequate nutrition and daily RDA vitamin B₁₂ supplements.
Children: 1 mcg P.O. daily as dietary supplement, or 1 to 30 mcg S.C. or I.M. daily for 5 to 10 days, depending on severity of deficiency. Maintenance dosage is at least 60 mcg/month I.M. or S.C. For subsequent prophylaxis, advise adequate nutrition and daily RDA vitamin B₁₂ supplements.
Pernicious anemia or vitamin B₁₂ malabsorption—
Adults: initially, 100 to 1,000 mcg I.M. daily for 2 weeks, then 100 to 1,000 mcg I.M. once monthly for life. If neurologic complications are present, follow initial therapy with 100 to 1,000 mcg I.M. once q 2 weeks before starting monthly regimen.
Children: 1,000 to 5,000 mcg I.M. or S.C. given over 2 or more weeks in 100-mcg increments; then 60 mcg I.M. or S.C. monthly for life.
Methylmalonic aciduria—
Neonates: 1,000 mcg I.M. daily for 11 days with a protein-restricted diet.
Diagnostic test for vitamin B₁₂ deficiency without concealing folate deficiency in patients with megaloblastic anemias—
Adults and children: 1 mcg I.M. daily for 10 days with diet low in vitamin B₁₂ and folate. Reticulocytosis between days 3 and 10 confirms diagnosis of vitamin B₁₂ deficiency.
Schilling test flushing dose—
Adults and children: 1,000 mcg I.M. in a single dose.

ADVERSE REACTIONS
CV: peripheral vascular thrombosis.
GI: transient diarrhea.
Skin: itching, transitory exanthema, urticaria.
Local: pain, burning at S.C. or I.M.

---

injection sites.
Other: *anaphylaxis,* anaphylactoid reactions.

INTERACTIONS
Neomycin, colchicine, para-aminosalicylic acid and salts, chloramphenicol: malabsorption of vitamin B_{12}. Don't use together.

NURSING CONSIDERATIONS
• Parenteral administration contraindicated in hypersensitivity to vitamin B_{12} or cobalt. Alternate use of large oral doses of vitamin B_{12} is controversial and should not be considered routine; combined with intrinsic factor increases risk of hypersensitive reactions and should be avoided. Therapeutic dosage contraindicated before proper diagnosis; vitamin B_{12} therapy may mask folate deficiency.
• I.V. administration may cause anaphylactoid reactions. Use cautiously and only if other routes are ruled out.
• Use cautiously in anemic patients with coexisting cardiac, pulmonary, or hypertensive disease; in early Leber's disease; in severe vitamin B_{12}–dependent deficiencies, especially those receiving cardiotonic glycosides (monitor closely the first 2 to 3 days for hypokalemia, fluid overload, pulmonary edema, CHF, and hypertension); and in gouty conditions (monitor serum uric acid for hyperuricemia).
• Don't mix parenteral liquids in same syringe with other medications.
• Protect from light and heat.
• Infection, tumors, or renal, hepatic, and other debilitating diseases may reduce therapeutic response.
• Deficiencies are more common in strict vegetarians and their breast-fed infants.
• Stress need for patients with pernicious anemia to return for monthly injections. Although total body stores may last 3 to 6 years, anemia will recur if not treated monthly.

• May cause false-positive intrinsic factor antibody test.
• Hydroxocobalamin is approved for I.M. use only. Only advantage of hydroxocobalamin over vitamin B_{12} is its longer duration.
• 50% to 98% of injected dose may appear in urine within 48 hours. Major portion of drug is excreted within first 8 hours after injection.
• Closely monitor serum potassium for first 48 hours. Give potassium if necessary.
• Physically incompatible with dextrose solutions, alkaline or strongly acidic solutions, oxidizing and reducing agents, and many other drugs.

folic acid (vitamin B_9)
Folvite♦, Novofolacid♦♦
Pregnancy Risk Category: A (C if > RDA)

MECHANISM OF ACTION
Necessary for normal erythropoiesis and nucleoprotein synthesis.

INDICATIONS & DOSAGE
Megaloblastic or macrocytic anemia secondary to folic acid or other nutritional deficiency, hepatic disease, alcoholism, intestinal obstruction, excessive hemolysis—
Pregnant and lactating women: 0.8 mg P.O., S.C., or I.M. daily.
Adults and children over 4 years: 1 mg P.O., S.C., or I.M. daily for 4 to 5 days. After anemia secondary to folic acid deficiency is corrected, proper diet and RDA supplements are necessary to prevent recurrence.
Children under 4 years: up to 0.3 mg P.O., S.C., or I.M. daily.
Prevention of megaloblastic anemia of pregnancy and fetal damage—
Women: 1 mg P.O., S.C., or I.M. daily throughout pregnancy.
Nutritional supplement—
Adults: 0.1 mg P.O., S.C., or I.M. daily.

Children: 0.05 mg P.O. daily.
Treatment of tropical sprue—
Adults: 3 to 15 mg P.O. daily.
Test of megaloblastic anemia patients to detect folic acid deficiency without masking pernicious anemia—
Adults and children: 0.1 to 0.2 mg P.O. or I.M. for 10 days while maintaining a diet low in folate and vitamin B_{12}.
(Reticulosis, reversion to normoblastic hematopoiesis, and return to normal hemoglobin indicate folic acid deficiency.)

ADVERSE REACTIONS
Skin: allergic reactions (rash, pruritus, erythema).
Other: *allergic bronchospasms,* general malaise.

INTERACTIONS
Chloramphenicol: antagonism of folic acid. Monitor for decreased folic acid effect. Use together cautiously.

NURSING CONSIDERATIONS
• Contraindicated in normocytic, refractory, or aplastic anemias; as sole agent in treating pernicious anemia (because it may mask neurologic effects); in treating methotrexate, pyrimethamine, or trimethoprim overdose; and in undiagnosed anemia (because it may mask pernicious anemia).
• Patients with small-bowel resections and intestinal malabsorption may require parenteral administration routes.
• Don't mix with other medications in same syringe for I.M. injections.
• Protect from light and heat.
• May use concurrent folic acid and vitamin B_{12} therapy if supported by diagnosis.
• Proper nutrition is necessary to prevent recurrence of anemia.
• Peak folate activity occurs in the blood in 30 to 60 minutes.
• Patients with pernicious anemia

should avoid multivitamins containing folic acid.
• Hematologic response to folic acid in patients receiving chloramphenicol concurrently with folic acid should be carefully monitored.

leucovorin calcium (citrovorum factor or folinic acid)
Wellcovorin

Pregnancy Risk Category: C

MECHANISM OF ACTION
A reduced form of folic acid that is readily converted to other folic acid derivatives.

INDICATIONS & DOSAGE
Overdose of folic acid antagonist—
Adults and children: P.O., I.M., or I.V. dose equivalent to the weight of the antagonist given.
Leucovorin rescue after high methotrexate dose in treatment of malignancy—
Adults and children: dose at doctor's discretion within 6 to 36 hours of last dose of methotrexate.
Toxic effects of methotrexate used to treat severe psoriasis—
Adults and children: 4 to 8 mg I.M. 2 hours after methotrexate dose.
Hematologic toxicity caused by pyrimethamine therapy—
Adults and children: 5 mg P.O. or I.M. daily.
Hematologic toxicity caused by trimethoprim therapy—
Adults and children: 400 mcg to 5 mg P.O. or I.M. daily.
Megaloblastic anemia caused by congenital enzyme deficiency—
Adults and children: 3 to 6 mg I.M. daily, then 1 mg P.O. daily for life.
Folate-deficient megaloblastic anemia—
Adults and children: up to 1 mg of leucovorin I.M daily. Duration of treatment depends on hematologic re-

sponse.

ADVERSE REACTIONS
Skin: allergic reactions (rash, pruritus, erythema).
Other: *allergic bronchospasms.*

INTERACTIONS
None significant.

NURSING CONSIDERATIONS
• Contraindicated in treating undiagnosed anemia, since it may mask pernicious anemia. Use cautiously in pernicious anemia; a hemolytic remission may occur while neurologic manifestations remain progressive.
• Do not confuse leucovorin (folinic acid) with folic acid.
• Follow leucovorin rescue schedule and protocol closely to maximize therapeutic response. Generally, leucovorin should not be administered simultaneously with systemic methotrexate.
• Treat overdosage of folic acid antagonists; administer within 1 hour if possible; usually ineffective after 4-hour delay.
• Protect from light and heat, especially reconstituted parenteral preparations.
• Since allergic reactions have been reported with folic acid, the possibility of allergic reactions to leucovorin should be considered.

---

niacin (vitamin B₃, nicotinic acid)◇
Niac, Nico-400, Nicobid, Nicolar**, Ni-Span

niacinamide (nicotinamide)◇

Pregnancy Risk Category: A (C if > RDA)

MECHANISM OF ACTION
Necessary for lipid metabolism, tissue respiration, and glycogenolysis.

Also (niacin only) decreases synthesis of low-density lipoproteins and inhibits lipolysis in adipose tissue.

INDICATIONS & DOSAGE
Pellagra—
Adults: 10 to 20 mg P.O., S.C., I.M., or I.V. infusion daily, depending on severity of niacin deficiency. Maximum daily dosage recommended is 500 mg; should be divided into 10 doses, 50 mg each.
Children: up to 300 mg P.O. or 100 mg I.V. infusion daily, depending on severity of niacin deficiency.
  After symptoms subside, advise adequate nutrition and RDA supplements to prevent recurrence.
Peripheral vascular disease and circulatory disorders—
Adults: 250 to 800 mg P.O. daily in divided doses.
Adjunctive treatment of hyperlipidemias, especially with hypercholesterolemia—
Adults: 1.5 to 3 g daily in three divided doses with or after meals, increased at intervals to 6 g daily.

ADVERSE REACTIONS
Most adverse effects are dose-dependent.
CNS: dizziness, transient headache.
CV: *excessive peripheral vasodilation (especially niacin).*
GI: *nausea, vomiting, diarrhea,* possible activation of peptic ulcer, epigastric or substernal pain.
Hepatic: hepatic dysfunction.
Metabolic: hyperglycemia, hyperuricemia.
Skin: *flushing,* pruritus, dryness.

INTERACTIONS
Antihypertensive drugs (sympathetic blocking type): may have an additive vasodilating effect and cause postural hypotension. Use together cautiously. Warn patient about postural hypotension.

Italicized side effects are common or life-threatening.
*Liquid form contains alcohol.   **May contain tartrazine.

NURSING CONSIDERATIONS

• Contraindicated in hepatic dysfunction, active peptic ulcer disease, severe hypotension, or arterial hemorrhage. Use with caution in gallbladder disease, diabetes mellitus, and gout.
• Monitor hepatic function and blood glucose early in therapy.
• Give with meals to minimize GI side effects.
• Aspirin may reduce the flushing response to niacin.
• Timed-release niacin or niacinamide may avoid excessive flushing effects with large doses. Give slow I.V. (no faster than 2 mg/minute). Explain harmlessness of flushing syndrome to ease patient's mind.
• Stress that medication used to treat hyperlipoproteinemia or to dilate peripheral vessels is not "just a vitamin." Explain importance of adhering to therapeutic regimen.

pyridoxine hydrochloride (vitamin B₆)◇

Beesix, Hexa-Betalin♦, Hexacrest

Pregnancy Risk Category: A (C if > RDA)

MECHANISM OF ACTION

Acts as coenzyme for various metabolic functions. Required for amino acid metabolism.

INDICATIONS & DOSAGE

Dietary vitamin B₆ deficiency—
Adults: 10 to 20 mg P.O., I.M., or I.V. daily for 3 weeks, then 2 to 5 mg daily as a supplement to a proper diet.
Children: 100 mg P.O., I.M., or I.V. to correct deficiency, then an adequate diet with supplementary RDA doses to prevent recurrence.
Seizures related to vitamin B₆ deficiency or dependency—
Adults and children: 100 mg I.M. or I.V. in single dose.
Vitamin B₆–responsive anemias or dependency syndrome (inborn errors of metabolism)—
Adults: up to 600 mg P.O., I.M., or I.V. daily until symptoms subside, then 50 mg daily for life.
Children: 100 mg I.M. or I.V., then 2 to 10 mg I.M. or 10 to 100 mg P.O. daily.
Prevention of vitamin B₆ deficiency during isoniazid therapy—
Adults: 25 to 50 mg P.O. daily.
Children: at least 0.5 to 1.5 mg daily.
Infants: at least 0.1 to 0.5 mg daily.
If neurologic symptoms develop in pediatric patients, increase dosage as necessary.
Treatment of vitamin B₆ deficiency secondary to isoniazid—
Adults: 100 mg P.O. daily for 3 weeks, then 50 mg daily.

ADVERSE REACTIONS

CNS: drowsiness, paresthesias.

INTERACTIONS

None significant.

NURSING CONSIDERATIONS

• Contraindicated in hypersensitivity to parenteral pyridoxine and in doses larger than 5 mg for patients also receiving levodopa. Caution patient to check dosage, especially in multivitamins.
• Protect from light. Do not use injection solution if it contains a precipitate. Slight darkening is acceptable.
• Excessive protein intake increases daily pyridoxine requirements.
• If sodium bicarbonate is required to control acidosis in isoniazid toxicity, do not mix in same syringe with pyridoxine.
• If prescribed for maintenance therapy to prevent deficiency recurrence, stress importance of compliance and of good nutrition. Explain that pyridoxine in combination therapy with isoniazid has a specific therapeutic purpose and is not "just a vitamin." Explain importance of adhering to therapeutic regimen.

• Patients receiving levodopa alone (not with carbidopa) shouldn't take pyridoxine.
• Used to treat seizures and coma as a result of acute isoniazid overdosage. Dosage equal to amount of isoniazid ingested.

riboflavin (vitamin B₂)◊

Pregnancy Risk Category: A (C if > RDA)

MECHANISM OF ACTION
Converted to two other coenzymes that are necessary for normal tissue respiration.

INDICATIONS & DOSAGE
Riboflavin deficiency or adjunct to thiamine treatment for polyneuritis or cheilosis secondary to pellagra—
Adults and children over 12 years: 5 to 50 mg P.O., S.C., I.M., or I.V. daily, depending on severity.
Children under 12 years: 2 to 10 mg P.O., S.C., I.M., or I.V. daily, depending on severity.
For maintenance, increase nutritional intake and supplement with vitamin B complex.

ADVERSE REACTIONS
GU: high doses turn urine bright yellow.

INTERACTIONS
None significant.

NURSING CONSIDERATIONS
• Protect from light.
• Stress proper nutritional habits to prevent recurrence of deficiency.
• Riboflavin deficiency usually accompanies other vitamin B complex deficiencies and may require multivitamin therapy.
• Since food increases absorption of riboflavin, encourage patient to take with meals.

thiamine hydrochloride (vitamin B₁)◊
Apatate Drops, Thia

Pregnancy Risk Category: A (C if > RDA)

MECHANISM OF ACTION
Combines with adenosine triphosphate to form a coenzyme necessary for carbohydrate metabolism.

INDICATIONS & DOSAGE
Beriberi—
Adults: 10 to 500 mg, depending on severity, I.M. t.i.d. for 2 weeks, followed by dietary correction and multivitamin supplement containing 5 to 10 mg thiamine daily for 1 month.
Children: 10 to 50 mg, depending on severity, I.M. daily for several weeks with adequate dietary intake.
Anemia secondary to thiamine deficiency; polyneuritis secondary to alcoholism, pregnancy, or pellagra—
Adults: 100 mg P.O. daily.
Children: 10 to 50 mg P.O. daily in divided doses.
Wernicke's encephalopathy—
Adults: up to 500 mg to 1 g I.V. for crisis therapy, followed by 100 mg b.i.d. for maintenance.
"Wet beriberi," with myocardial failure—
Adults and children: 100 to 500 mg I.V. for emergency treatment.

ADVERSE REACTIONS
CNS: restlessness.
CV: *hypotension after rapid I.V. injection,* angioneurotic edema, cyanosis.
EENT: tightness of throat (allergic reaction).
GI: nausea, hemorrhage, diarrhea.
Skin: feeling of warmth, pruritus, urticaria, sweating.
Other: *anaphylactoid reactions,* weakness, pulmonary edema.

INTERACTIONS
None significant.

NURSING CONSIDERATIONS
• Contraindicated in hypersensitivity to thiamine products. I.V. push is contraindicated, except when treating life-threatening myocardial failure in "wet beriberi." Use with caution in I.V. administration of large doses; give patient skin test if he has a history of hypersensitivity before therapy. Have epinephrine on hand to treat anaphylaxis should it occur after a large parenteral dose.
• Thiamine malabsorption is most likely in alcoholism, cirrhosis, or GI disease.
• Use parenteral administration only when P.O. route is not feasible.
• Clinically significant deficiency can occur in approximately 3 weeks of totally thiamine-free diet. Thiamine deficiency usually requires concurrent treatment for multiple deficiencies.
• Doses larger than 30 mg t.i.d. may not be fully utilized. After tissue saturation with thiamine, it is excreted in urine as pyrimidine.
• If beriberi occurs in a breast-fed infant, both mother and child should be treated with thiamine.
• Unstable in alkaline solutions; should not be used with materials that yield alkaline solutions.

---

vitamin C (ascorbic acid)◊
Ascorbicap, Ascorbineed, Cecon, Cemill, Cenolate, Cetane, Cevi-Bid, Ce-Vi-Sol♦*, Cevita, C-Syrup-500, Redoxon♦♦, Solucap C

*Pregnancy Risk Category: A (C if >
RDA)*

MECHANISM OF ACTION
Necessary for collagen formation and tissue repair; involved in oxidation-reduction reactions throughout the body.

INDICATIONS & DOSAGE
Frank and subclinical scurvy—
Adults: 100 mg to 2 g, depending on severity, P.O., S.C., I.M., or I.V. daily, then at least 50 mg daily for maintenance.
Children: 100 to 300 mg, depending on severity, P.O., S.C., I.M., or I.V. daily, then at least 35 mg daily for maintenance.
Infants: 50 to 100 mg P.O., I.M., I.V., or S.C. daily.
Extensive burns, delayed fracture or wound healing, postoperative wound healing, severe febrile or chronic disease states—
Adults: 200 to 500 mg S.C., I.M., or I.V. daily.
Children: 100 to 200 mg P.O., S.C., I.M., or I.V. daily.
Prevention of vitamin C deficiency in those with poor nutritional habits or increased requirements—
Adults: at least 45 mg P.O., S.C., I.M., or I.V. daily.
Pregnant and lactating women: at least 60 mg P.O., S.C., I.M., or I.V. daily.
Children: at least 40 mg P.O., S.C., I.M., or I.V. daily.
Infants: at least 35 mg P.O., S.C., I.M., or I.V. daily.
Potentiation of methenamine in urine acidification—
Adults: 4 to 12 g P.O. daily in divided doses.

ADVERSE REACTIONS
CNS: faintness or dizziness with fast I.V. administration.
GI: diarrhea, epigastric burning.
GU: acid urine, oxaluria, renal calculi, renal failure.
Skin: discomfort at injection site.

INTERACTIONS
None significant.

NURSING CONSIDERATIONS
• Use cautiously in G6PD deficiency.
• Administer I.V. infusion cautiously

---

in patients with renal insufficiency.
- Avoid rapid I.V. administration.
- When administering for urine acidification, check urine pH to ensure efficacy.
- Protect solution from light.

vitamin D◇
cholecalciferol (vitamin D₃)◇
ergocalciferol (vitamin D₂)◇

Calciferol♦, Drisdol♦, Radiostol♦♦,
Radiostol Forte♦♦

*Pregnancy Risk Category: A (D if >
RDA)*

MECHANISM OF ACTION

Promotes absorption and utilization of calcium and phosphate. Helps to regulate calcium concentration.

INDICATIONS & DOSAGE

*Rickets and other vitamin D deficiency
diseases; renal osteodystrophy—*
Adults: initially, 12,000 IU P.O. or
I.M. daily, increased as indicated by
response up to 500,000 IU daily in
most cases and up to 800,000 IU daily
for vitamin D–resistant rickets.
Children: 1,500 to 5,000 IU P.O. or
I.M. daily for 2 to 4 weeks, repeated
after 2 weeks, if necessary. Alternatively, a single dose of 600,000 IU
may be given.
 Monitor serum calcium daily to
guide dosage. After correction of deficiency, maintenance includes adequate dietary nutrition and RDA supplements.
Hypoparathyroidism—
Adults and children: 50,000 to
200,000 IU P.O. or I.M. daily, with
4-g calcium supplement.

ADVERSE REACTIONS

Side effects listed are usually seen in
vitamin D toxicity only.
CNS: headache, dizziness, ataxia,
weakness, somnolence, decreased libido, overt psychosis, seizures.
CV: calcifications of soft tissues, in-
cluding the heart.
EENT: dry mouth, metallic taste,
rhinorrhea, conjunctivitis (calcific),
photophobia, tinnitus.
GI: anorexia, nausea, constipation,
diarrhea.
GU: polyuria, albuminuria, hypercalciuria, nocturia, impaired renal function, renal calculi.
Metabolic: hypercalcemia, hyperphosphatemia.
Skin: pruritus.
Other: bone and muscle pain, bone
demineralization, weight loss.

INTERACTIONS

Mineral oil, cholestyramine resin: inhibited GI absorption of oral vitamin
D. Space doses. Use together cautiously.

NURSING CONSIDERATIONS

- Contraindicated in hypercalcemia,
hypervitaminosis A, or renal osteodystrophy with hyperphosphatemia.
- If I.V. route is necessary, use only
water-miscible solutions intended for
dilution in large-volume parenterals.
Use cautiously in cardiac patients, especially those receiving digitalis glycosides.
- Monitor eating and bowel habits;
dry mouth, nausea, vomiting, metallic taste, and constipation may be
early signs and symptoms of toxicity.
- Patients with hyperphosphatemia
require dietary phosphate restrictions
and binding agents to avoid metastatic
calcifications and renal calculi.
- When high therapeutic dosages are
used, serum and urine calcium, potassium, and urea should be monitored
frequently.
- Malabsorption from inadequate bile
or hepatic dysfunction may require
addition of exogenous bile salts to oral
vitamin D.
- I.M. injection of vitamin D dispersed in oil is preferable in patients
who are unable to absorb the oral
form.

Italicized side effects are common or life-threatening.
*Liquid form contains alcohol.   **May contain tartrazine.

• This vitamin is fat-soluble. Warn patient of the dangers of increasing dosage without consulting the doctor.
• Dosages of 60,000 units per day can cause hypercalcemia.
• Patients taking vitamin D should restrict their intake of magnesium-containing antacids.

vitamin E◇
Aquasol E♦*, Eprolin, Pertropin, Solucap E, Tocopher

Pregnancy Risk Category: A (C if > RDA)

MECHANISM OF ACTION
Acts as a cofactor and an antioxidant.

INDICATIONS & DOSAGE
Vitamin E deficiency in premature infants and in patients with impaired fat absorption—
Adults: 60 to 75 IU, depending on severity, P.O. or I.M. daily. Maximum dosage is 300 IU daily.
Children: 1 mg equivalent/0.6 g of dietary unsaturated fat P.O. or I.M. daily.

ADVERSE REACTIONS
None reported.

INTERACTIONS
Mineral oil, cholestyramine resin: inhibited GI absorption of oral vitamin E. Space doses. Use together cautiously.

NURSING CONSIDERATIONS
• Water-miscible forms more completely absorbed in GI tract than other forms.
• Adequate bile is essential for absorption.
• Requirements increase with rise in dietary polyunsaturated acids.
• May protect other vitamins against oxidation.
• Megadoses can cause thrombophlebitis.

• This vitamin is fat-soluble. Discourage patient from self-medication with megadoses, as they can cause undesirable adverse effects.

menadione/menadiol sodium diphosphate (vitamin K₃)
Synkavite♦♦, Synkayvite

Pregnancy Risk Category: C (X near term)

MECHANISM OF ACTION
Promotes hepatic formation of active prothrombin.

INDICATIONS & DOSAGE
Hypoprothrombinemia secondary to vitamin K malabsorption or drug therapy, or when oral administration is desired and bile secretion is inadequate—
Adults: 5 to 15 mg menadiol sodium diphosphate P.O. or parenterally, titrated to patient's requirements.

ADVERSE REACTIONS
CNS: headache, kernicterus.
GI: nausea, vomiting.
Skin: allergic rash, pruritus, urticaria.
Local: pain, hematoma at injection site.

INTERACTIONS
Mineral oil, cholestyramine resin: inhibited GI absorption of oral vitamin K. Space doses. Use together cautiously.

NURSING CONSIDERATIONS
• Contraindicated in treatment of hereditary hypoprothrombinemia (because vitamin K₃ can paradoxically worsen it); in hepatocellular disease, unless it is caused by biliary obstruction; in treatment of heparin-induced bleeding; and during last weeks of pregnancy to avoid toxic reactions in neonates. Use cautiously in G6PD de-

---

Unmarked trade names available in the United States only.
♦ Also available in Canada.   ♦♦ Available in Canada only.   ◇ Also available OTC.

ficiency to avoid hemolysis. In severe bleeding, do not delay other measures, such as giving fresh frozen plasma or whole blood. Use large dosages cautiously in severe hepatic disease.

• Failure to respond to vitamin K_3 may indicate coagulation defects.

• Excessive use of vitamin K_3 may temporarily defeat oral anticoagulant therapy. Higher doses of oral anticoagulant or interim use of heparin may be required.

• Protect parenteral products from light.

• When I.V. route must be used, rate shouldn't exceed 1 mg/minute.

• Effects of I.V. injections are more rapid but shorter lived than S.C. or I.M. injections.

• Monitor prothrombin time to determine dosage effectiveness.

• Observe for signs of adverse effects and report them to doctor.

• Use caution in handling bulk menadione powder. It is irritating to the skin and the respiratory tract.

• This vitamin is fat-soluble.

phytonadione (vitamin K_1)
AquaMEPHYTON♦, Konakion♦, Mephyton

Pregnancy Risk Category: C

MECHANISM OF ACTION
Promotes hepatic formation of active prothrombin.

INDICATIONS & DOSAGE
Hypoprothrombinemia secondary to vitamin K malabsorption, drug therapy, or excess vitamin A—
Adults: 2 to 25 mg, depending on severity, P.O. or parenterally, repeated and increased up to 50 mg, if necessary.
Children: 5 to 10 mg P.O. or parenterally.
Infants: 2 mg P.O. or parenterally.

I.V. injection rate for children and infants should not exceed 3 mg/m²/minute or a total of 5 mg.
Hypoprothrombinemia secondary to effect of oral anticoagulants—
Adults: 2.5 to 10 mg P.O., S.C., or I.M., based on prothrombin time, repeated, if necessary, within 12 to 48 hours after oral dose or within 6 to 8 hours after parenteral dose. In emergency, give 10 to 50 mg slow I.V., rate not to exceed 1 mg/minute, repeated q 4 hours, p.r.n.
Prevention of hemorrhagic disease in neonates—
Neonates: 0.5 to 1 mg S.C. or I.M. immediately after birth, repeated within 6 to 8 hours, if needed, especially if mother received oral anticoagulants or long-term anticonvulsant therapy during pregnancy.
Differentiation between hepatocellular disease or biliary obstruction as source of hypoprothrombinemia—
Adults and children: 10 mg I.M. or S.C.
Prevention of hypoprothrombinemia related to vitamin K deficiency in long-term parenteral nutrition—
Adults: 5 to 10 mg S.C. or I.M. weekly.
Children: 2 to 5 mg S.C. or I.M. weekly.
Prevention of hypoprothrombinemia in infants receiving less than 0.1 mg/liter vitamin K in breast milk or milk substitutes—
Infants: 1 mg S.C. or I.M. monthly.

ADVERSE REACTIONS
CNS: dizziness, seizure-like movements.
CV: transient hypotension after I.V. administration, rapid and weak pulse, cardiac irregularities.
GI: nausea, vomiting.
Skin: sweating, flushing, erythema.
Local: pain, swelling, and hematoma at injection site.
Other: bronchospasms, dyspnea, cramp-like pain, *anaphylaxis and*

Italicized side effects are common or life-threatening.
*Liquid form contains alcohol.   **May contain tartrazine.

anaphylactoid reactions (usually after rapid I.V. administration).

INTERACTIONS
Mineral oil, cholestyramine resin: inhibited GI absorption of oral vitamin K. Space doses. Use together cautiously.

NURSING CONSIDERATIONS
• Contraindicated in hereditary hypoprothrombinemia; bleeding secondary to heparin therapy or overdose; hepatocellular disease, unless caused by biliary obstruction (vitamin K can paradoxically worsen the hypoprothrombinemia). Oral administration is contraindicated if bile secretion is inadequate, unless supplemented with bile salts. Use cautiously, if at all, during last weeks of pregnancy to avoid toxic reactions in neonates and in G6PD deficiency to avoid hemolysis. Use large dosages cautiously in severe hepatic disease.
• Failure to respond to vitamin K may indicate coagulation defects.
• In severe bleeding, don't delay other measures, such as fresh frozen plasma or whole blood.
• Protect parenteral products from light. Wrap infusion container with aluminum foil.
• Effects of I.V. injections more rapid but shorter lived than S.C. or I.M. injections.
• Monitor prothrombin time to determine dosage effectiveness.
• Observe for signs of adverse effects and report them to the doctor.
• Phytonadione therapy for hemorrhagic disease in infants causes fewer adverse reactions than do other vitamin K analogs.
• Check brand name labels for administration route restrictions.
• Administer I.V. by slow infusion (over 2 to 3 hours). Mix in normal saline solution, dextrose 5% in water, or dextrose 5% in normal saline solution. Observe patient closely for signs

of flushing, weakness, tachycardia, and hypotension; may progress to shock.
• This vitamin is fat-soluble.
• Weekly addition of 5 to 10 mg to TPN solutions may be ordered.

multivitamins◊
Available by many brand names. Contain vitamins A, B complex, C, D, and E in varying amounts.
Pregnancy Risk Category: A

MECHANISM OF ACTION
Source of vitamins.

INDICATIONS & DOSAGE
Prevention of vitamin deficiencies in patients with inadequate diets or increased daily requirements; treatment of multivitamin deficiencies and prevention of recurrence; additions to parenteral nutrition solutions to meet patient's normal or increased requirements—
Adults and children: dosage depends on nature and severity of deficiencies and composition of multivitamin preparation.

ADVERSE REACTIONS
None reported.

INTERACTIONS
Refer to each component of the multivitamin combination.

NURSING CONSIDERATIONS
• A single discovered vitamin deficiency usually coexists with others. After initial deficiencies are corrected, stress need for adequate nutrition and multivitamin supplements, if appropriate.
• Tell patient about possible interactions of vitamins in combinations and what precautions to take to avoid problems.
• Stress need to follow doctor's orders regarding daily dosages and fol-

low-up therapy.
• Avoid excessive use of large-volume parenteral solutions of multivitamin supplements containing fat-soluble vitamins to prevent hypervitaminosis. I.V. solutions of water-soluble multivitamins may be used more frequently.
• Chewable flavored multivitamins are available for children. Prevent use of these drugs as candy.
• Liquid preparations may contain varying percentages of alcohol. Check label; alert patient to content.
• Warn against overdosing. Encourage patient to eat a well-balanced diet. Stress hazards of self-administered megadoses of vitamins. These medications are drugs, not just harmless vitamins. Explain possible adverse effects.
• Multivitamin preparations with ordinary doses of each component are usually nontoxic.
• Megavitamin combinations may promote significant accumulation of fat-soluble vitamins, with resultant toxicity.
• Multivitamins containing therapeutic doses of folic acid may mask pernicious anemia. Unless prescribed otherwise by doctor, patient should avoid folic acid in undiagnosed but suspected pernicious anemia.
• Other adverse effects depend on specific components and concentrations in each multivitamin preparation.
• Store vitamins in a cool place in light-resistant containers to limit loss of potency.

sodium fluoride◦
Fluor-A-Day◆◆, Fluoritab, Flura Drops, Karidium◆, Luride, Pediaflor
Pregnancy Risk Category: C

MECHANISM OF ACTION
May catalyze bone remineralization.

INDICATIONS & DOSAGE
Aid in the prevention of dental caries—
Oral:
Children over 3 years: 1 mg daily.
Children under 3 years: 0.5 mg daily.
Topical:
Adults and children over 12 years: 10 ml of 0.2% solution. Use once daily after thoroughly brushing teeth and rinsing mouth. Rinse around and between teeth for 1 minute, then spit out.
Children 6 to 12 years: 5 ml of 0.2% solution.

ADVERSE REACTIONS
CNS: headaches, weakness.
GI: gastric distress.
Skin: hypersensitivity reactions, such as atopic dermatitis, eczema, and urticaria.

INTERACTIONS
None significant.

NURSING CONSIDERATIONS
• Contraindicated when fluoride intake from drinking water exceeds 0.7 parts/million.
• Chronic toxicity (fluorosis) may result from prolonged use of higher-than-recommended doses.
• Advise patient to notify dentist if tooth mottling occurs.
• Tablets may be dissolved in mouth, chewed, or swallowed whole.
• Drops may be administered orally undiluted or mixed with fluids or food.
• Topical forms (rinses and gels) should not be swallowed. Most effective when used immediately after brushing teeth.
• Tell patient to dilute drops or rinses in plastic containers rather than glass.
• The presence of fluoride in prenatal vitamins has been shown to produce healthier teeth in infants.
• Used investigationally in treating

Italicized side effects are common or life-threatening.
*Liquid form contains alcohol.   **May contain tartrazine.

osteoporosis.

trace elements
chromium, copper, iodine (as
iodide), manganese, selenium, zinc
Pregnancy Risk Category: C

MECHANISM OF ACTION
Participate in synthesis and stabiliza-
tion of proteins and nucleic acids in
subcellular and membrane transport
systems.

INDICATIONS & DOSAGE
*Prevention of individual trace element
deficiencies in patients receiving long-
term total parenteral nutrition—*
Chromium—
Adults: 10 to 15 mcg I.V. daily.
Children: 0.14 to 0.20 mcg/kg I.V.
daily.
Copper—
Adults: 0.5 to 1.5 mg I.V. daily.
Children: 0.05 to 0.2 mg/kg I.V.
daily.
Iodine—
Adults: 1 mcg/kg I.V. daily.
Manganese—
Adults: 1 to 3 mg I.V. daily.
Selenium—
Adults: 40 to 120 mcg/day.
Children: 3 mcg/kg/day.
Zinc—
Adults: 2 to 4 mg I.V. daily.
Children: 0.05 mg/kg I.V. daily.

ADVERSE REACTIONS
None reported.

INTERACTIONS
None significant at recommended
dosages.

NURSING CONSIDERATIONS
• Check serum levels of trace elements in patients who have received
total parenteral nutrition for 2 months
or longer. Give supplement if ordered.
Call doctor's attention to low serum
levels of these elements.

• Normal serum levels are 0.07 to
0.15 mg/ml copper; 0.05 to 0.15 mg/
100 ml zinc; 4 to 20 mcg/100 ml manganese; selenium 0.1 to 0.19 mcg/ml.
• Solutions of trace elements are
compounded by pharmacy for addition to total parenteral nutrition solutions according to various formulas.
One common trace element solution is
Shil's solution, which contains copper
1 mg/ml, iodide 0.06 mg/ml, manganese 0.4 mg/ml, and zinc 2 mg/ml.
• Trace element solutions are now
also commercially available.

zinc sulfate◊
Orazinc♦
Pregnancy Risk Category: C

MECHANISM OF ACTION
Source of zinc.

INDICATIONS & DOSAGE
*Treatment of zinc deficiency or ad-
junct to treatment of disorders related
to low serum zinc levels, including
oral and decubitus leg ulcers, acne,
idiopathic hypogeusia, anosmia; also,
as adjunct to vitamin A therapy when
patient fails to respond to vitamin A
alone and in acrodermatitis entero-
pathica—*
Adults: 200 to 220 mg P.O. t.i.d.
(equivalent to 135 to 150 mg elemental zinc daily, 9 times the adult RDA
of 15 mg daily).
Children: dosages not established.
RDA is 0.3 mg/kg daily.

ADVERSE REACTIONS
GI: distress and irritation, nausea,
vomiting with high doses, gastric ulceration.

INTERACTIONS
None significant.

NURSING CONSIDERATIONS
• Beneficial only if patient is zinc-
deficient.

• Normal serum levels may not reliably show absence of zinc deficiency.
• Results may not appear for 6 to 8 weeks in zinc-depleted patients.
• Decreasing dosage to 100 mg b.i.d. may ease nausea or other GI adverse reactions; zinc is thought to irritate gastric mucosa.
• Take with meals to prevent possible gastric distress. However, dairy products may hinder zinc absorption.

102

Calorics

amino acid injection
amino acid solution
corn oil
dextrose (D-glucose)
essential crystalline amino acid
    solution
fat emulsions
fructose (levulose)
invert sugar
medium-chain triglycerides

COMBINATION PRODUCTS
Various products contain dextrose, fructose, or invert sugar in combination with electrolytes.

---

amino acid injection
FreAmine HBC, HepatAmine

Pregnancy Risk Category: C

MECHANISM OF ACTION
Provides a substrate for protein synthesis or enhances conservation of existing body protein.

INDICATIONS & DOSAGE
Treatment of hepatic encephalopathy in patients with cirrhosis or hepatitis; nutritional support—
Adults: 80 to 120 g of amino acids (12 to 18 g of nitrogen)/day. Typically, 500 ml is mixed with 500 ml dextrose 50% in water and administered over a 24-hour period. Add electrolytes, vitamins, and trace elements p.r.n.

ADVERSE REACTIONS
CNS: mental confusion, unconsciousness, headache, dizziness.

CV: hypervolemia related to CHF (in susceptible patients), *pulmonary edema,* exacerbation of hypertension (in predisposed patients).
GI: nausea, vomiting.
GU: glycosuria, osmotic diuresis.
Hepatic: fatty liver.
Metabolic: *rebound hypoglycemia* (when long-term infusions are abruptly stopped), *hyperglycemia,* metabolic acidosis, alkalosis, hypophosphatemia, *hyperosmolar syndrome, hyperosmolar hyperglycemic nonketotic syndrome,* hyperammonemia, *electrolyte imbalances,* dehydration (if hyperosmolar solutions are used).
Skin: chills, flushing, feeling of warmth.
Local: tissue sloughing at infusion site due to extravasation, *catheter sepsis, thrombophlebitis,* thrombosis.
Other: allergic reactions.

INTERACTIONS
None significant.

NURSING CONSIDERATIONS
• Contraindicated in anuria and in those with inborn errors of amino acid metabolism, especially involving branched-chain amino acid metabolism, such as maple syrup urine disease and isovaleric acidemia.
• Monitor serum electrolytes, and glucose, BUN, and renal and hepatic function.
• Administer cautiously to diabetic patients. To prevent hyperglycemia, insulin may be required. Administer cautiously in cardiac insufficiency.

Unmarked trade names available in the United States only.
♦ Also available in Canada.   ♦♦ Available in Canada only.   ◊ Also available OTC.

May cause circulatory overload. Patients with fluid restriction may only tolerate 1 to 2 liters.
• Monitor for extraordinary electrolyte losses that may occur during nasogastric suction, vomiting, or drainage from GI fistula.
• Control infusion rate carefully with infusion pump.
• If infusion rate falls behind, do not attempt to catch up. Notify doctor.
• Peripheral infusions should be limited to 2.5% amino acids and dextrose 10%. Check infusion site frequently for erythema, inflammation, irritation, tissue sloughing, necrosis, and phlebitis. Change peripheral I.V. sites routinely to prevent irritation and infection. If a subclavian catheter is used, the solution is administered into the midsuperior vena cava.
• Check fractional urine every 6 hours for glycosuria initially, then every 12 to 24 hours in stable patients. Abrupt onset of glycosuria may be an early sign of impending sepsis.
• Assess body temperature every 4 hours; elevation may indicate sepsis or infection.
• If patient has chills, fever, or other signs of sepsis, replace I.V. tubing and bottle, and send them to the laboratory to be cultured.

---

amino acid solution
(crystalline amino acid solution)
Aminosyn II♦, FreAmine III ♦,
Novamine, Travasol♦

Pregnancy Risk Category: C

MECHANISM OF ACTION
Used for protein synthesis of the viscera and skeletal muscles in the protein-depleted patient.

INDICATIONS & DOSAGE
Total, supportive, or supplemental and protein-sparing parenteral nutrition when gastrointestinal system must rest during healing, or when patient can't, shouldn't, or won't eat at all or eat enough to maintain normal nutrition and metabolism—
Adults: 1 to 1.5 g/kg I.V. daily.
Children: 2 to 3 g/kg I.V. daily. Individualize dosage to metabolic and clinical response as determined by nitrogen balance and body weight corrected for fluid balance. Add electrolytes, vitamins, and nonprotein caloric solutions as needed.

ADVERSE REACTIONS
CNS: mental confusion, unconsciousness, headache, dizziness.
CV: hypervolemia related to CHF (in susceptible patients), *pulmonary edema,* exacerbation of hypertension (in predisposed patients).
GI: nausea, vomiting.
GU: glycosuria, osmotic diuresis.
Hepatic: fatty liver.
Metabolic: *rebound hypoglycemia* (when long-term infusions are abruptly stopped), *hyperglycemia,* metabolic acidosis, alkalosis, hypophosphatemia, *hyperosmolar syndrome, hyperosmolar hyperglycemic nonketotic syndrome,* hyperammonemia, *electrolyte imbalances,* dehydration (if hyperosmolar solutions are used).
Skin: chills, flushing, feeling of warmth.
Local: tissue sloughing at infusion site due to extravasation, *catheter sepsis, thrombophlebitis, thrombosis.*
Other: allergic reactions.

INTERACTIONS
None significant.

NURSING CONSIDERATIONS
• Contraindicated in severe uncorrected electrolyte or acid-base imbalances, hyperammonemia, and decreased circulating blood volume. Use cautiously in renal insufficiency or failure, cardiac disease, and hepatic impairment. Long-term use for infants and children must be closely

---

Italicized side effects are common or life-threatening.
*Liquid form contains alcohol.   **May contain tartrazine.

monitored.
• Monitor serum electrolytes, magnesium, and glucose; BUN; and renal and hepatic function. Check serum calcium frequently to avoid bone demineralization in children.
• If long-term therapy is needed, doctor may order trace element and vitamin supplements. Avoid overuse of fat-soluble vitamins A and D—can cause toxic hypervitaminosis.
• Don't mix medications, except electrolytes, vitamins, and trace elements, with total parenteral nutrition solution without first consulting pharmacist.
• Control infusion rate carefully with infusion pump.
• If infusion rate falls behind, do not attempt to catch up. Notify doctor.
• Peripheral infusions should be limited to 2.5% amino acids and dextrose 10%. Check infusion site frequently for erythema, inflammation, irritation, tissue sloughing, necrosis, and phlebitis. Change I.V. sites routinely to prevent irritation and infection. I.V. catheter is usually introduced into subclavian vein.
• Watch closely for signs of fluid overload. Notify doctor promptly.
• Some crystalline amino acid solutions contain large amounts of acetates and lactates; use cautiously in alkalosis or hepatic insufficiency.
• Most adverse effects result from mixing amino acids with hypertonic dextrose solutions.
• Initially, check every 12 to 24 hours in stable patients, check fractional urines every 6 hours for glycosuria (if present, the doctor may order insulin coverage).
• Assess body temperature every 4 hours; elevation may indicate sepsis or infection.
• If patient has chills, fever, or other signs of sepsis, replace I.V. tubing and bottle, and send them to the laboratory to be cultured.

corn oil
Lipomul
Pregnancy Risk Category: C

MECHANISM OF ACTION
Source of calories.

INDICATIONS & DOSAGE
To increase caloric intake—
Adults: 45 ml P.O. b.i.d. to q.i.d. after or between meals, alone or with proteins, milk, or other energy sources.
Children: 30 ml P.O. daily to q.i.d. after or between meals, alone or with proteins, milk, or other energy sources.

ADVERSE REACTIONS
GI: nausea, vomiting, diarrhea.

INTERACTIONS
Griseofulvin: increased GI absorption of griseofulvin. A beneficial interaction.

NURSING CONSIDERATIONS
• Contraindicated in gallbladder calculi or complete GI obstructions. Use cautiously in steatorrhea, partial GI obstruction, and enterostomies.
• To minimize nausea, diarrhea, and vomiting, give more frequent, smaller doses with meals or mixed with milk.
• The dosage varies greatly with individual requirements; 30 ml of the emulsion provides 180 calories.

dextrose (D-glucose)
Pregnancy Risk Category: C

MECHANISM OF ACTION
Minimizes glyconeogenesis and promotes anabolism in patients who can't receive sufficient oral caloric intake.

INDICATIONS & DOSAGE
Fluid replacement and caloric supplementation in patient who can't main-

---

tain adequate oral intake or who is restricted from doing so—
Adults and children: dosage depends on fluid and caloric requirements. Use peripheral I.V. infusion of 2.5%, 5%, or 10% solution, central I.V. infusion of 20% solution for minimal fluid needs. Use 50% solution to treat insulin-induced hypoglycemia. Solutions from 40% to 70% are used diluted in admixtures, normally with amino acid solutions, for total parenteral nutrition given through a central vein.

ADVERSE REACTIONS
CNS: mental confusion, unconsciousness in hyperosmolar syndrome.
CV: (with fluid overload) pulmonary edema, exacerbated hypertension, and CHF in susceptible patients. *Prolonged or concentrated infusions may cause phlebitis, venous sclerosis, especially with peripheral route of administration.*
GU: glycosuria, osmotic diuresis.
Metabolic: (with rapid infusion of concentrated solution or prolonged infusion) hyperglycemia, hypervolemia, hyperosmolarity. Rapid termination of long-term infusions may cause hypoglycemia from rebound hyperinsulinemia.
Skin: sloughing and tissue necrosis, if extravasation occurs with concentrated solutions.

INTERACTIONS
None significant.

NURSING CONSIDERATIONS
• Contraindicated in hyperglycemia, diabetic coma, intracranial or intraspinal hemorrhage, or delirium tremens. Use cautiously in cardiac or pulmonary disease, hypertension, renal insufficiency, urinary obstruction, and hypovolemia.
• Control infusion rate carefully. Maximal rate for dextrose infusion is 0.5 g/kg hourly. Use infusion pump when infusing dextrose with amino

acids for total parenteral nutrition.
• Never infuse concentrated solutions rapidly; may cause hyperglycemia and fluid shift.
• Monitor serum glucose carefully. Prolonged therapy with dextrose 5% in water solution can cause depletion of pancreatic insulin production and secretion.
• Never stop abruptly. If necessary, have dextrose 10% in water solution available to treat hypoglycemia if rebound hyperinsulinemia occurs.
• Take care to prevent extravasation. Check injection site frequently to prevent irritation, tissue sloughing, necrosis, and phlebitis.
• Watch closely for signs of fluid overload, especially if fluid intake is restricted.
• Monitor intake/output and weight carefully, especially when renal function is impaired.
• Check vital signs frequently. Report adverse effects promptly.
• Don't give dextrose solutions without saline solution in blood transfusions; may cause clumping of red blood cells. Use central veins to infuse dextrose solutions with concentrations greater than 10%.

essential crystalline amino acid solution
Aminosyn-RF, Nephramine, Ren-Amine 6.5

Pregnancy Risk Category: C

MECHANISM OF ACTION
Enhances conservation of existing body protein.

INDICATIONS & DOSAGE
Management of potentially reversible renal decompensation—
Adults: 0.3 to 0.5 g/kg I.V., up to 26 g total daily (250 ml with 500 ml dextrose 70% injection), and infuse through central I.V. line at initial rate of 20 to 30 ml/hour, increased in steps

of 10 ml/hour q 24 hours, to a maximum of 60 to 100 ml/hour. Individualize dosage and infusion rate to patient's tolerance for glucose, fluid, and nitrogen. Add electrolytes and vitamins p.r.n.

Children: up to 1 g/kg daily, individualized to patient's tolerance for glucose, fluid, and nitrogen. Add electrolytes, trace elements, and vitamins p.r.n.

ADVERSE REACTIONS
CNS: mental confusion, dizziness, unconsciousness, headache.
CV: hypervolemia related to CHF (in susceptible patients), *pulmonary edema,* exacerbation of hypertension (in predisposed patients).
GI: nausea, vomiting.
GU: glycosuria, osmotic diuresis.
Metabolic: *rebound hypoglycemia* (when long-term infusions are abruptly stopped), *hyperglycemia,* metabolic acidosis, alkalosis, hypophosphatemia, hyperosmolar syndrome, *hyperosmolar hyperglycemic nonketotic syndrome,* hyperammonemia, *electrolyte imbalances,* dehydration (if hyperosmolar solutions are used).
Skin: chills, flushing, feeling of warmth.
Local: tissue sloughing at infusion site due to extravasation, *catheter sepsis, thrombophlebitis.*
Other: allergic reactions.

INTERACTIONS
None significant.

NURSING CONSIDERATIONS
• Contraindicated in severe uncorrected electrolyte or acid-base imbalances, hyperammonemia, and decreased circulating blood volume.
• Monitor serum electrolytes, magnesium, and glucose; BUN; and renal and hepatic function. Check serum calcium frequently to avoid bone demineralization in children.

• In long-term therapy, doctor may order trace element and vitamin supplements. Avoid overuse of fat-soluble vitamins.
• Refrigerate solution until half an hour before it will be infused.
• Don't mix medications, except electrolytes, vitamins, and trace elements with total parenteral nutrition solution without first consulting pharmacist.
• Control infusion rate carefully with infusion pump.
• If infusion rate falls behind, do not attempt to catch up. Notify doctor.
• Peripheral infusions should be limited to 2.5% amino acids and dextrose 10%. Check infusion site frequently for erythema, inflammation, irritation, tissue sloughing, necrosis, and phlebitis. Change I.V. sites routinely to prevent irritation. I.V. catheter is usually placed in subclavian vein.
• Watch closely for signs of fluid overload. Notify doctor promptly.
• Essential amino acid solution is used identically to other crystalline amino acid solutions, except that it contains only the essential amino acids. By controlling amino acid content, patients with impaired renal function have decreases in BUN and minimized deterioration of serum potassium, magnesium, and phosphorus balances. May lead to earlier return of renal function in patients with potentially reversible acute renal failure and may decrease morbidity associated with acute renal failure.
• Most adverse effects result from mixing essential crystalline amino acid solution with hypertonic dextrose solutions.
• Check blood glucose every 6 hours. Doctor may need to order insulin.
• Assess body temperature every 4 hours; elevation may indicate sepsis or infection.
• If patient has chills, fever, or other signs of sepsis, replace I.V. tubing and bottle, and send them to the laboratory to be cultured.

---

fat emulsions

Intralipid 10%♦, Intralipid 20%,
Liposyn 10%, Liposyn 20%,
Liposyn II 10%, Liposyn II 20%,
Soyacal 10%, Soyacal 20%,
Travamulsion 10%, Travamulsion
20%

*Pregnancy Risk Category: B for
Soyacal 10%; C for all others*

MECHANISM OF ACTION
Provides neutral triglycerides, predominantly unsaturated fatty acids.

INDICATIONS & DOSAGE
Intralipid:
*Source of calories adjunctive to total
parenteral nutrition—*
Adults: 1 ml/minute I.V. for 15 to 30
minutes (10% emulsion); 0.5 ml/min-
ute I.V. for 15 to 30 minutes (20%
emulsion). If no adverse reactions, increase rate to deliver 500 ml over 4 to
8 hours. Total daily dosage should not
exceed 2.5 g/kg.
Children: 0.1 ml/minute for 10 to 15
minutes (10% emulsion), 0.05 ml/
minute I.V. for 10 to 15 minutes (20%
emulsion). If no adverse reactions, increase rate to deliver 1 g/kg over 4
hours. Daily dosage should not exceed
4 g/kg. Equals 60% of daily caloric
intake. Protein-carbohydrate total
parenteral nutrition should supply remaining 40%.
Fatty acid deficiency—
Adults and children: 8% to 10% of
total caloric intake I.V.
Liposyn:
Prevention of fatty acid deficiency—
Adults: 500 ml (10% emulsion) I.V.
twice weekly. Infuse initially at a rate
of 1 ml/minute for 30 minutes. Rate
may be increased but should not exceed 500 ml over 4 to 6 hours.
Children: 5 to 10 ml/kg (10% emulsion) I.V. daily. Infuse initially at a
rate of 0.1 ml/minute for 30 minutes.
Rate may be increased but should not
exceed 100 ml/hour.

ADVERSE REACTIONS
Early reactions of fat overload:
Blood: hyperlipemia, hypercoagula-
bility, thrombocytopenia in neonates
(rare).
CNS: headache, sleepiness, dizzi-
ness.
EENT: pressure over eyes.
GI: nausea, vomiting.
Skin: flushing, diaphoresis.
Local: irritation at infusion site.
Other: fever, dyspnea, chest and back
pains, cyanosis, allergic reactions, de-
position of I.V. fat.
Delayed reactions:
Blood: thrombocytopenia, leuko-
penia, leukocytosis.
CNS: focal seizures.
CV: *shock.*
Hepatic: transient increased liver
function test, hepatomegaly.
Other: fever, splenomegaly, fat accu-
mulation in lungs.

INTERACTIONS
None significant.

NURSING CONSIDERATIONS
• Contraindicated in hyperlipemia,
lipid nephrosis, or acute pancreatitis
accompanied by hyperlipemia. Use
cautiously in severe hepatic disease,
pulmonary disease, anemia, blood coagulation disorders, and in patients at
risk for fat embolism.
• Lipids support bacterial growth.
Change all I.V. tubing at each infusion. Check injection site daily. Report signs of inflammation or infection promptly.
• Use cautiously in premature infants, as they are susceptible to I.V.
fat overload. Carefully monitor triglycerides and free fatty acids in these
infants.
• May be mixed with amino acid solution, dextrose, electrolytes, and vitamins in the same I.V. container.
Check with pharmacist for acceptable
proportions and compatibility information.

Italicized side effects are common or life-threatening.
*Liquid form contains alcohol.   **May contain tartrazine.

- Do not use an in-line filter when administering this drug because the fat particles are larger than the 0.22-micron cellulose filter.
- Do not use fat emulsion if it separates or becomes oily.
- Refrigeration is not necessary.
- Avoid rapid infusion. Use an infusion pump to regulate rate.
- Watch closely for adverse effects, especially during first half hour of infusion.
- Monitor serum lipids closely when patient is receiving fat emulsion therapy. Lipemia must clear between dosing.
- Check platelet count frequently in neonates receiving fat emulsions I.V.
- Monitor hepatic function carefully in long-term use.
- Intralipid, Travamulsion, and Liposyn differ mainly by their fatty acid components.

fructose (levulose)
Pregnancy Risk Category: C

MECHANISM OF ACTION
Minimizes glyconeogenesis and promotes anabolism in patients who can't receive sufficient oral caloric intake.

INDICATIONS & DOSAGE
Source of carbohydrate calories primarily when fluid replacement is also indicated and as a dextrose substitute for patients with diabetes—
Adults and children: dosage depends on caloric needs. I.V. infusion rate should not exceed 1 g/kg hourly. Single liter 10% solution yields 375 calories.

ADVERSE REACTIONS
CV: increased pulse rate, precipitation or exacerbation of CHF in susceptible patients, *pulmonary edema*.
Hepatic: hepatomegaly.
Metabolic: metabolic acidosis, hypervolemia.

Local: extravasation at infusion site may cause sloughing of skin, thrombophlebitis.
Other: increased respiratory rate.

INTERACTIONS
None significant.

NURSING CONSIDERATIONS
- Contraindicated in hereditary fructose intolerance, in gout, or in patients receiving therapy for hypoglycemia. Use cautiously in cardiac disease, hypertension, pulmonary disease, hypervolemia, renal insufficiency, and urinary tract obstructions.
- Control infusion rate carefully. Make sure rate does not exceed 1 g/kg hourly for infants.
- Change infusion sites regularly to avoid irritation with prolonged therapy. Take care to avoid extravasation.
- Don't use unless the solution is clear and the seal is intact.
- Watch closely for signs of fluid overload, pulmonary edema, or CHF.

invert sugar
Travert
Pregnancy Risk Category: C

MECHANISM OF ACTION
Minimizes glyconeogenesis and promotes anabolism in patients who can't receive sufficient oral caloric intake.

INDICATIONS & DOSAGE
Nonelectrolyte fluid replacement and caloric supplementation solution—
Adults and children: dosage depends on patient's age, weight, and clinical need. I.V. infusion rate should not exceed 1 g/kg hourly. A single liter of 5% invert sugar yields 375 calories.

ADVERSE REACTIONS
CNS: mental confusion.
CV: increased pulse rate, precipitation or exacerbation of CHF in susceptible patients, *pulmonary edema,*

hypertension.

GU: glycosuria, osmotic diuresis.

Metabolic: metabolic acidosis, hypervolemia, hyperglycemia, hypoglycemia.

Local: extravasation at infusion site may cause sloughing of skin, thrombophlebitis.

Other: increased respiratory rate.

INTERACTIONS
None significant.

NURSING CONSIDERATIONS
• Contraindicated in hereditary fructose intolerance, hyperglycemia, diabetic coma, intracranial or intraspinal hemorrhage, or delirium tremens. Use cautiously in cardiac disease, hypertension, pulmonary disease, hypervolemia, renal insufficiency, and urinary tract obstructions.

• Control infusion rate carefully. Make sure rate does not exceed 1 g/kg hourly for infants.

• Change infusion sites regularly to avoid irritation with prolonged therapy. Take care to avoid extravasation.

• Watch closely for signs of fluid overload, pulmonary edema, or CHF. Monitor blood pressure frequently.

• Monitor serum glucose closely. Prolonged therapy can cause depletion of pancreatic insulin production and secretion.

• Monitor intake/output and weight closely, especially if renal function is impaired.

• Check vital signs frequently. Tell doctor promptly if adverse effects occur.

medium-chain triglycerides
M.C.T. Oil♦

Pregnancy Risk Category: C

MECHANISM OF ACTION
Source of rapidly hydrolyzable lipid.

INDICATIONS & DOSAGE
Inadequate digestion or absorption of food fats—
Adults: 15 ml P.O. t.i.d. or q.i.d. Maximum of 100 ml/day.

ADVERSE REACTIONS
CNS: reversible coma in susceptible patients.

GI: *nausea, vomiting, diarrhea, abdominal distention, cramps.*

INTERACTIONS
None significant.

NURSING CONSIDERATIONS
• Contraindicated in advanced hepatic disease or abetalipoproteinemia. Use cautiously in patients with portacaval shunts.

• To minimize GI side effects, give smaller doses more frequently with meals or mixed with salad dressing or chilled fruit juice.

• More easily absorbed than long-chain fats; not dependent on bile salts for emulsification.

• Rapid metabolism provides quick energy.

• May be useful in lowering cholesterol levels. Also used in patients with short-bowel syndrome.

• Provides 7.7 calories/ml. No essential fatty acids are provided.

103

Immune serums

antirabies serum, equine
hepatitis B immune globulin,
  human
immune globulin
rabies immune globulin, human
Rh₀(D) immune globulin, human
tetanus immune globulin, human
varicella-zoster immune globulin
  (VZIG)

COMBINATION PRODUCTS
None.

---

antirabies serum, equine
Pregnancy Risk Category: C

MECHANISM OF ACTION
Provides passive immunity to rabies.

INDICATIONS & DOSAGE
Rabies exposure—
Adults and children: 40 to 55 units/
kg at time of first dose of rabies vaccine. Use half of dose to infiltrate
wound area. Give remainder I.M.
Don't give rabies vaccine and antirabies serum in same syringe or at same
site.
    For wounds, including mucous
membranes, the entire dose should be
administered I.M.

ADVERSE REACTIONS
Local: pain at injection site.
Systemic: within 6 to 12 days serum
sickness occurs in 15% to 25% of patients. Symptoms are skin eruptions,
arthralgia, pruritus, lymphadenopathy, fever, headache, malaise, abdominal pain, *anaphylaxis.*

INTERACTIONS
*Corticosteroids and immunosuppres-
sive agents:* interferes with response.
Avoid during postexposure immunization period.

NURSING CONSIDERATIONS
• In hypersensitivity to equine serum,
use rabies immune globulin, human,
instead. If unavailable, desensitize
before giving. Consult doctor or pharmacist.
• Do sensitivity test on all patients
before giving. Dilute serum 1:100 or
1:1,000 with normal saline solution
for injection. Inject intradermally on
inner forearm. Inject other arm with
0.1 ml of normal saline solution for
injection intradermally as a control.
Read within 20 minutes. Positive reaction: wheal 10 mm or more and erythematous flare 20 × 20 mm.
• Use only when rabies immune globulin, human, is not available.
• Obtain history of animal bite, allergies (especially to equine serum and
to eggs), and reaction to immunizations.
• Epinephrine solution 1:1,000
should always be available when administering this drug.
• This immune serum provides immediate passive immunity (short-
term).
• Do not confuse this drug with rabies vaccine, which is a suspension of
attenuated or killed microorganisms
used to confer long-term active immunity. These two drugs are often administered together prophylactically
after exposure to known or suspected

rabid animals.
• Ask patient when he received last tetanus immunization, since many doctors order a booster at this time.

hepatitis B immune globulin, human
H-BIG, Hep-B-Gammagee, HyperHep♦

Pregnancy Risk Category: C

MECHANISM OF ACTION
Provides passive immunity to hepatitis B.

INDICATIONS & DOSAGE
Hepatitis B exposure—
Adults and children: 0.06 ml/kg I.M. within 7 days after exposure. Repeat 28 days after exposure.
Neonates born to women who test positive for hepatitis B surface antigen (HB$_s$Ag): 0.5 ml within 24 hours of birth. Repeat dose at age 3 months and 6 months.

ADVERSE REACTIONS
Systemic: *anaphylaxis.*

INTERACTIONS
Other vaccines: Hepatitis B immune globulin may interfere with response to live virus vaccines. Defer administration for 3 months.

NURSING CONSIDERATIONS
• Anterolateral aspect of thigh or deltoid areas are the preferred injection sites in adults; anterolateral aspect of thigh is preferred for neonates and children under 3 years.
• Nurse should receive immunization if exposed to hepatitis B (for example, needle-stick, direct contact).
• Obtain history of allergies and reaction to immunizations.

immune globulin
Gamastan, Gamimune, Gammagard, Gammar, Sandoglobulin

Pregnancy Risk Category: C

MECHANISM OF ACTION
Provides passive immunity by increasing antibody titer.

INDICATIONS & DOSAGE
Agammaglobulinemia or hypogammaglobulinemia—
Adults: 30 to 50 ml I.M. monthly. Alternatively, administer 100 mg/kg I.V. (Gamimune) once a month. Infuse at 0.01 to 0.02 ml/kg/min for 30 minutes. For Sandoglobulin, administer 200 mg/kg I.V. once a month. Infuse at 0.5 to 1 ml/min. After 15 to 30 minutes, increase infusion rate to 1.5 to 2.5 ml/min.
Children: 20 to 40 ml I.M. monthly.
Hepatitis A exposure—
Adults and children: 0.02 to 0.04 ml/kg I.M. as soon as possible after exposure. Up to 0.1 ml/kg may be given after prolonged or intense exposure.
Post-transfusion hepatitis B—
Adults and children: 10 ml I.M. within 1 week after transfusion and 10 ml I.M. 1 month later.
Measles exposure—
Adults and children: 0.02 ml/kg within 6 days after exposure.
Modification of measles—
Adults and children: 0.04 ml/kg I.M. within 6 days after exposure.
Measles vaccine complications—
Adults and children: 0.02 to 0.04 ml/kg I.M.
Poliomyelitis exposure—
Adults and children: 0.3 to 0.4 ml/kg I.M. within 7 days after exposure.
Chicken pox exposure—
Adults and children: 0.2 to 1.3 ml/kg I.M. as soon as exposed.
Rubella exposure in first trimester of pregnancy—

Italicized side effects are common or life-threatening.
*Liquid form contains alcohol.   **May contain tartrazine.

Women: 0.2 to 0.4 ml/kg I.M. as soon as exposed.
Prophylaxis in primary immunodeficiencies—
Adults and children: 100 mg/kg by I.V. infusion monthly (Gamimune only). Infusion rate is 0.01 to 0.02 ml/kg/minute for 30 minutes. Rate can then be increased to 0.04 ml/minute for remainder of infusion.
Idiopathic thrombocytopenic purpura—
Adults: 0.4 g/kg Sandoglobulin I.V. for 5 consecutive days.

ADVERSE REACTIONS
Skin: urticaria.
Local: pain, erythema, muscle stiffness.
Systemic: angioedema, headache, malaise, fever, nephrotic syndrome, *anaphylaxis*.

INTERACTIONS
Live virus vaccines: don't administer within 3 months after administration of immune globulin.

NURSING CONSIDERATIONS
• Obtain history of allergies and reaction to immunizations.
• Have drugs available for anaphylactoid reaction.
• Two brands of I.V. immune globulin are now available (Gamimune and Sandoglobulin). They're especially useful in patients with clotting abnormalities or in those with small muscle mass.
• Inject into different sites, preferably anterolateral aspect of thigh or deltoid muscle for adults and anterolateral aspect of thigh for neonates and children under 3 years. Do not inject more than 3 ml per injection site.
• Do not give for hepatitis A exposure if 6 weeks or more have elapsed since exposure or after onset of clinical illness.

rabies immune globulin, human
Hyperab, Imogam
Pregnancy Risk Category: C

MECHANISM OF ACTION
Provides passive immunity to rabies.

INDICATIONS & DOSAGE
Rabies exposure—
Adults and children: 20 IU/kg at time of first dose of rabies vaccine. Use half of dose to infiltrate wound area. Give remainder I.M. Don't give rabies vaccine and rabies immune globulin in same syringe or at same site.

ADVERSE REACTIONS
Local: pain, redness, induration at injection site.
Other: slight fever, *anaphylaxis*.

INTERACTIONS
Corticosteroids and immunosuppressive agents: interferes with response. Avoid during postexposure immunization period.

NURSING CONSIDERATIONS
• Repeated doses contraindicated after rabies vaccine is started.
• Use only with rabies vaccine and immediate local treatment of wound. Give regardless of interval between exposure and initiation of therapy.
• Obtain history of animal bites, allergies, and reaction to immunizations.
• Don't administer more than 5 ml I.M. at one injection site; divide I.M. doses greater than 5 ml, and administer at different sites.
• This immune serum provides passive immunity.
• Do not confuse this drug with rabies vaccine, which is a suspension of attenuated or killed microorganisms used to confer active immunity. These two drugs are often given together

prophylactically after exposure to known or suspected rabid animals.
• Ask the patient when he received his last tetanus immunization, since many doctors order a booster at this time.

Rh₀(D) immune globulin, human

$Rh_o(D)$ immune globulin, human

Gamulin Rh, HypRho-D, MICRhoGAM, Mini-Gamulin Rh, Rhesonativ, RhoGAM♦

Pregnancy Risk Category: C

MECHANISM OF ACTION
Suppresses the active antibody response and formation of anti-Rh_o (D) in Rh_o (D)-negative, D^u-negative individuals, exposed to Rh-positive blood.

INDICATIONS & DOSAGE
Rh exposure—
Women (postabortion, postmiscarriage, ectopic pregnancy, or postpartum): transfusion unit or blood bank determines fetal packed red blood cell (RBC) volume entering woman's blood, then gives one vial I.M. if fetal packed RBC volume is less than 15 ml. More than one vial I.M. may be required if there is large fetomaternal hemorrhage. Must be given within 72 hours after delivery or miscarriage.
Transfusion accidents—
Adults and children: consult blood bank or transfusion unit at once. Must be given within 72 hours.
Postabortion or postmiscarriage to prevent Rh antibody formation—
Women: consult transfusion unit or blood bank. Ideally should be given within 3 hours, but may be given up to 72 hours after abortion or miscarriage.

ADVERSE REACTIONS
Local: discomfort at injection site.
Other: slight fever.

INTERACTIONS
Live virus vaccines: may interfere with response. Defer vaccination for 3 months after administration of Rh_o (D) immune globulin.

NURSING CONSIDERATIONS
• Contraindicated in Rh_o (D)-positive or D^u-positive patients and those previously immunized to Rh_o (D) blood factor.
• Immediately after delivery, send a sample of infant's cord blood to laboratory for typing and cross matching. Confirm if mother is Rh_o (D)-negative and D^u-negative. Infant must be $Rh_o(D)$-positive or D^u-positive.
• Obtain history of allergies and reaction to immunization.
• MICRhoGAM is recommended for every woman undergoing abortion or miscarriage up to 12 weeks' gestation unless she is Rh_o (D)-positive or D^u-positive, has Rh antibodies, or the father and/or fetus is Rh-negative.
• Store at 36° to 46° F. (2° to 8° C.).
• This immune serum provides passive immunity to the woman exposed to Rh_o-positive fetal blood during pregnancy. Prevents formation of maternal antibodies (active immunity), which would endanger future Rh_o-positive pregnancies.
• Explain to the patient how drug protects future Rh_o-positive infants.

tetanus immune globulin, human

Homo-Tet, Hu-Tet, Hyper-Tet♦

Pregnancy Risk Category: C

MECHANISM OF ACTION
Provides passive immunity to tetanus.

INDICATIONS & DOSAGE
Tetanus exposure—
Adults and children: 250 to 500 units I.M.
Tetanus treatment—
Adults and children: single doses of

Italicized side effects are common or life-threatening.
*Liquid form contains alcohol.   **May contain tartrazine.

3,000 to 6,000 units have been used. Optimal dosage schedules have not been established. Don't give at same site as toxoid.

ADVERSE REACTIONS
Local: pain, stiffness, erythema.
Other: slight fever, allergy, *anaphylaxis*.

INTERACTIONS
None significant.

NURSING CONSIDERATIONS
• Use tetanus immune globulin only if wound is over 24 hours old or patient has had less than two previous tetanus toxoid injections.
• Obtain history of injury, tetanus immunizations, last tetanus toxoid injection, allergies, and reaction to immunizations.
• Thoroughly cleanse and remove all foreign matter from wound.
• Antibodies remain at effective levels for 3 weeks or longer, which is several times the duration of antitoxin-induced antibodies. Protects the patient for the incubation period of most tetanus cases.
• Human globulin is not a substitute for tetanus toxoid, which should be given at the same time to produce active immunization.
• Inject into the deltoid muscle for adults and children 3 years and older and into the anterolateral aspect of the thigh in neonates and children under 3 years.
• Do not confuse this drug with tetanus toxoid.

---

varicella-zoster immune globulin (VZIG)
Pregnancy Risk Category: C

MECHANISM OF ACTION
Provides passive immunity to varicella-zoster virus.

INDICATIONS & DOSAGE
Passive immunization of susceptible immunodeficient patients after exposure to varicella (chicken pox or herpes zoster)—
Children to 10 kg: 125 units I.M.
Children 10.1 to 20 kg: 250 units I.M.
Children 20.1 to 30 kg: 375 units I.M.
Children 30.1 to 40 kg: 500 units I.M.
Adults and children over 40 kg: 625 units I.M.

ADVERSE REACTIONS
Local: discomfort at injection site, rash.
Systemic: gastrointestinal distress, malaise, headache, respiratory distress, *anaphylaxis*.

INTERACTIONS
Live virus vaccines: may interfere with response. Defer vaccination for 3 months after administration of VZIG.

NURSING CONSIDERATIONS
• Contraindicated in patients with a history of severe reaction to human immune serum globulin or severe thrombocytopenia.
• For maximum benefit, administer as soon as possible after presumed exposure.
• VZIG is not recommended for non-immunosuppressed patients.
• VZIG should not be administered indiscriminately because supplies are limited.
• Although usually restricted to children under 15 years, VZIG may be administered to adolescents and adults if necessary.
• Not commercially distributed. Available only from 20 regional distribution centers throughout the United States. These centers will distribute to Canada and overseas. Call the Centers for Disease Control for the distribution center in your area: Monday to

Friday, 8 a.m. to 4:30 p.m. (E.S.T.),
(404) 329-3670; weekends, nights,
and holidays (emergencies only),
(404) 329-2888.
• Should be administered only by
deep I.M. injection. Never administer
I.V.
• Store vial in refrigerator.

104

Acidifiers and alkalinizers

Acidifiers
ammonium chloride
dilute hydrochloric acid

Alkalinizers
sodium bicarbonate◇
sodium lactate
tromethamine

COMBINATION PRODUCTS
None.

---

ammonium chloride
Pregnancy Risk Category: B

MECHANISM OF ACTION
Increases free hydrogen ion (H^+) concentration. Also acts as an expectorant by causing reflex stimulation of bronchial mucous glands.

INDICATIONS & DOSAGE
Metabolic alkalosis—
Adults and children: I.V. dose (in mEq) is equal to the serum chloride deficit (in mEq/ml) multiplied by the extracellular fluid volume (estimated as 20% of the body weight in kilograms). One-half the calculated volume should be given, then patient should be reassessed.
As an acidifying agent—
Adults: 4 to 12 g P.O. daily in divided doses.
Children: 75 mg/kg P.O. daily in four divided doses.
As expectorant—
Adults: 250 to 500 mg P.O. q 2 to 4 hours.

ADVERSE REACTIONS
Side effects usually result from ammonia toxicity or too-rapid I.V. administration.
CNS: headache, confusion, progressive drowsiness, excitement alternating with coma, hyperventilation, *calcium-deficient tetany, twitching, hyperreflexia, EEG abnormalities.*
CV: bradycardia.
GI: (with oral dose) *gastric irritation, nausea, vomiting,* thirst, anorexia, retching.
GU: glycosuria.
Metabolic: *acidosis, hyperchloremia, hypokalemia,* hyperglycemia.
Skin: rash, pallor.
Local: pain at injection site.
Other: irregular respirations with periods of apnea.

INTERACTIONS
Spironolactone: systemic acidosis. Use together cautiously.

NURSING CONSIDERATIONS
• Contraindicated in severe hepatic or renal dysfunction. Use cautiously in pulmonary insufficiency or cardiac edema and in infants.
• Dilute concentrated form (26.75%) before administration. Add 100 to 200 mEq (20 to 40 ml of the 26.75% solution) to 500 or 1,000 ml of normal saline injection. Administer via infusion pump not exceeding 5 ml/min in adults.
• Give oral form after meals to decrease GI adverse reactions. Enteric-coated tablets may also minimize GI symptoms but are absorbed errati-

---

Unmarked trade names available in the United States only.
♦ Also available in Canada.　　　　♦♦ Available in Canada only.　　　◇ Also available OTC.

cally.
- Do not administer drug with milk or other alkaline solutions because they are not compatible.
- Pain of I.V. injection may be lessened by decreasing infusion rate.
- Determine CO_2 combining power and serum electrolytes before and during therapy to prevent acidosis.
- Monitor urine pH and output. Diuresis is normal for first 2 days.
- Monitor rate and depth of respirations frequently.
- When using as an expectorant, give with full glass of water.

---

dilute hydrochloric acid
Pregnancy Risk Category: C

MECHANISM OF ACTION
Increases free hydrogen ion (H^+) concentration.

INDICATIONS & DOSAGE
Metabolic alkalosis—
pharmacy prepares (0.1 normal HCl solution in sterile water) 100 mEq hydrogen and 100 mEq chloride/liter.

ADVERSE REACTIONS
None confirmed.

INTERACTIONS
None significant.

NURSING CONSIDERATIONS
- Not available commercially; prepared in pharmacy.
- Administer I.V. solution slowly through a central venous line.
- Monitor pH, blood gases, and serum electrolytes at 4- to 6-hour intervals.

---

sodium bicarbonate◊
Pregnancy Risk Category: C

MECHANISM OF ACTION
Restores buffering capacity of the body. Also neutralizes excess acid.

INDICATIONS & DOSAGE
Cardiac arrest—
Adults and children: as a 7.5% or 8.4% solution, 1 mEq/kg followed by 0.5 mEq/kg every 10 minutes depending on blood gases. Further dosages based on blood gases. If blood gases unavailable, use 0.5 mEq/kg q 10 minutes until spontaneous circulation returns.
Infants up to 2 years: 4.2% solution, I.V. infusion. Rate not to exceed 8 mEq/kg daily.
Metabolic acidosis—
Adults and children: dosage depends on blood CO_2 content, pH, and patient's clinical condition. Generally, 2 to 5 mEq/kg I.V. infused over 4- to 8-hour period.
Systemic or urinary alkalinization—
Adults: 325 mg to 2 g P.O. q.i.d.
Children: 12 to 120 mg/kg daily.
Antacid—
Adults: 300 mg to 2 g tablets chewed and taken with glass of water.

ADVERSE REACTIONS
GI: gastric distention, belching, flatulence.
GU: renal calculi or crystals.
Metabolic: (with overdose) alkalosis, hypernatremia, hyperkalemia, hyperosmolarity.

INTERACTIONS
None significant.

NURSING CONSIDERATIONS
- No contraindications for use in life-threatening emergencies. Contraindicated in hypertension, in patients with tendency toward edema, in patients who are losing chlorides by vomiting or from continuous GI suction, in patients receiving diuretics known to produce hypochloremic alkalosis, and in patients on sodium-restricted diets or with renal disease.
- May be added to other I.V. fluids.

Italicized side effects are common or life-threatening.
*Liquid form contains alcohol.   **May contain tartrazine.

• Because sodium bicarbonate inactivates such catecholamines as norepinephrine and dopamine, do not mix with I.V. solutions of these agents.
• To avoid risk of alkalosis, determine blood pH, PaO_2, $PaCO_2$, and serum electrolytes. Keep doctor informed of serum laboratory results.
• Tell patient not to take with milk. May cause hypercalcemia, alkalosis, and possibly renal calculi.
• Discourage use as an antacid. Offer a nonabsorbable alternative antacid if it is to be used repeatedly.
• May cause enteric-coated drugs to be prematurely released in the stomach.
• Sodium bicarbonate is not routinely recommended for use in cardiac arrest because it may produce a paradoxical acidosis from CO_2 production. It should not be routinely administered during the early stages of resuscitation unless preexisting acidosis is clearly present. May be used at team leader's discretion after such interventions as defibrillation, cardiac compression, and administration of first-line drugs.

sodium lactate
Pregnancy Risk Category: C

MECHANISM OF ACTION
Metabolized to sodium bicarbonate. Then produces buffering effect.

INDICATIONS & DOSAGE
Alkalinize urine—
Adults: 30 ml of ⅙ molar solution/kg of body weight given in divided doses over 24 hours.
Metabolic acidosis—
Adults: usually given as $1/_6$ molar injection (167 mEq lactate/liter). Dosage depends on degree of bicarbonate deficit.

ADVERSE REACTIONS
Metabolic: (with overdose) alkalosis, hypernatremia, hyperosmolarity.

INTERACTIONS
None significant.

NURSING CONSIDERATIONS
• Contraindicated in severe hepatic and renal disease, respiratory alkalosis, or acidosis associated with congenital heart disease with persistent cyanosis.
• Monitor serum electrolytes to avoid alkalosis.

tromethamine
Tham♦
Pregnancy Risk Category: C

MECHANISM OF ACTION
Combines with hydrogen ions and associated acid anions; the resulting salts are excreted.

INDICATIONS & DOSAGE
Metabolic acidosis (associated with cardiac bypass surgery or with cardiac arrest)—
Adults: dosage depends on bicarbonate deficit. Calculate as follows: ml of 0.3 M tromethamine solution required = wt in kg × bicarbonate deficit (mEq/liter). Additional therapy based on serial determinations of existing bicarbonate deficit. Concentration of tromethamine should not exceed 0.3 M.
Children: calculate dosage as above. Give slowly over 3 to 6 hours. Additional therapy based on degree of acidosis. Total 24-hour dosage should not exceed 33 to 40 ml/kg. Concentration of tromethamine should not exceed 0.3 M.

ADVERSE REACTIONS
CNS: respiratory depression.
Metabolic: hypoglycemia, hyperkalemia (with decreased urine output).
Local: venospasm; I.V. thrombosis; inflammation, necrosis, and sloughing if extravasation occurs.

INTERACTIONS
None significant.

NURSING CONSIDERATIONS
• Contraindicated in anuria, uremia, chronic respiratory acidosis, or pregnancy (except in acute, life-threatening situations). Use cautiously in renal disease and poor urine output. Monitor ECG and serum potassium in these patients.
• To prevent blood pH from rising above normal, adjust dosage carefully.
• Give slowly through large needle (18G to 20G) into largest antecubital vein or by indwelling I.V. catheter.
• Before, during, and after therapy make the following determinations: blood pH; carbon dioxide tension; bicarbonate, glucose, and electrolyte levels.
• Mechanical ventilation should be readily available. Use when giving drug to patient with associated respiratory acidosis.
• Except in life-threatening situations, do not use longer than 1 day.
• If extravasation occurs, infiltrate area with 1% procaine and hyaluronidase 150 units; may reduce vasospasm and dilute remaining drug in local area.

Uricosurics

probenecid
sulfinpyrazone

COMBINATION PRODUCTS
COLBENEMID: probenecid 500 mg
and colchicine 0.5 mg.
PROBEN-C: probenecid 500 mg and
colchicine 0.5 mg.

---

probenecid
Benemid♦, Benn, Benuryl♦♦,
Probalan, Robenecid

Pregnancy Risk Category: B

MECHANISM OF ACTION
Blocks renal tubular reabsorption of
uric acid, increasing excretion. Also inhibits active renal tubular secretion of
many weak organic acids (for example,
penicillins and cephalosporins).

INDICATIONS & DOSAGE
*Adjunct to penicillin or cephalosporin
therapy—*
Adults and children over 50 kg: 500
mg P.O. q.i.d.
**Children 2 to 14 years or under 50
kg:** initially, 25 mg/kg P.O., then 40
mg/kg divided q.i.d.
Single-dose treatment of gonorrhea—
Adults: 3.5 g ampicillin P.O. with 1 g
probenecid P.O. given together; or 1 g
probenecid P.O. 30 minutes before
dose of 4.8 million units of aqueous
penicillin G procaine I.M., injected at
two different sites.
*Treatment of hyperuricemia of gout,
gouty arthritis—*
Adults: 250 mg P.O. b.i.d. for first
week, then 500 mg b.i.d., to maximum of 2 g daily. Maintenance dosage is 500 mg daily for 6 months.

ADVERSE REACTIONS
Blood: *hemolytic anemia.*
CNS: *headache,* dizziness.
CV: hypotension.
GI: anorexia, nausea, vomiting, *gas-
tric distress.*
GU: urinary frequency.
Skin: dermatitis, pruritus.
Other: flushing, sore gums, fever.

INTERACTIONS
Salicylates: inhibited uricosuric effect
of probenecid, causing urate retention. Do not use together.
Indomethacin: decreased indomethacin excretion. Lower indomethacin
dosages may be required.

NURSING CONSIDERATIONS
• Contraindicated in blood dyscrasias; acute gout attack; penicillin therapy in presence of known renal impairment; gouty nephropathy; urinary
tract stones or obstruction; and azotemia or hyperuricemia secondary to
cancer chemotherapy, radiation, or
myeloproliferative neoplastic diseases. Use cautiously in peptic ulcer
and renal impairment.
• Usually preferred over sulfinpyrazone because probenecid produces
fewer and less severe GI and hematologic adverse reactions.
• Contains no analgesic or anti-inflammatory agent, and is of no value
during acute gout attacks. Don't initiate therapy until acute attack subsides.

Unmarked trade names available in the United States only.
♦ Also available in Canada.   ♦♦ Available in Canada only.   ◊ Also available OTC.

• Suitable for long-term use; no cumulative effects or tolerance.
• Not effective with chronic renal insufficiency (glomerular filtration rate less than 30 ml/minute).
• Periodic BUN and renal function tests recommended in long-term therapy.
• May increase frequency, severity, and length of acute gout attacks during first 6 to 12 months of therapy. Prophylactic colchicine or another anti-inflammatory agent is given during first 3 to 6 months.
• Tell patient to avoid alcohol; it increases urate level.
• Patient should avoid all medications that contain aspirin. These may precipitate gout.
• Force fluids to maintain minimum daily output of 2 to 3 liters. Alkalinize urine with sodium bicarbonate or potassium citrate as ordered by doctor. These measures will prevent hematuria, renal colic, urate stone development, and costovertebral pain.
• Give with milk, food, or antacids to minimize GI distress. Continued disturbances might indicate need to lower dosage.
• Restrict foods high in purine: anchovies, liver, sardines, kidneys, sweetbreads, peas, and lentils.
• Instruct patient and his family that drug must be taken regularly as ordered or gout attacks may result. Tell him to visit doctor regularly so uric acid can be monitored and dosage can be adjusted if necessary. Lifelong therapy may be required in patients with hyperuricemia.
• May produce false-positive glucose tests with Benedict's solution or Clinitest, but not with glucose oxidase method (Clinistix, Diastix, Tes-Tape).
• Decreases urinary excretion of 17-ketosteroids, Bromsulphalein (BSP), aminohippuric acid, and iodine-related organic acids, interfering with laboratory procedures.

sulfinpyrazone
Anturan◆◆, Anturane
Pregnancy Risk Category: C

MECHANISM OF ACTION
Blocks renal tubular reabsorption of uric acid, increasing excretion. Also inhibits platelet aggregation.

INDICATIONS & DOSAGE
Inhibition of platelet aggregation, increase of platelet survival time in treatment of thromboembolic disorders, angina, myocardial infarction, transient cerebral ischemic attacks, peripheral arterial atherosclerosis—
Adults: 200 mg P.O. q.i.d.
Maintenance therapy for common gout: reduction, prevention of joint changes and tophi formation—
Adults: 100 to 200 mg P.O. b.i.d. first week, then 200 to 400 mg P.O. b.i.d. Maximum dosage is 800 mg daily.

ADVERSE REACTIONS
Blood: *agranulocytosis,* blood dyscrasias (rare).
CNS: dizziness, vertigo, tinnitus.
GI: *nausea, dyspepsia,* epigastric pain, blood loss, reactivation of peptic ulcers.
Skin: rash.

INTERACTIONS
Probenecid: inhibited renal excretion of sulfinpyrazone. Use together cautiously.
Salicylates: inhibited uricosuric effect of sulfinpyrazone. Do not use together.

NURSING CONSIDERATIONS
• Contraindicated in hypersensitivity to pyrazole derivatives (including oxyphenbutazone and phenylbutazone); active peptic ulcer; gouty nephropathy; urolithiasis or urinary obstruction; bone marrow suppression; azotemia, hyperuricemia secondary

to cancer chemotherapy, radiation, or myeloproliferative neoplastic diseases; blood dyscrasias; and during or within 2 weeks after gout attack. Use cautiously in diminished hepatic or renal function.

• Use in treating thromboembolic conditions is investigational and is most often directed at prevention of recurrent myocardial infarction.

• Recommended for patients unresponsive to probenecid. Suitable for long-term use; neither cumulative effects nor tolerance develops.

• Contains no analgesic or anti-inflammatory agent and is of no value during acute gout attacks.

• Periodic BUN, CBC, and renal function studies advised during long-term use.

• May increase frequency, severity, and length of acute gout attacks during first 6 to 12 months of therapy. Prophylactic colchicine or another anti-inflammatory agent is given during first 3 to 6 months.

• Therapy, especially at start, may lead to renal colic and formation of uric acid stones. Until acid levels are normal (about 6 mg/100 ml), monitor intake/output closely.

• Force fluids to maintain minimum daily output of 2 to 3 liters. Alkalinize urine with sodium bicarbonate or other agent ordered by doctor.

• Give with milk, food, or antacids to minimize GI disturbances.

• Restrict foods high in purine: anchovies, liver, sardines, kidneys, sweetbreads, peas, and lentils.

• Instruct patient and his family that drug must be taken regularly as ordered or gout attacks may result. Tell him to visit doctor regularly so blood levels can be monitored and dosage adjusted if necessary.

• Lifelong therapy may be required in patients with hyperuricemia.

• Decreases urinary excretion of aminohippuric acid, interfering with laboratory test results.

• Alkalinizing agents are used therapeutically to increase sulfinpyrazone activity, preventing urolithiasis.

• Warn patient not to take any aspirin-containing medications.

• Monitor patients taking oral hypoglycemic agents; these drugs' effects may be potentiated by sulfinpyrazone, causing hypoglycemia.

chymopapain
fibrinolysin and
desoxyribonuclease
hyaluronidase

COMBINATION PRODUCTS
CHYMORAL-100: 100,000 units enzymatic activity; trypsin and chymotrypsin in ratio of 6:1.
GRANULEX AEROSOL: trypsin 0.1 mg, balsam Peru 72.5 mg, and castor oil 650 mg/0.82 ml.
ORENZYME BITABS ENTERIC-COATED TABLETS: 100,000 units trypsin and 8,000 units chymotrypsin.

---

chymopapain
Chymodiactin, Discase

Pregnancy Risk Category: C

MECHANISM OF ACTION
Hydrolyzes noncollagenous proteins in the chondromucoprotein of the nucleus pulposus.

INDICATIONS & DOSAGE
Treatment of herniated lumbar intervertebral disk—
Adults: 2,000 to 4,000 units per disk injected intradiskally. Maximum dosage in a single patient with multiple disk herniation is 10,000 units. (Should be administered in the hospital by doctors experienced and trained in diagnosis of lumbar disk disease.)

ADVERSE REACTIONS
Local: *back pain, stiffness, back spasm.*
Systemic: *anaphylaxis, paraplegia, cerebral hemorrhage, acute transverse myelitis,* nausea, headache, dizziness, leg weakness, paresthesias, numbness of legs and toes.

INTERACTIONS
None significant.

NURSING CONSIDERATIONS
• Contraindicated in patients with history of allergy to papaya or meat tenderizer; patients who have previously received an injection of chymopapain; severe spondylolisthesis in addition to spinal stenosis; severe progressing paralysis; or evidence of spinal cord tumor or a cauda equina lesion.
• Should be used only by doctors qualified by training and experience to perform laminectomy, diskectomy or other spinal procedures, and who have received specialized training in chemonucleolysis. Drug shouldn't be injected in any region other than the lumbar spine. Chymopapain is extremely toxic if injected into the subarachnoid space.
• A new test (ChymoFAST) can detect allergic sensitivity to chymopapain.
• Monitor very closely for anaphylactoid reaction (0.5% of patients). Can be immediate or delayed up to 1 hour after injection and can last for minutes to several hours or longer. Watch for hypotension and bronchospasm. These may lead to laryngeal edema, dysrhythmias, cardiac arrest, coma, and death. Other signs of allergic response include erythema, pilomotor

---

Italicized side effects are common or life-threatening.
*Liquid form contains alcohol.   **May contain tartrazine.

erection, rash, pruritic urticaria, conjunctivitis, vasomotor rhinitis, angioedema, or various GI disturbances.
• Keep an I.V. line open to permit rapid management of anaphylaxis. Keep epinephrine and steroids readily available.
• Instruct patient to anticipate the possibility of delayed allergic reactions, such as rash, urticaria, or itching, which may occur as late as 15 days after injection. Patient should report these to doctor immediately.
• Patients may experience back pain or involuntary muscle spasm in the lower back for several days after injection. Reassure patient that this is common and will not be chronic.
• Use within 60 minutes after reconstitution. Discard unused drug.

---

fibrinolysin and desoxyribonuclease
Elase♦

Pregnancy Risk Category: C

MECHANISM OF ACTION
Desoxyribonuclease attacks DNA and fibrinolysin attacks fibrin of blood clots and fibrinous exudates. Enzymatic action produces clean surfaces and promotes healing.

INDICATIONS & DOSAGE
Debridement of inflammatory and infected lesions (surgical wounds, ulcerative lesions, second- and third-degree burns, circumcision, episiotomy, cervicitis, vaginitis, abscesses, fistulas, and sinus tracts)—
Intravaginally:
Adults and children: 5 ml ointment may be inserted using applicator supplied, once daily for vaginitis or cervicitis.
Topical use:
Adults and children: apply ointment at intervals as long as enzyme action is desired.
Irrigating agent for infected wounds,

empyema cavities, abscesses, otorhinolaryngologic wounds, subcutaneous hematomas—
Adults and children: dilution for irrigation depends on extent and severity of wound.

ADVERSE REACTIONS
Local: hyperemia with high doses, allergic reactions.

INTERACTIONS
None significant.

NURSING CONSIDERATIONS
• Contraindicated for parenteral use.
• Dense, dry eschar must be removed surgically before enzymatic debridement. Enzyme must be in constant contact with substrate. Accumulated necrotic debris must be removed periodically and the enzyme replenished at least once daily.
• Cleanse wound with water, normal salines, or peroxide and dry gently; cover with thin layer of Elase. Cover with nonadhering dressing.
• Change dressing at least once and preferably two to three times daily. Flush away necrotic debris and reapply ointment. Frequency of application may be more important than the amount of drug used.
• Solution as wet to dry dressing: mix 1 vial of Elase powder with 10 to 50 ml saline solution; saturate strips of fine gauze with solution. Pack ulcerated area with Elase gauze. Allow gauze to dry in contact with ulcerated lesion for about 6 to 8 hours. Remove dried gauze and repeat 3 to 4 times daily.
• Solution as irrigating agent: Drain cavity and replace Elase every 6 to 10 hours to reduce amount of by-product accumulation and to minimize loss of enzyme activity. Although parenteral use is contraindicated, Elase is used as an irrigating agent in certain specific conditions.
• Prepare solution just before use.

Discard after 24 hours.

hyaluronidase
Wydase♦

Pregnancy Risk Category: C

MECHANISM OF ACTION
Hydrolyzes hyaluronic acid, thereby promoting diffusion of fluids in the tissues.

INDICATIONS & DOSAGE
Adjunct to increase absorption and dispersion of other injected drugs—
Adults and children: 150 units to injection medium containing other medication.
Hypodermoclysis—
Adults and children over 3 years: 150 units injected S.C. before clysis or injected into clysis tubing near needle for each 1,000 ml clysis solution.
Subcutaneous urography—
Adults and children: with patient in a prone position, give 75 units S.C. over each scapula, followed by injection of contrast medium at same sites.

ADVERSE REACTIONS
Skin: rash, urticaria.
Local: irritation.

INTERACTIONS
Local anesthetics: increased potential for toxic local reaction. Use together cautiously.

NURSING CONSIDERATIONS
• Use with caution in patients with blood-clotting abnormalities, severe hepatic or renal disease.
• Do not inject into acutely inflamed or cancerous areas.
• In hypodermoclysis, adjust dosage, rate of injection, and type of solution according to patient's response.
• Administration precautions: Perform a skin test for sensitivity. Avoid injecting into diseased areas (may spread infection). Observe injection site for local reactions.
• Avoid getting solution in eyes. If solution does get in eyes, flush with water at once.
• Protect from heat. Do not use cloudy or discolored solution.
• For children, 15 units are added to each 100 ml of solution. The drip rate should not exceed 2 ml/minute.
• Hyaluronidase is incompatible with epinephrine and heparin. Don't add to any solutions containing these drugs.

107

Oxytocics

carboprost tromethamine
dinoprostone
ergonovine maleate
methylergonovine maleate
oxytocin, synthetic injection
oxytocin, synthetic nasal
　solution

COMBINATION PRODUCTS
None.

carboprost tromethamine
Prostin/15 M

MECHANISM OF ACTION
Produces strong, prompt contractions
of uterine smooth muscle, possibly
mediated by calcium and cyclic $3',5'$-
adenosine monophosphate. A prostaglandin.

INDICATIONS & DOSAGE
*Abort pregnancy between 13th and
20th weeks of gestation—*
Adults: initially, 250 mcg is administered deep I.M. Subsequent doses of
250 mcg should be administered at intervals of 1½ to 3½ hours, depending
on uterine response. Increments in
dosage may be increased to 500 mcg
if contractility is inadequate after several 250-mcg doses. Total dosage
should not exceed 12 mg.
*Postpartum hemorrhage caused by
uterine atony that has not responded
to conventional management—*
Adults: 250 mcg by deep I.M. injection. May administer repeat doses at
15- to 90-minute intervals. Maximum
total dosage is 2 mg.

ADVERSE REACTIONS
GI: *vomiting, diarrhea,* nausea.
Other: *fever,* chills.

INTERACTIONS
None significant.

NURSING CONSIDERATIONS
• Contraindicated in pelvic inflammatory disease or active cardiac, pulmonary, renal, or hepatic disease. Use
cautiously in history of asthma; hypertension; cardiovascular, renal, or
hepatic disease; anemia; jaundice;
diabetes; epilepsy; and previous uterine surgery.
• I.M. injection of this drug is techni-
cally less difficult and poses fewer potential risks than other prostaglandin
abortifacients.
• Unlike other prostaglandin abortifacients, carboprost tromethamine is
administered by I.M. injection. Injectable form avoids risk of expelling
vaginal suppositories, which may occur in the presence of profuse vaginal
bleeding.
• Should be used only in a hospital
setting by trained personnel.

dinoprostone
Prostin E₂◆

MECHANISM OF ACTION
Produces strong, prompt contractions
of uterine smooth muscle, possibly
mediated by calcium and cyclic $3',5'$-
adenosine monophosphate. A prostaglandin.

INDICATIONS & DOSAGE

Abort second trimester pregnancy, evacuate uterus in cases of missed abortion, intrauterine fetal deaths up to 28 weeks of gestation, or benign hydatidiform mole—

Adults: insert 20 mg suppository high into posterior vaginal fornix. Repeat q 3 to 5 hours until abortion is complete.

ADVERSE REACTIONS

CNS: headache, *dizziness.*
CV: hypotension (in large doses).
GI: *nausea, vomiting, diarrhea.*
GU: vaginal pain, vaginitis.
Other: *fever, shivering, chills, joint inflammation, nocturnal leg cramps, bronchospasm.*

INTERACTIONS

Alcohol (I.V. infusions of 500 ml of 10% over 1 hour): inhibited uterine activity.

NURSING CONSIDERATIONS

• Contraindicated in pelvic inflammatory disease or history of pelvic surgery, incisions, uterine fibroids, or cervical stenosis. Use cautiously in asthma, epilepsy, anemia, diabetes, hypertension or hypotension, jaundice, and cardiovascular, renal, or hepatic disease.
• Administer only when critical care facilities are readily available.
• Patient may be pretreated with an antiemetic and an antidiarrheal agent.
• Just before use, warm dinoprostone suppositories in their wrapping to room temperature.
• After administration, patient should remain supine for 10 minutes.
• Store suppositories in freezer at temperature of $-20°$ C. ($-4°$ F.).
• Dinoprostone-induced fever is self-limiting and transient and occurs in approximately 50% of all patients. Treat with water or alcohol sponging and increased fluid intake rather than with aspirin.

• Check vaginal discharge daily.
• Abortion should be complete within 30 hours.

---

ergonovine maleate
Ergotrate Maleate♦

MECHANISM OF ACTION

Increases motor activity of the uterus by direct stimulation. Prolonged uterine contraction helps control hemorrhage.

INDICATIONS & DOSAGE

Prevent or treat postpartum and post-abortion hemorrhage from uterine atony or subinvolution—

Adults: 0.2 mg I.M. q 2 to 4 hours, maximum of 5 doses; or 0.2 mg I.V. (only for severe uterine bleeding or other life-threatening emergency) over 1 minute while blood pressure and uterine contractions are monitored. I.V. dose may be diluted to 5 ml with normal saline injection. After initial I.M. or I.V. dose, may give 0.2 to 0.4 mg P.O. q 6 to 12 hours for 2 to 7 days. Decrease dosage if severe uterine cramping occurs.

ADVERSE REACTIONS

CNS: dizziness, headache.
CV: hypertension, chest pain.
EENT: tinnitus.
GI: *nausea, vomiting.*
GU: uterine cramping.
Other: sweating, dyspnea, hypersensitivity.

INTERACTIONS

Regional anesthetics, dopamine, I.V. oxytocin: excessive vasoconstriction. Use together cautiously.

NURSING CONSIDERATIONS

• Contraindicated for induction or augmentation of labor, before delivery of placenta, in threatened spontaneous abortion, and in patients with allergy or sensitivity to ergot prepara-

---

Italicized side effects are common or life-threatening.
*Liquid form contains alcohol.   **May contain tartrazine.

tions. Use cautiously in hypertension, cardiac disease, venoatrial shunts, mitral valve stenosis, obliterative vascular disease, sepsis, and hepatic or renal impairment.
• Monitor blood pressure, pulse rate, and uterine response. Report sudden changes in vital signs, frequent periods of uterine relaxation, and/or character and amount of vaginal bleeding.
• If hypertension occurs, it may respond to chlorpromazine or hydralazine.
• Hypocalcemia may decrease patient response. If patient is not also taking digitalis, cautious administration of calcium gluconate I.V. may produce desired oxytocic action.
• Contractions begin 5 to 15 minutes after P.O. administration; immediately after I.V. injection. May continue 3 hours or more after P.O. or I.M. administration; 45 minutes after I.V. injection.
• Keep patient warm.
• Store in tightly closed, light-resistant container. Discard if discolored.
• Store I.V. solutions below 8° C. (46.4° F.). Daily stock may be kept at cool room temperature for 60 days.
• Have drug ready for immediate use if it is to be given postpartum.
• I.V. ergonovine is used to diagnose coronary artery spasm (Prinzmetal's angina).

methylergonovine maleate
Methergine

MECHANISM OF ACTION
Increases motor activity of the uterus by direct stimulation.

INDICATIONS & DOSAGE
Prevent and treat postpartum hemorrhage caused by uterine atony or subinvolution—
Adults: 0.2 mg I.M. q 2 to 5 hours for maximum of 5 doses; or I.V. (excessive uterine bleeding or other

emergencies) over 1 minute while blood pressure and uterine contractions are monitored. I.V. dose may be diluted to 5 ml with normal saline solution. Following initial I.M. or I.V. dose, may give 0.2 to 0.4 mg P.O. q 6 to 12 hours for 2 to 7 days. Decrease dosage if severe cramping occurs.

ADVERSE REACTIONS
CNS: dizziness, headache.
CV: hypertension, transient chest pain, dyspnea, palpitation.
EENT: tinnitus.
GI: *nausea, vomiting.*
Other: sweating, hypersensitivity.

INTERACTIONS
Regional anesthetics, dopamine, I.V. oxytocin: excessive vasoconstriction.

NURSING CONSIDERATIONS
• Contraindicated for induction of labor; before delivery of placenta; in patients with hypertension, toxemia, or sensitivity to ergot preparations; and in threatened spontaneous abortion. Use cautiously in sepsis, obliterative vascular disease, and hepatic, renal, or cardiac disease.
• Drug should not be routinely administered I.V. If it must be given by this route, administer slowly over 1 minute with careful blood pressure monitoring.
• Monitor and record blood pressure, pulse rate, and uterine response; report any sudden change in vital signs or frequent periods of uterine relaxation, and character and amount of vaginal bleeding.
• Contractions begin 5 to 15 minutes after P.O. administration; 2 to 5 minutes after I.M. injection; immediately following I.V. injection. May continue 3 hours or more after P.O. or I.M. administration; 45 minutes after I.V.
• Store in tightly closed, light-resistant containers. Discard if discolored.
• Store I.V. solutions below 8° C. (46.4° F.). Daily stock may be kept at

room temperature for 60 to 90 days.

---

oxytocin, synthetic injection
Oxytocin♦, Pitocin♦, Syntocinon♦

MECHANISM OF ACTION
Causes potent and selective stimulation of uterine and mammary gland smooth muscle.

INDICATIONS & DOSAGE
Induction or stimulation of labor—
Adults: initially, 1 ml (10 units) ampule in 1,000 ml of dextrose 5% injection or normal saline solution I.V. infused at 1 to 2 milliunits/minute. Increase rate at 15- to 30-minute intervals until normal contraction pattern is established. Maximum is 1 to 2 ml (20 milliunits)/minute. Decrease rate when labor is firmly established.
Reduction of postpartum bleeding after expulsion of placenta—
Adults: 10 to 40 units added to 1,000 ml of dextrose 5% in water or normal saline solution infused at rate necessary to control bleeding, usually 20 to 40 milliunits/minute. Also, 1 ml (10 units) can be given I.M. after delivery of the placenta.
Incomplete or inevitable abortion—
Adults: I.V. infusion with 10 units of oxytocin in 500 ml of normal saline solution or dextrose 5% in normal saline solution. Infuse at rate of 20 to 100 milliunits/minute.

ADVERSE REACTIONS
Maternal—
Blood: afibrinogenemia; may be related to increased postpartum bleeding.
CNS: subarachnoid hemorrhage resulting from hypertension; *seizures or coma resulting from water intoxication.*
CV: hypotension; increased heart rate, systemic venous return, and cardiac output; dysrhythmias.

GI: nausea, vomiting.
Other: hypersensitivity, tetanic contractions, abruptio placentae, *impaired uterine blood flow, increased uterine motility.*
Fetal—
Blood: hyperbilirubinemia.
CV: bradycardia, tachycardia, premature ventricular contractions.
Other: *anoxia, asphyxia.*

INTERACTIONS
Cyclopropane anesthetics: less pronounced bradycardia; hypotension.
Thiopental anesthetics: delayed induction reported.
Vasoconstrictors: severe hypertension if oxytocin is given within 3 to 4 hours of vasoconstrictor in patient receiving caudal block anesthetic.

NURSING CONSIDERATIONS
• Contraindicated in cases of cephalopelvic disproportion or where delivery requires conversion, as in transverse lie; fetal distress, when delivery isn't imminent; severe toxemia; and other obstetric emergencies. Use cautiously in history of cervical or uterine surgery, grand multiparity, uterine sepsis, traumatic delivery, or overdistended uterus, and in primiparas over 35 years. Use with extreme caution during first and second stages of labor because cervical laceration, uterine rupture, and maternal and fetal death have been reported.
• Don't give by I.V. bolus injection. Must administer by infusion; give by piggyback infusion so the drug may be discontinued without interrupting the I.V. line.
• Used to induce or reinforce labor only when pelvis is known to be adequate, when vaginal delivery is indicated, when fetal maturity is assured, and when fetal position is favorable. Should be used only in hospital where critical care facilities and doctor are immediately available.
• Oxytocin should never be given si-

Italicized side effects are common or life-threatening.
*Liquid form contains alcohol.   **May contain tartrazine.

multaneously by more than one route.
• Do the following every 15 minutes: monitor and record uterine contractions, heart rate, blood pressure, intrauterine pressure, fetal heart rate, and character of blood loss.
• May produce an antidiuretic effect; fluid overload can lead to seizures and coma. Monitor fluid intake/output.
• If contractions occur less than 2 minutes apart and if contractions above 50 mm Hg are recorded, or if contractions last 90 seconds or longer, stop infusion, turn patient on her side, and notify doctor.
• Not recommended for routine I.M. use. However, 10 units may be given I.M. after delivery of placenta to control postpartum uterine bleeding.
• Should have magnesium sulfate (20% solution) available for relaxation of the myometrium.

oxytocin, synthetic nasal solution

MECHANISM OF ACTION
Stimulates impaired milk ejection.

INDICATIONS & DOSAGE
To promote initial milk ejection; may relieve postpartum breast engorgement—
Adults: 1 spray or 3 drops into one or both nostrils 2 or 3 minutes before breast-feeding or pumping breasts.

ADVERSE REACTIONS
None reported.

INTERACTIONS
None significant.

NURSING CONSIDERATIONS
• Instruct patient to clear nasal passages first. With patient's head in vertical position, hold squeeze bottle upright and eject solution into nostril.
• To administer as nose drops, invert the squeeze bottle and exert gentle

pressure on it.

108

Spasmolytics

aminophylline
  (theophylline ethylenediamine)
dyphylline
flavoxate hydrochloride
oxtriphylline
oxybutynin chloride
theophylline
theophylline sodium glycinate

COMBINATION PRODUCTS

BRONCHIAL CAPSULES: 150 mg theophylline and 90 mg guaifenesin.
BRONDECON TABLETS: 200 mg oxtriphylline and 100 mg guaifenesin.
DILOR-G TABLETS: 200 mg dyphylline and 200 mg guaifenesin.
DYFLEX-G TABLETS: 200 mg dyphylline and 200 mg guaifenesin.
DYLINE-GG TABLETS: 200 mg dyphylline and 200 mg guaifenesin.
GLYCERYL-T CAPSULES: 150 mg theophylline and 90 mg guaifenesin.
LANOPHYLLIN-GG CAPSULES: 150 mg theophylline and 90 mg guaifenesin.
NEOTHYLLINE-GG TABLETS: 200 mg dyphylline and 200 mg guaifenesin.
QUIBRON CAPSULES: 150 mg theophylline and 90 mg guaifenesin.

---

aminophylline (theophylline ethylenediamine)

Aminophyllin, Corophyllin♦♦, Phyllocontin, Somophyllin-DF

Pregnancy Risk Category: C

MECHANISM OF ACTION

Inhibits phosphodiesterase, the enzyme that degrades cyclic AMP. Results in relaxation of smooth muscle of the bronchial airways and pulmonary blood vessels.

INDICATIONS & DOSAGE

Symptomatic relief of bronchospasm—
Patients not currently receiving theophylline who require rapid relief of symptoms: Loading dose is 6 mg/kg (equivalent to 4.7 mg/kg anhydrous theophylline) I.V. slowly (less than or equal to 25 mg/kg minute), then maintenance infusion.
Adults (nonsmokers): 0.7 mg/kg/hour for 12 hours; then 0.5 mg/kg/hour.
Otherwise healthy adult smokers: 1 mg/kg/hour for 12 hours; then 0.18 mg/kg/hour.
Older patients and adults with cor pulmonale: 0.6 mg/kg/hour for 12 hours; then 0.3 mg/kg/hour.
Adults with CHF or liver disease: 0.5 mg/kg/hour for 12 hours; then 0.1 to 0.2 mg/kg/hour.
Children 9 to 16 years: 1 mg/kg/hour for 12 hours; then 0.8 mg/kg/hour.
Children 6 months to 9 years: 1.2 mg/kg/hour for 12 hours; then 1 mg/kg/hour.
Patients currently receiving theophylline: Aminophylline infusions of 0.63 mg/kg (0.5 mg/kg anhydrous theophylline) will increase plasma levels of theophylline by 1 mcg/ml. Some clinicians recommend a dose of 3.1 mg/kg (2.5 mg/kg anhydrous theohpylline) if no obvious signs of theophylline toxicity are present.
Chronic bronchial asthma—
Adults: 600 to 1,600 mg P.O. daily

Italicized side effects are common or life-threatening.
*Liquid form contains alcohol.   **May contain tartrazine.

divided t.i.d. or q.i.d.
Children: 12 mg/kg P.O. daily divided t.i.d. or q.i.d.

ADVERSE REACTIONS

CNS: *restlessness, dizziness,* headache, *insomnia,* light-headedness, *seizures,* muscle twitching.
CV: *palpitations, sinus tachycardia,* extrasystoles, flushing, marked hypotension, increase in respiratory rate.
GI: *nausea, vomiting, anorexia,* bitter aftertaste, dyspepsia, heavy feeling in stomach, diarrhea.
Skin: urticaria.
Local: *rectal suppositories may cause irritation.*

INTERACTIONS

Alkali-sensitive drugs: reduced activity. Do not add to I.V. fluids containing aminophylline.
Beta-adrenergic blockers: antagonism. Propranolol and nadolol, especially, may cause bronchospasm in sensitive patients. Use together cautiously.
Troleandomycin, erythromycin, cimetidine: decreased hepatic clearance of theophylline; elevated theophylline levels. Monitor for signs of toxicity.
Barbiturates, phenytoin: enhanced metabolism and decreased theophylline blood levels. Monitor for decreased aminophylline effect.

NURSING CONSIDERATIONS

• Contraindicated in hypersensitivity to xanthine compounds (caffeine, theobromine) and in preexisting cardiac dysrhythmias, especially tachydysrhythmias. Use cautiously in young children; in elderly patients with CHF or other cardiac or circulatory impairment, cor pulmonale, or hepatic disease; in active peptic ulcer, because drug may increase volume and acidity of gastric secretions; and in hyperthyroidism or diabetes mellitus.
• Individuals metabolize xanthines at different rates. Adjust dosage by monitoring response, tolerance, pulmonary function, and serum theophylline levels. Theophylline concentrations should range from 10 to 20 mcg/ml; toxicity has been reported with levels above 20 mcg/ml.
• Plasma clearance may be decreased in patients with CHF, hepatic dysfunction, or pulmonary edema. Smokers show accelerated clearance. Dosage adjustments are necessary.
• I.V. drug administration can cause burning; dilute with 5% dextrose in water solution.
• Monitor vital signs; measure and record intake/output. Expected clinical effects include improvement in quality of pulse and respiration.
• Warn elderly patient of dizziness, a common adverse reaction at start of therapy.
• GI symptoms may be relieved by taking oral drug with full glass of water at meals, although food in stomach delays absorption. Enteric-coated tablets may also delay and impair absorption. No evidence that antacids reduce GI adverse reactions.
• Suppositories are slowly and erratically absorbed; retention enemas may be absorbed more rapidly. Rectally administered preparations can be given if patient cannot take drug orally. Schedule after evacuation, if possible; may be retained better if given before meal. Advise patient to remain recumbent 15 to 20 minutes after insertion.
• Question patient closely about other drugs used. Warn him that OTC remedies may contain ephedrine in combination with theophylline salts; excessive CNS stimulation may result. Tell him to check with doctor or pharmacist before taking *any* other medications.
• Before giving loading dose, check that patient has not had recent theophylline therapy.
• Supply instructions for home care

Unmarked trade names available in the United States only.
♦ Also available in Canada. ♦♦ Available in Canada only. ◊ Also available OTC.

and dosage schedule. Some patients may require an around-the-clock dosage schedule.

• Warn patients with allergies that exposure to allergens may exacerbate bronchospasm.

dyphylline
Brophylline, Dilin, Dilor*, Dyflex, Dylline*, Emfabid, Lufyllin*, Protophylline♦♦

Pregnancy Risk Category: C

MECHANISM OF ACTION
Inhibits phosphodiesterase, the enzyme that degrades cyclic adenosine monophosphate. Results in relaxation of smooth muscle of the bronchial airways and pulmonary blood vessels.

INDICATIONS & DOSAGE
For relief of acute and chronic bronchial asthma and reversible bronchospasm associated with chronic bronchitis and emphysema—
Adults: 15 mg/kg P.O. q 6 hours. I.M. route is rarely used, but patients may receive 250 to 500 mg I.M. injected slowly at 6-hour intervals. Dosage should be decreased in renal insufficiency.

ADVERSE REACTIONS
CNS: *restlessness, dizziness,* headache, *insomnia,* light-headedness, *seizures,* muscle twitching.
CV: *palpitations, sinus tachycardia,* extrasystoles, flushing, marked hypotension, increase in respiratory rate.
GI: *nausea, vomiting, anorexia,* bitter aftertaste, dyspepsia, heavy feeling in stomach.
Skin: urticaria.

INTERACTIONS
Beta-adrenergic blockers: antagonism. Propanolol and nadolol, especially, may cause bronchospasm in sensitive patients. Use together cautiously.

Troleandomycin, erythromycin, cimetidine: decreased hepatic clearance of theophylline; elevated theophylline levels. Monitor for signs of toxicity.
Barbiturates, phenytoin: enhanced metabolism and decreased theophylline blood levels. Monitor for decreased theophylline effect.

NURSING CONSIDERATIONS
• Contraindicated in hypersensitivity to xanthine compounds (caffeine, theobromine); preexisting cardiac dysrhythmias, especially tachycardias. Use cautiously in young children; in elderly patients with CHF, any impaired cardiac or circulatory function, cor pulmonale, renal or hepatic disease; and in peptic ulcer, hyperthyroidism, or diabetes mellitus.
• Do not administer I.V.
• Dyphylline is metabolized faster than theophylline; dosage intervals may have to be decreased to ensure continual therapeutic effect. Higher daily dosages may be needed.
• Monitor vital signs; measure and record intake/output. Expected clinical effects include improvement in quality of pulse and respiration.
• Warn elderly patient of dizziness, a common adverse effect at start of therapy.
• Gastric irritation may be relieved by taking oral drug after meals; there is no evidence that antacids reduce this adverse effect. May produce less gastric discomfort than theophylline.
• Discard dyphylline ampule if precipitate is present. Protect from light.
• Question patient closely about other drugs used. Warn him that OTC remedies may contain ephedrine in combination with theophylline salts; excessive CNS stimulation may result. Tell him to check with doctor or pharmacist before taking *any* other medications.
• Supply instructions for home care and dosage schedule.

Italicized side effects are common or life-threatening.
*Liquid form contains alcohol.   **May contain tartrazine.

flavoxate hydrochloride
Urispas
Pregnancy Risk Category: C

MECHANISM OF ACTION
Has a direct spasmolytic effect on smooth muscles of the urinary tract. It also provides some local anesthesia and analgesia.

INDICATIONS & DOSAGE
Symptomatic relief of dysuria, frequency, urgency, nocturia, incontinence, and suprapubic pain associated with urologic disorders—
Adults and children over 12 years: 100 to 200 mg P.O. t.i.d. to q.i.d.

ADVERSE REACTIONS
CNS: *mental confusion* (especially in elderly), nervousness, dizziness, headache, drowsiness, difficulty with concentration.
CV: tachycardia, palpitations.
EENT: *dry mouth and throat, blurred vision,* disturbed eye accommodation.
GI: abdominal pain, constipation (with high doses), nausea, vomiting.
Skin: urticaria, dermatoses.
Other: fever.

INTERACTIONS
None significant.

NURSING CONSIDERATIONS
• Contraindicated in pyloric or duodenal obstruction, obstructive intestinal lesions or ileus, achalasia, GI hemorrhage, or obstructive uropathies of lower urinary tract. Use cautiously in patients suspected of having glaucoma.
• Check history for other drug use before giving drugs with anticholinergic side effects.
• Warn about possible drowsiness, mental confusion, and blurred vision.
• Tell the patient to report adverse effects or lack of response to drug.

oxtriphylline
Choledyl♦*, Theophylline Choline
Pregnancy Risk Category: C

MECHANISM OF ACTION
Inhibits phosphodiesterase, the enzyme that degrades cyclic adenosine monophosphate. Results in relaxation of smooth muscle of the bronchial airways and pulmonary blood vessels.

INDICATIONS & DOSAGE
To relieve acute bronchial asthma and reversible bronchospasm associated with chronic bronchitis and emphysema—
Adults and children over 12 years: 200 mg P.O. q 6 hours, then adjust dosage based upon serum theophylline levels.
Children 2 to 12 years: 4 mg/kg P.O. q 6 hours. Adjust as needed to maintain therapeutic levels of theophylline (10 to 20 mcg/ml).

ADVERSE REACTIONS
CNS: *restlessness, dizziness,* headache, *insomnia,* light-headedness, *seizures,* muscle twitching.
CV: *palpitations, sinus tachycardia,* extrasystoles, flushing, marked hypotension, increase in respiratory rate.
GI: *nausea, vomiting, anorexia,* bitter aftertaste, dyspepsia, heavy feeling in stomach.
Skin: urticaria.

INTERACTIONS
Erythromycin, troleandomycin, cimetidine: decreased hepatic clearance of theophylline; increased plasma level. Monitor for signs of toxicity.
Barbiturates, phenytoin: enhanced metabolism and decreased theophylline blood levels. Monitor for decreased effect.
Beta-adrenergic blockers: antagonism. Propranolol and nadolol, especially, may cause bronchospasms in sensitive patients. Use together cau-

tiously.

NURSING CONSIDERATIONS

• Contraindicated in hypersensitivity to xanthines (caffeine, theobromine); preexisting cardiac dysrhythmias, especially tachydysrhythmias.

• Tell patient to report GI distress, palpitations, irritability, restlessness, nervousness, or insomnia; may indicate excessive CNS stimulation.

• Administer drug after meals and at bedtime.

• Store at 15° to 30° C. (59° to 86° F.). Protect elixir from light and tablets from moisture.

• Equivalent to 64% anhydrous theophylline.

• Monitor therapy carefully.

• Combination products that contain ephedrine are not recommended; excessive CNS stimulation may result (nervousness, tremors, akathisia).

---

oxybutynin chloride
Ditropan♦

Pregnancy Risk Category: C

MECHANISM OF ACTION
Has both a direct spasmolytic effect and an atropine-like effect on urinary tract smooth muscles. It increases urinary bladder capacity and provides some local anesthesia and mild analgesia.

INDICATIONS & DOSAGE
Antispasmodic for neurogenic bladder—
Adults: 5 mg P.O. b.i.d. to t.i.d., to maximum of 5 mg q.i.d.
Children over 5 years: 5 mg P.O. b.i.d., to maximum of 5 mg t.i.d.

ADVERSE REACTIONS
CNS: *drowsiness,* dizziness, insomnia, *dry mouth,* flushing.
CV: *palpitations, tachycardia.*
EENT: *transient blurred vision,* mydriasis, cycloplegia.

GI: nausea, vomiting, *constipation,* bloated feeling.
GU: impotence, *urinary hesitance or urine retention.*
Skin: urticaria, severe allergic reactions in patients sensitive to anticholinergics.
Other: decreased sweating, fever, suppression of lactation.

INTERACTIONS
None significant.

NURSING CONSIDERATIONS
• Contraindicated in myasthenia gravis, GI obstruction, glaucoma, adynamic ileus, megacolon, severe or ulcerative colitis, obstructive uropathy, or in elderly or debilitated patients with intestinal atony. Use cautiously in elderly patients and in autonomic neuropathy, reflux esophagitis, and hepatic or renal disease.

• May aggravate symptoms of hyperthyroidism, coronary artery disease, CHF, cardiac dysrhythmias, tachycardia, hypertension, or prostatic hypertrophy.

• Therapy should be stopped periodically to determine whether patient can get along without it. Minimizes tendency toward tolerance.

• Rapid onset of action, peaks at 3 to 4 hours, and lasts 6 to 10 hours.

• Neurogenic bladder should be confirmed by cystometry before oxybutynin is given. Evaluate patient response to therapy periodically by cystometry.

• Rule out partial intestinal obstruction in patients with diarrhea, especially those with colostomy or ileostomy, before giving oxybutynin.

• If urinary tract infection is present, patient should receive antibiotics concomitantly.

• Warn patient that drug may impair alertness or vision.

• Since oxybutynin suppresses sweating, its use during very hot weather may precipitate fever or heatstroke.

Italicized side effects are common or life-threatening.
*Liquid form contains alcohol.   **May contain tartrazine.

- Store in tightly closed containers at 59° to 86° F. (15° to 30° C.).

---

theophylline

Immediate-release tablets and capsules: Bronkodyl, Elixophyllin, Slo-Phyllin, Somophyllin-T
Immediate-release liquids: Accurbron*, Aerolate, Aquaphyllin, Asmalix*, Bronkodyl*, Elixicon, Elixomin*, Elixophyllin♦*, Lanophyllin*, Lixolin, Slo-Phyllin, Theolair♦, Theon*, Theophyl*
Timed-release capsules: Aerolate, Bronkodyl S-R, Elixophyllin SR, Lodrane, Slo-bid Gyrocaps, Slo-Phyllin, Somophyllin-CRT, Theo-24, Theobid Duracaps, Theobid Jr., Theochron, Theo-Dur Sprinkle, Theophyl-SR, Theospan SR, Theovent Long-acting
Timed-release tablets: Constant-T, Duraphyl, Quibron-T/SR, Respbid, Sustaire, Theo-Dur♦, Theolair-SR, Theo-Time, Uniphyl

theophylline sodium glycinate

Acet-Am♦♦, Synophylate

Pregnancy Risk Category: C

MECHANISM OF ACTION
Inhibits phosphodiesterase, the enzyme that degrades cyclic adenosine monophosphate. Results in relaxation of smooth muscle of the bronchial airways and pulmonary blood vessels.

INDICATIONS & DOSAGE
Prophylaxis and symptomatic relief of bronchial asthma, bronchospasm of chronic bronchitis and emphysema—
Adults: 6 mg/kg P.O. followed by 2 to 3 mg/kg q 4 hours for 2 doses. Maintenance dosage is 1 to 3 mg/kg q 8 to 12 hours.
Children 9 to 16 years: 6 mg/kg P.O. followed by 3 mg/kg q 4 hours for 3 doses. Maintenance dosage is 3 mg/kg q 6 hours.

Children 6 months to 9 years: 6 mg/kg P.O. followed by 4 mg/kg q 4 hours for 3 doses. Maintenance dosage is 4 mg/kg q 6 hours.
  Most oral timed-release forms are given q 8 to 12 hours. Several products, however, may be given q 24 hours.
Symptomatic relief of bronchial asthma, pulmonary emphysema, and chronic bronchitis—
Adults: 330 to 660 mg (sodium glycinate) P.O. q 6 to 8 hours, after meals.
Children over 12 years: 220 to 330 mg (sodium glycinate) P.O. q 6 to 8 hours.
Children 6 to 12 years: 330 mg (sodium glycinate) P.O. q 6 to 8 hours.
Children 3 to 6 years: 110 to 165 mg (sodium glycinate) P.O. q 6 to 8 hours.
Children 1 to 3 years: 55 to 110 mg (sodium glycinate) P.O. q 6 to 8 hours.

ADVERSE REACTIONS
CNS: *restlessness, dizziness,* headache, *insomnia,* light-headedness, *seizures,* muscle twitching.
CV: *palpitations, sinus tachycardia,* extrasystoles, flushing, marked hypotension, increase in respiratory rate.
GI: *nausea, vomiting, anorexia,* bitter aftertaste, dyspepsia, heavy feeling in stomach, diarrhea.
Skin: urticaria.

INTERACTIONS
Erythromycin, troleandomycin, cimetidine: decreased hepatic clearance of theophylline; increased plasma levels. Monitor for signs of toxicity.
Barbiturates, phenytoin: enhanced metabolism and decreased theophylline blood levels. Monitor for decreased effect.
Beta-adrenergic blockers: antagonism. Propranolol and nadolol, especially, may cause bronchospasms in sensitive patients. Use together cau-

---

Unmarked trade names available in the United States only.
♦Also available in Canada.   ♦♦Available in Canada only.   ◊Also available OTC.

tiously.

NURSING CONSIDERATIONS
• Contraindicated in hypersensitivity to xanthine compounds (caffeine, theobromine); preexisting cardiac dysrhythmias, especially tachydysrhythmias. Use cautiously in young children; in elderly patients with CHF or other circulatory impairment, cor pulmonale, renal or hepatic disease; and in peptic ulcer, hyperthyroidism, or diabetes mellitus.
• Individuals metabolize xanthines at different rates; determine dosage by monitoring response, tolerance, pulmonary function, and serum theophylline levels. Serum theophylline concentrations should range from 10 to 20 mcg/ml; toxicity has been reported with levels above 20 mcg/ml.
• Monitor vital signs; measure and record intake/output. Expected clinical effects include improvement in quality of pulse and respiration.
• Warn elderly patients of dizziness, a common adverse reaction at start of therapy.
• GI symptoms may be relieved by taking oral drug with full glass of water after meals, although food in stomach delays absorption.
• Question patient closely about other drugs used. Warn him that OTC remedies may contain ephedrine in combination with theophylline salts; excessive CNS stimulation may result. Tell him to check with doctor or pharmacist before taking *any* other medications.
• Supply instructions for home care and dosage schedule.
• Daily dosage may need to be decreased in patients with CHF or hepatic disease, or in elderly patients, since metabolism and excretion may be decreased. Monitor carefully, using blood levels, observation, examination, and patient interview. Give drug around the clock, using sustained-release product at bedtime.

• Drug dosage may need to be increased in cigarette smokers because smoking causes the drug to be metabolized faster.
• Be careful not to confuse sustained-release dosage forms with standard-release dosage forms.
• Warn patient not to dissolve, crush, or chew slow-release products. Small children unable to swallow these can ingest (without chewing) the contents of bead-filled capsules sprinkled over soft food.
• Warn patients to take the drug regularly, as directed. Patients tend to want to take extra "breathing pills."
• Patients taking Theo-24 brand of theophylline should take it on an empty stomach because food accelerates the drug's absorption.

Italicized side effects are common or life-threatening.
*Liquid form contains alcohol.   **May contain tartrazine.

109

Heavy metal antagonists

deferoxamine mesylate
dimercaprol
edetate calcium disodium
edetate disodium
D-penicillamine
trientine hydrochloride

COMBINATION PRODUCTS
None.

---

deferoxamine mesylate
Desferal♦

Pregnancy Risk Category: C

MECHANISM OF ACTION
Chelates iron by binding ferric ions.

INDICATIONS & DOSAGE
Adjunctive treatment of acute iron intoxication—
Adults and children: 1 g I.M. or I.V. followed by 500 mg I.M. or I.V. for two doses, q 4 hours; then 500 mg I.M. or I.V. q 4 to 12 hours. Infusion rate shouldn't exceed 15 mg/kg hourly. Don't exceed 6 g in 24 hours.
Chronic iron overload resulting from multiple transfusions—
Adults and children: 500 mg to 1 g I.M. daily and 2 g slow I.V. infusion in separate solution along with each unit of blood transfused. Maximum dosage is 6 g daily. I.V. infusion rate shouldn't exceed 15 mg/kg hourly. S.C.: 1 to 2 g via a subcutaneous infusion pump over 8 to 24 hours.

ADVERSE REACTIONS
Local: pain and induration at injection site.

Other: *after rapid I.V. administration: erythema, urticaria, hypotension, shock.*
With long-term use: sensitivity reaction (cutaneous wheal formation, pruritus, rash, *anaphylaxis), diarrhea, leg cramps, fever, tachycardia, blurred vision, dysuria, abdominal discomfort, cataracts.*

INTERACTIONS
None significant.

NURSING CONSIDERATIONS
• Contraindicated in severe renal disease or anuria. Use cautiously in impaired renal function.
• Monitor intake/output carefully.
• I.M. route preferred.
• Use I.V. only when patient has cardiovascular collapse or shock. For I.V. use, dissolve as for I.M. use; dilute in normal saline solution, dextrose 5% in water, or lactated Ringer's solution.
• If giving I.V., change to I.M. as soon as possible.
• For reconstitution, add 2 ml of sterile water for injection to each ampule. Make sure drug is completely dissolved. Reconstituted solution is good for 1 week at room temperature. Protect from light.
• Warn patient that urine may be red.
• Have epinephrine 1:1,000 readily available in case of allergic reaction.
• Recommend regular eye exams during long-term therapy.

---

dimercaprol
BAL in Oil♦

Pregnancy Risk Category: D

MECHANISM OF ACTION
Forms complexes with heavy metals.

INDICATIONS & DOSAGE
Adults and children:
Severe arsenic or gold poisoning—
3 mg/kg deep I.M. q 4 hours for 2
days, then q.i.d. on 3rd day, then
b.i.d. for 10 days.
Mild arsenic or gold poisoning—
2.5 mg/kg deep I.M. q.i.d. for 2
days, then b.i.d. on 3rd day, then once
daily for 10 days.
Mercury poisoning—
5 mg/kg deep I.M. initially, then 2.5
mg/kg daily or b.i.d. for 10 days.
*Acute lead encephalopathy or lead
level more than 100 mcg/ml—*
4 mg/kg deep I.M. injection, then q 4
hours with edetate calcium disodium
(12.5 mg/kg I.M.). Use separate
sites. Maximum dosage is 5 mg/kg
per dose.

ADVERSE REACTIONS
CNS: pain or tightness in throat,
chest, or hands; headache; paresthesias; muscle pain or weakness.
CV: *transient increase in blood pressure, returns to normal in 2 hours;
tachycardia.*
EENT: blepharospasm, conjunctivitis, lacrimation, rhinorrhea, excessive
salivation.
GI: *halitosis; nausea; vomiting; burning sensation in lips, mouth, and
throat; abdominal pain.*
GU: *dysuria;* renal damage if alkaline
urine not maintained.
Metabolic: decreased iodine uptake.
Local: sterile abscess, pain at injection site.
Other: *fever (especially in children),*
sweating, pain in teeth.

INTERACTIONS
131I uptake thyroid tests: decreased;
don't schedule patient for this test
during course of dimercaprol therapy.
Iron: forms toxic metal complex; concurrent therapy contraindicated. Wait
24 hours after last dimercaprol dose.

NURSING CONSIDERATIONS
• Contraindicated in hepatic dysfunction (except postarsenical jaundice),
or in acute renal insufficiency. Use
cautiously in hypertension.
• Should not be used in pregnancy except to treat life-threatening poisoning.
• Don't use for iron, cadmium, or selenium toxicity. Complex formed is
highly toxic, even fatal.
• Ephedrine or antihistamine may
prevent or relieve mild adverse reactions.
• Ineffective in arsine gas poisoning.
• Solution with slight sediment usable.
• Keep urine alkaline to prevent renal
damage. Oral sodium bicarbonate
may be ordered.
• Don't give I.V.; give by deep I.M.
route only. The injection site can be
massaged after drug is given.
• Drug has an unpleasant, garlic-like
odor.
• Be careful when preparing and administering drug not to let drug come
in contact with skin, as it may cause a
skin reaction.

edetate calcium disodium
Calcium Disodium Versenate,
Calcium EDTA

Pregnancy Risk Category: C

MECHANISM OF ACTION
Forms stable, soluble complexes with
metals, particularly lead.

INDICATIONS & DOSAGE
*Lead poisoning (blood levels greater
than 50 mcg/dl)—*

Italicized side effects are common or life-threatening.
*Liquid form contains alcohol.   **May contain tartrazine.

Adults and children: 1 g/m² in dextrose 5% in water or normal saline solution I.V. over 1 to 2 hours daily.
Acute lead encephalopathy or lead levels above 100 mcg/dl—
Adults and children: 1.5 g/m² daily for 3 to 5 days, usually in conjunction with dimercaprol. A second course may be administered at least 4 days later, but preferably 2 to 3 weeks should elapse between courses.

ADVERSE REACTIONS
CNS: headache, paresthesias, numbness.
CV: cardiac dysrhythmias, hypotension.
GI: anorexia, nausea, vomiting.
GU: *proteinuria, hematuria; nephrotoxicity with renal tubular necrosis leading to fatal nephrosis.*
Other: arthralgia, myalgia, hypercalcemia.
   4 to 8 hours after infusion: sudden fever and chills, fatigue, excessive thirst, sneezing, nasal congestion.

INTERACTIONS
None significant.

NURSING CONSIDERATIONS
• Contraindicated in severe renal disease or anuria.
• I.V. use contraindicated in lead encephalopathy; may increase intracranial pressure. Use I.M. route instead.
• Force fluids to facilitate lead excretion in all patients except those with lead encephalopathy.
• Monitor intake/output, urinalysis, BUN, and ECGs daily.
• To avoid toxicity, use with dimercaprol.
• Procaine hydrochloride may be added to I.M. solutions to minimize pain. Watch for local reactions.
• Avoid rapid I.V. infusions. I.M. route preferred, especially for children.
• Do not confuse this drug with edetate disodium, which is used for treating hypercalcemia.

edetate disodium
Disodium EDTA, Disotate, Endrate
Pregnancy Risk Category: C

MECHANISM OF ACTION
Chelates with metals, such as calcium, to form a stable, soluble complex.

INDICATIONS & DOSAGE
Hypercalcemic crisis—
Adults: 50 mg/kg by slow I.V. infusion added to 500 ml of dextrose 5% in water or normal saline solution. Maximum dosage is 3 g/day.
Children: 40 to 70 mg/kg by slow I.V. infusion, diluted to a maximum concentration of 30 mg/ml in dextrose 5% in water or normal saline solution. Maximum dosage is 70 mg/kg/day.

ADVERSE REACTIONS
CNS: circumoral paresthesias, numbness, headache, malaise, fatigue, muscle pain or weakness.
CV: hypertension, thrombophlebitis.
GI: nausea, vomiting, diarrhea, anorexia, abdominal cramps.
GU: in excessive doses—nephrotoxicity with urgency, nocturia, dysuria, polyuria, proteinuria, renal insufficiency and failure, tubular necrosis.
Metabolic: *severe hypocalcemia,* decreased magnesium.
Local: pain at site of infusion, erythema, dermatitis.

INTERACTIONS
None significant.

NURSING CONSIDERATIONS
• Contraindicated in anuria, known or suspected hypocalcemia, significant renal disease, active or healed tubercular lesions, history of seizures or intracranial lesions, and generalized arteriosclerosis associated with aging. Use cautiously in limited cardiac re-

---

serve, CHF, hypokalemia, and diabetes.
- Avoid rapid I.V. infusion; profound hypocalcemia may occur, leading to tetany, seizures, cardiac dysrhythmias, and respiratory arrest.
- Monitor ECG, and test renal function frequently.
- Obtain serum calcium after each dose.
- Keep I.V. calcium available.
- Monitor blood pressure closely.
- Keep patient in bed for 15 minutes after infusion to avoid postural hypotension.
- Don't use to treat lead toxicity; use edetate calcium disodium instead.
- Record I.V. site used, and try to avoid repeated use of the same site, as this increases likelihood of thrombophlebitis.
- Generalized systemic reactions may occur 4 to 8 hours after drug administration; these include fever, chills, back pain, emesis, muscle cramps, and urinary urgency. Report such reactions to doctor. Treatment is usually supportive. Symptoms generally subside within 12 hours.
- Edetate disodium not currently drug of choice for treatment of hypercalcemia; other treatments are safer and more effective.
- EDTA chelation therapy has been inappropriately recommended for treatment of atherosclerosis and related disorders. There's no scientific evidence that the drug is either safe or effective for these indications.

D-penicillamine
Cuprimine♦, Depen♦
Pregnancy Risk Category: D

MECHANISM OF ACTION
Mechanism of action in rheumatoid arthritis is unknown but is probably from inhibition of collagen formation. Also chelates heavy metals.

INDICATIONS & DOSAGE
Wilson's disease—
Adults: 250 mg P.O. q.i.d. 30 to 60 minutes before meals. Adjust dosage to achieve urinary copper excretion of 0.5 to 1 mg daily.
Children: 20 mg/kg P.O. daily divided q.i.d. before meals. Adjust dosage to achieve urinary copper excretion of 0.5 to 1 mg daily.
Cystinuria—
Adults: 250 mg P.O. q.i.d. before meals. Adjust dosage to achieve urinary cystine excretion of less than 100 mg daily when renal calculi present, or 100 to 200 mg daily when no calculi present. Maximum dosage is 5 g daily.
Children: 30 mg/kg P.O. daily divided q.i.d. before meals. Adjust dosage to achieve urinary cystine excretion of less than 100 mg daily when renal calculi present, or 100 to 200 mg daily when no calculi present.
Rheumatoid arthritis—
Adults: 125 to 250 mg P.O. daily initially, with increases of 250 mg q 2 to 3 months if necessary. Maximum dosage is 1 g daily.

ADVERSE REACTIONS
Blood: *leukopenia, eosinophilia, thrombocytopenia, monocytosis, granulocytopenia,* elevated sedimentation rate, lupus-like syndrome.
EENT: tinnitus.
GU: *nephrotic syndrome, glomerulonephritis, proteinuria.*
Hepatic: hepatotoxicity.
Metabolic: *decreased pyridoxine (may cause optic neuritis),* decreased zinc and mercury.
Skin: friability, especially at pressure spots; wrinkling; erythema; urticaria; ecchymoses.
Other: reversible taste impairment, especially of salts and sweets; hair loss. *About ⅓ of patients develop allergic reactions (rash, pruritus, fever), arthralgia, lymphadenopathy, or pneumonitis.* With long-term use,

---

Italicized side effects are common or life-threatening.
*Liquid form contains alcohol.   **May contain tartrazine.

myasthenia gravis syndrome.

INTERACTIONS
Oral iron: decreased effectiveness of D-penicillamine. If used together, give at least 2 hours apart.

NURSING CONSIDERATIONS
• Contraindicated in pregnant women with cystinuria. Use cautiously in penicillin allergy; cross-sensitivity may occur. However, most penicillin-allergic patients can receive penicilla-mine.
• Report to doctor if fever or other allergic reactions occur.
• Patient should receive supplemental pyridoxine daily.
• Handle patient carefully to avoid skin damage.
• Dose should be given on empty stomach to facilitate absorption, preferably 1 hour before or 3 hours after meals.
• Patient should drink large amounts of fluid, especially at night.
• Tell patient that therapeutic effect may be delayed up to 3 months in treatment of rheumatoid arthritis.
• Monitor CBC and renal and hepatic function regularly throughout therapy (every 2 weeks for the first 6 months, then monthly).
• Monitor urinalysis regularly for protein loss.
• Withhold drug and notify doctor if WBC count falls below 3,500/mm³ and/or platelet count falls below 100,000/mm³ (these are indications to stop drug). A progressive decline in platelet or WBC count in three successive blood tests may necessitate temporary cessation of therapy, even if these counts are within normal limits.
• Advise patient to report fever, sore throat, chills, bruising, and increased bleeding time; may be early signs of granulocytopenia.
• Provide appropriate health teaching for patients with Wilson's disease and

cystinuria.
• Antihistamines may be tried to manage skin reactions.
• Taste impairment usually resolves in 6 weeks without changes in dosage.

trientine hydrochloride
Cuprid

Pregnancy Risk Category: C

MECHANISM OF ACTION
Chelates copper and increases its urinary excretion.

INDICATIONS & DOSAGE
Treatment of Wilson's disease in patients who cannot tolerate penicilla-mine—
Adults: 750 to 2,000 mg daily in two, three, or four divided doses.
Children: 500 to 1,500 mg daily in two, three, or four divided doses.
   The optimal long-term maintenance dosage should be determined q 6 to 12 months, according to serum copper analysis.

ADVERSE REACTIONS
Blood: iron deficiency anemia.
Skin: rash.
Other: hypersensitivity, fever.

INTERACTIONS
Mineral supplements (including iron): may block trientine absorption. Administer at least 2 hours apart.

NURSING CONSIDERATIONS
• Patients (especially women) should be closely monitored for evidence of iron deficiency anemia throughout therapy.
• Observe patient for signs of hypersensitivity, such as skin rash.
• Tell patient to take trientine on an empty stomach at least 1 hour before meals or 2 hours after meals, and at least 1 hour apart from any other drug, food, or milk.
• Capsules should be swallowed

whole with water and should not be opened or chewed.

• Exposure to capsule contents may cause contact dermatitis. If capsule is accidentally opened and contents spilled on the skin, tell patient to wash the site thoroughly.

• Trientine should only be prescribed for patients who cannot tolerate penicillamine, the standard treatment for Wilson's disease.

• Urge your patient to faithfully follow his trientine regimen and low-copper diet as prescribed.

110

Gold salts

auranofin
aurothioglucose
gold sodium thiomalate

COMBINATION PRODUCTS
None.

---

auranofin
Ridaura

Pregnancy Risk Category: C

MECHANISM OF ACTION
Unknown. Anti-inflammatory effects
in rheumatoid arthritis are probably
caused by inhibition of sulfhydryl systems, which alters cellular metabolism. Auranofin may also alter enzyme function and immune response
and suppress phagocytic activity.

INDICATIONS & DOSAGE
Rheumatoid arthritis—
Adults: 6 mg P.O. daily, administered
either as 3 mg b.i.d. or 6 mg once
daily. After 6 months, may be increased to 9 mg daily.

ADVERSE REACTIONS
Blood: *thrombocytopenia* (with or
without purpura), *aplastic anemia,
agranulocytosis,* leukopenia, eosinophilia.
GI: *diarrhea, abdominal pain, nausea, vomiting, stomatitis, enterocolitis,* anorexia, metallic taste, dyspepsia, flatulence.
GU: *proteinuria,* hematuria.
Hepatic: jaundice, elevated liver enzymes.
Respiratory: interstitial pneumonitis.

Skin: *rash, pruritus, dermatitis, exfoliative dermatitis.*

INTERACTIONS
None significant.

NURSING CONSIDERATIONS
• Contraindicated in patients with
history of necrotizing enterocolitis,
pulmonary fibrosis, exfoliative dermatitis, bone marrow aplasia, or severe hematologic disorders. Use cautiously with other drugs that cause
blood dyscrasias. Use cautiously in
patients who have preexisting renal
disease, liver disease, inflammatory
bowel disease, and skin rash.
• Remind patients to see their doctors
on schedule for monthly platelet
counts. Auranofin should be stopped
if platelet count falls below 100,000/
mm^3.
• Reassure patient that beneficial
drug effect may be delayed as long as
3 months. However, if response is inadequate after 3 months, doctor will
probably discontinue auranofin.
• Encourage patient to take the drug
as prescribed and not to alter the dosage schedule.
• Diarrhea is the most common adverse reaction. Tell patient to continue
taking this drug if he experiences mild
diarrhea; however, if he notes blood
in his stool he should contact the doctor immediately.
• Tell patient to continue taking concomitant drug therapy, such as
NSAIDs, if prescribed.
• Dermatitis is a common adverse reaction. Advise patient to report any

---

Unmarked trade names available in the United States only.
♦Also available in Canada.　　♦♦Available in Canada only.　　◊Also available OTC.

rashes or other skin problems immediately. Pruritus often precedes dermatitis and should be considered a warning of impending skin reactions. Any pruritic skin eruption while a patient is receiving auranofin should be considered a reaction to this drug until proven otherwise. Therapy is stopped until reaction subsides.

• Stomatitis is another common adverse reaction. Tell patient that stomatitis is often preceded by a metallic taste. Advise him to report this symptom to his doctor immediately. Careful oral hygiene is recommended during therapy.

• Auranofin, like injectable gold preparations, should be prescribed only for selected rheumatoid arthritis patients. Warn your patient *not* to give the drug to others.

• Patient should receive a copy of the patient information supplied by the manufacturer.

---

aurothioglucose
Solganal

gold sodium thiomalate
Myochrysine♦

Pregnancy Risk Category: C

MECHANISM OF ACTION
Unknown. Anti-inflammatory effects in rheumatoid arthritis are probably caused by inhibition of sulfhydryl systems, which alters cellular metabolism. Gold salts may also alter enzyme function and immune response and suppress phagocytic activity.

INDICATIONS & DOSAGE
Rheumatoid arthritis—
Adults: initially, 10 mg (aurothioglucose) I.M., followed by 25 mg for second and third doses at weekly intervals. Then, 50 mg weekly until 1 g has been given. If improvement occurs without toxicity, continue 25 to 50 mg at 3- to 4-week intervals indefi-

nitely as maintenance therapy.
Children 6 to 12 years: ¼ usual adult dosage. Alternatively, 1 mg/kg I.M. once weekly for 20 weeks.
Rheumatoid arthritis—
Adults: initially, 10 mg (gold sodium thiomalate) I.M., followed by 25 mg in 1 week. Then, 50 mg weekly until 14 to 20 doses have been given. If improvement occurs without toxicity, continue 50 mg q 2 weeks for 4 doses; then, 50 mg q 3 weeks for 4 doses; then, 50 mg q month indefinitely as maintenance therapy. If relapse occurs during maintenance therapy, resume injections at weekly intervals.
Children: 1 mg/kg I.M. weekly for 20 weeks. If response is good, may be given q 3 to 4 weeks indefinitely.

ADVERSE REACTIONS
Adverse reactions to gold are considered severe and potentially life-threatening. Report any side effects to the doctor at once.
Blood: *thrombocytopenia* (with or without purpura), *aplastic anemia, agranulocytosis,* leukopenia, eosinophilia.
CNS: *dizziness,* syncope, sweating.
CV: bradycardia.
EENT: corneal gold deposition, corneal ulcers.
GI: *metallic taste, stomatitis,* difficulty swallowing, nausea, vomiting.
GU: *albuminuria, proteinuria, nephrotic syndrome,* nephritis, acute tubular necrosis.
Hepatic: hepatitis, jaundice.
Skin: *rash and dermatitis in 20% of patients. (If drug is not stopped, may lead to fatal exfoliative dermatitis.)*
Other: *anaphylaxis,* angioneurotic edema.

INTERACTIONS
None significant.

NURSING CONSIDERATIONS
• Contraindicated in severe uncontrollable diabetes, renal disease, he-

---

Italicized side effects are common or life-threatening.
*Liquid form contains alcohol.   **May contain tartrazine.

patic dysfunction, marked hypertension, heart failure, systemic lupus erythematosus, Sjögren's syndrome, skin rash, and drug allergies or hypersensitivities. Use cautiously with other drugs that cause blood dyscrasias.

• Indicated only in active rheumatoid arthritis that has not responded adequately to salicylates, rest, and physical therapy.

• Should be administered only under constant supervision of a doctor who is thoroughly familiar with the drug's toxicities and benefits.

• Most adverse reactions are readily reversible if drug is stopped immediately.

• Administer all gold salts I.M., preferably intragluteally. Color of drug is pale yellow; don't use if it darkens.

• Observe patient for 30 minutes after administration because of possible anaphylactoid reaction.

• Inform patient that benefits of therapy may not appear for 3 to 4 months or longer.

• Increased joint pain may occur for 1 to 2 days after injection. This usually subsides after a few injections.

• Gold therapy may alter liver function studies.

• Aurothioglucose is a suspension. Immerse vial in warm water and shake vigorously before injecting.

• When giving gold sodium thiomalate, advise patient to lie down and to remain recumbent for 10 to 20 minutes after injection to minimize adverse effects of hypotension.

• CBC, including platelet count, should be performed before every second injection for the duration of therapy.

• Dermatitis is the most common adverse reaction of these drugs. Advise patient to report any skin rashes or problems immediately. Pruritus often precedes dermatitis and should be considered a warning of impending skin reactions. Any pruritic skin erup-

tion while a patient is receiving gold therapy should be considered a reaction until proven otherwise. Therapy is stopped until reaction subsides.

• Exposure to sunlight or artificial ultraviolet light should be minimized.

• Stomatitis is the second most common adverse reaction of gold therapy. Advise patient that stomatitis is often preceded by a metallic taste. This warning should be reported to the doctor immediately.

• Careful oral hygiene is recommended during therapy.

• Advise patient of the importance of close medical follow-ups and the need for frequent blood and urine tests during therapy.

• Urine should be analyzed for protein and sediment changes before each injection.

• Platelet counts should be performed if patient develops purpura or ecchymoses.

• If adverse reactions are mild, some rheumatologists may order resumption of gold therapy after 2 to 3 weeks' rest.

• Dimercaprol should be kept on hand to treat acute toxicity.

111

Diagnostic skin tests

coccidioidin
histoplasmin
mumps skin test antigen
tuberculin purified protein
   derivative (PPD)
tuberculosis multiple-puncture
   tests

COMBINATION PRODUCTS
None.

coccidioidin
Spherulin

Pregnancy Risk Category: C

MECHANISM OF ACTION
Causes a cell-mediated immune response.

INDICATIONS & DOSAGE
Suspected coccidioidomycosis; to assess cell-mediated immunity—
Available as either a 1:100 or 1:10 dilution. The more dilute is always tried first.
Adults and children: 0.1 ml intradermally into the flexor surface of the forearm. Use tuberculin syringe with 26G or 27G ⅝″ to ½″ needle.

ADVERSE REACTIONS
Local: hypersensitivity (vesiculation, ulceration, necrosis).
Other: *anaphylaxis,* Arthus reaction.

INTERACTIONS
None significant.

NURSING CONSIDERATIONS
• Test is read at 24 and 48 hours. In-duration of 5 mm or more indicates a positive reaction (cell-mediated immune response). Erythema is not considered indicative of a delayed hypersensitivity reaction or positive response.
• Obtain history of allergies and reactions to skin tests. Patients allergic to Merthiolate and thimerosal should not receive this skin test.
• Tell the patient not to wash off the circle marked on the the skin for serial skin tests, since this aids in the reading of the test results.
• Obtain history of any recent residence or travel to endemic areas—southern California, Arizona, New Mexico, and western Texas.
• Keep epinephrine 1:1,000 available.
• If a patient is suspected of having coccidioidomycosis because of clinical manifestations or X-ray findings and the 1:100 dilution is negative, the 1:10 dilution may be applied.
• Reactivity to this test may be depressed or suppressed for as long as 4 to 6 weeks in individuals who have received concurrent or recent immunization with certain virus vaccines (for example, measles or influenza), in those who are receiving corticosteroid or immunosuppressive agents, in malnourished patients, and in those who have had viral infections (rubeola, influenza, mumps, and probably others).

histoplasmin
Histolyn-CYL

Pregnancy Risk Category: C

MECHANISM OF ACTION
Causes a cell-mediated immune response.

INDICATIONS & DOSAGE
Suspected histoplasmosis; to assess cell-mediated immunity—
Adults and children: 0.1 ml intradermally into the flexor surface of the forearm. Use tuberculin syringe with 26G or 27G ⅝″ to ½″ needle.

ADVERSE REACTIONS
Local: urticaria, ulceration or necrosis in highly sensitive patients.
Other: *anaphylaxis.*

INTERACTIONS
None significant.

NURSING CONSIDERATIONS
• Read test within 24 to 48 hours. Induration of 5 mm or more is positive response. In some instances, maximum reactions may not be present until the fourth day.
• A positive reaction may indicate a past infection or a mild subacute or chronic infection with histoplasmosis or such immunologically related organisms as coccidioidomycosis or blastomycosis.
• Obtain history of allergies and reactions to skin tests.
• Histoplasmin should not be administered to known positive reactors because of severity of reaction.
• Cold packs or topical corticosteroids may relieve pain and itching if severe local reaction occurs.
• Serologic titers are often boosted by previous skin test. Draw serologic sample between 48 to 96 hours after skin test administration.
• Tuberculin skin test is advisable concurrently with histoplasmin test.

• Obtain history of any residence or recent travel to endemic areas—central (Ohio Valley) and eastern United States and Africa.
• Reactivity to this test may be depressed or suppressed for as long as 4 to 6 weeks in individuals who have received concurrent or recent immunization with certain virus vaccines (for example, measles or influenza), in those who are receiving corticosteroid or immunosuppressive agents, in malnourished patients, and in those who have had viral infections (rubeola, influenza, mumps, and probably others).

mumps skin test antigen
MSTA

MECHANISM OF ACTION
Causes a cell-mediated immune response.

INDICATIONS & DOSAGE
To assess cell-mediated immunity—
Adults and children: 0.1 ml intradermally into the flexor surface of the forearm. Use tuberculin syringe with 26G or 27G ⅝″ to ½″ needle.

ADVERSE REACTIONS
Local: hypersensitivity (vesiculation, ulceration).
Other: *anaphylaxis,* Arthus reaction.

INTERACTIONS
None significant.

NURSING CONSIDERATIONS
• Test is read at 48- and 72-hour intervals. A positive reaction (cell-mediated immune response) is 5 mm or more of induration. Erythema is not considered indicative of a delayed hypersensitivity reaction.
• Obtain history of allergies and reactions to skin tests. In patients hypersensitive to eggs, feathers, and chicken, a severe reaction may follow

administration.
- Don't administer to patients allergic to thimerosal.
- Keep epinephrine 1:1,000 available.
- Store vials in refrigerator.
- Mumps skin test antigen is *not* used to assess exposure to mumps. This antigen is used in assessing T cell function for immunocompetence.
- Reactivity to this test may be depressed or suppressed for as long as 4 to 6 weeks in individuals who have received concurrent or recent immunization with certain virus vaccines (for example, measles or influenza), in those who are receiving corticosteroid or immunosuppressive agents, in malnourished patients, and in those who have had viral infections (rubeola, influenza, mumps, and probably others).

tuberculin purified protein derivative (PPD)
Aplisol, PPD-stabilized Solution (Mantoux test), Tubersol

Pregnancy Risk Category: C

MECHANISM OF ACTION
Causes a cell-mediated immune response.

INDICATIONS & DOSAGE
Diagnosis of tuberculosis, evaluation of immunocompetence in patients with cancer, malnutrition—
Adults and children: 5 tuberculin units (0.1 ml) intradermally into flexor surface of the forearm. Suspected sensitivity dose use is 1 tuberculin unit. First strength equals 1 tuberculin unit/0.1 ml; intermediate strength, 5 tuberculin units/0.1 ml. Second strength equals 250 tuberculin units/0.1 ml. Use tuberculin syringe with 26G or 27G ⅝″ to ½″ needle.

ADVERSE REACTIONS
Local: pain, pruritus, vesiculation, ulceration, necrosis.
Other: *anaphylaxis,* Arthus reaction.

INTERACTIONS
None significant.

NURSING CONSIDERATIONS
- Contraindicated in known tuberculin-positive reactors; severe reactions may occur.
- Read test within 48 to 72 hours. An induration of 10 mm or greater indicates a significant reaction (formerly called positive reaction). Significance of a reaction is determined not only by the size of the reaction but by circumstances. For example, a reaction of 5 mm or more may be considered significant in a close relative of a person with known tuberculosis. A reaction of 2 mm or more may also be considered significant in infants and children. The amount of induration at the site—not erythema—determines the significance of the reaction.
- Report all known cases of tuberculosis to the appropriate public health agency.
- Obtain history of allergies and reactions to skin tests.
- Reactivity to this test may be depressed or suppressed for as long as 4 to 6 weeks in individuals who have received concurrent or recent immunization with certain virus vaccines (for example, measles or influenza), in those who are receiving corticosteroid or immunosuppressive agents, in malnourished patients, and in those who have had viral infections (rubeola, influenza, mumps, and probably others).
- Keep epinephrine 1:1,000 available.
- S.C. injection invalidates test results. Bleb (6 to 10 mm in diameter) must form on skin upon intradermal injection.
- Cold packs or topical corticosteroids may relieve pain and itching of severe local reaction.

- Strongly positive tests can result in scarring at test site.
- Never give initial test with second test strength (250 tuberculin units). Use only when a patient has negative response to a 5–tuberculin unit PPD but has the clinical signs and symptoms of tuberculosis.

---

tuberculosis multiple-puncture tests
Aplitest (dried purified protein derivative [PPD]),
Mono-Vacc Test (liquid Old Tuberculin [OT]), Sclavo Test (dried PPD), Tine Test (dried OT, dried PPD)

Pregnancy Risk Category: C

MECHANISM OF ACTION
Causes a cell-mediated immune response.

INDICATIONS & DOSAGE
Screening for tuberculosis—
Adults and children: cleanse skin thoroughly with alcohol; make skin taut on flexor surface of forearm and press points firmly into selected site. Hold device at injection site for about 3 seconds. This will ensure stabilizing the dried tuberculin B in tissue lymph. All multiple-puncture tests are equivalent to 5 tuberculin units of PPD Mantoux.

ADVERSE REACTIONS
Local: hypersensitivity (vesiculation, ulceration, necrosis).
Other: *anaphylaxis.*

INTERACTIONS
Virus vaccine: tuberculosis skin-test reaction may be suppressed if test is given within 4 to 6 weeks after immunization with live or attenuated virus vaccines.

NURSING CONSIDERATIONS
- Contraindicated in known tuberculin-positive reactors.
- False-positive reaction can occur in sensitive patients.
- Reactivity to this test may be depressed or suppressed for as long as 4 to 6 weeks in individuals who have received concurrent or recent immunization with certain virus vaccines (for example, measles or influenza), in those who are receiving corticosteroid or immunosuppressive agents, in malnourished patients, and in those who have had viral infections (rubeola, influenza, mumps, and probably others), or miliary tuberculosis.
- Minimal bleeding can occur at the puncture site. This occurs infrequently and does not interfere with interpretation of the test results.
- Read test within 48 to 72 hours. Questionable or positive reactions to any multiple-puncture test must be verified by the Mantoux test. The amount of induration—not erythema—at the site determines significance of the reaction.
- Induration of 1 to 2 mm is significant.
- If vesiculation is present, the test may be interpreted as positive.
- All tuberculin multiple puncture tests are equivalent to 5 tuberculin units of PPD.
- Obtain history of allergies, especially to acacia (contained in the Tine Test as a stabilizer), and reactions to skin tests.
- Keep epinephrine 1:1,000 available.
- Report all known cases of tuberculosis to appropriate public health agency.
- Cold packs or topical corticosteroids may relieve pain and itching if severe local reaction occurs after test.

112

Uncategorized drugs

acetohydroxamic acid
allopurinol
alpha-1 proteinase inhibitor
 (human)
alprostadil
bromocriptine mesylate
carbidopa-levodopa
clomiphene citrate
colchicine
cromolyn sodium
diazoxide, oral
disulfiram
L-carnitine
levodopa
mesalamine
mesna
methoxsalen
nicotine resin complex
octreotide acetate
pentoxifylline
pralidoxime chloride
ritodrine hydrochloride
sodium benzoate and sodium
 phenylacetate
sodium cellulose phosphate
tiopronin

COMBINATION PRODUCTS
COLBENEMID: probenecid 500 mg
and colchicine 0.5 mg.
PROBENECID WITH COLCHICINE: probenecid 500 mg and colchicine 0.5
mg.

---

acetohydroxamic acid
Lithostat

Pregnancy Risk Category: X

MECHANISM OF ACTION
Prevents formation of renal stones by
inhibiting bacterial urease activity.

INDICATIONS & DOSAGE
*Treatment of infection-related kidney
stones—*
Adults: 250 mg P.O. t.i.d. or q.i.d.
Administer at 6- to 8-hour intervals at
a time when the stomach is empty.
Maximum daily dosage is 1.5 g.
Children: 10 mg/kg/day in two or
three divided doses.

ADVERSE REACTIONS
Blood: *hemolytic anemia.*
CNS: *mild headache, depression,*
anxiety, nervousness.
CV: phlebitis, palpitations.
GI: *nausea, vomiting, diarrhea, con-
stipation, anorexia.*
Skin: *nonpruritic, macular rash on
arms and face.*
Other: alopecia, deep vein thrombo-
sis, malaise.

INTERACTIONS
Oral iron supplements: reduce absorption of acetohydroxamic acid.
Check with doctor; he may request
that iron be administered I.M.
Methenamine: may produce synergistic effects.

NURSING CONSIDERATIONS
• Contraindicated in patients whose
physical state and disease are amena-
ble to surgery and appropriate antibiotics; in patients whose urine is infected by nonurease-producing organisms in pregnancy; and in poor renal
function.
• Use cautiously in patients predis-

Italicized side effects are common or life-threatening.
*Liquid form contains alcohol. **May contain tartrazine.

posed to deep vein thrombosis.
• Coombs'-negative hemolytic anemia has occurred in patients receiving acetohydroxamic acid.
• Monitor CBC, including a reticulocyte count, after 2 weeks of therapy. Thereafter, monitor at 3-month intervals for the duration of treatment. If laboratory findings indicate hemolytic anemia, discontinue drug.
• Skin rash more common during prolonged use and with concomitant use of alcoholic beverages. The rash appears 30 to 45 minutes after ingestion of alcoholic beverages; disappears spontaneously in 30 to 60 minutes. Although skin rash doesn't usually require treatment, advise patient to avoid alcohol.
• Reduced dosage may be necessary in renal impairment.
• Experience with acetohydroxamic acid is limited. About 150 patients have been tested, most for periods longer than 1 year.

---

allopurinol
Lopurin, Zyloprim♦

Pregnancy Risk Category: C

MECHANISM OF ACTION
Reduces uric acid production by inhibiting the biochemical reactions preceding its formation.

INDICATIONS & DOSAGE
Gout, primary or secondary to hyperuricemia; secondary to diseases such as acute or chronic leukemia, polycythemia vera, multiple myeloma, and psoriasis—
Dosage varies with severity of disease; can be given as single dose or divided, but doses larger than 300 mg should be divided.
Adults: mild gout, 200 to 300 mg P.O. daily; severe gout with large tophi, 400 to 600 mg P.O. daily. Same dosage for maintenance in secondary hyperuricemia.

Hyperuricemia secondary to malignancies—
Children 6 to 10 years: 300 mg P.O. daily or divided t.i.d.
Children under 6 years: 50 mg P.O. t.i.d.
Impaired renal function—
Adults: 200 mg P.O. daily if creatinine clearance is 10 to 20 ml/minute; 100 mg P.O. daily if creatinine is less than 10 ml/minute; 100 mg P.O. more than 24 hours apart if clearance is less than 3 ml/minute.
To prevent acute gouty attacks—
Adults: 100 mg P.O. daily; increase at weekly intervals by 100 mg without exceeding maximum dose (800 mg), until serum uric acid falls to 6 mg/100 ml or less.
To prevent uric acid nephropathy during cancer chemotherapy—
Adults: 600 to 800 mg P.O. daily for 2 to 3 days, with high fluid intake.
Recurrent calcium oxalate calculi—
Adults: 200 to 300 mg P.O. daily in single dose or divided doses.

ADVERSE REACTIONS
Blood: *agranulocytosis*, anemia, *aplastic anemia.*
CNS: drowsiness.
EENT: cataracts, retinopathy.
GI: nausea, vomiting, diarrhea, abdominal pain.
Hepatic: altered liver function studies, hepatitis.
Skin: *rash, usually maculopapular; exfoliative,* urticarial, and purpuric lesions; erythema multiforme; severe furunculosis of nose; ichthyosis, *toxic epidermal necrolysis.*

INTERACTIONS
Alcohol, bumetanide, diazoxide, ethacrynic acid, furosemide, triamterene, mecamylamine, pyrazinamide: increased serum uric acid concentration; adjust dosage of allupurinol.
Ampicillin, bacampicillin, hetacillin: increased possibility of skin rash.
Anticoagulants: potentiation of anti-

coagulant effect. Dosage adjustments may be necessary.
Antineoplastic agents: increased potential for bone marrow suppression. Monitor patient carefully.
Chlorpropamide: possible increased hypoglycemic effect.
Uricosuric agents: additive effect; may be used to therapeutic advantage.
Urinary acidifying agents (ammonium chloride, ascorbic acid, potassium or sodium phosphate): may increase the possibility of kidney stone formation.
Xanthines: increased serum theophylline. Adjust dosage of theophyllines.

NURSING CONSIDERATIONS
• Contraindicated in hypersensitivity and in idiopathic hemochromatosis. Use cautiously in cataracts and hepatic or renal disease.
• Obtain accurate patient history.
• Discontinue at first sign of rash, which may precede severe hypersensitivity reaction or any other adverse reaction. Tell patient to report all adverse reactions immediately. Skin rash is more common in patients taking diuretics and in those with renal disorders.
• Monitor intake/output; daily urine output of at least 2 liters and maintenance of neutral or slightly alkaline urine are desirable. Patient should be encouraged to drink plenty of fluids while taking this drug unless otherwise contraindicated.
• If renal insufficiency exists at any time during treatment, allopurinol dosage should be reduced.
• Periodically check CBC and hepatic and renal function, especially at start of therapy.
• If patient is taking allopurinol for treatment of recurrent calcium oxalate stones, advise him to also reduce his dietary intake of animal protein, sodium, refined sugars, oxalate-rich foods, and calcium.
• Acute gouty attacks may occur in first 6 weeks of therapy; concurrent

use of colchicine may be prescribed prophylactically.
• Minimize GI adverse reactions by administering with meals or immediately after.
• Evaluate effectiveness, using serum uric acid level.
• Allopurinol may predispose patient to ampicillin-induced rash.
• Allopurinol may cause rash even weeks after discontinuation.
• Since drug may cause drowsiness, advise patient to refrain from driving car or performing tasks requiring mental alertness until CNS effects of the drug are known.

alpha-1 proteinase inhibitor (human)
Prolastin
Pregnancy Risk Category: C

MECHANISM OF ACTION
Replaces alpha$_1$-proteinase in patients with alpha$_1$-antitrypsin deficiency.

INDICATIONS & DOSAGE
Chronic replacement therapy in patients with congenital alpha$_1$-antitrypsin deficiency and demonstrable panacinar emphysema—
Adults: 60 mg/kg I.V. once weekly. May be given at the rate of 0.08 ml/kg/minute or greater.

ADVERSE REACTIONS
Blood: possible viral transmission.

INTERACTIONS
None reported.

NURSING CONSIDERATIONS
• Explain to the patient that the product has been treated to minimize the risk of transmission of hepatitis and AIDS.
• Many commercial assays for alpha$_1$-proteinase inhibitor measure immunoreactivity of the protein and not inhibitor activity. Monitoring serum

level may not accurately reflect clinical response.

alprostadil
Prostin VR Pediatric♦

MECHANISM OF ACTION
A prostaglandin derivative which relaxes the smooth muscle of the ductus arteriosus.

INDICATIONS & DOSAGE
Palliative therapy for temporary maintenance of patency of ductus arteriosus until surgery can be performed—
Infants: 0.05 to 0.1 mcg/kg/minute by I.V., intraarterial, or intraaortic infusion. When therapeutic response is achieved, reduce infusion rate to give lowest dosage that will maintain response. Maximum dosage is 0.4 mcg/kg/minute. Alternatively, administer through umbilical artery catheter placed at ductal opening.

ADVERSE REACTIONS
Blood: disseminated intravascular coagulation.
CNS: seizures.
CV: *flushing,* bradycardia, hypotension, tachycardia.
GI: diarrhea.
Other: *apnea, fever, sepsis.*

INTERACTIONS
None reported.

NURSING CONSIDERATIONS
• Contraindicated in neonatal respiratory distress syndrome.
• Because drug inhibits platelet aggregation, use cautiously in neonates with bleeding tendencies.
• Monitor arterial pressure by umbilical artery catheter, auscultation, or Doppler transducer. Slow rate of infusion if arterial pressure falls significantly.
• In infants with restricted pulmonary blood flow, measure drug's effec-

tiveness by monitoring blood oxygenation. In infants with restricted systemic blood flow, measure drug's effectiveness by monitoring systemic blood pressure and blood pH.
• Drug must be diluted before being administered. Fresh solution must be prepared daily. Discard any solution more than 24 hours old.
• Apnea and bradycardia may reflect drug overdose. If the signs occur, stop infusion immediately.
• CV and CNS adverse reactions are more frequent in infants weighing less than 2 kg and in those receiving infusions for longer than 48 hours.
• Keep respiratory support available.
• Use a constant rate infusion pump to administer.
• If flushing occurs from peripheral vasodilation, reposition catheter.
• Reduce infusion rate if fever or significant hypotension occurs.
• Do not use diluents that contain benzyl alcohol. Fatal toxic syndrome may occur.

bromocriptine mesylate
Parlodel♦

Pregnancy Risk Category: C

MECHANISM OF ACTION
Inhibits secretion of prolactin. It acts as a dopamine-receptor agonist by activating postsynaptic dopamine receptors.

INDICATIONS & DOSAGE
To treat amenorrhea and galactorrhea associated with hyperprolactinemia; treatment of female infertility—
2.5 mg P.O. b.i.d. or t.i.d. with meals for 14 days, but for no longer than 6 months.
Prevention of postpartum lactation—
2.5 mg P.O. b.i.d. with meals for 14 days. Treatment may be extended for up to 21 days, if necessary.
Treatment of Parkinson's disease—
1.25 mg P.O. b.i.d. with meals. Dos-

age may be increased q 14 to 28 days, up to 100 mg daily.
Treatment of acromegaly—
Adults: 1.25 to 2.5 mg P.O. for 3 days. An additional 1.25 to 2.5 mg may be added q 3 to 7 days until patient receives therapeutic benefit.

ADVERSE REACTIONS
CNS: confusion, hallucinations, uncontrolled body movements, *dizziness, headache,* fatigue, mania, delusions, nervousness, insomnia, depression.
CV: *hypotension,* syncope.
EENT: nasal congestion, tinnitus, blurred vision.
GI: *nausea,* vomiting, *abdominal cramps,* constipation, diarrhea.
GU: urine retention, urinary frequency.
Other: *pulmonary infiltration and pleural effusion,* coolness and pallor of fingers and toes.

INTERACTIONS
Antihypertensive drugs: increased hypotensive effects. Adjust dosage of antihypertensive agent.
Haloperidol, loxapine, phenothiazines, methyldopa, metoclopramide, MAO inhibitors, reserpine: may interfere with bromocriptine's effects.
Levodopa: additive effects. Adjust dosage of levodopa.
Oral contraceptives, estrogens, progestins: interfere with effects of bromocriptine. Concurrent use not recommended.

NURSING CONSIDERATIONS
• Contraindicated in hypersensitivity to ergot derivatives.
• Use cautiously in preexisting psychiatric disorders.
• Patient should be examined carefully for pituitary tumor (Forbes-Albright syndrome). Use of Parlodel will not affect tumor size although it may alleviate amenorrhea or galactorrhea.

• May lead to early postpartum conception. Test for pregnancy every 4 weeks or whenever period is missed after menses are reinitiated.
• Advise patient to use contraceptive methods other than oral contraceptives during treatment.
• Patients with impaired renal function may require dosage adjustments.
• Incidence of adverse effects is high, particularly at beginning of therapy. Orthostatic hypotension is common. Adverse effects can be minimized by gradually titrating doses to effective levels. Advise patients to avoid dizziness and fainting by rising slowly to an upright position and avoiding sudden position changes.
• Monitor blood pressure closely in women who receive bromocriptine for suppression of postpartum lactation. In such patients, transient hypotension is common; however, hypertension, seizures, and stroke have also been reported.
• Incidence of adverse effects is high (68%); however, most are mild to moderate, and only 6% of patients discontinue drug for this reason. Nausea is the most common adverse reaction.
• Recurrence rates when used to treat amenorrhea or galactorrhea associated with hyperprolactinemia are high (70% to 80%).
• Advise the patient that it may take 6 to 8 weeks or longer for menses to be reinstated and galactorrhea to be suppressed.
• Patient may experience mild to moderate rebound breast secretion, congestion, or engorgement when therapy is discontinued.
• Should be given with meals.
• When used to treat Parkinson's disease, bromocriptine is usually given in addition to either levodopa alone or levodopa-carbidopa combination (Sinemet).
• Adverse reactions are more frequent when drug is used for Parkinson's disease.

Italicized side effects are common or life-threatening.
*Liquid form contains alcohol.   **May contain tartrazine.

- Also prescribed to treat hyperpro-lactinemia associated with pituitary adenomas.

carbidopa-levodopa
Sinemet♦

Pregnancy Risk Category: C

MECHANISM OF ACTION
Levodopa is decarboxylated to dopamine, countering the depletion of striatal dopamine in extrapyramidal centers. Carbidopa inhibits the peripheral decarboxylation of levodopa without affecting levodopa's metabolism within the CNS. Therefore, more levodopa is available to be decarboxylated to dopamine in the brain.

INDICATIONS & DOSAGE
Treatment of idiopathic Parkinson's disease, postencephalitic parkinsonism, and symptomatic parkinsonism resulting from carbon monoxide or manganese intoxication—
Adults: 3 to 6 tablets of 25 mg carbidopa/250 mg levodopa daily given in divided doses. Do not exceed 8 tablets of 25 mg carbidopa/250 mg levodopa daily. Optimum daily dosage must be determined by careful titration for each patient.

ADVERSE REACTIONS
Blood: hemolytic anemia.
CNS: *choreiform, dystonic, dyskinetic movements; involuntary grimacing, head movements, myoclonic body jerks, ataxia,* tremors, muscle twitching; bradykinetic episodes; psychiatric disturbances, memory loss, nervousness, anxiety, disturbing dreams, euphoria, malaise, fatigue; severe depression, suicidal tendencies, dementia, delirium, hallucinations (may necessitate reduction or withdrawal of drug).
CV: *orthostatic hypotension,* cardiac irregularities, flushing, hypertension, phlebitis.

EENT: blepharospasm, blurred vision, diplopia, mydriasis or miosis, widening of palpebral fissures, activation of latent Horner's syndrome, oculogyric crises, nasal discharge.
GI: nausea, vomiting, anorexia, weight loss may occur at start of therapy; constipation; flatulence; diarrhea; epigastric pain; hiccups; sialorrhea; dry mouth; bitter taste.
GU: urinary frequency, urine retention, urinary incontinence, darkened urine, excessive and inappropriate sexual behavior, priapism.
Hepatic: hepatotoxicity.
Other: dark perspiration, hyperventilation.

INTERACTIONS
Antihypertensives: additive hypotensive effects.
Papaverine, phenothiazines and other antipsychotics, phenytoin: may antagonize antiparkinsonian actions. Use together cautiously.
Sympathomimetics: increased risk of cardiac dysrhythmias.

NURSING CONSIDERATIONS
- Contraindicated in narrow-angle glaucoma, melanoma, or undiagnosed skin lesions. Use cautiously in cardiovascular, renal, hepatic, pulmonary disorders, in history of peptic ulcer, psychiatric illness, myocardial infarction with residual dysrhythmias, bronchial asthma, emphysema, and endocrine disease.
- Carefully monitor patients also receiving antihypertensive medication, hypoglycemic agents. Discontinue MAO inhibitors at least 2 weeks before therapy is begun.
- Dosage is adjusted according to patient's response and tolerance to drug. Therapeutic and adverse reactions occur more rapidly with levodopa-carbidopa than with levodopa alone. Observe and monitor vital signs, especially while dosage is being adjusted; report significant changes.

Unmarked trade names available in the United States only.
♦Also available in Canada.   ♦♦Available in Canada only.   ◊Also available OTC.

• Instruct patient to report adverse reactions and therapeutic effects.

• Warn patient of possible dizziness and orthostatic hypotension, especially at start of therapy. Patient should change position slowly and dangle legs before getting out of bed. Elastic stockings may control this adverse reaction in some patients.

• Muscle twitching and blepharospasm (twitching of eyelids) may be an early sign of drug overdosage; report immediately.

• Patients on long-term therapy should be tested regularly for diabetes and acromegaly; blood tests, liver and kidney function studies should be repeated periodically.

• If patient is being treated with levodopa, discontinue at least 8 hours before starting levodopa-carbidopa.

• This combination drug usually reduces the amount of levodopa needed by 75%, thereby reducing the incidence of adverse reactions.

• Pyridoxine (vitamin B_6) does not reverse the beneficial effects of Sinemet. Multivitamins can be taken without fear of losing control of symptoms.

• If therapy is interrupted temporarily, the usual daily dosage may be given as soon as patient resumes oral medication.

• Available as tablets with carbidopa-levodopa in a 1:10 ratio (Sinemet 10/100 and Sinemet 25/250); also in a 1:4 ratio (Sinemet 25/100).

• Sinemet 25/100 may reduce many adverse reactions seen with 1:10 ratio strengths.

• Carbidopa (Lodosyn) as a single agent is available from Merck Sharp & Dohme on doctor's request.

• Warn the patient and his family not to increase dosage without doctor's order.

clomiphene citrate
Clomid•

Pregnancy Risk Category: X

MECHANISM OF ACTION
Appears to stimulate release of pituitary gonadotropins, follicle-stimulating hormone, and luteinizing hormone. This results in maturation of the ovarian follicle, ovulation, and development of the corpus luteum.

INDICATIONS & DOSAGE
To induce ovulation—
50 to 100 mg P.O. daily for 5 days, starting any time; or 50 to 100 mg P.O. daily starting on day 5 of menstrual cycle (first day of menstrual flow is day 1). Repeat until conception occurs or until 3 courses of therapy are completed.

ADVERSE REACTIONS
CNS: headache, restlessness, insomnia, dizziness, light-headedness, depression, fatigue, tension.
CV: hypertension.
EENT: blurred vision, diplopia, scotoma, photophobia (signs of impending visual toxicity).
GI: nausea, vomiting, bloating, distention, increased appetite, weight gain.
GU: urinary frequency and polyuria; ovarian enlargement and cyst formation, which regress spontaneously when drug is stopped.
Metabolic: hyperglycemia.
Skin: urticaria, rash, dermatitis.
Other: *hot flashes,* reversible alopecia, *breast discomfort.*

INTERACTIONS
None significant.

NURSING CONSIDERATIONS
• Contraindicated in undiagnosed abnormal genital bleeding, ovarian cyst, or hepatic disease or dysfunction, or in patients with a history of thrombo-

---

Italicized side effects are common or life-threatening.
*Liquid form contains alcohol.   **May contain tartrazine.

phlebitis or thromboembolism. Use cautiously in hypertension, mental depression, migraines, seizures, diabetes mellitus, and gonadotropin sensitivity. Report the development or worsening of these conditions to doctor. May require stopping drug.
• Patient with visual disturbances should report symptoms to doctor immediately.
• Tell patient possibility of multiple births exists with this drug. Risk increases with higher doses.
• Teach patient to take basal body temperature and chart on graph to ascertain whether ovulation has occurred.
• Advise patient to stop drug and contact doctor immediately if abdominal symptoms or pain occurs because these indicate ovarian enlargement or ovarian cyst.
• Reassure patient that response (ovulation) generally occurs after the first course of therapy. If pregnancy does not occur, course of therapy may be repeated twice.
• Since drug may cause dizziness or visual disturbances, caution patient not to perform hazardous tasks until CNS effects of the drug are known.
• Advise patient to stop drug and contact doctor immediately if she suspects she is pregnant (drug may have teratogenic effect).

colchicine
Colsalide, Novocolchicine♦♦
Pregnancy Risk Category: D

MECHANISM OF ACTION
As antigout agent, apparently decreases leukocyte motility, phagocytosis, and lactic acid production, thus decreasing urate crystal deposits and reducing inflammation. As antiosteolytic agent, apparently inhibits mitosis of osteoprogenitor cells and decreases the activity of osteoclasts.

INDICATIONS & DOSAGE
To prevent acute attacks of gout as prophylactic or maintenance therapy—
Adults: 0.5 or 0.6 mg P.O. daily; or 1 to 1.8 mg P.O. daily for more severe cases.
To prevent attacks of gout in patients undergoing surgery—
Adults: 0.5 to 0.6 mg P.O. t.i.d. 3 days before and 3 days after surgery.
To treat acute gout, acute gouty arthritis—
Adults: initially, 1 to 1.2 mg P.O., then 0.5 or 0.6 mg q hour, or 1 to 1.2 mg q 2 hours until pain is relieved or until nausea, vomiting, or diarrhea ensues. Or 2 mg I.V. followed by 0.5 mg q 6 hours if necessary. Total I.V. dosage over 24 hours (one course of treatment) not to exceed 4 mg.
Note: Give I.V. by slow I.V. push over 2 to 5 minutes. Avoid extravasation. Don't dilute colchicine injection with dextrose 5% injection or any other fluid that might change pH of colchicine solution. If lower concentration of colchicine injection is needed, dilute with normal saline solution or sterile water for injection and administer over 2 to 5 minutes by direct injection. Preferably, inject into the tubing of a free-flowing I.V. solution. However, if diluted solution becomes turbid, don't inject.
Familial mediterranean fever suppression—
Adults: Acute attack: 0.6 mg. hourly for 4 doses, then q 2 hours for 4 doses on the first day. Then, give 1.2 mg q 12 hours for 2 days. Maintenance dosage is 0.5 to 0.6 mg b.i.d. to t.i.d.
Antiosteolytic treatment—
Adults: 0.6 mg t.i.d. Instruct patient in the proper methods of oral hygiene, including the use of a toothbrush, dental floss, and toothpicks.

ADVERSE REACTIONS
Blood: *aplastic anemia and agranulocytosis with prolonged use;* nonthrom-

---

bocytopenic purpura.
CNS: peripheral neuritis.
GI: *nausea, vomiting, abdominal pain, diarrhea.*
Skin: urticaria, dermatitis.
Local: severe local irritation if extravasation occurs.
Other: alopecia.

INTERACTIONS
Alcohol: may impair efficacy of colchicine prophylaxis.
Loop diuretics: may decrease efficacy of colchicine prophylaxis.
Phenylbutazone: may increase risk of leukopenia or thrombocytopenia.
Vitamin B$_{12}$: impaired absorption of vitamin B$_{12}$.

NURSING CONSIDERATIONS
• Use cautiously in hepatic dysfunction, cardiac disease, blood dyscrasias, renal disease, GI disorders, and in elderly or debilitated patients.
• Reduce dosage if weakness, anorexia, nausea, vomiting, or diarrhea appears. First sign of acute overdosage may be GI symptoms, followed by vascular damage, muscle weakness, and ascending paralysis. Delirium and seizures may occur without the patient losing consciousness.
• Discontinue drug as soon as gout pain is relieved or at the first sign of GI symptoms.
• Colchicine has no effect on nongouty arthritis.
• A course of I.V. colchicine should not be repeated for several weeks to avoid cumulative toxicity.
• Do not administer I.M. or S.C.; severe local irritation occurs. Administer I.V. over 2 to 5 minutes.
• As maintenance therapy, give with meals to reduce GI effects. May be used with uricosuric agents.
• Baseline laboratory studies, including CBC, should precede therapy and be repeated periodically.
• Monitor fluid intake/output. Keep output at 2,000 ml daily.

• Store in tightly closed, light-resistant container.
• Change needle before making direct I.V. injection.

cromolyn sodium
Intal♦**, Intal Inhaler, Intal Spincaps♦♦, Nalcrom, Nasalcrom, Opticrom, Rynacrom♦♦
Pregnancy Risk Category: B

MECHANISM OF ACTION
Inhibits the degranulation of sensitized mast cells that occurs after a patient's exposure to specific antigens. It also inhibits release of histamine and slow-reacting substance of anaphylaxis (SRS-A).

INDICATIONS & DOSAGE
Adjunct in treatment of severe perennial bronchial asthma—
Adults and children over 5 years: contents of 20-mg capsule inhaled q.i.d. at regular intervals. Or administer 2 metered sprays using inhaler q.i.d. at regular intervals. Also available as an aqueous solution administered through a nebulizer.
Prevention and treatment of allergic rhinitis—
Adults and children over 5 years: 1 spray in each nostril t.i.d or q.i.d. May give up to 6 times daily.
Prevention of exercise-induced bronchospasm—
Adults and children over 5 years: contents of 20-mg capsule or 2 metered sprays inhaled no more than 1 hour before anticipated exercise.
Allergic ocular disorders—
Adults and children 4 years and older: 1 to 2 drops in each eye 4 to 6 times daily at regular intervals.
Systemic mastocytosis—
Adults: 100 to 200 mg P.O. q.i.d.
Food allergy—
Adults: 200 mg P.O. q.i.d. 15 to 20 minutes before meals. Dosage may be doubled in 2 to 3 weeks if results are

---

Italicized side effects are common or life-threatening.
*Liquid form contains alcohol.   **May contain tartrazine.

not satisfactory.
Children 2 to 13 years: 100 mg P.O.
q.i.d. 15 to 20 minutes before meals.
Dosage may be doubled in 2 to 3
weeks if results are not satisfactory.
Do not exceed 40 mg/kg daily.
Children under 2 years: up to 20
mg/kg P.O. daily.
Inflammatory bowel disease—
Adults: 200 mg P.O. q.i.d. 15 to 20
minutes before meals.
Children 2 to 14 years: 100 mg P.O.
q.i.d. 15 to 20 minutes before meals.

ADVERSE REACTIONS
CNS: dizziness, headache.
EENT: *irritation of the throat and
trachea, cough, bronchospasm following inhalation of dry powder; esophagitis;* nasal congestion; pharyngeal irritation; wheezing.
GI: nausea.
GU: dysuria, urinary frequency.
Skin: rash, urticaria.
Other: joint swelling and pain, lacrimation, swollen parotid gland, angioedema, *eosinophilic pneumonia.*

INTERACTIONS
None significant.

NURSING CONSIDERATIONS
• Contraindicated in acute asthma attacks and status asthmaticus.
• Use cautiously in coronary artery
disease or history of cardiac dysrhythmias.
• Should be discontinued if patient
develops eosinophilic pneumonia.
• Capsule not to be swallowed; insert
capsule into inhaler provided; follow
manufacturer's directions.
• Watch for recurrence of asthmatic
symptoms when dosage is decreased,
especially when corticosteroids are
also used.
• Use only when acute episode has
been controlled; airway is cleared;
and patient is able to inhale.
• Patient considered for cromolyn
therapy should have pulmonary func-

tion tests to show significant broncho-
dilator-reversible component to his
airway obstruction.
• Teach correct use of Spinhaler: insert capsule in device properly, exhale
completely before placing mouthpiece
between lips, then inhale deeply and
rapidly with a steady, even breath; remove inhaler from mouth, hold breath
a few seconds, and then exhale. Repeat until all powder has been inhaled.
• Store capsules at room temperature
in a tightly closed container; protect
from moisture and temperatures
higher than 40° C. (104° F.).
• Instruct patient to avoid excessive
handling of capsule.
• Esophagitis may be relieved by antacids or a glass of milk.

---

diazoxide, oral
Proglycem
Pregnancy Risk Category: C

MECHANISM OF ACTION
Inhibits the release of insulin from the
pancreas and decreases peripheral utilization of glucose.

INDICATIONS & DOSAGE
*Management of hypoglycemia from a
variety of conditions resulting in hyperinsulinism—*
Adults and children: 3 to 8 mg/kg
P.O. daily, in three equally divided
doses q 8 hours.
Infants and newborns: 8 to 15 mg/
kg P.O. daily, in two or three equally
divided doses q 8 to 12 hours.

ADVERSE REACTIONS
Blood: *leukopenia, thrombocyto-
penia.*
CV: *cardiac dysrhythmias.*
EENT: diplopia.
GI: nausea, vomiting, anorexia, taste
alteration.
Metabolic: sodium and fluid reten-
tion, ketoacidosis and hyperosmolar

nonketotic coma, hyperuricemia.
Other: *severe hypertrichosis (hair growth) in 25% of adults and higher percentage of children.*

INTERACTIONS
Alpha-adrenergic blocking agents: antagonize inhibition of insulin release by diazoxide.
Anticoagulants: increased anticoagulant effect. Adjust dosage of anticoagulant.
Antigout agents: increased serum uric acid. Adjust dosage of antigout agent.
Antihypertensive agents, peripheral vasodilators: additive hypotensive effects.
Beta-adrenergic blocking agents: increased hypotensive effect.
Hydantoin anticonvulsants: decreased anticonvulsant effects and decreased hyperglycemic effect of diazoxide. Don't use together.
Thiazide diuretics: may potentiate hyperglycemic, hyperuricemic, and hypotensive effects. Monitor appropriate laboratory values.

NURSING CONSIDERATIONS
• Contraindicated in thiazide hypersensitivity and functional hypoglycemia.
• Oral diazoxide does not significantly lower blood pressure in dosages used to treat hypoglycemia.
• Most important use is in management of hypoglycemia from hyperinsulinism in infants and children.
• Monitor urine regularly for glucose and ketones; report any abnormalities to doctor.
• If not effective after 2 or 3 weeks, drug should be stopped.
• Reassure patient that hair growth on arms and forehead is a common adverse reaction that subsides when drug treatment is completed.
• Explain importance of following dietary restrictions for successful therapy.
• Advise patient to report any adverse

effects, including excessive thirst, fruity breath odor, or urinary frequency.
• Available in capsules and oral suspension.

disulfiram
Antabuse♦, Cronetal, Ro-Sulfiram-500

Pregnancy Risk Category: X

MECHANISM OF ACTION
Blocks oxidation of alcohol at the acetaldehyde stage. Excess acetaldehyde produces a highly unpleasant reaction in the presence of even small amounts of alcohol.

INDICATIONS & DOSAGE
Adjunct in management of chronic alcoholism—
Adults: maximum of 500 mg q P.O. morning for 1 to 2 weeks. Can be taken in evening if drowsiness occurs. Maintenance: 125 to 500 mg P.O. daily (average dose 250 mg) until permanent self-control is established. Treatment may continue for months or years.

ADVERSE REACTIONS
CNS: drowsiness, headache, fatigue, delirium, depression, neuritis.
EENT: optic neuritis.
GI: metallic or garlic-like aftertaste.
GU: impotence.
Skin: acneiform or allergic dermatitis.
Other: disulfiram reaction, which may include flushing, throbbing headache, dyspnea, nausea, copious vomiting, sweating, thirst, chest pain, palpitations, hyperventilation, hypotension, syncope, anxiety, weakness, blurred vision, confusion. In severe reactions, respiratory depression, cardiovascular collapse, dysrhythmias, myocardial infarction, acute CHF, seizures, unconsciousness, and even death can occur.

INTERACTIONS

Alfentanil: prolonged duration of effect.

Anticoagulants: increased anticoagulant effect. Adjust dosage of anticoagulant.

Ascorbic acid: may interfere with disulfiram-alcohol interaction.

Bacampicillin: use with caution, because its metabolism produces low concentrations of alcohol and acetaldehyde.

CNS depressants: increased CNS depression.

Isoniazid (INH): ataxia or marked change in behavior. Don't use together.

Metronidazole: psychotic reaction. Do not use together.

Midazolam: increased plasma levels of midazolam.

Paraldehyde: toxic levels of the acetaldehyde. Don't use together.

Tricyclic antidepressants, especially amitriptylene: transient delirium.

NURSING CONSIDERATIONS

• Contraindicated in alcohol intoxication, psychoses, myocardial disease, coronary occlusion, or in patients receiving metronidazole, paraldehyde, alcohol, or alcohol-containing preparations; and in pregnancy. Use cautiously in diabetes mellitus, hypothyroidism, epilepsy, cerebral damage, nephritis, hepatic cirrhosis or insufficiency, abnormal EEG, and multiple drug dependence.

• Used only under close medical and nursing supervision. Patient should clearly understand consequences of disulfiram therapy and give permission. Drug should be used only in patients who are cooperative, well motivated, and are receiving supportive psychiatric therapy.

• Complete physical examination and laboratory studies, including CBC, Sequential Multiple Analysis—12-channel biochemical profile, and transaminase, should precede therapy

and be repeated regularly.

• Warn patient to avoid all sources of alcohol (for example, sauces and cough syrups). Even external application of liniments, shaving lotion, and back-rub preparations may precipitate disulfiram reaction. Tell him that alcohol reaction may occur as long as 2 weeks after single dosage of disulfiram; the longer the patient remains on drug, the more sensitive he will become to alcohol.

• Patient should wear a bracelet or carry a card supplied by drug manufacturer identifying him as disulfiram user.

Note: Mild reactions may occur in sensitive patients with blood alcohol level of 5 to 10 mg/100 ml; symptoms are fully developed at 50 mg/100 ml; unconsciousness usually occurs at 125 to 150 mg/100 ml level. Reaction may last half an hour to several hours, or as long as alcohol remains in blood.

• Caution patient's family that disulfiram should never be given to the patient without his knowledge; severe reaction or death could result if such a patient then ingested alcohol.

• Reassure patient that disulfiram-induced adverse reactions, such as drowsiness, fatigue, impotence, headache, peripheral neuritis, and metallic or garlic taste, subside after about 2 weeks of therapy.

L-carnitine
Carnitor, Vitacarn

Pregnancy Risk Category: B

MECHANISM OF ACTION
Facilitates the transport of fatty acids into cellular mitochondria. The fatty acids are then used to produce energy.

INDICATIONS & DOSAGE
Primary systemic carnitine deficiency—
Adults: 990 mg (three tablets) P.O. b.i.d. or t.i.d. Alternatively, may give

enteral liquid 10 to 30 ml (1 to 3 g) daily.
Children: 50 to 100 mg/kg/day in divided doses of either the tablet or enteral liquid form.

All dosages depend upon the clinical response. Higher dosages may be given. However, for children, the maximum dosage is 3 g/day.

ADVERSE REACTIONS
GI: *nausea, vomiting, cramps, diarrhea.*
Other: body odor.

INTERACTIONS
D,L-carnitine (sold as vitamin B_T in vitamin stores): inhibits L-carnitine and can cause deficiency.
Valproic acid: increased requirement for carnitine.

NURSING CONSIDERATIONS
• Monitor patient's tolerance during the 1st week of therapy and after increasing dosage.
• May give enteral liquid alone or dissolved in drinks or liquid food.
• Space doses evenly every 3 to 4 hours if possible. Best to give with or after meals.
• Tell patient to consume enteral liquid slowly to minimize GI distress. If GI intolerance persists, dosage may have to be reduced.
• Warn patient to avoid so-called "vitamin B_T" in health food stores. This will interact with the drug and render it ineffective.
• Caution patient not to share drug with others. Some people have used it to improve athletic performance.
• The entire or partial contents of the containers of liquid should be used immediately after opening. Discard any unused contents of opened containers.
• Do not refrigerate solution.

levodopa
Dopar, Larodopa♦, Levopa, Parda, Rio-Dopa
Pregnancy Risk Category: C

MECHANISM OF ACTION
Levodopa is decarboxylated to dopamine, countering the depletion of striatal dopamine in extrapyramidal centers, which is thought to produce parkinsonism.

INDICATIONS & DOSAGE
Treatment of idiopathic parkinsonism, postencephalitic parkinsonism, and symptomatic parkinsonism after carbon monoxide or manganese intoxication; or in association with cerebral arteriosclerosis—
administered orally with food in dosages carefully adjusted to individual requirements, tolerance, and response.
Adults and children over 12 years: initially, 0.5 to 1 g P.O. daily, given b.i.d., t.i.d., or q.i.d. with food; increase by no more than 0.75 g daily q 3 to 7 days, until usual maximum of 8 g is reached. Higher dosage requires close supervision.

ADVERSE REACTIONS
Blood: hemolytic anemia, leukopenia.
CNS: *aggressive behavior, choreiform, dystonic, and dyskinetic movements, involuntary grimacing, head movements, myoclonic body jerks, ataxia, tremors, muscle twitching, bradykinetic episode, psychiatric disturbances, memory loss, mood changes, nervousness, anxiety, disturbing dreams, euphoria, malaise, fatigue, severe depression, suicidal tendencies, dementia, delirium, hallucinations (may necessitate reduction or withdrawal of drug).*
CV: *orthostatic hypotension,* cardiac irregularities, flushing, hypertension, phlebitis.

Italicized side effects are common or life-threatening.
*Liquid form contains alcohol.   **May contain tartrazine.

EENT: blepharospasm, blurred vision, diplopia, mydriasis or miosis, widening of palpebral fissures, activation of latent Horner's syndrome, oculogyric crises, nasal discharge.
GI: *nausea, vomiting, anorexia,* weight loss may occur at start of therapy, constipation, flatulence, diarrhea, epigastric pain, hiccups, sialorrhea, dry mouth, bitter taste.
GU: urinary frequency, retention, incontinence; darkened urine; excessive and inappropriate sexual behavior; priapism.
Hepatic: hepatotoxicity.
Other: dark perspiration, hyperventilation.

INTERACTIONS
Antacids: increased absorption of levodopa.
Antihypertensives: additive hypertensive effect.
High-protein foods: decreased absorption of levodopa.
Metoclopramide: accelerated gastric emptying of levodopa.
Papaverine, phenothiazines and other antipsychotics, phenytoin: watch for decreased levodopa effect.
Pyridoxine: reduced efficacy of levodopa. Examine vitamin preparations and nutritional supplements for content of vitamin B_6 (pyridoxine).
Sympathomimetics: increased risk of cardiac arrhythmias.

NURSING CONSIDERATIONS
• Contraindicated in narrow-angle glaucoma, melanoma, or undiagnosed skin lesions. Use cautiously in cardiovascular, renal, hepatic, and pulmonary disorders, peptic ulcer, psychiatric illness, myocardial infarction with residual dysrhythmias, bronchial asthma, emphysema, and endocrine disease.
• Carefully monitor patients also receiving antihypertensive medication and hypoglycemic agents. Stop MAO inhibitors at least 2 weeks before therapy is begun.
• Adjust dosage according to patient's response and tolerance. Observe and monitor vital signs, especially while adjusting dose. Report significant changes.
• Instruct patient to report adverse reactions and therapeutic effects.
• Warn patient of possible dizziness and orthostatic hypotension, especially at start of therapy. Patient should change position slowly and dangle legs before getting out of bed. Elastic stockings may control this adverse reaction in some patients.
• Muscle twitching and blepharospasm (twitching of eyelids) may be early signs of drug overdosage; report immediately.
• Patients on long-term use should be tested regularly for diabetes and acromegaly; repeat blood tests and liver and kidney function studies periodically.
• Advise patient and family that multivitamin preparations, fortified cereals, and certain OTC medications may contain pyridoxine (vitamin B_6), which can reverse the effects of levodopa.
• If therapy is interrupted for a long time, drug should be adjusted gradually to previous level.
• Therapeutic response usually occurs following each dose and disappears within 5 hours but varies considerably.
• Patient who must undergo surgery should continue levodopa as long as oral intake is permitted, generally 6 to 24 hours before surgery. Drug should be resumed as soon as patient is able to take oral medication.
• Protect from heat, light, and moisture. If preparation darkens, it has lost potency and should be discarded.
• Coombs' test occasionally becomes positive during extended use. Expect uric acid elevations with colorimetric method but not with uricase method.
• Alkaline phosphatase, AST

(SGOT), ALT (SGPT), lactate dehydrogenase, bilirubin, BUN, and protein-bound iodine show transient elevations in patients receiving levodopa; WBC, hemoglobin, and hematocrit show occasional reduction.

• A doctor-supervised period of drug discontinuance (called a drug holiday) may reestablish the effectiveness of a lower dosage regimen.

• Combination of levodopa-carbidopa usually reduces amount of levodopa needed by 75%, thereby reducing incidence of adverse reactions.

• Pills may be crushed and mixed with applesauce or baby food fruits for patients who have difficulty swallowing pills.

• Warn patient and family not to increase dosage without the doctor's orders (they may be tempted to do this as disease symptoms of parkinsonism progress). Daily dosage should not exceed 8 g.

mesalamine
Rowasa

Pregnancy Risk Category: B

MECHANISM OF ACTION
Exact mechanism unknown; mesalamine is one of the active metabolites of sulfasalazine. Probably acts topically by inhibiting prostaglandin production in the colon.

INDICATIONS & DOSAGE
Treatment of active mild to moderate distal ulcerative colitis, proctitis, or proctosigmoiditis—
Adults: 1 rectal unit (4 g/60 ml) as a retention enema once daily (preferably h.s.). Drug should be retained overnight (for about 8 hours). Usual course of therapy is 3 to 6 weeks.

ADVERSE REACTIONS
CNS: headache, dizziness, fatigue, malaise.
GI: abdominal pain, cramps, discomfort, flatulence, diarrhea, rectal pain, bloating, nausea, *pancolitis*.
Skin: hives, itching, rash, urticaria, hair loss.
Other: wheezing, *anaphylaxis* (rare), fever.

INTERACTIONS
None significant.

NURSING CONSIDERATIONS
• Contraindicated in patients sensitive to the drug or its components.
• Mesalamine may rarely cause allergic reactions in patients sensitive to sulfites, becasue it contains potassium metabisulfite.
• Patients intolerant of sulfasalazine may also be hypersensitive to mesalamine. Instruct these patients to discontinue drug if they have a fever or rash.
• Use cautiously in renal impairment. Problems have not been documented, but the nephrotoxic potential from absorbed mesalamine exists. Patients on long-term mesalamine therapy should have periodic renal function studies.

mesna
Mesnex

Pregnancy Risk Category: B

MECHANISM OF ACTION
Prevents ifosfamide-induced hemorrhagic cystitis by reacting with urotoxic ifosfamide metabolites.

INDICATIONS AND DOSAGE
Prophylaxis of hemorrhagic cystitis in patients receiving ifosfamide—
Adults: Dosage varies with amount of ifosfamide administered. Usual dosage is 240 mg/m² administered as an I.V. bolus with administration of ifosfamide. Repeat dosage at 4 hours and 8 hours after administration of ifosfamide.

Italicized side effects are common or life-threatening.
*Liquid form contains alcohol.   **May contain tartrazine.

ADVERSE REACTIONS
Note: Because it is used concomitantly with ifosfamide and other chemotherapeutic agents, it is difficult to determine adverse effects attributable solely to mesna.
EENT: dysgeusia.
GI: soft stools, nausea, vomiting, diarrhea.

INTERACTIONS
None reported.

NURSING CONSIDERATIONS
• Contraindicated in patients with hypersensitivity to mesna or thiol-containing compounds. Not effective in preventing hematuria from other causes (such as thrombocytopenia). Although formulated to prevent hemorrhagic cystitis from ifosfamide, it will not protect against other toxicities associated with ifosfamide therapy.
• Monitor urine samples in patients receiving mesna for hematuria daily.
• Up to 6% of patients may not respond to the drug's protective effects.
• May interfere with diagnostic tests for urine ketones.
• Prepare I.V. solutions by diluting commercially available ampules with dextrose 5% in water solution, dextrose 5% and normal saline injection, normal saline injection, or lactated Ringer's solution.
• Diluted solutions are stable for 24 hours at room temperature, but they should be refrigerated after preparation and used within 6 hours. After the ampule is opened, any unused drug should be discarded because it decomposes quickly into an inactive compound.
• Mesna I.V. is incompatible with cisplatin.

methoxsalen
Oxsoralen♦, Oxsoralen-Ultra
Pregnancy Risk Category: C

MECHANISM OF ACTION
May enhance melanogenesis, either directly or secondarily, to an inflammatory process.

INDICATIONS & DOSAGE
To induce repigmentation in vitiligo; psoriasis—
Adults and children over 12 years:
0.6 mg/kg P.O. 1.5 to 2 hours before measured periods of high-intensity long-wave ultraviolet exposure, 2 to 3 times weekly at least 48 hours apart.
Topical solution:
Apply to small, well-defined vitiliginous lesions and allow to dry (1 to 2 minutes) and reapply: 2 to 2.5 hours before measured periods of long-wave ultraviolet exposure. After exposure, wash lesions with soap and water. Protect area with opaque sunscreen. Although manufacturer recommends treatment weekly, some clinicians may treat q 3 to 5 days.

ADVERSE REACTIONS
CNS: nervousness, insomnia, depression, vertigo, headache.
GI: *discomfort, nausea, diarrhea.*
Skin: edema, erythema, painful blistering, burning, peeling, pruritus.

INTERACTIONS
Photosensitizing agents: do not use together. May increase toxicity.

NURSING CONSIDERATIONS
• Contraindicated in hepatic insufficiency, porphyria, acute lupus erythematosus, or hydromorphic and polymorphic light eruptions. Use with caution in patients with familial history of sunlight allergy, GI diseases, and chronic infection.
• Regulate therapy carefully. Overdosage or overexposure to light can

cause serious burning or blistering. Patients should avoid excessive sunlight during therapy.
• Drug should be taken with meals or milk. Patient should avoid the following foods: limes, figs, parsley, parsnips, mustard, carrots, and celery.
• During light exposure treatments, protect eyes and lips.
• Monthly liver function tests should be done on patients with vitiligo (especially at beginning of therapy).

nicotine resin complex
Nicorette

Pregnancy Risk Category: X

MECHANISM OF ACTION
Stimulates receptors in the CNS and causes the release of catecholamines from the adrenal medulla.

INDICATIONS & DOSAGE
Temporary aid to the cigarette smoker seeking to give up smoking while participating in a behavior modification program under medical supervision—
Adults: Chew one piece of gum slowly and intermittently for 30 minutes whenever the urge to smoke occurs. Most patients require approximately 10 pieces of gum daily during the first month. Don't exceed 30 pieces of gum daily.

ADVERSE REACTIONS
CNS: dizziness, light-headedness.
CV: atrial fibrillation.
EENT: throat soreness, jaw muscle ache (from chewing).
GI: nausea, vomiting, indigestion.
Other: hiccups.

INTERACTIONS
None significant.

NURSING CONSIDERATIONS
• Contraindicated in nonsmokers, during the immediate postmyocardial infarction period; in life-threatening dysrhythmias, severe or worsening angina pectoris, and active temporomandibular joint disease; or in pregnancy.
• Use cautiously in with hyperthyroidism, pheochromocytoma, or insulin-dependent diabetes.
• Nicotine resin complex is the only smoking cessation aid that has been proven safe and effective.
• Smokers most likely to benefit from nicotine gum are those with a high "physical" nicotine dependence. Such smokers show the following characteristics: smoke more than 15 cigarettes daily; prefer brands of cigarettes with high nicotine levels; usually inhale the smoke; smoke the first cigarette within 30 minutes of arising; find the first morning cigarette the hardest to give up; smoke most frequently during the morning; find it difficult to refrain from smoking in places where it's forbidden; or smoke even when they are so ill that they are confined to bed during the day.
• Instruct patient to chew gum slowly and intermittently for about 30 minutes to promote slow and even buccal absorption of nicotine. Fast chewing tends to produce more adverse reactions.
• Successful abstainers will begin gradually withdrawing gum usage after 3 months. Use of the gum for longer than 6 months is not recommended.
• Emphasize the importance of withdrawing the gum gradually.
• The gum is sugar-free and usually doesn't stick to dentures.
• Patient who stops smoking may require dosage adjustments of propoxyphene, propranolol, beta-blocking agents, and xanthine bronchodilators because decreased metabolism of these agents may increase their therapeutic effects.
• A patient instruction sheet is included in the package dispensed to the patient.

Italicized side effects are common or life-threatening.
*Liquid form contains alcohol.   **May contain tartrazine.

octreotide acetate
Sandostatin

Pregnancy Risk Category: B

MECHANISM OF ACTION
Mimics the action of naturally occurring somatostatin.

INDICATIONS AND DOSAGE
Symptomatic treatment of flushing and diarrhea associated with carcinoid tumors—
Adults: Initially 100 to 600 mcg daily S.C. in two to four divided doses for the first 2 weeks of therapy (usual daily dosage is 300 mcg). Subsequent dosage is based upon individual response.
Symptomatic treatment of watery diarrhea associated with vasoactive intestinal peptide secreting tumors (VIPomas)—
Adults: Initially 200 to 300 mcg daily S.C. in two to four divided doses for the first 2 weeks of therapy. Subsequent dosage is based upon individual response, but usually will not exceed 450 mcg daily.

ADVERSE REACTIONS
CNS: dizziness, light-headedness, fatigue.
GI: nausea, diarrhea, abdominal pain or discomfort, loose stools, vomiting, fat malabsorption.
Metabolic: hyperglycemia, hypoglycemia, hypothyroidism.
Skin: flushing, edema, wheal, erythema or pain at injection site.

INTERACTIONS
Cyclosporine: may decrease plasma levels of cyclosporine.

NURSING CONSIDERATIONS
• Contraindicated in patients with hypersensitivity to the drug or any of its components.
• Octreotide therapy may be associated with the development of cholelithiasis by either altering gallbladder motility or fat absorption. Monitor patient regularly for gallbladder disease, and tell patient to report any signs of abdominal discomfort.
• Half-life may be altered in patients in end-stage renal failure who are receiving dialysis.
• Baseline and periodic tests of thyroid function are advised because of the drug's metabolic effects.
• Laboratory tests that are frequently monitored during therapy include urine 5-hydroxyindole acetic acid (5-HIAA), plasma serotonin, and plasma substance P (for carcinoid tumors); plasma vasoactive intestinal peptide for VIPomas.
• Mild, transient hypoglycemia or hyperglycemia may occur during octreotide therapy. Monitor closely for symptoms of glucose imbalance during therapy.
• Insulin-dependent diabetics and patients receiving oral hypoglycemics (sulfonylureas) or oral diazoxide may require dosage adjustments during therapy.
• Octreotide therapy may alter fluid and electrolyte balance and may require adjustment of other drugs used to control symptoms of the disease (such as beta blockers).

pentoxifylline
Trental

Pregnancy Risk Category: C

MECHANISM OF ACTION
Improves capillary blood flow by increasing erythrocyte flexibility and lowering blood viscosity.

INDICATIONS & DOSAGE
Treatment of intermittent claudication caused by chronic occlusive vascular disease—
Adults: 400 mg P.O. t.i.d. with meals.

Unmarked trade names available in the United States only.
♦ Also available in Canada.　　♦ ♦ Available in Canada only.　　◊ Also available OTC.

ADVERSE REACTIONS
CNS: headache, dizziness.
GI: dyspepsia, nausea, vomiting.

INTERACTIONS
Antihypertensives: increased hypotensive effect. Dosage adjustments may be necessary.

NURSING CONSIDERATIONS
• Contraindicated in patients who are intolerant to methylxanthines such as caffeine, theophylline, and theobromine.
• Pentoxifylline should be taken for a minimum of 8 weeks to achieve clinical effects. Tell patient not to discontinue the drug during this period unless directed by doctor.
• Advise patient to take with meals to minimize GI upset.
• Patient should report any GI or CNS adverse reactions. Doctor may reduce dosage.
• Pentoxifylline therapy is useful in patients who are not good surgical candidates.
• Patient should avoid smoking because nicotine causes vasoconstriction that can worsen the condition.
• Patient should swallow medication whole, without breaking, crushing, or chewing.
• Elderly patients may be more sensitive to this drug's effects.

---

pralidoxime chloride
Protopam Chloride♦

Pregnancy Risk Category: C

MECHANISM OF ACTION
Reactives cholinesterase that has been inactivated by organophosphorus pesticides and related compounds. It permits degradation of accumulated acetylcholine and facilitates normal functioning of neuromuscular junctions.

INDICATIONS & DOSAGE
Antidote for organophosphate poisoning—
Adults: I.V. infusion of 1 to 2 g in 100 ml of saline solution over 15 to 30 minutes. If pulmonary edema is present, give drug by slow I.V. push over 5 minutes. Repeat in 1 hour if muscle weakness persists. Additional doses may be given cautiously. I.M. or S.C. injection can be used if I.V. is not feasible; or 1 to 3 g P.O. q 5 hours.
Children: 20 to 40 mg/kg I.V.
To treat cholinergic crisis in myasthenia gravis—
Adults: 1 to 2 g I.V., followed by increments of 250 mg I.V. q 5 minutes.

ADVERSE REACTIONS
CNS: dizziness, headache, drowsiness, excitement, and manic behavior following recovery of consciousness.
CV: tachycardia.
EENT: blurred vision, diplopia, impaired accommodation, laryngospasm.
GI: nausea.
Other: muscular weakness, muscle rigidity, hyperventilation.

INTERACTIONS
None significant.

NURSING CONSIDERATIONS
• Contraindicated in poisoning with Sevin, a carbamate insecticide, since it increases drug's toxicity. Use with extreme caution in renal insufficiency or myasthenia gravis (overdosage may precipitate myasthenic crisis); also in asthma or peptic ulcer.
• Use in hospitalized patients only; have respiratory and other supportive measures available. Obtain accurate medical history and chronology of poisoning if possible. Give as soon as possible after poisoning.
• I.V. preparation should be given slowly, as diluted solution.
• Initial measures should include removal of secretions, maintenance of patent airway, and artificial ventila-

---

Italicized side effects are common or life-threatening.
*Liquid form contains alcohol.   **May contain tartrazine.

tion if needed. After dermal exposure to organophosphate, patient's clothing should be removed and his skin and hair should be washed with sodium bicarbonate, soap, water, and alcohol as soon as possible. A second washing may be necessary. When washing the patient, wear protective gloves and clothes to avoid exposure.
• Drug relieves paralysis of respiratory muscles but is less effective in relieving depression of respiratory center.
• Atropine along with pralidoxime should be given I.V., 2 to 4 mg, if cyanosis is not present. If cyanosis is present, atropine should be given I.M. Give atropine every 5 to 6 minutes until signs and symptoms of atropine toxicity appear (flushing, tachycardia, dry mouth, blurred vision, excitement, delirium, and hallucinations); maintain atropinization for at least 48 hours.
• Dilute with sterile water without preservatives.
• Not effective against poisoning due to phosphorus, inorganic phosphates, or organophosphates with no anticholinesterase activity.
• Difficult to distinguish between toxic effects produced by atropine or by organophosphate compounds and those resulting from pralidoxime. Observe patient for 48 to 72 hours if poison was ingested. Delayed absorption may occur from lower bowel.
• Caution patients treated for organophosphate poisoning to avoid contact with insecticides for several weeks.
• Patients with myasthenia gravis treated for overdose of cholinergic drugs should be observed closely for signs of rapid weakening. These patients can pass quickly from a cholinergic crisis to a myasthenic crisis, and require more cholinergic drugs to treat the myasthenia. Keep edrophonium (Tensilon) available in such situations for establishing differential diagnosis.
• Although not approved, subcon-

junctival injection of pralidoxime has been used to reverse adverse ocular effects resulting from splashing into the eye or systemic overdose of organophosphates.
• Treatment is most effective if initiated within 24 hours after exposure.
• Draw blood for cholinesterase levels before giving pralidoxime.

ritodrine hydrochloride
Yutopar♦

Pregnancy Risk Category: B

MECHANISM OF ACTION
A beta-receptor agonist that stimulates the beta$_2$-adrenergic receptors in uterine smooth muscle, inhibiting contractility.

INDICATIONS & DOSAGE
Management of preterm labor—
I.V. therapy: dilute 150 mg (3 ampuls) in 500 ml of fluid, yielding a final concentration of 0.3 mg/ml. Usual initial dose is 0.1 mg/minute, to be gradually increased according to the results by 0.05 mg/minute q 10 minutes until desired result obtained. Effective dosage usually ranges from 0.15 and 0.35 mg/minute.
Note: I.V. infusion should be continued for 12 to 24 hours after contractions have stopped. Oral maintenance: 1 tablet (10 mg) may be given approximately 30 minutes before termination of I.V. therapy. Usual dosage for first 24 hours of oral maintenance is 10 mg q 2 hours. Thereafter, usual dosage is 10 to 20 mg q 4 to 6 hours. Total daily dosage should not exceed 120 mg.

ADVERSE REACTIONS
Intravenous:
CNS: nervousness, anxiety, headache.
CV: *dose-related alterations in blood pressure, palpitations, pulmonary edema, tachycardia,* ECG changes.

GI: nausea, vomiting.
Metabolic: *hyperglycemia,* hypokalemia.
Other: erythema.
Oral:
CNS: tremors, nervousness.
CV: palpitations.
GI: nausea, vomiting.
Skin: rash.

INTERACTIONS

Corticosteroids: may produce pulmonary edema in mother. When these drugs are used concomitantly, monitor closely.
Beta blockers: may inhibit ritodrine's action. Avoid concurrent administration.
Inhalational anesthetics: potentiated adverse cardiac effects, dysrhythmias, hypotension.
Sympathomimetics: additive effects. Use together cautiously.

NURSING CONSIDERATIONS

• Contraindicated before 20th week of pregnancy and in the following conditions: antepartum hemorrhage, eclampsia, intrauterine fetal death, chorioamnionitis, maternal cardiac disease, pulmonary hypertension, maternal hyperthyroidism, or uncontrolled maternal diabetes mellitus.
• Because cardiovascular responses are common and more pronounced during I.V. administration, cardiovascular effects—including maternal pulse rate and blood pressure, and fetal heart rate—should be closely monitored. A maternal tachycardia of over 140 or persistent respiratory rate of over 20/minute may be a sign of impending pulmonary edema.
• Monitor blood glucose concentrations during ritodrine infusions, especially in diabetic mothers.
• Discontinue drug if pulmonary edema develops.
• Monitor amount of fluids administered I.V., to prevent circulatory overload.

• Ritodrine decreases intensity and frequency of uterine contractions.
• Don't use ritodrine I.V. if solution is discolored or contains a precipitate.

---

sodium benzoate and sodium phenylacetate
Ucephan

Pregnancy risk category: C

MECHANISM OF ACTION
Activates metabolic pathways that are ineffective in patients with urea cycle enzymopathies, resulting in decreased ammonia formation.

INDICATIONS AND DOSAGE
Prevention or treatment of hyperammonemia in patients with urea cycle enzymopathy—
Children: 2.5 ml/kg P.O. daily in three to six equally divided doses. Total daily dosage should not exceed 100 ml.

ADVERSE REACTIONS
GI: nausea and vomiting.

INTERACTIONS
Penicillin, probenecid: may impair renal excretion of conjugated metabolites.

NURSING CONSIDERATIONS
• Contraindicated in patients with hypersensitivity to sodium benzoate or sodium phenylacetate. Use cautiously in neonates with hyperbilirubinemia.
• Benzoic acid may compete with bilirubin for binding sites on serum albumin.
• Not intended as sole therapy for patients with urea cycle enzymopathies. Most effective when combined with dietary modification (low-protein diet) and amino acid supplementation.
• Dilute each dose in 4 to 8 oz of infant formula or milk and administer with meals. Inspect the mixture for compatibility if other liquids are

---

Italicized side effects are common or life-threatening.
*Liquid form contains alcohol.   **May contain tartrazine.

used. The drug may precipitate in some solutions (especially acidic solutions like fruit juice), depending upon concentration and pH.
• Carefully measure the required dosage because the stock solution is very concentrated (10 g of sodium benzoate and 10 g of sodium phenylacetate per 100 ml).
• Avoid getting the solution on skin or clothing. The lingering odor of the drug may be offensive.
• Benzoic acid is structurally similar to salicylates.
• Watch for adverse effects associated with salicylates, including mild respiratory alkalosis and exacerbation of peptic ulcers.

sodium cellulose phosphate
Calcibind

Pregnancy Risk Category: C

MECHANISM OF ACTION
Binds calcium in the GI tract and decreases the amount absorbed.

INDICATIONS & DOSAGE
Treatment of absorptive hypercalciuria type I with recurrent calcium oxalate or calcium phosphate renal stones—
Adults: 15 g/day (5 g with each meal) in patients with urine calcium greater than 300 mg/day. When urine calcium declines to less than 150 mg/day, reduce dosage to 10 g/day (5 g with dinner, 2.5 g with two remaining meals).

ADVERSE REACTIONS
CNS: drowsiness, mood or mental changes, seizures, trembling.
GI: anorexia, nausea, vomiting, discomfort, diarrhea, dyspepsia.
GU: hyperoxaluria, hypomagnesuria.
Other: acute arthralgias.

INTERACTIONS
Magnesium-containing products: may bind drug. Separate doses by at least 1 hour.

NURSING CONSIDERATIONS
• Contraindicated in primary or secondary hyperparathyroidism, including renal hypercalciuria; hypomagnesemic states; bone disease; hypocalcemic states; normal or low intestinal absorption; renal excretion of calcium; or enteric hyperoxaluria.
• Use cautiously in CHF or ascites.
• Recommended only for the type of absorptive hypercalciuria in which both intestinal calcium absorption and urine calcium remain abnormally high even with a calcium-restricted diet. When administered inappropriately, it can cause hypocalciuria. This could stimulate parathyroid function and lead to parathyroid bone disease.
• Patient should maintain a calcium-restricted diet and avoid all dairy products.
• Patient taking sodium cellulose phosphate may develop hyperoxaluria and hypomagnesuria, which predispose him to stone formation. Therefore, advise patient to restrict dietary intake of oxalate (found in spinach, rhubarb, chocolate, and tea).
• Avoid vitamin C because it can increase urine oxalate.
• Encourage fluid intake. Urine output should be at least 2 liters/day.
• Patient can mix the powder with 8 oz of fruit juice, water, or a soft drink and take it with meals. Patient should rinse glass and drink all of the fluid to get the full dose.
• Encourage a low-sodium diet. Tell patient to avoid salty foods and to avoid adding salt at the table.
• Because of the difficulty involved in managing sodium cellulose phosphate therapy, many doctors prefer to treat hypercalciuria with a low-calcium diet, high fluid intake, and thiazides, when necessary.

tiopronin
Thiola

Pregnancy Risk Category: C

MECHANISM OF ACTION
Forms a water-soluble chemical complex with cysteine in the urine, increasing cysteine solubility and preventing the formation of urinary cysteine stones.

INDICATIONS AND DOSAGE
Prevention of urinary cysteine stone formation in patients with severe homozygous cysteinuria (urinary cysteine excretion exceeding 500 mg/day) unresponsive to other therapies—
Adults: 800 mg P.O. daily, divided t.i.d.
Children: 15 mg/kg P.O. daily, divided t.i.d.

ADVERSE REACTIONS
EENT: hypogeusia.
Skin: rash, pruritus, wrinkling and friability.
Other: drug fever, lupus erythematous-like reaction.

INTERACTIONS
None reported.

NURSING CONSIDERATIONS
• Contraindicated in patients with a history of agranulocytosis, aplastic anemia, or thrombocytopenia with tiopronin therapy.
• Dosage is usually adjusted to keep urine cysteine levels below 250 mg/liter.
• Conservative measures to treat cysteinuria should be attempted before tiopronin is administered. Patients should drink at least 3 liters of fluid daily, including at least two 8-oz glasses of water at each meal and at bedtime. Patient's urine output should be at least 3 liters daily, and urine pH should be 6.5 to 7. Excessive alkalization of urine may precipitate calcium stones. Urine pH should not exceed 7.
• Whenever possible, tiopronin should be administered at least 1 hour before or 2 hours after meals.
• Routine monitoring tests are recommended at 3- to 6-month intervals during treatment, including CBC, platelet counts, hemoglobin, serum albumin, liver functions tests, 24-hour urine protein, and routine urinalysis.
• Urine cysteine should be frequently monitored during the first 6 months of treatment (to identify optimal dosage level) and then at least every 6 months.
• An abdominal X-ray is advised annually to assess for the presence of stones.
• Tell patient to report any signs or symptoms of hematological abnormalities, including fever, sore throat, bleeding or bruising, and chills. Blood dyscrasias have been reported in patients receiving other drugs for cysteinuria.
• Rare complications to watch for include Goodpasture's syndrome (evidenced by abnormal urine findings, pulmonary infiltrates, and hemoptysis), myasthenia (evidenced by severe muscle weakness), and pemphigus-like reactions (bullous skin eruptions).
• Drug fever may develop, especially during the first month of therapy. Discontinue drug until fever subsides, then therapy will probably be reinstituted at lower dosages.
• Skin rashes have been noted with tiopronin therapy. A generalized rash with mild pruritus that develops in the first few months of therapy may be controlled with antihistamines, and disappears after discontinuing the drug. A less common rash that appears after at least 6 months of therapy appears on the trunk and is accompanied by intense pruritus. This form of rash disappears slowly after

---

Italicized side effects are common or life-threatening.
*Liquid form contains alcohol.   **May contain tartrazine.

discontinuing the drug.

• Some clinicians prefer to use penicillamine for cysteinuria therapy, but patients may not tolerate it well. Studies indicate about two-thirds of patients who cannot tolerate penicillamine will tolerate tiopronin.

113

Investigational drugs

azacytidine (5-azacytidine)
clomipramine
domperidone
enoxacin
gancyclovir
hexamethylmelamine (HMM, HXM)
israpidine
ketotifen fumarate
loratidine
metformin
nedocromil sodium
omeprazole
propafenone
selegiline
semustine (methyl CCNU)
sorbinil
tolrestat
trimebutine maleate
vindesine sulfate

COMBINATION PRODUCTS
None.

azacytidine (5-azacytidine)

MECHANISM OF ACTION
An antimetabolite that disrupts the translation of nucleic acid sequences into protein.

INDICATIONS & DOSAGE
Acute lymphocytic and acute myelogenous leukemia—
Adults and children: 200 to 300 mg/m² I.V. daily for 5 to 10 days. Repeated at 2- to 3-week intervals.

ADVERSE REACTIONS
Blood: *leukopenia (usually dose-limiting adverse reaction), thrombocytopenia.*
CNS: infrequent neurologic toxicities, including generalized muscle pain and weakness.
CV: *hypotension from rapid infusion.*
GI: *severe nausea and vomiting, diarrhea.*
Other: rare hepatotoxicity and drug fever.

INTERACTIONS
None significant.

NURSING CONSIDERATIONS
• Information based upon current literature. Dosage, indications, and adverse effect profile may change with additional clinical experience.
• Contraindicated in liver disease.
• For stability reasons, azacytidine should be infused only in lactated Ringer's solution.
• After the drug is diluted for infusion, it is stable for 8 hours.
• The drug should be given by slow I.V. infusion to prevent severe hypotension.
• Blood pressure should be monitored before infusion and at 30-minute intervals during infusion. If systolic blood pressure falls below 90 mm Hg, stop infusion and notify doctor.
• Nausea and vomiting may be reduced with continuous infusions. Tolerance to nausea and vomiting develops during extended course of treatment.
• Instruct patient to report any signs

of neurotoxicity; for example, muscle pain and weakness.
• If necessary, the drug may be given S.C. The drug should be mixed in a smaller quantity of diluent (3 to 5 ml for a 100-mg vial) for S.C. administration.
• Monitor temperature, CBC, and liver function tests.

clomipramine
Anafranil♦♦

MECHANISM OF ACTION
A tricyclic antidepressant that blocks serotonin and norepinephrine reuptake into presynaptic nerve terminals in the CNS. Also has anticholinergic effects.

INDICATIONS & DOSAGE
Depressive illness, especially if associated with an accompanying anxiety obsessive-compulsive neurosis—
Adults: 25 mg t.i.d. initially, increasing to a maximum of 150 mg. daily as needed and tolerated. Severely depressed hospitalized patients may receive up to 300 mg daily.
Elderly and debilitated patients: 20 to 30 mg daily in divided doses, with gradual increases in dosage as needed and tolerated.

ADVERSE REACTIONS
Blood: *agranulocytosis.*
CNS: drowsiness, fatigue, insomnia, nightmares, restlessness, agitation, excitement, hypomanic or manic episodes, disturbances of concentration, anxiety, impaired memory, disorientation, delusions, visual hallucinations, dizziness, extrapyramidal reactions, headache, convulsions, paresthesias.
EENT: blurred vision, difficulties with accomodation, mydriasis.
GI: dry mouth, constipation, nausea, vomiting, diarrhea, abdominal pain, changes of appetite.

GU: impotence, testicular swelling, urine retention.
Metabolic: menstrual irregularity, breast enlargement and galactorrhea in females, gynecomastia in males, changes in blood sugar levels, increases in prolactin levels, decreased hepatic function, jaundice.
Skin: photosensitivity, rash.
Other: changes of libido, weight changes, excessive sweating, hyperpyrexia, allergic reactions.

INTERACTIONS
Alcohol, CNS depressants: increased CNS depression. Avoid concomitant use.
Antihypertensive agents: decreased hypotensive effect. Monitor closely.
MAO inhibitors, sympathomimetics: enhanced sympathetic response. Don't use together.
Thyroid medications: increased risk of dysrhythmias. Monitor closely.

NURSING CONSIDERATIONS
• Information based upon current literature. Dosage, indications, and adverse effect profile may change with additional clinical experience.
• Contraindicated in patients with liver or kidney failure, glaucoma, congestive heart failure, and myocardial infarction (during the recovery phase). Avoid use in patients who have received a MAO inhibitor within preceeding 14 days, and in those with a history of blood dyscrasias. Use with caution in patients with risk of suicide.
• Monitor for urine retention and constipation. Suggest a stool softener, if needed.
• Clomipramine appears to have a mild sedating effect that may be helpful in treating depressive illness associated with anxiety.
• Warn patient to avoid hazardous activities requiring alertness or good psychomotor coordination until the CNS response to the drug is known.

• Dry mouth may be relieved with sugarless hard candy or gum.
• Advise patient not to take any OTC medications without first consulting the doctor.

domperidone
Motilium♦♦

MECHANISM OF ACTION
Blocks peripheral dopamine receptors, including those in the medullary chemoreceptor trigger zone (located outside the blood brain barrier). In the GI tract, it enhances motility in the stomach and small intestine.

INDICATIONS & DOSAGE
Symptomatic treatment of upper GI motility disorders associated with gastritis and diabetic gastroparesis; prevention of nausea and vomiting caused by antiparkinsonian medications—
Adults: 10 mg P.O. t.i.d. to q.i.d. 30 minutes before meals and h.s. Maximum dose is 20 mg P.O. q.i.d.

ADVERSE REACTIONS
CNS: headache.
GI: dry mouth.
Metabolic: galactorrhea, gynecomastia, menstrual irregularities, hot flashes.
Skin: rash.

INTERACTIONS
Antacids, H₂ antagonists: may impair absorption of domperidone.
Anticholinergic agents: decreased domperidone effectiveness.

NURSING CONSIDERATIONS
• Information based upon current literature. Dosage, indications, and adverse effects profile may change with additional clinical experience.
• Contraindicated in patients with hypersensitivity to the drug, mechanical obstruction of the GI tract, or gastrointestinal hemorrhage.

• Parenteral domperidone has also been tested as an antiemetic for patients receivin chemotherapy. Dosage up to 1 mg/kg appears to be effective and well tolerated.
• Because domperidone enhances gastric emptying and small intestine motility, it may alter the absorption of other drugs orally administered and may require dosage adjustments.

enoxacin
Comprecin

MECHANISM OF ACTION
Inhibits bacterial DNA gyrase, preventing bacterial replication.

INDICATIONS & DOSAGE
Mild to moderate urinary tract infections—
Adults: 200 mg P.O. b.i.d. for 5 days.
Complicated to severe urinary tract infections—
Adults: 400 mg P.O. b.i.d. for 14 days.
Skin and skin structure infections—
Adults: 400 mg P.O. b.i.d. for 7 to 14 days.
Uncomplicated genital tract infections (urethral or endocervical gonorrhea caused by Neisseria gonorrhoeae*)—*
Adults: 400 mg P.O. for one dose.

ADVERSE REACTIONS
CNS: headache, insomnia, tremors, restlessness.
GI: nausea, vomiting, diarrhea.

INTERACTIONS
Antacids containing aluminum or magnesium: decreased enoxacin absorption. Separate administration times as far as possible.
NSAIDs: possible increased risk of seizures.
Theophylline, caffeine: decreased metabolism and clearance of these drugs.

Italicized side effects are common or life-threatening.
*Liquid form contains alcohol.   **May contain tartrazine.

NURSING CONSIDERATIONS

• Contraindicated during pregnancy and in children because similar compounds have been shown to cause arthropathy in immature animals.

• Crystalluria has been reported with other compounds of this class. Dehydration, alkaline urine, and high doses may be contributing factors.

• Photosensitivity and skin rashes have been reported with other quinolones. Advise patient to avoid unnecessary exposure to sunlight and to use a sunscreen.

• Use cautiously with known or suspected CNS conditions that may predispose the patient to seizures, including epilepsy and severe cerebral arteriosclerosis.

• Encourage the patient to drink caffeine-free beverages while taking enoxacin because the drug impairs the metabolism of caffeine, which may lead to such adverse effects as tachycardia, nausea, and agitation.

• Obtain specimens for culture and sensitivity before starting therapy. First dose may be given before laboratory results are completed.

gancyclovir

MECHANISM OF ACTION
Inhibits viral DNA polymerase of cytomegalovirus (CMV) and herpes simplex viruses.

INDICATIONS & DOSAGE
Treatment of CMV retinitis—
Adults: 2.5 to 5 mg/kg I.V. every 8 hours for 10 to 14 days, followed by a maintenance dosage of 5 to 7.5 mg once or twice daily for 5 to 7 days per week.

ADVERSE REACTIONS
Blood: neutropenia, thrombocytopenia, anemia.
CNS: disorientation, confusion, seizures, dizziness, headaches.
GI: nausea, vomiting, diarrhea.
Skin: rash.
Other: hepatotoxicity, fever.

INTERACTIONS
Zidovudine: possibly increased neutropenia.

NURSING CONSIDERATIONS
• Information based upon current literature. Dosage, indications, and adverse effects profile may change with additional clinical experience.

• Available through a treatment investigational new drug (IND) protocol to treat CMV retinitis, which will cause blindness if untreated. Patients with AIDS and recipients of marrow transplants appear to be at risk of CMV infections. Gancyclovir is also under investigation for other forms of CMV infections, including pneumonitis and GI disease.

• Administer the drug over 1 hour.

• Maintenance infusions are necessary to prevent recurrence of the disease.

• Monitor CBC to detect neutropenia, which may occur in as many as 40% of patients who take the drug. It usually appears after about 10 days of therapy and may be associated with higher dosages (15 mg/kg/day). Neutropenia is reversible, but may necessitate discontinuation of therapy. Patients may restart the drug when blood counts return to normal.

• Patients with renal failure will probably need dosage adjustments to prevent toxicity.

hexamethylmelamine (HMM, HXM)

MECHANISM OF ACTION
Unknown.

INDICATIONS & DOSAGE
Ovarian carcinomas, lung cancer—
Adults: 4 to 8 mg/kg/day continu-

---

ously, or 240 to 320 mg/m² daily for
21 days repeated q 6 weeks.

ADVERSE REACTIONS
Blood: *mild leukopenia,* thrombocytopenia.
CNS: *paresthesias, numbness,* sleep disturbances, confusion, hallucinations, seizures, and parkinsonian syndrome with ataxia.
GI: *severe GI toxicity including nausea and vomiting, anorexia,* and occasional abdominal cramps and diarrhea.

INTERACTIONS
None significant.

NURSING CONSIDERATIONS
• Information based upon current literature. Dosage, indications, and adverse effects profile may change with additional clinical experience.
• GI toxicity may be decreased by giving the daily dosage in four divided doses. Antiemetics may be useful.
• Neurotoxicity is most common in patients receiving continuous daily therapy for longer than 3 months.
• Concomitant administration of pyridoxine 100 mg t.i.d. may decrease neurotoxicity.
• Instruct patient to report any signs of central nervous system or peripheral neuropathy.
• Monitor CBC.

israpidine
DynaCirc

MECHANISM OF ACTION
Decreases calcium ion movement across cardiac and smooth muscle cells. Israpidine appears to be selective for vascular smooth muscle.

INDICATIONS & DOSAGE
Mild to moderate hypertension—
Adults: 2.5 mg P.O. b.i.d. Early

studies indicate that doses of 2.5 to 10 mg b.i.d. are effective, but most patients respond to 7.5 mg b.i.d. or less.

ADVERSE REACTIONS
CNS: headache, dizziness, fatigue.
CV: peripheral edema, flushing, tachycardia.
GI: abdominal discomfort, constipation.

INTERACTIONS
None reported.

NURSING CONSIDERATIONS
• Information is based upon current literature and may change with further clinical experience.
• Israpidine is similar to nifedipine in many respects, but it may produce less reflex tachycardia because of drug's direct effect on the SA node.
• Food may delay the rate, but not the extent, of absorption.
• Drug is secreted in breast milk.

ketotifen fumarate
Zaditen

MECHANISM OF ACTION
Like cromolyn, ketotifen stabilizes mast cells. However, it has a number of other pharmacologic effects that may contribute to its action, including antihistamine, phosphodiesterase-inhibiting, and calcium channel blocking effects. It may also have some activity on beta₂-adrenergic receptors.

INDICATIONS & DOSAGE
Asthma prophylaxis; treatment of allergic rhinitis and conjunctivitis—
Adults: 1 mg P.O. b.i.d. with food. May be increased to 2 mg b.i.d.

ADVERSE REACTIONS
CNS: sedation, tiredness, dizziness, headache.
GI: dry mouth, nausea.
Other: increased appetite and weight

gain, exacerbation of asthma, *bronchospasm, status asthmaticus.*

INTERACTIONS
Alcohol: may potentiate adverse reactions.
Oral antidiabetic agents: reversible fall in platelet count has been reported. Avoid concomitant use.

NURSING CONSIDERATIONS
• Information is based upon current literature and may change with further clinical experience. Ketotifen is currently available in Europe.
• Long-term therapy is necessary for asthma prophylaxis. Studies lasting less than 4 weeks have not shown consistent benefits, but patients taking the drug for 3 months or more consider the drug effective.
• Ketotifen may produce drowsiness. Warn patients not to perform hazardous activities requiring alertness (such as operating heavy machinery or driving) until the adverse CNS effects of the drug are known.

loratidine
Claritin

MECHANISM OF ACTION
A selective histamine₁-receptor antagonist that has minimal CNS activity. A nonsedating antihistamine.

INDICATIONS & DOSAGE
Symptomatic treatment of seasonal and allergic rhinitis and of chronic urticaria—
Adults: 5 to 10 mg P.O. once daily. Preliminary trials have studied dosages as high as 40 mg daily.

ADVERSE REACTIONS
Early clinical trials indicate that the drug is well tolerated. Further study is necessary to obtain a complete adverse effects profile.

INTERACTIONS
None reported.

NURSING CONSIDERATIONS
• Information is based upon current literature and may change with further clinical experience.
• Loratidine appears to be well tolerated in early trials with no sedation or performance impairment with dosage up to 20 mg/day and only minimal performance impairment with 40 mg/day. It may have a more rapid onset of action than other nonsedating antihistamines.
• Once a day dosing may be an advantage.
• Some studies indicate that loratidine with pseudoephedrine is an effective combination.

metformin
Glucophage♦♦

MECHANISM OF ACTION
A substituted biguanide that produces its antidiabetic effects only in the presence of insulin. It facilitates insulin's action on peripheral receptor sites and may increase the number of insulin receptors. It has no effect on pancreatic beta cells.

INDICATIONS & DOSAGE
To control diabetes in stable, mild, nonketosis-prone type II diabetics—
Adults: Initially, 500 mg P.O. t.i.d., preferably with food. Adjust dosage upward as necessary, not to exceed 2.5 g daily.

ADVERSE REACTIONS
EENT: metallic taste.
GI: epigastric discomfort, nausea, vomiting, diarrhea, anorexia.
Other: *lactic acidosis.*

INTERACTIONS
Anticoagulants: metformin may increase the elimination of oral antico-

agulants. Monitor prothrombin times carefully during changes in metformin dosage.

Diuretics, corticosteroids, oral contraceptives, nicotinic acid: may produce hyperglycemia and reduce effectiveness of metformin therapy.

NURSING CONSIDERATIONS

• Information is based upon current literature and may change with further clinical experience.

• Contraindicated in patients allergic to the drug. It is also contraindicated in insulin-dependent diabetes; a history of ketoacidosis; liver disease; during periods of acute stress (surgery, severe infections, or trauma); lactic acidosis or a history of lactic acidosis; renal dysfunction; pregnancy; and in patients undergoing examinations that may involve pyelography or angiography, which may precipitate a temporary functional oliguria.

• Lactic acidosis is a potentially fatal complication of biguanide therapy. Phenformin (DBI), a similar compound, was withdrawn from the U.S. market in the mid 1970's after it was associated with this adverse effect. If vomiting occurs, drug should be discontinued immediately and patient assessed for the presence of lactic acidosis.

• Metformin should be discontinued 2 days before elective surgery or angiographic exams. Renal function should be assessed before the drug is restarted.

• Some patients may only need transient metformin therapy during periods of transient loss of blood glucose control.

• Metformin will not prevent the development of complications from diabetes mellitus.

• Patients should be advised of the importance of good dietary management to control their diabetes. Metformin therapy should not be used in place of good diet.

• Advise the patient to take metformin with food to minimize gastric irritation.

• Advise patients to avoid excessive alcohol consumption while taking metformin to prevent excessive elevation of blood lactate.

• Impaired absorption of vitamin B_{12} and folic acid have been reported in some patients on long-term therapy. Serum levels of these co-factors should be measured every 1 or 2 years.

• The drug should be temporarily discontinued once or twice a year to assess the patient's need for continued therapy.

nedocromil sodium
Tilade

MECHANISM OF ACTION
Inhibits activation and mediator release from inflammatory cells, such as mast cells. It may also act in the lung to attenuate local axon reflexes that are responsible for bronchoconstriction and edema.

INDICATIONS & DOSAGE
Prevention of symptomatic airway obstruction in patients with asthma—
Adults and children over age 12: 4 mg by inhalation (using metered-dose inhaler) two to four times a day.

ADVERSE REACTIONS
CNS: headache, dizziness.
EENT: unpleasant taste.
GI: nausea, vomiting.

INTERACTIONS
None reported.

NURSING CONSIDERATIONS
• Information is based upon current literature and may change with further clinical experience.
• Like cromolyn, nedocromil is con-

Italicized side effects are common or life-threatening.
*Liquid form contains alcohol.   **May contain tartrazine.

traindicated during an acute asthmatic attack. Beneficial effects are derived from regular daily use of the drug to prevent symptoms from appearing.

• Early studies indicate that nedocromil has both antiallergic and antiinflammatory properties. Some patients have been able to reduce (but not eliminate) the use of both bronchodilators and inhaled corticosteroids without increasing asthma symptoms.

omeprazole
Losec

MECHANISM OF ACTION
Decreases gastric hydrochloric acid secretion by inhibiting $H+/K+$ ATPase, a gastric parietal cell enzyme that is the proton pump responsible for HCl secretion.

INDICATIONS & DOSAGE
Short-term management of gastric and duodenal ulcer—
Adults: 20 mg P.O. once daily, preferably before breakfast.
Reflux esophagitis—
Adults: 40 mg P.O. once daily before breakfast.
Zollinger-Ellison syndrome—
Adults: 20 to 100 mg P.O. daily in one or more doses. Dosages as high as 360 mg daily have been used.

ADVERSE REACTIONS
CNS: dizziness, weakness, headache, numbness.
GI: dry mouth, diarrhea, nausea.
Metabolic: transient elevations of hepatic enzymes.

INTERACTIONS
Diazepam, phenytoin: decreased metabolism. Monitor for toxicity.

NURSING CONSIDERATIONS
• Information based upon current literature. Dosage, indications, and adverse effects profile may change with additional clinical experience.

• Dosages that exceed 120 mg daily should be given in divided doses.

• Morning administration is recommended to achieve maximal gastric acid suppression.

• Omeprazole is unstable in acid. Various pharmaceutical preparations have been tried to improve absorption and effectiveness, including encapsulation with sodium bicarbonate, enteric coating, and preparation of an alkaline suspension. Dosage will vary depending upon formulation.

• Because it will decrease stomach acidity, repeated dosing is expected to improve bioavailability. Further studies are necessary to confirm this effect.

• Instruct the patient not to take omeprazole with meals, because food appears to decrease this drug's bioavailability.

• Additional drug interactions with omeprazole are possible because it inhibits hepatic drug–metabolizing enzymes.

propafenone
Rhythmol♦♦

MECHANISM OF ACTION
A class Ic antiarrhythmic agent, propafenone stabilizes cardiac cell membranes, probably by decreasing sodium influx. It also has weak beta-adrenergic blocking properties.

INDICATIONS & DOSAGE
Suppression of ventricular dysrhythmias, such as episodic ventricular tachycardia—
Adults: initially, 150 mg P.O. q 8 hours. Dosage may be increased to 300 mg q 12 hours, then 300 mg q 8 hours. Maximum daily dosage is 900 mg.

Unmarked trade names available in the United States only.
♦Also available in Canada.   ♦♦Available in Canada only.   ◊Also available OTC.

ADVERSE REACTIONS
CNS: dizziness or light-headedness, headache.
CV: prodysrhythmic events (ventricular tachycardia, premature ventricular contractions), conduction disturbances, new or worsened CHF.
EENT: unusual taste.
GI: nausea, vomiting, constipation.

INTERACTIONS
Antiarrhythmics: increased potential for CHF.
Cimetidine: decreased metabolism of propafenone.
Digitalis glycosides, oral anticoagulants: propafenone may increase serum levels of these agents, resulting in toxicity.
Local anesthetics: increased risk of CNS toxicity.

NURSING CONSIDERATIONS
• Dosage information is based upon current literature and may change with further clinical experience.
• Contraindicated in severe or uncontrolled CHF; cardiogenic shock; SA, AV, or intraventricular disorders of impulse conduction; sinus node dysfunction in the absence of a pacemaker; severe bradycardia (50 beats/minute or less); marked hypotension; severe obstructive pulmonary disease; severe electrolyte imbalance; severe hepatic failure; and known hypersensitivity to the drug.
• Use cautiously in patients with CHF because propafenone can exert a negative inotropic effect on the heart. Use cautiously with other cardiac depressant drugs and in hepatic or renal failure.
• Because plasma levels do not increase linearly with dose, dosage should be increased stepwise at 3- to 4-day intervals.
• Some patients metabolize propafenone rapidly, and early studies indicate that the drug may have a plasma half-life of 5 to 6 hours in fast metabolizers and 17 hours or more in slow metabolizers.
• Continuous cardiac monitoring is recommended during initiation of therapy and during dosage adjustments. If PR interval or QRS duration increase by more than 25%, a reduction in dosage may be necessary.
• Administer drug with food to minimize adverse GI reactions.
• During concomitant use with digoxin, frequently monitor ECG and serum digoxin levels because propafenone increases serum digoxin levels by 35% to 85%.

selegiline
Eldepryl

MECHANISM OF ACTION
Inhibits monoamine oxidase in the brain (MAO-B), increasing the activity of dopamine in the CNS.

INDICATIONS & DOSAGE
Adjunct to therapy with levodopa or carbidopa-levodopa in patients with Parkinson's disease—
Adults: 10 mg P.O. daily, either as a single morning dose or 5 mg b.i.d.

ADVERSE REACTIONS
Investigators have found it difficult to distinguish adverse effects of selegiline from those associated with levodopa because these drugs are given together.
CNS: dyskinesia, hallucinations, confusion, agitation, anxiety, dizziness, insomnia.
CV: postural hypotension.
GI: nausea, vomiting.

INTERACTIONS
None reported.

NURSING CONSIDERATIONS
• Information is based upon current literature and may change with further clinical experience.

Italicized side effects are common or life-threatening.
*Liquid form contains alcohol.   **May contain tartrazine.

• Early studies indicate that selegiline decreases parkinsonian symptoms while allowing levodopa-carbidopa dosage to be reduced by up to 30%.

• Dosage adjustment of selegiline is usually not necessary because it irreversibly inhibits MAO-B, preventing loss of efficacy with prolonged use.

• Adverse effects of selegiline therapy may reflect levodopa-induced dopamine levels and may be reduced by decreasing levodopa dosage.

• Studies suggest that dosages above 20 mg/day may have an antidepressant effect.

• Early studies show that selegiline does not induce a hypertensive response in patients who consume foods and beverages high in tyramine (such as cheeses and red wines).

• Drug may slow progression of Parkinson's disease.

---

semustine
(methyl CCNU)

MECHANISM OF ACTION
A nitrosourea compound that probably acts as an alkylating agent. The drug cross-links DNA and also inhibits several key enzymatic processes.

INDICATIONS & DOSAGE
Advanced GI tumors, brain tumors, Hodgkin's and non-Hodgkin's lymphomas—
Adults: 150 to 200 mg/m² P.O. q 6 to 8 weeks.

ADVERSE REACTIONS
Blood: *delayed thrombocytopenia (about 4 weeks) and leukopenia (about 6 weeks). Myelosuppression may be cumulative.*
GI: *acute nausea and vomiting 2 to 6 hours after administration, anorexia.*
GU: *renal toxicity.*
Hepatic: elevated liver enzymes.
Other: pulmonary fibrosis with pro-

longed use.

INTERACTIONS
None significant.

NURSING CONSIDERATIONS
• Use cautiously when other nephrotoxic drugs are also being administered.

• Monitor renal and liver function tests.

• Capsules are usually stored in the refrigerator but are stable for 1 year at room temperature. Avoid storage in high temperatures and excessive moisture.

• The drug should be taken on an empty stomach to ensure complete absorption.

• Monitor CBC for delayed myelosuppression, up to 4 weeks for the onset of thrombocytopenia and 6 weeks for leukopenia.

---

sorbinil

MECHANISM OF ACTION
Blocks the enzyme aldose reductase, and prevents the intracellular formation of sorbitol from glucose and galactitol from galactose. This metabolic pathway is active in patients with diabetes and may be responsible for late diabetic complications.

INDICATIONS & DOSAGE
Prevention of late complications of diabetes, including diabetic retinopathy and neuropathy—
Adults: 250 mg P.O. once daily.

ADVERSE REACTIONS
Blood: transient leukopenia and thrombocytopenia.
Skin: rash.
Other: fever, oral ulcers.

INTERACTIONS
None reported.

NURSING CONSIDERATIONS
• Information is based upon current literature and may change with further clinical experience.
• Aldose reductase inhibitors have no effect on blood glucose, and patients must continue antidiabetic agents as instructed. The purpose of sorbinil therapy is to prevent late complications of diabetes that may be secondary to chronic elevation of blood sugar.
• The benefits of sorbinil therapy have been difficult to establish because of the slow onset of complications of diabetes. Some studies have shown objective improvement in such tests as nerve conduction velocity; others have reported pain relief in some patients.

tolrestat
Alderase

MECHANISM OF ACTION
Blocks the enzyme aldose reductase, and prevents the intracellular formation of sorbitol from glucose and galactitol from galactose. This metabolic pathway is active in patients with diabetes and may be responsible for late diabetic complications.

INDICATIONS & DOSAGE
Prevention of late complications of diabetes, including diabetic retinopathy and neuropathy—
Adults: dosage not clearly established. Early studies have used 50 to 200 mg P.O. once or twice daily.

ADVERSE REACTIONS
CNS: dizziness.
Skin: rash.
Other: elevations of liver enzymes.

INTERACTIONS
Salicylates, tolbutamide: increased plasma levels of active tolrestat by displacing the drug from protein-binding sites.

NURSING CONSIDERATIONS
• Information is based upon current literature and may change with further clinical experience.
• Aldose reductase inhibitors have no effect on blood glucose, and patients must continue antidiabetic agents as instructed. The purpose of therapy is to prevent late complications of diabetes that may be secondary to chronic elevation of blood sugar.
• The benefits of tolrestat therapy have been difficult to establish because of the slow onset of complications of diabetes. The drug appears to be well tolerated in clinical trials.

trimebutine maleate
Modulon ♦♦

MECHANISM OF ACTION
Acts on intestinal opiate and serotonin receptors to regulate normal intestinal motility.

INDICATIONS & DOSAGE
Symptomatic relief of irritable bowel syndrome—
Adults: 100 to 200 mg P.O. t.i.d. before meals.
Treatment of postoperative paralytic ileus—
Adults: 50 to 100 mg I.M. t.i.d. May also be given by slow I.V. push, or infused I.V. over 1 hour.

ADVERSE REACTIONS
CNS: dizziness, syncope, drowsiness, tiredness, headache.
CV: hypotension.
GI: constipation, diarrhea, nausea, vomiting, abdominal pain.

INTERACTIONS
Antihypertensives: possibly excessive hypotension, especially after rapid I.V. injection of trimebutine maleate.

Use together cautiously.
Tubocurarine: Animal studies have shown that trimebutine maleate may prolong neuromuscular blockade.

NURSING CONSIDERATIONS
• Information is based upon current literature and may change with further clinical experience.
• I.V. infusions may be mixed with normal saline solution or 5% dextrose in water.
• Rapid I.V. injection may cause hypotension. Inject drug over 1 minute.

vindesine sulfate
Eldisine♦

MECHANISM OF ACTION
Arrests mitosis in metaphase, blocking cell division.

INDICATIONS & DOSAGE
Acute lymphoblastic leukemia, breast cancer, malignant melanoma, lymphosarcoma, non–small cell lung carcinoma—
Adults: 3 to 4 mg/m² I.V. q 7 to 14 days, or continuous I.V. infusion of 1.2 to 1.5 mg/m² daily for 5 days q 3 weeks.

ADVERSE REACTIONS
Blood: *leukopenia, thrombocytopenia.*
CNS: *paresthesias, decreased deep tendon reflex, muscle weakness.*
GI: *constipation, abdominal cramping,* nausea, vomiting.
Local: *phlebitis,* necrosis on extravasation.
Other: *acute bronchospasm, reversible alopecia,* jaw pain, fever with continuous infusions.

INTERACTIONS
None significant.

NURSING CONSIDERATIONS
• Do not give as a continuous infusion unless patient has a central I.V. line.
• After administering, monitor for life-threatening acute bronchospasm reaction. If this occurs, notify doctor immediately. Reaction most likely to occur in patient who is also receiving mitomycin.
• To prevent paralytic ileus, encourage patient to drink fluids, increase ambulation, and use stool softeners.
• Instruct patient to report any symptoms of neurotoxicity: numbness and tingling of extremities, jaw pain, constipation (may be an early symptom).
• Assess for depression of Achilles tendon reflex, footdrop or wristdrop, and slapping gait (late signs of neurotoxicity).
• Neuropathy may be assessed by recording patient signatures before each course of therapy and observing for deterioration of handwriting.
• Monitor CBC.
• Avoid extravasation. Drug is a painful vesicant. Give 10-ml normal saline solution flush before drug to test vein patency, and 10-ml normal saline solution flush to remove any remaining drug from tubing after drug is given.
• When reconstituted with the 10-ml diluent provided or normal saline solution, the drug is stable for 30 days under refrigeration.
• Do not mix vindesine with other drugs; compatibility with other drugs has not yet been determined.

Appendices

Recommended drug dosage in renal failure

This table lists recommended dosage adjustments in mild, moderate, and severe renal failure. These adjustments are necessary because impaired renal function may modify a drug's bioavailability, distribution, pharmacologic action, or elimination, thereby predisposing the patient to drug toxicity. For example, digoxin toxicity can follow impaired renal function because digoxin is eliminated from the body almost exclusively by the kidneys (via glomerular filtration).

Drug	Mild renal impairment (GFR* > 50 ml/min)		Moderate renal impairment (GFR 10 to 50 ml/min)		Severe renal impairment (GFR < 10 ml/min)	
	% of normal dose	Interval	% of normal dose	Interval	% of normal dose	Interval
acetaminophen	100%	q 4 hr	100%	q 6 hr	100%	q 8 hr
acetazolamide	100%	q 6 hr	100%	q 12 hr	Avoid	Avoid
acetohexamide	100%	q 12 hr	Avoid	Avoid	Avoid	Avoid
acyclovir	100%	q 8 hr	100%	q 24 hr	100%	q 48 hr
allopurinol	100%	q 8 hr	75%	q 8 hr	50%	q 8 hr
amantadine	100%	q 12 to 24 hr	100%	q 48 to 72 hr	100%	q 7 days
amikacin	60% to 90%	q 8 to 12 hr	30% to 70%	q 12 hr	20% to 30%	q 24 hr
amoxicillin	100%	q 6 hr	100%	q 6 to 12 hr	100%	q 12 to 16 hr
amphotericin B	100%	q 24 hr	100%	q 24 hr	100%	q 24 to 36 hr
ampicillin	100%	q 6 hr	100%	q 6 to 12 hr	100%	q 12 to 16 hr
aspirin	100%	q 4 hr	100%	q 4 to 6 hr	Avoid	Avoid
atenolol	100%	q 24 hr	100%	q 48 hr	100%	q 96 hr
azathioprine	100%	q 24 hr	100%	q 24 hr	100%	q 36 hr
azlocillin	100%	q 4 to 6 hr	100%	q 6 to 8 hr	100%	q 8 hr
bleomycin	100%	Varies	100%	Varies	50%	Varies
bretylium	100%	Continuous infusion	25% to 50%	Continuous infusion	Avoid	Avoid
captopril	100%	t.i.d.	100%	t.i.d.	50%	t.i.d.
carbamazepine	100%	q 6 to 8 hr	100%	q 6 to 8 hr	75%	q 6 to 8 hr
carbenicillin	100%	q 8 to 12 hr	100%	q 12 to 24 hr	100%	q 24 to 48 hr
cefaclor	100%	q 6 hr	50% to 100%	q 6 hr	33%	q 6 hr

*glomerular filtration rate

Recommended drug dosage in renal failure *(continued)*

Drug	Mild renal impairment (GFR* > 50 ml/min)		Moderate renal impairment (GFR 10 to 50 ml/min)		Severe renal impairment (GFR < 10 ml/min)	
	% of normal dose	Interval	% of normal dose	Interval	% of normal dose	Interval
cefadroxil	100%	q 8 hr	100%	q 12 to 24 hr	100%	q 24 to 48 hr
cefamandole	100%	q 6 hr	100%	q 6 to 8 hr	100%	q 8 hr
cefazolin	100%	q 8 hr	100%	q 12 hr	100%	q 24 to 48 hr
cefotaxime	100%	q 6 to 8 hr	100%	q 8 to 12 hr	100%	q 12 to 24 hr
cefoxitin	100%	q 8 hr	100%	q 8 to 12 hr	100%	q 24 to 48 hr
cephalexin	100%	q 6 hr	100%	q 6 to 8 hr	100%	q 12 hr
cephalothin	100%	q 6 hr	100%	q 6 hr	100%	q 8 to 12 hr
cephapirin	100%	q 6 hr	100%	q 6 to 8 hr	100%	q 12 hr
cephradine	100%	q 6 hr	50%	q 6 hr	25%	q 6 hr
chloral hydrate	100%	At bedtime	Avoid	Avoid	Avoid	Avoid
chlorpropamide	100%	q 24 hr	Avoid	Avoid	Avoid	Avoid
chlorthalidone	100%	q 24 hr	100%	q 24 hr	100%	q 48 hr
cimetidine	100%	q 6 hr	100%	q 8 hr	100%	q 12 hr
cisplatin	100%	Varies	75%	Varies	50%	Varies
clofibrate	100%	q 6 to 12 hr	100%	q 12 to 18 hr	100%	q 24 to 48 hr
clonidine	100%	b.i.d.	100%	b.i.d.	50% to 75%	b.i.d.
colchicine	100%	Varies	100%	Varies	50%	Varies
cyclacillin	100%	q 6 hr	100%	q 6 to 12 hr	100%	q 12 to 24 hr
cyclophosphamide	100%	q 12 hr	100%	q 12 hr	100%	q 18 to 24 hr
diflunisal	100%	q 12 hr	100%	q 12 hr	50%	q 12 hr
digitoxin	100%	q 24 hr	100%	q 24 hr	50% to 75%	q 24 hr
digoxin	100%	q 24 hr	100%	q 36 hr	100%	q 48 hr
diphenhydramine	100%	q 6 hr	100%	q 6 to 9 hr	100%	q 9 to 12 hr
disopyramide	100%	q 6 hr	100%	q 12 to 24 hr	100%	q 24 to 40 hr

*glomerular filtration rate

(continued)

Recommended drug dosage in renal failure *(continued)*

Drug	Mild renal impairment (GFR* > 50 ml/min)		Moderate renal impairment (GFR 10 to 50 ml/min)		Severe renal impairment (GFR < 10 ml/min)	
	% of normal dose	Interval	% of normal dose	Interval	% of normal dose	Interval
doxycycline	100%	q 12 hr	100%	q 12 to 18 hr	100%	q 18 to 24 hr
ethacrynic acid	100%	q 6 hr	100%	q 6 hr	Avoid	Avoid
ethambutol	100%	q 24 hr	100%	q 24 to 36 hr	100%	q 48 hr
ethosuximide	100%	q 12 hr	100%	q 12 hr	75%	q 12 hr
flucytosine	100%	q 6 hr	100%	q 12 to 24 hr	100%	q 24 to 48 hr
gemfibrozil	100%	b.i.d.	50%	b.i.d.	25%	b.i.d.
gentamicin	60% to 90%	q 8 to 12 hr	30% to 70%	q 12 hr	20% to 30%	q 24 hr
guanethidine	100%	q 24 hr	100%	q 24 hr	100%	q 24 to 36 hr
hydralazine	100%	q 8 hr	100%	q 8 hr	100%	q 8 to 16 hr (fast acetylators) q 12 to 24 hr (slow acetylators)
hydroxyurea	100%	Varies	100%	Varies	50%	Varies
isoniazid	100%	q 24 hr	100%	q 24 hr	66% to 75%	q 24 hr
kanamycin	60% to 90%	q 8 to 12 hr	30% to 70%	q 12 hr	20% to 30%	q 24 hr
lincomycin	100%	q 6 hr	100%	q 12 hr	100%	q 24 hr
lithium carbonate	100%	t.i.d. to q.i.d.	50% to 75%	t.i.d. to q.i.d.	25% to 50%	t.i.d. to q.i.d.
lorazepam	100%	t.i.d. to q.i.d.	100%	t.i.d. to q.i.d.	50%	t.i.d. to q.i.d.
meprobamate	100%	q 6 hr	100%	q 9 to 12 hr	100%	q 12 to 18 hr
methadone	100%	q 6 to 8 hr	100%	q 6 to 8 hr	50% to 75%	q 6 to 8 hr
methenamine mandelate	100%	q.i.d.	Avoid	Avoid	Avoid	Avoid
methicillin	100%	q 4 hr	100%	q 4 to 8 hr	100%	q 8 to 12 hr
methotrexate	100%	Varies	50%	Varies	Avoid	Avoid

*glomerular filtration rate

Recommended drug dosage in renal failure *(continued)*

Drug	Mild renal impairment (GFR* > 50 ml/min)		Moderate renal impairment (GFR 10 to 50 ml/min)		Severe renal impairment (GFR < 10 ml/min)	
	% of normal dose	Interval	% of normal dose	Interval	% of normal dose	Interval
methyldopa	100%	q 6 hr	100%	q 9 to 18 hr	100%	q 12 to 24 hr
metoclopramide	100%	Varies	75%	Varies	50%	Varies
metronidazole	100%	q 8 hr	100%	q 8 to 12 hr	100%	q 12 to 24 hr
mezlocillin	100%	q 4 to 6 hr	100%	q 6 to 8 hr	100%	q 8 hr
mithramycin	100%	Varies	75%	Varies	50%	Varies
mitomycin C	100%	Varies	100%	Varies	75%	Varies
moxalactam	100%	q 8 hr	100%	q 12 hr	100%	q 12 to 24 hr
nadolol	100%	q 24 hr	50%	q 24 hr	25%	q 24 hr
nalidixic acid	100%	q.i.d.	Avoid	Avoid	Avoid	Avoid
neostigmine	100%	q 6 hr	100%	q 6 hr	100%	q 12 to 18 hr
netilmicin	60% to 90%	q 8 to 12 hr	30% to 70%	q 12 hr	20% to 30%	q 24 hr
nicotinic acid	100%	t.i.d.	50%	t.i.d.	25%	t.i.d.
nitrofurantoin	100%	q.i.d.	Avoid	Avoid	Avoid	Avoid
oxazepam	100%	q.i.d.	100%	q.i.d.	75%	q.i.d.
penicillin G	100%	q 6 to 8 hr	100%	q 8 to 12 hr	Avoid over 10 million units/day	q 12 to 16 hr
phenobarbital	100%	t.i.d.	100%	t.i.d.	100%	q 12 to 16 hr
phenylbutazone	100%	t.i.d. to q.i.d.	100%	t.i.d. to q.i.d.	Avoid	Avoid
piperacillin	100%	q 4 to 6 hr	100%	q 6 to 8 hr	100%	q 8 hr
primidone	100%	q 8 hr	100%	q 8 to 12 hr	100%	q 12 to 24 hr
probenecid	100%	q.i.d.	Avoid	Avoid	Avoid	Avoid
procainamide	100%	q 4 hr	100%	q 6 to 12 hr	100%	q 8 to 24 hr
propoxyphene	100%	q 4 hr	100%	q 4 hr	25%	q 4 hr
reserpine	100%	q 24 hr	100%	q 24 hr	Avoid	Avoid
spironolactone	100%	q 6 to 12 hr	100%	q 12 to 24 hr	Avoid	Avoid

*glomerular filtration rate

(continued)

Recommended drug dosage in renal failure *(continued)*

Drug	Mild renal impairment (GFR* > 50 ml/min)		Moderate renal impairment (GFR 10 to 50 ml/min)		Severe renal impairment (GFR < 10 ml/min)	
	% of normal dose	Interval	% of normal dose	Interval	% of normal dose	Interval
streptomycin	100%	q 24 hr	100%	q 24 to 72 hr	100%	q 72 to 96 hr
sulfamethoxazole	100%	q 12 hr	100%	q 18 hr	100%	q 24 hr
sulfisoxazole	100%	q 6 hr	100%	q 8 to 12 hr	100%	q 12 to 24 hr
sulindac	100%	b.i.d.	100%	b.i.d.	50%	b.i.d.
terbutaline	100%	t.i.d.	50%	t.i.d.	Avoid	Avoid
thiazides	100%	Daily to b.i.d.	100%	Daily to b.i.d.	Avoid	Avoid
ticarcillin	100%	q 8 to 12 hr	100%	q 12 to 24 hr	100%	q 24 to 48 hr
tobramycin	60% to 90%	q 8 to 12 hr	30% to 70%	q 12 hr	20% to 30%	q 24 hr
triamterene	100%	q 12 hr	100%	q 12 hr	Avoid	Avoid
trimethoprim	100%	q 12 hr	100%	q 18 hr	100%	q 24 hr
vancomycin	100%	q 1 to 3 days	100%	q 3 to 10 days	100%	q 10 days
vidarabine	100%	Continuous infusion	100%	Continuous infusion	75%	Continuous infusion

*glomerular filtration rate

Orphan drugs and biologicals

As defined by the Orphan Drug Act, an orphan drug is one that is useful for the diagnosis, treatment, or prevention of a rare disease or disorder. This act defines a rare disease as one that affects fewer than 200,000 persons in the United States, or one for which the expected sales will not recover the cost of developing and making the drug available. The following list includes the drugs and biologicals that have received orphan drug designation.*

GENERIC NAME	TRADE NAME	DESIGNATED USE
Drugs		
acetylcysteine	Mucomyst, Mucomyst 10 I.V.	Intravenous treatment of patients presenting moderate to severe acetaminophen overdose.
aconiazide		Treatment of tuberculosis.
allopurinol	Zyloprim	Ex vivo preservation of cadaveric kidneys for transplantation.
allopurinol riboside		Treatment of cutaneous and visceral leishmaniasis and Chagas' disease.
amsacrine	Amsidyl	Treatment of acute adult leukemia.
anagrelide		Treatment of polycythemia vera, essential thrombocytopenia, or thrombocytosis in chronic myelogenous leukemia.
antipyrine		Antipyrine test as an index of hepatic drug-metabolizing capacity.
AS-101		Treatment of AIDS.
bacitracin	Altracin	Treatment of antibiotic-associated pseudomembranous enterocolitis caused by toxins A and B and elaborated by *Clostridium difficile*.
baclofen (intrathecal)	Liorasal	Treatment of intractable spasticity caused by spinal cord injury or multiple sclerosis.
benzoate/ phenylacetate	Ucephan	Adjunct in prevention and treatment of hyperammonemia in patients with urea cycle enzymopathy (UCE) due to carba-mylphosphate synthetase, ornithine, transcarbamylase, or arginosuccinate synthetase deficiency.
bethanidine		Treatment of primary ventricular fibrillation.
BW B759U		Treatment of severe human cytomegalovirus (HCMV) infections in immunosuppressed patients (bone marrow transplant recipients and AIDS patients).

Federal Register 54(31): 7100-08, 1989.   (continued)

Orphan drugs and biologicals (continued)

GENERIC NAME	TRADE NAME	DESIGNATED USE
Drugs (continued)		
BW 12C		Treatment of sickle cell disease crisis.
caffeine		Treatment of apnea of prematurity.
calcitonin (human)	Cibacalcin	Treatment of symptomatic Paget's bone disease (osteitis deformans).
calcium acetate	Phos-Lo	Treatment of hyperphosphatemia in end-stage renal disease (ESRD).
ceramide trihexosidase/ alpha-galactosidase		Treatment of Fabry's disease.
cetiedal citrate		Treatment of sickle cell disease crisis.
chenodiol	Chenix	For treatment of patients with radiolucent stones in well-opacifying gallbladders and increased surgical risk associated with systemic disease or advanced age.
chlorhexidine gluconate mouth rinse	Peridex	Amelioration of oral mucositis associated with cytoreductive therapy used in conditioning patients for bone marrow transplantation therapy.
clindamycin	Cleocin	Treatment of *Pneumocystis carinii* pneumonia (PCP) associated with AIDS.
clofazimine	Lamprene	Treatment of lepromatous leprosy, including dapsone-resistant lepromatous leprosy and lepromatous leprosy complicated by erythema nodosum leprosum.
colchicine		Arresting progression of neurologic disability caused by chronic progressive multiple sclerosis.
copolymer 1 (COP1)		Treatment of multiple sclerosis.
cromolyn sodium	Cromoral, Gastrocrom	Treatment of mastocytosis.
cromolyn sodium 4% ophthalmic solution	Opticrom 4% Ophthalmic Solution	Treatment of vernal keratoconjunctivitis.
cyclosporine ophthalmic	Optimmune	Treatment of severe keratoconjunctivitis sicca.
cyproterone acetate	Cyproteron, Androcur	Treatment of severe hirsutism.
cysteamine (2-aminoethanethiol)		Treatment of nephropathic cystinosis.

Orphan drugs and biologicals (continued)

GENERIC NAME	TRADE NAME	DESIGNATED USE
Drugs (continued)		
dantrolene sodium	Dantrium	Treatment of the neuroleptic malignant syndrome.
defibrotide		Treatment of thrombotic thrombocytopenic purpura.
dextran sulfate sodium (UA001)		Treatment of AIDS.
diaziquone		Treatment of primary brain cancers (grade III and IV astrocytomas).
diethyldithiocarbonate	Imuthiol	Treatment of AIDS.
dimethyl sulfoxide (DMSO)	Sclerosol	Treatment of cutaneous manifestations of scleroderma.
dipalmitoyl-phosphatidylcholine (DPPC)/ phosphatidylglycerol (PG)	ALEC (Artificial Lung Expanding Compound)	Prevention and treatment of neonatal respiratory distress syndrome (RDS).
disodium silibinin dihemisuccinate	Legalon	Treatment of hepatic intoxication by *Amanita phalloides* (mushroom poisoning).
d,1-sotalol HCl		Prevention and treatment of life-threatening ventricular tachydysrhythmias.
eflornithine HCl (DFMO)	Ornidyl	Treatment of *Trypanosoma brucei gambiense* sleeping sickness, and of *Pneumocystis carinii* pneumonia in AIDS patients.
epidermal growth factor (human)		Acceleration of corneal epithelial regeneration and healing of stromal incisions from corneal transplant surgery; acceleration of corneal epithelial regeneration and the healing of stromal tissue in non-healing corneal defects; promotion of cutaneous wound healing in extreme burn treatment protocols.
epoprostenol	Cyclo-Prostin	Replacement of heparin in patients who require hemodialysis and who are at increased risk of hemorrhage.
epoprostenol/ prostacyclin/PGI$_2$/PGX	Flolan	Replacement of heparin in patients who require hemodialysis and are at increased risk of hemorrhage; treatment of primary pulmonary hypertension (PPH).

(continued)

Orphan drugs and biologicals (continued)

GENERIC NAME	TRADE NAME	DESIGNATED USE
Drugs (continued)		
etidronate disodium	Didronel	Treatment of hypercalcemia of a cancer inadequately managed by dietary modification and/or oral hydration.
ethanolamine oleate	Ethanolin	Treatment of bleeding esophageal varices.
ethinyl estradiol		Treatment of Turner's syndrome.
fibronectin (human plasma–derived)		Treatment of nonhealing corneal ulcers or epithelial defects that have been unresponsive to conventional therapy when the underlying cause has been eliminated.
fludarabine monophosphate		Treatment of chronic lymphocytic leukemia (CLL).
flumecinol	Zixoryn	Treatment of neonatal hyperbilirubinemia unresponsive to phototherapy.
flunarizine	Sibelium	Treatment of alternating hemiplegia.
gallium nitrate		Treatment of hypercalcemia of cancer.
ganciclovir (DHPG)		Treatment of serious life- or sight-threatening cytomegalovirus (CMV) infections in immunocompromised patients.
gangliosides as sodium salts	Cronassial	Treatment of retinitis pigmentosa.
glucocerebrosidase/ beta-glucosidase (placenta-derived)		Replacement therapy in patients with Gaucher's disease type 1.
gonadotropin-releasing hormone (Gn-RH)		Induction of ovulation in women with hypothalamic amenorrhea due to abnormal pattern of endogenous Gn-RH secretion.
guanethidine monosulfate	Ismelin I.V.	Treatment of moderate to severe reflex sympathetic dystrophy and causalgia.
histrelin		Treatment of central precocious puberty.
HPA-23		Treatment of AIDS.
hexamethylmelamine	Hexastat	Treatment of advanced ovarian adenocarcinoma.
hydroxycobalamin/ sodium thiosulfate		Treatment of severe acute cyanide poisoning.

Orphan drugs and biologicals (continued)

GENERIC NAME	TRADE NAME	DESIGNATED USE
Drugs (continued)		
idarubicin HCl		Treatment of acute myelogenous leukemia (AML), also referred to as acute nonlymphocytic leukemia (ANLL).
ifosfamide	Ifex	Treatment of soft tissue sarcoma and bone sarcoma. Used with other approved antineoplastic agents for third-line chemotherapy of germ cell testicular cancer. Should be used with a prophylactic agent for hemorrhagic cystitis, such as mesna.
inosine pranobex	Isoprinosine	Treatment of subacute sclerosing panencephalitis.
iodine ^{131}I meta-iodobenzylguanidine		Diagnostic adjunct in patients with pheochromocytoma.
iodine [131]I 6B-iodomethyl 19-norcholesterol		Adrenal cortical imaging.
L-alpha-acetyl-methadol (LAAM)		Treatment of heroin addicts suitable for maintenance on opiate agonists.
L-carnitine	Vita Carn	Treatment of genetic carnitine deficiency and manifestations of carnitine deficiency in patients with end-stage renal disease (ESRD) who require dialysis.
L-carnitine	Carnitor	Primary and secondary carnitine deficiency of genetic origin.
L-leucine, L-isoleucine, L-valine		Treatment of amyotrophic lateral sclerosis (ALS).
leucovorin	Leucovorin Calcium, Wellcovorin	Treatment of a metastatic adenocarcinoma of the colon and rectum (with 5-fluorouracil).
leuprolide acetate	Lupron injection	Treatment of central precocious puberty.
levocabastine HCl		Treatment of vernal keratoconjunctivitis (VKC).
LHRH [(DES-GLY[10])-D-Tri[8]-Pro[9]-N-Ethylamide)]		Treatment of central precocious puberty.
1-5 hydroxytryp-tophan (L-5HTP)		Treatment of postanoxic intention myoclonus.
mazindol	Sanorox	Treatment of Duchenne muscular dystophy (DMD).

(continued)

Orphan drugs and biologicals *(continued)*

GENERIC NAME	TRADE NAME	DESIGNATED USE
Drugs *(continued)*		
mefloquine HCl	Mephaquin	Treatment and prevention of chloroquine-resistant falciparum malaria.
megestrol acetate	Megace	Treatment of patients with anorexia, cachexia, or significant weight loss and confirmed diagnosis of AIDS.
mesna	Mesnex	Inhibition of urotoxic effects induced by ifosfamide and oxazaphosphorine compounds, such as cyclophosphamide.
methotrexate sodium	Methatrexate	Treatment of osteogenic sarcoma.
metronidazole (topical)	MetroGel	Treatment of acne rosacea.
metronidazole (topical)	Flagyl	Topical treatment of Grade III and IV anaerobically infected decubitus ulcers.
midodrine HCl	Midamine, Amatine	Treatment of idiopathic orthostatic hypotension.
mitoxantrone HCl	Novantrone	Treatment of acute myelogenous leukemia (AML), also referred to as acute nonlymphocytic leukemia (ANLL).
monooctanoin	Moctanin	Dissolution of cholesterol gallstones retained in the common bile duct.
morphine sulfate concentrate (preservative-free)	Duramorph	For administration via microinfusion devices in repeated doses or constant infusion; for *epidural* use in the treatment of severe and refractory chronic pain or when epidural administration is preferable to systemic administration; and for *intrathecal* use in patients with refractory pain due to cancer.
nafarelin acetate		Treatment of central precocious puberty.
naltrexone HCl	Trexan	Blockade of the pharmacologic effects of exogenously administered opioids as an adjunct to the detoxification of opioid-dependent individuals.
oxymorphone HCl	Numorphan H.P.	Relief of severe, intractable pain in narcotic-tolerant patients.
PEG-adenosine deaminase (PEG-ADA)	Imudon	Enzyme replacement therapy for ADA deficiency in patients with severe combined immunodeficiency (SCID).

Orphan drugs and biologicals (continued)

GENERIC NAME	TRADE NAME	DESIGNATED USE
Drugs (continued)		
pentamidine isethionate	Pentam 300	Treatment of *Pneumocystis carinii* pneumonia.
pentamidine isethionate (inhalation)	Aeropent, Pneumopent	Prevention of *Pneumocystis carinii* pneumonia in patients at high risk of developing this disease.
pentostatin		Treatment of hairy cell leukemia.
phosphocysteamine		Treatment of cystinosis.
physostigmine salicylate	Antilirium	Treatment of Friedreich's and other inherited ataxias.
piracetam	Nootropil	Treatment of myoclonus.
piritrexim isethionate		Treatment of infections caused by *Pneumocystis carinii*, *Toxoplasma gondii*, and *Mycobacterium avium-intracellulare*.
potassium citrate	Urocit-K	Prevention of calcium renal stones in patients with hypocitraturia and patients with uric acid nephrolithiasis.
potassium citrate/citric acid	Polycitra-K	Dissolution and control of uric acid and cystine calculi in the urinary tract.
praziquantel	Cysticide	Treatment of neurocysticercosis.
prednimustine	Sterecyt	Treatment of malignant non-Hodgkin's lymphomas.
propamidine isethionate	Brolene Eye Drops	Treatment of acanthamoeba keratitis.
protirelin (TRH)	Thymone	Treatment of amyotrophic lateral sclerosis (ALS).
pulmonary surfactant replacement		Prevention and treatment of respiratory distress syndrome (RDS).
quinacrine HCl		Prevention of recurrence of pneumothorax in patients at high risk.
rifampin	Rifadin I.V.	Antituberculosis treatment when use of the oral form of the drug is not feasible.
rifampin/isoniazid/ pyrazinamide	Rifater V	Short-course treatment of tuberculosis.
selegiline HCl	Deprenyl	Adjuvant to levodopa or levodopa and carbidopa treatment of idiopathic Parkinson's disease (paralysis agitans), postencephalitic parkinsonism, and symptomatic parkinsonism.

(continued)

Orphan drugs and biologicals (continued)

GENERIC NAME	TRADE NAME	DESIGNATED USE
Drugs (continued)		
sermorelin acetate [GRF (1-29) NH2]		Treatment of idiopathic and organic growth hormone deficiency in children with growth failure.
sodium monomercap-toundecahydro-*closo*-dodecaborate	Borolife	Treatment of glioblastoma multiforme as an alternative to conventional photon therapy.
sodium oxybate (sodium gamma hydroxybutyrate)		Treatment of narcolepsy and the auxiliary symptoms of cataplexy, sleep paralysis, hypnagogic hallucinations, and automatic behavior.
sodium pentosan polysulphate	Elmiron	Treatment of interstitial cystitis.
sodium tetradecyl sulfate	Sotradecol	Treatment of bleeding esophageal varices.
somatostatin	Reducin	Adjunct to the nonoperative management of secreting cutaneous fistulas of the stomach, duodenum, small intestine (jejunum and ileum), and pancreas.
somatrem	Protropin, Humatrope, Protropin II	Long-term treatment of children with growth failure resulting from inadequate secretion of endogenous growth hormone; treatment of short stature associated with Turner's syndrome.
somatropin	Saizen	Treatment of idiopathic or organic growth hormone deficiency in children with growth failure.
somatropin	Norditropin	Treatment of growth failure in children with inadequate secretion of growth hormone; adjunct in the induction of ovulation in women with infertility resulting from hypogonadotropic hypogonadism as well as bilateral tubal occlusion or unexplained infertility, who are undergoing in vivo fertilization procedures or in vitro fertilization with embryo transfer, respectively, and who fail to ovulate in response to gonadotropin therapy alone; treatment of short stature associated with Turner's syndrome.

Orphan drugs and biologicals (continued)

GENERIC NAME	TRADE NAME	DESIGNATED USE
Drugs (continued)		
spiramycin	Rovamycine	Symptomatic relief and parasitic cure of chronic cryptosporidiosis in patients with immunodeficiency.
superoxide diamutase (human)		Protection of donor organ tissue from damage or injury mediated by oxygen-derived free radicals that are generated during the necessary periods of ischemia (hypoxia, anoxia) and reperfusion.
surface active extract of saline lavage of bovine lungs	Infasurf	Prevention and treatment of respiratory failure due to pulmonary surfactant deficiency in preterm infants.
surfactant (human) (amniotic fluid derived)	Human Surf	Prevention and treatment of neonatal respiratory distress syndrome (RDS).
surfactant TA (modified bovine lung surfactant extract)	Survanta	Prevention and treatment of neonatal respiratory distress syndrome (RDS).
teniposide (VM-26)		Treatment of refractory childhood acute lymphocytic leukemia (ALL).
teriparatide	Parathar	Diagnostic agent in patients with clinical and laboratory evidence of hypocalcemia due to either hypoparathyroidism or pseudohypoparathyroidism.
terlipressin	Glypressin	Treatment of bleeding esophageal varices.
thalidomide		Prevention and treatment of graft-versus-host disease (GVHD) in patients receiving bone marrow transplantation (BMT); treatment and maintenance of reactional lepromatous leprosy.
thymoxamine		Reversal of phenylephrine-induced mydriasis in patients with narrow anterior angles, who are at risk of developing an acute attack of angle-closure glaucoma after mydriasis.
tiopronin	Thiola	Prevention of cystine nephrolithiasis in patients with homozygous cystinuria.
tocophersolan oral solution [(Vitamin E/d-alpha tocopheryl polylene glycol-1000 succinate (TPGS)]		Treatment of Vitamin E deficiency resulting from malabsorption due to prolonged cholestatic hepatobiliary disease.

(continued)

Orphan drugs and biologicals (continued)

GENERIC NAME	TRADE NAME	DESIGNATED USE
Drugs (continued)		
tranexamic acid	Cyklokapron	Treatment of hereditary angioneurotic edema; treatment of patients undergoing prostatectomy who risk hemorrhage as a result of increased fibrinolysis or fibingenolysis; treatment of surgical patients with congenital coagulopathies.
tretinoin		Treatment of squamous metaplasia of the ocular surface epithelia (conjunctive and/or cornea) with mucous deficiency and keratinization.
trientine HCl	Cuprid	Treatment of patients with Wilson's disease who cannot tolerate or are inadequately responsive to penicillamine.
trimetrexate glucuonate		Treatment of metastatic colorectal adenocarcinoma, metastatic carcinoma of the head and neck, and pancreatic adenocarcinoma; treatment of *Pneumocystis carinii* pneumonia (PCP) in AIDS patients.
urofollitropin	Metrodin	Induction of ovulation in patients with polycystic ovarian disease who have an elevated LH/FSH ratio and who have failed to respond to adequate clomiphene citrate therapy.
viloxazine hydrochloride	Vivalan	Treatment of narcolepsy and cataplexy.
zidovudine (AZT)	Retrovir	Treatment of AIDS and AIDS-related complex (ARC) in certain patients.
zinc acetate		Treatment of Wilson's disease.
4-aminopyridine (4-AP)		Relief of symptoms of multiple sclerosis.
5-AZA-2'-deoxycy-tidine		Treatment of acute leukemia.
2'-3'-dideoxy-adenosine		Treatment of AIDS.
2'-3'-dideoxycytidine		Treatment of AIDS.
2,3-dimercaptosuccinic acid (DMSA)		Treatment of lead poisoning in children.
24,25 dihydroxy-cholecalciferol		Treatment of uremic osteodystrophy.

Orphan drugs and biologicals (continued)

GENERIC NAME	TRADE NAME	DESIGNATED USE
Biologicals		
alpha-1 antitrypsin (recombinant DNA origin)		Treatment of alpha-1 antitrypsin deficiency in the ZZ phenotype population.
alpha-1 proteinase inhibitor (alpha-1 PI)	Prolastin	Treatment of alpha-1 PI congenital deficiency.
anti-J5mAb		Treatment of patients with gram-negative bacteremia that has progressed to endotoxin shock.
antimelanoma antibody XMMME-001-RTA		Treatment of Stage III melanoma not amenable to surgical resection.
anti-TAP-72 immunotoxin	XOMAZYME-791	Treatment of metastatic colorectal cancer adenocarcinoma.
antithrombin III (AT-III)		Replacement therapy in hereditary deficiency of AT-III for prevention and treatment of thrombosis and pulmonary emboli.
antithrombin III concentrate I.V.	Kybermin	Prophylaxis and treatment of thromboembolic episodes in patients with hereditary AT-III deficiency.
antithrombin III (human)	Antithrombin	Treatment of hereditary AT-III deficiency; prevention or arrest of thrombotic episodes in patients with hereditary AT-III deficiency; prevention of thrombosis in patients with AT-III deficiency after trauma or before surgery or parturition.
benzylpenicillin, benzylpenicilloic acid, and benzylpenilloic acid	Pre-Pen, MDM	Assessment of risk in administering penicillin when it is the drug of choice in adults with a history of hypersensitivity to it.
botulinum A toxin	Oculinum	Treatment of strabismus and blepharospasm.
botulinum toxin	Ortholinum	Treatment of spasmodic torticollis.
CD5-T lymphocyte immunotoxin	XOMAZYME-H65	Ex vivo treatment to eliminate mature T cells from potential bone marrow grafts; in vivo treatment of bone marrow recipients to prevent graft rejection and graft-versus-host disease (GVHD); treatment of GVHD and/or rejection in patients who have received bone marrow transplants.

(continued)

Orphan drugs and biologicals (continued)

GENERIC NAME	TRADE NAME	DESIGNATED USE
Biologicals (continued)		
cytomegalovirus immune globulin (human)		Prevention or attenuation of primary cytomegalovirus disease in immunosuppressed recipients of organ transplants.
digoxin immune fab (ovine)	Digidote, Digibind	Treatment of potentially life-threatening digitalis intoxication in patients who are refractory to conventional management.
erwinia 1-asparaginase		Treatment of acute lymphocytic leukemia and acute lymphoblastic leukemia.
erythropoietin (recombinant-human)	EPOCH	Treatment of anemia associated with end-stage renal disease (ESRD).
factor VIIa		Treatment of patients with hemophilia A & B with and without antibodies against factor VII/IX; treatment of patients with von Willebrand's disease.
factor XIII	Fibrogammin	Treatment of congenital factor XIII deficiency.
heme arginate	Normosang	Treatment of symptomatic stage of acute porphyria.
hemin	Panhematin	Amelioration of recurrent attacks of acute intermittent porphyria temporally related to the menstrual cycle in susceptible women and similar symptoms in other patients with acute intermittent porphyria, porphyria variegata, and hereditary coproporphyria.
indium in 111 antimelanoma antibody XMMME-0001-DTPA		Diagnostic imaging of systemic and nodal melanoma metastasis.
interferon alfa-n1	Wellferon	Treatment of AIDS-related Kaposi's sarcoma; treatment of human papillomavirus (HPV) in patients with severe resistant or recurrent respiratory (laryngeal) papillomatosis.
interferon alfa-2a (recombinant)	Roferon-A	Treatment of AIDS-related Kaposi's sarcoma.
interferon alfa-2b (recombinant)	intron A	Treatment of chronic myelogenous leukemia (CML), metastatic renal cell carcinoma, AIDS-related Kaposi's sarcoma, and ovarian carcinoma.

Orphan drugs and biologicals (continued)

GENERIC NAME	TRADE NAME	DESIGNATED USE
Biologicals (continued)		
interleukin-2 (recombinant)	Proleukin	Treatment of metastatic renal cell carcinoma.
iodine ^{123}I murine monoclonal antibody to human alpha-fetoprotein		Detection of hepatocellular carcinoma hepatoblastoma; detection of alpha-fetoprotein–producing germ cell tumors.
iodine ^{123}I murine monoclonal antibody to human chorionic gonadotropin (hCG)		Detection of hCG-producing tumors, such as germ cell and trophoblastic cell tumors.
iodine [131]I Lym-1 monoclonal antibody		Treatment of B-cell lymphoma.
monoclonal antibodies (murine or human) recognizing B-cell lymphoma idiotypes		Treatment of B-cell lymphoma.
monoclonal antiendotoxin antibody XMMEN-OE5		Treatment of gram-negative sepsis that has progressed to shock.
monoclonal antibody 17-1A	Panorex	Treatment of pancreatic cancer.
pentastarch	Pentaspan	Adjunct in leukapheresis, to improve the harvesting and increase the yield of leukocytes by centrifugal means.
polyribonucleotide	Ampligen	Treatment of AIDS.
serratis marcescens extract (polyribosomes)	ImuVert	Treatment of primary brain cancers.
ST1-RTA immunotoxin (SR 44163)		Prevention of acute graft-versus-host disease (GVHD) in allogenic bone marrow transplantation and treatment of patients with chronic lymphocytic leukemia (CLL).
technetium 99m (Tc 99m) anti-melanoma murine monoclonal antibody kit		Imaging detection of metastases of malignant melanoma.
trisaccharides A and B		Treatment of neonatal hemolytic disease arising from placental transfer of antibodies against blood group substances A and B; treatment of ABO-incompatible solid organ transplantation; treatment of transfusion reactions arising from ABO-incompatible transfusion of blood products.

Index

Index

Page numbers in boldface refer to major entries.

Page numbers in boldface refer to major entries.

990

O

998

X

Y

Z

Page numbers in boldface refer to major entries.

In the future as in the past...

You can rely on *Nursing* magazine to keep your skills sharp and your practice current—with award-winning nursing journalism.

Each monthly issue is packed with expert advice on the legal, ethical, and personal issues in nursing, plus up-to-the-minute...

- Drugs—warnings, new uses, and approvals
- Assessment tips
- Emergency and acute care advice
- New treatments, equipment, and disease findings
- Photostories and other skill sharpeners
- AIDS updates
- Career tracks and trends

Enter your subscription today

SAVE 38%

TABLE OF EQUIVALENTS

Frequently used equivalents in the metric system

Metric Weight
1 kilogram = 1,000 grams (g or gm)
1 gram   = 1,000 milligrams (mg)
1 milligram = 1,000 micrograms (μg or mcg)

Metric Volume
1 liter (l or L) =1,000 milliliters (ml)*
1 milliliter   =1,000 microliters (μl)

Frequently used equivalents in the apothecary system

Apothecary Weight
20 grains (gr)	=	1 scruple (℈)
3 scruples	=	1 dram (ȝ)
8 drams	=	1 ounce (ȝ)
12 ounces	=	1 pound (lb)

Apothecary Volume
60 minims (†)	=	1 fluidram (fȝ)
8 fluidrams	=	1 fluidounce (fȝ)
16 fluidounces	=	1 pint (pt)
2 pints	=	1 quart (qt)
4 quarts	=	1 gallon (gal)

Approximate metric and apothecary weight equivalents

Metric		Apothecary	Metric		Apothecary
1 gram (g) (1000 mg)	=	15 grains	0.05 g (50 mg)	=	¾ grain
0.6 g (600 mg)	=	10 grains	0.03 g (30 mg)	=	½ grain
0.5 g (500 mg)	=	7½ grains	0.015 g (15 mg)	=	¼ grain
0.3 g (300 mg)	=	5 grains	0.001 g (1 mg)	=	1/60 grain
0.2 g (200 mg)	=	3 grains	0.6 mg	=	1/100 grain
0.1 g (100 mg)	=	1½ grains	0.5 mg	=	1/120 grain
0.06 g (60 mg)	=	1 grain	0.4 mg	=	1/150 grain

Approximate household, apothecary, and metric volume equivalents

Household		Apothecary		Metric
1 teaspoon (tsp)	=	1 fluidram (fȝ)	=	4 or 5 ml‡
1 tablespoon (T or tbs)	=	½ fluidounce (fȝ)	=	15 ml
2 tablespoons	=	1 fluidounce	=	30 ml
1 measuring cupful	=	8 fluidounces	=	240 ml
1 pint (pt)	=	16 fluidounces	=	473 ml
1 quart (qt)	=	32 fluidounces	=	946 ml
1 gallon (gal)	=	128 fluidounces	=	3,785 ml

Conversions

Temperature	Centigrade (°C. x 9/5)	+	Fahrenheit 32 = °F.	Fahrenheit (°F. − 32)	x	Centigrade 5/9 = °C.
Weight	1 oz = 30 g		1 lb = 453.6 g	2.2 lb = 1 kg		

*1 ml = 1 cubic centimeter (cc); however, ml is the preferred measurement term today.

†A minim is *almost equal* to a drop. When a drug is prescribed in minims, it is best to measure it in minims. The minim is measured with a minim glass; a drop, with a medicine dropper.

‡Although the fluidram is approximately 4 ml, in prescriptions it is considered equivalent to the teaspoon (which is 5 ml).